Applying the Nursing Process

Resources

Quick Reference

Community Health Nursing

Theory and Practice

Community Health Nursing

Theory and Practice

Claudia M. Smith, R.N., C., M.P.H.
Assistant Professor
University of Maryland School of Nursing
Baltimore, Maryland

Frances A. Maurer, R.N., C., M.S.
Instructor
University of Maryland School of Nursing
Baltimore, Maryland

W.B. SAUNDERS COMPANY
A Division of
Harcourt Brace & Company
Philadelphia London Toronto Montreal Sydney Tokyo

W.B. SAUNDERS COMPANY
A Division of Harcourt Brace & Company

The Curtis Center
Independence Square West
Philadelphia, Pennsylvania 19106

Library of Congress Cataloging-in-Publication Data

Community health nursing: theory and practice / [editors], Claudia M. Smith, Frances A. Maurer.
p. cm.
ISBN 0-7216-2742-0
1. Community health nursing. I. Smith, Claudia M. II. Maurer, Frances A.
[DNLM: 1. Community Health Nursing—United States. WY 106 C73567 1995]
RT98.C65623 1995
610.73′43—dc20
DNLM/DLC 94-13122

COMMUNITY HEALTH NURSING: Theory and Practice ISBN 0–7216–2742–0

Printed in the United States of America.

Last digit is the print number: 9 8 7 6 5 4 3

This book is dedicated

to a vision of healthful families and communities,

to all community health nurses, students, educators, and community members who contribute to this vision,

and

to our families—

my parents, Claude and Gerry Smith, who helped me develop a foundation for integrity, excellence, caring, and fairness and who introduced me to primary prevention

my husband, Tony Langbehn, who is a true partner

my husband, Dick, and daughter, Jennifer Maurer, who provide support, encouragement, and honest review of all my endeavors

my sisters, brother and the memory of my parents, Francis and Anna May Rees, who taught me the value of critical inquiry and spirited debate.

Contributors

Adrianne E. Avillion, M.S., R.N., C.R.R.N., C.N.A.
Director, Professional Development, Montebello Rehabilitation Hospital, Baltimore, Maryland.
Rehabilitation Clients in the Community

Penny S. Brooke, R.N., M.S., J.D.
Assistant Dean, Associate Professor, University of Utah College of Nursing, Salt Lake City; Intermountain Health Care Board of Trustees, Salt Lake Valley Hospitals, Board of Governors, University Hospital Collaborative Council, Salt Lake City, Utah.
Legal Context for Community Health Nursing

Angeline Bushy, R.N., Ph.D.
Associate Professor, University of Utah College of Nursing, Division of Community Health, Salt Lake City, Utah.
Rural Health

Marcia Cooley, R.N., Ph.D. (A.A., M.S., C.S., Ph.D.)
Assistant Professor, University of Maryland School of Nursing, Baltimore, Maryland.
A Family Perspective in Community Health Nursing; The Nursing Process and Families; Multiproblem Families

Mary Ann Walsh Eells, R.N., Ed.D., C.S.
Associate Professor and Program Director, Community Addictions Nursing Project, University of Maryland School of Nursing, Baltimore, Maryland.
Common Addictions

Gail A. DeLuca Havens, R.N.,C., M.S.
Doctoral Candidate, Nursing Ethics, University of Maryland School of Nursing, Baltimore, Maryland.
Ethics Boxes I through IX

Gail L. Heiss, R.N., M.S.N.
Instructor, The Johns Hopkins University School of Nursing, Baltimore, Maryland.
Health Teaching

Kathryn Hopkins Kavanagh, R.N., M.S., Ph.D.
University of Maryland School of Nursing, Baltimore, Maryland.
The Relevance of Culture and Values for Community Health Nursing

Joan Kub, R.N., Ph.D.
Assistant Professor, The Johns Hopkins University, Baltimore, Maryland.
School Health

Mary Ellen Lashley, R.N., Ph.D., C.R.N.P., C.S.
Assistant Professor, Department of Nursing, Towson State University, Towson, Maryland.
Health Promotion and Risk Reduction in the Community; Screening and Referral; Elderly Persons in the Community

Lucile H. Maher, R.N., B.S.N., M.P.H.
Formerly Nursing Director, Akron Health Department, Akron, Ohio, Adjunct Faculty, Akron University College of Nursing, Clinical Faculty, Department of Community Health, Case Western Reserve University School of Nursing, Cleveland, Ohio.
Local Health Departments

Linda K. Matocha, R.N., Ph.D.
Associate Professor, College of Nursing, University of Delaware, Newark, Delaware; Visiting Professor, Beijing Medical University, Beijing, People's Republic of China.
Communicable Diseases

Frances A. Maurer, R.N.,C., M.S.
Instructor, University of Maryland School of Nursing, Baltimore, Maryland.
The U.S. Health Care System; Financing of Health Care: Context for Community Health Nursing; The Relevance of Culture and Values for Community Health Nursing; Community Assessment; Community Planning and Intervention; Violence: A Social and Family Problem; Teenage Pregnancy

Paula Milone-Nuzzo, R.N., Ph.D.
Assistant Professor and Program Director, Home Health Care Concentration, Yale School of Nursing, New Haven, Connecticut.
Home Health Care

Maggie T. Neal, R.N., Ph.D.
Assistant Professor, University of Maryland School of Nursing, Baltimore, Maryland.
Epidemiology: Unraveling the Mysteries of Disease and Health

Janet Primomo, R.N., Ph.D.
Assistant Professor, University of Washington, Tacoma, Washington.
Environmental Issues: At Home, at Work, and in the Community

Mary K. Salazar, R.N., Ed.D.
Assistant Professor, School of Nursing, University of Washington, Seattle, Washington.
Environmental Issues: At Home, at Work, and in the Community

Barbara Santamaria, R.N., B.S.N., C.F.N.P., M.P.H.
Nursing Associate, School of Nursing, University of Maryland; Nurse Practitioner, Hospital Based Home Care, Baltimore Veterans Administration Medical Center, Baltimore, Maryland.
Nursing in a Disaster

Alwilda Scholler-Jaquish, R.N., M.N., M.S., C.S.-P.
Instructor, University of Maryland School of Nursing, Baltimore; Director, Paul's Place Nurse's Clinic, Baltimore, Maryland.
Homelessness in America

Janie B. Scott, B.S., O.T.R./L.
Occupational Therapy Consultant, Maryland Department of Health and Mental Hygiene, Baltimore, Maryland.
Rehabilitation Clients in the Community

Janice Selekman, R.N., D.N.Sc.
Professor and Chairperson, College of Nursing, University of Delaware, Newark, Delaware.
Children in the Community

Claudia M. Smith, R.N.,C., M.S.
Assistant Professor, University of Maryland School of Nursing, Baltimore, Maryland.
Responsibilities for Care in Community Health Nursing; Origins and Future of Community Health Nursing; The Home Visit: Opening Doors for Family Health; Community Assessment; Community Planning and Intervention; Evaluation of Nursing Care with Communities

Shirley A. Steel, R.N., M.S.
Formerly Coordinator, Office of Health Services, Baltimore County Public Schools, Towson, Maryland.
School Health

Judith A. Strasser, R.N., D.N.Sc.
Associate Professor, Community Health Nursing, University of Maryland, Baltimore, Maryland.
The Relevance of Culture and Values for Community Health Nursing

Jean O. Trotter, R.N.,C., M.S.
Undergraduate Faculty, The Johns Hopkins University School of Nursing, Baltimore, Maryland.
Community Assessment; Community Planning and Intervention

Reviewers

Elizabeth A. Amos, Ph.D., R.N.C.S.
School of Nursing
University of Texas Health Science Center
Houston, Texas

Barbara M. Artinian, Ph.D, R.N.
School of Nursing
Azusa Pacific University
Azusa, California

Kathleen J. Brinker, M.S.N., R.N.C.
School of Nursing
Northern Kentucky University
Highland Heights, Kentucky

Cindy A.L. Burbach, Dr.P.H., R.N.
School of Nursing
Wichita State University
Wichita, Kansas

Rena Burnfield, M.S.N., R.N., C.R.R.N.
School of Nursing
Hahnemann University
Philadelphia, Pennsylvania

Linda Dennis Busl, M.Ed., B.S.N., R.N.
School of Nursing
Good Samaritan Hospital
Cincinnati, Ohio

Marian A. Conway, M.S.N., R.N.C.
School of Nursing
Armstrong State College
Savannah, Georgia

Becky Damazo, M.S.N., R.N., P.H.N.
School of Nursing
California State University
Chico, California

Mary V. Dooling, M.S.N., R.N.
U.S. Public Health Service Consultant
St. Louis, Missouri

Deborah L. Finfgeld, Ph.D., R.N.
School of Nursing
Illinois Wesleyan University
Bloomington, Illinois

Susan Gaskins, D.N.S., M.P.H., B.S.N., R.N.
School of Nursing
University of Alabama
Tuscaloosa, Alabama

Elizabeth J. Glassman, M.A., R.N.
School of Nursing
Mount St. Mary College
Newburgh, New York

Ella Herriage, Ph.D., R.N.
School of Nursing
Texas Technical University Health Science Center
Permian Basin, Odessa, Texas

Linda A. Jacobs, M.S.N., B.S.N., R.N., C.N.S.
School of Nursing
University of Pennsylvania
Philadelphia, Pennsylvania

Mary Agnes Kendra, Ph.D., M.S.N., B.S.N., R.N.
School of Nursing
Ursuline College
Pepper Pike, Ohio

P. Lea Monahan, Ph.D., M.S.N., B.S.N., R.N.
School of Nursing
Cardinal Stritch College
Milwaukee, Wisconsin

Sharon C. Posey, M.S.Ed., M.S.N., R.N.C.
School of Nursing
Purdue University
West Lafayette, Indiana

Catherine L. Powell, Ed.D., M.S.P.H., M.S., B.S.N., R.N.
School of Nursing
Armstrong State College
Savannah, Georgia

Cathleen M. Shultz, Ph.D., R.N., F.A.A.N.
School of Nursing
Harding University
Searcy, Arkansas

Lilyan Snow, Ph.D., R.N.
School of Nursing
Seattle Pacific University
Seattle, Washington

Alison H. Sweatt, M.S., R.N.
School of Nursing
University of New Hampshire
Durham, New Hampshire

Myra S. Tillis, M.S.N., R.N.C.
Loewenberg School of Nursing
Memphis State University
Memphis, Tennessee

Eunice N.-M. Warren, M.S., R.N.
School of Nursing
Baylor University
Dallas, Texas

Preface

In 1993, we celebrated the 100th anniversary of modern community health nursing in the United States. Among our historic roots are ethical values, commitments, principles, theories and concepts, experiences, models for nursing and health care delivery, and research findings that inform our current nursing practice. The arrival of the 21st century in the year 2000 brings both practical and symbolic implications for the future of community health nursing. Anniversaries and transitions offer time to reflect on the past and present, as well as to help clarify directions and strategies for the future.

Throughout this text, emphasis is placed on the core of "what a community health nurse needs to know" to practice effectively in the context of a nation, society, and health care system that are ever changing. This text is intended for baccalaureate nursing students taking courses related to community health nursing, including R.N.s returning for their baccalaureate degrees. Beginning practitioners in community health nursing will also find much useful information.

Unlike 100 years ago, the major causes of death in the United States today are not communicable diseases. Rather, the causes today are chronic diseases, such as heart disease, cancer, stroke, pulmonary diseases, and diabetes, and, at all ages, injury. Much of the premature death and disability is preventable through control of environmental and personal risk factors. Health promotion and prevention have been historic aims of community health nursing. Today, the National Health Objectives for the year 2000 identify measurable targets for reduction in death and disability. Because community health nurses are in the forefront of helping families and communities identify and reduce their risk factors, the ***Healthy People 2000*** **objectives are included in all appropriate chapters.**

Health and illness are unevenly distributed among people. The relevance of population-focused nursing emerges when the unmet health needs of various aggregates and groups are recognized. For example, numbers of homeless, chronically mentally ill, and poor persons are increasing. The poor have higher rates of illness, disability, and premature death. The cost of health care and absent or inadequate health insurance coverage combine to also increase the numbers of medically indigent, such as survivors of accidental head and spinal trauma. This text explores the commitments and activities of **community health nursing in improving the health of such vulnerable families, aggregates, and groups.**

To identify the health-related strengths and problems of a community, it is necessary to assess the demographic and health statistics of the community's population and to explore the existing community structures, functions, and resources. In this text we stress the importance of developing partnerships with community members, present a **community assessment tool,** with several case studies showing its application, and discuss varied perspectives for planning and evaluating nursing care within communities.

Community health nurses recognize that much of a person's health attitudes and behavior is learned initially in his or her own family. **Family-focused health promotion and prevention** is an important community health nursing strategy. As was true 100 years ago, some families today experience multiple problems with unhealthy environments, disabled or chronically ill members, developmental issues, breakdowns in family communication, and weak support systems.

The text reflects the increasing demand for community health nursing in **home health care for the ill.** Hospital cost-containment measures that began in the 1980s have resulted in a decrease in the average length of stay of patients in hospitals. As was true 100 years ago, families today are caring for ill members at home and are requiring assistance from community health nurses. In response to client needs, newer structures of nursing care delivery also have emerged, including hospice and medical daycare centers. Family-focus and care for clients in their daily settings—homes, schools, and worksites—are traditional aspects of community health nursing. Knowledge of community health nursing helps us recognize the importance of caring for the family caregivers as well as for ill family members and of strengthening community support services.

The community health nurse's involvement with **contemporary public health problems**—addictions, sexually transmitted diseases (including AIDS), and violence—is thoroughly covered. Teen pregnancy is explored as a health risk for adolescents and their infants. Toxic substances in home, work, and community environments are identified as special health risks.

Changes in the age composition of our country's residents poses concerns related to the ratio of dependent persons. More elderly persons and, in selected subpopulations, more children make up the population. Special emphasis is given in the text to a discussion of the support networks with which community health nurses work as they provide **nursing care with elderly people, children, and persons with disabilities.**

Level of Learner

This book is intended as a basic text for baccalaureate students in community health nursing. It is appropriate for basic baccalaureate students, R.N.s returning for baccalaureate degrees, and baccalaureate graduates who are new to community health employment.

Additionally, the text can benefit R.N.s without baccalaureate degrees who are changing their practice settings because of health care system changes. For example, in some places, R.N.s with strong technological medical-surgical or pediatric skills are being employed in home care. This text can be used by them, their supervisors, and/or in-service education directors to provide background information, especially in relation to the context of practice, family-focused care, home visiting, and scope of community resources.

The text has a descriptive focus, including both changes in practice historically and the relative magnitude of community health nursing problems and solutions today. The text also is structured to promote further inquiry related to each subject and to connect information with examples of practice. Thus, the text includes abstractions and concepts, as well as questions and examples, to promote application of the information.

This text builds on prerequisite knowledge and skills related to application of the nursing process, interpersonal relationships, and nurse/client communication skills. Other prerequisites are knowledge of human development, basic concepts of stress and adaptation, and nursing care with individuals. While a basic general systems language is used with family and community theory, terms are defined for those who have not had formal instruction in these concepts.

Organization of Text

The text is organized into seven units. Unit I, *The Role and Context of Community Health Nursing Practice,* describes the ethical commitments underlying community health nursing practice as well as the scope and context of community health nursing practice. We explore how the structure and function of our complex health care system and legal, economic, and cultural factors influence communities and community health nursing practice.

Unit II, *Family as Client,* presents a broad theory base related to family development, structure, functioning, and health. A family assessment tool is provided and sources for additional tools are identified. Specific case studies demonstrate the application of the nursing process with families. Special emphasis is given to working with families in crisis and "multiproblem" families.

Nurses with baccalaureate degrees belong to one of a few professions whose members learn to care for people at home as a part of their educational experiences. Many nurses without baccalaureate degrees who desire to transfer from hospital to home care settings must learn on the job. Consequently a chapter is devoted to home visiting, the fastest growing facet of community health nursing.

Unit III, *Community as Client,* presents the community and population approach that is unique to community health nursing. Epidemiology is the science used to study the distribution of health and illness among human populations. We introduce epidemiological statistics and methods. Current epidemiological data that describe patterns of death, disability, and illness within the United States are presented for age groups throughout the lifespan and for ethnic and/or racial minorities. Varieties of tables and figures are presented to demonstrate the way in which population and epidemiological data are published for use by community health nurses.

Communities may be characterized as geopolitical or phenomenological (communities of belonging). Assessment tools are presented for each type of community and case examples provided to illustrate the application of the nursing process with communities. Numerous measures for evaluating the outcomes of community health nursing programs are discussed. Additionally, process and management evaluations are examined.

Last in this unit, nursing care in community disasters is explored.

Unit IV, *Tools for Practice,* develops three strategies for intervention used frequently by community health nurses:

- Health promotion and risk reduction
- Screening and referral
- Health teaching

Specific tools are included that can be used to help individuals identify risk factors for illness and identify more healthful personal behavior. Detailed instructions are provided for conducting health screening. Also included are the current recommended schedules for health screening for males and females of various age groups. These specific practice skills may be applied with individuals, families, and populations.

Unit V focuses on contemporary problems encountered in community health nursing practice. A chapter is devoted to each of the following:

- Communicable disease, including HIV and AIDS
- Family violence
- Alcohol and drug addiction
- Teenage pregnancy

Homelessness is explored in depth, as are societal and personal factors contributing to homelessness; psychological and family stress related to homelessness; and health risks of the homeless. A never-before-published model presents nursing interventions appropriate for three levels of homelessness.

A chapter on environmental issues at home, at worksites, and in geopolitical communities identifies specific health risks. Responsibilities of occupational health nurses are included.

Unit VI discusses three vulnerable populations: persons with disabilities, children, and elderly persons. Prevalence of health problems, common nursing interventions, and importance of community support services are discussed.

Unit VII, *Settings for Community Health Nursing Practice,* describes schools, home health agencies, local health departments, and rural communities as settings for community health nursing practice. Each chapter includes either a day or a week in the life of a community health nurse to help students experience the reality of working in that setting.

Chapter Organization to Promote Learning

Each chapter has the following features:

- Outline
- Focus Questions
- Chapter narrative
- Key Ideas
- Application of the Nursing Process or Case Study
- Guidelines for Learning
- References
- Recommended Readings

Focus Questions at the beginning of each chapter and **Key Ideas** at the end help the reader focus on the material presented. The questions encourage the reader to approach learning from the perspective of inquiry. Key Ideas summarize the important ideas.

Application of the chapter material is encouraged. Most chapters provide an example of the nursing process being applied with a family or community or a case study in which the chapter concepts may be applied.

Guidelines for Learning in each chapter are designed to foster student learning through inquiry and a variety of ways of knowing—empirical knowledge and logic, interpersonal learning experiences, ethics, and greater awareness of personal preferences (aesthetics). Guidelines may promote reflection and self-awareness, observation, analysis, and synthesis. Each chapter includes guidelines for learning appropriate to most students as well as suggestions for those who are interested in further evaluation and creativity.

Recommended Readings have been selected with the level of student in mind. Some readings expand on concepts and tools of practice mentioned in the chapter. Where possible, other readings provide descriptions of community health nursing programs or nurses' experiences related to their professional practice.

Where appropriate, epidemiological data are presented to describe the magnitude of the health problems and the populations in which they occur more frequently.

Ethics Boxes are a special feature of each chapter in Units V and VI. A situation involving a community health nurse is used to identify ethical questions, related ethical principles, and the actions of the specific nurse. These situations provide the opportunity for student/faculty dialogue to explore one's own ethical decision-making. Several of the situations demonstrate the tension between the rights of individuals and the rights of the public at large; other situations depict competing values.

Resource lists exist in each chapter within Units IV through VII. Addresses and phone numbers allow the reader to contact national resources or their regional and local chapters to obtain further information and materials.

An **Instructor's Manual** for qualified instructors accompanies the text. The manual includes short answers to chapter **Focus Questions,** for convenience, teaching suggestions, and multiple-choice test questions. Contact your local W.B. Saunders representative for a copy.

Claudia M. Smith
Frances A. Maurer

Acknowledgments

Many people have contributed to our exploration of community health nursing practice: colleagues, former faculty and mentors, students, and clients. Antonia Fuller, Maggie Neal, Doris Scott, and Barbara Kern have contributed to our personal growth through their friendship and dialogue. Louise Berman and Francine Hultgren have encouraged exploration of interpretive, ethical, and critical ways of knowing and have role-modeled inquiry-based learning.

We are grateful for our relationships with community health nursing students, graduates, and community health nurses who have taught us much. We especially thank the community health nurses with Anne Arundel County Health Department, Prince George's County Health Department, and Bon Secours Home Health in Baltimore, who are friends and colleagues.

Without the contributors and their expertise, this book could never have been written. They have shared their knowledge, beliefs, experiences, and visions. Our conscientious reviewers affirmed our strengths; challenged us when we were unclear, inaccurate, parochial, or too narrow in our focus; and made constructive suggestions.

Colleagues and staff, especially our department chairpersons, Elizabeth Arnold and Mildred Kreider, at the University of Maryland have supported us in our endeavor. Ann Caverly worked many evenings typing manuscripts and retyping tables in various formats; without her, many deadlines would have been missed. Tanya Jones and Mary Alimo helped us unscramble our computer disks.

Our families have been extremely supportive, cooking meals, doing the shopping, organizing holiday events when we did not have time to do so, being willing to spend time without us, missing vacations, and taking pride in our accomplishment.

Ilze Rader, Acquisitions Editor, provided the opportunity, encouragement, patience, and sense of humor that allowed us to stay the course and complete this book. Her creativity and flexibility matches that of the best community health nurse. Dave Prout, Developmental Editor, did more than was required to organize the many pages and pieces of the manuscript. His attention to detail and commitment to quality kept us focused on accomplishing our goals and he provided hope when we were bogged down. The copy editing and production staff at W.B. Saunders transformed our manuscripts into a coherent publication.

Thank you.

Contents in Brief

Contents

UNIT I

The Role and Context of Community Health Nursing Practice 1

CHAPTER 3

The U.S. Health Care System 53

Frances A. Maurer

CHAPTER 4

Legal Context for Community Health Nursing Practice 88

Penny S. Brooke

CHAPTER 5

Financing of Health Care: Context for Community Health Nursing 110

Frances A. Maurer

CHAPTER 12

CHAPTER 13

CHAPTER 14

CHAPTER 15

UNIT IV

CHAPTER 16

CHAPTER 17

CHAPTER 18

UNIT V

Contemporary Problems in Community Health Nursing *471*

CHAPTER 19

CHAPTER 20

CHAPTER 21

CHAPTER 22

CHAPTER 23

CHAPTER 24

UNIT VI

CHAPTER 25

CHAPTER 26

CHAPTER 27

Unit I

The Role and Context of Community Health Nursing Practice

Chapter 1

Responsibilities for Care in Community Health Nursing

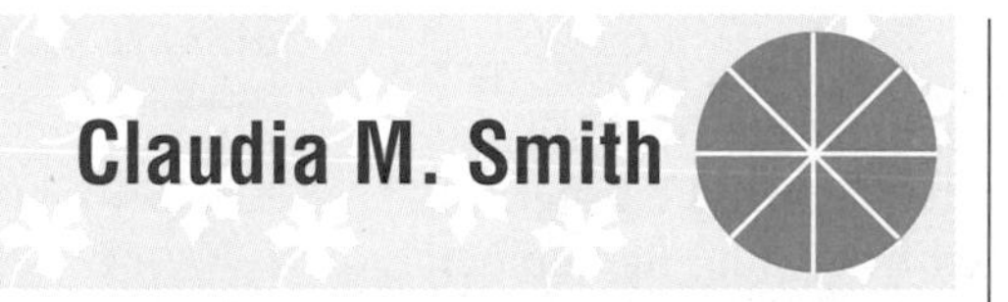

Claudia M. Smith

Continued

Focus Questions

What is the nature of community health nursing practice?

What values underlie community health nursing?

How is empowerment important in community health nursing?

What health-related goals are of concern to community health nurses?

Who are the clients of community health nurses?

What are the basic concepts and assumptions of general systems theory?

What is meant by the terms population-focused and aggregate-focused care?

What are the responsibilities of community health nurses?

What competencies are expected of beginning community health nurses?

How are community health nurse generalists and specialists similar and different?

EXPECTED COMPETENCIES OF BACCALAUREATE-PREPARED COMMUNITY HEALTH NURSES
Direct Care with Individuals
Direct Care with Families
Direct Care with Groups
Direct Care with Aggregates

LEADERSHIP IN COMMUNITY HEALTH NURSING
Professional Certification
Quality Assurance
Community Health Nursing Research

Imagine that you, dressed in navy and white, are knocking on the door of a residential trailer, seeking the mother of an infant who has been hospitalized because of low birth weight; you are interested in helping the mother to prepare her home for the hospital discharge of the infant. Or imagine that you are conducting a nursing clinic in a high-rise residence for the elderly. People have come for blood pressure screening, to inquire whether tiredness is a side effect of their antihypertensive medication, or to validate whether their diets this past week have reduced their sodium intake. Or picture yourself sitting at an office desk; you are telephoning a physical therapist to discuss the progress of a school-aged child who has mobility problems secondary to cerebral palsy.

Now imagine yourself at a school PTA meeting as a member of a panel discussion on the prevention of human immunodeficiency virus (HIV) transmission. Think about developing a blood pressure screening and dietary education program for a group of predominantly black male employees of a publishing company. Picture yourself reviewing the statistics for patterns of death in your community and contemplating with others the value of a hospice program.

Who would you be, to participate in all these activities, with people of all ages and all levels of health, in such a variety of settings: homes, clinics, schools, workplaces, community meetings? It is likely you would be a community health nurse and you would have specific knowledge and skills in public health nursing.

Notice that we have used two terms—*community health nursing* and *public health nursing*. In the literature and in practice there is often lack of clarity in the use of these terms. Both the American Nurses' Association (ANA, 1980a) and the Public Health Nurses' Section of the American Public Health Association (APHA, 1980) agree that the type of involvement previously described is a synthesis of nursing practice and public health practice. What the ANA called "community health nursing," the APHA called "public health nursing" (Table 1–1).

TABLE 1–1
Current Definitions of Community Health Nursing

ANA
Community health nursing is a synthesis of nursing practice and public health practice applied to promoting and preserving the health of populations. The practice is general and comprehensive. It is not limited to a particular age group or diagnosis, and is continuing, not episodic. The dominant responsibility is to the population as a whole; nursing directed to individuals, families, or groups contributes to the health of the total population. . . . The focus of community health nursing is on the prevention of illness and the promotion and maintenance of health.
APHA
Public health nursing synthesizes the body of knowledge from the public health sciences and professional nursing theories. The implicit overriding goal is to improve the health of the community by identifying sub-groups (aggregates) within the community population which are at high risk of illness, disability, or premature death and directing resources toward these groups. This lies at the heart of primary prevention and health promotion. Public health nursing accomplishes its goal by working with groups, families, and individuals.

Data from American Nurses' Association (ANA). *A conceptual model of community health nursing.* Washington, DC, ANA, 1980a, pp. 2, 11; and American Public Health Association, Public Health Nursing Section (APHA). *The definition and role of public health nursing in the delivery of health care.* Washington, D.C., APHA, 1980.

In 1984, the Division of Nursing, Bureau of Professions of the Health Resources and Services Administration of the U.S. Department of Health and Human Services (USDHHS), sponsored a national consensus conference, with participants invited from the APHA, the ANA, the Association of State and Territorial Directors of Nursing, and the National League for Nursing, for the purposes of clarifying the educational preparation needed for public health nursing and discussing the future of public health nursing. It was agreed that "the term 'community health nurse' is . . . an umbrella term used for all nurses who work in a community, including those who have formal preparation in public health nursing [Table 1–2]. In essence, public health nursing requires specific educational preparation and community health nursing denotes a setting for the practice of nursing" (USDHHS, 1985, p. 4). The consensus conference further agreed that educational preparation for beginning practitioners in public health nursing should include the following: (1) epidemiology, statistics, and research; (2) orientation to health care systems; (3) identification of high-risk populations; (4) application of public health concepts to the care of groups of culturally diverse persons; (5) interventions with high-risk populations; and (6) orientation to regulations affecting public health nursing practice (USDHHS, 1985, p. 9). This educational preparation is assumed to be complementary to a basic education in nursing.

Following the logic of the consensus statements, a registered nurse who works in a noninstitutional setting and has either received a diploma or completed an associate degree nursing education program can be called a com-

TABLE 1–2

Where Are Community Health Nurses Employed?

1. There are more than 250,000 registered nurses employed in community health in the United States (Fig. 1–1), which constitutes 13.5% of all employed registered nurses.
2. Between 1988 and 1992 the numbers of nurses employed in community health nursing settings increased by 30% compared with an increase of 11% in hospital settings.
3. The number of nurses employed in home health care almost doubled between 1988 and 1992. Home health care was the fastest growing area of nursing.
4. The largest percentage (37%) of community health nurses work in home health and hospice agencies to provide nursing care to ill, injured, or disabled individuals and their families.
5. Approximately one in four community health nurses are employed by local and state health departments or community health centers. They provide primary care services, promote health, and prevent illnesses, injury, and premature death.
6. Other community health nurses work with populations associated with a specific age group or type of organization: youth in public and parochial schools, students in colleges and universities, and adults at worksites.
7. However, it is *not* the place of employment that determines whether a nurse is a community health nurse. Instead, community health nurses are distinguished by their education and the community focus of their practice.

Data from USDHHS. *Registered nurse population 1992: Findings from the National Sample Survey of Registered Nurses.* Washington, DC, Division of Nursing, Bureau of Health Professions, Health Resources and Services Administration, 1993.

munity health nurse. However, this nurse would *not* have had any formal education in public health nursing.

Increasing numbers of registered nurses are being employed in home health agencies to provide home care for clients who are ill. This text can assist those without formal preparation in public health nursing to expand their thinking and practice to incorporate knowledge and skills from public health nursing.

For those currently enrolled in a baccalaureate nursing education program, this text can assist in integrating public health practice with nursing practice as part of the formal educational preparation for community health nursing.

The term *community health nurse* is used in this text to denote a nurse with formal public health nursing preparation.

Visions and Commitments

In describing something, we often discuss what the thing looks like, what its component parts are, how it works, and how it relates to other things. Although knowledge of structure and function is important, in interpersonal activities, the exact form is not as important as the purpose of the exchange. And the quality of our specific, purposeful relationships derives from our visions of what might be, as well as our commitments to work toward these visions.

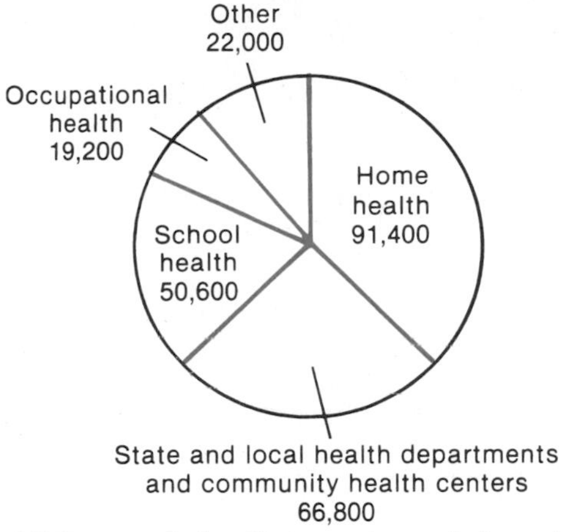

Figure 1–1 ● Community health nurses by worksites—1992 (total community health nurses = 250,000). (Data from United States Department of Health and Human Services. (1993). *Registered nurse population 1992: Findings from the National Sample Survey of Registered Nurses.* Washington, DC: Division of Nursing, Bureau of Health Professions, Health Resources and Services Administration.)

Visions are broad statements of what we desire something to be like; they derive from the ability of human beings to imagine that which is not. *Commitments* are agreements we make with ourselves that pledge our energies for or toward our visions.

As a synthesis of nursing and public health practice, community health nursing accepts the historical commitments of both. By definition and practice, our caring for clients who are ill *is* part of the essence of nursing. Likewise, we bring from nursing our commitment to help the client take responsibility for his or her own well-being and wholeness, through our genuine interest and caring. We add from public health practice our role as health teacher to provide individuals and groups the opportunity to see their own responsibility in moving toward health and wholeness.

Community health nurses are concerned with the development of human beings, families, groups, and communities. Nursing provides us our commitment to assist individuals developmentally, especially at the times of birth and death. Public health expands our commitment beyond individuals to consider the development and healthy functioning of families, groups, and communities.

Public health practice makes its unique contribution to community health nursing through adding to our commitments. These include ensuring (1) an equitable distribution of health care, (2) a basic standard of living that supports the health and well-being of all persons, and (3) a healthful physical environment. These commitments require our involvement with the public and private political and economic environments.

Tables 1–3 and 1–4 list commitments of nursing and public health, respectively, that are grounded in their historical developments. These commitments are the

TABLE 1–3

Commitments of Nursing

1. Patterning an environment of safety and asepsis that promotes health and protects patients
2. Promoting healthy individuals by caring for them when they are not able to do so themselves because of age, illness, disability, or dysfunction
3. Promoting health for individuals and support for families related to developmental stages (pregnancy, labor and delivery, and care of newborns; care of dependent family members; care of dependent elderly; care of the dying)
4. Promoting wellness and integration during illness, disability, and dying
5. Treating patients equitably without bias related to age, race, gender, socioeconomic class, religion, or cultural preferences
6. Calling forth the patient's commitment to his or her own well-being and wholeness

TABLE 1–4

Commitments of Public Health

1. Patterning of an environment that promotes health
2. Promotion of healthy families
3. Equitable, just distribution of health care to all
4. A just economic environment to support health and vitality of individuals, families, and groups
5. Prevention of physical and mental illnesses as a support to the wholeness and vitality of individuals, families, and groups
6. Providing the greatest good for the greatest number—thinking collectively on behalf of human beings
7. Educating others to be aware of their own responsibility to move toward health, wholeness, and vitality

foundations on which specific professional practices, projects, goals, and activities can be created.

Because our culture is biased toward "doing" (being active, being busy, and producing), we often are not conscious of our visions of what might be. We study, exercise, go out with friends, cook, clean, play with children, invest money, and shop. We can even get bogged down in "doing" the activities and projects appropriate to our commitments. For example, if you are committed to having relationships with friends, recall a time when a meeting with friends felt like a duty and obligation. You were going through the motions of being together, but you were not genuinely relating to one another. At that moment you were not creating the relationship from your commitment; you probably felt burdened rather than enlivened.

Likewise, it is possible to get bogged down professionally by doing the "right" things that community health nurses are supposed to do but not feeling satisfied. We are disappointed that results do not show up quickly enough or that suffering persists. We create too many professional projects and feel spread too thin. We burn out.

Working on activities directed toward the commitments underlying community health nursing does not guarantee that we will achieve our visions. But not working toward our visions and giving up on our commitments guarantees that we are part of the problem rather than part of the solution in our communities. Not working toward our visions also results in dissatisfaction and disconnectedness.

Remaining in touch with the reasons we are doing something empowers us. Our vision of healthy, whole, vital individuals, families, and communities and our related commitments can be a renewing source of energy. And it is hope and energy that we draw on to empower our professional practice and bring vitality to our relationships with individuals, families, and groups.

Expressing our visions and commitments to others provides them an opportunity to become partners in working *for* what might be. By having partners we gain support not only for our visions, but also for specific projects. For example, the mother of a young family, consisting of the mother, the father, and a 2-year-old son with cerebral palsy, called the health department during her second pregnancy. She requested a nurse to assist her in having a healthy second child. No one could guarantee that vision, but the mother's willingness to seek a partner in the commitment provided an opportunity for a nurse-client relationship that would increase the likelihood of a healthy newborn. The nurse and mother developed specific projects related to, among other things, financial access to prenatal care, nutrition, prenatal monitoring, and anxiety management.

Community health nurses often have visions about health that others do not know are possible. Nurses can educate and speak about visions of health and specific commitments that can increase the likelihood of particular health possibilities. For example, a married couple in their 60s were committed to remaining self-sufficient. Both husband and wife had diabetes, and the wife had had a stroke that resulted in right hemiparesis and expressive aphasia. When the wife had to retire from her job, their income declined dramatically. The husband worked two jobs and was rarely home as a companion to his wife. The couple fought about money, and because verbal communication was so slow and unclear, they resorted to expressing frustration and anger by hitting each other for the first time in their marriage. Initially the family did not ask the community health nursing student for assistance. On one visit the student recognized that the wife was angry and began to explore the family stressors. The student's vision that families can solve problems through communication made it possible to discuss the problem with the spouses and solicit their commitment to explore alternatives with her. The family eventually agreed to turn to their extended family, social services, and a bank for additional sources of revenue. In this situation it was the nurse who initiated the discussion of her vision and enlisted the family members' commitment to exploring possibilities.

We have discussed two examples of expressing visions as a basis for creating commitments in nurse-client relationships and in relationships between the nurse and other service providers. It is helpful for each nurse to express his or her visions and commitments to peers and supervisors. As nurses, we need colleagues to encourage us, work with us, and coach us. Work groups whose members can identify some visions common to their individual practices and can agree on some common commitments have a vital source of energy. When we know what we are *for,* we can assertively invite others to participate with us. When others are working with us, more possibilities are created for synergistic effects.

Distinguishing Features of Community Health Nursing

Community health nurses are expected to use the nursing process in their relationships with individuals, families, groups, populations, and aggregates (ANA, 1980a; APHA, 1980). Community health nursing is the care provided by educated nurses in a particular place and time and directed toward promoting, restoring, and preserving the health of the total population or community. Families are recognized as an important social group in which values and knowledge are learned and health-related behaviors are practiced.

HEALTHFUL COMMUNITIES

What aspects of this definition are different from definitions of nursing in general? The explicit naming of families, groups, and aggregates as the client is a major focus. Individuals are cared for by community health nurses; however, they are cared for in the context of a vision of a healthful community. Beliefs underlying community health nursing are summarized from Chapter 2 in Table 1–5. Community health nursing is nursing for social betterment.

Community health nurses seek to empower individuals, families, and groups to participate in creating healthful communities. The prevailing theory about how healthful communities develop has been that individuals and social groups clarify their identities first and then protect their own rights while also considering the rights of others. More recent studies on the moral development of women in the United States suggest that women first participate in a network of relationships of caring for others and then consider their own rights (Gilligan, 1982).

The ideal for a healthful community is a balance of individuality and unity. Community health nurses seek to promote healthful communities in which there is individual freedom *and* responsible caring for others.

It is impossible for an individual to consider only his or her desires without infringing on the freedoms of others. For collective well-being to exist, we must also be concerned about caring accountability. We must "ask about justice, about . . . each person having space in which to grow and dream and learn and work" (Brueggemann, 1982, p. 50). We must ask about the conditions that promote health.

TABLE 1–5

Beliefs Underlying Community Health Nursing

- Human beings have rights and responsibilities.
- Promoting and maintaining family independence is healthful.
- Environments have an impact on human health.
- Nurses can make a difference and promote change toward health for individuals, families, and communities. Vulnerable and at-risk populations/groups/families need special attention, especially the aged, infants, and disabled, ill, and poor persons.
- Poverty and oppression are social barriers to achievement of health and human potential.
- Interpersonal relationships are essential to caring for others.
- Hygiene, self-care, and prevention are as important as care of the sick.
- Community health nurses can be leaders and innovators in developing programs of nursing care and programs for adequate standards of living.
- Community health nursing care should be available to all, not just the poor.

EMPOWERMENT FOR HEALTH PROMOTION

Because community health nurses often work with persons who are *not* ill, emphasis is placed on promoting and preserving health in addition to assisting people to respond to illnesses. Although not all illnesses can be prevented, nor can death be eliminated, community health nurses seek to empower human beings to live in ways that strengthen resilience; decrease preventable diseases, disability, and premature death; and relieve experiences of illness, vulnerability, and suffering.

Empowerment is the process of assisting others to uncover their own inherent abilities, strengths, vigor, wholeness, and spirit. Empowerment depends on the presence of hope. Power is not actually provided by the community health nurse. Empowerment is a process by which possibilities and opportunities for the expression of an individual's being and abilities are revealed. Nurses can assist this process by fostering hope and by removing barriers to expression.

Community health nurses use the information and skills from their education and experiences in medical-surgical, parent-child, and psychiatric–mental health nursing in assisting individuals, families, and groups to have *opportunities* to make choices that promote health and wholeness. In community health nursing, nurses rarely make the choices for others. Instead, as a means of expanding opportunities for others, community health nurses provide information about interpersonal relationships and alternative ways of doing things. This is especially true when community health nurses instruct others to care for those with illnesses or to generally support growth and development of other members of families or groups. For example, a husband may be shown how to safely transfer his wife from the bed to a chair or a young father may be taught how to praise his son and set limits without resorting to threats and frequent punishment.

Being related to people can invite them to risk being connected and to trust in the face of their fears. This is particularly true for those who have experienced intense or patterned isolation, abuse, despair, or oppression. A nurse "is present" with a client when the nurse is both physically near and psychologically "being with" the person (Gilje, 1993). The "presence" of a community health nurse is revealed in the case study at the end of the chapter.

Theory and Community Health Nursing

Nursing practice is based on our understanding of the concepts of human beings, health and illness, problem-solving and creative processes, and the human-environment relationship (Hanchett, 1988; Marriner-Tomey, 1989). Our environment includes physical, social, cultural, spiritual, economic, and political facets.

Our knowledge of these concepts evolves from several routes, including personal experience, logic, a sense of right and wrong (ethics), empirical science, aesthetic preferences, and an understanding of what it means to be human (Marriner-Tomey, 1989). Concepts are labels or names that we give to our perceptions of living beings, objects, or events. Theories are a set of concepts, definitions, and hypotheses that help us describe, explain, or predict the interrelationships among concepts (Marriner-Tomey, 1989).

Although Florence Nightingale began the formal development of nursing theory, most theory development in nursing has occurred since the 1960s (Choi, 1989). Marriner-Tomey (1989) describes the work of 26 nursing theorists. (Obviously, we cannot discuss all of them here.) In community health nursing, general systems theory provides a way to link many of the concepts related to nursing. The nursing theories of Johnson (1980), King (1971), Neuman (1982), and Roy (1984) rely in part on general systems theory. Perspectives on client-environment relationships from these theories are discussed later in the chapter.

GENERAL SYSTEMS THEORY

An *open system* is a set of interacting elements that must exchange energy, matter, or information with the external environment to exist (Katz and Kahn, 1966; von Bertalanffy, 1968). Open systems include individuals as well as

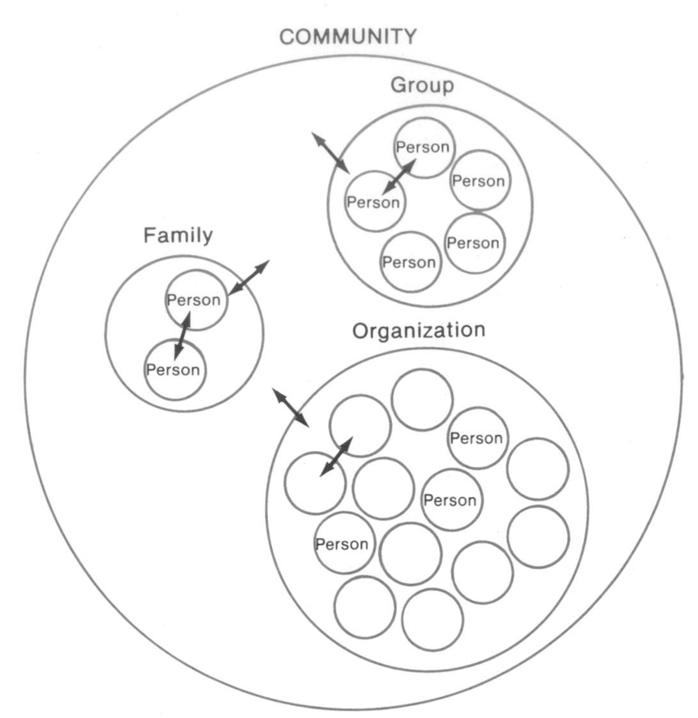

Figure 1–2 ● Social systems.

social systems such as families, groups, organizations, and communities with whom the community health nurse must work (Fig. 1–2). Systems theory is especially useful in exploring the numerous and complex client-environment interchanges.

For example, a community health nurse may provide postpartum home visits to a woman and her newborn, simultaneously focusing on the adjustment of the entire family to the birth. The same nurse may also teach teen parenting classes in a high school and monitor the birth rates in the community, identifying those populations at statistical risk of low birth weight.

Compared with inpatient settings, the environments in community health nursing practice also are more variable and less controllable (Kenyon et al., 1990). General systems theory provides an umbrella for assessing and analyzing the various clients and their relationships with dynamic environments. In this text, family and community assessment are approached from a general systems framework.

Each open system has the same basic structures (Smith and Rankin, 1972) (Fig. 1–3*A*). Figure 1–3*B* is an example of the open systems model applied to a specific organization. The *boundary* separates the system from its environment and regulates the flow of energy, matter, and information between the system and its environment. The *environment* is everything outside the boundary of the system. The skin acts as a physical boundary for human beings. A person's preference for relatedness is a more abstract boundary that helps determine the pattern of interpersonal relationships. Family boundaries may be determined by law and culture, such as a rule that a family consists of blood relatives. A family may have more open

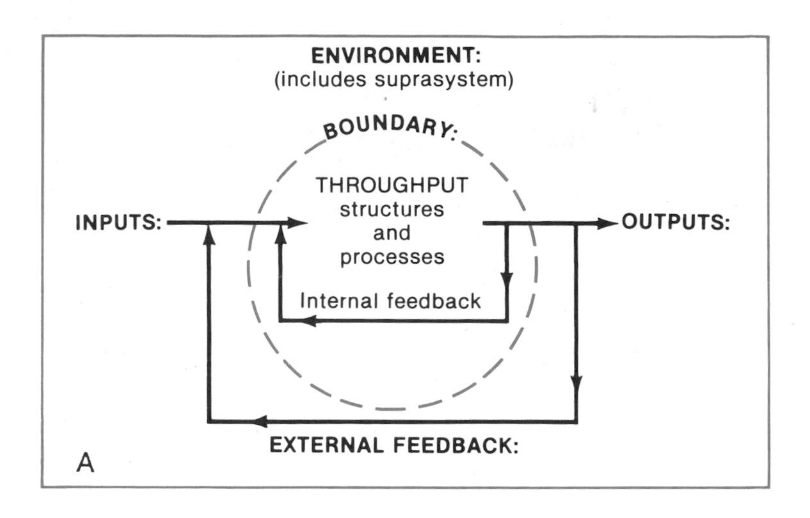

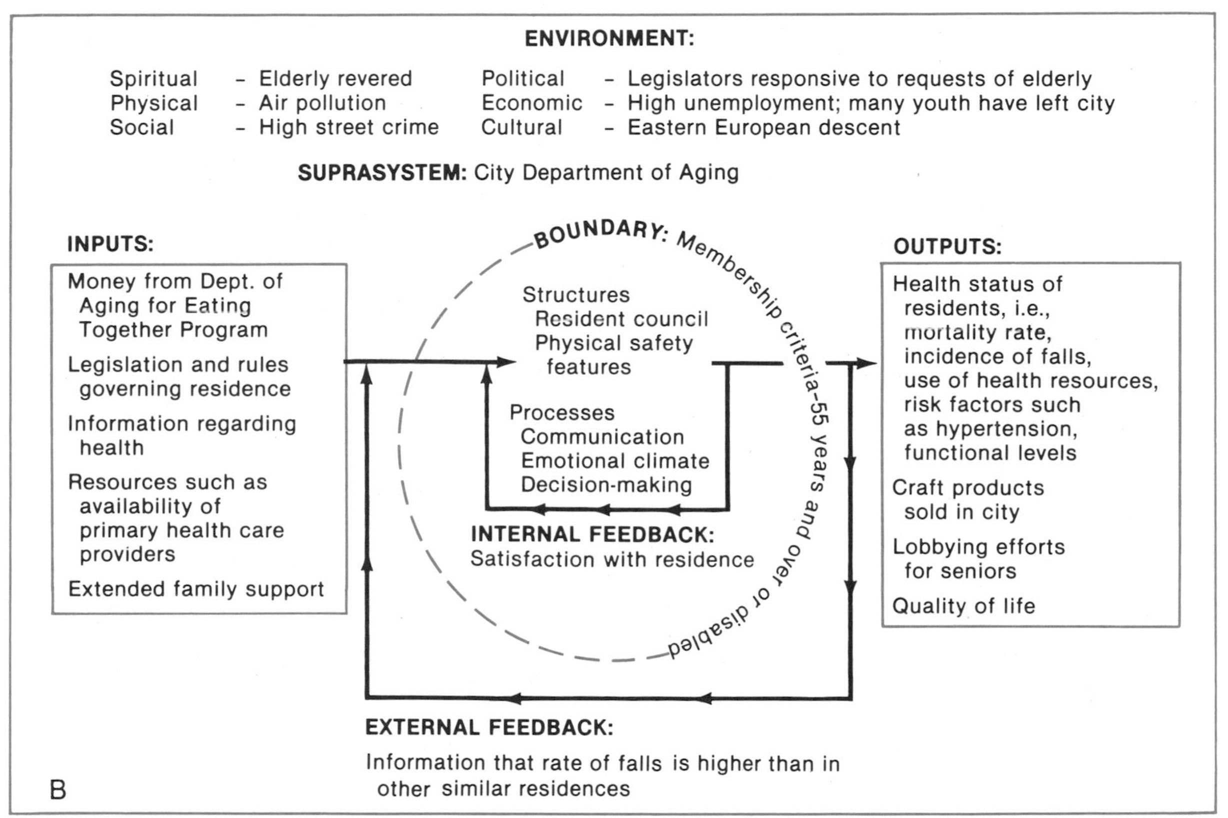

Figure 1–3 ● *A,* Model of an open system. *B,* Residence for the elderly viewed as an open system.

boundaries and define itself by including others as family members. Groups, organizations, and some communities have membership criteria that assist in defining their boundaries. Other community boundaries may be geographical and political, such as the city limits.

Outputs are the created products, energy, and information that emerge from the system into the environment. Health behaviors and health status are examples of outputs. *Inputs* are the matter, energy, and information that come from the environment into the system. Inputs may be resources or stressors to the system. Each system uses the inputs together with internal resources to achieve its purposes and goals. *Feedback* is information channeled back into the system from its environment that describes the condition of the system. When a nurse tells a mother that her child's blood pressure is higher than the desired range, the nurse is providing health information as feedback to the mother. Feedback provides an opportunity to modify system functioning. The mother can then decide when and where to seek medical evaluation.

Each system is composed of parts called *subsystems.* Subsystems have their own goals and functions and exist in relationship with the other subsystems. In a human being, the gastrointestinal system is an example of a subsystem. In social systems, the subsystems may be structural or functional. Structural subsystems relate to organization. Examples of structural subsystems are a mother-child dyad in a family or the nursing department in a local health department. Functional subsystems are more abstract and relate to specific purposes. For example, the subsystems of organizations have been conceptualized as production, maintenance, integration, and adaptation (Katz and Kahn, 1966). Subsystems of a community are often named by their function, such as the health care subsystem, the educational subsystem, and the economic subsystem.

Systems may relate as separate entities that interact or they may create a variety of partnerships and confederations. Systems may be hierarchical. The *suprasystem* is the next larger system in a hierarchy. For example, the suprasystem of a county is the state; the suprasystem of a parochial school may be the church or the diocese that sponsors the school.

The assumptions that relate to all open systems (von Bertalanffy, 1968) are similar to those underlying holism in nursing (Allen, 1991).

1. A system is greater than the sum of its parts. One cannot understand a system by studying its parts in isolation. For example, we cannot make inferences about the health of a family unless we inquire about the health status of each member. However, knowing the health history and present status of individual members does not tell us how the family addresses its health concerns. Knowing the parts is necessary, but not sufficient, to describe the health of the family system.
2. The primary focus of systems theory is the relationship of the parts, not the parts per se. Life is dynamic. When nurses assess a family or community at a specific time, the assessment is more like a photograph than a movie. Exploring how the system has changed, how the individual members affect each other, and how the system interacts with the environment helps our assessment to become more like a movie.
3. A change in one part of a system affects the whole system. Change is a part of life. It may be accompanied by suffering because of either the type of change (an accident) or the quality of the change (too many changes exceed the resources). At other times change brings relief and strengthened resources.
4. Elements of one system may also be parts of another system. For example, a college student also belongs to a family, social groups, and, perhaps, a religious organization.
5. Exchanges between a system and its environments tend to be circular or cyclical. Interaction exists between the system and its environment. For example, in a community with a high percentage of hazardous occupations, a high accident rate may increase the disabilities and unemployment within families. The unemployed pay less income tax, and money available to develop services for the disabled within the community is therefore reduced. Because the community has fewer resources, new businesses may find it a less attractive location. Although a single cause-and-effect relationship cannot usually be established, health problems are interconnected with social concerns. In the community just described, accident rates are related to unemployment and economics.
6. Human beings and social systems seek to survive and to avoid disorganization and randomness (or *entropy*). As social systems develop they tend to become more complex, with specialized structures and functions. Organizations often change their goals rather than disband when they have achieved their original goals. A multitude of health care professions, services, programs, and equipment have developed within U.S. health care. Community health nurses must recognize the complexity to assist others to access health care and to propose changes.
7. Systems operate with *equifinality,* meaning that the same end point can be reached from a variety of starting points and through various paths. There is not one right way. Culture influences child-rearing among families, for example, and local communities organize their health services differently.

NURSING THEORY

Nursing theories are based on a range of perspectives about the nature of human beings, health, nursing, and the environment. Most nursing theories have been developed with individual clients in mind (Hanchett, 1988). However, many concepts from the different nursing theories are applicable to nursing with families and communities. The concepts of self-care and environment are introduced here.

Self-care

Self-care is "the production of actions directed to self or to the environment in order to regulate one's functioning in the interests of one's life, integrated functioning, and well-being" (Orem, 1985, p. 31). Self-care depends on knowledge, resources, and action (Erickson et al., 1983). The concept of self-care is consistent with the community nursing focus on empowerment of persons and groups to promote health and to care for themselves.

Although each person is responsible for his or her own health habits, the family and community have responsibilities to support self-care (USDHHS, 1990). The family is the immediate source of support and health information. The community has responsibilities to provide safe food, water, air, and waste disposal; enforce safety standards; and create and support opportunities for individual self-care (USDHHS, 1990). When the focus is on self-care, the family and community are viewed primarily as suprasystems to individuals.

TABLE 1–6

Perspectives on Client-Environment Relationships in Selected Nursing Theories

Theorist	Relationship of Client and Environment
Dorothy Johnson	Clients attempt to adjust to environmental factors. Strong inputs from the environment may cause imbalance and require excess energy to the point of threatening the existence of the client. Stable environments help clients conserve energy and function successfully.
Sister Callista Roy	Clients attempt to adjust to immediate environmental excesses or absences within a background of other stimuli. Successful adaptation allows survival, growth, and improved ability to respond to the environment.
Imogene King	Clients interact purposefully with other people and the environment. Health is the continuous process of using resources to function in daily life and to grow and develop.
Betty Neuman	Clients continuously interact with people and other environmental forces and seek to defend themselves against threats. Health is balance and harmony within the whole person.

Data from Marriner-Tomey, A. (1989). *Nursing theorists and their work,* (ed. 2). St. Louis: Mosby–Year Book.

Client-Environment Relationships

Nursing theories acknowledge that humans live within an environment (Marriner-Tomey, 1989). Nurses are caring professionals within the clients' environments who influence the clients through direct physical care, provision of information, interpersonal presence, and environmental management. Nursing theories that build on general systems theory tend to place more emphasis on the environment than do other nursing theories (Hanchett, 1988). The continuously changing environment requires that the client expend energy to survive, perform activities of daily living, grow, develop, and maintain harmony or balance. Clients must adapt within a dynamic environment (Table 1–6).

PUBLIC HEALTH THEORY

Public health theory is concerned with the health of populations of human beings. Public health is a practice discipline that applies knowledge from the physical, biological, and social sciences to prevent disease, injury, disability, and premature death. Epidemiology is the study of health in human populations and is explored in more detail in Chapter 11. Population, prevention, risk, and social justice are among the concepts from public health theory that are important to community health nursing. The first three concepts are discussed here, and justice is discussed later in the chapter.

Populations and Risk

Population has two meanings: people residing in an area and a group or set of persons under statistical study. The word group is used here to mean a set or collection of persons, not a system of individuals who engage in face-to-face interactions, which is the definition of group used for discussion of systems theory. The fact that there are multiple definitions for population and group leads to lack of clarity and necessitates debate.

Both definitions of population are used in public health and community health nursing. The initial goal of public health has been to prevent or control communicable diseases that were the major causes of death within human populations (i.e., the people living in specific geographical or political areas). Today, for example, a director of nursing in a city health department is concerned with the health of the population within the city limits. When used in this way, population means all the people in the area or community. The noun *public* is often used as a synonym for this definition of population.

Because not everyone has the same health status, the second definition of population is especially important in public health practice: a set of persons under statistical study. Using this definition, a population is a set of persons having a common personal or environmental characteristic. The common characteristic may be anything thought to relate to health, such as age, race, sex, social class, medical diagnosis, level of disability, exposure to a toxin, or participation in a health-seeking behavior, such as smoking cessation. It is the researcher or health practitioner who identifies the characteristic and set of persons that make up this population. In epidemiology, numerous sets of persons are studied clinically and statistically to identify the causes, methods of treatment, and means of prevention of diseases, accidents, disabilities, and premature deaths. In community health nursing, epidemiological information is used to identify populations at higher risk for specific preventable health conditions. *Risk* is a statistical concept based on probability. Community health nursing is concerned with human risk of disease, disability, and premature death. Therefore, community health nurses work with persons within the population to reduce their risk of developing a health condition.

Aggregate is a synonym for the second definition of population. Aggregates are a number of people who do not have the relatedness necessary to constitute an interpersonal group (system), but who have one or more characteristics in common, such as pregnant teenagers (Schultz, 1987). Williams (1977) focused attention on the aggregate as an additional type of client with whom community health nurses apply the problem-solving process. For example, aggregates may be identified by virtue of setting (those enrolled in a well-baby clinic), demographic characteristic (women), or health status (smokers or those with hypertension) (APHA, 1980). It is the community health nurse who identifies the aggregate by naming one or more common characteristics.

The terminology regarding statistical groups and aggregates is confusing. Although there are subtle differences, the terms *at-risk population, specified population,* and *population group* are used to mean aggregate. The APHA (1980) uses the term *at-risk population* in place of the term aggregate. In its description of community health nursing, the ANA (1980a) uses the term *specified population.* Others use *population group* to mean a population that shares similar characteristics but limited face-to-face interaction (Porter, 1987). It is important to remember that whichever of these terms is used, such a population is not a system. The individuals within these populations are not classified because of interaction or common goals. It is the community health nurse who conceptually classifies, collects, or aggregates the individuals into such a population. The individuals within such a population may often not even know one another. The nurse has identified the population to focus intervention efforts toward health promotion and prevention.

Prevention

Prevention is a complex concept that also evolved from an attempt to control diseases among the public. Epidemiology is a science that helps to describe the natural history of specific diseases, their causes, and their treatments. The natural history of a disease involves a presymptomatic period, a symptomatic period, and a resolution (death, disability, complications, or recovery) (Friedman, 1987). The broad concept of prevention has three levels: primary, secondary, and tertiary. The goal of *primary prevention* is the prevention of the occurrence of the disease. Activities of primary prevention include environmental protection (such as asepsis) and personal protection (such as immunizations and avoiding smoking). The goal of *secondary prevention* is the detection (screening) and treatment of the disease as early as possible during the natural history of the disease. For example, Papanicolaou's smears allow cervical cancer to be detected earlier in the disease process so that cure is more likely. *Tertiary prevention* is geared toward preventing disability, complications, and death from the disease. Tertiary prevention includes rehabilitation.

All levels of prevention may be accomplished through work with individuals, families, and groups. Prevention may also be accomplished by targeting changes in the behaviors of specified populations, changes in social functioning of communities (law, social mores), and changes in the physical environment (waste disposal). The well-being and health of the entire population within the community is the ultimate goal of public health.

Goals for Community Health Nursing

Care is always in the here and now, responsive to the needs of specific persons, in a specific place, at a specific time. It is always personal and intimate. Even when community health nurses work with other professionals and community groups, the care is expressed through recognition of the uniqueness of each of the others.

TABLE 1–7

Major Goals for Community Health Nursing

- Care of the ill, disabled, and suffering in nonhospital settings
- Support of development and well-being throughout the life cycle
- Promotion of human relatedness and mutual caring
- Promotion of self-responsibility regarding health and well-being
- Promotion of relative safety in the environment while conserving resources

Smith, C. M. (1985). Unpublished data. Baltimore: University of Maryland School of Nursing.

There are several major goals for community health nursing (Table 1–7). Table 1–8 identifies examples of health outcomes for each of the goals, for each category of client.

All nurses address these goals but most do so with individuals, hospitalized individuals and their families or friends, and small groups. In addition to formulating these goals with individuals, community health nurses do the same with families, groups, aggregates, and organizations within the community.

Nursing Ethics and Social Justice

The goals of community health nursing reflect the values and beliefs of both nursing and public health. Each profession has an ideology, or set of values, concepts, ideas, and beliefs, that defines its responsibilities and actions (Hamilton and Keyser, 1992). Ideologies are linked closely with ethics—the study and thinking about what one ought to do (i.e., right conduct).

Public health and nursing are based on the same ethical principles: respecting autonomy, doing good, avoiding harm, and treating people fairly (Fry, 1983; Last, 1992) (Table 1–9). These principles are sometimes in conflict. Issues related to application of these principles are discussed in case examples in Ethics Boxes I through IX (Chapters 19 through 27).

ETHICAL PRIORITIES

The ANA Code for Nurses (1985, p. 2) states that the most important ethical principle of nursing practice is the "respect for the inherent dignity and worth . . . of human existence and the individuality of all persons" (Table 1–10). However, because public health is concerned with the well-being of the entire population, the foremost ethical principle of public health practice is doing good for the greatest number of persons with the least harm. Consequently, in community health nursing there is a tension

TABLE 1–8

Examples of Health Outcomes Related to Goals of Community Health Nursing

	Care of the Ill	Support of Development	Support of Relatedness	Promotion of Self-responsibility	Promotion of Healthful Environment
Individual	Individual learns self-management of diabetes mellitus	Teenage mother adjusts to newborn care	Retarded adult joins group for socialization	Adult child of alcoholic seeks counseling	Homeless person seeks shelter
Family	Family cares for member with terminal cancer	Extended family decides how best to care for aging grandparents	Family with disabled child seeks out other such families	Family identifies preferences of members	Elderly couple improves safety in home
Group	Children with physical disabilities are cared for in school	Junior high school students explore responsibility regarding sexual activity	Several women in a residence start a sharing group	Women at a mother and children's center take on responsibilities in the center	Mothers Against Drunk Driving advocates laws against driving while intoxicated
Aggregate	Barriers are identified in a number of patients regarding failure to return for tests of cure after antibiotics	Worksite program regarding preretirement planning is established	*	Worksite program for counseling for health risk reduction is initiated	Curriculum is developed for schools regarding burn prevention
Community	A hospice program is initiated in a city	Regulations for safe daycare are passed as county ordinance	A network of case management is established for discharged psychiatric patients	Crisis hotline is established	A waste recycling program is established

*By definition, aggregates are individuals or families with common characteristics who are identified as such by the community health nurse or other professional. If such clients become known to one another and develop a sense of belonging or support, the aggregate would become a group or community.

between an individual-focused ethic and a society-focused ethic (Fry, 1983; Hamilton and Keyser, 1992). Community health nurses consider both ethical perspectives.

How does a nurse respect the autonomy of individuals while securing health for many? There is not one "right" answer. The question needs to be asked often and answered anew as circumstances change. At times, the community health nurse's decision will be to protect the autonomy of an individual while working for environmental changes that seek to protect many. For example, a community health nurse honors a teenager's autonomy and does not force him or her to avoid cigarette use. However, the nurse can lobby for higher cigarette taxes that decrease consumption, for enforcement of laws prohibiting cigarette sales to minors, and for substance-free recreation centers. Both nursing and public health ideologies value education and environment modifications over coercion.

TABLE 1–9

Basic Ethical Principles in Health

Principle	Definition	Example
Altruism	Concern for the welfare of others	Being present
Beneficence	Doing good	Providing immunizations
Nonmaleficence	Avoiding harm	Not abandoning client
Respect for autonomy	Honoring self-determination, i.e., right to make one's own decisions; respecting privacy	Allowing client to refuse treatment, informed consent; maintaining confidentiality
Veracity	Truth-telling	Communicating authentically and not lying
Fidelity	Keeping promises	Arriving on time for home visit
Justice	Treating people fairly	Providing nursing services to all, regardless of ability to pay

Data from American Association of Colleges of Nursing (AACN). (1989). *Essentials of College and University Education for Professional Nursing:* Washington, DC: Author; and Beauchamp T., Childress, J. (1989). *Principles of biomedical ethics,* (ed. 3). New York: Oxford University Press.

TABLE 1–10

Code for Nurses

1. The nurse provides services with respect for human dignity and the uniqueness of the client, unrestricted by considerations of social or economic status, personal attributes, or the nature of health problems.
2. The nurse safeguards the client's right to privacy by judiciously protecting information of a confidential nature.
3. The nurse acts to safeguard the client and the public when health care and safety are affected by the incompetent, unethical, or illegal practice of any person.
4. The nurse assumes responsibility and accountability for individual nursing judgments and actions.
5. The nurse maintains competence in nursing.
6. The nurse exercises informed judgment and uses individual com petence and qualifications as criteria in seeking consultation, accepting responsibilities, and delegating nursing activities to others.
7. The nurse participates in activities that contribute to the ongoing development of the profession's body of knowledge.
8. The nurse participates in the profession's efforts to implement and improve standards of nursing.
9. The nurse participates in the profession's efforts to establish and maintain conditions of employment conducive to high-quality nursing care.
10. The nurse participates in the profession's effort to protect the public from misinformation and misrepresentation and to maintain the integrity of nursing.
11. The nurse collaborates with members of the health professions and other citizens in promoting community and national efforts to meet the health needs of the public.

From ANA. (1985). *Code for nurses with interpretive statements.* Washington, DC: Author.

The ANA (1985) acknowledges that there are "situations in which individual rights to autonomy in health care may be temporarily overridden to preserve the life of the human community" (p. 3). For example, in an airplane disaster one individual already close to death may be allowed to die in order to save several others. Individual autonomy may also be curtailed by involuntary confinement if a person is threatening to commit suicide or to abuse or kill another.

DISTRIBUTIVE JUSTICE

A more difficult issue emerges when we consider the number of individuals with competing interests and needs. Does everyone have a right to health care? If so, what kind and how much health care? Nursing is working to "ensure the availability and accessibility of high quality health services to all persons whose health needs are unmet" (ANA, 1985, p. 16). Our public health ethic goes further. Not only is health care considered a right, but "a basic standard of living necessary for health" is also a right (Winslow, 1984).

How are health care, nursing, and other social services to be distributed within the population? *Justice* is an ethical concept concerned with treating human beings fairly. Nurses are to provide competent, personalized care regardless of an individual client's financial, social, and personal characteristics (ANA, 1985). Because the nursing code of ethics focuses on care with individuals, community health nurses also need other perspectives of justice in helping to provide ethical care with populations (Fry, 1985).

There are two perspectives for determining justice when working with populations: egalitarian (equal) and utilitarian (Fry, 1985). In an egalitarian system of justice, each person has equal access to equal health services. Providing every person in this country with access to basic health services is an example of egalitarian justice. In a utilitarian system of justice, resources are distributed to provide the greatest good for the greatest number with the least amount of harm. When resources are limited, the utilitarian perspective is helpful. At times, individuals may be harmed under the utilitarian perspective. The airplane disaster mentioned earlier is an example of utilitarian decision-making. With utilitarian justice, it is important to try to determine the benefits and risks of an action (Last, 1992). If health care services are provided only to those who can pay, that health care system does not meet a criterion for justice. Instead, health care is provided unequally (only to those who can afford it) and the good of the entire population is not considered.

Creating a just health care system in a context of limited resources is a major challenge as we enter the 21st century. Questions that are being asked to determine health care priorities for populations are, for example: Who decides what is good? What are the benefits and risks? How do we weigh the short-term and long-term benefits and risks? How do we determine who has a reasonable chance of benefiting? In our democratic society, there are competing interests and the process is ongoing. Potentially, all community members, government leaders, nurses, and other health care professionals contribute to priority-setting. Community health nursing practice and research contribute information to help answer these questions. An ethic that includes social justice also helps to focus priorities.

There is a constant tension between facilitating the freedom of individuals and nurturing a community in which people feel connected enough to care for one another. One of our challenges as community health nurses is to foster communities in which people experience their interconnection and treat one another justly. In the rest of this chapter, the specific responsibilities and competencies that assist community health nurses in working for social betterment are explored.

The Nursing Process in Community Health

The ANA Standards of Community Health Nursing (1986) are developed in concert with the steps of the nursing process and indicate that community health nurses are to apply the entire nursing process with individuals,

TABLE 1–11

Standards of Community Health Nursing Practice

Standard I: Theory

The nurse applies theoretical concepts as a basis for decisions in practice.

Standard II: Data Collection

The nurse systematically collects data that are comprehensive and accurate.

Standard III: Diagnosis

The nurse analyzes data collected about the community, family, and individual to determine diagnoses.

Standard IV: Planning

At each level of prevention, the nurse develops plans that specify nursing actions unique to client needs.

Standard V: Intervention

The nurse, guided by the plan, intervenes to promote, maintain, or restore health, to prevent illness, and to effect rehabilitation.

Standard VI: Evaluation

The nurse evaluates responses of the community, family, and individual to interventions to determine progress toward goal achievement and to revise the data base, diagnoses, and plan.

Standard VII: Quality Assurance and Professional Development

The nurse participates in peer review and other means of evaluation to assure quality of nursing practice. The nurse assumes responsibility for professional development and contributes to professional growth of others.

Standard VIII: Interdisciplinary Collaboration

The nurse collaborates with other health care providers, professionals, and community representatives in assessing, planning, implementing, and evaluating programs for community health.

Standard IX: Research

The nurse contributes to theory and practice in community health nursing through research.

From ANA. (1986). *Standards of community health nursing practice.* Washington, DC: Author.

families, and groups to promote health and wellness throughout the entire life span (Table 1–11). These standards describe both a competent level of nursing care provided to clients and a competent level of behavior within the profession. Thus, standards of clinical community health nursing practice help define the scope and quality of community health nursing care; they also help to distinguish community health nursing from other nursing specialties. One of the particular features of the specialty is that community health nurses are concerned with the health of communities.

How do community health nurses work with communities? Community health nurses use demographic and epidemiological data to identify health problems of families, groups, and aggregates; community health nurses comprehend community structure, organization, and resources in developing solutions to meet the needs of families, groups, and aggregates (ANA, 1980a; ANA, 1986). From this point of view, the community may be seen as part of the environment or suprasystem of the families, groups, and aggregates.

The ANA (1980a) makes a distinction between direct and indirect care in community health nursing. Direct community health nursing care is the application of the nursing process with individuals, families, and groups and involves face-to-face relationships. Direct care includes management and coordination of care. For example, a community health nurse who performs a developmental assessment of an infant, teaches the mother about age-appropriate play, and administers immunizations is engaged in direct care.

Indirect community health nursing does not involve interpersonal relationships with all persons who benefit from care. The nurse collaborates in interpersonal relationships with others to promote the health and well-being of the community. Priorities are determined after assessing the health status of the entire population and aggregates, the existing resources, the environment, and the social mechanisms for solving problems (AACN, 1986). Goals include promotion of self-help and appropriate use of health resources by community members, development of new services, and provision of effective, adequate direct nursing care services (ANA, 1980a). Indirect care also includes the use of political, social, and economic means to ensure a basic standard of living for community members. A nurse who writes a grant proposal for providing primary health care to a rural population is engaged in indirect community health nursing care.

All professional nurses are expected to collaborate with their peers to improve nursing care and to collaborate with others to develop new health resources and "ensure safe, legal and ethical health care practices" (American Association of Colleges of Nursing [AACN], 1986, p. 18). So we might ask, how is community health nursing distinct from other specialties? One distinction is that community health nursing has a broader perspective and is concerned with the health of the entire community and all of the aggregates within it. A second difference is that the direct care in community health is *targeted* toward individuals, families, groups, and aggregates based on those at risk (APHA, 1980). Care is not just provided to those who seek it. It is the responsibility of community health nurses to identify those who might benefit from health promotion and health prevention as well as those with illnesses and disabilities who are not receiving care.

Responsibilities of Community Health Nurses

The traditional historical responsibilities of community health nurses (see Chapter 2) are summarized in Table 1–12. While many of these are responsibilities of *all* nurses today, several strategies stand out as being of great impor-

TABLE 1–12

Responsibilities of Community Health Nurses

1. Providing care to the ill and disabled in their homes, including teaching of caregivers.
2. Maintaining healthful environments.
3. Teaching about health promotion and prevention of disease and injury.
4. Identifying those with inadequate standards of living and untreated illnesses and disabilities and referring them for services.
5. Preventing and reporting neglect and abuse.
6. Advocating for adequate standards of living and health care services.
7. Collaborating to develop appropriate, adequate, acceptable health care services.
8. Caring for oneself and participating in professional development activities.
9. Ensuring quality nursing care and engaging in nursing research.

tance in community health nursing: (1) identification of unmet needs and referral, (2) teaching, (3) environmental management, (4) collaboration and coordination, and (5) political action for adequate standards of living and health care services and resources. In the following discussion of nursing responsibilities in community health, direct care of the clients who are ill is discussed first because it is the responsibility nurses are most familiar with.

DIRECT CARE OF ILL, INFIRM, SUFFERING, AND DISABLED CLIENTS

"Doing for" those who cannot do for themselves, because of illness, infirmity, suffering, or disability, is a historical basis of nursing. Hospitals and nursing homes have been the places where most nursing care has been provided in the United States during this century. However, home care of ill persons by nurses preceded hospital care. Since the mid-1960s, the significance of care for ill clients in the home has re-emerged. Reasons for this include the aging of the population, the relative magnitude of chronic diseases, reimbursement for skilled nursing care in the home (see Chapter 29), and the decreased length of hospital stays resulting from efforts to reduce hospital costs.

Care of individuals in the home today builds on care that nurses have learned to provide in institutional settings. Whatever theoretical framework is used for viewing the needs and health problems of individuals, with creativity it can be transferred to the home setting. Generally speaking, a family's access to 24-hour home nursing care for sick family members depends on the family's ability to pay for such services. Most insurance policies limit payment for nursing care for the ill in their homes to the intermittent performance of specific treatment procedures and to the nurse's instructing a family member or other caretaker in 24-hour care.

As is discussed in Unit II, a distinguishing feature of community health nursing is that care in the home is provided from a family-focused model, which is broader than and qualitatively different from an individual-focused model. The community health nurse is concerned not only with the health of the identified patient but also with the health of other family members and the family as a unit.

REFERRAL AND ADVOCACY

Community health nurses often encounter individuals who have significant concerns, untreated diseases, or unmet needs related to a basic standard of living (food, clothing, shelter, transportation) or who have experienced oppression such as neglect or abuse. The community health nurse is not expected to independently solve all existing problems. When problems cannot be managed by the nurse and client, the community health nurse assists the client in seeking appropriate resources.

Referral is the process of directing someone to another source of assistance. The community health nurse is expected to make assessments with clients, discuss the possible significance of such findings, explore the meaning of the experience with the client, and refer the client to appropriate resources. This process is discussed in more depth in Chapter 17.

To facilitate a match between the client's need and the available resources, the community health nurse must be aware of the channels for accessing that help. Assessing the presence and quality of other health and social resources is a skill that community health nurses learn. There are some resources such as welfare departments, churches, and schools that exist to serve all geopolitical areas. There are other resources such as drug detoxification units that do not exist within easy traveling distance or have waiting lists. A community health nurse should not be surprised if it takes up to 6 months to feel knowledgeable about the resources in specific communities. Keeping abreast of the changes in the resources, their services, and contact persons is an ongoing activity.

Unless a service requires that a referral be initiated by a health professional, clients are usually encouraged to initiate the contact. At times, clients will be reluctant to pursue a referral because they are afraid or do not know how to make requests for themselves. Others may be unable to pursue the referral because of limits in functioning or inadequacy of means (such as absence of a telephone). In such instances, community health nurses attempt to empower the client to overcome barriers and initiate referrals.

Community health nurses have the option of advocating for the client. *Advocacy* is an instance of speaking or writing on behalf of someone else, and using persuasion in support of another. This requires the skill of assertive communication and the knowledge of communication channels within and among organizations. Especially in large bureaucratically administered programs, special channels for complaints and appeals exist if services have been denied. Clients have general legal rights as health consumers that can be inquired about through the state attorney general's office. Additionally, administrators of health programs can provide information about client rights related to specific programs (such as Medicare insurance for the elderly).

In some circumstances, families, groups, or aggregates do not have access to a health or social service. Community health nurses can advocate for a population by networking with others for the development of such services. For example, a community health nurse may work with other professionals, religious leaders, welfare-rights advocates, and homeless persons to develop a primary health care site for the homeless. Advocacy is linked with being a leader in collaborating with others.

TEACHING

Teaching is the process of imparting cognitive knowledge, skills, and values. Nurses have information and skills that make them specialists in caring for the ill; preventing disease, illness, disability, suffering, and premature death; and promoting well-being. "Self-determination, independence, and choice in decision-making in health matters" is of "highest regard" to nurses (ANA, 1980a, p. 18). Because community health nurses work with people in various stages of wellness, community health nurses have special opportunities to foster human development and capabilities through client education. The teaching process is discussed in more depth in Chapter 18. *Anticipatory guidance* is education that occurs before the client is expected to need to act on the information.

Following Nursing and Medical Plans

Community health nurses have always imparted information and demonstrated to family members how to care for the ill at home, especially in relation to nutrition, comfort, and maintaining a healthful, clean home. For practical reasons, it is mandatory that family members or other caretakers both provide nursing care and follow the medical treatment plan of the sick person. Community health nurses have provided this teaching and continue to do so today, especially in home health care. For example, individuals newly diagnosed with hypertension and their families or significant others are taught about taking multiple medications, modifying dietary intake, and employing relaxation techniques.

Preventing Illness and Injury

All life involves risk of disease, injury, and premature death. However, individuals have choices that affect their risks; these depend on the existing knowledge about natural history of diseases, epidemiology, modalities for early detection and treatment, methods of protection and prevention, and determinants of human behavior. Community health nurses apply this information in education for prevention of disease, injury, and premature death.

For example, we know that smoking is a risky behavior related to cancer, heart disease, and lung disease, and that alcohol consumption harms the fetus. Treatment of childhood asthma reduces the number of days missed from school. Use of bicycle helmets and automobile seat belts reduces head injuries. Safer sex and sexual abstinence reduce the likelihood of transmission of human immunodeficiency virus (HIV). A basic truth about the teaching-learning process is that information alone is *not* sufficient to change human behavior. Telling someone what to do or how to do it will not result in modified behavior unless the person sees the relevance of the behavior to his or her values and goals and believes that the behavior change will contribute to the achievement of aspirations. Consequently, values clarification is a primary strategy in identifying and changing people's health-related attitudes (see Chapter 6).

Promoting Wellness and Transcending Suffering

A primary responsibility of community health nurses is teaching to promote health (see Chapter 16). Each of us has a perception of what is necessary to promote health, which depends in part on our definition of health (Benner and Wrubel, 1989). If health is viewed as the ability to fulfill our social roles, then we will be interested in learning about what will support us in performing activities of daily living, communicating, thinking, problem-solving, and relating to others. If we define health as a commodity, we will be interested in learning what will repair or replace our deficiencies, what will cure or "fix" us. If we define health as the ability to adapt, we will be interested in learning about stress-reduction techniques, what resources are available for support, and methods of environmental control. If we view health as well-being we will be interested in learning to create meaning and a sense of belonging in our lives, and to accept that total control and autonomy are not possible. For example, a family with a child who has severe developmental delays may focus on providing loving care for each family member even though they cannot predict exactly what the child may be able to learn to do as he or she develops.

Nurses working in acute care settings with the critically ill and dying have opportunities to promote well-being by assisting clients and family members to find meaning and interpersonal connectedness. Community health nurses also have opportunities to address well-being with those dying at home or in hospices. Steeves and Kahn (1987, p. 116) discuss ways to reduce suffering by establishing conditions for "experiences of meaning." Meaning cannot be imparted through providing information or skills; rather, meaning may be discovered as a possibility by the client through discussions. When the nurse attends carefully to the verbal and nonverbal messages of the client and family members, the nurse may help to discover what will provide meaning within the experience of suffering and death (Callanan and Kelley, 1993).

In community health nursing there are circumstances besides illness and a client's impending death that evoke the need for meaning. The devastation from death of a loved one, divorce, abuse by a family member, unemployment, neglect, loss of one's home by fire, and acts of prejudice are examples.

MONITORING AND EVALUATION

Community health nurses monitor the health of individuals, families, and communities. *Monitoring* is the verification of the state or condition of health and *evaluation* is the determination of the significance or value of this information. *Assessment* also denotes determination of the state of health and involves the collection and analysis of data; *reassessment* may occur at a later time. A distinction between monitoring and reassessment is that monitoring implies either a continuous process or short intervals between episodes of data collection and evaluation.

Monitoring the health of individuals in their homes and clinics differs from monitoring patients in hospitals. In inpatient settings, many individual clients are monitored continuously because of the acuteness and instability of their diseases and illness. When sick persons are cared for at home, the family is taught what to monitor and what is significant to report to the nurse or other health professional. The nurse, in collaboration with the physician and other health professionals, determines the frequency of monitoring by the health professionals.

In clinics, protocols are often used to schedule the next appointment. For example, individuals receiving antibiotics are often scheduled to return after 10 days for evaluation of treatment effectiveness; women are rescheduled annually for Papanicolaou's smears.

When providing family-centered care, the community health nurse determines the frequency of monitoring based on the health status of the family, the preferences of the family, and agency policy. When determining the frequency of contact with families the nurse must always consider any life-threatening situation and the family's perception of priorities.

Monitoring the health of groups, aggregates, and communities involves collecting and evaluating information about populations. Demographic and epidemiological data are used to determine age distributions, mortality, morbidity, and risky behavior of populations. Unit III discusses data important for determining the availability, accessibility, and acceptability of health and other community resources. Community health nurses often monitor data collected by others and can participate in data collection, especially as regards the need for and client responses to nursing care. Monitoring the health of communities is an interdisciplinary process.

Both objective and subjective information are collected during monitoring. Because nursing is concerned with "human responses" (ANA, 1980b, p. 9), it is insufficient for community health nurses to monitor objective information such as physiological outcomes, patterns of death and illness, health-related behavior, and the presence and quality of community resources. Subjective meaning and life experiences also must be explored. What do clients think about their health status? What health concerns are foremost? Interviews, conversations, and surveys are some of the ways community health nurses learn how clients view their own health needs.

ENFORCEMENT

Because our culture values individual autonomy highly, and because nursing and public health both value human growth and self-actualization, most health-related interventions do not involve coercion. However, there are instances in which the rights of the majority take precedence over the rights of individuals. The health of the family or community is protected by limiting individual autonomy. Most states have laws that protect nurses from liability for reporting neglect, abuse, and threats of bodily harm by clients to themselves or others. Many states also provide for forced treatment or curtailed behavior for individuals who have a specified communicable disease, such as tuberculosis, and who refuse to protect others from exposure. In these circumstances, community health nurses develop skill in balancing persuasion with enforcement, empowerment with coercion (Zerwekh, 1992b).

Community health nurses who are employed by local or state health departments have special responsibilities as agents of the government to enforce selected public health laws. For example, if the source of food poisoning has been attributed to an infected food handler, it will likely be the community health nurse who explains to the restaurant employee why stool cultures (negative for specific microorganisms) are required prior to their return to work.

ENVIRONMENTAL MANAGEMENT

Environmental management means the control of those things in the immediate surroundings to protect human beings from disease and injury or the promotion of a place conducive to healing and well-being. Environmental management also includes the conservation of resources and limitation of pollution in the environment. Providing asepsis and safety are basic ethical and legal responsibilities of all nurses in managing the physical aspects of environment. The ANA code of ethics (1985) also calls for nurses to relate to clients in ways that promote their dignity and respect their religious, cultural, and political preferences. Nurses are to foster interpersonal and social environments that recognize cultural differences and promote the dignity of all persons.

Institutional Environments

Some community health nurses are employed by local or state governments to inspect daycare centers (for children and adults), nursing homes, and residential care settings as part of quality control of the environments. School nurses, employed by health departments or school boards, also seek to promote healthful environments, especially to prevent communicable diseases, injuries, substance abuse, and violence.

Home Environments

Community health nurses who make home visits and those who work in clinics have special responsibility for assisting families to provide safe home environments. The kind of injuries depend in part on the age of the family members, the characteristics of housing structures, limitations in activities of daily living, knowledge of prevention by family members, and presence of specific hazards. Falls, burns, poisoning, and gunshot wounds are prevalent injuries in U.S. homes.

Clean, orderly physical environments and safe, adequate food, water, and waste disposal are to be provided in hospitals and other institutions. In homes, families have that immediate responsibility. Some families may need information on what constitutes safe preparation and storage of food. For example, parents may not realize that their infants may become ill from microorganisms growing in improperly stored formula. Community health nurses can provide information about proper formula preparation and storage. At other times, families may not have sufficient food because of chronic poverty or an emergency. Community health nurses assist the family in obtaining the necessary resources in such circumstances.

To promote development and well-being, community health nurses instruct family members in such tasks as providing stimulation for infants, communicating with bed-bound family members, and exploring the meaning of health and well-being with those who suffer from pain or isolation.

Occupational Environments

Chapter 24 describes occupational health nursing as a subspecialty of community health nursing. As part of their practice, occupational health nurses seek to limit hazards in the workplace and to promote safer working habits.

Community Environments

The environmental responsibilities of community health nurses do not stop at the physical boundaries of homes or institutions. Through observations in communities and discussion with numbers of clients, community health nurses are in special positions to observe hazards and the environmental concerns of community members. Community health nurses can collaborate with others, such as sanitarians, environmental scientists, and environmental advocacy groups.

The view of the environment primarily as a suprasystem to be controlled and used for human consumption is evolving to a view that human survival as a global community is inextricably linked with the environment. There is more focus on living not in, but in relationship with, the environment. Rather than focusing solely on the use of environmental resources for humans, the need to focus on conservation and regeneration of natural resources where possible has been recognized.

Health professionals are recognizing that the social environment is especially important when considering such concerns as teenage pregnancy, poverty, homicide, suicide, and substance abuse. Community health nurses are exploring ways to strengthen human connectedness, promote a basic standard of living, and reduce dependence on violence as a means of conflict resolution.

COORDINATION OF CARE

Coordination is bringing together the parts or agents of a plan or process into a common whole. Community health nurses work within complex community networks of resources to coordinate care for clients in a variety of ways. Community health nurses coordinate or manage care through case management, caseload management, site management, and coordination of teams.

Case management refers to the development and coordination of a plan of care for a selected client, usually an individual or family. This is similar to the concept of primary nursing in the hospital. Case management depends on the nurse's ability to accurately assess client needs and community resources. The community health nurse works with the client and the other disciplines and resources involved to create and manage a coherent plan of care that neither overwhelms the client nor results in some needs being overlooked. Goals of case management include promoting client self-care, facilitating access to resources, and creating new services (Bower, 1992).

Caseload management refers to the coordination of care for a number of clients for whom the community health nurse is accountable. Caseload management involves the community health nurse's self-management, time management, and resource management for numerous clients during a specified period. Community health nurses often schedule their own workdays and determine who will receive home visits, who will be scheduled for clinic appointments, when phone calls and meetings will be held, and how much time will be devoted to each. Travel time must also be considered. Community health nurses need to make certain that they have sufficient equipment, such as forms for documentation, health teaching materials, and biologicals for immunization.

Site management refers to the coordination of nursing effort at a specific geographic place, such as a clinic, school, or office for community health nurses where nursing care is planned and provided. While community health nursing supervisors usually manage nursing administrative offices, community health nurses may be responsible for the equipment, cleanliness, and efficiency of clinic sites and nursing areas in schools.

Community health nurses are often the *coordinators of direct care teams.* Management of nursing teams refers to the coordination of care provided by nurses, nursing assistants, licensed practical nurses (called licensed vocational nurses in some states), nurse practitioners, homemakers, and parent aides. This is identical to the concept of team nursing in inpatient settings, except that the community health nurse is not always immediately available to the nursing team member. Management often occurs via telephone calls, meetings, and intermittent on-site supervisory visits.

Coordinating multiple disciplines can occur within a single organization. For example, within a health department well-child clinic, there may be nurses, secretaries or receptionists, social workers, and dietitians. The community health nurse may be the designated coordinator of services. At other times, the community health nurse may emerge as coordinator because he or she is the one who initiates the interdisciplinary communications across two or more organizations. The latter often occurs because the community health nurse has frequent contact with the client and has developed a meaningful relationship. Coordination occurs through phone calls, meetings, and sharing of written patient records. As coordinator, the nurse needs to assure that written records of discussions and decisions are kept and shared with team members.

COLLABORATION

Collaboration means working together and denotes that the participants have relatively equal influence. Collaboration can occur informally or formally; it takes place among nursing peers, community members, and interdisciplinary professional teams.

Peer sharing occurs when nurses share their experiences with successes and disappointments in providing care. It is a means of giving and receiving support and an educational process.

Networking means the establishing and maintaining of relationships with other professionals and community leaders for the purpose of solving common problems, creating new projects or programs, identifying experts for future consultation, maintaining mutual support, or enrolling others to work toward common ground.

Community health nurses may be *team members* of multidisciplinary teams that plan and provide direct care. The care is organized but not through one coordinator. Rather, each team member is seen as having something to contribute of equivalent value and the team is accountable for results. In practice, influence varies among the members, but influence is not dependent on a designated leader or coordinator.

Membership in community planning groups is critical for collaborating with interagency and communitywide planning groups. Such groups exist to assess the health status and needs of the entire community or aggregates, to target recipients of direct care, to develop additional health care services, and to evaluate the quality of existing care. Individuals who are seen as influential in their respective fields are usually included as members. They are expected to contribute their perspective to collaborative planning. Community health nurses have relevant contributions because they know about nursing and they can advocate for client needs as well.

CONSULTATION

Consultation means the seeking of advice, especially from an expert or professional. Community health nurses are experts in community health nursing by virtue of education and experience. Community health nurses also are experts on the health status and needs of families, population groups, aggregates, and the community with which they work; this is especially true in regard to the needs for nursing care services. Community health nurses have special knowledge of the meaning of health to the people they serve.

Legally, community health nurses may be called as *expert witnesses* to testify in courts about the quality of care rendered by other community health nurses. Some state nurses' associations establish criteria for expert witnesses and maintain lists of qualified nurses (Kelly, 1991) (see Chapter 4).

Community health nurses seek expert opinion from nurses, other professionals, agency representatives, key leaders or informants, and clients themselves. For example, if a parent is giving his or her child a chemical home remedy, the nurse may consult with a registered pharmacist about the clinical compounds and their actions and, perhaps, with a community elder regarding the cultural meaning of the remedy.

SOCIAL, POLITICAL, AND ECONOMIC ACTIVITIES

The American Nurses' Association asserts that all of nursing derives from a social contract that permits autonomy within the profession as long as "responsibility to society as a whole is exercised" (ANA, 1980b, p. 8).

Community health nurses were the first nurses to make a concerted effort to identify the health needs of populations, promote adequate standards of living, and facilitate and encourage people to care for themselves.

Community health nurses, by virtue of their special commitment to the health of communities, are called on to be involved with the social power structures in the health care system and the larger community. What would be a more healthful balance of individual choices and social responsibility in our culture? How can nurses model and advocate for a more humane society? Community health nurses may work for change within existing systems and work to change the systems themselves. *Social action* is the influencing of decisions in community.

Change within Existing Power Structures

Change is a continuous process. There is room for change within the existing organizations and governmental structures. Assessment of unmet health needs and creation of nursing services through social planning is one example (see Unit III). Identification of population groups at special risk and development of outreach, screening, and educational programs for them is another example. Nurses exert influence to promote change.

Such changes can also be encouraged through political and economic strategies. *Political action* depends on the use of power to influence decisions. Many public health decisions are made by governments. Community health nurses can support the election of those sympathetic to community needs. Nurses can also influence the development of legislation and administrative rules and regulations. This can be done by testifying at hearings, participating on task forces, supplying written testimony, and personally visiting legislators. Initiating lawsuits can be attempts to influence judicial decisions. For example, the APHA and the ANA worked together to challenge President Bush's executive order that temporarily prohibited health professionals from discussing abortion in clinics that received federal funding. (The order was rescinded by President Clinton.)

Political action also includes attempts to influence decisions made by nongovernmental groups. For example, a community health nurse employed by the health department may assist the local mental health association to obtain grant money from a private foundation to establish a substance abuse hotline.

Economic action depends on the use of money to influence social decisions. Money is contributed to political action committees (PACs) to support those candidates for political office who espouse specific values and health programs. For example, the ANA-PAC of the American Nurses' Association contributes money to the campaigns of those supportive of the nursing profession. Financial decisions also can affect business policy. For example, some professionals boycotted imaging equipment made by a major company because it also made nuclear bombs; the boycott was ended when the company sold its defense business.

Becoming Part of Power Structures

Obtaining membership in decision-making groups is another way to increase influence. Nurses in political office and as members of planning bodies increase the influence of the nursing profession's voice. Community health nurses can recognize imbalances of power that oppress individuals and groups. Nurses can empower disenfranchised people, such as the poor, cultural minorities, and disabled, to become members of influential groups or to form their own organizations.

Since the 1980s, nurses have become better educated in business and economic areas so that they can participate as full partners in the business of health care. Equality in a flawed health care system has value and it has its limits (Reverby, 1987). While business participation increases nurses' power within existing structures, it is important that nursing also seeks to make the health care system more equitable and caring for clients.

Changing Power Structures

According to a chief of nursing of the World Health Organization, the values underlying health for a community should include equity, empowerment, and cooperation (Maglacas, 1988). While these values are inherent in care and responsibility, they are not dominant values in our culture. Dominant values within the United States culture include preferences for quick fixes, action, production and technology, material goods, control of natural resources, individual autonomy, and hierarchical power structures. What would it take to transform our current structures of power to allow currently subordinate values to emerge? How can speaking about our values, and what we are for, transform the current structure into a more balanced and caring community? The specific answers to these questions are still being created.

Many nurses are speaking for more human connectedness and caring in our communities (Aroskar, 1987; Benner and Wrubel, 1989; Leininger, 1984; Maglacas, 1988; Moccia, 1988; Watson, 1988). National interest in health care reform provides an opportunity for nurses to advocate for equitable health care for all, and to apprise policymakers of the contributions of community health nurses.

> The process of "enabling people to increase control over and to improve their health" represents a mediating strategy between people and the environments in which they live, synthesizing personal choice and social responsibility to create a healthier future. (Maglacas, 1988, p. 68)

> Nursing's role was always to extract from the bureaucracy its hidden humanity and use it to "civilize the system," to bring caring into interpersonal relations. (Jessie Scott quoted in Moccia, 1988, p. 31)

A contextual question for each community health nurse might be, how does my practice further a more caring community?

In summary, all nursing is concerned with public and nongovernmental decisions that shape the health care services and delivery system and affect access to care. Community health nurses have special concerns related to adequate standards of living, appropriate and adequate health care and social services for the underserved and at-risk populations, environmental management and preservation, and empowerment of community members.

EMPOWERMENT FOR CREATIVITY

Empowerment depends on the presence of hope, or an expectation that what is not could actually be. Empowerment is blocked by magical thinking, in which a desire or wish itself is held as the solution to a problem. Rather, empowerment involves the creation of a vision of what is desired and the development of a plan to work toward the vision. The plan needs to consider the reality of the circumstances.

Empowerment consists of more than solving problems or fixing what does not work. For example, a paraplegic man living in the community has hope that he can be more mobile and envisions himself as a participant in sports. A plan is created, depending on what sports he is interested in, and involves creation of equipment adapted to his physical capabilities and limitations. There is no ready-made means to achieve his vision, and he may not be able to achieve exactly what he envisioned. Yet, were it not for the original vision, even the current degree of exercising and participating in sports would not have come about.

Empowerment provides for creation of new ways of being and doing and for transformation—that is, going beyond the next obvious step to radical shifts. Fritz (1989) discusses how individuals can move from reaction and response to the circumstances of life to creativity. Wheeler and Chinn (1993) describe a process by which caring communities can be created in groups. The possibility of a culture more balanced between autonomy and relatedness exists for the future.

Changing the structures of power and the dominant culture of our society depends on empowerment of ourselves and others to envision an equitable, cooperative society in which individuals have an opportunity to develop their uniqueness regardless of age, race, gender, culture, sexual orientation, or economics, and "to be" in a caring community. Does this sound like a magical wish? It may be, or it can be a vision of community to live toward.

SELF-CARE AND DEVELOPMENT

Professional development is a lifelong process. To continue to give accurate information to others we must stay informed. To continue to stay in touch with our own concerns and commitments we need caring professional partners and persons who will listen to and coach us when we have forgotten our calling. To continue to competently perform therapeutic treatments we must have opportunities to learn from other nurses and practice new skills. To assist others in finding meaning in life's circumstances, we must continue to face our own imperfections, vulnerabilities, and mortality and to re-create meaning for our lives.

As humans we are social beings; to care for others we must be cared for. To be cared for we must be in relationships with others who are able and willing to give to us, and we must be willing to receive (Karl, 1992). Nurses often are so committed to caring for others that a conscious effort must be made to include sufficient being-cared-for. In our own lives we must address the issues that also confront families and communities. Given the specific circumstances, what is a workable balance between your own individuality and "being in community"? You can ask yourself what balance you want to establish between professional and personal aspects of your life. There is no right way to work toward knowing ourselves and developing our empirical, experiential, and moral knowledge.

Carper (1978) proposed four patterns of knowing: empirical or factual knowledge; knowledge that emerges from experiential acquaintance with others; self-knowledge; and ethical knowledge, involving moral judgments. There are other schemes for thinking about knowing.

Table 1–13 describes some ways in which nurses can develop different patterns of knowing to promote professional development. Table 1–14 provides specific examples of knowledge that emerge from different ways of knowing.

> Nursing thus depends on the scientific knowledge of human behavior in health and in illness, the aesthetic perception of significant human experiences, a personal understanding of the unique individuality of the self, and the capacity to make choices within concrete situations involving particular moral judgments (Carper, 1978, p. 22).

Expected Competencies of Baccalaureate-prepared Community Health Nurses

Generalists in community health nursing are those prepared at the baccalaureate level (ANA, 1986). Such community health nurses are expected to be able to apply the entire nursing process with individuals, families, and groups to promote health and wellness. The individuals,

TABLE 1–13

Ways of Developing Patterns of Knowing*

Factual	Experiential	Ethical	Self-Knowledge
• Reading • Studying logic and analysis • Continuing education • Extending formal education • Participating in quantitative research • Participating in study groups • Observing and describing	• Joining peer sharing groups, interest groups regarding professional experiences • Studying art, music, dance • Perceiving own experiences • Participating in qualitative research • Exploring meaning with clients • Seeking cross-cultural experiences, traveling • Becoming aware of own creativity • Envisioning what you desire • Continuing education regarding creativity	• Studying human rights • Studying codes of ethics • Exploring values underlying goals and actions • Studying philosophy • Studying ethical frameworks • Participating on ethics panels • Continuing education/formal education regarding ethics • Exploring own ethical decisions	• Participating in counseling • Clarifying values • Spiritual study and worship • Clarifying commitments • Accepting uncertainty

*Categories of knowing from Carper B. (1978). Fundamental patterns of knowing in nursing. *Advances in Nursing Science, 1*(1), 13–23.

TABLE 1–14

Ways of Knowing Related to the Example of Infant Feeding

Knowledge Route*	Example
Experiential	
Personal and interpersonal experience	You have cared for a newborn and experienced your own alertness and anxiety when the infant cried. You have felt satisfaction when the infant quieted during feeding.
Factual	
Logic	You use knowledge of nutrition and physiology to assist infant in rooting and sucking formula or breast milk.
Empirical science	You ask whether there are different types of cries. You systematically observe infant crying patterns and read research reports.
Ethical	
Ethics	You wonder whether crying is good/helpful or bad/unhealthy for the infant.
Self	
Aesthetic preferences	You prefer a quiet environment, without infant crying.
Understanding of what it means to be human	You recognize that every culture has a way of caring for human infants, but the specific details may differ.

*Knowledge routes adapted from Carper B. (1978). Fundamental patterns of knowing in nursing. *Advances in Nursing Science, 1*(1), 13–23; and Marriner-Tomey, A. (1989). *Nursing theorists and their work,* (ed. 2). St Louis: Mosby–Year Book.

families, and groups targeted for direct community health nursing care are to be selected on the basis of the results of a communitywide analysis. Baccalaureate-prepared nurses are expected to assist master's degree–prepared community health nurses, interdisciplinary teams, and community members in conducting communitywide data collection, analyses, and priority-setting. It is the generalist community health nurses who often implement the interventions that emerge from such community planning. Generalist community health nurses also participate in collecting data used for evaluation of nursing care.

DIRECT CARE WITH INDIVIDUALS

Related to the direct care of individuals in nonhospital settings, new baccalaureate graduates are expected to apply the nursing process with limited supervision, that is, they have already learned to provide such care and need to validate their judgments and interventions with a nursing supervisor (AACN, 1986). Most employers of new community health nurses will provide a more experienced nurse who is available to validate adaptations to nonhospital settings; this is especially important when resources and environments are severely compromised, as occurs in some household settings. New baccalaureate-prepared community health nurses are expected to independently and proficiently use numerous skills and to adapt them to client needs. Such skills include those related to medication, treatment, management of the environment, asepsis, recording, and providing assistance with activities of daily living (AACN, 1986).

The AACN expects recent baccalaureate graduates to seek supervision (validation of performance) when performing the following skills (AACN, 1986, pp. 20–23):

1. Administering developmental, functional, and psychosocial screening tools
2. Using consultation skills
3. Monitoring psychological crises and using crisis intervention skills
4. Analyzing results of evaluation tools, such as surveys of client satisfaction with nursing care
5. Resolving conflict
6. Using change strategies as a coordinator of care and as a member of the profession

DIRECT CARE WITH FAMILIES

Beginning community health nurses with baccalaureate degrees are expected to apply the nursing process with limited supervision while adapting care to families' "preferences and needs" (AACN, 1986). Goals of family care include support during a family member's dying, fostering "family growth during developmental transitions," and promoting "family integrity and autonomy" (AACN, 1986, pp. 11–12).

Through conducting interviews and taking family histories, community health nurses are to collect and analyze the following information about the family system (AACN, 1986, p. 9):

- Family development
- Structure and function
- Communication patterns
- Decision-making
- Family dynamics and behavior
- Family dysfunction

Family assessment is the competency ranked as most important by community health nursing educators in baccalaureate programs (Blank and McElmurry, 1986).

The predominant intervention strategies with families are providing primary care, health teaching (including anticipatory guidance), referral, and collaborating and coordinating care (AACN, 1986). In their survey of all National League for Nursing–accredited baccalaureate programs, Blank and McElmurry (1986) determined that these competencies are emphasized by educators regardless of geographic location and size or type of curriculum. Ability to perform these intervention strategies is consistent with the responsibilities of community health nurses in caseload management. Family care is explored further in Unit II.

DIRECT CARE WITH GROUPS

Application of the nursing process with groups is also expected of baccalaureate-prepared community health nurses; limited supervision is to be available (AACN, 1986). Required nursing skills include the ability to assess group dynamics and group dysfunction, to facilitate group process, to teach groups, and to solve coordination problems (AACN, 1986). Some emphasis on group leadership is provided in most baccalaureate community health nursing curricula, although it is not emphasized to the degree that it is stressed by professional organizations' definitions of community health nursing (Blank and McElmurry, 1986).

DIRECT CARE WITH AGGREGATES

As more community health nurses have become employed in agencies that serve a specific population, rather than agencies with a broad public health mandate, direct care of aggregates has become a more prevalent form of delivering community health nursing care since the early 1970s. It is the responsibility of nurses in such settings to assess the entire caseload or clinic enrollment for common health needs and to plan interventions accordingly (APHA, 1980).

For example, a nurse employed in a home health agency recognized that many of the elderly she visited had limited socialization and recreation. She joined with a social worker and neighborhood groups to develop a more systematic survey of the elderly. Eventually a senior center was established in the urban neighborhood, and the baccalaureate-prepared nurse was appointed to the board of directors, where she continued to assess the health-related needs of the center members. Besides assessing the unmet affiliation needs of the elderly and determining that inadequate resources existed, she collaborated to develop services such as health screening.

The same nurse did not stop at serving the elderly enrolled in the home health agency or senior center. She knew that many elderly are at risk of social isolation and participated with others in publicizing the senior center and finding elderly who could benefit from attendance at the center. She was reaching out to those who were eligible for the program but were not using it; such *outreach* is another distinguishing feature of community health (APHA, 1980). In business language this practice might be called *capturing market share;* however, the primary motivation of outreach is not revenue but provision of health care to the previously underserved.

Population-based care and aggregate-based care are ranked among the top ten concepts that constitute the basis for baccalaureate-prepared community health nursing education (Blank and McElmurry, 1986). Community assessment is one of the basic competencies expected of baccalaureate-prepared community health nurses (AACN, 1986; Blank and McElmurry, 1986). Community health nurses are to collect and analyze information about communities such as the following (AACN, 1986, p. 10):

- Epidemiology
- Risk factors
- Resources
- Environmental factors
- Social organization

Such nurses are expected to apply the nursing process with aggregates with limited supervision. Baccalaureate-prepared community health nurses are expected to be able to collaborate with others to assess the entire population and multiple aggregates in a geopolitical community. Unit III provides more in-depth discussion of working with communities and aggregates.

Leadership in Community Health Nursing

Leaders in community health nursing have demonstrated a common set of concerns, skills and actions (Table 1–15). Leaders are sensitive to the needs of others, are able to respond, and are willing to work toward their visions of what might be. All community health nurses have opportunities to be leaders for healthful communities. Specialists in community health nursing provide orientation, staff development, consultation, and professional leadership to nurse generalists. The ANA reserves the term *nurse specialist* for those who have graduate degrees in specific areas of nursing. Generalists are licensed professional nurses with a baccalaureate degree in nursing.

Community health nursing specialists usually have a master's degree in community health nursing/public health nursing from a school of nursing, or a master's degree in public health from a school of public health. Community health nurse specialists are capable of and may perform the functions of a community health nursing generalist and are competent to provide care with families and groups. However, community health nursing specialists usually focus their practice with communities, the entire population, or multiple aggregates. Such specialists are proficient in assessing the health of an entire community or population and in planning, implementing, and evaluating population-focused health programs (ANA, 1980a). Community health nursing specialists structure systems of data collection and evaluation. They target intervention strategies toward the health care delivery system, institutions, and organizations (ANA, 1980b), including health and social policy development, development and evaluation of health programs, and research and theory development (ANA, 1986).

All community health nurses can contribute to improving the quality of community health nursing practice by meeting qualifications for professional certification, participating in quality-assurance programs, and generating and disseminating new knowledge through nursing research.

TABLE 1–15

Leadership Characteristics in Community Health Nursing

1. An ability to recognize and be present to human suffering
2. Creation of a vision of improvement in the health and well-being of people
3. Commitment to action
4. Identification of specific health problems and sources of suffering within a specific time and place
5. Openness to possibilities to alleviate and prevent suffering and ability to develop a plan
6. Ability to communicate with other people to enlist support and enroll partners
7. Ability to create opportunities for people to help themselves
8. Commitment to advocacy to affect social policy
9. Patience and persistence

PROFESSIONAL CERTIFICATION

A program of certification for community health nurses is conducted by the ANA. *Certification* is a process that validates an individual registered nurse's qualifications, nursing practice, and knowledge in a defined area of nursing (ANA, 1993) and acknowledges that the nurse's education, experiences, and knowledge meet standards determined by the profession. Certification is voluntary.

Nurse generalists may become certified as the following:

- Community Health Nurse
- School Nurse
- College Health Nurse
- Home Health Nurse

Nurse specialists may become certified as the following:

- Clinical Specialist in Community Health Nursing
- School Nurse Practitioner

Currently, only those with a master's degree or a more advanced degree in nursing with a specialization in community/public health nursing are eligible for the clinical specialist certification. However, in 1998, nurses with "a baccalaureate or higher degree in nursing *and* a master's degree in Public Health with a specialization in community/public health nursing" also may become certified clinical specialists (ANA, 1993).

Certification expires in 5 years and may be renewed. The nurse needs at least 1500 hours of practice during the previous 5 years and documentation of continuing education or reexamination to become recertified (ANA, 1992).

QUALITY ASSURANCE

Community health nurses have a responsibility to maintain and improve the quality of community health nursing practice. Community health nurses are expected to maintain requirements for relicensure and participate in self-evaluation, continuing education, and peer review. In peer review, nurses "appraise the quality of nursing care in a given situation in accordance with established standards of practice" (ANA, 1980a, p. 18).

COMMUNITY HEALTH NURSING RESEARCH

Community health nurse generalists identify questions for investigation and participate in agency-based research under the supervision of nurse researchers (ANA, 1986). Generalists need to keep up with nursing and other research findings that are relevant to their practice.

Community health nurse specialists collaborate or consult with researchers with doctoral degrees to engage in all phases of the research process (ANA, 1986). Community health nursing specialists ensure that research findings are disseminated and assist nurse generalists in interpreting and applying the research findings in their nursing practice.

The National Institute of Nursing Research collaborates with other nurses to identify a national agenda for nursing research. The agenda for the next 5 years focuses on both nursing care delivery and specific nursing interventions. Many of the priorities within the national agenda are of relevance to community health nurses. Nurse researchers are challenged to study ways to improve the health of the underserved as well as those with HIV and AIDS, cognitive impairment, and chronic illness.

1995—*Community-based nursing models:* Creating and testing community-based nursing models to improve the health care access of rural and other underserved populations.
1996—*Effectiveness of nursing intervention in HIV and AIDS:* Evaluate the effectiveness of nursing interventions to improve the health behaviors of those at risk of HIV infection and to reduce the suffering of those infected.
1997—*Cognitive impairment:* Develop and test interventions for memory loss and confusion, especially among the elderly.
1998—*Living with chronic illness:* Evaluate interventions to strengthen personal coping with chronic illnesses.
1999—*Biobehavioral factors related to immunocompetence:* Identify and test interventions to improve immunocompetence.

Federal funding for nursing research is not limited to these priorities.

Nursing research also helps to describe the scope of practice and to strengthen nursing theory. Often, nurses take much of their practice for granted and do not describe explicitly what they are doing and how they are relating to clients. Studies of the practice of community health nurses can uncover the details of nursing practice (Zerwekh, 1991, 1992a, 1992b). Community health nursing practice can be improved only when nurses are clear about their practice and how interventions explicitly relate to human health and client satisfaction.

Much research is needed to explore what encourages health-promoting and risk-reducing behavior. Even when interventions are based on existing scientific knowledge, attempts at assisting others, such as intravenous drug users, to modify their behavior have not been very successful. Community health nurses need to study what works with specific aggregates and to learn more about "personalizing" care with different populations.

Because cost containment in health care continues to be a national goal, it is important for community health nurses to continue to demonstrate the savings that nursing care can provide. Home care expanded because nurses demonstrated that quality care can be provided for some patients in the home at a lower cost than in the hospital (Brooten et al., 1986).

One example of cost savings involves maternal and infant health promotion. A prenatal and infancy home visitation program not only led to healthier infants, fewer injuries, less abuse, and improved maternal social outcomes, but also resulted in a net savings in government expenditures such as Aid to Families with Dependent Children and food stamps (Olds et al., 1993).

A second example of cost savings relates to tuberculosis control. When community health nurses visit tuberculosis patients to directly administer antibiotics at home, worksites, or shelters, it is less expensive than hospitalization. Furthermore, the percentage of clients who complete a course of antibiotic therapy is increased, drug-resistant strains of tuberculosis are thereby prevented, and mortality is reduced (Lewis and Chaisson, 1993). When nurses are involved, health outcomes are better than when clients self-administer medications obtained from clinics or private physicians.

Nurses are concerned with people's health responses as they seek to restore or promote health (ANA, 1980b). Community health nursing research needs to consider the degree to which clients become healthier (epidemiological measures of outcomes) as well how much nursing care costs. Additionally, community health nursing research needs to describe the specific interventions that best facilitate modification of behavior and promote health. What helps to prevent illness and injury and to promote well-being? What helps people work collaboratively to improve their physical and social environments? Community health nurses will continue to be challenged by this inquiry during the 21st century.

KEY IDEAS

1. Community health nurses synthesize their knowledge of nursing and public health to promote the health of communities. Nursing knowledge helps in the understanding of problem-solving and creative empowerment, of human beings and their responses to health and illness, and of relationships between people and their environment. Public health knowledge helps make clear the magnitude of disease, disability, and premature death in human populations and suggests methods of prevention.
2. Community health nurses seek to empower persons in families, groups, organizations, and communities to achieve their individual potentials *and* to care for one another.
3. Empowerment is accomplished by using interpersonal relationships to create opportunities for people to promote their own health.

4. Health promotion involves decreasing preventable diseases, disability, and premature death; reducing experiences of illness, vulnerability, and suffering; and fostering experiences of human caring, connectedness, and self-fulfillment.
5. Baccalaureate-prepared community health nurses (generalists) apply the nursing process with individuals, families, groups, and populations or aggregates as guided by the Standards for Community Health Nursing Practice.
6. Generalists work with community health nurse specialists, other professionals, and community members to identify the populations or aggregates at greatest risk of compromised health.
7. General systems theory is useful in studying clients at multiple hierarchical levels. Individuals, families, groups, organizations, and communities are open systems that exchange energy with their environment to survive and develop. Population aggregates are not systems because the members are not related interpersonally. Instead, they have one or more health-related characteristic in common.
8. Physical, social, cultural, spiritual, economic, and political facets of our environment all have impact on community health. Community health nurses need to be broadly educated to recognize human-environment interactions. Community health nurses seek healthful environments while preserving natural resources.
9. Prevention is a complex public health concept linked with the natural history of diseases. Primary prevention activities preclude the occurrence of a disease or injury. Secondary prevention activities focus on early identification and treatment of diseases. Tertiary prevention seeks to reduce negative consequences of illness and restore health as much as possible.
10. Community health nurses use a variety of nursing interventions. Identifying and referring persons with health and social problems, teaching, providing and coordinating direct care, and participating with others to influence community decisions are especially important to community health nurse generalists.
11. Concern for the "greatest good for the greatest number" sometimes allows community health nurses to force clients to do something (take antituberculosis medications), or not to do something (abuse a spouse), to protect others. However, education and empowerment are preferred to enforcement and coercion.
12. Mechanisms to ensure the quality of nursing care include licensure, continued professional development, certification, quality assurance, and research.
13. Social justice is important in the promotion of community health.

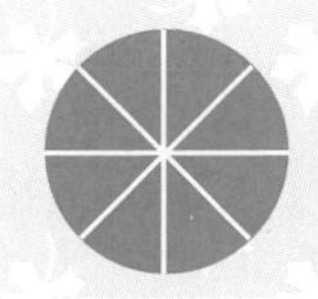

CASE STUDY

Being Present

The community health nurse greets the 30-year-old mother at the door of the apartment. They had met numerous other times. The mother has a history of "crack" use, although she denies current use. She has had difficulty feeding her 2-year-old son because of his almost constant seizures. The relationship between the mother and the community health nurse had developed slowly. The nurse was aware that the child's pediatrician would not prescribe strong antiseizure medication because he did not trust the mother to give it appropriately and feared resultant liver damage in the child. The mother had refused to return to the pediatrician. The nurse knew that the only health service the mother had attended with regularity was the health department "well-child" clinic where the nurse worked, which provided screening, education, and immunizations. The child's immunizations were also delayed because of the seizures.

The nurse spoke the mother's name, seated herself quietly, and took in what was happening in the room. The mother was ironing and had age-appropriate toys next to her developmentally delayed son. The nurse said hello to the boy, commenting that he seemed to be interested in the toy the mother had placed with him. She followed the mother's lead as they discussed how the mother was providing stimulation for her son's development. The nurse said that it must be difficult to feed a child with frequent seizures; the mother replied that she could not take all day to feed him because she had two other children to care for and she was afraid he would choke. The nurse realized that she would have similar feelings if the child were hers. She acknowledged the mother's request to get seizure medication and indicated that she might find another pediatrician for the child.

Because of her resourcefulness and persistence, the nurse was able to find a second pediatric neurologist in another city, 40 miles away. With transportation arranged through volunteers, the mother and son were seen. He was hospitalized for regulation of the seizure medication regimen and the mother agreed to implantation in the child of a gastrostomy tube for feedings. Three months after the home visit described earlier, the mother had been taught to feed the child and his seizures were sufficiently controlled for him to be accepted into a special education program in the public school system. The mother was beginning to talk about seeking job training.

The nurse could have judged the mother for having used cocaine, which may have caused her child's health problems. The nurse could have labeled the mother as noncompliant when she refused to return to the first pediatrician. Instead, the community health nurse was "present" to the mother; she was physically present in the home several times and psychologically present to acknowledge the mother's strengths and perspective of the circumstances. Additionally, the community health nurse was spiritually there and could honestly say that she liked the mother, despite all of her troubles. She felt genuine positive regard for the mother as a human being, while not forgetting that her primary professional goal as a "child health nurse" was to promote the well-being of the child. Her presence demonstrated her genuine caring and led to new possibilities for this family.

GUIDELINES FOR LEARNING

1. Look through several copies of a major newspaper to find articles related directly or indirectly to human health. Describe any inequalities in access to health care and inequalities in access to a basic standard of living. Identify implications for community health nursing practice.
2. Express your vision of a healthy family and of a healthy community. List some of your commitments related to your choice of nursing as a profession. As your experience in community health nursing broadens, consider modifying your list of commitments.
3. Express your vision of an empowering work environment. If you are a student, consider what an empowering clinical practice environment would be like for you. Identify what commitments you are willing to make *for* this vision. Share your visions and commitments with your work group or learning group in an attempt to identify some common visions and commitments as a basis for partnership.
4. Select a public health problem of interest to you, such as falls among the elderly, and describe primary, secondary, and tertiary prevention strategies.
5. Using the same health problem discuss how interventions may be directed toward individuals, families, groups, and the public. To whom would you target interventions and why?
6. Interview or accompany a community health nurse to identify his or her professional responsibilities. To what degree does the nurse provide care with individuals, families, or groups? How does the nurse use data about the public or aggregates to target care? How does the nurse participate in continuing professional development and improvement of nursing care?

REFERENCES

Allen, C. (1991). Holistic concepts and the professionalization of public health nursing. *Public Health Nursing, 8*(2), 74–80.

American Association of Colleges of Nursing. (1986). *Essentials of college and university education for professional nursing: Final report.* Washington, DC: Author.

American Nurses' Association (ANA). (1980a). *A conceptual model of community health nursing.* Washington, DC: Author.

ANA. (1993). *American Nurses Credentialing Center certification catalog.* Washington, DC: Author.

ANA. (1992). *American Nurses Credentialing Center recertification catalog.* Washington, DC: Author.

ANA. (1985). *Code for nurses with interpretive statements.* Washington, DC: Author.

ANA. (1980b). *Nursing: A social policy statement.* Washington, DC: Author.

ANA. (1986). *Standards of community health nursing practice.* Washington, DC: Author.

American Public Health Association, Public Health Nursing Section. (1980). *The definition and role of public health nursing in the delivery of health care.* Washington, DC: Author.

Aroskar, M. A. (1987). The interface of ethics and politics in nursing. *Nursing Outlook, 35*(6), 268–272.

Beauchamp, T., & Childress, J. (1989). *Principles of biomedical ethics* (3rd ed.). New York: Oxford University Press.

Benner, P., & Wrubel, J. (1989). *The primacy of caring.* Menlo Park, CA: Addison-Wesley.

Blank, J., & McElmurry, B. (1986). An evaluation of consistency in baccalaureate public health nursing education. *Public Health Nursing, 3*(3), 171–182.

Bower, K. (1992). *Case management by nurses.* Washington, DC: ANA.

Brooten, D., Kumar, S., Brown, L., Butts, P., Finkler, S., Bakewell-Sachs, S., Gibbons, A., Delivoria-Papadopoulos, M. (1986). A randomized clinical trial of early hospital discharge and home follow-up of very-low-birth-weight infants. *New England Journal of Medicine, 315(15),* 934–938.

Brueggemann, W. (1982). *Living toward a vision.* New York: United Church Press.

Callanan, M., & Kelley, P. (1993). *Final gifts.* New York: Bantam Books.

Carper, B. A. (1978). Fundamental patterns of knowing in nursing. *Advances in Nursing Science, 1*(1), 13–23.

Choi, E. (1989). Evolution of nursing theory development. In A. Marriner-Tomey (Ed.). *Nursing theorists and their work* (pp. 51–61). St. Louis: Mosby–Year Book.

Erickson, H., Tomlin, E., & Swain, M. (1983). *Modeling and role-modeling: A theory and paradigm for nursing.* Englewood Cliffs, NJ: Prentice-Hall.

Friedman, G. (1987). *Primer of epidemiology.* New York: McGraw-Hill.

Fritz, R. (1989). *The path of least resistance: Learning to become the creative force in your own life.* New York: Fawcett Columbine.

Fry, S. (1983). Dilemma in community health ethics. *Nursing Outlook, 31*(3), 176–179.

Fry, S. (1985). Individual vs aggregate good: Ethical tension in nursing practice. *International Journal of Nursing Studies, 22*(4), 303–310.

Gilje, F. (1993). Being there: An analysis of the concept of presence. In D. Gaut (ed.). *The presence of caring in nursing* (pp. 53–67). New York: National League for Nursing.

Gilligan, C. (1982). *In a different voice.* Cambridge, MA: Harvard University Press.

Hamilton, P., & Keyser, P. (1992). The relationship of ideology to developing community health nursing theory. *Public Health Nursing, 9*(3), 142–148.

Hanchett, E. (1988). *Nursing frameworks and community as client: Bridging the gap.* Norwalk, CT: Appleton & Lange.

Johnson, D. (1980). The behavioral system model for nursing. In J. Riehl & C. Roy (Eds.). *Conceptual models for nursing practice* (2nd ed.). New York: Appleton-Century-Crofts.

Karl, J. (1992). Being there: Who do you bring to practice? In D. Gaut (Ed.). *The presence of caring in nursing* (pp. 1–13). New York: National League for Nursing Press.

Katz, D., & Kahn, R. (1966). *The social psychology of organizations.* New York: John Wiley & Sons.

Kelly, L. (1991). *Dimensions of professional nursing* (6th ed.). New York: Pergamon Press.

Kenyon, V., Smith, E., Vig Hefty, L., Bell, M., McNeil, J. & Martaus, T. (1990). Clinical competencies for community health nursing. *Public Health Nursing, 7*(1), 33–39.

King, I. (1971). *Toward a theory for nursing: General concepts of human behavior.* New York: John Wiley & Sons.

Last, J. (1992). Ethics and public health policy. In J. Last & R. Wallace (Eds.). *Public health and preventive medicine* (pp. 1187–1196). Norwalk, CT: Appleton & Lange.

Leininger, M. (1984). Care: A central focus of nursing and health care services. In M. Leininger (Ed.). *Care: The essence of nursing and health* (pp. 45–59). Thorofare, NJ: Slack.

Lewis, J., & Chaisson, R. (1993, September). *Tuberculosis: The reemergence of an old foe.* Paper presented at the Baltimore City Health Department 200th Anniversary Celebration Conference, Baltimore, MD.

Maglacas, A. (1988). Health for all: Nursing's role. *Nursing Outlook, 36*(2), 66–71.

Marriner-Tomey, A. (1989). *Nursing theorists and their work* (2nd ed.). St. Louis, Mosby–Year Book.

Moccia, P. (1988). At the faultline: Social activism and caring, *Nursing Outlook, 36*(1):30–33.

Neuman, B. (1982). *The Neuman systems model: Application to nursing education and practice.* Norwalk, CT: Appleton-Century-Crofts.

Olds, D., Henderson, C., Phelps, C., Kitzman, H., Hanks, C. (1993). Effect of prenatal and infancy nurse home visitation on government spending. *Medical Care, 31*(2), 155–174.

Orem, D. (1985). *Nursing: Concepts of practice.* New York: McGraw-Hill.

Porter, E. (1987). Administrative diagnosis—implications for the public's health. *Public Health Nursing, 4,* 247–256.

Reverby, S. (1987). *Ordered to care: The dilemma of American nursing 1850–1945.* Cambridge, England: Cambridge University Press.

Roy, C. (1984). *Introduction to nursing: An adaptation model* (2nd ed.). Englewood Cliffs, NJ: Prentice-Hall.

Schultz, P. (1987). When client means more than one: Extending the foundational concept of person. *Advances in Nursing Science, 10,* 71–86.

Smith, C. M. (1985). Unpublished data. Baltimore: University of Maryland School of Nursing.

Smith, C., & Rankin, E. (1972). *General systems theory and systems analysis* (audiotape and study guide). Baltimore, MD: University of Maryland School of Nursing.

Steeves, R. H. & Kahn, D. L. (1987). Experience of meaning in suffering. *Image: Journal of Nursing Scholarship, 19*(3), 114–116.

U.S. Department of Health and Human Services (USDHHS). (1985). *Consensus Conference on the Essentials of Public Health Nursing Practice and Education: Report of the Conference.* Rockville, MD: Author.

USDHHS. (1990). *Healthy People 2000: National health promotion and disease prevention objectives. Summary report.* Washington, DC, Government Printing Office.

USDHHS. (1993). *Registered nurse population 1992: Findings from the National Sample Survey of Registered Nurses.* Washington, DC. Division of Nursing, Bureau of Health Professions, Health Resources and Services Administration.

von Bertalanffy, L. (1968). *General systems theory.* New York: George Brazziller.

Watson, J. (1988). *Nursing: Human science and human care.* New York: National League for Nursing.

Wheeler, C., & Chinn, P. (1993). *Peace and power* (Publication No. 15–2301) (3rd ed.). New York: National League for Nursing.

Williams, C. (1977). Community health nursing—what is it? *Nursing Outlook, 25*(64), 251.

Winslow, C.-E. A. (1984). *The evolution and significance of the modern public health campaign.* South Burlington, VT: Journal of Public Health Policy. (Originally published in 1923 by Yale University Press.)

Zerwekh, J. (1991). A family caregiving model for public health nursing. *Nursing Outlook, 39*(5), 213–217.

Zerwekh, J. (1992a). Laying the ground work for family self-help: Locating families, building trust, and building strength. *Public Health Nursing, 9*(1), 15–21.

Zerwekh, J. (1992b). The practice of empowerment and coercion by expert public health nurses. *Image: Journal of Nursing Scholarship, 24*(2), 101–105.

SUGGESTED READINGS

American Nurses' Association (ANA). (1985). *Code for nurses with interpretive statements.* Washington, DC: Author.

ANA. (1986). *Standards of community health nursing practice.* Washington, DC, Author.

Beauchamp, D. (1985, December). Community: The neglected tradition of public health. *Hastings Center Report,* pp. 28–36.

Faherty, B (1993). Now is the time to advocate. *Nursing Outlook, 41*(6), 248–249.

Graham, K. (1992). Health care reform and public health nursing. *Public Health Nursing, 9*(2), 73.

Hefty, L., Kenyon, V., Martaus, T., Bell, M., & Snow, L. (1992). A model skills list for orienting nurses to community health agencies. *Public Health Nursing, 9*(4), 228–233.

Reverby, S. (1993). From Lilliam Wald to Hillary Rodham Clinton: What will happen to public health nursing? *American Journal of Public Health, 83*(12), 1662–1663.

Salmon, M. (1993). Public health nursing—the opportunity of a century [Editorial]. *American Journal of Public Health, 83*(12), 1674–1675.

Schorr, L. (1989). *Within our reach: Breaking the cycle of disadvantage.* New York: Doubleday.

Zerwekh, J. (1993). Going to the people—public health nursing today and tomorrow [Commentary]. *American Journal of Public Health, 83*(12), 1676–1678.

Zlotnick, C. (1992). A public health quality assurance system. *Public Health Nursing, 9*(2), 133–137.

Chapter 2

Origins and Future of Community Health Nursing

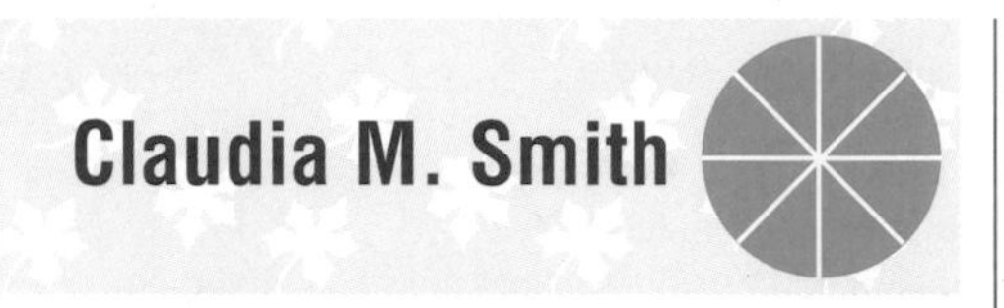

Continued

Focus Questions

What are distinctions among visiting nursing, district nursing, public health nursing, home health care nursing, and community health nursing?

What are some historical roots of such nursing?

How did nursing leaders, such as Florence Nightingale and Lillian Wald, merge public health practice with nursing to create public health nursing?

What led to the renaming of public health nursing as community health nursing?

How have subspecialties in community health nursing emerged from aggregate-focused care?

What stimulated the expansion of community health nursing into rural areas of the United States?

How did the government sponsorship of community health nursing contribute to the field's dichotomy?

How does health care reform offer the opportunity for community health nursing to regain its holistic perspective for human health?

How can *Healthy People 2000* goals and objectives for health promotion and disease prevention help to guide community health nursing practice?

What unresolved issues persist in defining practice?

Because community health nursing is a synthesis of nursing and public health, an exploration of the evolution of each of these will strengthen our understanding of the roots of practice. The care of the sick has always been influenced by the meaning given to illnesses, injuries, and human suffering by members of a given culture. Types and prevalence of injuries and illnesses have also influenced care. Other roots of community health nursing include health promotion and disease prevention and population-focused care from public health. Both nursing and public health have been concerned with the interrelationships among people and their physical and social environments.

This chapter traces the evolution of community health nursing in the United States. Visiting nursing and district nursing became public health nursing, which includes home health nursing. Public health nursing today is often called community health nursing.

Community health nursing in the United States has generally evolved from several programs developed in Western Europe, particularly Great Britain. Many people have influenced the development of community health nursing. A synopsis of their commitments, ideas, and activities provides an understanding of the foundation of contemporary community health nursing. Where possible, the names of specific nurses are included to demonstrate that the history of nursing is the result of the collective efforts of individual nurses. Other community leaders are identified to demonstrate that early community health nurses worked in partnerships to create services and obtain financial support. Inclusion of their names allows further research for interested readers.

Roots of Community Health Nursing

Visiting nursing originated when concerned laypersons provided care to the sick in their homes. In Europe the Catholic Sisters of Charity and Protestant deaconesses evolved from groups of such layperson nurses. In the United States, organized visiting nursing tended to be provided by nonreligious organizations such as benevolent and ethical societies.

District nursing was started in England in 1859 by William Rathbone, who proposed to Florence Nightingale that visiting nurses who had graduated from nursing school be assigned within a parish or district. In the United States district nurses often worked in conjunction with physicians who worked in the local dispensary. This was the forerunner of neighborhood or city block nursing.

In the 1880s nonprofit visiting nursing associations were formed in several U.S. cities to provide care to ill persons and to teach health promotion and disease prevention. Some associations assigned nurses by geographic districts and others did not.

Lillian Wald included visiting nursing and district nursing within her broader concept of public health nursing. Public health nursing is nursing for social betterment and includes nursing in schools, in clinics, at worksites, and in community centers, as well as in homes. Whether it is called public health nursing or community health nursing, the practice combines caring and activism to promote the health of the public (Backer, 1993).

VISITING NURSING IN EUROPE BEFORE 1850

During the Middle Ages warfare, famine, and plagues persisted in Europe and the Middle East. Hospitals existed for military personnel, and wealthy patients were cared for at home. In 1617 in France Vincent de Paul established the Society of Missionaries, whose members were priests especially trained to work among poor persons. His concept of charity expanded the idea that rich and powerful persons could alleviate the suffering of poor persons through material relief alone. He asserted that human sympathy and personal service were of value as well, that the causes of poverty must be remedied, and that poor persons might be better able to care for themselves if they were employed (Brainard, 1985).

Simultaneously Vincent de Paul created the Dames de Charité (Sisters of Charity), who provided visiting nursing among sick poor people. The association was a voluntary one, and the women did not take religious vows. Ten years later the need for care continued to exceed the resources and "girls of the humbler class" were recruited as Filles de Charité (Brainard, 1985). These caring women made beds, prepared medicines, fed sick persons, and comforted dying and grief-stricken persons.

From the 1600s through the 1900s isolated endeavors to alleviate human suffering emerged throughout Europe and gradually converged in a "great movement for human welfare" (Brainard, 1985, p. 47). Brainard, former president of the Visiting Nurse Association of Cleveland, attributed three revolutions with having provided the cultural opportunity for the proliferation of visiting nurse services:

> The Intellectual Revolution [Age of Enlightenment], which opened up new avenues of thought and showed the deeper relation between cause and effect, opportunity and growth, poverty and disease; the French Revolution, which together with the American Revolution, spread the doctrine of independence and the rights of man, and taught that all men are born free and equal and are entitled to life, liberty, and the pursuit of happiness; and finally, the Industrial Revolution . . . which . . . brought about conditions of poverty, over-crowding and disease. . . . (p. 49).

Scientific knowledge and concern for the well-being of individuals provided the intellectual and philosophical bases for responding to the dehumanizing conditions of industrialized, urban Europe.

After being appointed pastor in 1822 at a small village, Kaiserwerth, Germany, Theodor Fliedner toured richer Protestant parishes to seek financial aid for his poor parishioners. In Holland he was impressed by the deaconesses' groups established by the Mennonites. His wife, Frederika Fliedner, started a women's society for visiting and nursing sick poor persons in their homes. In 1836 he started a hospital and 3-year training school for deaconesses. The students were at least 25 years old, of good character and health, and from the working class. Protestants feared he was setting up convents; Roman Catholics feared he was trying to convert Catholic parishioners.

By 1850 several institutes for training deaconesses were established in Paris, Austria, and Switzerland. In England Mrs. Fry, a prison reformer, founded the Society of Protestant Sisters of Charity to supply nurses to the sick of *all classes,* including poor persons, in their homes. In 1841 a physician in a British dispensary requested a nurse to

> instruct the poor people how to perform the ordinary duties of the sick room, how to stop bleeding from leech bites and how to make poultices, determine whether children were vaccinated [for smallpox], report cases of blindness or idiocy and teach cheap cooking (Brainard, 1985, pp. 79–80).

WORKHOUSE AND HOSPITAL NURSING IN ENGLAND: 1825–1850

Social change had a profound effect on nursing for the poor in England in the mid-19th century (White, 1978). The middle and upper classes continued to be cared for by physicians and nurses privately employed in their homes. By 1825 there were 154 hospitals in England maintained by private membership subscriptions. Because the hospitals were used for teaching, admissions tended to be of persons with uncommon illnesses and those with good prognoses. However, "hospitals still were regarded as death houses and their fatality rates were high" (White, p. 14). For example 70% of patients with compound fractures, 50% of those with amputations, 70% of non–breast-fed infants, and 60% of breast-fed infants died. (It was not until after 1870 that Lister advocated antisepsis in surgery to reduce infection) (Roemer, 1988).

Hospital nurses were "ward maids" supervised by sisters. It was the sisters who gave medications, applied poultices, and oversaw patient feedings. Both nurses and sisters resided in the hospital and worked under the supervision of matrons who were equivalent to housekeepers in private domestic service.

Continuing until 1834 in England, each parish had its own poorhouse in which sick persons were looked after by other "inmates." Usually the houses were small cottages. Under English law "the aged, infirm, handicapped, orphans, widows and poor sick were traditionally accepted as being valid candidates for poor relief." Local physicians were employed by the local overseers. In 1834 amendments to the Poor Law attempted to control the money spent on poor persons. "No one could receive relief if he had any resources at all, including an article of furniture. Relief was therefore reserved for the destitute. . . . [To receive care] the sick poor had to be admitted to workhouses together with their families" (White, 1978, p. 7).

By the mid-1800s more than 50,000 sick and elderly persons lived in the workhouses, some of which were large enough to house 300 people. Tuberculosis was rampant. Sickness was the basis for 70% of instances of pauperism (poverty) (White, 1978, pp. 17–19). There were no longer sufficient able-bodied residents to care for elderly and ill persons.

The "pauper nurses" were themselves residents of the workhouses, were untrained, and cared for people throughout the entire residence. In the 1834 Poor Law Amendments, nurses were listed with masters and matrons as personnel of workhouses (White, 1978). In the 1850s there were 500 pauper nurses, half of whom were older than 50 years.

By 1850 248 paid nurses in England and Wales were employed in workhouses. They had no formal training because none existed, and most had some experience in hospitals. In 1848 the Poor Law Board redefined the duties of paid nurses to be more like the duties of ward sisters in hospitals. There was medical resistance to a plan proposed in 1856 by the Epidemiological Society for instructing nurses for care of sick persons in the workhouse infirmaries (White, 1978).

Concurrently the total population in England doubled between 1800 and 1850, and overcrowding occurred in cities as a result of urban migration for employment in industries (White, 1978). Common lodgings also became centers for disease among factory workers and their families. It was in this environment that reformers sought to prevent deaths through improvement of living conditions for residents of jails, workhouses, and urban slums. Reforms for treatment of sick poor persons were also sought.

For some the motivation for reform came as a result of attempts to reconcile Christian principles with poverty, suffering, and premature deaths of poor persons at the time. Businessmen were beginning to realize that a sick work force affected production, so economics provided another motivation.

THE BIRTH OF DISTRICT NURSING IN ENGLAND: 1859

Rathbone, a Quaker, merchant, and philanthropist, is considered the originator of district nursing (Brainard, 1985; Gardner, 1936; Monteiro, 1985). Rathbone was a visitor for the District Provident Society in Liverpool, England, and went to the homes of members of his district every week. He believed that personal contact with the poor could assist people out of poverty and that financial relief alone was insufficient. He persuaded the Liverpool Relief Society to adopt a system whereby the town was divided into districts and subdivided into sections; after a paid relief worker had assessed the situation initially, the "case" was turned over to the friendly visitor in the district for ongoing assistance.

During his wife's long illness, Rathbone employed a nurse, Mary Robinson, to comfort and care for her. After his wife's death in 1859 Rathbone realized that if nursing care could be such an asset to his wealthy family, it could be an even greater asset to families whose suffering was compounded by poverty and ignorance. His idea was to provide nursing care by district as welfare relief was provided. He employed Robinson for a 3-month experiment in nursing sick poor persons in their own homes in a district of Liverpool (Brainard, 1985). Additionally, she was to instruct the families to care for their own sick members and to provide personal and home cleanliness. Brainard reports that at the end of a month, Robinson felt hopeless about the intense "squalor" and asked to be relieved. Rathbone encouraged her to persist, and at the end of 3 months she was able to see relief from suffering and improved circumstances for some families. She continued in this new field of work and was the first "district nurse."

Rathbone sought to expand the district nursing model by employing additional nurses in other areas of Liverpool. Two barriers immediately emerged: public resignation to poverty and suffering and the absence of a sufficient number of trained nurses. In 1861 he wrote to Nightingale, who had started St. Thomas' School to train nurses in London in 1860, to request her assistance in training nurses for Liverpool. She was already engaged in a project for sanitary reform in India, which she directed from England, and so referred him to the Royal Liverpool Infirmary to request that they open a school to train nurses for both the infirmary and district nursing (Monteiro, 1985). With Rathbone's financial support, such a school was established the next year; a third objective was to provide nurses for care for the sick in private families (Brainard, 1985). By 1865 there were trained nurses in 18 districts of Liverpool (Brainard, 1985; Monteiro, 1985).

The district boundaries were often the same as parishes so that nursing care could be coordinated with the work of the clergy. When a new district was established, meetings were held among clergy, physicians, residents, and philanthropists to educate them about the proposal, to enlist cooperation, and to recommend those who needed care. The superintendent of each district was a "lady" who was responsible for securing money from philanthropists, managing accounts and records, and encouraging the nurse. Such positions were often handed down from mothers to daughters as civic duties (Brainard, 1985).

The district nurse visited numerous homes of the sick poor for 5 to 6 hours per day. Brainard (1985) summarizes the nurse's duties (Table 2–1). Generally, district nurses did not care directly for persons with communicable diseases, to avoid transmission from one household to another. Instead, nurses taught family members how to perform necessary care and provided equipment "at the door."

These duties are consistent with the principles of district nursing that emerged from the philosophy of Rathbone and the nursing reforms espoused by Nightingale. The nurse was to provide nursing to the sick, rather than to give relief in terms of money, food, clothes, or other charity. Nurses were not to make families dependent on them by providing the necessities that the head of the family would ordinarily provide (Brainard, 1985; Monteiro, 1985).

That nurses should be trained was an essential point advocated by Rathbone and Nightingale. Nightingale wrote, "a District Nurse must . . . have a fuller training than

TABLE 2–1

Duties of District Nurses Liverpool, England: 1865

- Investigate new referrals as soon as possible
- Report to the superintendent situations in which additional food or relief would improve recovery
- Report neglect of patients by family or friends to the superintendent
- Assist physicians with surgery in the home
- Maintain a clean, uncluttered home environment and tend fires for heat
- Teach the patient and family about cleanliness, ventilation, the giving of food and medications, and obedience to the physician's orders
- Set an example for "neatness, order, sobriety, and obedience"
- Hold family matters in confidence
- Avoid interference with the religious opinions and beliefs of patients and others
- Report facts to and ask questions of physicians
- Refer acutely ill to hospitals and the chronically ill, poor without family to infirmaries

From: Brainard, M. (1985). *The evolution of public health nursing* (pp. 120–121). New York: Garland. (Original work published in 1922. Philadelphia: W. B. Saunders.)

a hospital nurse, because she has no hospital appliances at hand at all" [and because she is the only one to make notes and report to the doctor] (Monteiro, 1985, p. 184).

The integration of the public health sanitary movement and nursing can also be seen in Nightingale's comments that a district nurse must "nurse the room" and report sanitary defects to the officer of health. Hygiene was seen as an empirical help for recovery from illness and prevention of disease.

Nightingale also believed that nurses should not have to do their own cooking and housekeeping after caring for patients all day in minimal environments. Nurses themselves needed to be restored and nurses' homes were eventually established as residences for district nurses. As a result an espirit de corps developed among nurses who otherwise worked separately.

In 1874 Rathbone persuaded Nightingale to expand district nursing throughout London. The Metropolitan Nursing Association was established in 1875 with Florence Lees, a Nightingale graduate, as president; its purpose was to provide "nursing to the sick poor at home" (Monteiro, 1985, p. 183). An evaluation of existing district nursing was undertaken. Surveys inquiring about nursing in their districts were sent to clergy and medical officers. Lees personally observed the nurses engaged in district nursing. Finding wide variability in nursing practice, the association sought to standardize the training for district nurses. Nurses were recruited from the class of "gentlewomen," and after a year of hospital training they received 6 months of supervised district training (Brainard, 1985).

In 1893 at the International Congress of Nursing in Chicago, Florence Craven (née Lees) spoke for district nursing as requiring nurses of intelligence, initiative, and responsibility, with the ability to teach and the commitment to reduce the suffering of poor persons. District nursing had crossed the Atlantic from London. Table 2–2 presents

TABLE 2–2

Dates in U.S. Community Health Nursing History

1813	Ladies Benevolent Society first organizes visitation by women to sick poor persons, Charleston, SC
1819	Hebrew Female Benevolent Society of Philadelphia organizes volunteer visiting nurses to the sick
1839	Nurse Society in Philadelphia assigns women visitors to care for ill poor persons at home
1861	Teachers Dorothea Dix, Clara Barton, and other women organize a system of supplies and visiting nurses during the Civil War
1877	Womens' Branch of the New York City Mission assigns first educated nurses to homes of sick poor persons
1885–1886	Visiting nurse associations established in Boston, Buffalo, and Philadelphia
1893	Nurses Lillian Wald and Mary Brewster organize Henry Street Settlement in New York
1895	First occupational health nurse, Ada Stewart, employed by Vermont Marble Works
1902	School nursing established in New York City
1903	First home care program for tuberculosis patients established by Visiting Nurse Association of Baltimore
1906	First infants' clinic established by Visiting Nurse Association of Cleveland
1908	First child health visitation program in a local health department, New York City
1909	National survey of visiting nursing associations conducted by Yssabella Waters: visits no longer limited to the poor; nurses work with patients of more than one physician
1909	Metropolitan Life Insurance Company employs visiting nurses for policy-holders
1910	Collegiate education in public health nursing established at Columbia University, New York
1912	National Organization for Public Health Nursing (NOPHN) formed
1912	Quarterly publication of the Cleveland Visiting Nurse Association and forerunner of the journal *Public Health Nursing* given to the NOPHN
1912	Red Cross Town and Country Nursing Service established
1916	First public health nursing text written by Mary Gardner
1918	National League for Nursing Education recommends that aspects of public health nursing be included in nursing education
1919	Red Cross manages more than 2900 rural public health nursing services providing both sick care and prevention through their Town and Country Nursing Service
1919	More than 1200 occupational health nurses employed by industries
1925	Frontier Nursing Service established by Mary Breckenridge in Kentucky
1934	First nurse (Pearl McIver) employed by U.S. Public Health Service
1952	NOPHN incorporated into the National League for Nursing (NLN)
1965	Public health pediatric nurse practitioner graduate program established by Loretta Ford at University of Colorado
1973	Federal Health Maintenance Organization Act recommends extended roles for nurses in primary care
1974	Formation of Nurses' Coalition for Action in Politics (N-CAP), political action committee of American Nurses' Association (ANA)
1975	Certification of community health nurses established by ANA
1980	ANA and the American Public Health Association publish statements about public health and community health nursing
1984	Consensus Conference on the Essentials of Public Health Nursing Practice and Education
1986	ANA *Standards for Community Health Nursing Practice* revised
1988	National Center for Nursing Research (NCNR) established at the National Institutes of Health
1991	ANA publishes *Nursing's Agenda for Health Care Reform*
1993	National Institute of Nursing Research replaces NCNR

milestones of U.S. community health nursing, many of which are discussed in greater detail throughout the chapter.

DISTRICT VISITORS AND VISITING NURSES IN THE UNITED STATES

The first organized lay visitors to sick poor persons in America were members of the Ladies' Benevolent Society of Charleston, South Carolina, founded in 1813 (Brainard, 1985). The society's formation was a response to the poverty and suffering brought about by a yellow fever epidemic and the trade embargoes during the War of 1812. The society adopted principles that did not appear in England until 40 years later. Membership transcended church and color lines, and the patient's religion was not interfered with. Although substantial amounts of food, clothing, fuel, bedding, and soap were distributed, money was not given out. The circumstances of sick poor persons were investigated and attempts were made to furnish work for unemployed persons. Charleston was divided into districts that corresponded to election wards; ladies visited for 3 months. The society existed until the Civil War; in 1881 it resumed work, and a trained nurse was employed in 1903.

In 1839 the Nurse Society in Philadelphia assigned lady visitors by districts; responsible women were assigned to *act* as nurses under the direction of physicians and lady visitors (Brainard, 1985). Although these nurses are considered the "first to systematically care for the poor in their homes" in the United States, they were not trained. Neither did they visit multiple homes; rather they stayed with one patient until discharged by the physician.

TRAINED VISITING NURSES IN THE UNITED STATES

Visiting nursing by *trained* nurses in the United States began in the industrialized cities of the northeast almost 20 years after its inception in Liverpool (Waters, 1912). In 1877 the Women's Branch of the New York City Mission sent trained nurses into the homes of poor persons; 2 years later the Society for Ethical Culture placed one nurse in a city dispensary for the purpose of home visiting. Both assigned nurses by districts (Brainard, 1985).

It is not known whether the New York City Mission spontaneously generated the idea of visiting nurses or whether members of their board had visited London (Brainard, 1985). Frances Root, a graduate of the first class of nurses trained at Bellevue Hospital, was the first *trained* visiting nurse in the United States. During the next year, the number of nurses expanded to five, and the salary of each was provided by a charitable lady. The philosophy of the New York City Mission focused on fulfilling a religious call, providing material relief, and caring for sick persons.

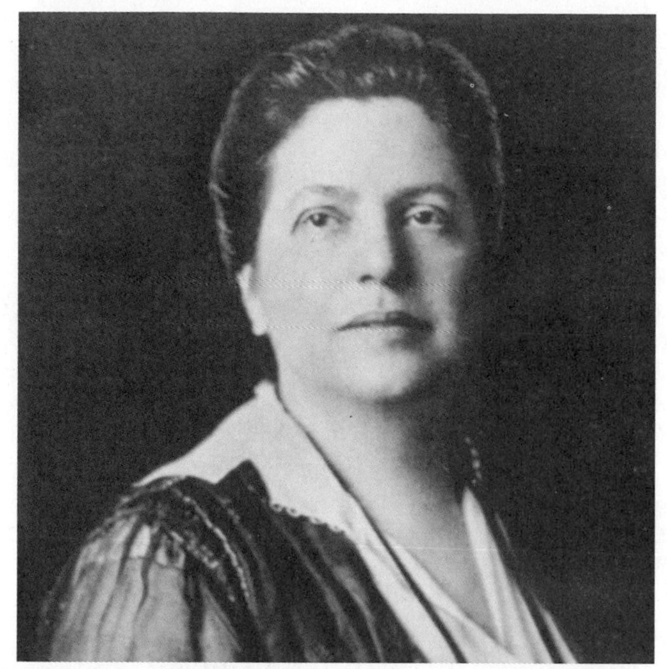

Figure 2–1 ● Lillian Wald (1867–1940), founder of the Henry Street Settlement and the Visiting Nurse Service of New York City, first coined the term *public health nurse.* (Courtesy of Visiting Nurse Service of New York City.)

There was little focus on instruction for hygiene, sanitation, or prevention.

Felix Adler, founder of the Ethical Society, was influenced by the New York City Mission but wanted nurses to provide care in a nonsectarian way. The nurses employed by the Ethical Society received their patients from physicians in dispensaries; each nurse visited in the district served by a dispensary. Teaching of cleanliness and proper feeding of infants and children were included as aspects of preventive care.

In 1893, Wald (age 26 years) and Mary Brewster organized the Nurses' Settlement in New York City, also known as the Henry Street Settlement. An 1891 graduate of the New York Hospital Training School for Nurses, Wald cared for neglected children for a year at the New York Juvenile Asylum (Kraus, 1980). She entered the Women's Medical College and was asked to teach home nursing to a group of immigrant women. When she went to the home of a young girl who requested aid for her sick mother, Wald had an experience that changed the direction of her life. She left the medical college and enrolled Brewster, a nursing school classmate, in the idea of living on the East Side, a poverty-stricken neighborhood of Jewish immigrants. Mrs. Solomon Loeb, the wife of a wealthy banker, agreed to support the two nurses and provided $60 per month for each nurse and money for emergencies. During the summer of 1893 they lived in the College Settlement (started in 1889).

Settlements were part of a movement of university-educated young adults to reside in communities, to study the problems through relationships with residents, and to reform the squalid conditions of urban workers (Kraus, 1980). Crowded tenements had insufficient ventilation and no toilets or baths; fire escapes were also crowded with sleeping people. A police census in 1900 identified more than 2900 persons living in an area smaller than two football fields—approximately 1724 persons per acre (Kraus, 1980, p. 180). In this environment, Wald was committed to provide nursing services to sick poor persons. By 1900 there were 15 nurses; by 1909 there were 47 nurses on call; and by 1914 there were 82 affiliated nurses (Kraus, 1980). In 1913 the Henry Street Settlement reached 22,168 persons, or 1,048 more than all persons admitted that year to Mt. Sinai Hospital, New York Hospital, and Presbyterian Hospital combined (Kraus, 1980, p. 176).

Alleviation of human suffering and illness was profound. The results in terms of creative nursing practice and the inception of new modes of health care delivery are with us today.

ASSOCIATIONS FOR VISITING NURSING AND DISTRICT NURSING

In 1886 two associations were founded that were the first in the United States to be organized for the sole purpose of providing care by trained nurses to sick poor persons in their homes (Gardner, 1936; Brainard, 1985). The associations in Boston and Philadelphia were started independently, but each was inspired by district nursing in England.

Abbie Howes and Phoebe Adam were members of the Womens' Education Association in Boston; they approached the association to support the new idea of district nursing. To convince the association that education, not charitable relief, would be a large part of the nursing work, the name *Instructive District Nursing Association of Boston* was adopted (Brainard, 1985).

Amelia Hodgkiss was the first nurse so employed in February 1886; during the first year three nurses visited 707 cases, making 7182 visits (Brainard, 1985, p. 207). Two lady managers were appointed to each district, similar to the English model. Each nurse obtained orders from and reported to the dispensary physician in her district each morning. Nurses worked 8 hours per day, 6 days per week.

The association adopted the more modern principles in working with the poor. Nurses were not to give money to the patients to relieve their financial plight or to interfere with the patients' religion. It was also explicitly stated for the first time that nurses were not to interfere with the political opinions of patients (Brainard, 1985). To prevent cross-infection, caring of patients with contagious diseases was limited. Instruction to families about hygiene, self-care, and prevention was held to be equal with care for sick poor persons. It was in 1890 that professional nursing supervisors were employed.

Each nurse worked with a local committee of residents in her district who were to publicize the work and raise money to support the service. By 1920 more than 36,000 patients were seen per year by the association's nurses; 23% were maternity cases.

Also in February 1886 Mrs. William Jinks called together other women active in Philadelphia charity work to raise $100 to employ a nurse to care for poor sick persons in their homes for a month's trial. She had heard of district nursing from an English guest. In March 1886 Sarah Haydock started her nursing experiment. Initially physicians did not refer patients and physicians and philanthropists resisted the new idea. They insisted that poor persons were to be cared for in hospitals and should not be "indulged a luxury" of home care that could not be continued (Brainard, 1985). After the support of leading physicians was sought and obtained, patients were referred.

Initially called the *District Nurse Society,* the name was changed to the *Visiting Nurse Society of Philadelphia* because it was difficult to limit the nurse's work to a particular geographic area. Nurses were on call 11 hours per day. Fees of $.50 to $1.00 were charged for each visit, although services were provided free to those unable to pay. A new idea was emerging: visiting nurses were available to all, not just poor persons. By 1919 a general pay service had been implemented ($.75 per visit), in which the nurse's visit was determined at the convenience of her work schedule, and an hourly service was available at a higher rate ($1.24 per hour), in which the nurse visited at the time requested by the patient and stayed as many hours as were needed, short of residency in the home (Brainard, 1985, p. 224). After 5 PM the hourly rate increased to $1.75.

Like the Boston Association, the Philadelphia Society had a twofold mission: to care for the sick and "to teach cleanliness and proper care of the sick" (Brainard, 1985, p. 219). The Philadelphia Society employed attendants as well as nurses, and within the first year the need for a supervisory nurse was recognized.

The idea of district nursing in England had been successfully transplanted to the United States and was generally known as visiting nursing (Brainard, 1985). The number of visiting nursing associations dramatically increased during the 1890s, especially in northeastern and midwestern cities, as word of their value spread (Brainard, 1985). The name *visiting nursing* was probably adopted because there were so many types of organizations that employed visiting nurses—nursing associations, churches, hospitals, industries, and charity organizations—and not all nurses were assigned by districts.

In 1909, Yssabella Waters, a nurse with the Henry Street Settlement, undertook a national survey of organizations that employed trained nurses as visiting nurses. A dramatic increase of visiting nursing associations and visiting nurses occurred between 1890 and 1909. Waters reported that poverty was no longer an indirect requirement for visitation and that visiting nurses could accept requests for their services from all physicians. A visiting nurse no longer worked primarily with one physician. An explicit rule now

TABLE 2–3

Rules for Nurses from the Instructive Visiting Nurse Association of Baltimore, MD

1. Each nurse shall pledge herself to give at least 6 months' service to the Association, and if desiring to withdraw, shall give a month's notice.
2. Each nurse shall give 8 hours' work daily, and shall be at the office twice daily for calls, at the hours of 9 AM and 1 PM; but on Sundays and legal holidays no calls to new patients will be received, although visits to critical cases under her care may be required.
3. Each nurse shall be entitled to 1 month's vacation during the year, and, as her salary is continued during this time, it is required that she shall not exercise her profession.
4. Nurses shall answer all calls in their districts, excepting those from disorderly houses.
5. Nurses shall not nurse contagious diseases, but in all cases give instruction and every possible assistance to the families.
6. Nurses are not allowed to prescribe treatment or to continue to attend cases which are not under the care of a physician.
7. Nurses are not expected to attend cases of labor, but may afterwards visit mother and infant until recovery.
8. Nurses, in addition to their care of patients, shall give suitable instruction in each case to some member of the family, or other available person, on ventilation, food, cleanliness, etc.
9. Nurses are not allowed to give material assistance, except in cases of real emergency, and then only until the need can be relieved by some other agency. They shall keep a record of all cases in which material assistance is given or which are referred to other agencies, and shall report them weekly to the Secretary. They are advised, in cases of doubtful emergency, to consult with the local agent of the Charity Organization Society.
10. Nurses shall not give or receive presents of any kind.
11. In lending articles to the sick, each nurse must keep a record of the date of loan and require all articles to be returned clean and in good order.
12. Nurses are instructed to collect at least ten cents for each professional visit, excepting when, in their judgment, the families are unable to make any payment.
13. There shall be no interference with the religious or political opinions of the patients.

From: Waters, Y. (1912). *Visiting nursing in the United States* (pp. 27–28). New York: Charities Publication Committee, The Russell Sage Foundation.

required that patients be under the care of a physician. Table 2–3 depicts rules for nurses that were included in Waters' book; they incorporate the principles that first appeared in district nursing.

PUBLIC HEALTH NURSING: NURSING FOR SOCIAL BETTERMENT

The demand for even more visiting nursing service led nursing leaders to consider the issue of standards for practice. There was concern that untrained nurses would be hired to meet the expanding demand and that nursing might revert to pre-Nightingale practices. In 1911 Ella Crandall, professor in the Department of Public Health and Nursing at Teachers College in New York, initiated correspondence with other nursing leaders to solicit their opinions about an "organization to protect the standards of visiting nursing" (Brainard, 1985, p. 326).

A joint committee appointed by the American Nurses' Association (ANA) and the Society of Superintendents of Training Schools and chaired by Wald met to consider the issue. They sent letters to more than 1000 organizations in the United States that employed visiting nurses, inviting each to send a representative to a special meeting at the next ANA meeting in June 1912. Eighty replies were received and 69 organizations agreed to send a delegate (Brainard, 1985; Fitzpatrick, 1975).

The report of the joint committee was accepted. A National Visiting Nurse Association was formed as a member of the ANA and recommended standards for organizations that employed visiting nurses were accepted (Brainard, 1985; Fitzpatrick, 1975).

The name of the association was debated at length because there had not been agreement within the joint committee; a majority had favored *The National Visiting Nurse Association,* and Crandall led a vocal minority advocating Wald's term *Public Health Nursing* (Brainard, 1985; Fitzpatrick, 1975). Reasons for selecting *visiting nursing* included the fact that it was the term commonly recognized by the public. *Public health nursing* was a broader term, which encompassed all nurses "doing work for social betterment," and was not limited to those who primarily did home visiting to provide bedside care (Brainard, 1985, p. 332). Public health nursing was general enough to include nurses in schools, tuberculosis programs, hospital dispensaries, factories, settlements, and child welfare organizations in addition to those providing bedside care through home visiting. Crandall asserted that the public health movement would expand, and that adoption of the term *public health nursing* provided a generic term under which new forms of practice could evolve. The organization was finally named the *National Organization for Public Health Nursing* (NOPHN). The word "for" was consciously selected to allow the participation of non-nurses in promoting the work of public health nursing (Brainard, 1985; Fitzpatrick, 1975). In 1952 the NOPHN merged with the National League for Nursing (NLN), which continues today.

A Definition of Public Health

C.-E.A. Winslow (1877–1957), the leading theoretician of the American public health movement, provided a definition of public health in 1920 (Table 2–4). He asserted that public health is a social activity that builds "a comprehensive program of community service" on the basic sciences of chemistry, bacteriology, engineering and statistics, physiology, pathology, epidemiology, and sociology (Winslow, 1984, p. 1).

Although his original definition of public health focused on the goal of physical health, by 1923 Winslow acknowl-

TABLE 2–4

Definition of Public Health

Public health is the science and the art of preventing disease, prolonging life, and promoting physical health and efficiency through organized community efforts for the following purposes:

1. Sanitation of the environment
2. Control of community infections
3. Education of the individual in principles of personal hygiene
4. Organization of medical and nursing service for the early diagnosis and preventive treatment of disease
5. Development of the social machinery that will ensure to every individual in the community a standard of living adequate for the maintenance of health

Data from Winslow, C.-E. A. (1984). *The evolution and significance of the modern public health campaign.* South Burlington, VT: Journal of Public Health Policy, p. 1. (Original work published in 1923. New Haven, CT: Yale University Press.)

edged that prevention and treatment of mental illness was an expanding sector of the public health movement (Winslow, 1984). In 1945 Winslow predicted that "Public health which was an engineering science and has now become a medical science must expand until it is in addition a social science" (p. x). In 1953 the American Public Health Association encouraged "collaboration between public health workers and social scientists to better promote the utilization of social science findings toward the solution of public health problems" (Suchman, 1963, p. 22). In 1963 Edward A. Suchman, Professor of Sociology at the University of Pittsburgh, described the application of sociology in the field of public health. He noted that both sociology and public health originated in the social reform movement, that both deal with populations of individuals, and that both employ statistical methods. The connection between social context and public health remains. It is especially important in the area of preventive mental health.

Winslow specifically named nursing services as being an essential part of the organized community efforts that will "prevent disease, prolong life and promote . . . health." He was an advocate for public health nursing, and in 1923 he agreed with Welch (the founder of The Johns Hopkins School of Public Health) that public health nursing was one of two unique contributions that the United States had made to public health. Winslow (1984) acknowledged public health nurses as "teachers of health par excellence" and recognized teaching as a responsibility additional to "care of the sick in their homes" (p. 56).

If the environment is healthful, if medical and nursing services are provided to assist ill persons, and if individuals are taught about health-related behavior and responsibilities, does a comprehensive community effort for health exist? "No," according to Winslow. There must also be "social machinery . . . [to] ensure a standard of living adequate for the maintenance of health." The science and art of public health is inherently concerned with the standard of living of others.

Public health nursing, as a composite of nursing and public health, is committed to the existence of standards of living sufficient to maintain health. The fields of public health and public health nursing originated in social reform that occurred as a result of the collective commitment of individuals to the health and well-being of others.

Acknowledging this commitment can provide renewed energy and clarity of purpose. Community health nurses who are empowered by this commitment, can continue to have an impact on the social and political power structures.

Nursing and Sanitary Reform

Prior to 1890 the primary public health measures to control communicable diseases in Europe and the United States were isolation of ill persons (quarantine) and enactment of laws governing food markets, water supplies, and sanitation (Duffy, 1990). As a result of the industrial revolution many people had moved to cities, where crowded conditions and poor sanitation helped to spread communicable diseases.

Descriptive epidemiological studies laid the groundwork for sanitary reforms in England and the United States (Duffy, 1990). In 1842 Edwin Chadwick published a report on the unsanitary conditions among poor persons in cities in Great Britain. Lemuel Shattuck founded the American Statistical Society in 1839 and identified high death rates among workers in Boston. His *Report of the Sanitary Commission of Massachusetts* in 1850 called for the government to improve sanitary and social conditions to reduce disease and death. In 1854 the English physician John Snow demonstrated that a cholera outbreak was linked to water from the same well. The germ theory of disease was only emerging. Table 2–5 lists other public health accomplishments in the United States.

During this time Nightingale in England and Dorothea Dix and Clara Barton, both teachers, in the United States confronted the unsanitary conditions and high death rates from disease among military personnel (Hays, 1989; Pryor, 1987). In the 1850s British troops entered the Crimean War in Turkey and occupied India. The Civil War (1861–1865) erupted in the United States.

Nightingale hypothesized that both environmental and behavioral factors increased the soldiers' risk of infectious disease (Hays, 1989). In Turkey she organized and managed the nurses who cared for wounded soldiers and she instituted reforms in sanitation, lifestyle, and data collection for monitoring disease. Sanitary reforms included improvements in drainage, laundries, hospital design, and kitchen cleanliness. She recommended a varied diet, reduced alcohol consumption, and activities to improve the soldiers' quality of life. As a result of her

TABLE 2–5

Dates in U.S. Public Health History

Year	Event
1793	First local health department in Baltimore, MD
1798	New York City establishes street cleaning system
1813	Federal law to encourage smallpox vaccination
1842	Massachusetts Registration Act provides for collecting vital statistics
1850	*Report of the Sanitary Commission of Massachusetts* by statistician Lemuel Shattuck
1855	First state quarantine board in Louisiana
1869	First state board of health in Massachusetts
1872	American Public Health Association (APHA) established
1878	Federal Marine Service Hospital established for sick and disabled seamen
1881	American Red Cross founded by Clara Barton
1890	Federal Marine Hospitals authorized to inspect immigrants
1894	First medical inspection of school children in New York City
1900	38 states have health departments
1910	Tuberculosis programs included in local and state health departments
1912	U.S. Public Health Service (USPHS) established
1912	National Safety Council formed
1935	Federal Social Security Act institutes Social Security retirement, disability, and survivors' benefits
1945	Federal Hill-Burton Act funds building of community hospitals
1963	Federal Community Mental Health Centers Act
1965	Amendments to Social Security Act provide financial mechanisms to pay for health care for poor (Medicaid) and elderly (Medicare) persons
1965	Regional Medical Program established to disseminate research findings to public regarding prevention and treatment of heart disease, cancer, and stroke
1966	Comprehensive Health Planning Amendments to Public Health Service Act
1974	National Health Resources Planning and Development Act provided for system of community-based health planning for entire nation
1980	First national health objectives published
1980	Smallpox eradicated throughout the world via leadership of World Health Organization
1983	Health Resources Planning and Development Act not renewed: national health planning abolished
1983	Prospective payment system instituted under Medicare
1988	Institute of Medicine of the National Academy of Sciences publishes *The Future of Public Health*
1990	*National Health Objectives for the Year 2000* published
1991	*Healthy Communities 2000: Model Standards* published by APHA
1993	National legislation introduced for health care reform

advocacy, libraries, athletic programs, and service projects were established for the troops in India.

Nightingale proposed new ways of reporting and analyzing biostatistics about the health of the British military. Although she never went to India, she established a uniform data collection system that she managed from England. She established population-based objectives and demonstrated that annual mortality rates dramatically declined from 70 per 1000 population to 19 per 1000 population after her reforms (Hays, 1989, p. 154).

Initially there was no system for battlefield care during the American Civil War. Even with surgery 90% of soldiers with abdominal wounds and 62% with other wounds died (Pryor, 1987, p. 94). More soldiers died of disease than of effects of wounds. The Sanitary Commission was a relief agency started by northerners to supply the Union Army with equipment. Newspapers advertised for surgeons and male nurses.

Although Nightingale's work was known in America, public roles for women remained limited. However, because of the magnitude of the need, numerous womens' groups traveled to the battlefields to care for the wounded. Dix led a group of nurses in the Christian Commission, a branch of the Young Mens' Christian Association (YMCA) (Pryor, 1987). She had gained national prominence for her work in reforming prisons and mental institutions, and was appointed head of the Department of Female Nurses. Most of the nurses worked in hospitals in Washington, DC.

Barton also organized volunteers at the battlefields. Although not a trained nurse, she found her life's purpose in caring for the wounded (Pryor, 1987). She tended wounds, cooked, and collected relief supplies for the troops. She was an excellent organizer and enrolled others in providing enough supplies to fill several warehouses. For a while during the war, she continued to receive her salary as one of only a few women employees of the U.S. Patent Office. She was committed to providing relief in times of war and disaster and became an advocate for the International Red Cross, a relief organization started in Switzerland. In 1881 Barton was one of the founders of the American branch of the Red Cross.

By the last quarter of the 19th century, the discovery of microbes had transformed the sanitary movement into the "golden age of public health" (1880–1910). General sanitary reforms were supplemented by specific actions aimed at preventing communicable diseases. These included pasteurization of milk, surgical asepsis, and immunization. The germ theory of disease also gave new impetus to campaigns for adequate housing, public water and sewage systems, pure food and drugs, and reporting systems for disease surveillance. Public health nurses continued to be leaders in educating the public about disease prevention. As the demand for public health nurses increased, specialization within community health nursing emerged.

Aggregate-Focused Care and Subspecialties

Public health nursing was for the entire public. Nurses in most rural communities and nurses assigned by districts in urban areas continued to practice as generalists. Generalists worked with families and incorporated health promotion and disease prevention with care of the sick.

At its first annual meeting in 1913, the NOPHN recognized seven specializations and interest areas within public health nursing: general visiting nursing, rural nursing, school nursing, tuberculosis nursing, infant welfare, mental hygiene, and industrial welfare (Fitzpatrick, 1975). No longer were urban poor persons and military personnel the only target population groups.

Two schemes of subspecialties emerged simultaneously in public health nursing, especially in urban areas. One scheme considered the aggregate of people served: school populations and industrial workers. The second scheme considered health problems: health supervision or preventive education, maternity, and illnesses (morbidity). Mental hygiene was not specifically mentioned in either scheme. By the early 1930s the NOPHN surveyed public health nurses according to these two classification systems (Gardner, 1936).

Health supervision overlapped with the population classification because some nurses worked with a specific age group to promote health and prevent illness. For example some nurses worked exclusively with mothers and children and others worked with school or employed populations. Maternity services encompassed prenatal care, labor and delivery (including home deliveries by physicians or midwives), and postpartum and neonatal care. As previously discussed, care of ill persons in their homes was the basis for visiting nursing care. Morbidity care expanded to include the care of those not confined to bed, especially those with tuberculosis, gonorrhea, and syphilis.

SCHOOL NURSING

As a specialty in visiting nursing, school health nursing evolved in London in 1892 and in New York in 1902 (Brainard, 1985; Gardner, 1936). In London the first school nurse visited a school weekly to oversee nutrition and remedy minor ailments. By 1898 the London School Nurses' Society was organized as a private charity. Five nurses served 500 elementary schools, with each visiting 4 schools per day and examining 100 children (Brainard, 1985, p. 264).

Medical inspection of schoolchildren in the United States was instituted in Boston in 1894, long after such systems were initiated in France (1837), Germany, England, Russia, Chile, and Egypt (Gardner, 1936). Physicians excluded from school children who had untreated communicable diseases.

Wald noticed that the children excluded from school often did not receive medical treatment and so remained out of school for long periods but transmitted microorganisms to other children while playing in the streets. Nurses from the Henry Street Settlement determined to prove that children could remain in school, receive treatment, and not increase the transmission of disease. In 1902 more than 10,000 children were excluded from New York City schools; in 1903 after the school health nursing services had been introduced, slightly more than 1000 children were excluded (Gardner, 1936). Daily treatment of illnesses such as ringworm and impetigo by the school nurses not only reduced illnesses but dramatically reduced absenteeism.

As a result of such success, the New York Board of Health employed 12 nurses to continue the work. Brainard (1985) reports that these nurses are "called the first Public Health Nurses" (p. 270).

The goal of protecting school-age children from communicable diseases expanded to include screening and examination for other treatable conditions such as deficits in growth, vision, and hearing. Children were taught hygiene in the schools by the nurses as they provided first aid. During the first quarter of the 20th century, school nurses worked with teachers and parent associations to incorporate more group health education.

Elementary schools remained the focus of school nursing because communicable diseases were more prevalent in younger children. Likewise it was important to correct potentially handicapping conditions at the earliest possible age. Nursing with high school populations was to emerge later.

School nursing was introduced in other cities, often because the local visiting nurse association would "loan" a nurse to demonstrate the value of the service (Brainard, 1985). Frequently either the health department or the board of education became interested in continuing the service.

INDUSTRIAL NURSING

Industrial nursing in the United States pre-dated industrial nursing in England. The Vermont Marble Works is credited with having employed Ada Stewart, a trained visiting nurse, to care for sick employees and their families in 1895 (Brainard, 1985; Gardner, 1936). Industrial nursing grew slowly and was started independently in firms by employer or employee associations, or both (Gardner, 1936).

With the start of World War I in 1914, industrial nursing positions increased (Brainard, 1985). Federal government contracts for war-related goods stimulated manufacturing businesses and industrial nursing positions. Productivity was important. The National Safety Council had been formed in 1912. Industrial nursing was beneficial because factory efficiency was improved if workers were at work and healthy (Gardner, 1936). Gardner (1936) suggests philanthropy, industrial justice, and fear of union movements were other motives for starting industrial nursing services. By 1919 there were more than 1200 industrial nurses in 871 industries in the United States (Brainard, 1985, p. 294).

Employee health was the initial concern and was addressed by providing advice and first aid to individual employees, teaching employees collectively about safety and sanitation, visiting at home to care for and instruct the ill employees and their families, and initiating other public health services in the communities (Gardner, 1936). Ella

Crandall in 1916 advocated that nurses also be involved directly with environmental safety and sanitation of plants and "social service for employees, including recreation, vacation homes, education, relief and general fitting of the man to the job" (Brainard, 1985, p. 295).

CHILD HEALTH NURSING

Among the humanitarian reforms during the 19th century was the beginning of concern for the health and welfare of infants and children. In 1817 the Englishman John Davis wrote a book in which he explored the causes of mortality in children and suggested that "benevolent ladies" visit homes to instruct mothers, inspect children, and report on their conditions (Brainard, 1985; Gardner, 1936). Little came of his idea. Concurrently he founded a dispensary especially for children in London.

In Paris in 1844 the first day nursery for infants (*la crèche*) was started. A nurse cared for 12 infants in a poor community and a physician visited daily (Brainard, 1985). In 1876 a society for nursing mothers established shelters in Paris to care for poor women during the last few weeks of their pregnancy: breast-feeding was promoted, infants were observed monthly, and social work services were provided (Brainard, 1985; Gardner, 1936). The rate of infant mortality persisted.

The pasteurization of milk allowed clean milk supplies for mothers who could not breast-feed. In 1892 milk stations were established in New York City and Hamburg, Germany, to provide sanitary milk supplies to sick infants (Brainard, 1985). Little accompanying instruction existed related to infant feeding.

In the same year in Paris, Boudin provided the foundation for the modern movement to combat infant mortality (Brainard, 1985). After infants were discharged from maternity hospitals, they were seen regularly on an outpatient basis for 2 years. Their growth was monitored, breast-feeding was encouraged, and hygienic bottle-feeding was taught to mothers who could not breast-feed. In 1894 Dufour prepared artificial feedings according to medical formulas and distributed them to the poor of Paris when breast-feeding could not be accomplished (Brainard, 1985).

From the beginning of district nursing in England and visiting nursing in the United States, the nurses devoted much effort to the care of women, infants, and children. This was a part of their generalized practice.

Specialized infant nursing began in the United States in 1902, the same year as school nursing. In that year special nurses were employed solely to visit sick children in a district of New York City, and other nurses visited infants born in the summer months of 1902 and 1903 (Brainard, 1985).

Following French and German models, the Infants' Clinic was established in 1906 by the Visiting Nurse Association of Cleveland and the Milk Fund Association (Brainard, 1985). Infants were examined until age 15 months by physicians in the dispensary; nurses provided home visits every 2 to 3 weeks to promote breast-feeding, supervise formula preparation and feeding when necessary, and support mothers to follow medical advice. These nurses specialized in teaching mothers to properly care for their infants. Visiting nurse associations around the country begin to hire nurses solely for infant welfare work.

Local government became involved in 1908 with the formation of the Division of Child Hygiene in the New York City Department of Health. Nurses visited all newborns and sick infants in 89 districts (Brainard, 1985).

After the annual meeting of the American Academy of Medicine in 1908, nurses met with physicians, social workers, and laypersons to form the American Association for the Study and Prevention of Infant Mortality (Brainard, 1985). Through the advocacy of Wald, visiting nurses were recognized as being qualified to work in infant dispensaries (the forerunners of well-child clinics) to instruct mothers how to prevent illness (Brainard, 1985).

In 1912 the federal government created the Children's Bureau, which sought to reduce morbidity and mortality in the children of the United States. This body established policy to promote prenatal care and home visits to mothers and children, vaccination and immunization, provision of sanitary milk, and prompt medical care, especially for physical defects (Gardner, 1936). With World War I, death rates of adult males increased and birth rates fell. Saving the lives of children became especially important for families (Gardner, 1936).

TUBERCULOSIS NURSING

Tuberculosis was a dread disease in the 1870s in the United States. It was known to be communicable and incurable. Tuberculosis was the primary cause of death among young and middle-aged adults (Gardner, 1936).

Fresh air, rest, and good food had been recommended by physicians throughout the 19th century, but no one knew why the treatments worked. When Robert Koch discovered in 1882 that tuberculosis was caused by a microorganism transmitted by sputum that could be killed by exposure to sunlight and boiling, prevention was possible. To prevent the spread of disease, persons with tuberculosis were instructed to collect sputum for proper disposal, avoid sleeping with others in close quarters, and avoid sharing eating utensils.

The tuberculosis nurse originated in the United States in 1903 when William Osler, Professor of Medicine at the Johns Hopkins Medical School, hired Reiba Thelin to provide home care and instruction to tuberculosis patients in Baltimore (Brainard, 1985). Thelin had never done visiting nursing before and resigned after a year to study at the Henry Street Settlement.

Mrs. Osler was also an ardent supporter of the antituberculosis movement; she sent letters to all the residents in

Baltimore, soliciting $1.00 to support tuberculosis nurses (Brainard, 1985). The money went to the visiting nurse association to pay for nurses especially assigned as tuberculosis nurses. Similarly the visiting nurse associations in other urban areas provided tuberculosis care.

The National Tuberculosis Association was founded in 1904. Its members soon recognized that there was much overlapping and confusion in the provision of tuberculosis care; some programs were privately sponsored and others were sponsored by municipalities. By 1910 coordination and standardization of tuberculosis programs was recommended and the cities and states took over sponsorship of the antituberculosis programs (Brainard, 1985). By the 1930s tuberculosis nursing had become a part of the generalized practice of nurses employed by health departments (Gardner, 1936), but more than 500,000 cases of tuberculosis still existed. Public health nurses cared for those with advanced disease, conducted tuberculin skin testing to identify infection in children, and taught good ventilation practices and sputum disposal as effective preventive actions.

Expansion into Rural America

Wald advocated that public health nursing services also be provided to rural Americans (Bigbee and Crowder, 1985; Hamilton, 1988; Haupt, 1953). Consequently the Visiting Nurse Service of the Metropolitan Life Insurance Company (1909) and the Red Cross Rural Nursing Service were established (1912). Economic support from business and private philanthropic sources now existed for nationwide systems of public health nursing.

THE RED CROSS RURAL NURSING SERVICE

Originally called the Town and Country Nursing Service, the Red Cross Rural Nursing Service (RNS) established more than 1000 local nursing services, one of which led to the establishment of public health nursing services on American Indian reservations (Bigbee and Crowder, 1985). The services were funded totally by local Red Cross chapters or by local chapters in partnership with other private and government agencies. Traveling nurses were sent by the National Red Cross to local communities for several months to stimulate interest.

The RNS supported high professional qualifications for its nurses, including graduation from a 2-year nursing school, registration (in states requiring it), prior public health experience or postgraduate education, and membership in a professional association (Bigbee and Crowder, 1985).

The National Red Cross provided scholarships and loans for nurses to obtain postgraduate education in public health nursing. The RNS designed a model curriculum for postgraduate courses in rural public health nursing (4 to 8 months' duration). The courses were first offered at Teachers College in New York City in 1913.

Financial support for the RNS dwindled during the 1920s because of economic depression and the emergence of public health nursing programs in local and state health departments. However, hundreds of rural counties still did not have public health nursing services (Bigbee and Crowder, 1985).

THE METROPOLITAN LIFE INSURANCE COMPANY VISITING NURSE SERVICE

The Visiting Nurse Service of the Metropolitan Life Insurance Company (MLIC) was the prototype for businesses to contract for public health nursing services (Hamilton, 1988). The MLIC insured poor, industrial workers who had high death rates. Lee Frankel of the company proposed that insurance agents provide health and safety teaching to their policy-holders. When Wald persuaded him that public health nurses would be better health teachers, a 44-year partnership began between the company and public health nurses. Insurance agents provided publicity.

The MLIC contracted with existing visiting nurse associations to avoid duplication of services and to strengthen community-based agencies (Haupt, 1953). During its peak year, in 1931, more than 750,000 policy-holders received more than 4 million home visits in more than 7000 cities in the United States and Canada (Hamilton, 1988; Haupt, 1953). Nurses also collected baseline health data in communities, started clinics, and gave immunizations (Hamilton, 1988). To stimulate the creation of nursing services where there were none, MLIC provided scholarships for nurses to attend college and university programs (Haupt, 1953). Statistics showed that public health nursing care resulted in decreased mortality and improved health among its policy-holders.

The MLIC service ended in 1953 because the diminishing outcomes no longer justified the rising costs (Hamilton, 1988). By then immunizations had reduced deaths from communicable diseases. The numbers of home visits had decreased because patients were now cared for in community hospitals, which were started as a result of the federal Hill-Burton Act (1945). Simultaneously the costs for home visits had risen, partially because of the increased education of nurses.

Funding from the Red Cross and the MLIC resulted in new instructive visiting nurses associations throughout the country. The nurses continued to combine preventive work with care for sick persons at home. Some visiting nurses associations entered contracts with MLIC. Other associations entered joint ventures and started demonstration projects (Buhler-Wilkerson, 1985). In joint ventures another voluntary organization, such as the Red Cross, provided finances; in demonstrations, experimental programs were piloted on a small scale until their worth was proved, at which point someone else, such as a local health department, would take over the project. Until the 1920s most public health nurses were employed by not-for-profit, nongovernmental agencies.

THE FRONTIER NURSING SERVICE

As a nurse midwife Mary Breckenridge made an extraordinary contribution to the health of women and children in the underserved, rural area of eastern Kentucky through the establishment of the Frontier Nursing Service in 1925. (See Table 2–6 for more details about her life and nursing leadership.)

Government Employment of Public Health Nurses

By 1900 38 states had established health departments (Hanlon and Pickett, 1984, p. 33). As the government took a more active role in public health, more nurses were employed by state and local governments—by local health departments and boards of education.

As previously discussed, public hygiene measures implemented during the golden age of public health had successfully reduced sickness and death rates from infectious diseases in urban areas. Water was filtered, milk was pasteurized, garbage was removed, and housing codes were instituted. The rural sanitation movement of the 1920s stimulated the development of local health departments.

C.-E.A. Winslow (1984, p. 58) asserted that "the new public health movement" was to be based on "hygienic instruction, plus the organization of medical service for the detection and early treatment of incipient disease." Some physicians advocated that a new kind of public health worker who possessed knowledge of health, education, and social work be developed as a "health visitor" to perform the preventive activities normally done by public health nurses (Fitzpatrick, 1975). Winslow advocated for the public health nurse, who was already established in the homes. "Unlike the social worker, she knew the human body," its reactions and "hygienic conduct of life;" unlike the physician who was focused on pathology, "she was trained to see the body as a whole" (Buhler-Wilkerson, 1985, pp. 1156–1157). The public health nurse was to be the educator for personal hygiene.

In 1916 the NOPHN supported "public health nursing under government auspices" as a means of extending health care services to more people (Fitzpatrick, 1975, p. 48). By the mid-1920s more than 50% of public health nurses were government employees. By the late 1930s all 48 states had public health nursing programs (Roberts and Heinrich, 1985). Many of the services provided by the Red

TABLE 2–6

Mary Breckenridge: A Public Health Nursing Leader

Mary Breckenridge initiated a study of the health needs of 29,000 people in three counties in eastern Kentucky in 1923. She rode more than 700 miles on horseback to interview 53 "granny women" or midwives, young mothers, schoolteachers, and those in charge of missions.

Her family had lived in Kentucky since 1790 and been in public service since the time of Thomas Jefferson. Her father was Minister to Russia under President Grover Cleveland. She spent 12 winters in Washington, DC, as a girl and 2 years in Russia with French and German governesses. A great aunt established schools for mountain children in the southern U.S. To prepare for service Mary "took the stiff training as a nurse at St. Luke's Hospital in New York."

After her husband died, her second marriage was unhappy and two children died. She went to France to care for children there during World War I. Her thoughts returned to Kentucky where neonatal and maternal deaths and epidemics of hookworm, diphtheria, smallpox, typhoid, and tuberculosis ravaged the population. Her assessment emerged from her commitment to demonstrate "what intelligent nursing could do to safeguard the lives of mothers and children on our many forgotten frontiers" in the United States. To be able to address the health needs she had identified, she studied in London to become licensed as a nurse-midwife. She returned to Kentucky in 1925 to provide trained nurse-midwives "to deliver women in childbirth and safeguard the lives of little children, to care for the sick of all ages and take measures to prevent disease, and to work for economic conditions less inimical to health."

The Frontier Nursing Service was thus created. By 1931 "the staff included two assistant directors, three supervisors, relief nurses, three nurses and a physician in a small hospital . . . , and 21 nurses in the field." One nurse's report indicated she had made rounds for 11 hours a day and during the week had visited 143 persons. Additionally, patients were seen at the centers. All services were provided for only $10.92 per year per individual served. In the year ending May 1931, 7806 persons in 1675 families were cared for; this included bedside nursing to 459 cases of serious illness.

The nurses at the outlying stations lived in comfortable quarters with two nurses per station and a housekeeper-cook. One nurse was assigned general duty and one midwifery. Each nurse was assigned a district and could cover 80 square miles per day. Six weeks of vacation were earned each year, preferably in two 3-week periods. The work itself was demanding; the nurse must be independent, capable of extensive horseback travel, unstopped by vagaries of weather, and available to respond to emergency illnesses. The nurses were committed to the people as well as their own professional practice.

Mary Breckenridge enlisted others to assist in addressing the multitude of problems. She organized a local committee of mountaineers so she could work with the people, rather than for them. She involved her relatives, physicians, experts in public health, and the Kentucky State Board of Health in planning the organization. The nurses avoided involvement in the mountaineer clan wars and served all who were wounded or in need. She collaborated with federal and state authorities, the Rockefeller Foundation, and The Johns Hopkins and Vanderbilt Universities; the American Child Health Association participated to cure hookworm. Graduates of the Forestry Department of Yale University were invited to survey logging practices and revitalize the forests to improve employment opportunities to reduce poverty.

Mary Breckenridge was a pioneer in community assessment, population- based planning, and partnership building. She created a system for rural nursing and used research to demonstrate its effectiveness. Her vision remains fulfilled in the Frontier Nursing Service that continues today.

Data from Poole, E. (1932). *Nurses on horseback.* New York: Macmillan.

Cross Nursing Service were taken over by local health departments.

The federal government also stimulated the increase in public health nurses. Growth of state health departments was a result of the federal Sheppard-Towner Act of 1921, which sought improved maternal and child health.

As a result of the Great Depression, many people were unemployed. The Federal Emergency Relief Act of 1933 identified bedside nursing care of poor persons as a relief service; federal money was made available for contracting with nongovernmental visiting nurse associations to provide such services. The Civil Works Administration included relief projects for unemployed nurses themselves. By employing nurses in governmental agencies, the Civil Works Administration stimulated tax-supported public health nursing programs (Fitzpatrick, 1975).

During World War II the U.S. Public Health Service temporarily employed 200 nurses and 35 supervisors to prevent disease and provide health education to families of servicemen near military installations (Fitzpatrick, 1975, p. 65). Emphases were on childhood immunization, control of sexually transmitted diseases, and maternity care.

As of 1984, 8.3% of all employed registered nurses in the United States were employed in community health (101,430 registered nurses) or occupational health (22,890 registered nurses) (ANA, 1987a, p. 101). Thirty-six percent were employed by local health departments, 30% by boards of education, and 21% by home health agencies. More than two thirds of nurses in community health were government employees.

Dichotomy in Public Health Nursing

Early in the 20th century competition began to exist between health departments and nongovernmental organizations. Visiting nursing associations feared that health departments might take over. There was simultaneous conflict between the public health practitioners in health departments and the medical profession. Private physicians feared loss of income if health departments engaged in treating patients in addition to preventing illnesses. Thus, health officers made decisions that limited "publicly supported nurses to the prevention of disease, leaving the care of the sick to the visiting nurse associations" (Buhler-Wilkerson, 1985, p. 1159).

These decisions obviously acknowledged a place for nursing in both health departments and visiting nurse associations. However, the tragedy of these decisions was that they split nursing care of sick persons from preventive nursing activities. Public health nursing was no longer whole. Buhler-Wilkerson (1985) asserts that it was this division that has prevented public health nursing from achieving its potential as a delivery system of comprehensive health care.

Many nursing leaders in the 1920s attempted to maintain a "framework that would allow the public health nurse to care for both the healthy and the sick" (Buhler-Wilkerson, 1985, p. 1159). In some communities, partnerships developed between the health department and the visiting nurse association to provide both types of nursing care through a "combined" administrative structure. Most of these structures did not survive.

In 1929 the NOPHN stressed that public health nursing was a nonprofit community service

> "Public health nursing is an organized community nonprofit service, rendered by graduate nurses to the individual, family and community. This service includes interpretation and application of medical, sanitary, and social procedures for the correction of defects, prevention of disease and the promotion of health; and may include skilled care of the sick in their homes (Fitzpatrick, 1975, p. 102)."

This definition included government-sponsored services as well as private, nonprofit services such as visiting nurse associations. Preventive services were a necessary component of public health nursing, and skilled care of sick persons in their homes was permitted but not required.

In 1934 the NOPHN and the APHA definition of public health nursing was more general and included all nursing services that assisted with the "public health program."

> "Public health nursing includes all nursing services organized by a community or an agency to assist in carrying out any or all phases of the public health program. Services may be rendered on an individual, family, or community basis in the home, school, clinics, business establishment, or the office of the agency (Fitzpatrick, 1975, p. 127)."

By then, however, most public health programs were government-sponsored.

The division in public health nursing in the United States occurred as a result of a basic schism within the health care system: the private sector vs. the government-sponsored (public) sector. To manage competition and conflict between the two sectors, diagnosis and treatment of ill persons remained the domain of private physicians, and health promotion and disease prevention were the domain of state and local health departments. This division of responsibility was relatively clear and remained so until 1965, when, with the enactment of Medicare and Medicaid legislation, the government sector began paying for the health care of ill elderly and poor persons.

Educational Preparation for Public Health Nurses

Prior to 1935 most public health nurses were trained nurses who learned about public health nursing from their on-the-job experience. By 1959 20% of public health nurses had an academic degree.

In the early 1900s some hospital schools placed students in private homes to provide nursing care and to increase revenues for the hospitals. However, most nurses in public health learned through apprenticeships with visiting nurse associations. In 1906 the Boston Instructive District Visiting Nurses Association developed a course for its nurses. For 4 months nurses were closely supervised in their practice, and received room and board but no salary (Brainard, 1985).

In 1910 Teacher's College of Columbia University established the Department of Nursing and Health for postgraduate work for trained nurses. Western Reserve University in Cleveland and Simmons College in Boston soon followed (Brainard, 1985). By 1922 there were 15 postgraduate schools of public health nursing (Goodnow, 1928, p. 240). Knowledge of hygiene and sanitation; prevention and control of health problems, such as tuberculosis and infant mortality; sociology; and social psychology were valuable to nurses promoting health (Brainard, 1985).

The NOPHN believed that effective nursing care for families was based on good general nursing. The National League for Nursing Education (NLNE) advocated that specialists in public nursing be prepared through university-sponsored courses for nurses who had graduated from training schools. The NLNE also advocated that training schools for nurses should prepare generalists in public health by affiliating with visiting nurse associations and adding lectures in sociology, psychology, and public health nursing (Fitzpatrick, 1975). Electives in public health nursing were also encouraged in training schools.

By 1918 the NLNE had agreed on a standard curriculum that incorporated "social aspects of nursing" into the third year of basic diploma training schools (Fitzpatrick, 1975). Field practice was resisted by training schools because the students were needed to staff hospitals.

The NLNE and the NOPHN divided the duties of overseeing the incorporation of public health nursing content into curricula. The NLNE oversaw basic training schools and the NOPHN was responsible for postgraduate and staff education (Fitzpatrick, 1975).

Despite the leadership's belief that additional knowledge and experience were necessary for public health nurses, few nurses working in public health had the extra education. Correspondence courses were developed for those working in the field who were academically unprepared; the NOPHN endorsed the courses as appropriate staff education for those who had had 4 months of public health nursing experience (Fitzpatrick, 1975). Most public health nurses received additional information about their practice from publications supported by the NOPHN.

After baccalaureate schools of nursing became more prevalent, Alma Haupt, Director of the MLIC Visiting Nurse Association and a member of the NOPHN Education Committee, proposed in 1924 that public health nursing content be integrated into undergraduate education as a part of each specialized course, such as obstetrical nursing. Each graduate would be able to "organize care, make nursing assessments, appreciate the home conditions of patients and learn about community resources [and] the concept of health as a community responsibility" (Fitzpatrick, 1975, p. 101). However, to avoid overburdening public health agencies with students, hospital schools were to place their students in clinics, with only observations in public health nursing agencies (Fitzpatrick, 1975).

Substantive increases occurred between 1935 and 1950 in the percentage of public health nurses having adequate academic preparation. Baccalaureate nursing programs were encouraged to have 8-week affiliations in public health agencies that met NOPHN standards; students were to "study health and sickness in one family over time" (Fitzpatrick, 1975, p. 129) and understand the neighborhood factors that "influenced a family's health and socio-economic situation." The number of postgraduate courses approved by the NOPHN increased from 16 in 1935 to 26 in 1940 (Roberts and Heinrich, 1985, p. 1164). By 1950, 1 in 5 of the 25,000 public health nurses had one or more academic degrees; 56% of all supervisors and 70% of state-employed supervisors had degrees (Fitzpatrick, 1975, p. 193).

Community Health Nursing: 1965 to the Present

Several forces converged to promote the emergence of the term *community health nursing*. Hanlon and Pickett (1984) attribute the use of the term to the fact that numerous private, not-for-profit agencies evolved in the 1960s to address health needs that were not being met by local governments (the publicly sponsored agencies). As discussed previously, public health nursing had come to be associated with government-sponsored services; now that others also were addressing health needs of neighborhoods and population groups, an expanded term was needed. The term *community health nursing* included nursing sponsored by both private, nonprofit organizations and governmental agencies (Hanlon and Pickett, 1984). For-profit agencies were not mentioned as being related to community health nursing.

Simultaneously the ANA began to develop the following divisions of nursing practice: community health; gerontological; maternal and child health; medical-surgical; and psychiatric and mental health. Each division was to describe its scope and standards of practice.

Creation of the Division of Community Health Practice promoted the widespread use of the term *community health nursing* (U.S. Department of Health and Human Services [USDHHS], 1985). The Division included nurses working within a variety of community-based settings including health departments; schools; worksites; private physicians' offices; private, nonprofit clinics; visiting nurses associations; and for-profit home health agencies. Thus, the term included nurses employed by governmental, private nonprofit, and private for-profit agencies.

For-profit (proprietary) home health agencies began to increase in number after 1965 when Medicare made skilled nursing care (home health care) financially accessible to homebound elderly persons (see Chapter 29). Today agencies providing visiting nurses to care for ill persons in their homes are no longer sponsored primarily by the government and nonprofit private agencies.

The term *community health nursing,* in some respects, has reunited nursing both for the promotion of health and prevention of disease and for the care of ill persons at home. The possibility exists for community health nursing in the 21st century to recapture the vitality and wholeness that existed in public health nursing in the late 1800s.

Community Health Nursing and the Future

The essence of public health is "organized community efforts" that ensure "conditions in which people can be healthy" (Institute of Medicine [IOM], 1988, pp. 7, 41). Safe environments; timely immunization; sound nutrition; attention to maternal and fetal health; responsible behaviors and self-care; and provision of health care services help create healthful conditions (Last, 1992). Social and health care needs cannot be met solely by making sure that everyone has financial access to medical care (IOM, 1988). Community health nurses as public health personnel are experts in "health problem identification, disease and disability prevention, and health promotion" (IOM, 1988, p. 153). Community health nurses are exemplars in "outreach and case finding, direct service delivery, and management of needs of multiproblem clients" (IOM, 1988, p. 153).

NATIONAL HEALTH CARE REFORM

Nursing's Agenda for Health Care Reform (ANA, 1991) calls for a health care system that supports more nurses as primary care providers. Primary health care includes essential health care that is universally accessible to individuals and families within communities (ANA, 1986b). Primary health care includes health promotion and disease prevention as well as a basic package of services for treatment of illnesses and injury.

Even when almost everyone has financial access to a basic package of health care services, people will still need to learn to gain access to that care, to cope with personal responses to their health status, and to understand how their own behavior can improve their well-being. These concerns are all within the domain of nursing practice. A variety of models for delivering nursing care in a changing health care system are under exploration (ANA, 1986a). Community health nurses, especially those employed by the government and charged with the health of entire populations, need to become more visible and vocal as leaders for health (Shalala, 1992; Ward, 1989).

We can look to nursing in other countries for nursing care delivery models that may fit our changing circumstances. For example since the 1970s some community health nurses in Canada and Britain have been employed by the government but "attached" to work with primary care physicians and their enrolled patients (Ciliska et al., 1992; Mc Clure, 1984). As more Americans join health plans in which they designate a primary care provider, similar nursing care delivery models may be appropriate in the United States.

In addition to universal access to primary health care services, public-focused care services continue to be needed. Philip Lee (1993), Assistant Secretary of Health and Human Services, challenged public health leaders to (1) help develop data systems to monitor how well primary health care services affect the health of populations, (2) engage in research about health care delivery and prevention, and (3) provide more primary health care workers (including community health nurses, nurse practitioners, and midwives) in underserved areas. He also called for more flexible outreach, support, and translation services to population groups that have previously been underserved. Communitywide services continue to be needed for the prevention and control of communicable diseases and environmentally induced illnesses and injuries, such as human immunodeficiency virus (HIV) infection and violence. Community health nurses can stand on a century of nursing history to create nursing services for the future.

Knowledge of the structure and financing of U.S. health care is necessary if quality nursing in a climate of cost containment is advocated (Hamilton, 1988) (see Chapters 3 and 5). Making health insurance coverage available to more people is not the same as transforming our health care system into one that advocates health promotion and social betterment (Anderson, 1991).

NATIONAL HEALTH OBJECTIVES

National health promotion and disease prevention objectives for the year 2000 provide a guide when community health nurses speak with people about healthy communities (USDHHS, 1990). Published in 1990, the objectives provide a vision for improved health of the nation in the new century. There are three goals:

1. **Increase the span of healthy life for Americans**
2. **Reduce health disparities among Americans**
3. **Achieve access to preventive services for all Americans.**

To achieve the goals almost 300 measurable objectives were developed to serve as the basis for action plans. Under the leadership of the U.S. Public Health Service, representatives from professional nursing organizations participated in the process with other health leaders and consumers (Mc Farlane, 1989). The objectives are based on a projected profile of the American people (Table 2–7) and knowledge of the current health status of the public. There are objectives for infants (younger than 1 year), children, adolescents and youth (15 to 24 years), adults, and older adults (65 years and older).

Objectives are organized in 22 priority areas, grouped into four categories (Table 2–8). Health promotion priorities rely heavily on individual responsibility to change behavior (such as exercising). Health protection priorities call for action plans dealing with environmental measures. Preventive priorities depend on the existence of health services that prevent disease (such as immunization) and that diagnose and treat illnesses. The fourth category deals with improving systems for collecting and monitoring health information.

Within each of the 22 priority areas, objectives address health status, risk reduction, and provision of services. Examples of the three kind of objectives follow (USDHHS, 1990, p. 114):

Health status: Slow the rise in lung cancer deaths to achieve a rate of no more than 42 per 100,000 people (without intervention, the rate in 2000 is expected to be 53 per 100,000).

Risk reduction: Reduce cigarette smoking to no more than 15% among persons aged 20 years and older (baseline: 29% in 1987).

Services: Increase to at least 75% the proportion of primary care providers who routinely counsel patients about tobacco cessation (baseline: 52% of internists reported counseling their smoking patients in 1986).

Within many priority areas, population groups (aggregates) are identified and targeted because they have higher rates of death, disease, or disability. For example, American Indians and Alaska Natives are targeted for special attention for reduction in cigarette smoking because their rates are much higher than the national baseline of 29%. Two warnings are provided that caution against the misuse of such information (USDHHS). First, it is possible that there are other groups that have higher smoking rates for whom we do not have data. Objectives were targeted to aggregates only when information on baseline rates had already been collected. Second, there are many variations within an aggregate. Not all people within an aggregate are alike. For example not all American Indians smoke, and some tribes have very low smoking rates. Community health nurses must be careful to validate whether a national health priority is actually a problem with the people with whom they are working.

There is not a single national plan for achieving the national objectives. An agency of the federal government is assigned to provide leadership for each of the 22 priority areas (Table 2–8). Government funding can be targeted toward regional and national priorities for health promotion and disease prevention (Lee, 1993). For example preventive mental health and other school-based services for children and adolescents can strengthen the overall health of adults in the future.

The objectives are being used by the federal, state, and local governments, as well as by nongovernmental groups interested in the health of communities. However, not all of the national objectives are relevant in every community. For instance some communities may already be achieving the objectives. *Healthy Communities 2000: Model Standards* (APHA, 1991) is a publication that helps community health nurses and others in state and local communities determine which priorities, objectives, and strategies are appropriate for the populations within their communities.

TABLE 2–7 HEALTHY PEOPLE 2000

Profile of the American People, the Year 2000

The total population of the United States will have grown to nearly 270 million people from 254 million in 1990. The rate of growth between 1995 and 2000 is expected to be the slowest in the nation's history.

Between 1990 and 2000, 6 million people will have migrated to the United States, primarily to the East and West Coasts.

The population will be older, with the median age being greater than 36 years (in 1975 it was 29 years). Persons 65 years and older will constitute 13% of the population; 4.6 million people will be older than 85 years.

There will be fewer children younger than 5 years of age (17 million, compared with 18 million in 1990).

Average household size will be smaller at 2.48 people (compared with 2.69 in 1985).

Racial and ethnic composition will be different. The proportion of whites will decline from 76% to 72% of the population. The proportion of blacks, Hispanics, and others (including American Indians, Alaska Natives, Asians, and Pacific Islanders) will increase to 28%. The Hispanic population will have grown at the fastest rate during the 1990s.

Data from U.S. Department of Health and Human Services. (1990). *Healthy People 2000: National health promotion and disease prevention objectives. Summary report* (pp. 2–3). Washington, DC: Government Printing Office.

AGGREGATES AND COMMUNITY HEALTH NURSING

To make progress toward our national vision of healthier people and communities, community health nurses must understand our historical roots. Earlier community health nurses recognized that people are whole human beings

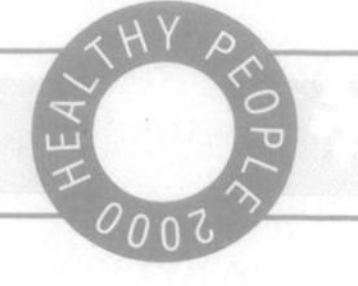

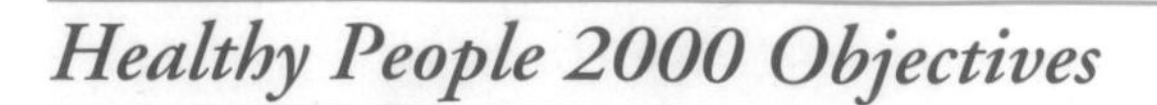

TABLE 2 – 8

Healthy People 2000 Objectives

Priority Area	Lead Agency
Health Promotion	
1. Physical activity and fitness	President's Council on Physical Fitness and Sports
2. Nutrition	National Institutes of Health Food and Drug Administration
3. Tobacco	Centers for Disease Control and Prevention
4. Alcohol and other drugs	Alcohol, Drug Abuse, and Mental Health Administration
5. Family planning	Office of Population Affairs
6. Mental health and mental disorders	Alcohol, Drug Abuse, and Mental Health Administration
Health Protection	
7. Violent and abusive behavior	Centers for Disease Control and Prevention
8. Educational and community-based programs	Centers for Disease Control and Prevention Health Resources and Services Administration
9. Unintentional injuries	Centers for Disease Control and Prevention
10. Occupational safety and health	Centers for Disease Control and Prevention
11. Environmental health	National Institutes of Health Centers for Disease Control and Prevention
12. Food and drug safety	Food and Drug Admnistration
13. Oral health	National Institutes of Health Centers for Disease Control and Prevention
Preventive Services	
14. Maternal and infant health	Health Resources and Services Administration
15. Heart disease and stroke	National Institutes of Health
16. Cancer	National Institutes of Health
17. Diabetes and chronic disabling conditions	National Institutes of Health Centers for Disease Control and Prevention
18. Human immunodeficiency virus infection	National AIDS Program Office
19. Sexually transmitted diseases	Centers for Disease Control and Prevention
20. Immunization and infectious diseases	Centers for Disease Control and Prevention
21. Clinical preventive services	Health Resources and Services Administration Centers for Disease Control and Prevention
Surveillance and Data Systems	
22. Surveillance and data systems	Centers for Disease Control and Prevention

Adapted from U.S. Department of Health and Human Services. (1990). *Healthy People 2000: National health promotion and disease prevention objectives. Summary report* (pp. 7, 143). Washington, DC: Government Printing Office.

within complex social and physical environments. The betterment of human communities remains the goal of community health nursing. However, our specific objectives change with social and environmental conditions, types of illnesses present, and needs of specific aggregates.

Elderly, adolescent, low-income, and homeless persons are just some of the populations that can benefit from community health nursing care (Riportella-Muller et al., 1991). More elderly persons will continue to make up a greater percentage of our national population. Elderly persons experience more illness than young persons and are in need of information on how to maintain their well-being and independence in the presence of chronic diseases and disabilities.

Attitudes and knowledge about health and health-promoting behaviors are learned within the family and community. Schools and peer groups are important social networks for children and adolescents. Even though children tend to be physically healthier than their elders, issues of spiritual and emotional well-being are important. Teen pregnancy, HIV infection, substance abuse, and violence are public health priorities for youth. Community health nurses working with families and in schools will continue to confront these challenges.

Poverty is stressful. Poor persons tend to have poorer health than their wealthier neighbors. The growing numbers of poor persons, especially women, children, and homeless persons, require coordinated assistance to meet their multiple needs. Sustained relationships are necessary for their empowerment (Schorr, 1989). Poverty rates tend to be higher in rural and inner-city communities, where health care services are fewer. Although the greatest number of poor in the United States are white, nonwhite populations suffer higher rates of poverty. Community health nurses have a long history of advocating for those who have not had equal access to health care and a basic standard of living, and are challenged to continue to pursue justice.

Neonatal and infant illness and deaths are an important measure of a community's health. Infant mortality continues to decline in the United States. However, infant mortality among blacks, Puerto Ricans, and some American Indian tribes is much higher than among whites. More than 100 years ago community health nurses demonstrated their ability to reduce mortality among newborns and infants. Although communicable diseases are no longer the primary causes of death, community health nurses have demonstrated their ability to work with parents to reduce low-birth-weight rates in neonates and to prevent child abuse and accidents (Brooten et al., 1986; Olds et al. 1993). Special research opportunities exist for community health nurses to identify interventions that work best to reduce infant mortality among various socioeconomic, racial, and cultural populations.

Population-focused health promotion and primary prevention will be provided in community sites where the individuals spend much of their time. Worksites will continue to be important places to assist people to change their lifestyles and reduce their risk of such diseases as heart disease, cancer, diabetes, obstructive lung disease, and alcoholism. Community health nurses and other public health professionals will have opportunity to promote more healthful work environments, including improvement of indoor air quality. Occupational health nurses will be instrumental in preventing worksite exposure to specific toxins and in teaching other nurses and the public about such hazards.

Community health nurses have demonstrated that nursing care can be provided in the variety of other settings in which various populations spend much of their day (ANA, 1986a), such as medical daycare centers, child daycare centers, homeless shelters, prisons, and churches. (Alexander-Rodriguez, 1983; ANA, 1985). Community health nurses also provide communicable disease and safety consultation to in-home daycare providers (Lie, 1992). With the expected increases in persons with acquired immunodeficiency syndrome and the numbers of elderly persons, hospice programs will become even more important (ANA, 1987b).

CONTINUING ISSUES

The challenge continues for community health nurses to reunite aspects of practice, with focus on all levels of prevention. What is a practical balance between providing care for sick people in homes and providing health promotion and primary prevention within the community?

Community health nurses continue to use their knowledge of epidemiology to identify vulnerable aggregates within the entire population. However, community health nursing care is provided to human beings as individuals and as members of families, groups, and organizations. It is the collective health of individual humans that contributes to the health of the entire public. It is also the network of social relationships that contributes to the degree of connected caring. In community health nursing, there is always a tension of perspective. Unlike some planners and statisticians, community health nurses can attach human faces and personal stories to the numbers. Unlike many other nurses who choose to focus predominantly on the health of individuals, community health nurses think in terms of the health of populations.

An increasing percentage of community health nurses are employed by private businesses rather than state and local governments. National health care reform is bringing changes in the organization and distribution of health care. Where will community health nurses fit in the scheme? Should community health nurses continue to be employed by others? Will more community health nurses consider starting private businesses and practices in which they contract with larger health care entities to provide community health nursing care?

How do we continue to provide quality community health nursing care? There are many nurses, especially in the subspecialty of home health care, without formal community health nursing education. How can technological competence be linked with competence in family-focused and aggregate-focused care? The questions are like those that the nurses in the 1920s asked themselves, "How do we best provide on-the-job training, apprenticeships, formal education, and continuing education?"

How can we work more effectively for social betterment in our communities? For vulnerable populations to become empowered, we must engage in sustained relationships that focus on the wholeness of persons and their communities (Schorr, 1989); community health nurses have known this for almost 150 years. Therefore, to truly improve the health of a community, community health nurses must provide holistic care, especially in underserved urban and rural communities.

More nurses may need to return to district or neighborhood nursing (Zerwekh, 1993). We also need to listen to people suffering and respond to their needs. We need to commit to stay in nurse-client relationships for awhile. We need to be more vocal and more visible in sharing our ideas about what works with other community leaders.

KEY IDEAS

1. Community health nursing has its roots in nursing and public health. The challenges of community health nursing evolve as changes occur in population characteristics, scientific knowledge and theory about health and illness, prevalent illnesses and causes of death, societal values, and economic and political systems.
2. Nursing's roots include visiting and district nursing to care for ill persons in their homes, health teaching and promotion with families, and "nursing the environment."
3. Public health's roots include the provision of a sanitary environment and the prevention of disease through immunization and personal responsibility for hygiene.
4. Aggregate-focused nursing started with an interest in urban poor populations and British and American military personnel during the mid-1800s.
5. In 1912, visiting nurses in the United States named themselves *public health nurses* because they provided care to all members of the community—to the entire public—and were committed to social betterment.
6. As additional aggregates were identified as being at risk of illnesses and in need of nursing care, subspecialties of public health nursing emerged. These included maternal and child health, school health, and occupational health.
7. Under the leadership of Lillian Wald, public health nursing expanded into rural communities with the creation of the Visiting Nurse Service of the Metropolitan Life Insurance Company (1909) and the Red Cross Town and Country Nursing Service (1912). In 1925, Mary Breckenridge founded the Frontier Nursing Service in Kentucky, which survives today.
8. Public health nursing was originally sponsored by financial donations from the wealthy. As public health nursing demonstrated its effectiveness, it became institutionalized in health departments of local and state governments.
9. The holism of community health nursing, with its focus on both sickness care and prevention, was broken when health departments sought not to threaten physician practices. Health departments took on the responsibility for health promotion and disease prevention and visiting nurse agencies continued with care of sick persons in their homes.
10. The term *public health nursing* had become associated primarily with those nurses employed by the government. Public health nurses working in new community centers and for-profit home health agencies also needed to be included. The term *community health nursing* emerged in the 1970s as the new name for public health nursing.
11. Expanded roles for nurses continue to emerge to provide primary health care. Nurse midwives, nurse practitioners, and clinical specialists are needed, especially to serve the urban poor and rural communities.
12. With health care reform and national health promotion goals, new opportunities exist to reunite the care and prevention within community health nursing. New models are emerging to deliver community health nursing to the public.
13. Issues of organizing and delivering community health nursing services are ongoing.

GUIDELINES FOR LEARNING

1. After reading Table 2–6 in this chapter regarding the work of Mary Breckenridge, describe how she displayed the leadership characteristics presented in Chapter 1.
2. Read a biography of a community health nurse. Identify the health problems and the communities that the community health nurse worked with. Reflect on the degree to which both care of ill persons and health promotion and primary prevention were included in the nurse's practice. Describe how the social and physical environment affected the clients and nursing practice. Identify the expressed and implied ethical commitments and values of the nurse.
3. Interview a retired community health nurse and compare his or her experiences with those of a contemporary community health nurse. Focus on similarities and differences.
4. Identify the *Healthy People 2000* objectives applicable to a population or aggregate to which you belong, such as young adult Asian women; urban African-American adult men; rural, low-income white women. Notice your thoughts and feelings as you consider the objectives.
5. Discuss which populations/aggregates should receive the most nursing attention. Is your answer different if you consider the community where you live, your state, or the entire nation?

⑥ Identify client needs that are not likely to be solved by financial access to medical care. Envision how community health nursing care might address these needs.

REFERENCES

Alexander-Rodriguez, T. (1983). Prison health—A role for professional nursing. *Nursing Outlook,31*(2), 115–118.

American Public Health Association (APHA). (1991). *Healthy communities 2000: Model standards* (3rd ed.). Washington, DC: Author.

ANA (1987a). *Facts about nursing 86–87.* Washington, DC: Author.

ANA (1987b). *Standards and scope of hospice nursing practice.* Washington, DC: Author.

ANA (1991). *Nursing agenda for health care reform.* Washington, DC: Author.

ANA Council of Community Health Nurses. (1985). *Standards of nursing practice in correctional facilities.* Washington, DC: ANA.

ANA Council of Community Health Nurses. (1986a). *Community-based nursing services: Innovative models.* Washington, DC: ANA.

ANA Council of Community Health Nurses. (1986b). *Standards of community health nursing practice.* Washington, DC: ANA.

Anderson, E. (1991). A call for transformation. *Public Health Nursing, 8*(1), 1.

Backer, B. (1993). Lillian Wald: Connecting caring with activism. *Nursing and Health Care, 14*(3),122–129.

Bigbee, J., & Crowder, E. (1985). The Red Cross Rural Nursing Service: An innovative model of public health nursing delivery. *Public Health Nursing,* 2(2), 109–121.

Brainard, A. M. (1985). *The evolution of public health nursing.* New York: Garland. (Original work published in 1922. Philadelphia: W.B. Saunders.)

Brooten, D., Kumar, S., Brown, L., et al. (1986). A randomized clinical trial of early hospital discharge and home follow-up of very-low-birth-weight infants. *New England Journal of Medicine, 315,* 934–938.

Buhler-Wilkerson, K. (1985). Public health nursing: In sickness or in health? *American Journal of Public Health, 75*(10), 1155–1161.

Ciliska, D., Woodcox, V., & Isaacs, S. (1992). A descriptive study of the attachment of public health nurses to family physicians' offices. *Public Health Nursing, 9*(1), 53–57.

Duffy, J. (1990). *The sanitarians: A history of American public health.* Urbana, IL: University of Illinois Press.

Fitzpatrick, M. L. (1975). *The national organization for public health nursing, 1912–1952: Development of a practice field.* New York: National League for Nursing.

Gardner, M. S. (1936). *Public health nursing.* (3rd ed.). New York: Macmillan.

Goodnow, M. (1928). *Outlines of nursing history* (4th ed.). Philadelphia: W.B. Saunders.

Hamilton, D. (1988). Clinical excellence, but too high a cost: The Metropolitan Life Insurance Company Visiting Nurse Service (1909–1953). *Public Health Nursing, 5*(4), 235–240.

Hanlon, J. J., & Pickett, G. E. (Eds.). (1984). *Public health: Administration and practice* (8th ed.). St. Louis, MO: Mosby.

Haupt, A. (1953). Forty years of teamwork in public health nursing. *American Journal of Nursing, 53*(1), 81–84.

Hays, J. (1989). Florence Nightingale and the India sanitary reforms. *Public Health Nursing, 6*(3), 152–154.

Institute of Medicine. (1988). *The future of public health.* Washington, DC: National Academy Press.

Kraus, H. P. (1980). *The settlement house movement in New York City, 1886–1914.* New York: Arno Press.

Last, J. (1992). Scope and methods of prevention. In J. Last & R. Wallace (Eds.). *Public health and preventive medicine.* Norwalk, CT: Appleton & Lange.

Lee, P. (1993, September). *Key note: Health care reform and public health.* Paper presented at the Baltimore City Health Department 200th Anniversary Celebration Conference, Baltimore, MD.

Lie, L. (1992). Health consultation services to family day care homes in Minneapolis, Minnesota. *Journal of School Health, 62*(1), 29–31.

McClure, L. (1984). Teamwork, myth or reality: Community nurses' experience with general practice attachment. *Journal of Epidemiology and Community Health, 38,* 68–74.

McFarlane, J. (1989). Year 2000 health objectives for the nation. *Public Health Nursing, 6*(2), 51–54.

Monteiro, L. A. (1985). Florence Nightingale on public health nursing. *American Journal of Public Health, 75*(2), 181–186.

Olds, D., Henderson, C., Phelps, C., Kitzman, H., & Hanks, C. (1993). Effect of prenatal and infancy nurse home visitation on government spending. *Medical Care, 31*(2), 155–174.

Poole, E. (1932). *Nurses on horseback.* New York: Macmillan.

Pryor, E. (1987). *Clara Barton: Professional angel.* Philadelphia: University of Pennsylvania Press.

Riportella-Muller, R., Selby, M., Salmon, M., Quade, D., & Legault, C. (1991). Specialty roles in community health nursing: A national survey of educational needs. *Public Health Nursing, 8*(2), 81–89.

Roberts, D., & Heinrich, J. (1985). Public health nursing comes of age. *American Journal of Public Health, 75*(10), 1162–1172.

Roemer, M. (1988). Resistance to innovation: The case of the community health center. *American Journal of Public Health, 78*(9), 1234–1239.

Schorr, L. (1989). *Within our reach: Breaking the cycle of disadvantage.* New York: Doubleday.

Shalala, D. (1992). Nursing and society—The unfinished agenda for the 21st century. In National League for Nursing: *Perspectives in nursing 1991–1993.* New York: National League for Nursing Press, pp. 3–8.

Suchman, E. A. (1963). *Sociology and the field of public health.* New York: Russell Sage Foundation.

U.S. Department of Health and Human Services (USDHHS). (1985). *Consensus Conference on the Essentials of Public Health Nursing Practice and Education: Report of the conference.* Rockville, MD: USDHHS.

USDHHS. (1990). *Healthy people 2000: National health promotion and disease prevention objectives. Summary report.* Washington, DC: Government Printing Office.

Ward, D. (1989). Public health nursing and the future of public health, *Public Health Nursing, 6*(4), 163–168.

Waters, Y. (1912). *Visiting nursing in the United States.* New York: Charities Publication Committee, The Russell Sage Foundation.

White, R. (1978). *Social change and the development of the nursing profession: A study of the poor law nursing service 1848–1948.* London: Henry Kimpton.

Winslow, C.-E. A. (1984). *The evolution and significance of the modern public health campaign.* South Burlington, VT: Journal of Public Health Policy, (Original work published in 1923. New Haven, CT: Yale University Press).

Zerwekh, J. (1993). Commentary: Going to the people—Public health nursing today and tomorrow. *American Journal of Public Health, 83*(12), 1676–1678.

BIBLIOGRAPHY

Reverby, S. (Ed.). (1984). *Lamps on the prairie: A history of nursing in Kansas.* New York: Garland. (Original work compiled by Works Projects Administration, Writer's Program, and published in 1942).

Rosen, G. (1955). *A history of public health.* New York: MD Publications.

SUGGESTED READINGS

Backer, B. (1993). Lillian Wald: Connecting caring with activism. *Nursing and Health Care, 14*(3), 122–129.

Barger, S., & Rosenfield, P. (1993). Models in community health care: Findings from a national study of community nursing centers. *Nursing and Health Care, 14*(8), 462–431.

Buhler-Wilkerson, K. (1993). Bringing care to the people: Lillian Wald's legacy to public health nursing. *American Journal of Public Health, 83*(12), 1778–1786.

Milio, N. (1971). *9226 Kercheval: The store front that did not burn.* Ann Arbor, MI: The University of Michigan Press.

Salmon, M. (1993). Editorial: Public health nursing — The opportunity of a century. *American Journal of Public Health, 83*(12), 1674–1675.

Salmon, M., Peoples-Sheps, M. (1989). Infant mortality and public health nursing: A history of accomplishments, a future of challenges. *Nursing Outlook, 37,* 6–7, 51.

Wald, L. (1936). *Windows on Henry Street.* Boston: Little, Brown.

Chapter 3

The U.S. Health Care System

Frances A. Maurer

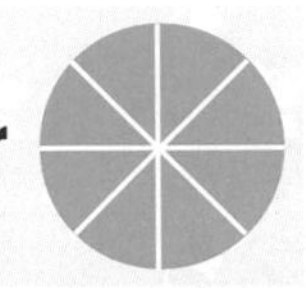

Continued

Focus Questions

What are the basic features and components of the U.S. health care system?

What distinguishes the U.S. health care system from those of other developed countries?

Why do community health nurses need to understand the health care system?

What are the differences between direct and indirect service and public and private sector health care services?

When did the focus of care shift toward prevention, and what were some of the reasons for the shift?

Which agencies have the most important role in health care issues at the federal, state, and local levels?

What is the priority focus of health care in the United States?

What are the major problems with the current health care delivery system?

How have problem-solving strategies had an impact on health care services, personnel, and cost?

What are some of the proposals for health care reform?

What do we mean by the term *health care system?* What kind of health care system does the United States have? What are its component parts? This chapter examines the structure of the present system and identifies the principal areas of concern associated with its operation. At the end of the chapter, potential directions for change are explored. The current political climate leans toward popular support for some change. If substantive, change could dramatically affect the delivery of health care as we presently know it.

Few people really stop to think about the health care system and the organizational structure that delivers care. Those who do so are usually responding to an unsatisfactory personal encounter. Dissatisfaction with treatment for an immediate need or emergency leads people to critically question the delivery system, identify areas for change, and think about how they might plan change.

Critical analysis of the system by most health professionals is a recent development. Although the organization of health care has an impact on practice, most professionals had not contemplated substantive change. Health care practitioners tended to view the system as static and inflexible, rather than a dynamic model—a model subject to review and evaluation which could be modified or discarded if an alternative seemed more complete. Health professionals, like most Americans, have simply not been in the habit of viewing the system as one open to influence or replacement at the behest of those it serves.

In fact the system is not impervious to outside influence (Fig. 3–1). Changes and modifications do occur, although most of the time change occurs slowly and incrementally because the system is so large. For example the expanded role of nurse practitioners was gradually accepted over a long period. Once in a while discontent builds to such a peak that significant change occurs in a relatively short time. For example dissatisfaction with the financial burdens and limited access to medical care for older Americans led to the passage of the Medicare program in 1965. At present the country is again experiencing significant dissatisfaction with the health care delivery system, and there is a window of opportunity for sweeping change to occur.

Health care professionals bear a responsibility to know and understand the system in which they function because it has considerable impact on both their behavior and the health behavior of the people they serve. Nurses should be cognizant of the issues that have an impact on their nursing practice both in the workplace and from the broader perspective of the entire health care system. Beyond the personal influence on nursing practice, community nurses must understand the impact of the system on individual clients, groups, and communities.

At present health care is neither available nor accessible to everyone. Millions lack health insurance and are unable to pay for basic services. Every day in their nursing practice, community health nurses see people who are denied basic services and people with serious illness who delay treatment because of cost. Because the professional practice of nursing is built around the promotion of health, the prevention of illness, and the restoration of health to all in need, it is hard for community health nurses to see people in need and know that for some, they can offer no solution to lack of access to health care.

Ultimately the real impact of any health care system must be measured in the people it serves: How healthy is our population? How does our health status compare with that of other nations? Does our health care system prevent premature death and disability and provide good care to

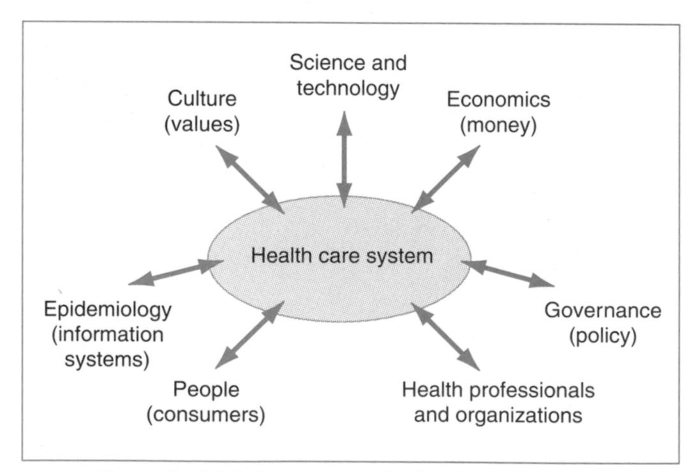

Figure 3–1 ● Influences on the health care system.

most of its citizens? Nurses need basic information about the health care system so they can make an informed judgment about the efficacy of the present system and the impact of suggested reforms.

Traditional Health Care System

When compared with health care systems in other developed countries, the delivery network in the United States seems disorganized and confusing (Tallan and Nathan, 1992). The U.S. health care system has been variously defined as a system without a system, a fragmented system, and a nonsystem (Smith and Kaluzny, 1986; Congressional Budget Office, 1992; Salloway, 1982). There is no central organization that plans and links the various elements into an integrated and purposeful whole. Others argue that as disjointed and decentralized as it may be, it is still a system (Jones, 1981; Rydman and Rydman, 1983; Roemer, 1991).

COMPONENTS OF THE HEALTH CARE SYSTEM

The U.S. health care system is complex, and it is difficult to reduce all of its elements, influences, and decision-makers into a simple diagram. Roemer (1991) provides a basic model that identifies essential components of a health care system (Fig. 3–2), which are the basis of the U.S. system as well. Each component is affected by and has impact on the others, and ultimately determines the health care services offered, and the people serviced, by the system.

KEY FEATURES OF THE U.S. SYSTEM

Among all of the developed countries, the U.S. system is unique. Roemer (1991) has identified three prominent features of the system that help to explain, to some degree, the structure of the system and the manner in which it evolved. These features include highly decentralized governance, a strong emphasis on laissez faire philosophy, and an abundance of economic resources. Each of these features is briefly examined in the following text. Key terms are listed in Table 3–1.

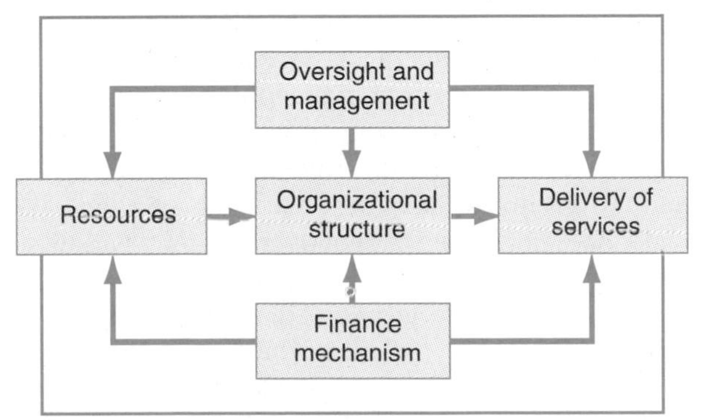

Figure 3–2 ● Components of a health care system. (Modified from Roemer, M. [1991]. *National health care systems of the world.* New York: Oxford University Press.)

Decentralization

Consistent with other aspects of governance in the United States, legal governance and regulation of the health care delivery system are highly decentralized. The government was designed by individuals whose previous experiences led them to mistrust a highly centralized, autocratic system. Their solution was a decentralized federated system with checks and balances at each level. Local communities, states, and the federal government share responsibilities for regulation and provision of services to the population; health care services are no exception. The United States has a delivery system in which funding, planning, regulation, and service delivery are influenced by city, county, state, and federal government policies, as well as the policies of no ngovernmental organizations, such as businesses.

Laissez Faire Philosophy

The free market economy of the United States encourages a laissez faire approach. In a free market, i.e., a laissez faire system, there is no centralized planning structure. Private enterprise is allowed to develop goods and services as it chooses, and to offer them to the clientele, or market, it selects. The health service market is no exception. Private individuals, groups, or corporations can plan, offer, and deliver health care to the target groups they wish to serve. Hospital owners or managers, physicians, and philanthropists, not the government, determine the organizational structure of U.S. health care. As with any business operation, payment is expected for service provided. In this country, a portion of the population cannot pay for service. For those unable to pay, the question of whether health care is a right or a privilege becomes critical. Debate on this

TABLE 3–1

Definition of Terms

GNP (gross national product)—A measure of all goods and services sold in the United States

Free market—In a capitalistic economy the method used to determine the number of products made and bought without any regulation or interference from government

Private sector—Term used to define the segment of the economy outside the government

Public sector—Segment of the economy that is provided by government at all levels: federal, state, or local

question has raged since the nation's inception (Lindblom, 1953; Wilensky, 1975; Anderson, 1985; Reinhardt, 1986).

Those who espouse a totally free market system support a laissez faire attitude toward health care services. They consider health care a privilege, rather than a right, and would not support government intervention to ensure health care for those who cannot pay. Those who consider health care a right, rather than a privilege, would support action aimed at providing health care services to all.

In this country health care is provided to the population by a combination of private and public means. Our bent toward a free market economy has encouraged development of a private, entrepreneurial delivery system and personal responsibility for medical expenses. This private subsystem serves middle- and upper-income Americans who can afford to pay for their care.

Public support, however, does not allow a totally laissez faire approach. Most Americans support the idea of basic health care services for all. The public health community's commitment to the ethical position of providing the greatest good for the greatest number supports universal access to care, rather than the laissez faire approach. The government has gradually undertaken to provide some support to those persons who cannot afford to pay for health care. The public subsystem tends to care primarily for the poor and special populations.

Abundant Resources

Even though the United States is a wealthy country, its economic resources for health care are limited. We spend more, in actual dollars, on health than most other countries. In 1993 the projected cost for health care was $903.3 billion, or 14% of the gross national product (Burner et al., 1992). The United States has devoted large sums of money to research and has led the way in development and employment of complex and expensive medical procedures and equipment, such as organ transplants, in vitro fertilization, and magnetic resonance imaging.

Decentralized governance, mass expenditures, and a free market philosophy have helped to shape the existing health care system. As various aspects of the system are examined in this chapter, it would be useful to attempt to identify how each of these elements has an impact on a particular area of practice or delivery of care to population subgroups.

COMPARISON OF HEALTH CARE SYSTEMS

Among industrialized countries only the United States and South Africa insist on an individualized free market approach to health care. The others have developed national health care systems that provide coverage to all, or nearly all, citizens. Each country's system varies in its organization and delivery of care. Roemer (1991) has identified two broad types: the welfare oriented and the comprehensive health care systems (Table 3–2).

TABLE 3–2

National Health Care Systems

	Welfare	Comprehensive
Financing	Indirect, through health insurance and government subsidies; may require co-payment	Direct, government provides and pays for care through taxes; may require co-payment
Planning (service, facilities)	Government	Government
Organization	Diversified Government owns most hospitals Some hospitals privately owned	Government
Delivery	Independent Private practice physicians and other providers) Some health care professionals are government employees	Government-organized Practitioners are salaried Teams provide comprehensive services, usually in health centers
Covers	Most individuals	All citizens

From Roemer, M. (1991). *National health care systems of the world.* New York: Oxford University Press.

In welfare-oriented systems, *most* persons have medical care protection. The national government assumes responsibility for financing and planning, but organizing and delivering care are shared with private enterprise. Care is paid for by health insurance, which is subsidized by the government. Providers usually remain in independent practice and consumers may choose health care providers. The government owns most, but not all, hospital facilities. Australia, Canada, the former West Germany, Japan, and France are examples of welfare-oriented health care systems.

Comprehensive health care systems provide a broad scope of health care services to *all* citizens. In contrast to welfare systems, both the finance mechanism and the organizational structure are directed by the government. The national government assumes the major role in planning, organizing, financing, and delivering care to all. Most health care providers are government employees and services are provided in government-operated health centers. Consumers have a choice of provider if the provider does not have a patient overload. Most allow some element of private practice by providers, but only a small percentage of citizens are served in this manner. Great Britain, New Zealand, and all of the Scandinavian nations are examples of countries with comprehensive health care systems.

Countries with national health care systems engage in more comprehensive health planning and provide all, or almost all, citizens with comprehensive health care ser-

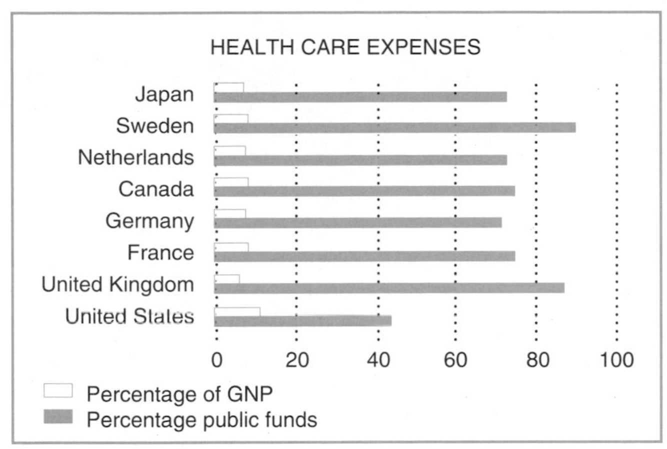

Figure 3–3 ● Health care expenses as a percentage of gross national product (GNP) and public funds for selected countries in 1989. (Data from Schieber, G. J., Pouiller, J. P., & Greenwald, L. M. [1991]. Health care systems in 24 countries. *Health Affairs,* 10(3), 23.)

vices. Central planning is possible because the government has the means to influence services either by providing direct care or by reimbursing the cost of care for most of its citizens.

In contrast, the United States has engaged in little central health planning. The federal government is becoming more involved in national health planning and has established national health objectives. These objectives are only guidelines and do not have the force of law. At the current time those segments of the health care system not directly under federal control are free to ignore or address the objectives as they choose.

The most frequent criticism of our health care system is that delivery of "basic" (primary care and preventive) services is not readily available to the entire population (Reinhardt, 1990; Holahan and Zedlewski, 1992). Despite large health care expenditures, a significant segment of the population does not receive care; at least 37 million Americans have no health coverage (Congressional Budget Office, 1992). The U.S. government provides fewer public monies for health care than any other developed country (Roemer, 1991). Most commit more public funds and provide more services while spending less of their gross national product (GNP) on health care (Fig. 3–3).

If the U.S. system provided a better standard of health than that of other countries, then the differences in expenditure of public funds would be more understandable. That is not the case. Figure 3–4 provides comparison data on infant mortality and life expectancy for eight selected countries; according to these data the United States ranks lowest in life expectancy and highest in infant mortality. In fact the United States ranks 20th of the 24 developed nations compared by the World Health Organization. Only Greece, New Zealand, Portugal, and Turkey have higher infant mortality rates (Schieber et al., 1991). Jonsson (1989) links the U.S. ranking to a lack of comprehensive planning for prenatal care—a characteristic not shared by countries with national health care systems.

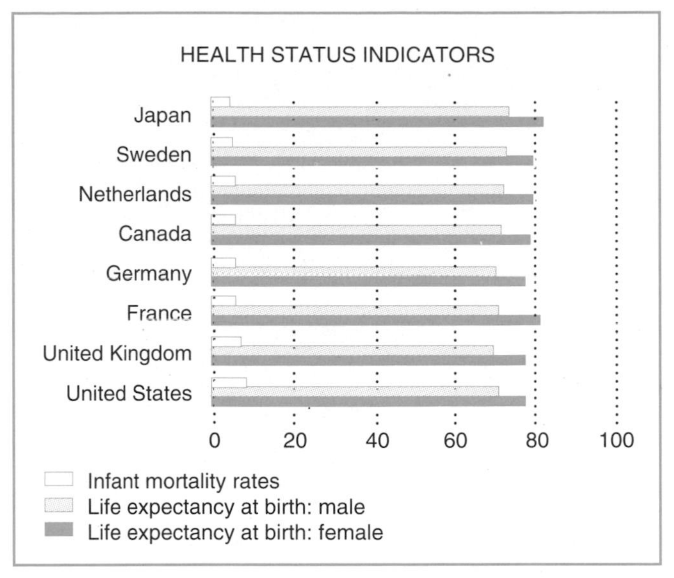

Figure 3–4 ● Health status indicators: infant mortality rates per 1000 live births and life expectancies for selected countries. (Data from Schieber, G. J., Pouiller, J. P., & Greenwald, L. M. [1991]. Health care systems in 24 countries. *Health Affairs,* 10(3), 23.)

Components of the U.S. Health Care System

In attempting to examine any health care system, identification of the components that make up the "whole" or "system" is useful. This is especially relevant, but difficult, in the U.S. system, which has a complex arrangement of component parts. Fig. 3–5 identifies important components of the health care system, attempts to illustrate some of the interrelationships between the segments, and shows how the system links the consumer to health care services.

ORGANIZATIONAL STRUCTURE

In health care, as in other systems, structure significantly influences function. Structure determines how goods or resources are acquired and how services are dispersed or provided. The organizational structure of U.S. health care is a disjointed combination of public and private agencies, including government (federal, state, county, city/local) and voluntary and charitable, entrepreneurial, and professional agencies and organizations (Fig. 3–6). All of these agencies are involved in decisions that have an impact on the delivery of health care. Agencies sometimes operate with competing or overlapping objectives and functions. Because of the absence of a central organization, gaps exist in services and in

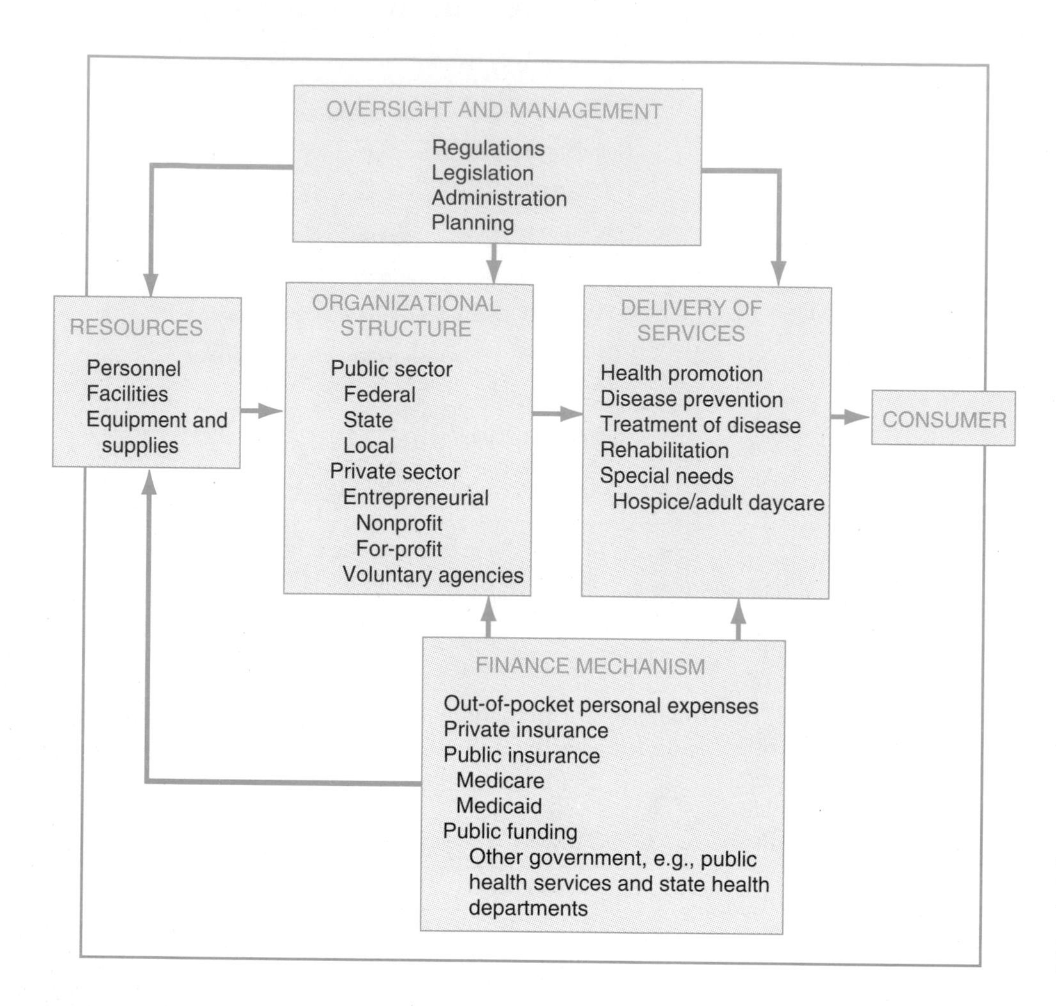

Figure 3–5 ● Components of the U.S. health care system. (Modified from Roemer, M. [1991]. *National health care systems of the world.* New York: Oxford University Press.)

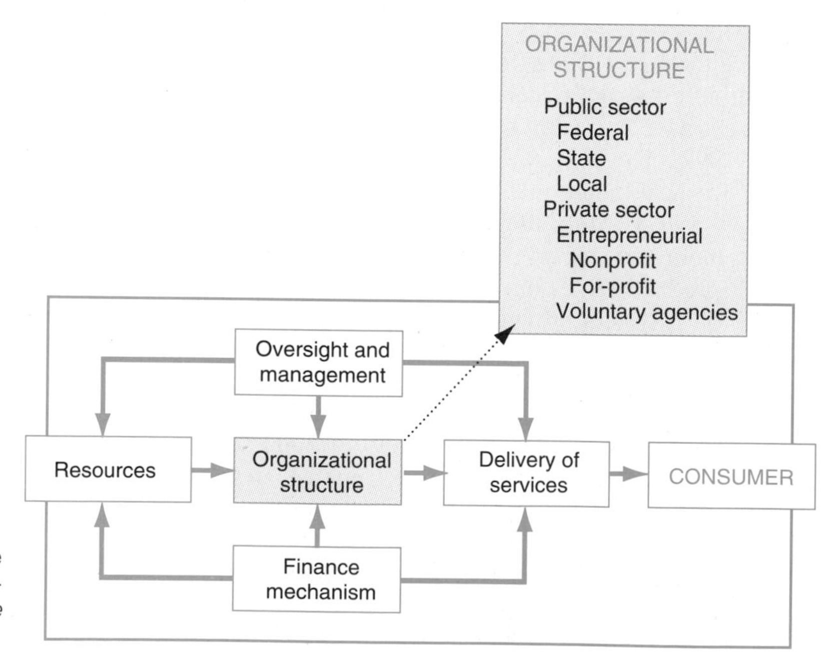

Figure 3–6 ● Components of the U.S. health care system: organizational structure. (Modified from Roemer, M. [1991]. *National health care systems of the world.* New York: Oxford University Press.)

population groups served. (It is helpful to keep this concept in mind as the discussion continues.)

MANAGEMENT AND OVERSIGHT

The three key features of our health care system were identified earlier. Two of these are important to the management aspect of health care. Both decentralized governance and a laissez-faire philosophy have created the environment within which oversight functions (Fig. 3–7). A single overseer or manager is lacking, as is a central plan for organizing and delivering health care. Instead, multiple levels of government interrelate and interact with multiple levels of private sector management in a bewildering arrangement.

Multiple Levels of Government

Within government itself there are planning, legislative, and regulatory management efforts at the federal, state, and county levels. City government lends yet another level in some instances. Each layer directs services within its scope of operation. Because of the decentralized nature of American government, federal agencies usually manage specific programs by designating day-to-day administration and oversight to local authorities. Federal agencies do so, however, only after devising guidelines or criteria that must be met by the specific program.

If one health program—the Women, Infant, and Children (WIC) Program—is taken as an example, multiple levels of managers and requirements for that program can be identified. The WIC Program managers in the field, who actually provide service to the target groups, must comply with criteria that have been set at the federal and state levels. The WIC Program field director (county, city, or geographic district operation) reports to the state agency responsible for the program. The state manager, in turn, reports to an official in the U.S. Department of Agriculture. That individual is, in turn, answerable to both the President (executive branch) and the Congress (legislative branch) to ensure that management directives and budgeting requirements are followed.

Variety of Private Management Styles

Management, planning, and oversight methods of private organizations vary widely and are not easily categorized. They include centralized and decentralized, democratic and autocratic, and laissez faire and extremely regulated management efforts. Most private facilities operate with a board of directors that influences the planning and administrative process. Generally, management and oversight of private facilities are not as decentralized as those of public facilities and programs, perhaps because the former are smaller.

Private facilities and organizations must comply with applicable federal, state, and local regulations, which place constraints on how they may operate, the types of services they may provide, and whether they may continue to offer services. State licensing is an example of regulatory activity. For example states conduct inspections and issue licenses for nursing homes and home care agencies. If the homes are not able to meet state standards, they are penalized either by being assessed fines or by closure. Failure to meet licensing standards may also result in loss of revenue, since some reimbursement mechanisms are tied to continued licensure.

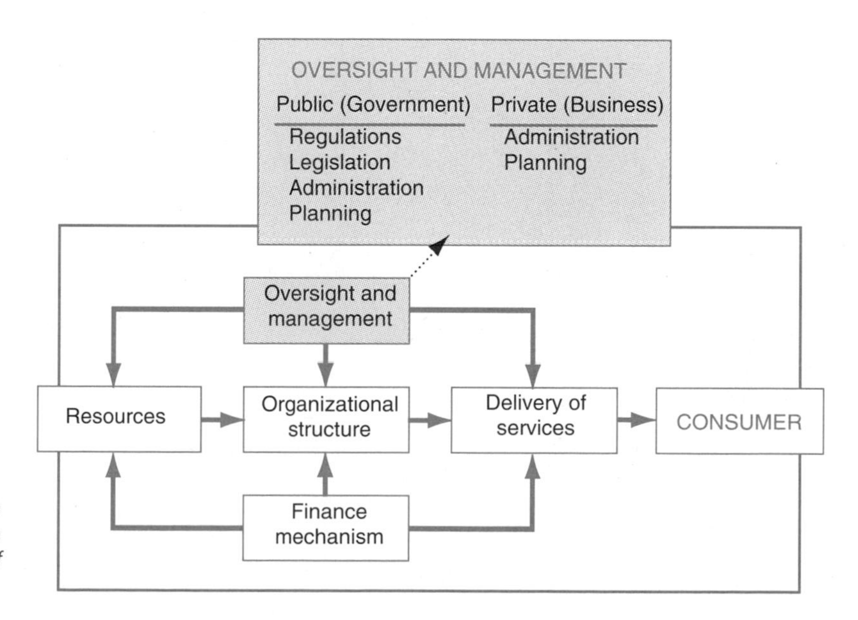

Figure 3–7 ● Components of the U.S. health care system: oversight and management. (Modified from Roemer, M. [1991]. *National health care systems of the world.* New York: Oxford University Press.)

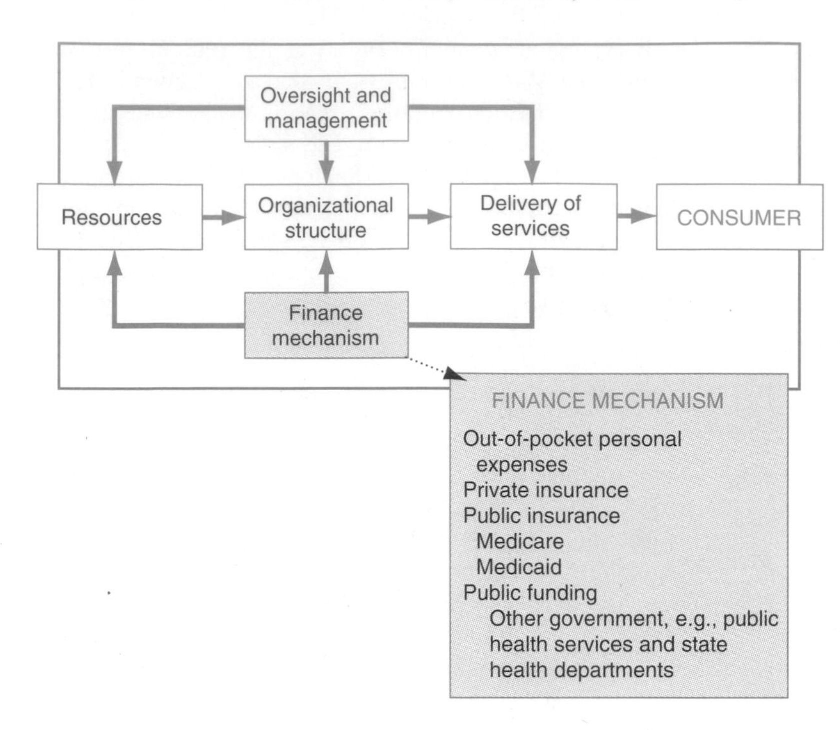

Figure 3–8 ● Components of the U.S. health care system: finance mechanism. (Modified from Roemer, M. [1991]. *National health care systems of the world.* New York: Oxford University Press.)

FINANCING MECHANISMS

The financing of health care services is discussed in detail in Chapter 5. In brief, financing support is derived from a variety of sources, both private and public (Fig. 3–8). Private sources include personal expenditures of individuals and families, private insurance payments, corporate expenditures, and charitable contributions. Public sources are composed of federal, state, and local government revenues directed toward health care services.

RESOURCES

Health resources are considered essential for health care system functioning (Fig. 3–9). These include (1) health professionals, who constitute the personnel who run the system; (2) facilities such as hospitals and other structural elements from which care is provided; and (3) health supplies and equipment. Since space is limited, this chapter highlights only some of the relevant resources to health care delivery. Community health nurses need to know about health care resources, including the supply of other health care professionals, because resources influence the availability and accessibility of health care services to those in need.

Personnel

People are a crucial health care resource. Health professionals display considerable variety in education,

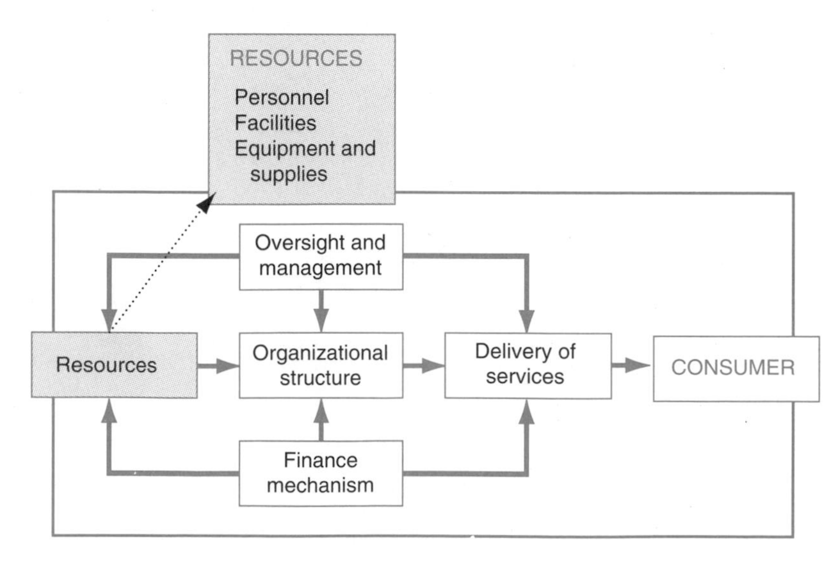

Figure 3–9 ● Components of the U.S. health care system: resources. (Modified from Roemer, M. [1991]. *National health care systems of the world.* New York: Oxford University Press.)

TABLE 3–3

Comparisons of Selected Health Professions

Profession	No.	Supply per 100,000 Population	Average Salary ($)
Physician	573,070	223.4	155,800
Dentist	137,817	58.0	80,000
Optometrist	37,000	10.8	75,000
Pharmacist	161,600	63.8	41,300
Physician assistant	53,000	20.7	40,000
Registered nurse	2,033,032	668.0	33,969

Data from U.S. Department of Labor Statistics. (1992). *Occupational outlook handbook: 1992–93 edition.* Washington, DC: Author and U.S. Public Health Service. (1990). *Seventh Report to the President and Congress on the status of health personnel in the U.S.* (DHHS Publication No. HRS–P–OD–90–1). Washington, DC: Government Printing Office.

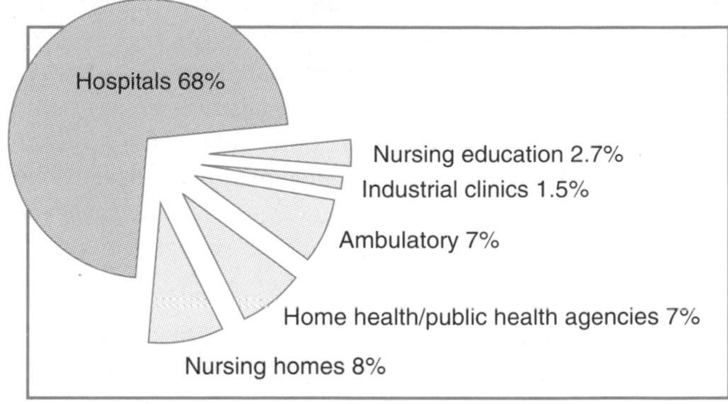

Figure 3–10 ● Registered nurse practice settings. (Data from Bureau of Health Professions, Division of Nursing (1986). *The registered nurse population: Findings from the National Sample of Registered Nurses November 1984.* Washington, DC: DHHS, Health Resources and Service Administration Publ. No. HRP-0906938.)

skill, and practice-setting. Table 3–3 presents some of the most common health care professions, their accessibility (supply), and average salary levels.

Physicians. Since the 1960s medical schools have received considerable financial support from both state and federal governments to increase the number of practicing physicians, improve chances of medical school admission for women and racial minorities, and increase access in underserved populations. As part of the effort to increase the physician supply, restrictive certification requirements for foreign-trained physicians were eased. These actions increased the supply of physicians.

Today there are more than 200 physicians per 100,000 population, and there is some concern about a pending physician surplus (Ginzberg, 1989). Through the year 2030 the projected supply is more than adequate to meet the needs of the population.

Despite an adequate supply of doctors, accessibility to primary care service is problematic for many people. Two factors combine to restrict patient access to primary care physicians: (1) geographic maldistribution and (2) specialization (Schoeder, 1992). Physicians tend to concentrate in urban rather than rural areas. The Northeast has the highest ratio of physicians to population, and the South has the lowest. Most physicians specialize (more than 70%); only 11% are engaged in primary care general practice (Schoeder, 1992). By contrast, other developed countries restrict specialty practice and 50% to 70% of physicians are engaged in primary care. Few American physicians specialize in community/public health medicine. According to the American Medical Association (AMA), only 0.3%—or roughly 1700—practice in that specialty (U.S. Public Health Service [USPHS], 1990).

Registered Nurses. Registered nurses constitute the largest group of health professionals. According to the U.S. Department of Labor there are more than 2 million licensed registered nurses. Most are salaried employees. Hospitals remain their largest single employer (Fig. 3–10).

Only about 7% (115,000) of registered nurses practice community/public health nursing, a slightly higher rate than that of physicians. Another 8% (125,800) are involved in ambulatory care facilities that offer some community-related services. Only 9088 registered nurses with advanced degrees (masters' degrees or higher) prepared as community health specialists (USPHS, 1990).

Federal government estimates project a decline in the proportion of registered nurses practicing in hospital settings and an increased need of registered nurses prepared in community-type practice, including public health and ambulatory care. The need is expected to increase 52% by the year 2000 (USPHS, 1990). If health care reform initiatives are successful, the need for community-based nursing services will create additional demand.

Physician Extenders/Substitutes. These professionals are trained to provide primary care in place of physicians and are either physician's assistants or advanced nurse practitioners.

Physician's assistants receive a minimum of 2 years of education and must pass a national certification examination, after which they must practice under the direct supervision of a physician.

Advanced nurse practitioners are registered nurses with advanced education and certification, such as nurse anesthetists, nurse clinical specialists, nurse practitioners, and nurse midwives. In most states, the Nurse Practice Act allows independent practice and direct reimbursement for nurse practitioners and nurse midwives (Levine et al., 1993). Clinical specialists and nurse anesthetists are usually salaried employees rather than independent practitioners.

Of the approximately 77,000 physician extenders, approximately 30% are nurse practitioners. Many serve populations that do not attract physicians, especially the poor and chronically ill (Sorkin, 1986). Advanced nurse practitioners are especially good at working with the chronically ill because of their background in health teaching and their interest in health promotion and health maintenance. Nurse practitioners and nurse midwives are commonly employed in community health agencies. Studies indicate that physician extenders compare favorably with physicians in quality of care delivered and patient satisfaction with service (see Chapter 5).

Dentists. Because of the selective demand for dental care at present, there is an ample supply of dentists to meet demand. Poor people, unfortunately, do not seek care frequently or in large numbers because dental care is expensive and most do not have dental insurance. Most dentists work in private practice; only a few work in the field of public health. The United States does have some publicly funded clinics, but not enough to serve the needs of the medically indigent. Dental care is one health service that is largely confined to serving persons with the ability to pay.

Pharmacists. In the United States pharmacists dispense medication prescribed by physicians, manage pharmacies, and are involved in public awareness health teaching programs. The supply of pharmacists is adequate to meet the demand for service. Most pharamacists do not work in the public health field. In a state that operates mental health clinics (e.g., Maryland), pharmacists are employed in low-cost drug programs, where their primary responsibility is to supervise the distribution of psychotropic medications to mental health clients.

Optometrists. Optometrists provide vision acuity services, and most are in group or private practice. Their public health participation is minimal.

Allied Health Professionals

Over the last several decades, a variety of new health care workers have emerged to assist the more established professional groups in providing care to the population. A list of selected allied health workers and the approximate numbers in each category can be found in Figure 3–11. Their specialized occupational activities are wide ranging.

Vocational/Practical Nurses. The allied health worker most often involved in substantial direct patient care is the practical nurse (these individuals may be called *vocational* or *practical nurse* depending on the state in which they practice). Licensure in some states is voluntary, but is more commonly mandated by the state practice board.

The role of the licensed vocational nurse or licensed practical nurse is ambiguous. Although defined by state practice acts, their actual duties vary with employers. Historically, the practical nurse assisted registered nurses, but licensed vocational and practical nurses have assumed responsibilities once thought to be the sole province of professional nurses. In some states and clinical situations they administer medications, manage units, and take verbal orders from physicians.

There are approximately 400,000 licensed vocational or practical nurses (Levine et al., 1993). Most are employed in nursing homes and hospitals. They have limited experience in public health settings, although some are employed in ambulatory care and home health agencies.

Facilities

Health care is provided in a wide variety of inpatient and outpatient facilities. Some of these are listed in Table 3–4. The types of care delivered in facilities can be limited or

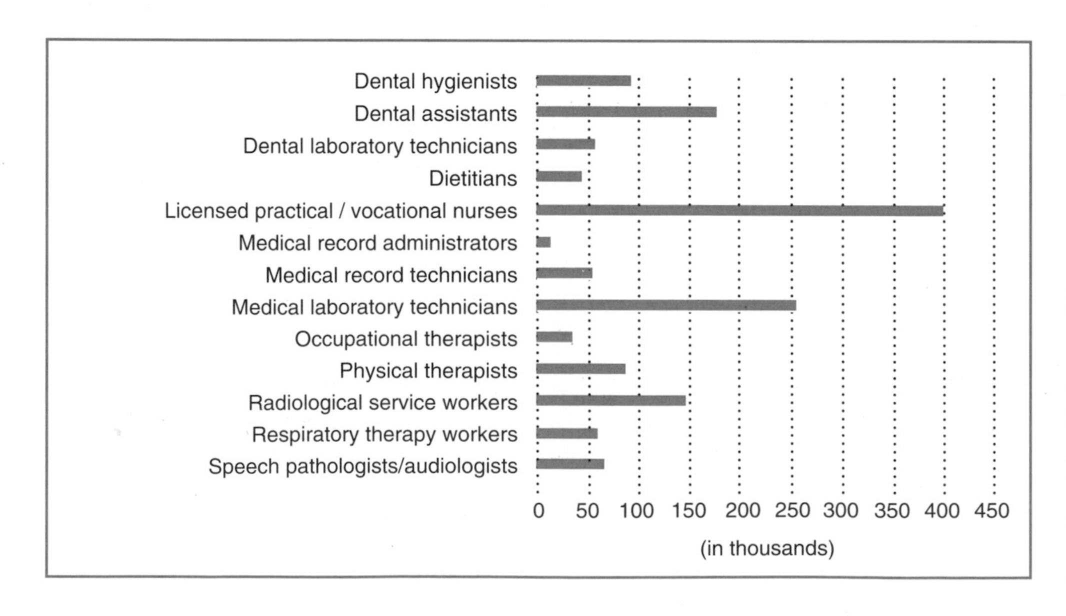

Figure 3–11 ● Supply of allied health professionals. (Data from *Occupational outlook handbook, 1992–93* (Bulletin 2400). (1992). Washington, DC: U.S. Dept. of Labor Statistics; and *Seventh Report to the President and Congress on the status of health personnel in the United States* (DHHS Publication No. HRS-P-OD-90-1). (1990). Washington, DC: Government Printing Office).

TABLE 3–4

Types of Health Care Facilities

Inpatient	Outpatient
General hospitals	Hospital-based clinics and emergency rooms
Special hospitals	Local health departments and clinics
Psychiatric residential treatment centers	Specialty programs and services
Nursing homes	Alcoholism programs and services
Skilled nursing facilities	Birth centers
Intermediate care facilities	Drug programs and services
Resident care facilities	Mental health programs and services
Other types of residential homes	Women's clinics
Adult homes	Family planning centers
Halfway houses	Ambulatory care walk-in facilities
	Physician practice
	Solo
	Group
	Partnership
	Professional corporation
	Short-stay surgical centers
	Renal dialysis centers
	Rehabilitation centers
	Hospice/respite care
	Home health agencies
	Wellness and health promotion centers
	Workplace health services

wide ranging, simple or complex, and tailored to specific conditions or to a broad scope of health concerns.

Hospitals. Hospitals may be short stay (average stay, 30 days or less) or long stay (more than 30 days) and provide generalized or specialized health care services. They are further differentiated by type of control or ownership: nonprofit, for-profit, or government owned.

Nonprofit hospitals are controlled by local communities or voluntary organizations (e.g., a religious or charitable organization). Their nonprofit status means they operate at no profit, and expenses must equal revenues each fiscal year. Most of these facilities do offer limited service to nonpaying patients.

Proprietary hospitals are privately owned, for-profit enterprises. They could be owned by an individual or set up with a corporate structure and a board of directors. Investors expect to see a return on their investments in the form of yearly dividends. Proprietary hospitals do not generally accept nonpaying patients.

Publicly owned hospitals, the third type, are owned and operated by various levels of government such as the state, county, or city; a few are run by federal agencies. Most were set up to serve indigent patients, although they accept paying patients. Some publicly owned hospitals, especially in larger cities, are teaching hospitals or hospitals with ties to medical schools. Two of the more widely known are Cook County Hospital in Chicago and Bellevue Hospital in New York City.

In 1991 there were 6700 hospitals in the United States. Approximately 82% of these were short-stay general hospitals (American Hospital Association, 1990). Slightly more than half of U.S. hospitals are nonprofit, although the trend is toward more for-profit institutions. The rise in for-profit corporate ownership of hospitals with an emphasis on commercial profit is a source of concern among health professionals (Roemer, 1986).

Long-term Care. Care of chronically ill persons or those needing rehabilitation after discharge from a general hospital is frequently provided in a long-term care facility. Patients with chronic illnesses can be transferred to long-term care hospitals, nursing homes, or rehabilitation centers. Nursing homes constitute the fastest-growing segment of this care market. Earlier hospital discharges and an ever-increasing population of elderly persons are the reasons for rapid growth of nursing homes. In 1991 there were 16,000 licensed nursing homes, triple the number of acute care hospitals (*Directory of Nursing Homes,* 1991). The bulk of nursing homes are proprietary, for-profit establishments.

Residential Care. A number of other residential care facilities have a health and social focus. Although not the largest group, these have also grown in number. Homes for aged persons, custodial residential schools for blind and deaf persons, hospice care for terminally ill persons, halfway houses for mentally ill persons, and alcohol and drug abuse treatment residential units are a few examples of the kinds of facilities that provide both a health and a social welfare focus.

Psychiatric Hospitals. Before 1960 mental care hospitals were separate facilities operated primarily by state and local governments. Starting in the 1960s, efforts to provide psychiatric patients with the least restrictive environment resulted in a large number of discharges from these institutions. Deinstitutionalization did not result in the closing of many facilities, but most state and local hospitals significantly reduced bed capacity.

Since 1960 there has been a growth in privately owned and operated psychiatric facilities; they now outnumber any other type of psychiatric facility. Service is directed primarily to persons who can afford to pay. State and local government facilities are left to provide the bulk of care for patients who cannot afford private care.

Ambulatory and Community Care. General hospitals usually operate outpatient facilities in addition to inpatient services. They provide primary care to patients who do not require hospital admission. Recently, to reduce costs and entice new customers, outpatient services have been promoted heavily as a substitute for inpatient care.

The delivery of primary health care in ambulatory care facilities has gained in popularity over the last several decades. Ambulatory care facilities provide a broad range of both services and health care professionals under one roof. Thus, they are convenient for the consumer. Some contend that these types of facilities will gradually replace the private practice of medicine.

Expansion of hospital-sponsored services has blurred the line between inpatient and outpatient facilities. Hospitals are now engaged in home health, rehabilitation, health promotion, and other enterprises to increase visibility and attract new clients (Lawrence and Jonas, 1990). Hospital-sponsored ambulatory services are located in hospitals or free-standing hospital-owned facilities. In addition to hospital outpatient clinics, Roemer (1986) identified seven different types of ambulatory facilities: (1) public health clinics, (2) industrial health service units, (3) school health clinics, (4) voluntary agency clinics, (5) private group medical practices, (6) clinics of other public agencies, and (7) clinics run by health maintenance organizations (HMOs).

Expanded Focus of Ambulatory Services. Primary care in clinics has always been used to serve poor populations but is now becoming popular with other consumer groups. The greatest number of new ambulatory care clinics have been those set up to attract middle-class consumers, rather than low-income or public assistance clients. Consumers who find the clinics particularly attractive are those with no regular physician who want quick treatment for a specific complaint. The new facilities are generally sponsored by hospitals, health corporations, or physicians in group partnership.

The expectation of payment at time of service is a common feature of the newer clinics; many do not process insurance forms as direct payment. Consumers are usually expected to file health insurance and Medicare claims to receive reimbursement for whatever out-of-pocket expenses are covered by their insurance carrier.

The advent of wellness or health promotion centers mirrors the national interest in disease prevention. There is growing professional interest in this area of health care. Whether hospital-based or free-standing, these programs offer primary and secondary prevention health-promoting activities. Some are narrowly focused on a single issue, such as smoking cessation, breast screening, or pregnancy (Scheffler et al., 1992). Those with a broader focus aim to identify all health risks to individuals and offer programs tailored to promote or enhance individual health. Some are geared toward certain groups such as the elderly (Rodgers et al., 1992). Wellness centers are a growing area in the health care market (Stifler, 1991).

Home-based care has surged as the number of elderly continues to grow. Home care is popular because it is cost efficient and often preferred to other types of care (see Chapter 5). Today there are more than 11,000 home care and hospice agencies in the United States (National Association for Home Care, 1989).

Equipment and Supplies

Health equipment and supplies are another health resource. Materials used in the diagnosis and treatment of specific illness, prosthetic devices, eyeglasses, hearing aids, and drugs constitute just a partial list of the types of equipment in this category. The industry is enormous. For example, in 1992 the cost of eyeglasses and medical appliances was $74.5 billion (Burner et al., 1992).

Medications are the largest single category. Drugs are a multimillion dollar industry. In 1992, $87 billion was spent on drugs and other nondurable medical supplies (Burner et al., 1992). Approximately three quarters of the drugs sold are prescription medications. Prescription drugs are protected by patent for 17 years. Drug companies derive greater profits from the sale of brand name (patent) drugs, so there is clear incentive to protect and maintain patent rights as long as possible. Most companies, although they could, do not manufacture generic versions of their own patent drugs until after the 17-year patent limit has expired. In community health and other settings, the use of generic (nonpatent) drugs is encouraged.

HEALTH SERVICES

Perhaps more important than the system is the final product. What does the system provide for consumers (Fig. 3–12)? A complete and comprehensive health system should provide certain essential health care services (Torrens, 1978):

- Public/preventive medicine
- Emergency medical care
- Nonemergency care
- Inpatient care
- Long-term continuing care and rehabilitation
- Care for social, emotional, and developmental problems
- Transportation
- Financial compensation for disability

The U.S. health care system contains most of these elements. However, not every community or individual has easy access to all elemental services, and health care services are not well integrated and coordinated. Critics contend that care and consumer needs do not match well, that care is often inappropriate, and that services are unevenly and unequally distributed (Raffel and Raffel, 1989; Congressional Budget Office, 1992).

The U.S. health care system has a strong business influence, and, as with any business, political and economic concerns take precedence over patient needs (Stevens, 1993). The interplay of business, philosophy, and other

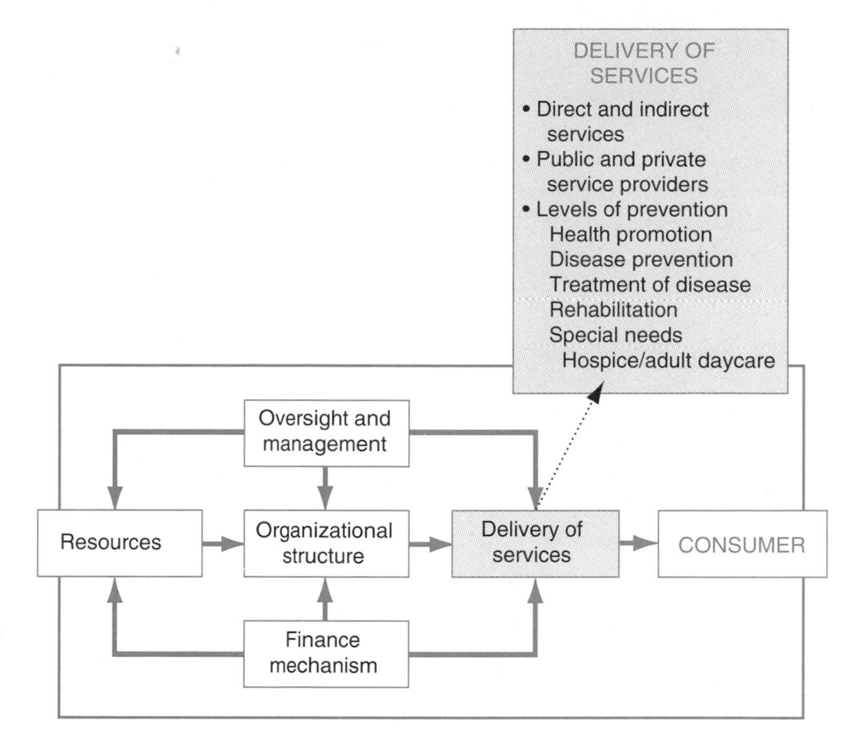

Figure 3–12 ● Components of the U.S. health care system: delivery of services. (Modified from Roemer, M. [1991]. *National health care systems of the world.* New York: Oxford University Press.)

influences has impact on all five components of our health care system.

CONSUMER

The consumer is the recipient of services delivered by the system. Ideally services should be planned and implemented to benefit the client. It is the consumer who is most affected by operational efficiency or inefficiency of health care delivery.

Some critics suggest that patient care is secondary to profit (Feldstein, 1993). Although the aim of basic health care is to maintain the health of populations, the health care system is a large business. Better health status for the population is not the primary value in determining the types of services rendered and to whom services will be provided. Profits and service are competing goals. Health care professionals and management often derive greater benefits than the consumer by way of generous salaries, benefits, stock profits, and professional prestige (Ehrenreich and Ehrenreich, 1971; Krausse, 1977; Congressional Budget Office, 1992).

The consumer and health care services should be the main focus of the health professions. The consumer is the most vulnerable, and is the most likely to be hurt by ineffective functioning of the system. For example, health care providers may relocate or refuse certain patients (Medicaid patients) to maintain an income or increase their profit margin; the consumers left behind or denied care are not the primary focus in the provider's decision process. (Refer to the section in Chapter 5 on free market failure for a discussion of how system shortcomings may have an impact on consumers.)

Direct and Indirect Services and Providers

In any delivery system there are direct and indirect services and direct and indirect providers. *Direct services* are those health services that are most personally experienced by the individual. Physical therapy, nursing care, or a doctor's visit are examples of direct services. Direct services are provided in a variety of settings including hospitals, public health clinics, and, in the case of home health, the home itself. The personnel who provide these types of services are considered direct service providers. The majority of health care personnel in the United States are engaged in direct care.

Indirect services are those health services that are not personally received by the individual, though they do influence health and welfare. Health planning by community agencies, monitoring and regulation of environmental hazards, and inspection of public use facilities are examples of indirect health services. Health is certainly affected by pollution of the food and water sources, or by community planning decisions regulating the number of hospital beds or the type of equipment employed in these facilities. The difference is that many of us are not consciously aware of indirect services and how they may affect our health.

Public- and Private-Sector Health Care Services Before 1965

Direct health care services developed in this country as a two-tiered or two-class system (Reinhardt, 1990). The private system was available to those with the ability to pay for care and concentrated on the delivery of direct services. Care providers were paid by private funds. Private hospitals expected payment for service. Some of these establishments, particularly hospitals managed by churches and other philanthropic endeavors, did provide a certain number of services to community members who could not pay.

The public system consists of those services provided by public funds and public organizations, and services are largely provided by some type of governmental agency. The public sector is concerned with both direct and indirect services. Involvement with direct services is an attempt to provide care for those who cannot pay and for certain other target groups for whom the government is legally required or feels compelled to provide health care. The large number of indirect services that are within the government's purview are there because the private sector is not interested in them. Funding for public services comes from local governments and communities and state and federal agencies. Charitable organizations provide limited public sector services.

THE PROVIDERS OF HEALTH CARE

Before 1965 personal health services in the United States for most people were largely available through private enterprise. Medical care was set up as a business on a fee-for-service basis. Initially physicians provided care in the home and office and nursing care was supplied by family members and visiting nursing services in the home. As other types of health professionals appeared (pharmacists, dentists, podiatrists, radiologists), they set up practice using a similar business model of reimbursement. The greatest exception was nursing. As the numbers of hospitals increased during the 1940s, nurses' services were controlled by other health professionals or providers, primarily physicians and hospitals. Nurses, for the most part, were neither engaged in independent practice nor paid directly by the recipient of their services.

Over time hospitals replaced the family as the principal caregiver for seriously ill patients. In 1960, most general hospitals were nonprofit community hospitals, primarily serving paying patients. Publicly owned hospitals provided health care for most nonpaying patients, and most were operated by state and local governments, not the federal government. In addition to providing general health care services, the state and local governments assumed the responsibility for most of the public health activities directed at citizens and communities as well as the bulk of inpatient psychiatric care for the poor mentally ill.

ROLE OF INSURANCE AND OTHER THIRD-PARTY PAYERS

By the 1920s escalating hospitals costs became a concern for middle-class Americans. The American Hospital Association (AHA) noted that care was provided by public sector funds for poor persons and was affordable for the rich, but was becoming unaffordable for the middle class. Technological advances (which increased hospital expenses), combined with the Great Depression (which caused a considerable drop in income for most Americans), created a financial crisis for hospitals and physicians. Fewer middle-class paying patients could afford care. Hospital admission rates dropped, and cash revenues from paying patients were reduced dramatically for both hospitals and physicians. In an effort to ensure survival and guarantee income, hospitals and state physician societies developed a prepayment health insurance plan for both hospital (Blue Cross) and doctor (Blue Shield) fees. These two plans grew rapidly. There were 6 million members by 1940 and 40 million by 1950 (Anderson, 1985). After Blue Cross/Blue Shield proved insurance to be a viable method of financing health care services, commercial insurance companies began to offer competing plans.

Health care financed by the insurance company rather than the individual is called *third-party reimbursement.* The federal and state governments also assume the role of a third-party reimburser when they pay health care providers through Medicare and Medicaid. It should be noted that Blue Cross and Blue Shield, although the first large-scale voluntary plans, did not pioneer the concept of third-party payment. Small groups of workers, single employers, and a few hospitals had experimented with various types of health insurance plans prior to the 1930s. By the 1960s, health insurance plans had become one of the largest payers of hospital and physician charges (see Chapter 5).

FOCUS OF CARE

An individual-centered focus on acute illness is the historical method of health care delivery in the United States (Haggerty, 1990). The health care industry, which developed around this concept of care, had little incentive to consider another approach. Physician practice and institutional health facilities depended on the treatment of patients with acute problems. Health economists assert that both had an economic stake in maintaining the focus on personalized health services (Relman, 1990; Feldstein, 1993), and that any other approach to health services might jeopardize their livelihood or place unwelcome restraints on their practice. Neither of these two possibilities was viewed with any favor by the most powerful interest groups in health care delivery: physicians, hospitals, and voluntary health insurance companies.

An individualized, acute-care focus in health care services meant that most of the energy was spent at the level of secondary and tertiary prevention, an emphasis that is evidenced by the growth of hospitals, clinics, and other facilities and services aimed at treating acute problems and minimizing disabilities.

At the same time community health officials and policies continued to emphasize primary prevention, which was aimed at avoiding accidents, illness, and disease before they occurred. However, support in terms of funding and public interest was not overwhelming for primary prevention activities. Ironically, some of the lack of interest can be attributed to past successes in public health prevention activities (Pickett and Hanlon, 1990). By the 1960s, public health efforts had significantly reduced the dangers of many life-threatening health problems. Sanitation, food inspection, and other environmental controls, combined with immunization efforts, ameliorated the more common hazards for a large percentage of the population. People became complacent, and the lower mortality rates were accepted as the norm.

Because they had startling success with few resources and little funding, public health administrators were now facing difficulties. The role of public health departments was no longer clear to the public. Since public health practitioners had practically eliminated major life-threatening dangers to the entire population, their new efforts needed to be directed at distinct blocks of people or target groups rather than the population at large. Success could not be expected to be as dramatic nor to affect as many people as previous campaigns. There was not as much public enthusiasm for funding these efforts. As a result, public health efforts increased their focus on the family. Family risk factors were identified and interventions were initiated that aimed to reduce the risks of illness and death from specific diseases among family members. Population-based efforts, while never really abandoned, were not as numerous during this period.

Public and Private Sector after 1965

The year 1965 is commonly viewed as a turning point in health care delivery services. In the 1960s two issues became of paramount importance: (1) public recognition that access and quality of care was disproportionate, particularly with respect to poor and elderly individuals, and (2) rising health care costs. Attempts to solve these two problems resulted in implementation of a number of strategies that, as time progressed, would prove to be somewhat at cross purposes.

MEDICARE AND MEDICAID

In 1965, in an attempt to facilitate access to care, federal legislation was passed that increased access for the elderly (Medicare) and the poor (Medicaid) (see Chapter 5.) Medicare and Medicaid were viewed as strategies that could facilitate access to care because they would provide new funding for services. The programs were intended to expand the number of potential providers for poor and elderly patients. It was the hope of program supporters that these federal programs would ameliorate the two-tiered structure of health care services. Providers who had formerly avoided the elderly and poor were encouraged to serve them because payment was now guaranteed. That is exactly what happened. As providers willingly mingled middle-class privately insured patients with government-insured patients, the boundaries of the two-tiered health care system began to blur.

Cost became an issue of increasing concern even as access and equity of care was being addressed. Personal health care expenditures had steadily increased since before World War II. This concern led to initial attempts at cost cutting. The driving force for cost saving was third-party payers (government and insurance companies), employers, and unions. These large organizations were immediately and directly affected by escalating costs (Califano, 1986).

In the beginning the general public and providers of care were not as concerned with cost. Insurance served as an insulation from the actual cost of care. The direct effect of out-of-pocket medical expenses was a greater concern. Health care providers were essentially satisfied, since they received adequate compensation from the insurance companies.

The enactment of Medicare and Medicaid in 1965 opened the way for federal efforts at cost containment. The Department of Health and Human Services (DHHS) had oversight of both programs and directed the Health Care Finance Administration (HCFA) to initiate efforts at containing costs (see Chapter 5). Subsequent amendments to these two acts expanded authority of the HCFA to contain costs.

Hospitals were the area in which increasing costs were especially dramatic and were the site of greatest effort at cost containment. According to HCFA, overall expenditures on hospital care rose from $8.09 to $179.6 billion between 1960 and 1986. A substantial portion of that increase was the result of improvements in treatment and technology. Innovations were not cheap. In less than 15 years the cost of an average inpatient day increased more than five times, from $83 to $460 (National Center for Health Statistics, 1987).

Efforts at cost reduction involved monitoring activities to validate physician decisions with respect to length of stay and type of care prescribed during hospitalization. Peer review involved physicians monitoring their compatriots. Utilization review involved oversight of medical practice by other interested parties, usually health insurance companies and government agencies. Peer review has been the less successful effort. The AMA acknowledged that the number of disciplinary actions in peer review are practically nil ("AMA Initiative," 1986). Review efforts were not popular with physicians because the efforts held professional judgment open to inspection and evaluation (Feldstein, 1993). Both methods have become a mainstay in attempts to reduce expenditures.

EFFORTS AT HEALTH PLANNING

Throughout the late 1960s and the 1970s Congress initiated efforts aimed at increasing the level of health planning for the country. Table 3–5 offers a brief synopsis of the two most important laws, which culminated in the conception of health systems agencies (HSAs).

Consumer input was considered so vital to success that a consumer majority was mandated on the planning boards. Although a minority, health providers attempted to dominate the direction and scope of planning activities.

Opposition to health planning boards was strong, especially among vested interest groups such as the AHA and the AMA (Pickett and Hanlon, 1990). With the advent of the Reagan administration, government support eroded. President Reagan was philosophically opposed to health planning because it set limits on the "free market" delivery system. Funding for HSAs was eliminated by the 1982 budget, effectively dampening the move toward national health planning. Most states have maintained some of the oversight and review functions, transferring these activities to other agencies.

TABLE 3–5

Federal Health Planning Efforts

PL 89–749: Community Health Planning and Public Health Service Amendment

Passed by Congress in 1966, this law focused health planning responsibilities at the state and local level. It authorized state and local agencies. The state agency assumed responsibility for coordinating efforts into one plan. It dictated membership criteria for the agencies. A majority had to be consumers and the characteristics of all members had to reflect the social characteristics of their communities (race, ethnicity, and socioeconomic class).

The law favored the establishment of new agencies rather than using preexisting state/local agencies. The active participation of state and local public health officials was not solicited and usually not volunteered. Funding for these agencies was voluntary; state and local municipalities could decide whether to fund and how much to fund. Agencies did not have authority over federal grant monies designated to communities within its jurisdiction.

PL 93–641: Comprehensive Health Planning and Public Health Amendments

Passed by Congress in 1974, this act was an attempt to legislate responsible health planning. It differed from previous efforts at health planning because it required a merger of planning and regulatory activities and was mandatory. Each state was required to have an operating program in place by 1978 or suffer federal funding cuts in other state-run health programs. Federal funds were provided to support the legislative effort.

The law stipulated the development of three agencies to plan and oversee health care: health systems agencies (HSAs); a state health coordinating council (SHCC); and a state health planning and development agency (SHPDA). The HSAs were responsible for local health planning. Each region was composed of 250,000 to 3 million people; HSAs were expected to plan for needed facilities and resources, review applications from hospitals and other health care institutions for major capital investments, and pass their recommendations on to the state.

The SHCC was to combine the individual HSA plans into one state health plan. The SHPDA was created to provide staff support for the SHCC. Each state's governor could designate an existing state agency to be the SHPDA or could create a new agency to handle the functions. The HSAs and SHCCs were directed to have a majority membership of consumers, with the remaining members being health care providers.

One of the most important state responsibilities was directed toward reviewing and deciding on capital investment requests through the certificate of need (CON) process. Capital investments by health care providers include, for example, facility expansion, new building construction, and upgrading or acquiring of new technological equipment. Input from HSA review was a part of the decision-making process. The idea was to regulate the state supply of health facilities and services to prevent duplication of services and to reduce excess capacity. The ultimate aim was reduction of health care costs.

In 1981, as part of the Reagan administration's emphasis on greater local autonomy and reduction in federal funding for state programs, PL 93-641 was diluted by legislative changes that weakened mandatory participation and reduced federal funding by 60%. Funding was eliminated in the 1982 federal budget.

A SHIFT IN FOCUS OF CARE

Another important effort was a reexamination of the usual strategy for providing care to populations. The emphasis on individuals and illness-oriented care was debated. Gradually support began to build for a different philosophy of care.

Consumer and Professional Support for Prevention Focus

Public health personnel had long argued for a more proactive approach, one that emphasized preventive health practices and identification of at-risk populations for selected interventions. It was not until cost factors became a significant concern that public opinion shifted again, to a more historical public health focus on planning and delivering health care (Walker, 1992).

A number of experimental programs proved to be cost effective. A few large employers implemented fitness and health teaching programs. These innovations resulted in an improvement in health status and a reduction in illness and sick days. Ultimately, they saved employers money on sick pay benefits and lower health insurance claims (Califano, 1986; Reed, 1991).

Coupled with employer efforts, an awakening of consumer interest in health status and health care services occurred. Consumer groups became active in monitoring and questioning standard medical practice, as well as espousing consumer responsibility for health-seeking behaviors (Illich, 1977).

Employees and labor unions drew public attention to the link between occupational exposures and hazards and certain illnesses and injuries. Their efforts helped the push toward laws intended to improve working conditions. Safety measures to eliminate or reduce illness and injury received broad support (Pickett and Hanlon, 1990; Roemer, 1991).

Comparison of Health Status Indicators

Information about models of care in other developed countries became more available to consumers, health professionals, sociologists, and economists. Instead of concentrating on physical care, political activists, economists, and sociologists argued it would be more efficient to correct poverty, because poor health was significantly associated with a deprived standard of living (McKeown, 1976; Blum, 1981). They pointed to evidence from developing countries that showed direct correlation between improvements in health status of the population and improved economic status.

Comparisons of standard measures of health among developed countries indicated that the U.S. performance was mediocre. People began to question this country's emphasis on acute care. Milio (1981; 1983) and others argued that health status should not be measured in terms of presence or absence of disease or death rates. In general, healthy people have a better quality of life than people who are not healthy. The aim should be to encourage health and maintain as many people as possible in a disease-free state. It is more cost-effective to place emphasis on prevention rather than on care or treatment of illness. A strong preventive component that would be directed toward eliminating or postponing illness for as long as possible is necessary to truly improve the health status of the population. Former Governor Lamm of Colorado offered a "ten commandments" proposal for improving the health care system. One of these was "Honor not only thy doctor and thy hospital, but thy public health nurse and thy sewage disposal plant worker" (Lamm, 1990, p. 126).

Support for Health Planning Increases

As support grew for this health concept, emphasis began to shift toward prevention. The HSAs and other health planning agencies were charged with assessing the health status of populations in their area, identifying specific health needs, and developing plans to ensure adequate services and treatment of expected health problems and to strengthen preventive measures to reduce the incidence of disease. A health plan for cardiac disease, for example, would include both an adequate supply of cardiac hospital beds and aggressive health teaching aimed at reducing the population's risk of developing heart disease. Support grew for increasing the emphasis on preventive measures aimed at target groups rather than illness care aimed at the individual.

The focus on prevention-related activities also increased at the federal level. Growing research evidence supported the idea that preventive measures were less costly than treatment of specific illnesses. National goals were developed that were intended to improve the health status of the population. Action plans were devised to meet these health goals; most actions were preventive in nature and aimed at reducing risks within specific age groups (USPHS, 1979). For example an immunization strategy targeted communicable childhood diseases, hepatitis among health care workers, and flu in elderly persons.

TWO PREVENTION EFFORTS

As the evidence of a link between disease and personal health habits grew, efforts toward effecting lifestyle changes within the population were increased. During the Reagan Administration, Surgeon General C. Everett Koop became a vocal proponent of preventive practices at the federal level. Two of his more controversial issues were cigarette smoking and acquired immunodeficiency syndrome (AIDS). In both instances he prodded the public to a growing awareness of how behavior patterns can affect the quality of life even to the extent of becoming life-threatening.

Cigarettes and Health

The link between smoking and health problems, combined with public interest in improving health, aided efforts to reduce this risky personal habit. Actions were gradual and incremental. Before Dr. Koop's efforts, the federal government's risk reduction methods were limited to warning labels on cigarette packs and the banning of cigarette advertisements on television. The focus shifted to reducing the number of smokers in the population, reducing exposure rates of the general public, and discouraging the entrance of new smokers into the risk group (Breslow, 1990).

Dr. Koop was an effective leader in this endeavor, publishing reports of the effects of secondary smoke on nonsmokers and instituting health teaching programs aimed at educating the public about the adverse effects of cigarette smoke on the human body. Legislation was enacted to establish clean air standards and to limit smoking in public places. The costs of these activities were minimal compared with the sums spent each year to treat patients with smoking-related illnesses such as lung cancer, chronic obstructive pulmonary disease, and heart disease. The relatively low monetary outlay made the campaign more palatable to cost-conscious legislators and federal administrators.

Public Education about AIDS

Strategies employed against the spread of the human immunodeficiency virus (HIV) were also primarily preventive. The Surgeon General took the lead, mailing a pamphlet to each household in the United States containing factual information about the disease, methods of transmission, and practices aimed at reducing or eliminating a person's risk of contracting HIV. Public service announcements were prevalent on radio and television and in newspapers; some announcements were made by Dr. Koop himself. Risk groups were targeted for extra effort and reinforcement of risk reduction behaviors. Condoms were made readily available to sexually active populations. Although controversial, some community programs initiated dissemination of clean syringes to intravenous drug users (Anderson, 1991), reasoning that AIDS prevention was more important than the appearance of condoning drug use (Guydish et al. 1991). Again, these activities were quite cost effective when measured against the cost of treatment of HIV infection.

Variable Public Support

It is worth noting that neither of these two campaigns had unanimous support. Cigarette manufacturers and some members of Congress from tobacco-producing states vigorously objected to the smoking reduction campaign. Businesses that were required to offer smoke-free seating were also opposed. With respect to AIDS, a vocal minority objected to providing sexually explicit information to minors or to discussing such topics in the media or in information provided to minors. The federal government, especially the executive branch, was criticized by many health professionals and organizations for its reluctance to identify AIDS as a major public health crisis. Data on the spread of this virus and related illness were ignored, and when those data became impossible to ignore, the seriousness of the disease's impact on the population was downplayed (Lee, 1990).

The new public attitude was an important reason for the success of strategies aimed at combatting these two health hazards. Consumer interest in personal responsibility and education about health-related issues and the relatively low cost of these campaigns were significant factors in their success. Anyone who doubts this need only consider whether a campaign to eliminate smoking would have been successful in the 1950s or early 1960s when prevention and costs were not important concerns.

Voluntary Component of the Private Sector

Voluntary agencies have long been a part of the U.S. health care scene. What exactly is a voluntary agency? Earlier the distinction was made between public- and private-sector organizations. All private-sector organizations are voluntary to some extent. They all originate through some sort of private initiative and are not compelled by government sanction to organize or to provide health care services. If we use these criteria to define "voluntary," then all private-sector agencies engaged in health care activities are voluntary agencies, regardless of whether they are for-profit or nonprofit. In more common usage, the term *voluntary,* with respect to health care agencies, usually applies to nonprofit agencies.

There are many hundreds of voluntary nonprofit agencies, thousands if voluntary nonprofit hospitals are included. This section concentrates on non-hospital–type voluntary agencies involved in health care.

GOALS AND TYPES OF VOLUNTARY AGENCIES

Voluntary agencies engage in a variety of health-related activities. The classic work by Gunn and Platt (1945) identified eight basic functions of voluntary agencies, which are still valid today. These basic functions are summarized in the following two basic concepts:

Creativity

- Efforts to address unmet health needs
- Efforts to improve or design new methods to meet recognized health needs
- Efforts to plan and coordinate health activities to avoid overlap and conflict between public and private initiatives

Advocacy

- Promotion of health legislation to benefit the public interest
- Promotion of public health programs and defense against political interference or funding reductions
- Provision of health education of the public and support for professional education

An agency may concentrate on one function or be involved in a number of different functions depending on its stated mission.

There are several types of health-related voluntary agencies. The most common are agencies supported by contributions from the general public (for example, the American Heart Association), philanthropic trusts (for example, The Robert Wood Johnson Foundation), and health professional organizations (for example, the American Public Health Association). The largest group and the most familiar to the general public consists of agencies that receive their support from citizen donations and fund-raising campaigns.

AGENCIES SUPPORTED BY PRIVATE FUNDS

The goals of publicly supported organizations vary greatly but many are clearly health related. Most have very specific purposes. Some examples are as follows:

- Agencies that concentrate on a specific illness, disease, or body organ (for example, the American Heart Association, the American Diabetes Association, or the American Cancer Society)
- Agencies concerned with providing services to specific target groups, such as children, elderly persons, or homeless persons (for example, the National Society for Crippled Children and Adults and the National Council on Aging)
- Hospice organizations that target terminally ill patients and their families
- Agencies that concentrate on a certain type of health-related service or phase of health (for example, Planned Parenthood Federation of America, the National Safety Council, and Visiting Nurse Association)

Specialized agencies usually rely on public donations from a large number of contributors. Most attempt some type of fund-raising campaigns including mail or media, door-to-door solicitations, and telethons. So many organizations have made public appeals for support that a number of charities have banded together in a united appeal process. The United Way and Community Chest efforts are an attempt to limit requests for contributions and consolidate efforts.

FOUNDATIONS AND PRIVATE PHILANTHROPY

Foundations are established and funded by private donations. These philanthropic organizations are involved in a number of health-related areas including basic research, professional education, efforts in international health, and assisting efforts of official health departments located primarily in rural or isolated areas. In addition to The Robert Wood Johnson Foundation, the Milbank Memorial Fund, the Rockefeller Foundation, the W.K. Kellogg Foundation, and the Carnegie Foundation are a few of the philanthropic organizations with a primary interest in health care. Their addresses and special interests are listed in Table 3–6.

TABLE 3–6

Sample List of Foundations Involved with Health Care Issues

Carnegie Foundation (interest in education, including health education)
Five Ivy Lane
Princeton, NJ 08540

The Robert Wood Johnson Foundation (interest in ambulatory care and health personnel)
P.O. Box 2316
Princeton, NJ 08543–2316

W. K. Kellogg Foundation (health delivery and education)
One Michigan Ave, East
Battle Creek, Michigan 49017–4508

Milbank Memorial Fund (health care and health statistics)
One East 75th St.
New York, NY 10021

Rockefeller Foundation (health issues)
1133 Avenue of the Americas
New York, NY 10036

PROFESSIONAL ORGANIZATIONS

The third group of voluntary agencies consists of health professional organizations. These are usually funded by membership dues. Professional associations are concerned with health issues, especially those that involve the well-being of their members, and are usually not involved in direct health care services. Some of the activities that they conduct include provision of continuing education, establishment and improvement of standards and qualifications for professional practice, encouragement of research, and safeguarding of the independence and the interests of the professional membership. The last is usually accomplished by lobbying and other types of activity aimed at governmental bodies that have the potential to affect professional practice.

DISTINCTIONS FROM OTHER TYPES OF ORGANIZATIONS

Voluntary agencies have operational freedoms that other types of organizations do not. They are less constrained by laws and regulations and are able to move quickly to initiate new programs or change existing ones. They enhance creativity in care and are often the initiator of new programs, research, or services to underserved groups. Although voluntary organizations contribute to health care, they play a very small role in the delivery of services to the nation's population. Using charitable efforts as an indirect measure of impact, their efforts provide a mere 1% of the total health care budget (Ginzberg, 1991).

Some functions of voluntary agencies have been assumed by public-sector organizations. Voluntary agencies have advocated a shift in public opinion toward the idea that health care is a right rather than a privilege (Banta, 1990). There is no danger that the public sector will take over all voluntary health-related activities in the near future. The current wave of budget reductions ensures an ongoing need for voluntary agencies.

Government's Authority and Role in Health Care

As previously noted each of the three levels of U.S. government assumes some of the responsibilities for health care. Indirect services make up a major portion of services provided by government. In keeping with a free market economy, government usually does not attempt to provide services in areas in which provision by private enterprise has been satisfactory. For the most part private enterprise provides direct services of personal health care for Americans able to pay, either directly (out of pocket) or through third-party payers (private health insurance plans).

Certain population groups not covered by private-sector services are provided care by the various levels of government. State and local governments are more involved in direct care. Federal, state, and local governmental agencies are frequently involved in administration of a single program or basic service, such as the WIC program discussed earlier. How they are involved, or the exact role each plays, is generally the distinguishing element.

THE FEDERAL GOVERNMENT

The authority for the federal government's involvement is derived from the Constitution of the United States. Although not explicitly stated, federal authority is assumed from the charge to provide for the general welfare and the federal role in the regulation of interstate commerce. The federal government has the power to collect and spend monies for general welfare and to regulate business and organizations that conduct operations in more than one state.

Since the 1930s the federal role in health care has expanded. Even so, federal health programs are frequently delegated to the states for actual implementation. The federal government does, however, assume overall responsibility for the health protection of its population.

Although all three branches of government make health-related decisions, the major policy decisions are made by the President and his or her staff (executive branch) and Congress (legislative branch). These two branches set the tone for delivery of care; they dictate which groups will be served and the manner of service. Both branches are subject to political pressures that influence the decision-making process. Health-related matters are the purview of numerous individuals and committees, as are many areas of federal activity.

Once policy is decided, other government agencies are responsible for oversight to ensure implementation. These agencies regulate and interpret health law, administer services mandated by law, and are responsible for supervision of compliance with health laws and regulation. Federal agencies are primarily involved in indirect services.

U.S. Department of Health and Human Services

The federal agency with the most health-related responsibilities is the U.S. Department of Health and Human Services (DHHS). Although DHHS is responsible for some direct services, most of its activities involve indirect care. Responsibilities include health planning and resource development, research, health care, financing, and regulatory oversight. The DHHS either carries out these services itself or delegates responsibility and funding for services to other public and private organizations. The organizational chart in Figure 3–13 illustrates some of the specific responsibilities of DHHS.

Because DHHS responsibilities are varied and complex, only two offices and their functions are outlined in this chapter. Public health and political science texts are two reference sources that can provide a more in-depth discussion of DHHS for those who wish to investigate this area.

The Health Care Finance Administration. The primary responsibility of HCFA is oversight of the Medicare and Medicaid programs, which constitute 80% of the federal budget for personal health care services (Lazerby and Letsch, 1990). Chapter 5 provides detailed program information and explores the role of HCFA in administering and ensuring the quality of care to individuals served by Medicare and Medicaid.

U.S. Public Health Service (PHS). This agency administers many of the most familiar federal health functions. The PHS is headed by the Surgeon General of the United States, a politically appointed position. President Clinton appointed Joycelyn Elders as Surgeon General in 1993.

Many of the administrative responsibilities of the PHS are managed by the Assistant Secretary of Health. This situation has created ambiguity in the role of the Surgeon General, who has little real power in terms of directing health policy. The last several Surgeons General have attempted to enhance their impact on health policy by publicizing selected health care issues. For example, C. Everett Koop emphasized public awareness of AIDS and Antonia Novella highlighted the effects of substance abuse, especially the effects of alcohol and tobacco on adolescents.

The PHS provides indirect care primarily. Figure 3–14 identifies the various agencies within PHS. A brief description of each is listed here:

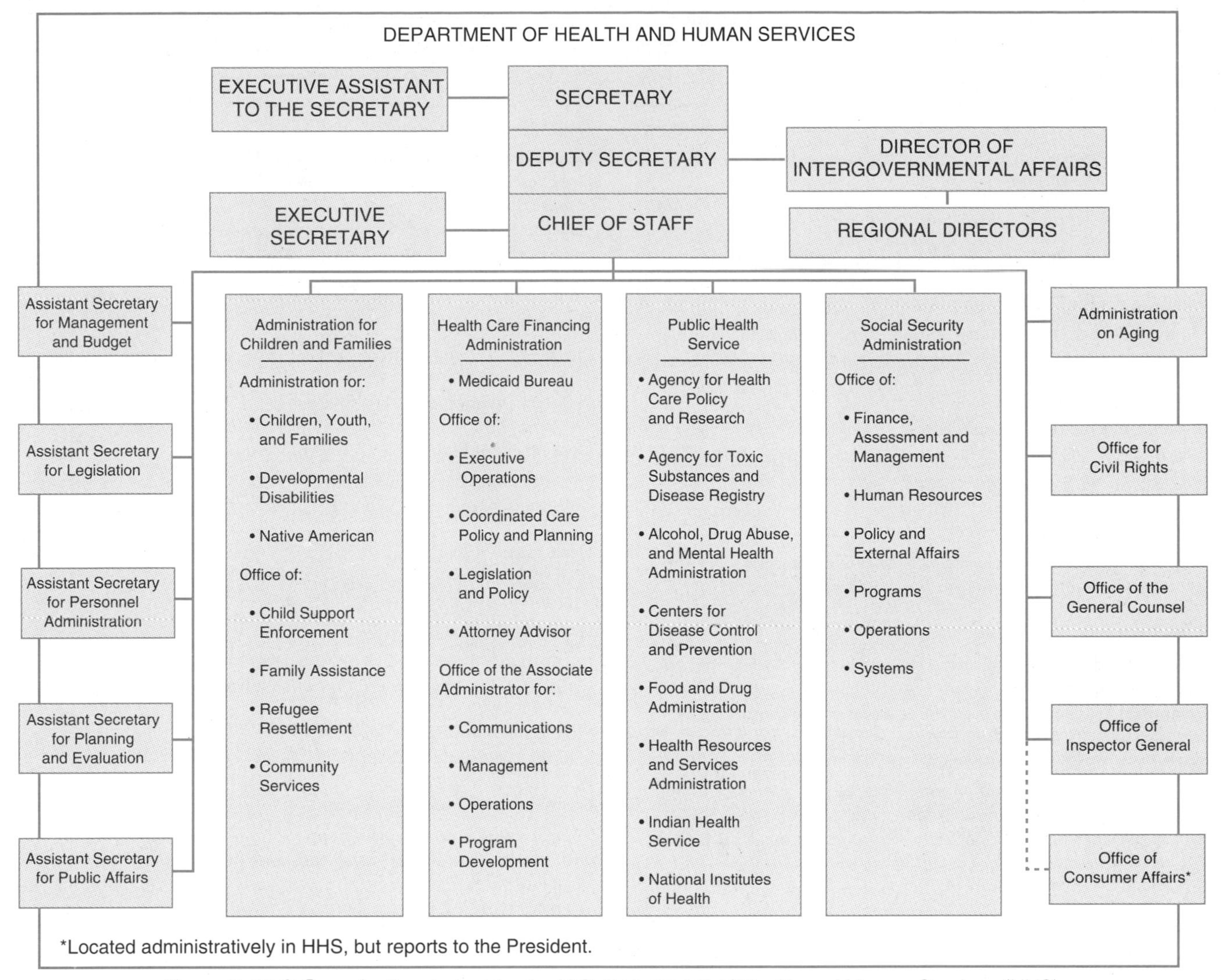

Figure 3–13 ● Organizational chart for the U.S. Department of Health and Human Services (HHS).

- The National Institutes of Health (NIH) funds and conducts research, including nursing research, which is primarily funded through the National Center for Nursing Research. The NIH may be used as a referral source for clients who require experimental care.
- Food and Drug Administration (FDA) establishes and enforces safe standards for food, drugs, and cosmetics. FDA approval is necessary before experimental drugs may be tested and marketed in the United States.
- Health Resource and Services Administration (HRSA)

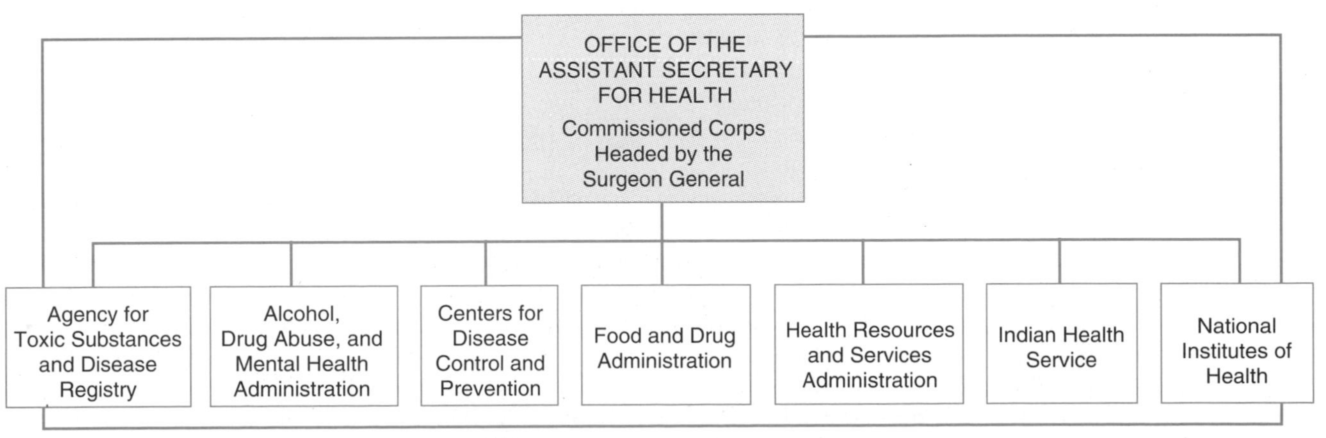

Figure 3–14 ● Organization of U.S. Public Health Service.

TABLE 3–7

Scope of Services for Centers for Disease Control and Prevention (CDC)

National Center for Chronic Disease Prevention and Health Promotion

- To prevent death and disability from chronic diseases and promote healthy personal behavior

National Center for Environmental Health

- To prevent death and disability due to environmental factors

National Center for Health Statistics

- To monitor the health of the American people, the impact of illness and disability, and factors affecting health and the nation's health care system

National Center for Infectious Diseases

- To prevent and control unnecessary disease and death caused by infectious diseases of public health importance

National Center for Injury Prevention and Control

- To prevent and control nonoccupational injuries, both those that are unintentional and those that result from violence

National Center for Prevention Services

- To prevent and control vaccine-preventable diseases, human immunodeficiency virus infection, sexually transmitted diseases, tuberculosis, dental diseases, and the introduction of diseases from other countries

National Institute for Occupational Safety and Health

- To prevent workplace-related injuries, illnesses, and premature death caused by trauma; toxic chemicals, dusts, and radiation; musculoskeletal and psychological stressors; noise; and other occupational hazards

Epidemiology Program Office

- To provide domestic and international epidemiological, communication, and statistical support and to train experts in epidemiology

International Health Program Office

- To strengthen the capacity of other nations to reduce disease, disability, and death

Public Health Practice Program Office

- To improve the effectiveness of public health delivery systems in health promotion and prevention

From CDC, Atlanta.

does health resource planning; funds training of health; and administers the Indian Health Service, the Federal Bureau of Prisons, and the Bureau of Health Professionals (which contains a division of nursing, a source of funding grants for nursing education and training).

- Alcohol, Drug Abuse, and Mental Health Administration coordinates and funds programs for each related area, most of which are community based and some of which are based in community health agencies.
- The Agency for Toxic Substance and Disease Registry is responsible for preventing health-related problems associated with toxic substances.
- Indian Health Service provides health care services to American Indian populations, primarily on reservations in the West.
- The Centers for Disease Control and Prevention (CDC) is the primary source of information on communicable diseases and is a vital resource for all public health personnel. Table 3–7 details the scope of services provided by CDC.

TABLE 3–8

Sample Listing of Other Federal Agencies Involved in Health Matters

Department of Agriculture

Develops dietary guidelines for national nutritional policy
Does research and provides prevention data in areas of improved crop and animal protection
National School Lunch Program enforces food safety regulations; grades meats and other foods
Food Stamp Program

Department of Defense

Provides direct and indirect medical services to military members and their families
Provides environmental health services to military communities

Department of Housing and Urban Development

Provides mortgage insurance for hospitals and long-term care facilities
Constructs rural hospitals and neighborhood clinics

Department of Justice

Operates facilities for the health care of federal prisoners

Department of Labor

Occupational Safety and Health Administration (OSHA)—provides technical assistance and enforces health and safety standards in the workplace
Mine Safety and Health Administration—inspects mines and enforces health and safety standards

Environmental Protection Agency

Controls air and water quality and pollution standards
Oversees solid waste and toxic substances disposal
Regulates pesticides
Oversees radiation hazard control
Oversees noise abatement

National Science Foundation

Provides money for health research

Other Federal Agencies

Several other federal agencies provide health-related services. Table 3–8 lists the most important of these and some of their health care responsibilities. Note that most provide indirect services that play an important role in the health and welfare of the population. Imagine the potential for outbreaks of food poisoning if there were no inspection of the food, meat, and poultry produced for public consumption. The current rash of environmental problems, such as air and water pollution, toxic dumps, and food pollutants, point to the need for continued, vigilant health monitoring.

Some federal agencies, including the Veterans Administration (VA) and the Department of Defense, provide direct health care to specific populations. The VA is an independent agency that reports directly to the President. It is responsible for providing direct health care to certain groups of military veterans, especially those who have service-connected injuries, receive veterans' pensions, are 65 years or older, and/or are medically indigent. Thus the VA serves as a source of care for veterans who have exhausted other health care resources.

The VA operates hospitals that provide inpatient and outpatient medical, surgical, and psychiatric services. It also operates satellite and independent clinics and offers limited nursing home and residential facilities. The VA is a large direct-care system with 172 hospitals, 17 domiciles, 229 outpatient clinics, and 117 nursing home units.

Some have questioned the need to operate a separate health care system for veterans. Recommendations to eliminate the VA and provide care in the private sector have surfaced from time to time. Veterans and VA employees have always been successful at resisting such efforts (Brecher, 1990).

The Department of Defense provides both direct and indirect care to active-duty military members and their dependents. It pays for indirect care of family members of military personnel and retirees through the Civilian Health and Medical Program of the Uniformed Services (CHAMPUS) insurance program. The Department of Defense operates hospitals and clinics in the United States as well as overseas and provides limited care to retired career military and their dependents based on availability of resources. Public/community health is emphasized, perhaps because the Department of Defense assumes responsibility for the health of all persons living on military bases. Environmental regulation (of food, water, etc.), preventive health practices, and health promotion activities are emphasized.

STATE GOVERNMENT

States derive their authority to govern from the Constitution, which reserved for the states all power not specifically given to the federal government. States play a broad role in health care. They finance care of the poor and disabled, primarily through the Medicaid program; operate state mental hospitals; ensure quality of service through licensure and regulation of health practitioners and facilities; and attempt to control health care costs and regulate insurance companies (Litman, 1990; Brecher, 1990). States play the major role in directing and supervising public health activities for their citizens, including disease control, sanitation, and environmental oversight.

Because state governments have diverse organizational structures there is no single way in which health care services are organized and supplied by the states. Health care concerns are spread throughout various state agencies.

The State Health Agency

Each state has a state health agency that is the principal agency for health care services for that state. Roles and responsibilities for state health agencies vary: some have vast authority over most health care issues, and others share power with a number of other agencies or organizations. Figure 3–15 represents an example of a hypothetical state health agency with considerable authority. Most states provide the listed health services either through state health or through other state agencies. In states where the state health agency is the state health department, the director may hold the title of health officer or health commissioner.

According to the Association of State and Territorial Health Officers (ASTHO), most state health agencies are actively involved in six areas: (1) personal health, (2) environmental health, (3) health resources, (4) laboratory, (5) general administration and services, and (6) funding to local health departments not allocated to program areas. Most of the personal care is aimed at poor people (Miller et al., 1977; Brecher, 1990). Local health departments may share in providing some of these services if directed to do so by the state authority (see Chapter 30).

Other Health-Related State Activities

Green and Anderson (1982) have identified approximately 36 state agencies outside the state health agency that have health-related responsibilities. Departments of education are responsible for school health programs and health education policy. Licensing of health professionals is usually the purview of the state board of licensing and examination for that specific profession. Vocational rehabilitation, occupational health, health planning, and selected environmental health responsibilities may also be found outside the scope of the state health agency.

The National Commission on Community Health Services (1967) recommended consolidation of all official health services into a single agency, which would result in streamlining bureaucracy, reducing duplication of efforts, and, potentially, cutting costs. Almost 30 years later there has been little progress toward this recommendation, and it is not likely that we will see substantial consolidation of health-related services in the near future (Koplin, 1990). As a result, the states' health care responsibilities are still divided over an extensive and bewildering number of departments, commissions, agencies, and boards.

LOCAL GOVERNMENT

Local governments are created by the states. Authority at the local level is delegated by state government. The local unit can be a city, village, township, county, or special

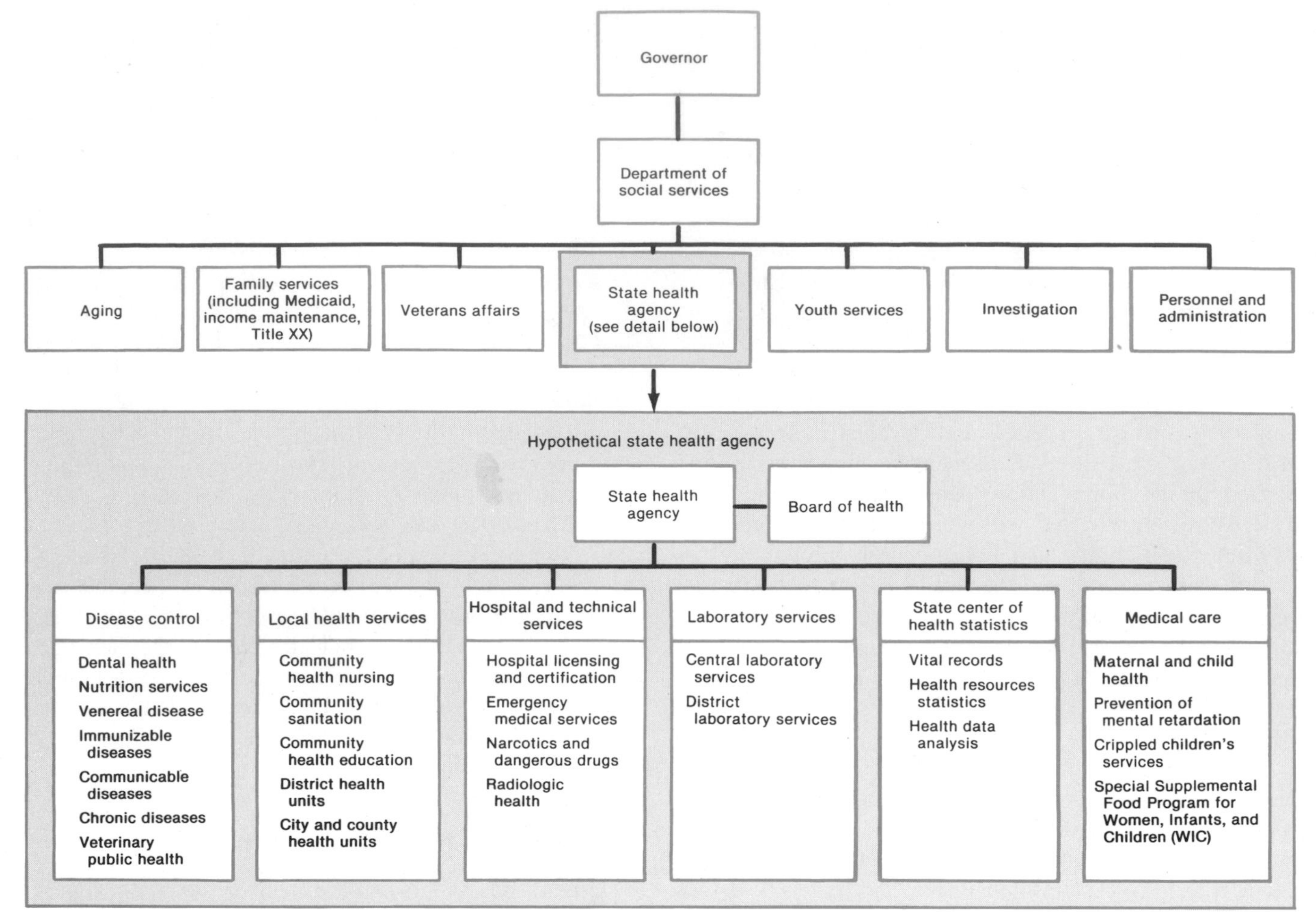

Figure 3–15 ● Hypothetical social services superagency. (Redrawn from National Public Health Reporting System. [1980]. *Public health programs.* Washington, DC: Association of State and Territorial Health Officials.)

district. State legislatures determine the responsibilities and roles of local units, including the definition of the units' role in health care.

Many of the direct personal services are performed by the local governments. Maternal and child health programs are examples of such endeavors. The WIC Program is an example of shared authority. Most of the responsibility for health care at the local level resides in the local health department. Some local health departments provide ambulatory health services for poor persons, especially in areas where other providers limit service to this group (Institute of Medicine, 1988; Pickett and Hanlon, 1990). Funding of local health departments is shared among local, state, and federal efforts. Federal funding is usually in the form of grants for specific programs. Most of the burden for operating local health departments is assumed by local governments (ASTHO, 1980; Koplin, 1990).

Like state governments, local units do not consolidate all health care services in the local health department. Many variants of organizational structure exist. Mental health and environmental health services, such as waste disposal and air pollution and water quality control, are commonly found under the auspices of other local agencies. School health programs may be the responsibility of the local school district rather than the local health department. Communities that operate general public hospitals and other such facilities frequently have seaparate organizational and funding structures for these facilities.

Relative Magnitude of Health Spending in the United States

Since 1965 national expenditures on health care have risen steadily and are a serious concern. By 1992 expenses were roughly $838.5 billion and represented 14% of the country's entire GNP.

PRIVATE- AND PUBLIC-SECTOR SHARES OF HEALTH EXPENSES

Government at all levels accounts for 42.4% of the total health care costs in 1990 (Congressional Budget Office,

1992). Two large programs, Medicare and Medicaid, account for almost one quarter of all health expenses.

In 1965, before Medicare and Medicaid, the federal share of health care expenses was roughly equal to the combined state and local contributions. By 1970 the federal share had doubled. By 1990 the federal government paid approximately 70% of public-sector costs, and state and local governments paid the remaining 30% (Congressional Budget Office, 1992).

In 1965 the private sector accounted for 74% of all health care expenses. By 1975, after Medicare and Medicaid were well established, the private sector share dropped to 57.5%, where it has remained ever since.

According to Mechanic (1986), the pattern of health expenditures is a reflection of age and social risk factors. Elderly and poor persons are at greater risk for accidents and illness. It is in these groups that the largest expenses occur, which became evident as social health programs made access and care available to these risk groups.

PRIORITIES IN HEALTH CARE EXPENDITURES

By far the largest amount of money is spent on personal health care, very little on public health. In Figure 3–16 expenditures for 1991 are broken down by type and source of funding. Personal health care services accounted for all but 7% of the entire health budget. Hospital care is the most costly category; physicians services and nursing homes are two other expensive areas. Other personal care expenses such as for drugs, eyeglasses, medical equipment, and dental services account for most of the remainder.

Public health, research, and construction together account for a mere 7% of the entire budget. Public health activities are subsidized wholly by the public sector. State and local governments bear the major costs of providing these services. Public health's share of funding has remained relatively stable since the early 1970s.

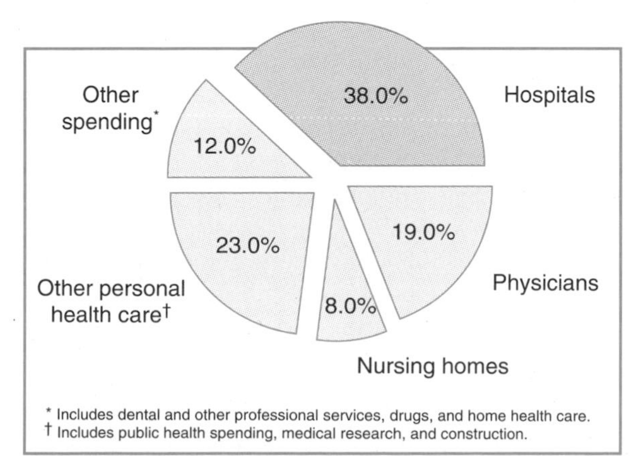

Figure 3–16 ● Where U.S. health care dollars were spent, 1991. (Redrawn from Health Care Financing Administration, Office of the Actuary; Office of National Health Statistics.)

Government, especially the federal government, bears the major responsibility for research. Most of these funds were used or distributed by the National Institutes of Health. The private sector invests much of the construction funds for building projects. Private costs were roughly double public sector outlays in the construction area.

Shifts in Federal and State Relationships

In the 1960s and 1970s the federal government assumed a greater role in the delivery and funding of health services. From the early 1980s there has been a federal effort to reduce service and responsibilities and to shift those duties to the states (Brecher, 1990). Federal tactics have included program cuts, funding cuts for special programs, and the use of block grants to shift responsibility. States have resisted these efforts, caught in a bind between federally mandated service requirements and shrinking federal funds (Congressional Budget Office, 1992).

Federal minimum standards for air and water quality and Medicaid services, for example, both have an impact on public health. In both areas federal regulations must be met by the states, even if that means states incur additional expenses. State and federal officials continue to pressure each other to assume a greater share of the health care burden.

Federal retrenchment and the financial hardships at the state and federal level have led to a weakening of public health agencies at all levels. State and local health departments have suffered severe funding cuts resulting in reductions in staff (including community health nurses), reductions in worker benefits, retention of stationary salary scales that have not kept pace with inflation, reductions in the amount and type of direct care provided to risk groups, and imposition of fees for services once provided for free (Koplin, 1990; Walker, 1992).

Remaining staff operate under increasing stress and pressure to produce. They are left to question the effectiveness and adequacy of their services. It is ironic that at a time of increasing emphasis on health promotion and disease prevention, which is the very essence of community health practice, the survival of some public health agencies is doubtful.

Emerging Health Care System

Evolution continues in our health care system as it reacts to changes and pressures from providers and consumers. Several issues have had an impact on health care delivery in the 1980s and 1990s. Escalating costs, tension between health professions, and a fragmented structure have been instrumental in variously impeding or expanding access to services as well as dictating the level of services available for selected groups within the population.

Cost Increases Have an Impact on the Entire Economy

Health care expenditures are particularly significant because they are so large. As health care expands its share of the country's GNP, other industries lose ground. For example, for every 1% increase in the health care GNP, there is a corresponding 1% loss in revenues to other industries. Eventually everyone is affected by increases in health costs. Government must pay for increases in services that they are pledged to provide. Governmental expenses are ultimately the responsibility of the taxpayer. As federal and state health care costs have escalated, the increased expense has been passed on to individual taxpayers via the income tax and other taxes.

Insurance coverage has also been influenced by inflated expenses. Insurance companies pass on expenses to employers. Employers, in turn, usually pass on the extra costs to their employees by increasing the employee's share of health insurance contributions. Those without health insurance pay more directly in out-of-pocket costs. No one escapes increases in the costs of health care services (see Chapter 5).

Power Conflicts within the System

Earlier in the chapter changes in a sector of the system were shown to produce changes in other sectors of the system. Change is not always beneficial to all concerned; thus some resistance and conflict can be expected. Conflicts are a part of any system, which is demonstrated precisely by the health care system. Cost increases, growing consumer awareness, and competing philosophies about the nature of health care delivery have produced some changes, which have created conflict among various participants (providers and consumers) as they struggle to gain or maintain power. We discussed funding and regulatory conflicts between federal and state/local governments. Many other power-related conflicts exist.

One particularly telling clash continues between hospital administrations and physicians. Administrators pressed to operate a hospital within ever-tightening budget restraints have initiated curbs on medical practice. Areas such as the number of days a patient remains in the hospital, the types of laboratory and radiological procedures ordered, the use of extra personnel or equipment, and choice of treatment modality are examples of decisions that are now open to administrative scrutiny. Physicians have vigorously resisted outside influences in practice decisions, pointing to the need for professional autonomy to ensure optimal patient care. Nevertheless, hospital administrators have gradually assumed some influence over practice decisions.

Nursing has engaged in numerous conflicts as the profession struggles toward greater respect and autonomy. These conflicts can be expected to continue because as nursing increases its voice and power, others must share in the decision-making process. A nursing voice on a hospital or home care board, for instance, means someone else is displaced or their influence is diluted by the addition of a new member.

Increased wages for hospital nurses means that administration must find ways to meet those salary concessions. Wage increases were historically passed on to the consumer, but current budgetary constraints do not always allow that possibility. Administrators must make shifts in the budget to accommodate nursing gains. Building or remodeling may be postponed, travel budgets for administrators and division chairs may be suspended or reduced, "perks" offered to some hospital employees may be withdrawn or reduced, investments in new equipment may be delayed or scrapped, and wage or benefit increases of other health care professionals may be canceled or postponed.

Historically, physicians have assumed the major role for making decisions in patient care and treatment. They have also had the most influence on policy decisions affecting health care (Roemer, 1991). Their premier status was the result of education: few other health workers were sufficiently educated to exert much influence on health care. This is no longer true. A large number of well-educated health professionals now demand a greater share in the decision-making process. Physicians account for only 14% of all educated medical professionals. Although physicians have resisted efforts at power sharing, other health professionals have gained a voice in shaping health policy and services. During the Clinton administration health care reform process, nurse leaders and professional nursing organizations have been clearly consulted. The President and the Health Reform Task Group made a point of acknowledging the importance of nursing's role in the health care delivery system.

Insurance companies, physicians, and state regulatory bodies struggle over treatment and cost issues. Malpractice frequently pits administration, physicians, nurses, other health care workers, and lawyers against one another as they struggle over issues of cost, liability, and jurisdiction. As consumer groups attempt to gain a greater voice in the delivery and organization of health care services, many of those already involved in the decision-making process work to retard or dilute consumer groups' influence. In the health care industry, power struggles have intensified and can be expected to continue as attempts to resolve the budget crisis continue.

Specialization and Fragmentation

More than 6 million people are employed in health care, which has seen a rapid increase in specialized workers. Health care workers have become more sophisticated and specialized. Technological advances have led to increasingly more complex facilities and care requirements, which have fueled demand for specialization. The result has been a bewildering array of individuals who can be involved in the care of a single patient. It takes special skills to handle a magnetic resonance imaging or computed tomography scanner or to prepare and maintain a heart-lung bypass machine. Add to this the myriad types of care and treatment options available and it is easy to see how specialization in health care has become so prolific.

Nurses and physicians have moved from general practice into specialty areas. Specialization is often viewed as more prestigious than general practice. This has been a particular problem for medicine. By the 1960s a dramatic imbalance existed between primary practitioners and specialists. Prestige, larger salaries, and fewer working hours lured many physicians away from general community practice. Alarm over decreasing numbers of general practitioners led to adoption of family practice as a specialty area in 1969, in an attempt to enhance the status of family practice. Specialty and geographic imbalances still exist in the distribution of physicians.

Up to this point specialization has not been problematic for nursing. Federal estimates of future needs point to a continuing demand for graduate nurses prepared as nurse practitioners and clinical specialists, including community health specialists (PHS, 1990).

Fragmentation remains a major feature of our health care. Roemer and colleagues (1975) identified the most important problems associated with fragmented health care as being poor access to care, gaps and inequities, inadequate prevention efforts, discontinuous and inappropriate care, poor responsiveness to consumer needs, inefficient use of scarce resources, ineffective planning and evaluation, escalating costs, inadequate quality controls, and fragmented policies. Although some attempts have been made to address these issues, they remain largely the same today.

Subspecialization of professions enhances the problem of fragmented care for individuals, since specialists tend to concentrate in their specialty, rather than take a holistic care view. It is easy to conceive of one person being seen by two or three specialists without coordination of overall care. In the community, patients are frequently seen who are taking medication prescribed by two or three physicians. Without coordination, a danger exists that medications may be counterproductive or even life-threatening in combination.

Subspecialization of a profession is only one example of this problem. Overall care for individual patients is divided among many separate individuals and agencies, each of whom has a specific purpose, without any integrated direction of purpose and coordination of services. Patients or their families are often expected to coordinate services. Many miss out on available resources because they lack the skill and information necessary to plan for care.

Consider some of the resources that might be needed to provide quality care to a stroke patient after hospital discharge: the primary doctor, a physician specialist, a nursing service, physical therapy and other rehabilitative services, respite workers to relieve family caregivers, Meals on Wheels, telephone monitoring, various assistive devices, home remodeling to accommodate physical deficits, and senior daycare. Most communities still have no coordination and oversight services for their citizens.

STRATEGIES TO ADDRESS PROBLEM AREAS

Since the early 1970s attempts have been made to address specific problems within the system. Efforts have been aimed at improving efficiency, coordinating planning, and controlling costs; some have been more successful than others. Following is a brief discussion of the most important strategies. Chapter 5 provides a more detailed discussion of selected cost-cutting strategies.

Methods to Decrease Costs

Major effort has been applied to seeking solutions to the cost issue. Hospital expenses seemed a logical place to initiate reforms, since hospitals accounted for approximately 50% of all personal health care expenditures in 1980.

Shorten Hospital Stays and Increase Home Health Care. The primary efforts at reducing hospital Medicare costs were federal actions. Prospective payment and diagnosis-related groups (DRGs) were imposed on hospitals who cared for Medicare patients. These reforms were an attempt to encourage hospitals to curb costs (see Chapter 5).

The net effect of federal reform was a reduction in the average length of hospital stay for Medicare patients and an increased demand for home health and other community care services. Transfers to after-hospital care facilities doubled. The largest growth was in home health care agencies, which increased 41% between 1983 and 1985 alone (Morrisey et al., 1988). Other community agencies, including public health departments, were similarly affected by the increased demand for community-related services (Walker, 1992).

Federal efforts did not eliminate cost increases significantly but seemed to have slowed the rate of increase. In 1982, the year before DRGs were implemented, Medicare expenses increased by 17.6%. According to HCFA, Medicare increases slowed to only 5.7% by the year 1986.

Implement Coordinated Care. The intent of coordinated care strategies is to include a mechanism for reviewing care prior to and during treatment to reduce costs and eliminate the use of unnecessary services.

Health maintenance organizations (HMOs), preferred-provider organizations (PPOs) and other types of coordinated care have expanded rapidly, primarily because they appear to be cost-effective at delivering care. Chapter 5 provides a discussion of how costs are affected by these health care service options.

Health maintenance organizations, the oldest model of coordinated care, began to grow in the 1970s. They offer a comprehensive service package for a fixed price. An individual's choice of provider is limited to those with HMO contracts. Almost 15% of the population, 37 million persons, are enrolled in HMOs (Porter et al., 1992).

Most of cost-savings with HMOs comes from efforts to reduce hospitalization rates among members. One study by Schlag and Piktialis (1987) found that HMOs had a hospital utilization rate approximately half that of traditional medical practice in the same geographic area. Providing HMO service to Medicare patients is a recent development. It remains to be seen whether HMOs can continue to operate as effectively as they increase the number of older, more medically needy members.

The PPOs have a looser organizational structure and are a more recent development. They contract with a network of providers (doctors, hospitals, and others) to provide service at a discounted rate to members. There is a fixed premium (insurance cost). Members may, in addition, be expected to pay a portion of the cost for selected services. Membership in PPO groups is growing, especially among employer-provided health plans (U.S. Department of Labor, 1990).

Coordinated or managed care also applies to other strategies aimed at controlling costs; these are almost always developed by third-party payers. Some of the current techniques include prior approval for hospital admission, second opinions for surgery and other costly treatment options, controls on the use of specialists, and case management of care provided to high-cost patients.

Promote Use of Generic Medication. One simple means of cutting costs is the use of generic medications. Insurance plans that pay the pharmacy directly for medications have specified the use of generic drugs whenever possible. Other plans simply put a cap on the amount reimbursed to the patient in an effort to encourage use of generics. There is also a widespread effort to educate consumers and health professionals about the cost savings associated with generic drugs.

Reduce Waste of Equipment. Because of emphasis on budget reduction, institutions have been more vigorous in attempts to encourage judicious use of disposable equipment. Some institutions have formalized their cost-benefit reviews to make more fiscally sound equipment decisions. A number of nurseries have returned to cloth diapers because their cost is less than disposables.

Health facilities managers are employing more rigorous review procedures in the decision-making process concerned with new equipment and costly new technologies. These actions were first encouraged by health planning legislation that attempted to reduce duplication of services. Now, because of tight budget restraints, administrators are continuing the practice.

Increase Productivity of Health Professionals

One method to reduce costs is judicious use of skilled workers and identification of techniques that increase efficiency.

Perform Health Teaching to Groups. Any activity that increases the number of persons affected by a given action is cost productive. Health teaching to groups is one such action, because it provides sound health information to a larger audience than does a one-on-one approach. Studies indicate that group teaching is effective in transmitting health-related information (Dodds et al., 1993).

Maintaining health is the goal of health teaching aimed at essentially well individuals. Corporations find that group teaching programs focused on health promotion and disease prevention are cost-effective both because they reach a wide audience and they save on illness-related expenses (Califano, 1986).

Institute Wider Use of Nurse Practitioners. First used as physician extenders, nurse practitioners are considered effective physician substitutes in certain settings. For health managers, economics is the major motivator. Nurse practitioners cost less than physicians, their care is of similar quality, and consumers are pleased with their service (Lenz and Edwards, 1992). The Medicare and Medicaid programs took the lead in expanded use of nurse practitioners (see Chapter 5). As emphasis shifts toward noninstitutional services, nurse practitioners are expected to assume responsibility for care of a large share of the elderly and persons with medically stable chronic illness or disability.

The trend toward expanded use of nurse practitioners could be reversed by an oversupply of physicians. As the supply of doctors increases, the potential exists that physician groups may attempt to reduce supply or limit practice of physician extenders. Physician assistants are more vulnerable to such a possibility because their practice is more dependent on physician sponsorship.

Increase Accountability of Provider Services. Oversight of services and costs is becoming tighter. Itemized bills are required and are carefully scrutinized by consumers and third-party payers. Both government and private insurers have instituted mechanisms to review patient service records for appropriateness of services and costs. Utilization review studies indicate that these mechanisms are cost effective (Scheffler et al., 1991). Nurses are often employed as reviewers because their expertise is an asset to the insurers.

Implement Health Care Planning: Public Law 93–641. As previously discussed, health planning gradually evolved from a voluntary into a mandatory process with stringent criteria.

Public Law (PL) 93–641 was not fully implemented until 1979. It is difficult to evaluate the effects of PL 93–461 because it operated as originally developed only for a short period of time. The program did produce modest successes in terms of cost containment by retarding the rate of increase in specific health care costs. It also allowed for greater local participation in the decision-making process (Lefkowitz, 1983).

Promote Continuity of Care. Ensuring that people get what they need to maintain or improve their health status requires the creation of some method to coordinate all necessary services. This is especially important in a system noted for fragmented care. The use of case managers has proved to be effective. Pilot studies sponsored by the DHHS have shown that the use of case managers to coordinate services to elderly clients has been beneficial. Clients received all necessary services, and the need for institutional care, the most costly service method, was delayed, therefore benefiting the entire system. Community nurses make excellent case managers because they are already familiar with many community resources and the referral process (Erkel, 1993). Case management has been a responsibility of community health nurses since the profession's inception.

A National Health Care System

So far, reform efforts have had little impact on cost and have proved unsuccessful at reaching underserved populations. In *Nursing's Agenda for Health Care Reform* (ANA, 1992), the ANA strongly advocates a national health care plan with universal access, community-based primary care, illness prevention, and health promotion initiatives. The country seems prepared to implement some type of national health care. Numerous plans have been proposed; they can be described as one of two types: a single-payer or an all-payer system (Table 3–9).

SINGLE-PAYER SYSTEM

In a single-payer system the government is the sole financer of health care. All citizens are covered and private health insurance is unnecessary. The monies to finance care come from tax revenues. Centralized control of costs and utilization of services are elements of such systems. Fixed fees are assigned for all health services. Administration can be either contained at the federal level or allocated to the states. A state-administered program would most closely resemble the Canadian health system.

In the Canadian model each province assumes management responsibilities for its district and the central government determines the minimum package of health services that each province must provide. The provinces are free to provide other services. There is some variation in services and management among the various provinces.

Since it has become apparent that the United States is seriously considering a national plan, criticism of the Canadian model has become more pronounced. Many of the complaints are accepted as factual, although detailed investigation reveals most to be untruths or half-truths. Table 3–10 lists some of the more prominent criticisms with a response to each.

ALL-PAYER SYSTEM

An all-payer system is one in which health care is financed by a number of sources, public and private. A wide variety of proposals fall into this category. Each has its own structure, but some common elements exist. Although all citizens would be covered, control would be more decentralized. Public financing would be from tax revenues, private financing through insurance and out-of-pocket expenses. Theoretically there would be some minimum standard of service that must be offered to all citizens, and providers will be free to add more. Costs and utilization of service would be less centralized and more difficult to manage. Because there are so many all-payer proposals, only representative samples are highlighted in Table 3–11. *Nursing's Agenda for Health Care Reform* (ANA, 1992) takes the position that an all-payer system is the one most likely to work for U.S. health care reform.

TABLE 3–9

National Health Care Proposals

	Insurer	Coverage	Finance	Payment
Single-payer system	Government	Universal	Combination of taxes (e.g., income and sales)	Payment fee set by government
All-payer systems	Mix of insurers, government and private	Universal, but there may be some differences in type of care	Combination of taxes and private monies (e.g., employer insurance and out-of-pocket)	Payment fees may be set by government for all or only for special groups

TABLE 3–10

Canadian Health Care System: Myths and Facts

Criticism	Response	Reason
It's socialized medicine.	No.	It is a social insurance plan similar to the U.S. Social Security System and Medicare. Doctors are not state employees, but have a private practice.
Health care is rationed.	Yes and no.	There may be a wait for hospital beds, specialists, and diagnostic tests. Canadians do not have to wait to see their primary physician. Health care is rationed through the primary physician by immediate need vs. delayed need for special services, not by ability to pay. In contrast, in the U.S. system care is rationed by ability to pay (refer to Chapter 5).
There are not enough doctors.	No.	The distribution of physicians is different; about 50% of physicians are primary care–family practice physicians and there is some oversupply in certain provinces. The United States is attempting to create a ratio of primary-care-to-specialist physicians similar to what is already found in Canada.
There are long waits for care.	Maybe.	There is no wait for a primary care physician. Certain high-technology procedures, e.g., lithotripsy, magnetic resonance imaging, and bypass surgery, usually require some waiting. Research into the actual waiting time dispels the notion that there are long gaps before treatment. Hospitals are closing beds, but not because of financial problems with the system. There is an excess of beds. Surveys in all provinces indicate that few hospitals operate at full-bed capacity.
The quality of health care is poor.	No.	As Figure 3–4 shows, during the 1992 Presidential campaign, President Bush cited a Canadian study that indicated surgical outcomes were poorer for Canadians than Americans. The study was misinterpreted. Of the 10 surgical procedures compared, Canadians fared better on 9. Poor results in 1 were a result of transportation problems, not the medical care received.
Administrative costs are greater.	No.	The provider bills the government directly for all services and is paid within a month. Patients neither pay nor are billed for services. Contrast this with the current waiting time for reimbursement from third parties and the amount of energy expended by the patient in filing insurance forms. Another aspect of the same argument is that government is inefficient and more expensive than private administrators. In this country, the administrative costs for Medicare and Medicaid are only 10% of the costs of private insurance administration (see Chapter 5).
The system is troubled by escalating costs.	Yes and no.	The Canadian system has experienced increasing costs, but they will remain below costs in the American system. A review of health care systems in developed countries reveals that all are experiencing rising costs, but that the United States remains well ahead of every other country in this area. Canada controls costs at the source; for example, physician fees are set by negotiation between the health ministry and the physician's organization; patients do not have out-of-pocket expenses. In the United States physicians still engage in balanced billing (in which the patient is billed directly for the difference between the charge and the insurance payment), although Medicare has outlawed this practice.
Physicians earn less.	Yes.	Physicians in all national health systems earn less than U.S. physicians; however, their overhead with respect to administrative costs is less.

Data from Barer, M. L., & Evans, R. G. (1992). Interpreting Canada: Models, mind-sets, and myths. *Health Affairs, 11*(1), 44–61; Roos, L. L., Fisher, E. S., Brazaukas, R., Sharp, S. M., & Shapiro, E. (1992). Health and surgical outcomes in Canada and the United States. *Health Affairs, 11*(2), 56–72; (1992, September). The search for solutions: Does Canada have the right answers? *Consumer Reports,* pp. 579–592.

No health care system is without problems. Each new proposal has advantages and disadvantages. As the country searches for an alternative delivery system it is imperative to examine and debate all plans, including the current model. Criticisms of each should not be taken at face value, but investigated for validity and relevance.

VESTED INTERESTS

Any new proposal has its critics. Among the most vocal are those who have a vested interest in maintaining the status quo. In health care the providers have a lot at stake. Any change will have an impact on practice, and some could reduce profits. The goal of each provider group is to minimize impact on its area of special interest. To that end, groups may engage in efforts to advance proposals with little or no impact on their own operations and defeat or drastically alter those with more stringent controls.

Perhaps because they have the most to lose, the biggest players in the debate over health care reform have been the drug and insurance companies, the AMA, and the hospital industry (Kennedy, 1990). Each works to advance favorable proposals and to defeat plans that have an impact on its own independence or profit. Insurance companies are

TABLE 3–11

National Health Care Selected All-Payer Proposals

Consumer Choice Plan for the 1990s

Provides for managed competition and encourages selection of HMO providers. Individuals would receive a set amount of money to invest in a health plan; the rest would be out-of-pocket expenses. Providers would have an incentive to offer the best benefit package for the least cost. Medicare and Medicaid would continue. Medicaid would pick up those not covered by other means (Enthoven and Kronick, 1989).

Health Access America

Proposed by the AMA. Expands Medicaid to unserved populations and increases reimbursement rates to the level of Medicare. Everyone else remains under current system (National Health Care Campaign, 1990).

"Pay or play" Model

Sets up a fund to provide health insurance (public or private) to the uninsured and underinsured. Employers would be required to provide employees with insurance or pay into the fund. All others would maintain their current insurance plan.

Pepper Commission Plan

Incorporates pay or play, eliminates Medicaid, and places everyone not covered by private plans under Medicare. Recognizes the problems of long-term care by including a program of nursing homes and home care for those in need (U.S. Commission on Comprehensive Health Care, 1990).

especially concerned about the single-payer system, although physician and hospital groups are also opposed.

Nursing and public health have traditionally been more active in supporting consumer rights and universal access to health care. The ANA supported Medicare and Medicaid long before other disciplines did so. Both the ANA and the APHA have been active in support of a national health care system. However, as no profession is completely altruistic, nursing, too, is concerned about protecting its interests (Hamric, 1992).

Several strategies exist to influence the political decision-making process: one is to contribute funds to support the election of sympathetic politicians in an effort to influence policy and regulation of health care. The health industry contributed $16.3 million to the 1990 congressional candidates; 60% of those funds came from a few organizations, including the ANA. The ANA share represented a mere 1.7% of the total (Table 3–12). Lobbying is another way to advance an agenda and is not as easy to track as campaign contributions. As the debate on national health care continues, pay particular attention to news accounts of lobbying activity. Look for each organization's budget for lobbying activities, and scan newspapers and television for organization-sponsored advertisements about health care plans.

Influencing the President, his or her task force, and Congress is an accepted part of the political process. Nurses need to become more astute in evaluating the impact of personal interests on any organization's position on specific delivery plans and on the information about those plans

TABLE 3–12

Campaign Contributions by Health Care Organization or Industry for 1990 Congressional Campaign

Group	Contribution ($)
Health insurance industry	4,871,001
American Medical Association	2,647,981
Pharmaceutical companies	990,000
American Hospital Association	680,989
American Nurses' Association	290,360
Total	9,480,331

Data from Makinson, L. (1992). Political contributions from the health and insurance industries. *Health Affairs, 11*(4), 119–144.

they supply to the general public. Nurses need to become very active in the political process and to make their voices heard, or risk being excluded.

Challenges for the Future

The health care system is at a crossroads. Public health practitioners have long advocated universal access to health care. Cost concerns point toward retrenchment in funding and service. At the same time the concept of health as a right has gained in popularity. The latter two issues have engendered concern about what direction to take. Supporters of the right to health care wish for expanded services. Supporters of funding reduction seem devoted to service cuts. Change in either direction is vigorously opposed by the other group. We appear to be headed toward either inertia and stalemate or a time of collective community in which we tackle the problem with creativity and drive.

The challenge is to find a way to cut or maintain cost levels and to simultaneously ensure a minimum standard of health for the entire population. The current structure is evolving to meet that expectation. A philosophical shift toward a more community-directed health promotion focus and away from an illness-oriented focus would make that goal more viable. To provide a higher quality of care, competing interests need to form a coalition rather than to concentrate on protecting vested interests.

The years ahead are an exciting time for community nurses. Nursing has always maintained a strong interest in health in addition to caring for the ill. As the emphasis shifts to community-based care with limitated institutional care, the need to maintain health and delay the progress of disease will create increased demand for community nursing service. Community nurses have always enjoyed greater autonomy than their hospital counterparts. The influx of nurses into community practice will assist the nursing profession's movement toward professional independence and integration as a full and equal partner in the health care team.

KEY IDEAS

1. The U.S. health care system is a fragmented, noncentralized arrangement consisting of multiple public and private providers.
2. The cost of health care is paid by a similar system of multiple sources.
3. Community health nurses need to know about both the structure of the health care system and how it operates, because it has significant impact on nursing practice and determines who has access to services and what types of services are available.
4. Although the United States has the most advanced medical technology, qualified personnel, and abundant resources, it does not lead in health status in comparison with other developed countries, and on some specific indicators (e.g., infant mortality) it compares poorly.
5. Acute care, rather than disease prevention or health promotion, has been the major focus of the health care delivery system in the United States.
6. Recognition is growing of the importance of disease prevention as an effective means of improving health status.
7. The crisis in federal, state, and local government budgets has severely decreased the ability of states and local governments to deliver public health services.
8. Cost-containment strategies have been only marginally successful, slowing the rate of increase rather than reducing the cost of care.
9. Cost-containment measures and recognition of the importance of community care will continue to increase the demand for community health services, including community health nursing.
10. Health care is at a crossroads; the nation is considering institution of a national health care system. The decision-making process will be influenced by many players. Vested interests are intent on tailoring change to their advantage.
11. To improve the health status of the country, any decision about the evolving structure of our health care system must ensure a reasonable standard of care for all citizens.

GUIDELINES FOR LEARNING

1. Develop your vision of the ideal health care system. List some of the characteristics which that constitute such a system. What would be the goal or goals of your ideal system?
2. Think about how you would go about implementing your ideal system. Consider some of the problems you are likely to encounter. Identify individuals/groups/organizations with a vested interest in the present system. How might you expect them to react to your proposal?
3. From your current practice identify a chronically ill individual and explore his or her thoughts on the present system. Explore his or her concerns about health care: how needs are being met, expectations of how the illness will affect life in the future, and ideas on what (if anything) should be changed about the current method of care delivery.
4. Investigate current health-related issues in your community. Arrange an interview, in person or by phone, with the legislator who represents your community in the state legislature, or with a staff member. Explore health-related issues, find out his or her position, and lobby for your position on the issue or issues.
5. Discover which agencies in your state are responsible for the public health of citizens. Do you have a centralized or decentralized management of state responsibilities? Determine some key indicators of health. Compare your state's indicators with those of surrounding states. How does your state fare?
6. You are a community health nurse in the public health department of Coty, a town of approximately 25,000 population on the outskirts of a major metropolitan city. Your health department provides primary obstetrical care to certain prenatal populations. You notice that your clients have a higher infant mortality rate than the national average. The director of public health has authorized you to explore the problem and design a plan that will reduce the infant mortality rate in your area.
   a. How would you start to locate information which might be helpful to your study? Determine if resources for prenatal care are available, accessible, acceptable, adequate, and effective.
   b. What other health issues could have an impact on your problem? Are the surrounding areas having similar problems or are you unique?
   c. What about the local providers of care? What would their concerns be with an intervention plan? If they are opposed how might you structure your plans to reduce opposition?
   d. What types of issues would be essential in constructing an evaluation plan? Can you anticipate potential barriers to an effective evaluation plan?

REFERENCES

AMA initiative on quality of medical care and professional self regulation. (1986). *Journal of the American Medical Association, 256,* 1036–1037.

American Hospital Association. (1990). *Hospital Statistics, 1990–1991.* Chicago: Author.

American Nurses' Association. (1987). *ANA facts about nursing '86–'87.* Kansas City, MO: Author.

American Nurses' Association (1992). *Nursing's agenda for health care reform: Executive summary.* Kansas City, MO: Author.

Anderson, O. W. (1985). *Health services in the United States: A growth enterprise since 1875.* Ann Arbor, MI: Health Administration Press.

Anderson, W. (1991). The New York needle trail: The politics of public health in the age of AIDS. *American Journal of Public Health, 81,* 1506–1517.

Annual Report of Administrator of Veterans Affairs, Directory of VA facilities. (1987). Washington, DC: U.S. Government Printing Office.

ASTHO. (1980). *The Association of State and Territorial Health Officials comprehensive national public health program reporting system report: Services, expenditures, and programs of state and territorial health agencies, fiscal year 1978.* Silver Springs, MD: Author.

Banta, H. D. (1990). What is health care? In A. R. Kovner (ed.). *Health care delivery in the United States.* New York: Springer Publishing Co.

Barer, M. L., & Evans, R. G. (1992). Interpreting Canada: Models, mind-sets, and myths. *Health Affairs, 11*(1), 44–61.

Bates, E. (1983). *Health systems and public scrutiny: Australia, Britain, and the United States.* New York: St. Martin's Press.

Blum, H. (1981). *Planning for health* (2nd ed.). New York: Human Sciences Press.

Brecher, C. (1990). The government's role in health care. In A. R. Kovner (Ed.). *Health care delivery in the United States.* New York: Springer Publishing Co.

Breslow, L. (1990). The future of public health prospects in the United States for the 1990s. *Annual Review of Public Health, 11,* 1–28.

Bureau of Health Professions, Division of Nursing (1986). *The registered nurse population: Findings from the National Sample of Registered Nurses, November 1984.* Washington, DC: DHHS, Resources and Service Administration, Publ. No. HRP-0906938.

Burner, S. T., Waldo, D. R., & McKusick, D. R. (1992). National health expenditures projections through 2030. *Health Care Financing Review, 14*(1), 1–29.

Califano, J. A., Jr., (1986). *America's health care revolution: Who lives? Who dies? Who pays?* New York: Random House.

Congressional Budget Office. (1992). *Economic implications of rising health care costs* (CBO study). Washington, DC: U.S. Government Printing Office.

Directory of nursing homes 1991–1992 (5th ed.). (1991). Phoenix, AZ: Oryx Press.

Ehrenreich, B., & Ehrenreich, J. (1971). *The American health empire: Power, profits, and politics.* New York: Vintage Books.

Enthoven, A., & Kronick, R. (1989). A consumer-choice health plan for the 1990s. *New England Journal of Medicine, 320,* 29–37; 94–101.

Erkel, E. A. (1993). The impact of case management in preventive services. *Journal of Nursing Administration, 23*(1), 27–32.

Feldstein, P. J. (1993). *Health care economics* (4th ed.). West Albany, NY: Delmar Publishers.

Ginzberg, E. (1989). Physician supply in the year 2000. *Health Affairs, 8*(2), 84–90.

Ginzberg, E. (1991). Philanthropy and nonprofit organizations in U.S. health care: A personal retrospective. *Inquiry, 28*(2), 179–186.

Green, L. W., & Anderson, C. L. (1982). Community health (4th ed.). St. Louis, MO: Mosby.

Gunn, S. M., & Platt, P. S. (1945). *Voluntary health agencies: An interpretative study.* New York: Ronald Press Co.

Guydish, J., Clark, G., Garcia, D., Downing, M., Case, P., & Sorensen, J. L. (1991). Evaluating needle exchange: Do distributed needles come back? *American Journal of Public Health, 81*(5), 617–619.

Haggerty, R. J. (1990). The boundaries of health care. In P. R. Lee & C. L. Estes (Eds.). *The nation's health* (3rd ed.). Boston: Jones and Bartlett.

Hamric, A.B. (1992). Resolving the health care crisis: Where is the CNS? *Clinical-Nurse-Specialist, 6*(2):105.

Holahan, J., & Zedlewski, S. (1992). Who pays for health care in the United States? Implications for health system reform. *Inquiry, 29*(2), 231–248.

Illich, I. (1977). *Medical nemesis: The expropriation of health.* Toronto: Bantam Books.

Institute of Medicine. (1988). *The future of public health.* Washington, DC: National Academy Press.

Jones, S. (1981). *Health care delivery in the United States* (2nd ed.). New York: Springer Publishing Co.

Jonsson, B. (1989). What can Americans learn from Europe? *Health Care Financing Review, Annual Supplement,* pp. 79–93.

Kennedy, E. M. (1990). The politics of health. In P. R. Lee & C. L. Estes (Eds.). *The nation's health* (3rd ed.). Boston: Jones and Bartlett.

Koplin, A. N. (1990). The future of public health: A local health department view. *Journal of Public Health Policy, 11*(4), 420–437.

Krausse, E. A. (1977). *Illness: Political sociology of health and medical care.* New York: Elsevier.

Lamm, R. D. (1990). The ten commandments of health care. In P. R. Lee & C. L. Estes (Eds.). *The nation's health* (3rd ed.). Boston: Jones and Bartlett.

Lawrence, R. S., & Jonas, S. (1990). Ambulatory care. A. R. Kovner (Ed.). In *Health care delivery in the United States* (4th ed.). New York: Springer Publishing Co.

Lazerby, H. C, & Letsch, S. W. (1990). National health expenditures 1989. *Health Care Financing Review, 12*(2), 1–26.

Lee, P. R. (1990). AIDS: Allocating resources for research and patient care. In P. R. Lee & C. L. Estes (Eds.). *The nation's health* (3rd ed.). Boston: Jones and Bartlett.

Lefkowitz, B. (1983). *Health planning lessons for the future.* Rockville, MD: Aspen.

Lenz, C. L., & Edwards, J. (1992). Nurse-managed primary care. Tapping the rural community power base. *Journal of Nursing Administration 22*(9), 57–61.

Levine, E., Leatt, P., & Poulton, K. (1993). *Nursing practice in the UK and North America.* London: Chapman and Hall.

Lindblom, C. E. (1953). *Politics, economics, and welfare.* New York: Harper Press.

Litman, T. J. (1990). *Government and health: The political aspects of health care — a sociopolitical overview.* In P. R. Lee & C. L. Estes (Eds.). *The nation's health* (3rd ed.). Boston: Jones and Bartlett.

Makinson, L. (1992). Political contributions from the health and insurance industries. *Health Affairs, 11*(4), 119–144.

McKeown, T. (1976). *The role of Medicare: Dream, mirage, or nemesis.* London: The Nutfield Provincial Hospitals Trust.

Mechanic, D. (1986). *From advocacy to allocation: The evolving American health care system.* New York: The Free Press.

Milio, N. (1981). *Promoting health through public policy.* Philadelphia: F. A. Davis.

Milio, N. (1983). *Primary care and the public's health.* Lexington, KY: Lexington Books.

Miller, C. A., Brooks, E. F., DeFriese, G. H., Gilbert, B. J., Sagar, C., & Kavaler, F. (1977). A survey of local public health departments and their directors. *American Journal of Public Health, 67,* 931–939.

Morrisey, M. A., Sloan, F. A., & Valvona, J. (1988). Shifting Medicare patients out of the hospital. *Health Affairs, 7*(5), 52–64.

National Association for Home Care (1989). *1990 National home care and hospital directory* (2nd ed.). Washington, DC: Author.

National Center for Health Statistics. (1988). *United States Health Status, 1987* (DHHS Publication No. (PHS) 88–1232). Washington, DC: U.S. Government Printing Office.

National Commission on Community Health Services. (1967). *Health administration and organization in the decade ahead.* Cambridge, MA: Harvard University Press.

National Health Care Campaign. (1990). *AMA—health access campaign* (summary). Washington, DC: Author.

Occupational outlook handbook, 1992–93 edition. (U.S. Department of Labor Statistics bulletin 2400) (1992). Washington, DC: U.S. Government Printing Office.

Pickett, G., & Hanlon, J. J. (1990). *Public health administration and practice.* St. Louis: Mosby–Year Book.

Porter, M., Ball, P., & Kraus, N. (1992). *The interstudy competitive edge* (Vol. 1, No. 2). Excelsion, MNL.

Public Health Service, Health Resources and Services Administration (1990). *Seventh Report to the President and Congress on the status of health personnel in the U.S.*

Raffel, M. W., & Raffel, N. K. (1989). *The U.S. health system: Origins and functions* (3rd ed.). New York: Wiley.

Reed, G. B. (1991). On-site health-monitoring program keeps "lifestyle" diseases in check. *Occupational Health and Safety, 60*(10), 56,59–62.

Reif, L., & Estes, C. L. (1984). Long term care: New opportunities for professional nursing. In P. R. Lee, C. L. Estes, & N. B. Ramsay (Eds.). *The nation's health* (2nd ed.). San Francisco: Boyd and Fraser.

Reinhardt, U. E. (1986). Rationing the health care surplus. *Nurse Economics, 4*(May/June), 101-108.

Reinhardt, U. E. (1990). Rationing the health care surplus: An American tragedy. In P. R. Lee & C. L. Estes (Eds.). *The nation's health* (3rd ed.). Boston: Jones and Bartlett.

Relman, A. S. (1990). The new medical-industrial complex. In P. R. Lee & C. L. Estes (Eds.). *The nation's health* (3rd ed.). Boston: Jones and Bartlett.

Rodgers, J., Grower, R., & Supino, P. (1992). Participant evaluation and cost of a community-based health promotion program for elders. *Public Health Reports, 107*(4), 417–426.

Rodwin, V. G. (1990). Competitive health systems: A policy perspective. In A. R. Kovner (Ed.). *Health care delivery in the United States* (4th ed.). New York: Springer Publishing Co.

Roemer, M. I. (1986). *An introduction to the United States health care system* (2nd ed.). New York: Springer Publishing Co.

Roemer, M. I. (1991). *National health care systems of the world.* New York: Oxford University Press.

Roemer, R., Kramer, C., & Frink, J. E. (1975). Planning urban health service: From jungle to system. New York: Springer Publishing Co.

Roos, L. L., Fisher, E. S., Brazaukas, R., Sharp, S. M., & Shapiro, E. (1992). Health and surgical outcomes in Canada and the United States. *Health Affairs, 11*(2), 56–72.

Rydman, L. D., & Rydman, R. J. (1983). The United States health care delivery system. In W. Burgess & E. C. Ragland (Eds.). *Community health nursing: Philosophy, process, and practice,* Norwalk, CT: Appleton-Century-Crofts.

Salloway, J. C. (1982). *Health care delivery systems.* Boulder, CO: Westview Press.

Scheffler, R., Sullivan, S., & Ko, T. (1991). The impact of Blue Cross and Blue Shield utilization management programs, 1980–1988. *Inquiry, 28*(3), 263–275.

Scheffler, R. M., Feuchtbaum, L. B., & Phibbs, C. S. (1992). Prevention: The cost-effectiveness of the California diabetes and pregnancy program. *American Journal of Public Health, 82*(2), 165–178.

Schieber, G. J., Poullier, J. P., & Greenwald, L. M. (1991). Health care systems in 24 countries. *Health Affairs, 10*(3), 23–38.

Schlag, W. A., & Piktialis, D. S. (1987). HMOs and the elderly: The potential for vertical integration of geriatric care. *Quality Review Bulletin 13*(4), 140–147.

Schoeder, S. S. (1992). Physician supply and demand in the U.S. medical marketplace. *Health Affairs, 11*(1), 235–243.

Smith, D. B., & Kaluzny, A. D. (1986). *The white labyrinth: A guide to the health care system* (2nd ed.). Ann Arbor, MI: Health Administration Press.

Sorkin, A. L. (1986). Health care and the changing economic environment. Lexington, MA: Lexington Books.

Stevens, P. E. (1993). Who gets health care: Access to health care as an arena for nursing action. In B.A. Kos-Munson (Ed.). *Who gets health care: An arena for nursing action.* New York: Springer Publishing Co.

Stifler, L. T. (1991). Preventive health programs attract industry. *Hospitals, 65*(5), 68.

Tallan, J. R., & Nathan, R. P. (1992). A federal/state partnership for health system reform. *Health Affairs, 11*(4), 7–16.

The search for solutions: Does Canada have the right answer? (1992, September). *Consumer Reports,* pp. 579–592.

Torrens, P. R. (1978). *The American health care system: Issues and problems.* St. Louis, MO: Mosby.

U.S. Bipartisan Commission on Comprehensive Health Care. (1990). *A call to action — final report.* Washington, DC: U.S. Government Printing Office.

U.S. Bureau of Labor Statistics. (1990). *Employee benefits in medium and large firms, 1989* (Bulletin No. 2363). Washington, DC: U.S. Government Printing Office.

U.S. Public Health Service. (1979). *Healthy people: The Surgeon General's Report on Health Promotion and Disease Prevention* (DHEW Publication No. 79–55071). Washington, DC: Office of Assistant Secretary for Health and Surgeon General.

U.S. Public Health Service, Health Resources and Services Administration. (1990). Seventh report to the President and Congress on the status of health personnel in the U.S. (DHHS Publication No. HRS–P–OD–90–1). Washington, DC: U.S. Government Printing Office.

Walker, B. (1992). The future of public health. *Public Health Policy Forum, 82*(1), 21–23.

Wilensky, H. L. (1975). *Welfare state and equality: Structural and ideological roots of public expenditures.* Berkeley: University of California Press.

Williams, S. J., & Torrens, P. R. (Eds.). (1993). *Introduction to health services* (4th ed.). Albany, NY: Delmar.

BIBLIOGRAPHY

Altman, S., & Jackson, T. (1991). Health care in Australia: Lessons from down under. *Health Affairs, 10*(3), 129–146.

Barer, M. L., Welch, W. P., & Anticoh, L. (1991). Canadian/U.S. health care: Reflections on the HIAA's analysis. *Health Affairs, 10*(3), 229–236; (discussion) 237–239.

Holahan, J., & Zedlewski, S. (1992). *Who pays for health care in the United States? Implications for health system reform.* Washington, DC: Health Policy Center, Urban Institute.

Hurst, J. W. (1991). Reforming health care in seven European countries. *Health Affairs, 10*(3), 7–21.

Ikegami, N. (1991). Japanese health care: Low cost through regulated fees. *Health Affairs, 10*(3), 87–109.

Inglehart, J. K. (1992). The American health care system. Managed care. *New England Journal of Medicine, 327,* 742–747.

Kover, A. R. (Ed.). (1990). *Health care delivery in the United States.* New York: Springer.

Lee, P. R., & Estes, C. L. (Eds.). (1990). *The nation's health.* Boston: Jones and Bartlett.

Lohr, K. N., Yordy, K., Harrison, P. F., & Gelinjs, A. C. (1992). Health care systems: Lessons from international comparisons. *Health Affairs, 11,* 238–241.

Roemer, M. I. (1991). *National health systems of the world.* New York: Oxford University Press.

Roemer, J. I. (1993). *National health systems of the world. Vol. II. The issues.* New York: Oxford University Press.

SUGGESTED READINGS

UNITED STATES HEALTH CARE SYSTEM

DeLaw, N., Greenberg, G., & Kinchen, K. (1992). A layman's guide to the U.S. health care system. *Health Care Financing Review, 14*(1), 151–169.

Lee, P. R., & Estes, C. L. (Eds.). (1990). *The nation's health.* Boston: Jones and Bartlett.

HEALTH CARE SYSTEM REFORM AND COMPARISON OF NATIONAL HEALTH CARE SYSTEMS

McMahon, J. A. (1992). The health care system in the year 2000: Three scenarios. *Academic Medicine, 67*(1), 1–7.

Schieber, G. J., Pouilier, J. P., & Greenwald, L. M. (1991). Health care reform in 24 countries. *Health Affairs, 10*(3), 22–38.

Tallon, J. R., & Nathan, R. P. (1992). A federal/state partnership for health system reform. *Health Affairs, 11*(4), 7–16.

CURRENT AND FUTURE STATUS OF PUBLIC HEALTH

Breslow, L. (1990). The future of public health: Prospects in the United States for the 1990s. *Annual Review of Public Health, 11,* 1–28.

Evans, C. A., Jr. The IOM report: The future of public health: Comments. *Journal of Public Health Policy, 11*(1): 254–256.

Hinman, A. R. (1990). 1889 to 1989: A century of health and disease. *Public Health Reports, 105,* 374–380.

Keck, C. W. (1990). The IOM report: The future of public health: Comments. *Journal of Public Health Policy, 11*(1): 257–258.

Koplin, A. N. (1990). The future of public health: A local health department view. *Journal of Public Health Policy, 11,* 420–437.

McBeath, W. H. (1991). Health for all: A public health vision. *American Journal of Public Health, 81,* 1560–1565.

McGinnis, J. M. (1990). Setting objectives for public health in the 1990s: Experience and prospects. *Annual Review of Public Health, 11,* 231–249.

Terris, M. (1992). Budget cutting and privatization: The threat to health. *Journal of Public Health Policy, 13*(1), 27–41.

Thorpe, K. E. (1992). Inside the black box of administrative costs. *Health Affairs, 11*(2), 41–55.

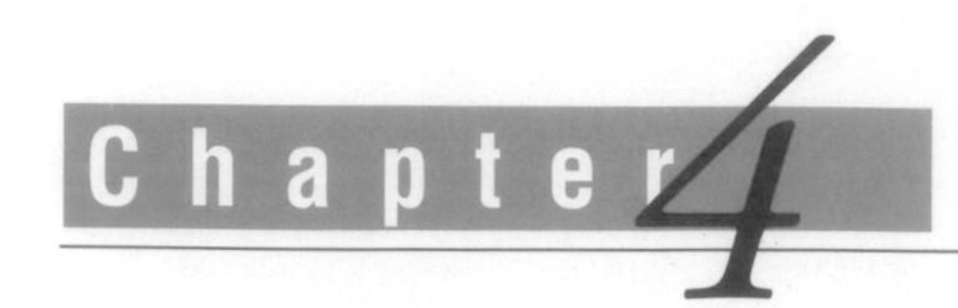

Legal Context for Community Health Nursing Practice

Penny S. Brooke

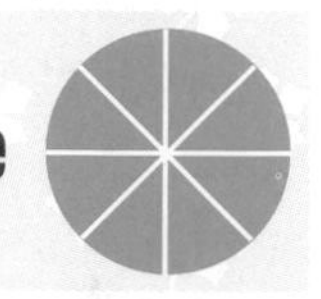

Continued

Focus Questions

How are basic legal issues relevant in community health nursing practice?

What are the sources and purposes of public health law?

What are the responsibilities or legal duties of community health nurses related to public health law?

When may a community health nurse not be covered by the employer's professional liability insurance?

What are the responsibilities of community health nurses in being accountable for their own practice?

How are legal and ethical issues alike and different?

Public Health Law

Public health law consists of all legislation, regulations, and court decisions enacted by federal, state, and local governments to protect the public's health. Public health laws identify the policies and procedures that guide the fair process of preventing disease and promoting health. The rights of individuals are balanced with the need to protect the entire public (Beauchamp, 1985).

Under the authority of the U.S. Constitution, federal public health law exists to promote the general welfare of society (Pickett and Hanlon, 1990). Because states retain those powers not delegated to the federal government, much of public health law remains under state jurisdiction. Therefore, there is variation among states regarding specific public health laws. A local jurisdiction, such as a county, a city, or a township, receives its authority from the state to enact public health law.

Each level of government (federal, state, and local) has a legislative, executive, and judicial branch. Each branch is a source of public health law.

Statutory law is enacted through the legislative branch and declares as lawful or prohibits certain behaviors or actions. Laws from the legislative branches of the federal and state governments are called *statutes.* Similar laws from local governments are usually called *ordinances.* Statutes often authorize new health initiatives and appropriate tax funds to implement the law. Community health nurses influence the political process by lobbying legislators for or against specific statutes and ordinances.

Administrative law consists of orders, rules, and regulations promulgated by the administrative branches of governments. As an example, the state board of nursing is the administrative body that regulates the practice of nursing. Other examples of administrative bodies are the U.S. Department of Health and Human Services and state and local health departments. Administrative law often spells out in more detail the policies and procedures necessary to implement statutes. Community health nurses influence the development of administrative law by initiating ideas and commenting on proposed regulations during periods for public review.

Judicial or common law is developed by means of court decisions (i.e., judge and jury decisions). The similarities and differences between the facts and law in previously decided cases are compared with the current factual situation before the court. The values and customs of society are reflected in court decisions.

Community Health Nurses and Public Health Law

"Everything that is done in a health agency has a basis in law and is subject to legal sanctions of one type or another" (Pickett and Hanlon, 1990, p. 158). Also, official (government) health agencies often enforce laws in addition to providing health services.

An "ounce of prevention" is as important for legal issues as health care issues. Community health nurses most often work very autonomously without the opportunity for on-site immediate collaboration with other nurses or members of the health care team. Nurses as professionals are accountable for the nursing judgments they make. It is wiser to admit that one does not have all of the answers to a client's health care questions than to give inaccurate responses. Consumers have begun to question their health care providers and are demanding a high standard of care. They still see nurses as trustworthy experts in their field and rely on what nurses tell them. Few lawsuits alleging negligence or malpractice have been brought against community health nurses (Brent, 1988; Northrop, 1985). However, if a client is harmed because of a nurse's action, inaction, or incorrect advice, the nurse can be held legally accountable for the resulting injury.

Not only do community health nurses need to understand the legal protections and rights of the public, they also need to be able to advocate for themselves. Protection of professional practice includes not allowing oneself to be placed in compromising positions wherein one is expected to practice outside the scope of nursing. The Nurse Practice Act in each state defines what is legally within the scope of nursing practice. Community health nurses are accountable for working within this legal framework. A copy of this statute should be available through employers, the state nurses' association, or the state board of nursing.

This chapter broadly describes legal issues in community health nursing; the rights of the public or clients and the rights of the nurse are discussed throughout. Laws are written to mutually protect the rights of both nurses and their clients. If nurses work within the guidelines of the law, safe care will be provided, benefiting both the client and the nurse. Federal laws and regulations apply to persons throughout the United States, whereas state and local laws apply within the respective state and local jurisdictions. It is important for nurses to become aware of the laws for which they will be held accountable in their state. For example state or public agencies may be protected by immunity statutes, whereas private agencies may not be included in these statutory protections. Specific facts and legal issues of case law are used to evaluate potential liability and are constantly changing. Therefore, it is impossible to rely solely on a chapter such as this to understand all of the liability issues associated with community health nursing. It is the responsibility of individual nurses to familiarize themselves with specific laws in their state, such as the Nurse Practice Act and the state board of nursing rules and regulations. Today's nurses have become more mobile, and it is not unusual for a nurse to have worked in several states very early in her or his career. Laws do differ from state to state, but ignorance is no defense for a violation of a statute, rule, or regulation.

Sources of Law

American society prides itself on the freedoms Americans enjoy and on the participation of its citizens in setting laws and policies. Citizens most often participate through voting for representatives or by serving as a jury member. However, law is not made only by legislators. When serving on a policy-making committee of a state board of nursing, the nurse has the opportunity to affect nursing practice much like a legislator. All law that governs society is designed to maintain order and to inform all who are accountable to the law exactly what is expected behavior, and what behavior will not be allowed.

Laws are written to carry out the wishes of the majority of the people and to protect the rights of the minority. Environmental and public health issues are of special concern and interest to communities. Therefore, laws in these areas are usually enacted by the legislative and administrative bodies of the individual states. Federal lawmakers provide the guidelines or the "umbrella" laws. States must abide by federal laws and must avoid enacting state statutes that conflict with federal guidelines. Both state and federal courts write case law or common law, which reflects society's current beliefs regarding what is in the best interest of public welfare. Sometimes the laws that nurses must work within lend themselves to varied interpretations. In these cases agencies must seek the opinion of their state's attorney general.

Rules, regulations, and statutes guide the community health nurse and are references with which the nurse must become familiar. A specific law cannot be read in isolation; a wider scope is needed to understand the nurse's total legal responsibilities. For example, when reporting communicable diseases, both state and federal laws must be considered.

In addition local ordinances and regulations also apply. Table 4–1 provides examples of public health law from all three levels of government that a community health nurse may encounter in caring for a family.

STATE AND LOCAL STATUTES

There are many public health statutes enacted by state legislatures that are of concern to community health nurses. Statutes seek to protect the rights of both the health care provider and the consumer. Nurse Practice Acts are broad frameworks within which the legal scope of nursing practice is defined. Many states also have statutes defining malpractice actions against health care providers that pertain to community health nurses. Within these statutes can be found the applicable statute of limitations for malpractice actions or the timeframe within which a legal action must be brought. Often, the specific procedures for bringing a lawsuit against a health care provider are also defined within these malpractice statutes. Statutes regarding informed consent require that the nurse explain significant risks, benefits, and available alternatives before immunizing clients at a clinic offered by a community health agency.

State legislatures also enact statutes under health codes that describe laws for reporting communicable diseases, laws regarding school immunizations, and additional laws directed toward promoting health and reducing health risks in the community. Even the records required to be kept by health care providers may be described within a state's health code. State laws also usually address actions to be taken in reporting child abuse or neglect and the penalties associated with failure to report known or suspected cases of abuse. A growing number of states have enacted confidential communications protections for sexual abuse acts. Immunity from legal action is afforded to health care providers who report, in good faith, suspected abuse of a client to a legal authority. Statutes also define penalties for not reporting known cases of abuse.

Statutes affording protection for privileged communication of confidential information learned in the professional role may, but do not always, include the community health nurse. It is important for nurses to be aware of the protections afforded in their state to nurse-client confidential communications. If a state's statutes do not entitle nurses to a nurse-client privilege, nurses will not be able to hold all communications with clients confidential. A court in such a state can demand that the nurse divulge information learned from a client. In most states, nurse-

TABLE 4–1

Examples of Law Affecting Clients and Nursing Practice

Community Health Situation: A student nurse is asked to assess a family of five: a mother, age 36, caring for a 2-month-old infant; a 6-yr-old child in school; a maternal grandmother, 65, with diabetes; and a son, 21, who works as a short-order cook. The mother receives Aid to Families with Dependent Children (AFDC) for the two youngest children. She desires to keep another youngster in her home. Neighbors have complained about the noisy dogs. The 21-yr-old has been diagnosed by stool culture as being infected with salmonella.

	Sources of Law Applicable		
Level of Government	Legislative Law	Administrative Law	Judicial Law
Federal	Medicare for grandmother	Forms and information necessary for clients to enroll; delegates authority to implement	Decisions regarding sexual discrimination in Social Security payments
	Medicaid for those on AFDC	Same as above	
	Food stamps	Same as above	
State	Daycare licensing needed	Details regarding who orients mothers for daycare and what is included	
	Immunization requirements for 6-yr-old	Interpretation of what constitutes "initial series" of immunizations for various ages	Court decisions regarding religious exemptions from immunizations
	Reportable diseases (Salmonella) under General Welfare; may detail that those with infectious diseases cannot handle food	Delegates authority to implement programs to protect the public's health	
	Nurse Practice Act enables students to practice	State board of nursing issues rules and regulations to allow student learners to practice nursing	
Local	Nuisances (dogs)	Procedure for hearings	Previous decisions regarding nuisances
	Leash laws; requirements for rabies vaccinations		

From Claudia M. Smith, RN, C, MPH, Assistant Professor, University of Maryland School of Nursing.

client communications do not have the privilege of confidentiality.

A community health nurse must be aware of the state's laws pertaining to family privacy matters, such as abortion, distribution of contraceptives to minors, and family violence. Clients may very likely seek advice on these matters. Community health nurses may also be asked to explain a living will statute, if one exists in their state, and the uses of a durable power of attorney (see Chapter 29). Statutes that require specific behaviors, such as the procedures for pronouncing a patient dead or reporting child abuse, vary among states. A practicing attorney from each state can clarify the specific expectations of a community health nurse in that state.

FEDERAL STATUTES

Federal statutes should also be of interest to community health nurses. The Public Health Service and the Centers for Disease Control and Prevention (CDC) were created by Congress specifically for the purpose of coordinating the collection, sharing, and analyzing of data from all of the states and the U.S. territories on certain diseases. Guidelines for dealing with legal issues pertaining to the reporting requirements, such as the importance of maintaining confidentiality, are issued by the CDC. The Occupational Safety and Health Administration (OSHA) also provides guidelines for safe and healthy work environments.

Examples of federal statutes that must be understood by community health nurses include the Social Security Act and its amendments. Within these Social Security amendments, the enactment of the Medicare and Medicaid programs is of specific interest to community health clients (see Chapter 5). Community health clients who are eligible for either Medicaid or Services for Children with Special Health Care Needs (formerly Crippled Children's Services) should also be made aware of the Early and Periodic Screening Diagnosis and Treatment (EPSDT) Program. These programs are discussed in detail in Chapter 26. Without an adequate knowledge base or understanding of federally enacted programs, community health nurses may neglect to inform a client of existing federal programs for which the client qualifies. Children who qualify for EPSDT are eligible to receive immunizations, eye examinations, hearing tests, and dental care. Countless previously undiagnosed conditions may be discovered and treated as a result of this early diagnosis and screening program. Other examples of federal statutory law are included in Table 4–2.

TABLE 4–2

Federally Legislated Public Health Laws

Title	Purpose	Impact of Law
Social Security Act and Amendments		
Social Security of 1935 (PL 74–271) Title I Grants to States for Old Age Assistance	To enable each state to furnish financial assistance to aged needy individuals.	Also created: Title II, Federal Old Age Benefit—payment to persons over 65 based on their wage; benefits are to be paid to the estate if the person dies before age 65; Title III, Unemployment Compensation; Title IV, Aid to Dependent Children; Title V, Maternal-Child Welfare—to promote health, especially rural health of women and children; Title VI, Public Health Work—established to maintain public health services, including training of personnel; Title VII, the Social Security Board; Title VIII, Taxes With Respect to Employment; Title IX, Tax on employers with eight or more employees; Title X, Grants to States for Aid to the Blind; Title XI, General Provisions.
Maternal and Child Health and Retardation Amendments of 1963 (PL 88–156)	Amends the Social Security Act to assist states and communities in preventing and combating retardation.	Expanded and improved maternal and child health in Services for Children with Special Health Care Needs; provides prenatal, maternity, and infant care to plan for comprehensive action to combat mental retardation.
Social Security Amendments of 1965 (PL 87–97), Title XIX: Grants to States For Medical Assistance Program	Provided funding to states to establish medical assistance for the needy as defined under the act.	Established a state plan to provide medical assistance to families with dependent children; the aged; the blind; and permanently and totally disabled individuals whose income and resources are insufficient to meet the costs of necessary medical care; also established rehabilitation services to assist clients in obtaining or retaining the capacity for independence or self-care.
Social Security Amendments of 1965 (PL 87–97), Title XVIII: Health Insurance for the Aged (known as Medicare). (Tied into Railroad Retirement Act of 1937)	Established hospital and medical insurance benefits for persons over the age of 65 who are residents of the U.S. (i.e., a citizen or lawful alien [permanent resident who has resided continually in the U.S. during the preceding 5 years]).	Provides access to health institutions of the patient's choice (agencies must qualify to be eligible for payment for patient services); patients retain the option to obtain other additional health insurance, as coverage period is limited and benefits may vary from year to year. A monthly premium is paid, and routine physical check-ups and hearing or sight aids are excluded.
Social Security Amendments of 1977—Health Clinic Services (PL 95–210)	Authorizes reimbursement for clinic services in rural areas designated as a "health manpower shortage area."	Clinics who employ physician assistants or nurse practitioners are eligible for reimbursement under Medicare or Medicaid if the patient population is below 3,000 or there are no physicians practicing within 5 miles of the clinic.
Public Health Services Act and Amendments		
Public Health Services Act of 1944 (PL 78–410)	Created federally coordinated departments to address the public health needs of the nation; established the office of the Surgeon General and the National Institutes of Health, The Bureau of Medical Services, and the Bureau of State Services. The divisions created are administered by the Surgeon General.	Power to establish divisions was given to the Surgeon General, who serves as the administrator of the Public Health Services Act.
Special Health Revenue Sharing Act of 1975 (PL 94–63)	Amended the Public Health Service Act and related health laws to revise and extend the health revenue sharing program, providing comprehensive public health services. Grants to state health and mental authorities were made to assist with the cost of providing care.	Programs affected by these block grants include family planning programs; community mental health center programs, including the requirements for the mental health centers; programs and centers for migrant worker health; community health centers; and miscellaneous home health services, mental health and illness of the elderly; the National Health Service Corps program; commissions on epilepsy, Huntington's disease, and hemophilia programs; assistance for nurse training and for other purposes such as the advanced nurse training and nurse practice programs, special projects, grants, and contracts.

TABLE 4–2

Federally Legislated Public Health Laws *Continued*

Title	Purpose	Impact of Law
Social Services		
Omnibus Budget Reconciliation Act of 1981 (PL 97–35) Block Grants for Social Services	Created to consolidate federal assistance to states for social services into a single grant to increase the states' flexibility in using grants to achieve the goals of preventing, reducing or eliminating dependency; achieving or maintaining self-sufficiency; or preventing or remedying neglect, abuse, and exploitation of children and adults unable to protect their own interests; to rehabilitate and reunite families and provide for community home-based care. Procurement of referrals for institutions when other forms of care are not appropriate are also a purpose under this title. The Maternal and Child Health Services Block Grant was created to ensure low-income persons with limited availability for health services access to quality maternal and child health services. Subtitle C block grants for social services consolidated federal assistance to the states for social services into a single grant to increase states' flexibility in using the grant money to achieve their goals.	Increased flexibility for states in coverage of and services for the medically needy. Human Services affected by Title VI include education of the handicapped; vocational rehabilitation programs; handicapped programs and services; older Americans' domestic volunteers and senior companion programs; child abuse prevention and treatment; the community services program; urban and rural special impact programs; supportive programs to Head Start; Title VIII, School Lunch and Nutrition Programs; Title IX, Health Services Facilities; rodent control; fluoridation programs; hypertension; developmental disabilities; research; health planning and maintenance; adolescent family; alcohol and drug programs; Title XXI Medicare, Medicaid, and maternal and child health reimbursement changes (changes in services and benefits). Title XXII Federal Old-Age Survivors and Disability Insurance Program newly defined benefits; Title XXIII, Aid to Families and Dependent Children (AFDC)—past-due child support can be collected from federal tax refunds.

Data from the *U.S. Code, Congressional and Administrative News* (1935, 1937, 1944, 1963, 1965, 1975, 1977, 1981). St. Paul, MN: West Publishers.

ADMINISTRATIVE RULES AND REGULATIONS

Rules and regulations are established by administrative bodies of government, such as licensing boards and regulatory agencies. Administrative bodies, including state nursing boards and health departments, are composed of experts in the field who are considered to be better prepared than the average layperson to make decisions regarding the specific rules and regulations of safe practice. The authority to promulgate rules and regulations is delegated to the administrative body from the legislative branch of government, such as Congress and state legislatures. Very often the rules and regulations enacted by the administrative body are intended to provide the details or clarification of a broader statute enacted by the legislature. As an example the Nurse Practice Act in most states provides broad guidelines defining the scope of nursing practice. The more specific rules and regulations promulgated by the state nursing board help to fill in the necessary details to give guidance to nurses in the state. Administrative rules and regulations cannot conflict with the statute they seek to interpret, yet the details that the rules and regulations provide can be very powerful in defining the scope of practice of nursing in the state. Regulations also provide guidelines for how to work within the health care system (e.g., how to make an application to receive Medicare or Medicaid and even who may apply).

Administrative law making, the promulgation of rules and regulations, is usually preceded by notice of the proposed rule or regulation. An opportunity to provide input is also given to those who will be affected. For example nurses are affected by the state board of nursing rules and regulations, and interested nurses may provide input in writing or attend a hearing specifically held to discuss the proposed rule or regulation.

Administrative law bodies are often empowered to revoke or suspend professional licenses. Suspected violations of the Nurse Practice Act or of administrative rules or regulations, or other charges brought against a nurse related to professional practice, are heard and decided by the state board of nursing. The decision of the administrative rule-making body may usually be appealed to the state court system. Community health nursing issues must be understood by the administrative bodies that regulate nursing practice.

If a community health nurse is required to perform a medical procedure that is beyond the scope of nursing practice, the nurse or supervisor can receive clarification from the state board of nursing. A nurse, for example, should not be asked to instruct school bus personnel or teachers of disabled children about replacement of an outer cannula for a tracheostomy. The nurse needs to consider safety factors and appropriateness of the information shared with untrained personnel. Refusal to perform questionable duties until clarification is received should be considered reasonable and safe practice, not insubordination.

An example of administrative rules and regulations that protect the public are those promulgated by OSHA. The occupational safety of workers is central to maintaining a healthy workforce, and employers must comply with the regulations that define a safe and healthy work environment. For example employers of health care workers are required to provide protective equipment and conduct inservice education regarding universal precautions to prevent the spread of human immunodeficiency virus (HIV) and hepatitis B virus.

JUDICIAL OR COMMON LAW

Common or judicial law is based on common usage, custom, and court rulings called *case precedents.* Case precedents are useful for interpreting statutory language and for comparative purposes. The facts of a current case and those of preexisting, previously ruled on, legal cases are evaluated for similarities and differences. The cases of most interest to community health nurses would be those lawsuits in their specific state that involve circumstances very similar to the practice of community health nursing in their institution or agency. For example court decisions may provide support for exemptions from immunizations based on a person's religious beliefs; nurses would need to understand the specific facts of a case to safely compare their own situation or likelihood of liability. Cases from other states or from federal District Court can also be used but do not usually carry the same weight as cases actually settled in the community health nurse's state.

In legal suits brought against community health nurses, an expert witness is called on to testify to the reasonableness of the professional behavior of the community health nurse who is the defendant in the case. Case precedent can be used to understand the standards expected in the community health nurse's practice. Case law involving community health nurses has dealt with communicable diseases; Medicaid regulations; medication administration, especially as related to immunizations; and the treatment provided directly by or under the supervision of the nurse. These cases involve negligence, product liability, and informed consent issues (Northrop and Kelly, 1987). A nurse's response to an asthmatic child in school demonstrates liability risks for school nurses; the case study later in this chapter serves as an example. The elements of negligence will be discussed in greater detail later in this chapter.

Existing cases have shown that community health nurses must become aware of informed consent legislation in their state. Because community health nurses work autonomously in the field, the acquisition of informed consent may become the nurse's responsibility. Consent to treat a child must be obtained from the parent or legal guardian or custodian of the child. However, to truly provide informed consent, the patient or parent must be given enough information to understand the consequences of his or her decision. For example the significant risks, benefits, and alternatives of immunizations must be disclosed prior to obtaining consent.

Roles that the community health nurse assumes become legally binding duties and must be undertaken responsibly. Some community health nurses may be required to perform laboratory tests such as phenylketonuria testing. Failure to adequately inform a patient or guardian or performing a test improperly may lead to a liability suit. Nursing judgments, such as the assessment of an individual's condition and the documentation of signs and symptoms supporting the nursing inferences, may be critical in deciding the severity of the illness or describing adverse reaction to prescribed treatments. For example, when providing home health care to ill persons, blood pressure readings that are outside normal parameters must be reported to the physician or nurse practitioner. The community health nurse may be the only person in actual physical contact with the community health client, and therefore, communication between the health department, physician, or other members of the health care team and the community health nurse is critical. The importance of accuracy and timeliness of communication has been tested in many legal cases involving nurses.

Community health nurses may find themselves involved in the process of judicial or common law in one of several roles. As a defendant, the nurse is accused of causing harm to another; as an expert witness, the nurse testifies as to the standard of care in community health nursing; and as a general witness, the nurse testifies regarding the specific facts at issue in a case. The facts of a case at trial are compared with the facts of existing case law. The standard in the jurisdiction is determined by previous case precedence. If the nurse is planning to rely on a previously decided case as a standard, it must be validated—legally called *shepardized*—to ensure that it is still current law in good standing. Case law reflects the changes in society's views; cases may be overturned or overruled and therefore no longer be safely relied on as the law in that state. The expertise of an attorney who practices specifically in health care law is recommended when evaluating the current validity of existing cases. Whether the political or social climate of a community is stable or changing, these community standards will usually be reflected in the case law of the courts.

Community health nurses currently enjoy greater autonomy and an expanded scope of nursing practice that brings additional professional accountability. Court cases relating to the practice of community health nursing will most likely increase as society recognizes the independent nursing judgments and the autonomous decision making that occur in community health nursing. Respondeat superior and vicarious liability (i.e., being responsible for another's actions), which transfers liability from the nurse to the physician or the health department, has been replaced by individual accountability for a nurse's own professional actions. Supervisory liability, as previously mentioned, is one of the few times that vicarious liability occurs in current case law. As a supervisor of nurse's aides or LPNs in an agency, a community health nurse must not delegate tasks to these workers that are beyond the scope of their knowledge base or the legal scope of their practice. If they harm a patient while providing nursing care, the community health nurse's professional judgment when delegating such tasks will be assessed to determine whether it was reasonable.

ATTORNEY GENERAL OPINIONS

In many states the attorney general for the state is the official legal counselor for public agencies, including health departments. If the public health nurse has questions pertaining to the legality of procedures or the scope of nursing practice within the state, the agency can clarify these issues with the attorney general. The state attorney general can provide both informal and formal opinions. If the legal issue is of such concern that the nurse believes the liability risks are great, a formal written opinion should be requested.

The state attorney general's opinions provide guidelines based on both statutory and common law interpretations. Sometime statutes are written in such vague terms that the application or interpretation of the law is difficult to ascertain. The attorney general's office evaluates the written law, including its legislative history, and provides an opinion as to how the law should be applied. If a legal issue arises and the community health nurse has a formal written attorney general's opinion offering an interpretation of a particular issue or statute, the court will most likely view the nurse or the agency as having acted reasonably and responsibly in seeking clarification of what behavior is legal. If the nurse or the agency responded in a manner in conformity with the attorney general's opinion, the court will usually consider this action favorably on behalf of the nurse or agency named as defendant in a lawsuit, when the reasonableness of the behavior is being evaluated.

The basic underlying principle is that a nurse should be able to rely on the professional advice of legal counsel. An attorney general's opinion may differ from a second opinion from the same office or an opinion from another attorney at a later date. Sometimes there are political influences in an attorney general's office, as this is an elected office and the legal staff is often chosen by the successful candidate. Political issues such as abortion and contraception for adolescents may receive differing interpretations by different individuals in the same office.

CONTRACTS

A contract is an agreement between two persons who have the legal capacity and are competent to join into a binding agreement that is recognized under the law. Contracts are based on the mutual promises of two or more parties. Community health nurses must be aware that promises made to clients, meant to be reassurances, may be interpreted by clients as binding promises of outcomes. It is best to avoid making promises about things that are outside one's control.

There are situations in community health nursing in which a formal contractual agreement is necessary. If one agency agrees to provide services to another agency, it is wise to have the understanding in writing. The purpose of a written contract is to provide evidence of what the parties are mutually agreeing to do. Contracts protect both clients' and the nurses' rights.

Employment contracts are an important issue for all nurses. The customary practice in nursing has been to hire a nurse without a formal written contract. In this situation the nurse often later learns that the policies and procedures describing the duties and responsibilities of the community health nurse are the agency's legally binding employment agreement. If an employment agreement requires duties that are beyond the legal scope of nursing practice in the state, nurses must not agree to provide these services. Responsibilities that extend beyond the scope of nursing practice, yet are regularly practiced by nurses in an agency, are not legal. If you question whether you should be performing some of the skills being required of you by your community health agency, bring these concerns to the attention of your supervisor and request a legal opinion as to whether this practice is within the scope of nursing.

If the policies and procedures of an agency are not safe or require revisions, the community health nurse should request to serve on the committee that revises and reviews policies and procedures. It is a good idea to update policies and procedures no less often than every 2 years. The fact that an agency may require a community health nurse to perform a procedure will not protect the nurse as an individual if this practice is found to be outside the scope of nursing as defined by the state's Nurse Practice Act. The law as written will overrule any agency policy or procedure. In a Texas case, a nurse testified that she was merely following the physician's direction and the agency's policy. The court ruled that the state statute or Nurse Practice Act was the rule of law the nurse should be following. The fact that she was relying on what the physician or her employer told her to do was not a good defense (*Lunsford vs. Board of Nurse Examiners,* 1983).

Before signing an employment or other contract, nurses should read the contract carefully. If anyone signs a contract without reading it, the court will not be sympathetic toward that person's ignorance of the agreement. Community health nurses must make certain that the terms of agreements are written out before asking clients for a signature.

Classification of Laws and Penalties

Laws are enacted by the state legislature or Congress, as described previously, and specific categories of laws have associated penalties. The authorities or bodies that enforce the laws are also unique to the particular classification of the laws, whether criminal or civil.

CRIMINAL LAWS

Laws enacted under the criminal code are written for the protection of the public welfare as a whole. For this reason, when a case is brought under the criminal code, the defendant finds himself or herself facing society or the community prosecutor instead of an individual plaintiff. Criminal cases are prosecuted by the government. The penalties attached to criminal violations are also more severe owing to the possibility of limiting one's freedom by incarceration. Examples of potential violations of the criminal code in community health nursing include the situation in which the nurse believes that her or his own judgment as to the worth of a person's life is the correct one and acts to hasten the death of that person. The criminal code would refer to this behavior as either murder or manslaughter. There have been cases involving nurses who saw themselves as "angels of mercy" and hastened death in hospitals and long-term care facilities.

A community health nurse who recklessly endangers others can be criminally prosecuted. Laws relating to theft and other property violations are also found under the criminal code. Laws that prohibit abuse of children or elderly people are criminal laws written to protect these segments of the public. Most states have statutes that require nurses to report suspected child or elder abuse.

It is not unusual to read about a nurse who has been convicted of a crime and later discover that the state board of nursing has scheduled a hearing to consider whether the nurse's license should be revoked or suspended. Certain crimes are considered to involve moral implications and can be grounds for the loss of one's professional license, if the behavior can be reasonably connected to the professional responsibilities of the nurse. Violations involving substance abuse may result in suspension of a community health nurse's license until such time as proof is offered that the nurse is no longer using the substance in question. Because nurses are in a position to affect the health and safety of consumers, nurses' own personal habits and behavior are linked to their professional license.

A conviction for a criminal violation may result in imprisonment, parole, the loss of privileges such as a nursing license, a fine, or a combination of any of these penalties. Criminal penalties are intended to deter others from unsafe or unlawful behavior and also to punish the violator.

CIVIL LAWS

Civil laws are written to regulate the conduct between private persons or businesses. For example, malpractice laws are civil laws written to protect consumers of health care against unsafe health care practices. A private group or individual may bring a legal action for a breach of a civil law; this private group or individual is called the *plaintiff*. The person charged with violating a law or legal right is called the *defendant*. The court's ruling will hopefully result in a plan to correct the wrong between the two parties and may include a monetary payment to the wronged party, commonly known as *damages*. The penalties associated with violations of civil laws are different from those associated with criminal laws because the grievance is between two individual members of society rather than between society and an unsafe individual. The penalties for most civil wrongs do not include incarceration. Some civil cases may discover violations of the criminal laws, which may then lead to criminal penalties such as a jail term.

There may be both civil and criminal components when behavior violates laws that govern the practice of any licensed professional. A violation of both civil and criminal statutes in community health nursing may occur when a state's Nurse Practice Act defines or restricts some functions of the nurse to acting under the directions of a physician or other licensed professional such as a pharmacist. To act as a professional, explicit legal authority must exist. Standing or written orders, such as for medication administration, give the nurse authorization to act if the behavior is dependent on the directions of another licensed professional. Custom or usual practice will not substitute for the specific authority required by law. A violation of a professional practice act may be prosecuted as a crime even if no actual harm occurs to a client. As stated previously, an agency's policies and procedures cannot give nurses authority to practice outside the scope of their license.

If a community health nurse does not have a standing order for a particular medication, yet knows the routine well and proceeds to call a pharmacy to order the necessary medication, the nurse could be both civilly and criminally liable for this action. Even if the nurse attempts and fails to reach the physician to obtain permission, this action is illegal. The Medical Practice Act gives physicians the authority to diagnose disease and prescribe medication. In a growing number of states, advanced practice nurses may now be licensed to prescribe medications. The nurse has violated the Medical Practice Act, practiced outside the scope of the Nurse Practice Act, and fraudulently and criminally ordered medication without a license to do so. If the patient is harmed by the nurse's actions, a civil action can be brought by the patient against the nurse for the injury or damages caused by the nurse's negligence. Thus, one action can lead to both civil and criminal liability. In one case, a nurse was charged with interfering with the physician-patient relationship when the nurse provided information to the patient that was outside the physician's prescribed treatment plan (*Tuma vs. Board of Nursing*, 1979). On a patient's request, nurse Tuma discussed alternative treatments for cancer with a hospitalized woman who was about to start chemotherapy. When the woman stopped chemotherapy, the son told the physician about the conversation, and the physician brought charges against the nurse (Kelly, 1991). The Idaho Board of Nurses suspended her license for 6 months for unprofessional conduct. The Idaho Supreme Court eventually ruled that she could not be found guilty of unprofessional conduct because the state's Nurse Practice Act did not define unprofessional conduct (Kelly, 1991). Nurse Tuma's behavior itself was not addressed by the court.

Civil law, under which medical or professional malpractice falls, is called *tort law*. The civil law describes both intentional and unintentional torts. An *intentional tort* is found when an outcome is planned, whereas an *unintentional tort* involves accidental or unintended behavior. In malpractice cases involving health care providers such as community health nurses, no intent to harm the patient is needed for the defendant to be found guilty of negligence or malpractice. *Negligence* is merely the failure to act as a reasonably prudent professional would have acted in a specific situation. *Malpractice* is a specific type of negligence. When an educated person, in the performance of his or her professional role, fails to act as a reasonably prudent professional would have acted, the civil violation of malpractice has occurred. If a nurse unintentionally harms a patient, a malpractice or negligence case under the civil statutes would be the most likely result. If a community health nurse intentionally plans an injurious outcome, a criminal case could result.

Purposes and Application of Public Health Law

Public health laws are written for several purposes or with expected outcomes, such as protecting the public's health, advocating for persons or vulnerable groups who otherwise may not be served, regulating health care delivery and financing, and regulating the professional accountability of health care providers.

PROTECTING THE PUBLIC'S HEALTH

One of the main purposes for laws that apply to community health nursing is to protect the public. Examples of existing laws that protect the public follow and are discussed in more detail in accompanying chapters as identified. Communicable disease reporting and control laws, as well as mandatory immunizations, are discussed in Chapter 19. Other laws written to protect the public include abuse and neglect laws, which are discussed in Chapter 20. Protection of the public health occasionally must override the personal rights of individuals. For example, immunizations help to protect groups of people, as well as the individual, from illness. Some people may not desire to be immunized, but the good of the group must take priority in most cases (see ethics box VIII in Chapter 26).

Involuntary and emergency psychiatric admission laws are important for community health nurses to understand. These laws are written to protect not only the public, but also the person who is a danger to himself or herself. The standards and procedure for involuntarily committing a client to a hospital must be understood. The nurse may be called on to provide evidence of the necessity for involuntarily hospitalizing a client for the client's own safety and protection. The safety and protection of the family or neighbors of an unstable client may also be good reason to request that a client be involuntarily admitted through a court procedure. Emergency psychiatric admissions against the client's will are time-limited. State statutes usually identify the particular procedure for such admissions. The nurse must balance the need to protect the client's autonomy when evaluating the need to initiate an involuntary hospitalization.

A growing number of laws focus on dangerous products. These laws seek to protect the public through imposing liability on the product's manufacturers. Producers of products are held to a high standard of care in an effort to protect the public from dangerous products. Environmental hazards and laws relating to occupational safety are discussed in Chapter 24.

ADVOCATING FOR RIGHTS

A second purpose of public health law is protecting the rights of groups of people. In Chapter 20 the rights of vulnerable children and elders are discussed. Examples of federal laws that are written to protect special groups include laws directed toward the rights and needs of disabled children in school (see Chapters 26 and 28), laws protecting disabled adults (see Chapter 25), and occupational health and safety laws protecting workers (see Chapter 24). Many occupational health and safety laws focus on environmental hazards. Some laws are written for the purpose of protecting both the public and the rights of specified members of society. For example, as stated earlier, laws that require parents to immunize their children protect both the child and the general public.

Other examples of federal laws enacted to protect the rights of groups of people include the Civil Rights Acts of 1964 and 1965 and The Americans with Disabilities Act of 1990. These laws and their amendments were created to advocate equality for all people. The right of all people to move freely throughout our country and the right to be treated equally and without discrimination in the provision of services or employment are protected by the Civil Rights Acts. If a community health agency has a limited supply of needed vaccines and decides to reserve these limited resources for only white male patients, a civil right's violation has occurred. Such a policy, whether written or in practice, would discriminate against all persons of other races as well as white females. Civil rights violations carry strong penalties. The Civil Rights Acts identify the rights and immunities created by or dependent on the Constitution of the United States. The acts are a statement that Congress will protect against discrimination and will provide for equal protection, equal immunities, and equal privileges for all persons.

REGULATING HEALTH CARE DELIVERY AND FINANCING

Another purpose of public health law is to regulate or provide health care delivery and financing. The federal government has greatly affected society with its initiation of federally regulated health care delivery and health care financing. The Social Security Act of 1935 and its 1965 amendments created both Medicare and Medicaid programs (see Chapter 5).

The Public Health Services Act and its amendments were created through a federal regulatory statute. The Public Health Service was created to both collect and analyze data on selected diseases from all of the states and territories of the United States. Efforts to control or regulate the control and spread of disease are organized by both the Public Health Service and the Centers for Disease Control and Prevention.

The 1975 amendments of the Public Health Services Act also provided grant funding to states for various categories or "blocks" of public health services (see Table 4–2). This funding is often called *block grant funding.*

Another important purpose and application of public health law includes appropriations for populations at risk. These populations may include vulnerable groups of persons who have been identified as needing special protection or groups with specific health care problems. Amendments to the Social Security Act of 1963 addressed specific needs of maternal and child health, as well as mental retardation planning. The Social Security Amendments of 1977 and the Rural Health Clinic Amendments are directed toward specific populations in rural communities. The Omnibus Budget Reconciliation Act of 1981 created block grants for both maternal child health and social services (see Table 4–2).

PROFESSIONAL ACCOUNTABILITY

The purposes of public health laws not only include protecting the health of our communities, advocating public rights and needs, and regulating health care standards and financing, but also serve to regulate the professional accountability of health care providers.

Accountability means being answerable for one's professional judgment and actions within one's realm of authority (Kelly, 1991). Community health nurses are held accountable to uphold public health laws and regulations. Whether a community health nurse is working for a state, federal, or private agency, a general understanding of the appropriate and applicable laws is needed. For specific interpretations of these laws as they apply to nursing practice or clients' rights, the advice and counsel of the agency's attorney is recommended. Professional accountability is further defined in policy manuals, accrediting body guidelines, and professional organizations' standards and ethical codes (see Chapter 1).

Because the duty of an employer's attorney is to protect the employer, nurses who are being sued need their own attorney in addition to that of their employer. An attorney may be provided by the nurse's own professional liability insurance company or selected by the nurse.

When selecting a personal legal counselor, it is important to choose an attorney who understands health care issues. A nurse-attorney or an attorney with a proven record of success in health care law, malpractice defense work, personal injury, or the specific area of expertise required can be the strongest advocate.

Legal Responsibilities of Community Health Nurses

The duties of all nurses become legally binding responsibilities for which the nurse is accountable. In addition the community health nurse has many responsibilities that are unique to public health–focused practice.

PRACTICE WITHIN THE SCOPE OF THE LAW

As stated earlier, community health nurses must practice within the scope of the Nurse Practice Act and all relevant statutes and administrative rulings. The Nurse Practice Act of the state and the standards of practice described by rules exist to minimize the potential for negligence. To be found guilty of negligence or malpractice, a nurse must have accepted a duty to the patient, the breach of which has injured the client. The commissions or omissions of the nurse must have actually and directly caused the injury to the client for malpractice to have occurred.

Community health nurses must also carefully follow the rules for reimbursable services under Medicaid and Medicare. Clients must be screened for financial eligibility, and the signatures of the client must be witnessed after explaining client rights and legal contracts for service.

The community health nurse must honor the contracts made with clients. Contracts may include both written and implied agreements between the client and the nurse. If a contract cannot be honored, written documentation in the nursing notes should state the reason why, and the client should be notified. If the client unilaterally ends the relationship either explicitly or by consistently not keeping appointments with the nurse, this should also be documented. The community health nurse or a designate should contact the client if the nurse must cancel an appointment, a clinic visit, or other service. Clients should also be notified about any substitutions of personnel (Brent, 1988).

The nurse may be charged with abandonment if follow through on contracted care is not completed. *Abandonment* is the "unilateral termination of a professional relationship without affording the patient reasonable notice and health care services" (Brent, 1988, p. 7). Planning for the client's discharge from services prevents abandonment. The individual or family should be given adequate notice and informed of resources for any continuing care that is needed. After obtaining the client's written permission, a copy of the health records, including the nursing plan of care, should be transferred to another provider.

INFORMED CONSENT

Permission to obtain or transfer medical records is only one example of informed consent. Informed consent means that clients understand the risks and benefits of potential treatment alternatives before they voluntarily consent to it. If clients are to be allowed to make informed decisions, they must have adequate information told to them in an understandable way. If informed consent for a medical procedure is being sought, the community health nurse may be limited to witnessing the client's signature only and insisting that the treating physician explain the necessary medical information. Nurses are not educationally prepared to know all of the potential risks, benefits, and options of medical treatment.

Many nursing procedures are performed through implied consent. Implied consent occurs when the patient has had the nursing procedure explained and the patient's actions, such as exposing an injection site, indicate a willingness to proceed. A good rule to follow in deciding whether to rely on implied consent or to require a written form is this: the more intrusive the procedure, the greater likelihood that a written and signed consent form will be in the client's and nurse's best interest. If a procedure is performed against the patient's will or without consent, charges of assault (the threat of touching) and battery (the actual touching of the patient) can be brought against the nurse.

Informed consent may be especially difficult to receive if the nurse is involving the client in research, because all the potential risks may not be known in many cases. Informed consent should be obtained by the actual researcher, who can also explain the benefits of the research.

Community health nurses may be asked to witness the signing of forms related to nursing services as well as to non–health-related matters (e.g., wills). Witnessing a signature means that the witness is stating that the individual signed voluntarily, understood the document, and intended his or her signature to mean agreement with the contents of the document (Connaway, 1985). "Witnessing to signature only" means that the witness has seen another sign his or her name and may be written in when witnessing a non–health-related document such as a will (Connaway, 1985). All forms signed by the patient, parent, or guardian, and the date each form was signed, should be listed on the health care record.

REFUSAL OF CARE AND LIMITS OF CARE

An issue of growing concern is the patient's right to refuse treatment. If a community health nurse is unaware that the patient has created a living will, a special directive, or a durable power of attorney, which specifically states that certain procedures such as resuscitation are not desired, the nurse may act without the patient's consent and in a manner that is not in the patient's desired best interest. A patient can deny consent to treatment or withdraw previously granted consent at any time. Even a verbal withdrawal of consent is valid and must be communicated immediately to members of the health care team. Documentation of the refusal or withdrawal of consent is also important.

PRIVACY

The legal right of the client to maintain privacy and confidentiality in the nurse-client relationship must also be protected. If a transfer of information regarding a client is requested, the community health nurse must obtain a signed release form from the client before transferring this information.

Release forms should identify exactly what information is allowed to be released, to whom, and the duration of the period for which the release is being granted (Fig. 4–1). Such releases are very common in community health nursing, because the nurse is often the case manager who coordinates care among a variety of health care and social providers and agencies.

In some jurisdictions the communications between nurse and client have a statutory legal privilege that

Name ______________________
H.D. No. ______________________
Service Unit ______________________

CONSENT TO OBTAIN OR RELEASE CLIENT MEDICAL RECORD INFORMATION

______________________ (Client full name), ☐ Male ☐ Female, born ______________ (Date of birth), residing at

______________________ (Address of client) ________ (City) ________ (State) ________ (Zip Code)

hereby requests that the following information ______________________ (Specific information requested)

____

be disclosed by ______________________ (Name of person, program and/or organization receiving information)

______________________ (Address) ________ (City) ________ (State) ________ (Zip Code)

TO: ______________________ (Name of person, program and/or organization receiving information)

______________________ (Address) ________ (City) ________ (State) ________ (Zip Code)

solely for the purpose of ______________________ (Be specific)

to apply both now and in the future. This consent expires on ______________________ (Date, event or condition)

> I voluntarily consent for Prince George's County Health Department, Cheverly, Md., to obtain or release medical record information for the purposes stated above.
>
> I understand that this consent can be revoked by me in writing at any time. I understand that this information may not be redisclosed without my permission.
>
> Signed (check one): ☐ Client
> ☐ Legal Guardian ______________________ (Signature) ____________ (Date)

Explained by: ______________________ (Health care provider or representative) ____________ (Date)

______________________ (Title) ____________ (Phone number)

Figure 4–1 ● Consent to obtain or release client medical record information. (Courtesy of Prince George's County Health Department, Cheverly, Md.)

protects the privacy of this communication. Not all states or jurisdictions have enacted statutes that attach this legal privilege to nurse-client communications. A *legal privilege* is a legislatively created protection that the nurse will not be forced to disclose confidential communications that occur between nurse and client. If a legal privilege does not exist in a state, the nurse can be called on to disclose conversations with the client. The philosophy behind creating a statutory legal privilege is to provide the safety of confidentiality, thereby encouraging a client to openly and honestly disclose even the most intimate necessary information to the professional. A legal privilege between a lawyer and his or her client is intended to encourage the client to be totally truthful about his or her participation in the case before the court. There may be instances where even statutorily created legal privileges do not apply. For instance, most child and elder abuse reporting laws require that the nurse disclose reasonable suspicions of abuse. It is important to be aware of any legal privileges for nurse-client communications that the nurse can rely on.

STANDING ORDERS

Additional duties of the community health nurse include care of the ill in the home, clinic, school, or workplace. Direct care can include dispensing medications, giving immunizations, and following physicians' standing orders. Community health nurses need to protect themselves by ensuring that standing orders are regularly reviewed and updated as well as by having the physician sign the standing order that is acted on by the nurse. The community health nurse must be especially cautious to clarify orders when following verbal and or standing orders.

Verbal orders can be a source of risk to the community health nurse. The dangers of miscommunication are greatly heightened when communicating verbally. The likelihood of a patient being injured increases when the nurse allows verbal orders to become a pattern within the agency. When a patient is injured and a verbal order has been acted on by the nurse, there is no written evidence of what the physician ordered, and the nurse will have difficulty attempting to demonstrate that the doctor's verbal order was followed accurately.

Written confirmation of verbal orders must be received as soon as reasonably possible. In practice, community health nurses often write the orders they verbally receive and mail them to the physician with a self-addressed envelope. The physician is requested to verify and sign the orders and mail them back to the community health nurse.

CLIENT EDUCATION

The nurse's duty in caring for the client in the home, clinic, school and other community settings always includes the duty to teach the client. Much like discharge teaching in a hospital, community-based teaching may include both preventive and self-care information. Community health nurses must remember that the individual client's ability to understand what is being taught is of utmost importance. If the client does not speak English, the nurse may need the assistance of an interpreter. If the nurse is not sure whether the client is capable of understanding the nurse's instructions, it is important to involve a family member or other persons who will be involved in providing the client's ongoing health care. If the client is a child, the parents should be fully informed about how to perform the care that the community health nurse is teaching. It is a good idea to have the client explain to the nurse his or her understanding or perception of what the nurse has explained. In this way the nurse can be sure that the client has understood the nurse's directions.

It is also very important that the community health nurse teach the client accurately. If the nurse needs references to provide correct information, she or he should postpone answering a question until the information has been gathered. Community health clients rely on the information provided to them by their community health nurse. It is therefore essential that the information taught be accurate and up-to-date. If the nurse is unsure about how to answer a question asked by the client, it is not unprofessional to tell the client that she or he will check and get back to the client with accurate information. It does not destroy a nurse's credibility to admit that she or he is not a walking textbook; it is far more important to provide a correct response to the client. If a nurse guesses at information and is wrong, an injury may result to the client for which the nurse is legally responsible.

DOCUMENTATION

It is important for the community health nurse to be consistent in recording the care provided to clients. Thorough, accurate, and timely recording demonstrates quality of care; helps ensure reimbursement for services; and reduces the risk of lawsuits (Morrissey, 1988). Information regarding client visits and care should be documented as soon as possible after the care. Especially when providing care in the home, the nurse may need to record some immediate brief notes that are then documented more thoroughly in the client's health record as soon as the nurse returns to the agency.

Documentation of teaching and other care provided is important not only as a means of communicating with other health care providers who may be working with a client, but also as the ongoing written memory of the nurse. If the client later develops a problem, accurate and timely documentation of the care provided to date will provide the nurse with a record of what has or has not been done for the client and why. If a lawsuit ensues, the documentation kept by the community health nurse will be reviewed to establish the reasonableness of the care provided by the nurse. Thus, accurate and up-to-date recording is essential. It is difficult, if not impossible, to later remember everything done for every client if thorough recording was not completed at the time of care delivery. The records of the community health nurse are documents that can be subpoenaed in a trial to determine whether the nurse has caused harm to the patient.

Documentation also provides an ongoing history for future health care providers to determine what care has been provided for the client and what still needs to be done. The nurse's records are usually a part of the client's health care history. In documentation, as in all other community health nursing procedures, it is important to comply with the employer's policies and procedures.

AGENCY POLICIES

Community health nurses have a duty to inform themselves about their employer's written policies and procedures. Deviation from these agency policies may be viewed as substandard care. If policies and procedures established by an employer do not comply with reasonable nursing care, it is important to become involved in changing them to conform to safe practice. Nurses can actively participate in policy-making committees to provide input regarding safe nursing care within the scope of the state's Nurse Practice Act. It is important to ensure that the employer's policies and procedures do not require practice outside the scope of the nursing license. Deviations from policies and procedures, which can often become common practice in an agency, do not make the practice legally sound. Shortcuts or ignorance about the standards set by an employer can increase the nurse's risk of a malpractice suit. The employing agency's policies and procedures are standards that the community health nurse's behavior will be measured against if a lawsuit develops. Therefore, it is important to follow the agency's policies and procedures and to ensure that these policies and procedures are legally sound. If the nurse has questions about the legality of any policies or procedures, she or he should consult the agency's attorney.

PUBLIC HEALTH LAW ENFORCEMENT

Community health nurses also have the legal responsibility to enforce laws, especially laws enacted to protect the public health. Whether the nurse is employed by a public or private agency may have an impact on the degree and the responsibility of the nurse for enforcing laws. Community health nurses may be hired by local, state, or federal authorities that have enacted rules and regulations requiring specific enforcement of laws in areas such as infection control and reportable events. The hiring agency's policies and procedures, as well as the employee manual, should notify the nurse of any special duties or responsibilities. Examples of public settings in which community health nurses work include public school nursing, health department–based nursing, and federal employee health programs. Community health nurses may also be found working in private schools, clinics, or organizations such as Planned Parenthood.

A community health nurse is an agent of her or his employer. The legal definition of *agency,* in this sense, means that the nurse, as an employee, represents the employer and has the delegated authority to carry out the purposes of the employer. For example, if a nurse is working for a state health department, the nurse is an agent of the state. The legal liability and responsibilities of the community health nurse vary depending on the employer.

Conditions that may be reportable by all community health nurses under law include suspected abuse and neglect of children, elderly persons, or persons being cared for by others. Other reportable conditions include communicable diseases. Selected immunizations are required by law for school attendance.

Community health nurses should also be familiar with the procedure for commitment to psychiatric care, as discussed previously. The community health nurse who is hired by a public agency may also be required to enforce laws for licensing and inspection of daycare facilities and nursing homes. For example licensed facilities must comply with regulations providing a safe environment for daycare or long-term care facility clients.

It is evident that the role of the community health nurse interfaces with public health laws frequently. Because laws are constantly being enacted and revised, it is impossible to cover all of the potential laws that community health nurses must be aware of to enforce the laws of their state and also to be of the greatest assistance to their clients.

REFERRALS AND ADVOCACY

Nurses need to be familiar with laws that have been enacted to protect their client's rights and with the legislated services their clients are likely to be eligible to receive. The community health nurse is often placed in the position of serving as the client's advocate. As an advocate the nurse should be able to identify available community resources and assist clients in pursuing the rights that are legally afforded them. As an example the community health nurse may become aware of a client being unduly harassed by a creditor and may be able to help by directing the client to a consumer protection agency that can assist the client in resolving his or her financial difficulties. Providing referrals to appropriate available community resources is a valuable responsibility of the community health nurse.

The nurse should be familiar with the legal aid services available for low-income clients. Providing referrals to appropriate legal services is a community nursing function. These services ensure that all of the public's rights are protected. People who could not otherwise afford legal services can be represented by legal aid staff.

SPECIAL AND VULNERABLE POPULATIONS

Laws related to special populations affect the community health nurse's clients. Such laws have been enacted specifically to protect the rights of disabled persons, foster children, elderly persons, and the abused (Lerner and Ross, 1991; Talley and Coleman, 1992). Access to health care may be the client's greatest problem. Laws written to protect the uninsured, persons who reside illegally in the U.S., the homeless, and migrant workers should be explored by the community health nurse. Laws related to housing and the rights of the renter or tenant are also important to understand. Many state legislatures have enacted laws to protect families from eviction under certain circumstances.

FAMILY LAW

The community health nurse very often will deal with laws considered to be family law. Issues of guardianship or the legal right and power to decide for another may arise, and it is important for the community health nurse to understand how to advise clients on how to obtain guardianship and the obligations that go along with being a guardian. If the nurse is obtaining consent for a procedure to be performed on a minor or on a person who is incompetent, the guardian must sign the consent for treatment. In the case of a divorced couple, the spouse who has been awarded custody of the children would be the legal guardian of those children and the person from whom consent must be obtained.

Issues surrounding family privacy and reproductive rights are also very relevant. Along with federal legislation and court rulings, many state legislatures and courts have created laws affecting the legality of providing information regarding contraception to minors. It is important for the community health nurse to be aware of the abortion laws in the state in which the nurse is practicing. The U.S. Supreme Court decisions have encouraged states to handle the abortion issue, within certain guidelines, in a manner that reflects their own community standards. Community health nurses must understand their own state's standards to advise and correctly inform community health clients.

END OF LIFE/SELF-DETERMINATION

With the movement toward shorter hospital stays and discharging persons to home for long-term care of terminal illnesses, a growing area of discussion between community health nurses and their clients involves the clients' wishes as they plan for their death. Most states have enacted living will statutes that define how clients may let their wishes be known when death is imminent. Clients must have the capacity to create a living will or, in other terms, be deemed competent to make these important decisions for themselves. However, most living will statutes apply only to terminally ill patients.

Many persons additionally assign a durable medical power of attorney to a trusted person, who then becomes empowered to act as a surrogate decision maker if the client becomes incompetent or is unable to make his or her desires known to health care providers (Montminy, 1990). Laws support the idea that patients should have the right to make choices and give consent for treatment. However, health care providers are often held legally responsible by family members when the patient's condition worsens because all that is medically possible is not provided to the patient. Community health nurses can be most supportive of their clients by informing them of their rights and of possible ways to formally document their wishes that care be provided or withheld under certain circumstances. Specific directives will be the most clear and convincing evidence of a client's wishes.

The Patient Self Determination Act of 1992 requires that facilities that receive federal funding (including hospitals, nursing homes, home health agencies, hospices, and prepaid health care organizations) inquire whether patients being admitted to their services have executed a living will or special directive. Sample forms for a living will and a durable power of attorney for health are included in Chapter 29.

ENVIRONMENTAL PROTECTION

Nurses can also encourage their clients to pursue their rights and to protect themselves through laws relating to environmental hazards. Laws related to the wearing of seat belts and infant car seats should be discussed with clients. Other environmental hazard laws include those pertaining to chemical use or waste disposal. Food preparation laws apply where food is being prepared for service to the public; community health nurses can help clients avoid unsuspected barriers to employment by helping them become aware of their rights, responsibilities, and liabilities as food handlers. Laws related to sanitation and other environmental issues are often managed under local and state health departments. A growing number of states are developing separate divisions to specifically address the environmental hazard laws that are increasingly being legislated.

NURSE LOBBYISTS

The practice of a community health nurse is greatly affected by legal responsibilities. When a health risk is identified for which there is little legal guidance, nurses should proceed cautiously and become actively involved as lobbyists through the legislative and administrative processes. Nurses serve as client advocates when they become involved as active lobbyists for improved health care (Faherty, 1993). A *lobbyist* is a person who informs decision makers and educates others who need to understand community health care issues. Nurses are informed providers of care who can serve as experts in teaching law makers and policy makers about the needs of the community and specific clients. Community health nurses also serve as expert witnesses in court cases, describing the standard of nursing care expected in their community. A thorough discussion of the nurse as an advocate in the legislative and administrative law-making process is discussed in Goldwater and Zusy (1990) and Mason and Talbott (1985).

How to Find Out about Laws

Laws have important ramifications for community health nursing practice. Nurses must become informed about the laws they are held accountable to. If a nurse is employed by a community health agency, the attorney who represents the agency should be the nurse's legal advisor. The agency's attorney will be able to direct the nurse to written health codes, as well as local or state health department policies that are written to conform to existing laws in the state. It is also wise to talk with one's supervisor before consulting with the agency's attorney. Agency protocols often dictate the appropriate channels of communication. Consult first with your supervisor or health officer regarding questions or concerns about existing policies or procedures.

To gain firsthand information, nurses can visit a law library. Law schools or the state attorney general's office generally provide excellent law library resources. The law librarian can be a great resource person for locating the sources and references desired for review. Legal aid services and state offices of consumer affairs can also be helpful to the nurse and the community health client.

There is a growing body of literature developed by advocacy groups concerned about the public's health and welfare. The community health nurse must be familiar with and continue to read updated materials on developing trends in health care law. Numerous continuing education programs related to community health nursing and the legal aspects of nursing are available in many communities. Attendance at these continuing education programs is highly recommended. Because laws continually change with the trends of society, it is not safe to rely on outdated information related to health care law. Changes and updates in the law are continuously occurring. Professional associations and the media often provide initial information about current or potential changes in laws that affect a community health nurse's practice. Nurses must continually update their knowledge of health-related laws.

Standards of Care

The standard of care defines the legal responsibility of the community health nurse. It serves as the "measuring rod" of what appropriate professional nursing care should include. There are both internal, self-set standards of care and externally created standards by which professional behavior is evaluated.

DEFINITION OF A STANDARD OF CARE

A *standard of care* is defined by the courts as the care that a reasonably prudent community health nurse would have performed under similar circumstances. If the nurse has an advanced nursing degree, a higher standard of competence will be expected. The standard of care is also related to what is called the *locality rule.* Specific geographic areas or similar communities are compared when setting the standards for nursing care. This locality rule is especially important to community health nursing. Whether a nurse works in an urban or a rural community health setting also helps to determine the standards that a nurse will be held accountable to practice.

INTERNAL AND EXTERNAL STANDARDS

The professional behavior of a community health nurse is measured by both internal and external standards of reasonableness. Internal standards include policies and procedures and may be viewed as self-set standards of the employing agency. The community health nurse's job description is an internal standard that she or he must work within. If the nurse's job description requires the nurse to practice outside the scope of nursing, then the Nurse Practice Act takes priority over this internal standard. Courts review these internal standards to evaluate what professionals in the field have determined desired performance to include. Hospital or agency rules are admissible as evidence of standards of care in the community. Other internal standards that may be used to evaluate the reasonableness of nursing practice include nursing care plans. If the nurse outlines a care plan for a client and then deviates from this plan, the court may determine that the nurse strayed from a reasonable standard of care. Nursing care plans are the most direct evidence of nursing care judgment. With national accreditation of most agencies and an increasingly mobile society, a national standard has also developed.

External standards of the reasonableness of the care provided by a community health nurse are determined by reviewing the nurse's actions in relation to the Nurse Practice Act or the rules and regulations of the state board of nursing. If a community health nurse believes that the state's Nurse Practice Act or nursing board rules and regulations do not adequately describe community health nursing practice, it is essential that she or he lobby to change these standards to which nurses are held accountable. Other external standards that courts use in evaluating the reasonableness of nursing care include the guidelines submitted by accrediting agencies and the nursing theories of recognized authorities. If a nurse recognizes the authority of an author, the nurse will be held accountable for the safe practice of community health nursing described by this author. It is a common court procedure to introduce authorities in the field to verify the standard of care.

ROLE OF THE EXPERT WITNESS

The standard of care serves as a means of comparing what an ordinarily prudent nurse would have reasonably done compared with the defendant's conduct. In a legal case involving professional behavior, an expert witness is required to explain to the jury and/or judge what reasonable community health nursing behavior entails. The practice of professionals such as nurses is deemed to be "beyond the ken" of the average person. This means that nurses' professional behavior is not commonly understood and is a very specific body of knowledge that must be explained to the common juror and judge.

The expert witness in a case must be truly qualified as an expert in the area of nursing in the case being decided. The expert witness must be certified by the court as holding the credentials and the knowledge to provide the court with an accurate and up-to-date evaluation of prudent community health nursing. Once the expert is recognized by the court, the expert's opinion or testimony is given no greater weight than the testimony of any other witness. Although juries may be influenced by the credentials and the expertise of an expert witness and may tend to give the testimony more weight than other witnesses, the rules of the court do not demand this.

Both parties to a suit are allowed to introduce expert witnesses and testimony. Very often the differing opinions of experts serve to reduce the credibility or impact of both experts' testimony. Plaintiffs, defendants, or their attorneys cannot buy or influence the opinion of the expert. They cannot tell the expert what they believe to be true; instead, both parties seek to find an expert who agrees with their views of the behavior of the nurse. For example, if a plaintiff's attorney hires an expert to evaluate a case and the expert returns an opinion that the defendant nurse acted reasonably and prudently as expected of a community health nurse, the plaintiff's attorney will not introduce this expert's testimony at the time of trial. However, if the defendant's attorney becomes aware of this expert's opinion, the defendant will likely want to hire this expert to testify on the defendant's behalf.

A community health nurse who is being sued deserves to have the nursing care provided analyzed by a community health nurse in a comparable setting. If the community health nurse holds a master's or doctoral degree, the expert witness most likely will also be required to have comparable educational preparation. A specialist is held to the standard of care for a member of the specialty. Therefore, a higher standard of care will be applied to community health nurses holding advanced degrees. Nurses are also held accountable for the knowledge they should have gained in their education, as well as for the materials presented in continuing education programs they attend.

Standards of care change with the growing body of knowledge and expectations of what care community health nurses will provide. The American Nurses' Association Standards of Care for Community Health Nurses are discussed in Chapter 1. Community health nurses must attend community education programs to stay abreast of current trends in community health nursing. The courts will not evaluate a nurse who received a degree 20 years previously by the standards of care taught in the nursing curriculum at that time. Changes in society continue to influence and affect the public's health. Examples of changes in the standards of care include the community health nurse's involvement in abortion and contraception advice and the care needed for communicable diseases such as hepatitis and acquired immunodeficiency syndrome.

Quality and Risk Management

Attention to minimizing the risks of injuring a client when providing care in the community benefits both patients and nurses. Quality management involves learning from past experiences and avoiding known risks to patients. By evaluating the care provided and the outcomes of care, an assessment of quality can be made. Risk management is a component of quality management and serves to indicate where special attention may be needed to both minimize risks and improve quality of care. Nurses can reduce the possibility that they will be financially and emotionally devastated by a lawsuit by utilizing quality management information to identify and reduce risks, thereby avoiding injury to clients. The responsibility for assuring quality care rests with the individual provider as well as the employer. A nurse who comes to work overly tired automatically increases the need for risk management. The nurse's role is too important to the patient's well-being to attempt to provide services while functioning in a diminished capacity, regardless of the reason. The employer's policies and procedures should also provide for a safe level of care.

CONTINUING EDUCATION

From a legal standpoint, one of the best ways to maintain quality assurance in community health practice is by enhancing knowledge through continuing education.

Nurses must keep up with new theories and advancements in patient care. The standards of care that are expected to be met are based on the most recent existing information, not on what one learned in one's nursing program. Nurses, like all members of society, are also held accountable for having knowledge of and functioning within the laws of the country and the states in which they practice. The fact that a nurse did not realize that she or he was breaking the law is not a sound defense. Ignorance of the law will not protect nurses from legal liability.

INCIDENT REPORTS

Incident reports are a means of risk management or quality assurance. They should be the community health care agency's internal source for identifying real and potential risks. They can be used to alter past patterns of care and even provide the basis for rewriting policies and procedures to enhance a high quality of care. An example of an incident that would need to be reported by a community health nurse would be giving the wrong immunization to a patient. This incident may encourage better labeling of vaccines and improvements in clarifying the client's identity before proceeding with any procedure.

Incident reports should be written carefully in compliance with an agency's procedures for reporting actual or potential harm to a client. Because public policy desires to encourage practices that reduce the risks of potential harm, incident reports have traditionally been protected from use in lawsuits against health care providers. However, a trend is developing in which incident reports are becoming available as evidence. It is therefore important that the statements in incident reports describing the occurrence be made in nonaccusatory terms. Nurses should describe the event in factual terms without pointing fingers at certain persons or assigning blame for the injuries that resulted. It is always safest to document facts rather than opinions. As with all documentation, incident reports should be reported truthfully and in a timely fashion, and nurses should follow the agency's policy when filing an incident report.

An incident report is an internal risk management document. However, if reference is made to its existence in the patient record, a plaintiff's attorney may then have access to the report. A growing number of jurisdictions are allowing incident reports to become "discoverable." This means that if an incident report exists, and is subpoenaed, it must be shared with the opposing side.

TIMELY DOCUMENTATION AND COMMUNICATION

A nurse's documentation can serve as proof that the nurse acted reasonably and safely. As discussed earlier, documentation should be accurate, thorough, and performed in a timely manner.

Documentation serves as communication to other members of the health care team regarding the client's status and the care that has been provided. If care is not documented in a timely manner, other health care providers may perform their services for clients based on inaccurate or incomplete information. It is also important that nurses, as members of the health care team, communicate verbally in a timely manner with other team members. When the potential for a lawsuit is being evaluated, the nurse's notes are very often the first record to be reviewed by the plaintiff's legal counsel. If the nurse's credibility becomes questionable as a result of these documents, a greater risk of liability exists for the nurse. The nurse's notes are a risk management and quality assurance tool not only for the employer, but also for the individual nurse.

PROFESSIONAL LIABILITY INSURANCE

Professional liability insurance may be considered a means of risk management. Liability insurance will not prevent the nurse from being sued, but will rather serve as a safety net to protect the nurse's personal resources and ability to defend against a lawsuit. Many nurses rely totally on their employer's professional liability insurance policy as their total coverage. If the employer and the nurse find themselves in the position of having a conflict of interest (e.g., the nurse did not follow the agency's policy and procedures), it is likely that the nurse will be less protected by the policy than the employer. It is recommended that nurses, as professionals, carry their own personal professional liability insurance in addition to that provided by their employer. A professional liability policy is a contract between the insured professional and the insurance company. If nurses carry their own liability coverage, they are buying the protection of the insurance company, provided they comply with all of the conditions of the policy.

When selecting a professional liability policy, it is suggested that the nurse seek an occurrence policy rather than a claims made policy. An occurrence policy will provide protection if the incident occurs while the nurse is insured by the policy. Under a claims made policy, not only would the incident have to occur while the nurse is insured by the company, but the policy would also have to still be in force at the time the plaintiff brings suit against the nurse. Statutes of limitations in various jurisdictions limit the time under which a plaintiff may bring suit against a health care provider. If the statute of limitations is 2 years, the nurse could be sued by a client who has not been seen for 2 years. Therefore, under a claims made policy the nurse would have to continuously maintain the same policy or buy tail coverage from the insurance company. Tail coverage extends the policy's protection beyond the term of the policy and can be very expensive.

Community health nurses may be asked to provide assistance that is not within the scope of their employment and therefore not within the coverage of the employer's liability insurance. While the nurse may be covered by the employer during travel between visits to clients, automobile trips to and from work are not within the scope of employer insurance. Another risk involves transporting clients in the community health nurse's automobile. It is not a wise practice for the nurse to chauffeur clients. If an accident occurs and the client is injured, the fact that the nurse is driving the client in the capacity of an employed professional affects the relationship defined and may diminish the nurse's protection. Also, if the nurse is participating in a health screening clinic that is sponsored by an agency other than the employer, the employer's liability insurance likely would not cover the nurse. The nurse's membership on community boards, if she or he is not acting as a representative of the employer, and any private nursing business would also not be covered under an employer's liability insurance policy.

PROFESSIONAL INVOLVEMENT

Professional involvement in organizations or on committees that define the standards of care for community health nursing is another means of risk management. Nurses also benefit their profession when they actively participate on community boards. Nursing input is very valuable when future planning or current community issues are being discussed. Nurses must be willing to represent nursing and patient perspectives regarding community needs and future directions. Membership in professional nursing organizations such as the American Nurses' Association, the National League for Nursing, and state nursing associations is also important. The viewpoint of nurses becomes more powerful when nurses work together to create an organized and cohesive profession.

Ethics and Law

Ethical and legal issues are closely related to many areas of concern for nurses. Legal and ethical issues surround the right to choose how one will live while dying, and who should have the right to make decisions regarding the treatment plan. Because nurses live in a society that is based on laws, they must work to change any laws that do not reflect nurses' ethical values. Ethical issues reflect moral ideas of right and wrong, whereas laws deal with the regulation of social behavior. Laws are passed to protect society as a whole or at least segments of the population that need special protection. The ethical implications of these laws are related to legal responsibilities in community health nursing. The community health nurse's moral and value-laden beliefs on the rights of family members to deal with privacy matters, including contraception and abortion, exist simultaneously with legal responsibilities for nurses. Abuse in society is also an ethical issue that imposes direct legal responsibilities on nursing practice.

Ethical decision making may be very difficult and emotionally charged. Decision makers with differing values attempt to be fair to the people involved while determining what is considered wrong or right or where the duties, obligations and responsibilities lie. Consensus is not easily achieved. When ethical issues become of great enough concern to society at large, they usually result in laws that provide guidance as to how society has determined nurses must respond. Because ethical issues are highly emotionally charged, the legal system does not intervene until there is a clear mandate from society to make a decision. Current court decisions on the patient's right to refuse or terminate lifesaving treatment are examples of how one ethical issue—the right to die—has become a legal issue with implications for nursing care delivery.

While ethics are influenced by attitudes, values, and beliefs that determine what is right, wrong, or fair, laws generally speak only to what is wrong in a particular society. It is not always possible or desirable to attempt to translate ethical principles into legal terms. Laws may restrict or protect personal freedoms. Ethics is a broader, more universal concept than law. Law is narrower and deals with the system of compliance in a given society. As advocates, nurses may provide a bridge between ethics and law. Justice, or the principles of fairness and equity, is needed in law and ethics.

KEY IDEAS

1. Community health nurses need a clear understanding of the laws that govern their nursing practice, including criminal law, civil law, and family law.
2. The majority of environmental and public health laws are enacted at the state level but must conform to broad directives in federal legislation.
3. Administrative bodies are responsible for formulating the rules and regulations that clarify and interpret the intent of legislation. The state board of nursing is an example of an administrative body that interprets the legislative intent of the state Nurse Practice Act.
4. Nurses interested in affecting or changing laws must understand the importance of lobbying administrative agencies as well as legislative representatives.
5. Community health nurses may incur both criminal and civil sanctions for acts performed in the course of their nursing practice. Civil malpractice is the most common action. Criminal prosecution is usually reserved for egregious acts such as mercy killing.

6. All community health nurses have a duty to be knowledgeable about and practice within the scope of their state's Nurse Practice Act. They should be clear about their responsibilities related to physician orders (both standing and verbal), documentation of services, and the relationship between their employing agency's policies and their own professional responsibilities.
7. Nurses must be aware of client rights, including the right to informed consent, the right to privacy, and the right to select or reject health care services as well as determine the limits of health care services desired.
8. Nurses whose practice includes vulnerable populations such as disabled persons, children, elderly persons, and victims of abuse have a duty to understand the law regarding their professional responsibilities and the rights of their clients.
9. The legal yardstick on which any nurse's professional competence is judged is the standard of care, or what a reasonably prudent nurse would do in a similar situation.
10. Community health nurses should be vigilant in monitoring and influencing laws that affect their professional practice and the health of individuals, families, and communities.

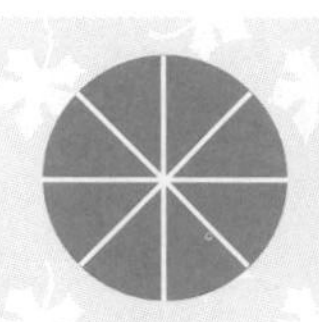

CASE STUDY
Understanding A CHN's Legal Responsibilities

In a case involving a community health nurse (CHN), the court determined that the nurse was negligent in failing to properly assess the seriousness of a school child's asthma attack.

The child came to the school nurse's office seeking help. The nurse gave another child's inhaler to the student and sent her back to class, but soon learned that her classmates were still concerned and believed their friend needed help. The nurse assessed the student and determined that an ambulance, supplemental oxygen, or a wheelchair was not needed for the student to travel to her physician's office. Within minutes the student collapsed and stopped breathing; she died following a brief comatose period.

The plaintiff presented expert testimony from a registered nurse and asthma specialist. Their opinions were that the defendant nurse deviated from the standard of care in the community for school nursing and directly caused the student's death. Three experts testified on the defendant's behalf expressing their opinions that the nurse did not deviate from the standard of care nor cause the death of the student.

The jury concluded the nurse was negligent and ordered the defendant to pay the child's family $142,289. The nurse's failure to provide the needed care in a timely fashion was found by the court to be directly related to the child's death. The nurse had also violated the school district's policy by not calling the student's parents.

The court found that the school nurse has a higher duty of care than a hospital nurse to make an assessment of the need for emergency medical services. The nurse was not expected to provide medical care, but rather to determine the need for emergency care. The nurse's action also fell below the required standard of reasonable judgment by authorizing the use of another student's asthma inhaler (*Schlussler vs. Independent School District,* 1989).

There are several nursing actions that might have assisted this community health nurse to provide safe, appropriate care in these circumstances:

1. Better physical assessment skills might have enabled the nurse to determine the severity of the student's signs and symptoms and to conclude that, without available medication, emergency care was appropriate.
2. The nurse might have consulted with other nurses and physicians to develop written criteria to be used to determine when emergency care is needed for selected circumstances.
3. The nurse might have followed the basic standard of care and laws governing prescription medications by not giving the student someone else's medication.
4. The nurse might have monitored the student for a longer period of time, recognized that the asthma attack was not abating, and then called for emergency services.
5. The nurse might have followed school policy and informed the parents of the student's illness, in which case the parents might have come to the school in time to initiate a request for emergency services.
6. The nurse might have instituted a health form to be completed by parents and, for those students with chronic illnesses, requested orders from the students' physicians regarding individualized treatment.

GUIDELINES FOR LEARNING

1. Review your state's procedure for enacting laws. You can contact your state legislature for a copy of the process or visit your local library for the information.
2. Identify your district representatives to your state legislature. Find out if any of them serve on committees that help to determine public health or professional practice legislation. If so, call or write, asking them for copies of the current issues before their committee and their position on those issues.
3. Contact your state board of nursing. Ask about pending hearings regarding a rule, regulation, or disciplinary matter. If possible, attend the hearing. If you are not able to attend, ask the board to send you information on a proposed change or new rule or regulation. Review the proposal and try to identify what impact it would have on your practice.
4. Courtrooms are open to the public. Attend a trial or hearing as an observer of the legal process. Ask a court clerk if there are any health-related cases on the court schedule. If so, attending the trial will give you some idea of how a health-related matter is handled within the court system.
5. Read the local newspaper. Identify a health-related issue that is under consideration either within the legislature or by an administrative agency. Follow the progress of the debate or hearings via the news. Try to identify the various interested parties and their positions on the issue. Write, call, or visit your legislator or the administrative agency and express your views on the issue.
6. Contact your state nurses' association and obtain a list of issues that are critical to nursing. Determine your association's position on the issues and its rationale for that position. Ask how your nursing organization lobbies for its positions with the legislature and administrative agencies.
7. Obtain a copy of your state's Nurse Practice Act. *READ IT.*
8. Review the policy and procedure manual from a community health nursing agency. Identify forms that must be signed by clients to receive services, transfer medical records, and authorize reimbursement.

REFERENCES

Beauchamp, D. (1985, December). Community: The neglected tradition of public health. *Hastings Center Report,* pp. 28–36.

Brent, N. (1988). Avoiding patient abandonment charges: Balancing the legal and ethical issues. *Home Healthcare Nurse, 7*(2), 7–8.

Connaway, N. (1985). Documenting patient care in the home—legal issues for the home health nurse—witnessing documents in the home. *Home Healthcare Nurse, 3*(6), 44–46.

Faherty, B. (1993). Now is the time to advocate. *Nursing Outlook, 41*(6), 248–249.

Goldwater, M., & Zusy, M. (1990). *Prescription for nurses: Effective political action.* St. Louis: Mosby.

Kelly, L. (1991). *Dimensions of professional nursing* (6th ed.). Elmsford, NY: Pergamon Press.

Lerner, H., & Ross, L. (1991). Community health nurses and high-risk infants: The current role of Public Law 99–457. *Infants and Young Children, 4*(1), 46–53.

Lunsford v Board of Nurse Examiners, 648 S.W. 2d 391 (Tex. App. 1983).

Mason, D., & Talbott, S. (Eds.). (1985). *Political action: Handbook for nurses.* Menlo Park, CA: Addison-Wesley.

Montminy, A. (1990). Decision-making authority for family caregivers of the cognitively impaired elderly. *Journal of Community Health Nursing, 7*(4), 215–221.

Morrissey, R. (1988). Documentation: If you haven't written it, you haven't done it. *Nursing Clinics of North America, 23*(2), 363–371.

Northrop, C. (1985). Legal responsibilities of public health nurses. *Nursing Outlook, 33*(6), 316.

Northrop, C. E., & Kelly, M. E. (1987). *Legal issues in nursing.* St. Louis: Mosby.

Pickett, G., Hanlon, J. J. (1990). *Public health administration and practice.* St. Louis: Mosby–Year Book.

Schlussler v Independent School District No. 200, et al. Case number MM89-14V, Minnesota Case Reports, 1989.

Talley, B., & Coleman, M. (1992). The chronically mentally ill: Issues of individual freedom versus societal neglect. *Journal of Community Health Nursing, 9*(1), 33–41.

Tuma v Board of Nursing, 593 P. 2nd 711 (ID, 1979).

U.S. Code, Congressional and Administrative News. (1935, 1937, 1944, 1963, 1965, 1975, 1977, 1981). St. Paul, MN: West Publishing.

BIBLIOGRAPHY

Benjamin, M., & Curtis J. (1986). *Ethics in nursing.* New York: Oxford University Press.

Cushing, M. (1988). *Nursing jurisprudence.* Norwalk, CT: Appleton & Lange.

Fiesta, J. (1988). *The law and liability—a guide for nurses.* New York: John Wiley & Sons.

Fiscina, S. R., Zimmerly, J. G., Seifert, J. B., & Connors, P. J. (1985). *A sourcebook for research in law and medicine.* Owing Mills, MD: National Health Publishing.

Fox, C. (1986). *Long term care and the law.* Owing Mills, MD: National Health Publishing.

Fromer, M. J. (1981). *Ethical issues in health care.* St. Louis: Mosby.

Goldstein, A., Perdew, S., & Pruitt, S. (1989). *The nurses legal advisor.* Philadelphia: J. B. Lippincott.

Hogue, E. (1985). *Nursing and informed consent.* Owing Mills, MD: National Health Publishing.

Hogue, E. (1985). *Nursing and legal liability.* Owing Mills, MD: National Health Publishing.

Murchison, I., Nicholes, T., & Hanson, R. (1982). *Legal accountability in the nursing process.* St. Louis: Mosby.

Thompson, J. B., Thompson, H. O. (1981). *Ethics in nursing.* New York: Macmillan.

SUGGESTED READING

Killion, S. (1993). Case commentary—*Bass v. Barksdale:* Implications for public health and home care nurses. *Public Health Nursing, 10*(2), 129–133.

Chapter 5

Financing of Health Care: Context for Community Health Nursing

Frances A. Maurer

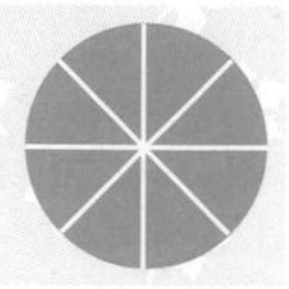

Continued

Focus Questions

What sources provide funding for health care in this country?

What has been the general pattern of expenditures for health care?

Are there groups who are at greater risk for diminished or no access to health care services?

How have Medicare and Medicaid affected health care delivery to the populations they serve?

What methods have been used to attempt cost containment in health care?

Has cost containment affected service? If so, in what ways?

How can nurses influence the cost and delivery of health care services?

Today's nurses need to have a clear understanding of the health care system, including the mechanisms for the distribution and reimbursement of services. In the past these topics were not considered relevant to the practice of nursing and were largely ignored by nurses involved in both service and education. The financial component was considered especially irrelevant to the planning and distribution of good nursing care. The expectation was that people should be provided with the best and most appropriate nursing care and medical treatments regardless of their ability to pay.

Although universal access is admirable, it has never been a reality in this country. While debate rages about potential rationing of health care, in actuality health care is already rationed by the ability to pay. A person's financial status affects the quality and quantity of care available. Current events have served to highlight that problem to health care providers, the public at large, and individual consumers.

Since the 1970s numerous attempts have been made to limit health care expenditures as concerns escalate over costs. Yearly costs rose from 12.7 billion in 1950 to $838.5 billion in 1992 (Fig. 5–1). Of even greater concern than escalating costs is the growth of health care as a portion of the national budget. Health care continues to increase its share of the gross national product (GNP) in comparison to other expenditures and currently outstrips the combined costs of both defense and education (Fig. 5–2).

The increasing proportion of the gross national product (GNP) (14%) devoted to health care means that individuals and families spend more on health care and have less to spend on food, clothing, housing, schooling, leisure, and

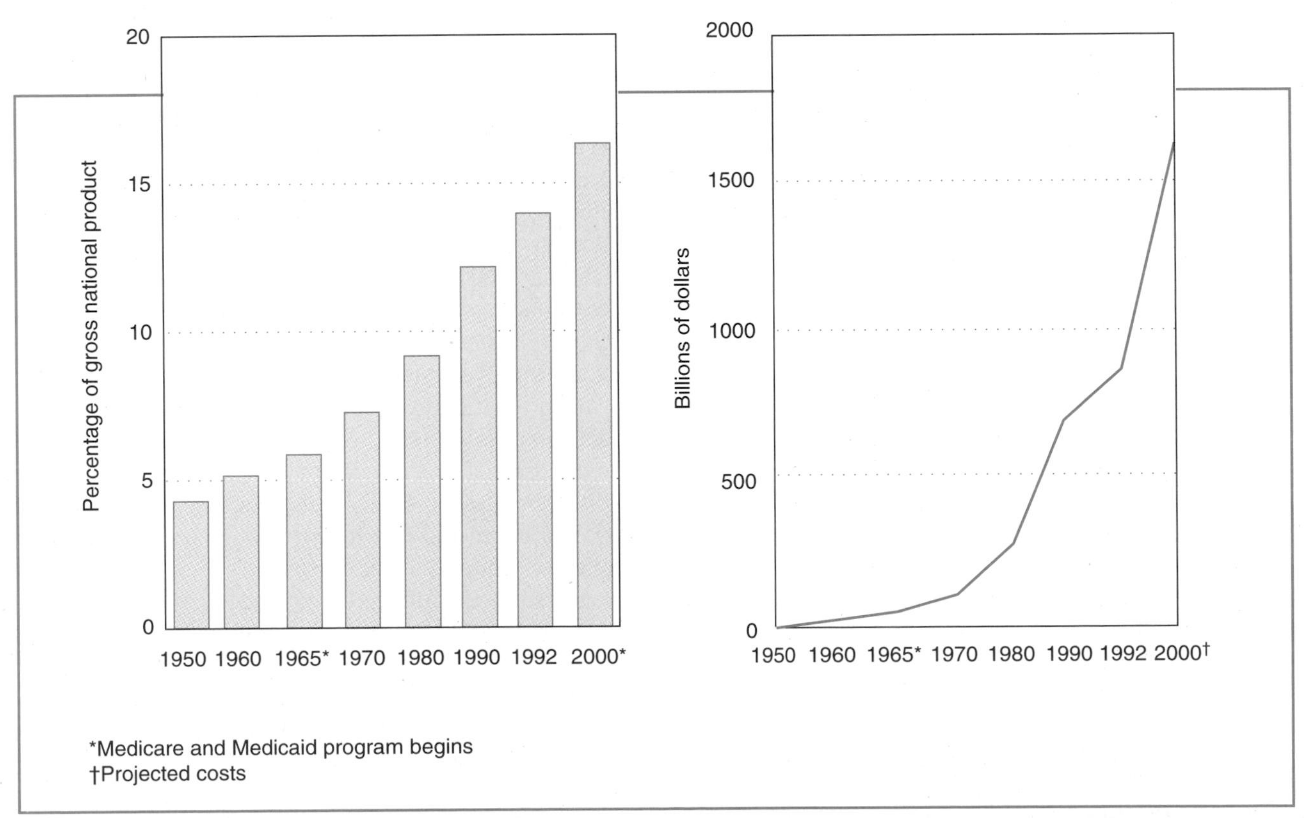

Figure 5–1 ● Health care costs for selected years, 1950–2000. (Data from Health Care Finance Administration, Office of the Actuary; and Office of National Estimates.)

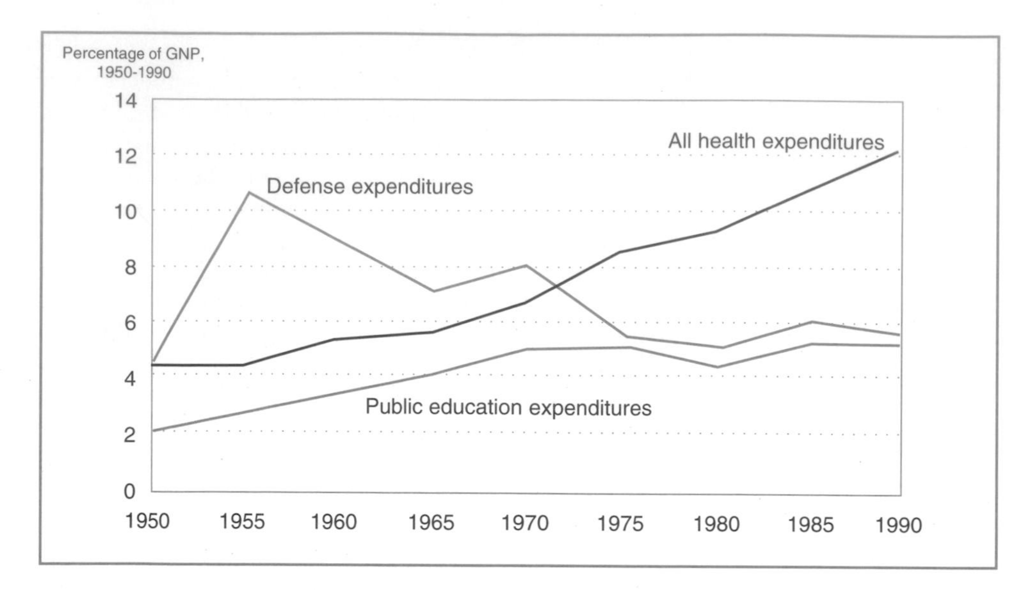

Figure 5–2 ● Health, education, and defense spending. (Redrawn from U.S. National Center for Education Statistics, Health Care Finance Administration, U.S. Office of Management and Budget.)

other needs or interests. The personal cost of health care—what each American spends on health care services and products such as insurance premiums, medications, physician and hospital services—has doubled every decade. In 1990, the average yearly cost for every American was $2518 (Letsch et al., 1992). By the year 2000, it is estimated that health care costs will average $5712 per year for each person in the country (Levit et al., 1991).

Reasons for the Increase in Health Care Costs

There are three basic factors responsible for escalating costs. The first is inflation. Inflation as a generic factor affects the costs of all types of goods and services and has played a significant role in cost increases. Between 1950 and 1990, there were several periods of heavy inflation. The net effect was a dramatic increase in the cost of basic goods and services such as food, fuel, electricity, telephone, construction, labor, and insurance. As inflation increased prices, the health care industry's costs for these goods and services also increased. As with any business, the higher expenses were passed on to the consumer.

Inflation helps to explain increases in the overall monetary expenditures for health care but does little to explain increases in the share of GNP. Increases in the health care market's share of GNP are more closely related to two other factors: escalating demand for health care services and technological advances in medical care.

Increased demand for services is primarily the result of federal programs (Medicare and Medicaid) and an aging population. Before these programs were instituted, cost was a rationing factor for poor and elderly patients in need of care. Medicare and Medicaid reduced the access barrier and created a greater demand for health care by previously restricted groups.

At the same time, the growth of the elderly population created its own additional demand for service. Even without Medicare, the number of elderly requiring services has grown, and as "baby boomers" reach old age, the need for health care services is expected to increase even more. By the year 2000 the elderly are expected to represent 14% of this country's population. By comparison, in 1991, 12% of the population, or 31.8 million persons, were age 65 years or older (*U.S. Bureau of the Census,* 1991).

Technological advances in medicine have been both enormous and expensive. Development costs of new procedures, drugs, and equipment is high, and new technologies generally require more skilled technicians and professionals to operate them. Advances in medical treatment have also created an increased demand for services, as refinements frequently increase the number of patients who can be successfully treated. The cost of technology is very difficult to isolate as it is integrally linked to service (Congressional Budget Office, 1992). Raffel and Raffel (1989) report one study that determined that technology accounted for approximately one fourth of the overall increases in health care expenditures in 1986.

One widely publicized myth is that malpractice reform would dramatically reduce the cost of health care. Malpractice premiums (i.e., what the health care provider pays for malpractice insurance) make up only 1% of the total health care budget. Individuals concerned with malpractice contend that in addition to malpractice premiums, there are expenses incurred by defensive medicine strategies performed solely to reduce the provider's risk of being sued. A Congressional Budget Office Study (1992) suggests that the costs of defensive medicine are highly exaggerated. It contends that most of the testing and procedures are done to reduce the uncertainty of medical diagnosis and these would continue with or without the risk of lawsuits.

As health care costs have escalated, government and private industry have made efforts to contain expenditures. These efforts have resulted in actions that have either limited access to health care or reduced available services to certain segments of the population.

Groups at Risk from Increasing Costs and Fewer Services

Three specific groups have been particularly hard hit by escalating costs and reductions in services: the elderly, poor children, and a growing population of medically indigent individuals. The medically indigent are those who do not have health insurance coverage, do not qualify for government health care assistance, and are unable to pay health care costs on their own.

The rapid expansion of the elderly population has increased the number of patients in need of health care services. In 1991, 42.4% of the aged were 75 years or older (U.S. Bureau of the Census, 1991). The elderly, especially frail elderly persons, are at increased risk of disability and chronic disease. As will be seen, the services they receive under Medicare are limited and require co-payments.

Children in low-income families are another risk group. From 1979 to 1989, the number of children at the poverty level increased 22% (Martin, 1992). During that same time, the social service and health care assistance programs designed to assist them were, in many instances, cut back (Pepper Commission, 1990). As a result, the number of children at risk for hunger and health problems rose significantly, so that currently one of every five children lives in poverty (Segal, 1991; Kliegman, 1992).

In 1992, there were approximately 37 million persons who were medically indigent. This group had no health insurance, including government-sponsored medical insurance (Chisman & Pifer, 1987; Ginsburg & Prout, 1990). They are the "working poor." Their income makes them ineligible for governmental assistance, but is not sufficient for them to purchase their own health care or insurance.

While the elderly, poor children, and the medically uninsured are the groups most prominently in the national spotlight, others have been affected by the rising cost of health services. As cost containment strategies are implemented by employers, many employees find their health insurance benefits reduced or eliminated. Others assume they are adequately covered until they experience a catastrophic illness or chronic disability and discover firsthand the personal cost of health care services.

Relevance of Health Care Financing to Community Health Nursing Practice

Why is the financing of health care services important to the community health nurse? Why not just continue providing appropriate care to a case load or community and leave others to worry about the financial costs and how to meet them? For one thing, nurses will find that nursing practice is shaped to some extent by those financial constructs. If a community health nurse is providing home visits to a newly diagnosed diabetic patient, the number of home visits allowed is limited by the government agency or private insurance company who finances the visits. A nurse assigned to provide skilled nursing care in the home to an individual (e.g., dressing changes), may find that the person requires other services, such as nutritional health teaching or medication monitoring. These services may not be covered by the payer, especially if they are not related to the specific medical condition for which the visits are made. If, while on a home visit, a community health nurse discovers that other household members need or would benefit from nursing care, these members may not be covered by the insurance company, or if they are covered, the problem identified may not be considered reimbursable by the payer.

Why should community health nurses care whether the needed services are paid for? Why not provide the service anyway while the nurse is already in the home? Although occasionally this solution is possible, more often time constraints will not allow the nurse to do this on a regular basis. The nurse's employing agency is reimbursed only for specific services provided to clients. Therefore, the agency will set a nurse's patient load for the day based on a reasonable time for those designated services. Any nurse who routinely provides additional services to clients or cares for other household members may fall behind in the agency's caseload expectation. Nurses may also find that they are not covered in case of a malpractice claim, because the additional service was not first sanctioned by the agency (Creighton, 1986). Thus, the community health nurse faces a dilemma: how to reconcile the ideals of good nursing care to the realities dictated by circumstances, the nurse's employer, and the financial reimbursement system.

Financial Reimbursement for Health Care in the United States

A review of the methods by which health care services are financed in the United States is an important first step in any effort to understand how health care services are currently funded in this country. The United States has a fragmented (some would say multifaceted) method of financing health care. It has even been called "the system that is no system." While most major developed countries have addressed the question of health care delivery by adopting some version of a national health care system, the United States, with its reliance on the free market system, decided to allow the private sector to provide insurance coverage. Those not covered under private insurance or

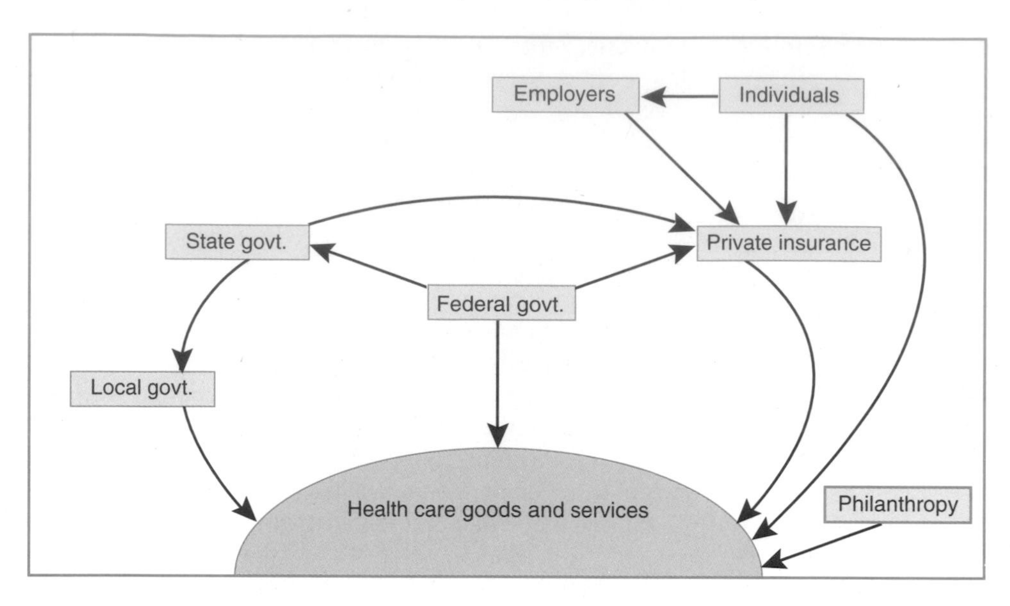

Figure 5–3 ● Funding sources for health care goods and services.

unable to pay for themselves receive aid through a variety of governmental programs. In the U.S. system, the government acts as the agent of last resort to insure care for certain groups of citizens.

At the present time, health care financing is very complex. Services are paid for by a variety of sources and methods, rather than by a single funding source (Fig. 5–3). Health insurance is a voluntary arrangement developed and managed by commercial insurance companies and Blue Cross and Blue Shield. Employers also provide a variety of health insurance plans. Health care for the poor is provided by local, state, and federal funding, primarily through Medicaid. State and local health departments provide some direct services, most of them concentrated in the area of preventive health services (well-baby clinics, family planning, immunizations). Senior citizens are usually covered under the Medicare program, and some may also have any of a variety of private insurance plans to supplement Medicare coverage. The federal government provides directly funded care to a variety of groups, including military personnel and their families, armed services veterans, and American Indians. Individuals may also purchase health care services directly rather than using health insurance or government-funded programs.

CONCERNS WITH THE PRESENT SYSTEM

Health care costs continue to spiral upward, generating concern at all levels of government and in the private sector and the public at large. Critics of the system say that it is cumbersome, too decentralized, and lacking in common purpose or goals. Publicly funded or government-supplied care has continued to expand since the 1960s. As a result, government's share of the cost of medical care has increased, while the private sector's share has declined, as shown in Figure 5–4. The creation of Medicare and Medicaid in 1965 rapidly increased public funding. Concern over governmental costs prompted the Reagan administration to institute cost-cutting measures; these have resulted in a stabilization of the government's share at around 42% of total cost. Current estimates expect the government's share to remain stable through 1993. Policy changes in response to increased public concern over access and quality of health care could lead to increasing costs if the government assumes more responsibility for health care coverage.

Why has the public sector's share expanded? The original intent was to allow the private sector to plan and implement care for most people. The government was to provide back-up care for those few groups not covered by the private sector. The answer to government's expanded role, economists believe, centers around the structure and function of the current health care system, an example of market failure.

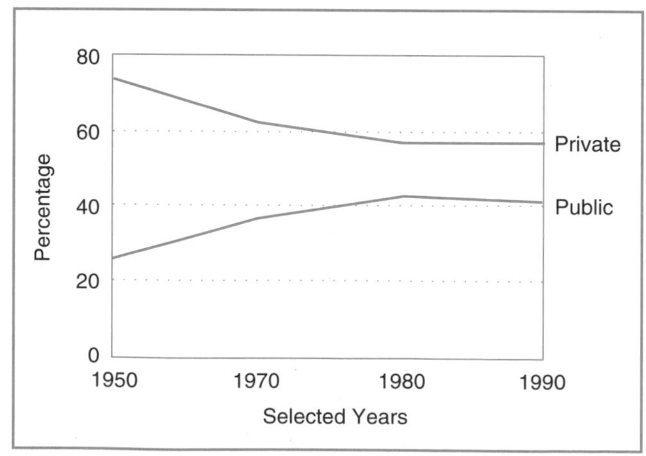

Figure 5–4 ● Public and private share of health care costs. (Data from Health Care Finance Administration.)

THE FREE MARKET ECONOMY AND CONSEQUENCES OF MARKET FAILURE

The United States economic system is biased toward a strong capitalistic or free market economy. This means that in general, business has traditionally been allowed to operate independently, without much governmental interference. That same inclination has been followed in the system or market that provides health care services. The result is that the private sector plays a substantial role in the delivery of health care.

In a theoretically pure free market economy, the price of a product determines how much will be produced (supply) and consumed (demand). In the health care system, products include all types of care (either services or goods) currently available. Thus, products include services such as physician office visits, nursing care, and dental care and goods such as medications, diagnostic tests, and prosthetics. Figure 5–5 shows how price influences both the production (supply) and the consumption (demand) of a specific good (in this case, golf balls).

According to economic theory, the capitalistic or free market will operate efficiently only under certain conditions. If any or all of these conditions are not present, the market will fail, and one of two situations will occur: either the market will not operate effectively, or it will cease to operate at all. In both situations, the consumer is generally at a disadvantage.

The main problem with the free market system of health care delivery is that it has not worked well in providing health care to the entire population. The reason it has not, critics argue, is because it is an example of market failure, violating tenets basic to the effective operation of a free market (Congressional Budget Office, 1992). In other words, the free market delivery of health care is impeded.

When market failure is present, the government can act to protect the consumer in several ways. The government can place restrictions or regulations on the producers in the market (i.e., regulate the market), or the government can take over the production and distribution of the market (i.e., the government becomes the supplier of services). Both types of actions have been taken with regard to the health care market in the United States. Government supervision of the health insurance industry is an example of regulation. The Medicare program is an example of government supplying a service to a specific group (i.e., Americans older than 65 years).

BARRIERS TO AN EFFICIENT FREE MARKET HEALTH CARE SYSTEM

A number of factors hamper effective free market enterprise in health care delivery. Foremost is the lack of strong incentives to encourage competition among providers of health care goods and services. Coupled with few incentives for competition, there has been a slow response of third-party payers (private insurers) to control or influence the price structure for health services.

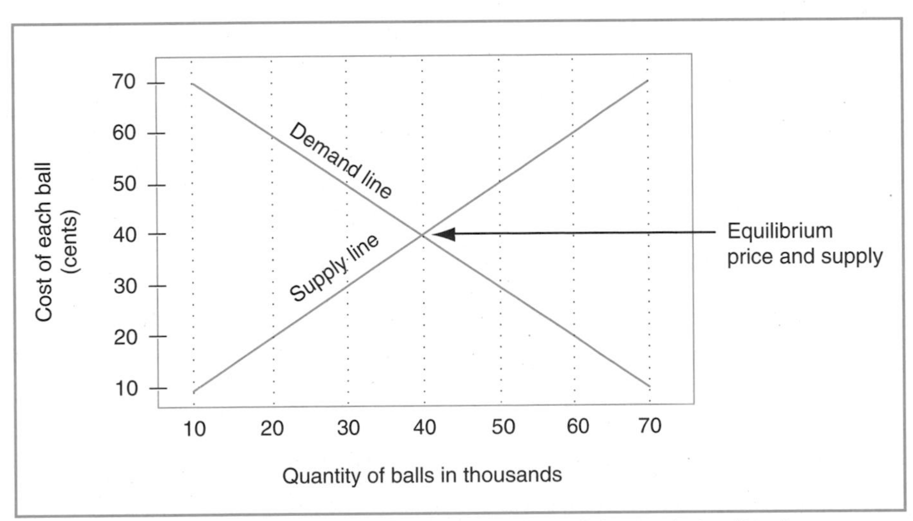

Figure 5–5 ● How price influences supply and demand of golf balls.

The supply line shows that as the price of an item increases, production and, therefore, the amount of goods produced increases. When the price is high, the producer is willing to make larger quantities, and as the price falls, the producer makes fewer balls. The demand line demonstrates how price affects the consumer's demand for golf balls. The greater the price, the less demand.

When the free market operates effectively, competition forces a balance between the amount supplied and the amount demanded. The price of goods produced at that point is called the equilibrium price, 40¢ per ball in this case.

If the price were higher, the producer would be willing to supply a greater quantity, but the consumer would not be willing (or would be unable) to purchase that quantity and there would be an oversupply. If the cost were lower, the consumer would be willing to buy a greater quantity, but the producer would not be willing (or able) to produce the quantity in demand at that price and there would be a shortage.

Reinhardt (1973), Battistella and Begun (1984), Feldstein (1993), and others have identified several additional conditions that make it hard for competition to balance the interests of suppliers and consumers. Consumers do not have good information with which to make decisions about selecting specific providers or types of care, because comparison information is hard to find or not available (Quinn, 1992). Some health care professionals have invested in laboratories, diagnostic equipment, and other health care facilities and thus have a financial interest that may affect their ability to offer impartial advice, treatment, or referrals to their clients (Brown, 1992). Finally, a true market economy is expected to operate in a cost-efficient manner. The operational framework of private nonprofit organizations requires a balanced budget, not cost efficiency. There are a large number of private nonprofit organizations, with few constraints to limit the manner in which their funds are spent. Many are cost efficient, but others can be very wasteful of financial resources. A more detailed discussion of the barriers to an efficient health care market is provided in Table 5–1.

HEALTH CARE AS A RIGHT OR PRIVILEGE

Perhaps the ultimate concern about the market system's ability to provide health care services revolves around the central philosophy that guides the provision of health care services. In a capitalistic market, not everyone may be able to purchase services. As the price of services goes up, the number of consumers who are unable to participate or purchase health care increases. If you believe that health care is a privilege based on the ability to pay, then there is no problem with providing care via the free market system. Those who can afford services receive them, and those who cannot do without.

The United States, like most industrialized nations, adheres to the idea that at least some measure of care should be considered the right of its citizens. Instead of allowing some people to go without any health care, the government has assumed responsibility for financing health care for selected aggregates of the population—namely, the elderly and the very poor. The government has in effect become the

TABLE 5–1

Barriers to a Free Market Economy in Health Care

Poor Consumer Information
If you were planning to buy a car, you would probably seek advice from friends or relatives; read the available literature on performance, cost, and safety of various models; and maybe seek out "expert" advice. When people deal with health care needs, their information sources are more limited and frequently imperfect. They are often under time constraints. Even when information is available, it frequently costs more than the consumer is able to spend. When faced with cancer and told of the need for immediate treatment, few people will take the time to seek multiple sources of information on all available treatment modalities, even if they know how to go about acquiring such information (Quinn, 1992).
Competition Hampered
Ineffective Pricing System: Pricing is based on "reasonable and customary" charges. The provider (seller) of care determines the "reasonable" price with little input from others. Critics argue that the suppliers usually expend efforts in attempts to increase the "allowable fees" for such a service (Feldstein, 1993). This strategy is usually successful. For example, the suppliers of a medical good or service (drugs, office visit, diagnostic test) increase the price in a given geographic region. After a time, this becomes the new "reasonable and customary" charge for reimbursement for that particular product. *Indirect Payment Structure Reduces Concern for Costs of Services:* Until relatively recently, the largest payers of service have been unable or unwilling to influence the pricing mechanism and have done little to encourage competition. Individual consumers have not had the clout to attempt to alter the payment mechanism.
Imperfect Agents to Represent Consumers' Best Interest
The free market has two mutually exclusive sets of actors: buyers and sellers. This is not true of the health care market, especially with respect to physicians. Physicians act as both suppliers of health care and demanders of patient services, many of which the physician may supply. In an economic sense this action places physicians in a conflict of interest, because their income source is derived in large measure from services they demand and frequently supply to their patients. As a result, physicians can be torn between their financial interests and the least costly mechanism of care. Thus, physicians are imperfect agents to represent the client's best interest. Studies by the Department of Health and Human Services and others indicate that physicians are more likely to require laboratory studies, radiographs, ultrasound, and physical therapy if they own such equipment or have an interest in a business that provides such services (Brown, 1992).
Suppliers of Service are not Always Motivated by Cost Efficiency
In the competition model, service providers are expected to be profit maximizers. They are expected to make every effort to operate efficiently and to make a profit. Feldstein (1993) argues that there are a large number of private nonprofit organizations that provide health care with little incentive to be cost efficient. By law, nonprofit organizations cannot make a profit. Their budgets must balance at the end of each year; expenditures must equal revenues. Within that constraint, nonprofit organizations may spend their revenues as they please. Many nonprofit organizations are cost conscious, striving to maximize health services and limit administrative costs. Others may have different preferences. Some examples include enhancing the organization's professional reputation with state-of-the-art equipment, regardless of need; enhancing the physical amenities and ambiance of the institution with plush lounges or sporting facilities; or extending benefits to administrative officers such as personal limousines, recreational trips with luxurious accommodations, or private boxes at sports stadiums. In 1992 both the national director of the United Way Campaign and several administrators of Blue Cross/Blue Shield were cited for just such actions (Crenshaw and Heath, 1992).

guarantor of last resort for specific risk groups. The most common government role is funding of care, either directly or through insurance companies. Health services are usually provided by the private sector rather than by government agencies.

Under these conditions a true market economy for health care does not apply, and, some would argue, with good reason. There has been increasing concern regarding the U.S. system of health care delivery. Critics charge that it is neither effective nor efficient and advocate a complete overhaul with increased governmental regulation as the only strategy that will provide the necessary funds and organization to deliver adequate care at a reasonable price. Chapter 3 identifies the most prominent alternatives for health care reform. While there are many critics of the current system, there are also supporters. Supporters generally argue that the current system meets the needs of most citizens and provides high-quality care. They contend that government action should be directed toward fine-tuning the system to ensure service to those not covered or with inadequate coverage. Nursing's Agenda For Health Care Reform supports a national health care system that ensures universal access and health care services to the entire population (American Nurses' Association, 1991).

Whatever your personal position on this issue, it is useful to examine the present financing system to determine how it operates. After identifying the individual components, discovering who has access, and examining what services are available and to whom they are available, you will be in a better position to evaluate how well the system operates in providing care to the entire population.

Health Care Financing Mechanisms

There are several methods by which people can finance health care services in the United States: self-payment, health care insurance, or health care assistance. The last two are examples of third-party payment, which simply means that a third party (i.e., someone other than the recipient of care) directly pays for all or part of the health services provided. The third party may be a private insurance company or the government. Frequently, the patient has no notion of the exact costs of the services provided and sometimes never sees the bills.

SELF-PAYMENT

In self-payment method, a person or a family essentially assumes the financial cost of all medical services. This was the most common method of purchasing services before the 1930s. Currently, however, it is the least common method

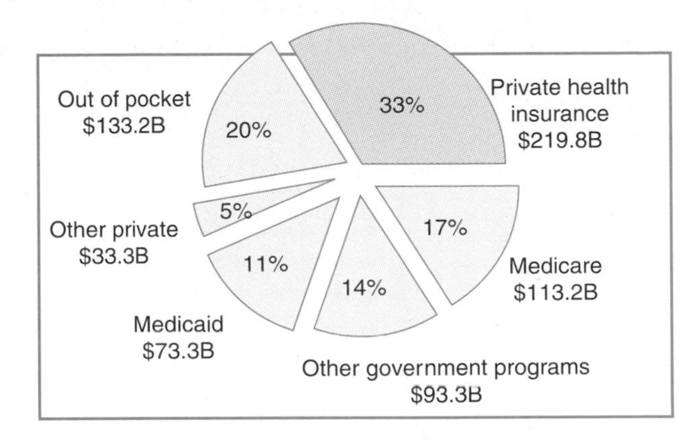

Figure 5–6 ● Funding sources for health care (1990) in billions of dollars (B) (total = $666.2 billion). The category "other private" includes industrial health services, nonpatient revenues, and privately financed construction. (Redrawn from Levit, K. R., Lazenby, H. C., Cowan, C. A., & Letsch, S. W. (1991). National health expenditures, 1990. *Health Care Financing Review, 13*(1), 29.)

of payment, primarily because individuals are very wary of the financial burden posed by chronic or catastrophic illness. Private self-payment makes up only 20% of the total nongovernmental expenditures for health care (Fig. 5–6).

HEALTH CARE INSURANCE

Gradually health insurance replaced self-payment and by 1970 was the most common means of paying medical costs. Currently, 45% of the total expenditures for health are paid by health insurance (private health insurance and Medicare). Premiums for health insurance were $216.8 billion in 1990, or 32.5% of the total health care budget for that year (Levit et al., 1991).

Employer-Provided Health Insurance

The most common form of health insurance is employer-provided insurance, in which employees and their families are covered through their employer. Usually the employer pays some or all of the cost of the premiums for workers. The employee receives health insurance benefits at no cost or at less than the actual cost of insurance premiums. Employer-provided health care insurance is an expected benefit for many employees, but it has never been a universal benefit of employment. This type of coverage appears to be eroding (Fig. 5–7). In 1990, approximately 2.1 million fewer workers were covered than in 1989 (Sullivan et al., 1992). Employees of small companies are less likely to have employer-sponsored health insurance. Only one third of firms with 10 or fewer employees offer health insurance plans, and almost all companies with 100 or more employees do so (Congressional Budget Office, 1992).

Employers' costs of contributions have risen over the years as premium costs have increased. In 1950 employers paid the equivalent of one half of 1% (0.5%) of their

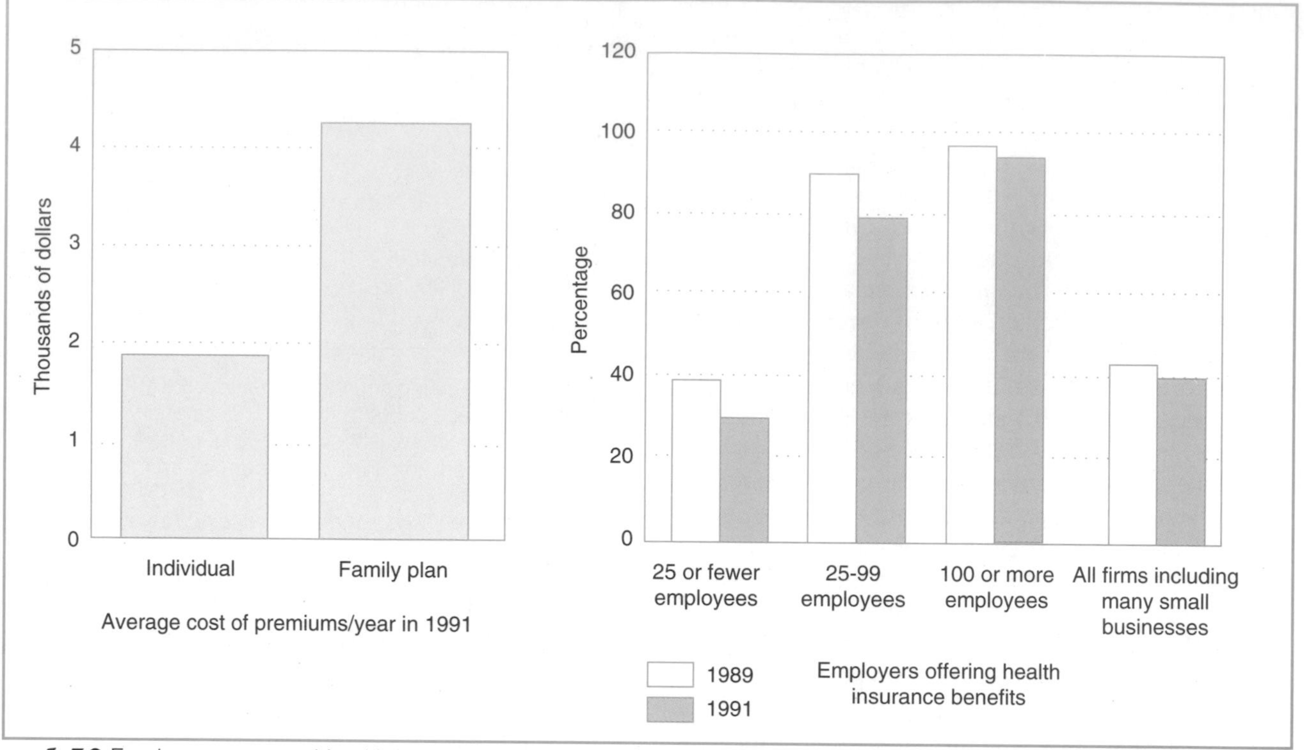

Figure 5–7 ● Employer-sponsored health insurance, 1989–1991. Average cost of premiums per year, 1991 (*left*). Employers offering health insurance benefits, 1989 and 1991 (*right*). (Redrawn from Sullivan, C. B., Miller, M., Feldman, R., & Dowd, B. (1992). Employer-sponsored health insurance in 1991. *Health Affairs 11*,(4), 172.)

employees' salaries (Freeland and Schendler, 1984). By 1991, however, premium costs were very substantial, forcing employers to examine the cost of offering health insurance benefits. Hefty premium increases between 1989 and 1991 were directly related to decreases in the number of employer-offered plans during the same period (see Fig. 5–7).

As employer costs have continued to increase, more and more cost-containment strategies have been initiated. Chrysler Corporation, for example, reviewed all its costs when the company experienced financial difficulty in 1981 and found that health care expenses were expected to be $460 million by 1984 and more than $1 billion by 1991, costing $16,000 per worker (Califano, 1986). In 1 year alone, Chrysler paid $12 million for laboratory tests and $4 million for physician first-day hospital admission visits. Chrysler's expenses are somewhat dramatic, because it is a very large corporation. Nevertheless, these figures underscore the concern all employers have with increasing health care costs and indicate a need for action.

Cost-containment strategies are becoming routine in employer-provided group health insurance plans. The Health Care Finance Administration (HCFA) reports common strategies employers use: reimbursement for generic-only prescriptions; increasing reliance on second opinions for surgery; provisions for preadmission testing to eliminate the larger costs incurred for these services on hospitalization; and increased reliance on outpatient surgery. Health maintenance organizations (HMOs) and other managed care plans are also being offered to employees as an alternative or exclusive health plan. By 1991, 54% of employees in employer-sponsored plans were in managed care (Sullivan et al., 1992).

Employers have also become more involved in their benefits programs, reducing their reliance on traditional insurers, increasing self-funding of health benefits, using non–insurance program administrators to monitor costs, and requiring employees to shoulder more of the cost of health insurance. On average, employees are required to pay 10% to 15% of the premium cost for individuals and 25% to 30% of the premium cost for a family plan (Sullivan et al., 1992).

The current political debate centers around whether health insurance coverage should be mandated for all firms with employees. Most small business leaders are opposed to employer-mandated health insurance, claiming the net effect would be a loss of jobs, increasing costs to consumers, and some business failures. Proponents argue that it is sound business practice to provide coverage, as it will attract a more stable work force. There have been some moves in the direction of employer-mandated health insurance for workers, and several states have passed legislation requiring such benefits. Hawaii, for example, has operated a health care plan with universal coverage for all employed citizens since the early 1980s.

Other Health Insurance

Medicare, another type of health insurance plan, is a government insurance program designed primarily for use by older Americans. Medicare will be addressed later in this chapter.

HEALTH CARE ASSISTANCE

There are a number of other ways care is funded for people who cannot afford to pay for services and do not have health insurance. Health care assistance is another third-party payment mechanism in which payment is provided by a governmental program (either federal or state) or private charity. The most familiar program of this type is Medicaid, which provides service to about 27.3 million persons at a cost of $96.5 billion, or 13% of the entire health care budget (Congressional Budget Office, 1991, unpublished data; Letsch et al., 1992). Details of this program are discussed later in the chapter.

Both state and local health departments provide a variety of health services. Most of these services are aimed at poor populations, and the majority are prevention oriented, although some direct services to ill persons may be available. Funds for these services are a mix of federal, state, and local monies (see Chapter 30).

Private charity provides a variety of services to the needy. Nonprofit organizations usually target special health needs or special risk groups. Philanthropic gifts to hospitals assist with payments for persons without insurance, and many health care providers offer some free care. Spontaneous fund raisers meet expensive special needs such as liver or heart transplants for certain individuals. It is difficult to quantify the actual dollars provided by charitable organizations and events for direct health services to individuals. The HCFA reports that philanthropic activities accounted for 2.8% of the total health budget in 1989, or $16.1 billion. That amount includes both direct care to individuals and contributions to research and facilities development. It is safe to say that charitable contributions make up a minuscule portion of the health care budget.

LACK OF HEALTH INSURANCE

More than 37 million persons are not covered by health insurance or assistance of any kind and are unable to pay for services on their own (Ginsburg and Prout, 1990). Most are workers attempting to provide a living for themselves and their dependents at low-paying jobs with few benefits. These are the "working poor." They and their dependents make up an estimated 60% to 80% of the medically indigent (Wilensky, 1987; Fuschs, 1991). The remainder are individuals who are currently unemployed or uninsurable and others who fall outside the eligibility requirements for Medicare or Medicaid (e.g., some of the homeless, some elderly, and children).

Employees with limited job skills have less bargaining power as employers attempt cost-cutting measures. Many of the uninsured work in a service industry such as food or janitorial service. Those jobs require few skills and little education, offer fewer benefits, and are generally low paying. Service type jobs are increasing, thus placing more workers at risk. By 1987 there were 31 million service jobs, an increase of 6 million from 1970 (Wilensky, 1987). The majority of those employed in service positions receive no health insurance benefits. When the uninsured need health care, they are limited in their options. They must pay at the time of service or find a health care provider who is willing to defer payment. Many delay seeking care, hoping they will improve on their own.

UNDERINSURED AND AT FINANCIAL RISK

In addition to those with no medical insurance, there are millions who are underinsured. These have insurance requiring large out-of-pocket expenses or limiting coverage of catastrophic illnesses. Ginsburg and Prout (1990) estimate that between 8% and 26% of all privately insured persons in the United States are underinsured. This translates to an estimated 30 to 60 million Americans who are underinsured (Knox, 1989; Jacobs, 1991).

LEVEL OF HEALTH RELATED TO MEDICAL INSURANCE

The medically indigent (uninsured) have greater health risks. These families have a harder time acquiring the basic necessities of food, clothing, shelter, and transportation, and medical needs force them to make hard choices regarding exactly what services they can afford. Studies show that the uninsured contain a larger number of people in fair to poor health, with a greater incidence of chronic illness. They are less likely to seek care early, make fewer visits to physicians, and are less likely to be hospitalized than insured individuals. There are at least 13.5 million Americans (6%) who do not seek or receive medical care for financial reasons (Chisman and Pifer, 1987; Freeman et al., 1987). The uninsured delay care, so when they finally seek care, their health problems are usually more severe than those of insured people. They are more likely to use the hospital emergency department because they have no personal health care provider, and hospitals are obliged to provide some care to indigent patients and treat all life-threatening conditions. The cost of such care either is assumed by the hospital or becomes a public expenditure. Emergency department care is a more costly form of service than clinics or physicians' offices. The American Hospital Association (AHA) reports that the cost of uncompensated care in hospitals doubled from 1980 to 1985, and the cost of such care in 1990 was $8.3 billion dollars (American Hospital Association, 1990).

Publicly Funded Programs for Health Care Services

Medicare and Medicaid are the two programs that provide a major portion of health care services to populations who have been identified as in greater need (elderly persons) or having fewer resources (the poor). Specific costs and benefits change periodically. Rather than concentrate on current benefits, the focus of this discussion will be on exploring each program's basic purpose, evolution, and beneficiaries. A brief comparison of covered and excluded services for each program is discussed, and examples and costs will be used to illustrate points under discussion. This information is important to community health nurses, because many of their clients are covered by these programs. Nurses need to know what services clients can expect if they are enrolled in these programs.

MEDICARE

Medicare was created in 1965. Before that time, the burden for providing health care for the elderly and chronically ill was borne by family members, friends, and charitable organizations. Medicare was an attempt to ensure that adequate medical care would be available to the aged and some chronically ill persons, and that the price of such services would not be so prohibitive that persons would have to forgo basic care. Its major strengths are that it has significantly improved access to health services for eligible persons and has helped reduce the number of elderly in poverty.

Medicare is federally funded and is financed by a tax on wages. Every citizen who is currently working provides a portion of his or her salary to the budget of the Medicare program. Employers and employees contribute an equal percentage of wages to fund Medicare. Formerly the contribution was tied to the Social Security contribution, but in 1991 Medicare was separated from Social Security contributions to include federal workers and others who did not contribute to Social Security. The contribution levels for both employer and employee have risen so that both pay 1.45% of the worker's salary into the Medicare Insurance Fund. The net effect is that all costs, for both worker and employer, have risen. Medicare's budget increased from $4.7 billion in 1967, the first full year of operation, to $132 billion in 1992, a 2800% increase.

Medicare has evolved into an important source of income for health care providers. It provides more than 30% of total income to hospitals and 21% of all income to physicians, although some hospitals and physicians receive even a greater portion of their income from Medicare. Califano (1986) reports that certain medical specialties commonly exceed the 21% average Medicare income level. Those include thoracic surgeons, internists, and radiologists.

Beneficiaries

The primary beneficiaries of Medicare are the elderly who have contributed to the system during their working life or those persons whose spouse contributed. In 1972, Congress extended coverage to persons under age 65 years with long-term disabilities or end-stage renal disease. By 1991, 30.5 million senior citizens and 3.25 million disabled persons received benefits (*Statistical Abstracts of the United States,* 1992).

Benefits

Medicare is divided into two parts: part A covers hospital insurance, and part B covers supplementary medical insurance (SMI). All contributors are covered by part A, but part B is voluntary and is limited to those who choose to participate and pay a premium deducted from their Social Security check. Most Medicare recipients (99%) do participate in part B coverage. The cost of premiums has steadily increased, and voluntary contributions currently pay for only 25% of the total cost of part B benefits; the rest is financed by the federal government. Benefits under part A and part B are listed in Table 5–2.

Criticisms

Several major concerns have been leveled against the program structure. Most criticisms have to do with institutional bias, service restrictions, or equity.

Institutional Bias. The Medicare payment structure previously was heavily weighted in favor of hospital care. Similar services provided in outpatient settings were not covered, and individuals were encouraged to elect inpatient rather than outpatient service. Califano (1986) notes that between 1970 and 1983, the rate of hospitalization of elderly persons rose 35%.

More recently, as a result of the need for cost-cutting measures, hospitals have sought to reduce the rate of inpatient services and have lobbied Congress to allow increased outpatient utilization. Outpatient services are cost effective because they are less labor intensive, take up little space, and cost less to operate than inpatient services. For example, outpatient clinics do not require the same amount of floor space, can operate with fewer employees, are not staffed 24 hours a day, and require much less high-technology equipment than inpatient units. Outpatient services are expected to continue to increase in the near future, with the HCFA projecting an annual growth rate of 6% in outpatient services at community hospitals (Freeland and Schendler, 1984). In fact, the use of hospital outpatient services grew from 13% of all hospital care in 1980 to 24% in 1990 (Levit et al., 1991).

Other types of outpatient services are also expected to grow, such as freestanding emergency care centers and preferred provider organizations (see Chapter 3).

TABLE 5–2

Medicare Benefits

Medicare (Part A): Hospital Insurance–Covered Services for 1994

Services	*Benefit*	*Medicare Pays*	*You Pay*
Hospitalization: Semiprivate room and board, general nursing and miscellaneous hospital services and supplies. (Medicare payments based on benefit periods).	First 60 days	All but $696	$696
	61st to 90th day	All but $174/day	$174/day
	91st to 150th day*	All but $348/day	$348/day
	Beyond 150 days	Nothing	All costs
Skilled Nursing Facility Care: Semiprivate room and board, general nursing, skilled nursing and rehabilitative services, and other services and supplies† (Medicare payments based on benefit periods).	First 20 days	100% of approved amount	Nothing
	Additional 80 days	All but $87/day	Up to $87 a day
	Beyond 100 days	Nothing	All costs
Home health care: Part-time or intermittent skilled care, home health aide services, durable medical equipment and supplies, and other services.	Unlimited as long as patient meets Medicare conditions	100% of approved amount; 80% of approved amount for durable medical equipment	Nothing for services; 20% of approved amount for durable medical equipment
Hospice care: Pain relief, symptom management, and support services for the terminally ill.	For as long as physician certifies need	All but limited costs for outpatient drugs and inpatient respite care	Limited cost sharing for outpatient drugs and inpatient respite care
Blood	Unlimited if medically necessary	All but first three pints per calendar year	For first three pints‡

1994 Part A monthly premium: None for most beneficiaries; either $245 or $184 if you must buy part A (premium may be higher if you enroll late).
*This 60-reserve-days benefit may be used only once in a lifetime.
†Neither Medicare nor private Medigap insurance will pay for most nursing home care.
‡Blood paid for or replaced under part B Medicare during the calendar year, does not have to be paid for or replaced under part A.

Medicare (Part B): Medical Insurance–Covered Services for 1994

Services	*Benefit*	*Medicare Pays*	*You Pay*
Medical Expenses: Physicians' services, inpatient and outpatient medical and surgical services and supplies, physical and speech therapy, ambulance, diagnostic tests, and durable medical equipment and other services.	Unlimited if medically necessary	80% of approved amount (after $100 deductible)	$100 deductible,* plus 20% of approved amount and limited charges above approved amount.†
Clinical Laboratory Services: Blood tests, biopsies, urinalyses, and more.	Unlimited if medically necessary	Generally100% of approved amount	Nothing for services
Home health care: Part-time or intermittent skilled care, home health aide services, durable medical equipment and supplies, and other services.	Unlimited for as long as patient meets conditions for benefits	100% of approved amount; 80% of approved amount for durable medical equipment	Nothing for services; 20% of approved amount for durable medical equipment
Outpatient hospital treatment: Services for the diagnosis or treatment of illness or injury.	Unlimited if medically necessary	Medicare payment to hospital based on hospital cost	20% of billed charges (after $100 deductible)
Blood	Unlimited if medically necessary	80% of approved amount (after $100 deductible and starting with 4th pint)	First 3 pints plus 20% of approved amount for additional pints (after $100 deductible).‡

1994 Part B monthly premiums: $41.10 (premium may be higher if you enroll late).
*Once patient has had $100 of expenses for covered services in 1994, the part B deductible does not apply to any further covered services received for the rest of the year.
†Unless your doctor does not accept assignments.
‡Blood paid for or replaced under part A. Medicare during the calendar year, does not have to be paid for or replaced under part B.
Source: The Medicare Handbook. (1994) Washington, DC: U.S. Department of Health and Human Service, Health Care Financing Adminstration.

Limited Access and Unequal Burden of Risk. Cost sharing is a requirement of the Medicare program. In addition to the voluntary contribution for part B coverage, recipients must pay a portion of the expenses of the services that they use. Critics charge that co-payments, especially for hospital care, have escalated until they are a major hardship for a large percentage of the covered population (Sidel, 1991).

Co-payments were instituted to save the government money and to encourage judicious use of services. Numerous studies support co-payments as a method that tends to reduce usage. There is an inverse relationship between services used and the rate of co-payment: a 20% or 25% co-payment significantly reduces the use of services (Scitovsky and Snyder, 1972; Snyder and McCall, 1977; Newhouse et al., 1981; CBO Study, 1992). In other words, as the amount of personal cost declines, people seek more health care, and as personal cost increases, people curtail the use of services.

Critics of cost sharing charge that it discourages people from receiving necessary medical care or encourages them to postpone care until the condition becomes more severe or even life threatening. While there are few data in controlled studies to support this argument, we do know that people who are living on small amounts of money tend to be sicker when they seek care and require more extensive care as a result (Anderson et al., 1987). It would appear logical to assume that the same condition holds true with persons whose co-payment levels are relatively high with respect to their incomes. Data to support or deny this position would be extremely useful in planning changes to the system.

Equity. A major concern of cost sharing is the question of equity. Medicare is a regressive cost program in which everyone, regardless of circumstances and finances, essentially pays the same amount or cost for similar benefits. Thus, greater cost burdens are placed on the poor, because their out-of-pocket expenses reflect a larger proportion of their income than those of persons with larger incomes. This disproportionate cost is illustrated in Figure 5–8. It can be seen that if three patients are hospitalized for the same number of days, with the same problem, and receive the same treatment, their costs (Medicare co-payments and deductibles) are essentially the same, but the impact on their finances is not. As income goes up, the impact of health care expenses is less. The greatest burden is to Mr. A, who has the lowest income.

Protection from Financial Hardship

Medicare does not protect the individual from financial destitution, the primary reason for creation of the program. Currently, the cost of co-payments and restrictions on coverage make it very difficult for many persons who face a major illness, particularly a long illness, to afford the health care services they need.

The chronically ill can easily have several hospital stays owing to complications and deteriorating health status. While in the hospital, a person can expect to see the primary physician and one or two specialists, either for consultation or for specific therapy, and undergo radiographs and other diagnostic examinations. With co-payments and deductibles for covered services and no ceiling on potential expenses, it is easy to see that a chronically ill person could quickly accrue a bill of several thousand dollars.

Often the elderly are faced with the prospect of "spending down" to qualify for another health coverage program, Medicaid. Spending down is the process whereby a person must first exhaust most assets to pay medical bills. When the person's assets are nearly gone, he or she will qualify for medical assistance care under the program that provides care to the poor, Medicaid.

Medigap Insurance

To insure against devastating financial loss, the majority of elderly (approximately 66%) have some additional health care insurance from private companies. Medigap policies are intended to reimburse out of pocket costs for Medicare covered services; additionally, some pay for services not covered by Medicare. Before 1990, wide variation in costs, covered services, eligibility requirements, and reimbursable amounts was normal, and some policies were comprehensive in scope, while many were not. The number and variety of policies available make benefit comparison difficult, and fraud and abusive sales tactics were common. The Advocates for Senior Alert (1990) reported that many elderly had purchased two or more policies with duplicate benefits.

Therefore, in 1990 Congress directed the National Association of Insurance Commissioners to standardize policies. This group developed 10 standardized plans (Fig. 5–9). Each Medigap insurance provider must offer the basic policy (A) and may choose to offer any or all of the remaining plans (B through J). These new insurance plans should ease comparison of costs and benefits for the elderly (Rice and Thomas, 1992).

The need for Medigap insurance places the elderly who can least afford it at the greatest financial risk. While two thirds of Medicare recipients carry extra coverage, one third do not, usually because they cannot afford coverage. Premiums for Medigap insurance are expensive, ranging

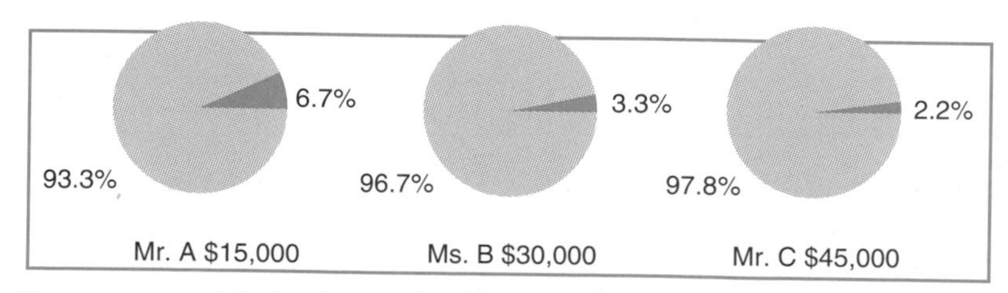

Figure 5–8 ● Percentage of income needed for health care for three individuals with different incomes and similar health care needs. All three persons have $1000 out-of-pocket expenses in deductibles and co-payments for Part A and B Medicare benefits.

Basic Benefits: Included in all plans.
Hospitalization: Part A co-insurance plus coverage for 365 additional days after Medicare benefits end.
Medical Expenses: Part B co-insurance (20% of Medicare-approved expenses).
Blood: First three pints of blood each year.

A	B	C	D	E	F	G	H	I	J
Basic Benefits	Basic Benefits	Basic Benefits	Basic Benefits	Basic Benefits	Basic Benefits	Basic Benefits	Basic Benefits	Basic Benefits	Basic Benefits
		Skilled Nursing Co-insurance	Skilled Nursing Co-insurance	Skilled Nursing Co-insurance	Skilled Nursing Co-insurance	Skilled Nursing Co-insurance	Skilled Nursing Co-insurance	Skilled Nursing Co-insurance	Skilled Nursing Co-insurance
	Part A Deductible	Part A Deductible	Part A Deductible	Part A Deductible	Part A Deductible	Part A Deductible	Part A Deductible	Part A Deductible	Part A Deductible
		Part B Deductible			Part B Deductible				Part B Deductible
					Part B Excess (100%)	Part B Excess (80%)		Part B Excess (100%)	Part B Excess (100%)
		Foreign Travel Emergency	Foreign Travel Emergency	Foreign Travel Emergency	Foreign Travel Emergency	Foreign Travel Emergency	Foreign Travel Emergency	Foreign Travel Emergency	Foreign Travel Emergency
			At-Home Recovery			At-Home Recovery		At-Home Recovery	At-Home Recovery
							Basic Drugs ($1,250 Limit)	Basic Drugs ($1,250 Limit)	Extended Drugs ($3,000 Limit)
				Preventive Care					Preventive Care

Figure 5–9 ● Ten standard Medigap insurance policies. (Reprinted by permission of the National Association of Insurance Commissioners (NAIC). (1990). *Medigap policy prototypes,* Kansas City, MO: NAIC.)

from $650 to $1500 or more per year. As costs increase, more elderly can be expected to be unable to afford coverage, thereby increasing their risk of financial destitution.

For example, an elderly couple living on a fixed income of $20,000 per year would pay 10% of their total income in Medigap premiums alone. In addition, they would pay the medical cost of part B Medicare premiums and a 20% co-payment on any medical services needed.

Services not Covered

The single most common misconception about Medicare is that it meets long-term care needs, including nursing home care. In fact, benefits are severely restricted. Skilled nursing home care is limited to 100 days per year with mandatory deductibles (Table 5–3).

Custodial nursing home care is not covered by Medicare or by many private insurance plans. Most elderly nursing home residents require custodial or intermediate skilled care, are not eligible for Medicare benefits, and are at financial risk. The average annual cost of nursing home care per patient exceeds $30,000 (Cohen et al., 1992), an amount that can rapidly deplete personal savings. In fact, many nursing home residents meet the income means test for Medicaid coverage. The Institute of Medicine (1986) reports that about half of the costs of nursing home care are paid by the individual, 47% by Medicaid, and 3% by Medicare or private insurance.

For example, Mrs. Jones had Alzheimer's disease and required custodial nursing care for 2 years before her death. The cost of 2 years of care was $60,000. The Jones family had to "spend down," using $15,000 of their savings before Medicaid paid for nursing care.

As the incidence of chronic illness increases with age, the probability of nursing home admission also increases.

TABLE 5–3

Services not Covered under Medicare

- Long-term care—custodial care over an extended period in the home, a custodial nursing home, or a residential care facility
- Limited nursing home coverage—only a skilled nursing home for limited periods of time
- Part A and part B deductible and co-payment obligations
- Prescription drugs
- Dental, eye, ear, and foot care, including eyeglasses, hearing aids, and dentures
- Limited home health services; does not cover unlimited nursing care or custodial care, Meals on Wheels or other food service programs, or homemaker services

The lifetime risk of needing institutional care exceeds 40%: two of every five elders can expect to stay in an extended care facility either as an intermediate step between hospital and home or at the end of their life (Cohen et al., 1992). This important and common need, one of considerable concern for elder individuals, is not covered by Medicare.

Other services and benefits that are not covered are also outlined in Table 5–3. The most burdensome of these are prescriptions and deductibles and co-payments, especially for the elderly with chronic illnesses and disabilities. In 1994, the part A hospitalization deductible increased to $696, and the monthly cost of part B coverage increased to $41.10, or $493 per person per year.

For example, Mr. and Mrs. Smith have an annual income of $30,000. Mr. Smith has a heart condition that requires $1488 per year in prescription drugs. Mrs. Smith has Parkinson's disease and pays another $1200 a year for medication. The total cost of their medications is $2688 per year. In addition, they pay $986 in premiums for Medicare part B coverage and $1200 per year in Medigap insurance. These medical expenses total $4974 per year, or approximately 17% of their annual income. Physician office visits, laboratory bills, and other medical costs, excluding hospitalization, if necessary, would be in addition to these expenses. The elderly often do not comply with prescribed medication therapy because the costs are more than their limited budgets can handle.

Recent Attempts at Program Change

In 1988, Congress attempted to improve Medicare coverage by easing the burden on patients with chronic and catastrophic illness. Key features of the proposal included the following:

- A flat annual deductible for part A benefits
- Limits on the personal liability of part B deductibles and co-payments ($1370/year)
- Prescription drugs added to coverage
- Increased financial protection for the spouses of persons with catastrophic illness.

These reforms were to be paid for by increasing monthly premiums and adding a surcharge for catastrophic insurance. The surcharge was tied to taxable income, with the more well-to-do elderly expected to contribute more for coverage than those less well off. Resistance to the financing proposal by senior citizens groups was well organized and massive (Rice et al., 1990), and Congress responded by rescinding the reforms before they were implemented.

Current Status of Medicare Coverage

Since the 1988 reform attempt, no substantial changes to Medicare have been made. A separate amendment was passed in 1990 limiting the financial depletion of spousal assets by debilitating illness.

Medicare remains a program with limited coverage, a program with increasing cost liabilities to the consumer that does not meet many of the most serious medical needs of the population it serves. The current concern is whether Medicare can address the needs of the chronically ill in a more comprehensive fashion, and if so, at what cost to the individual and to the nation.

MEDICAID

Medicaid, created in correlation with Medicare in 1965, has a different purpose and a different financing and administrative structure. It is a grant program designed to provide medical assistance to the poor and is funded by both federal and state governments. Medicaid has done a moderately competent job of providing care to limited segments of poor pregnant women and young children, but has been less successful in caring for the aged poor, the disabled, and adults and children not covered under the pregnant women and children programs.

The individual states administer the program. Overall, the federal government pays approximately 50% of the Medicaid budget, but the specific allotment for each state varies from 50% to 78% depending on criteria set by the federal government (Kaiser Family Foundation, 1993). The criteria used to determine the federal share include each state's per capita income and the percentage of Medicaid recipients in the state population. Poorer states receive a greater share from the federal government.

Medicaid is financed by income tax revenues at the federal level and by general tax revenues at the state level, with some contributions from local municipalities. Feldstein (1993) considers this a more equitable method for financing than that used for Medicare, because individual contributions to the program are based on income, so persons with greater income contribute more to the program than do those who have less income.

Like Medicare, Medicaid costs have risen dramatically (Fig. 5–10). In 1968 the program cost approximately $3.45 billion in both federal and state contributions; by 1996, it is expected to cost $158 billion. Medicaid expenditures represent an increasing burden on state budgets. In fact, expenses have often outpaced the rate of growth in state revenues creating a major concern for state administrators (Congressional Budget Office, 1992).

Beneficiaries

The number of persons that Medicaid served varied from time to time but had no dramatic changes until the recession of the early 1990s. In 1983 the number of persons receiving benefits was approximately 21.5 million, the same number as in 1979. Since the number of persons in poverty grew by approximately 10 million during that same time period, the

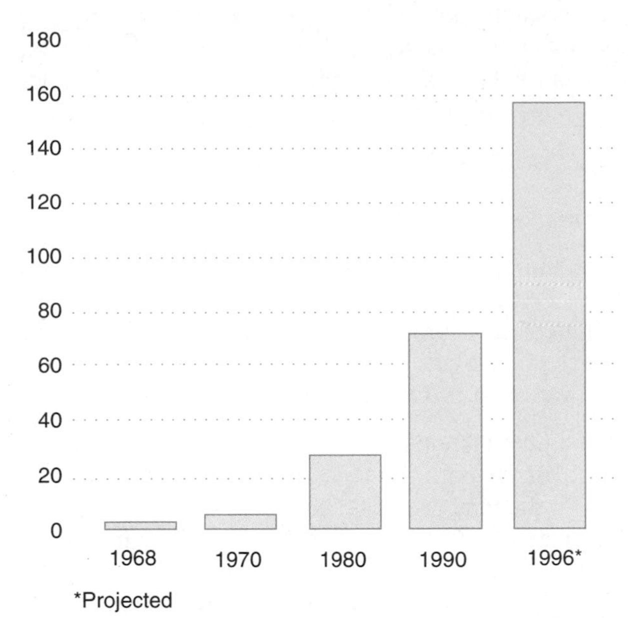

Figure 5–10 ● Medicaid costs for selected years, 1968–1996, in billions of dollars. (Data from Health Care Finance Administration.)

net effect was that approximately 55% fewer poor were covered by the program (Sorkin, 1986). The 1990s recession had the effect of substantially increasing the number of those eligible for Medicaid (Kaiser Family Foundation, 1993). In 1991, Medicaid enrolled 27 million people in the program. Past and current studies indicate that many more who are not enrolled in the program are also in need (Burwell and Rymer, 1987; Pepper Commission, 1990).

Mandated and Optional Recipients

The states are required by the federal government to provide services to certain groups and have the option of providing benefits to others (Table 5–4). The states have some control over the number of state residents covered under federally mandated programs, because they can establish most of the eligibility criteria. Each state establishes its own income and asset ceilings, as well as other criteria. Most states provide Medicaid coverage for families with children on welfare (Aid to Families with Dependent Children [AFDC]). However, not all poor families qualify for AFDC. In 1991, the Medicaid income eligibility level for an AFDC family ranged from 13% to 77% of the poverty level. Thirty-three states have income thresholds below 50% of the poverty level (Congressional Budget Office, May 1992). As an example, eligibility thresholds for an AFDC family of three are 14.1% of the poverty level, or $1,416 per year in Alabama; 26%, or $2,616 per year in Kentucky; and 47.1%, or $4,836 per year in South Carolina (Capilouto et al., 1992)

Family composition is another variant among state AFDC programs. A large majority of the states deny coverage to households if two parents reside in the home, regardless of the financial condition of the family. Single-parent families make up the overwhelming majority of recipients. Almost 90% of the parents in this program are female single parents (Capilouto et al., 1992). Some states allow coverage to two-parent households if the father is unemployed and not receiving unemployment compensation. Seventeen states cover children whose families meet the AFDC income eligibility levels, regardless of their family parental composition or employment status (Sorkin, 1986).

From time to time the federal government may mandate coverage for certain at-risk populations. This was done in

TABLE 5–4

Medicaid Beneficiaries and Services

Medicaid Recipients
Federally Dictated Recipients
• All persons in federal aide programs, including Supplemental Security Income (SSI) and Aid to Families with Dependent Children (AFDC)
• Pregnant women and children up to age 6 with a family income below 133% of the poverty level
• Children aged 18 and under, born after September 30, 1983, with a family income below the poverty level
• Medicare beneficiaries with income below the poverty level (but only for payment of Medicare premiums and cost sharing)
Optional Recipients
• Medically needy families with incomes above AFDC limits with sick children
• Medically needy elders not qualified for income assistance (welfare)
Major Benefits under Medicaid
Federally Required
• Inpatient and outpatient hospital care
• Physician services
• Diagnostic services (laboratory tests, radiographs)
• Skilled nursing home care
• Home health care
• Family planning
• Nurse midwife services
• Certified family or pediatric nurse practitioner services
• Ambulatory services provided in federally qualified health centers
• Early and Periodic Screening, Diagnosis, and Treatment (EPSDT) for people under 21 years of age
State-Determined Optional Services
• Drug therapy
• Dental care
• Physical therapy
• Eyeglasses
• Podiatry
• Optometry
• Clinic services
• Transportation
• Residential intermediate care facilities for the mentally retarded (ICF-MR)
• Nursing facility services for people under 21 years of age
• Prescription drugs
• Prosthetic devices

Note: Covered services are provided to those groups with federally required coverage. Mandated services to optional groups are less comprehensive.
Source: Congressional Budget Office Staff Memorandum, May 1992.

1984, 1985, 1986, 1989, and 1990 as a result of increased concern over the uneven coverage criteria for pregnant women and children. Medicaid coverage was extended in all states, first to pregnant women and children younger than 5 years in two-parent homes that met AFDC income eligibility standards, then to all pregnant women and children younger than 5 years who were at or below the nationally set poverty level, then to children younger than 6 years, then to pregnant women and eligible children at income levels 33% above the poverty level, and finally to all children younger than 19 years in families with income below the poverty level (Congressional Budget Office, May 1992).

The rationale for extended coverage was cost–benefit analysis. Simply stated, the cost of extending medical coverage for prenatal and pediatric care to these populations was significantly less than the cost of providing treatment for problems that would have resulted without care. It should be noted that the coverage expansion just discussed is limited. Nonpregnant females and children above the poverty level were not covered in the expansion and so are still subject to their state's established criteria.

In addition to those beneficiaries who are mandated at the federal level, states may extend care to other groups. The states may or may not receive federal matching funds for these additional groups. Many states have different eligibility requirements and offer optional programs. Thirty-six states cover medically needy families, but income and asset ceilings vary (Congressional Budget Office, May 1992). Some families may find that their income is too high to qualify initially, but extensive medical expenditures will reduce their assets to qualifying levels.

The following needy groups are excluded from Medicaid benefits altogether:

- Single persons and childless couples not aged or disabled
- Most two-parent families
- Most families with a father who works at a low-paying job
- Specific categories of people in states that do not provide voluntary portions of programs (e.g., certain children aged 6 years and over in certain low-income families or medically needy) (Schultz, 1985; Sorkin, 1992; Congressional Budget Office, May 1992).

Approximately 14 states chose not to extend coverage to medically needy families with optional programs.

Benefits

Medicaid benefits vary greatly depending on the state. The federal government requires certain minimum services for recipients, but the states are at liberty to expand the scope of services. Federal minimums and selected state optional benefits are listed in Table 5–4. Community health nurses need to become familiar with the benefits extended to participants in their state of residence.

Approximately half of Medicaid budgets are spent to provide federally mandated programs (Califano, 1986; Kaiser Family Foundation, 1993). Optional services account for most of the remainder of budget expenses.

Criticisms

Several important concerns with the program have been identified. Principal among these are concerns related to increasing costs, disproportionate distribution of services, the impact of cost-cutting measures on beneficiaries, and the wide variation in benefits and recipients covered.

Program Cost Increases. Escalating costs are creating a major burden for both the federal and state governments. Since 1972, the total Medicaid budget has risen an average of 17% annually (Califano, 1986; Congressional Budget Office, May 1992; Kaiser Family Foundation, 1993). Increases in program costs have been most dramatic at the state level (Burke, 1991). Medicaid costs represent a greater share of state budgets than of the federal budget (an average of 9% and 7%, respectively, in 1990) (Congressional Budget Office, May 1992). In addition, state Medicaid costs have risen at three to five times the rate of increases in state revenues. Medicaid costs consumed on average of 14% of state budgets in 1991 (Kaiser Family Foundation, 1993). The Congressional Budget Office estimates that by the year 2000, Medicaid costs will expand to 18% of each state's budget if the program continues as currently structured (Congressional Budget Office, May 1992). Certainly the states have reason for concern.

States must also contend with federal actions that have effectively reduced the expected federal share of the Medicaid budget. In 1981, as part of the Reagan administration's cost-cutting measure known as the Omnibus Budget Reconciliation Act, federal Medicaid grants to the states were reduced 11.5% (Inglehart, 1983). Federal actions did allow states more discretion in administering various portions of the program, but each new directive also placed additional burdens on state funds already straining to meet the demands of the program (Burke, 1991).

Disproportionate Distribution of Services to Beneficiaries. A relatively small group of people account for the majority of costs in the Medicaid program. The elderly and disabled, 27% of beneficiaries, receive care that accounts for 70% of the Medicaid budget (Congressional Budget Office, May 1992). According to the Kaiser Family Foundation (1993), the annual average Medicaid costs were almost eight times higher for the aged and disabled than for children and their parents ($1086 per child and $1844 per parent, compared with $8524 per aged patient and $7729 per disabled patient benefits per year). Faced with expanding numbers of aged and disabled participants, the program becomes increasing inefficient at serving the very people for whom Medicaid was originally intended.

TABLE 5–5

Examples of Specific Cost Containment Measures in the Medicaid Program

Reduction of Beneficiaries
• Federal criteria changes in 1981 eliminated 750,000 persons and saved an estimated $3.9 billion between 1982 and 1985 (Inglehart, 1983) • California eliminated services to medically indigent adults, dropping 270,000 people from service (Sorkin, 1986)
Cost Sharing or Co-payment Requirements
• Since 1982, the federal government has allowed states to require co-payments for services, excluding emergency care, family planning, and prenatal services. Some examples: co-payments for drugs, glasses, dental visits, and inpatient hospital care (Sorkin, 1986).
Control of Cost of Services Provided
• States are authorized by federal government to set Medicaid fee standards, usually at or below the prevailing rate in that state. For example, the average Medicaid payment for a physician visit is 35% below the standard fee to other patients (Sorkin, 1986).
Limited Choice or Selected Providers for Medicaid Recipients
• Managed care or prepaid plans. Twenty-three states have patients in prepaid plans such as PPOs and HMOs (Califano, 1986). • Contract services for drugs, laboratory tests, etc., to specific providers. California found that by contracting services to low bidders, $165 million or more could be saved each year (Califano, 1986).

Federal and State Cost Containment Effects on Beneficiaries. Implementation of cost-cutting measures has resulted in dropping some needy individuals or some necessary services to needy individuals (Table 5–5). Changing the eligibility requirements has been the major method used to reduce the number of eligible recipients. Lowering the income ceiling for Medicaid qualification has the effect of restricting the number of persons who can qualify for the program. Follow-up studies on dropped populations indicate that when services are terminated, there is a general worsening of health status, less satisfaction with health care, and increased inability to obtain other sources of care when compared with persons not terminated from programs (Lurie et al., 1984; Coburn and McDonald, 1993; Halfon and Newacheck, 1992). The long-term effects of restricting access can be costly, as people are sicker and require more intense treatment by the time they obtain care.

Most other methods of cost containment involve attempts at reducing the cost of services to the state and federal government. One method employed is cost sharing or co-payments. Although co-payments and deductibles in this program do not approach the costs of other co-payment programs (e.g., Medicare), they generally tend to have the same effect. People who can least afford it pay the most in terms of relative cost (i.e., a regressive tax situation). It is important for community health nurses to understand the economic burdens health care may impose and the impact cost may play on an individual's ability to access and utilize health care services.

Controlling the amount paid for a service by establishing set fees for services is another means of cost containment. Set fee schedules have resulted in an effort by some providers to limit service to Medicaid populations. For example, some physicians refuse to treat or place a limit on the number of Medicaid patients they will accept in their practice (Sloan et al., 1978; Schlesinger and Kronebusch, 1990; American Academy of Pediatrics, 1990; Yudkowsky et al., 1990). The willingness of physicians to accept Medicaid patients is tied to the level of payment received: lowering the fee any further will reduce access for a larger number of poor patients.

Another method of cost containment is to limit the choices or dictate the providers of service. The result of limited choice is that Medicaid recipients can be told where to go to obtain certain services and can be denied service if they do not comply with these restrictions. Some may argue that such limits deny patients the ability to seek compatible providers and in some cases may place an unnecessary or impossible burden on patients in terms of time and transportation. Nevertheless, there is a very real probability that more services will be controlled by such programs as states grapple with increases in their health care budgets.

Variable Program Qualifications among States. Eligibility standards for Medicaid are primarily state determined, and there is wide variation in the services offered and recipients covered. Because states have discretion over optional services and groups they can elect to cover, benefits are uneven and not comparable from state to state. Table 5–4 lists both required and optional services and identifies groups that may be served.

States also affect the services provided by the criteria they establish for federally assisted programs. Each state sets its own limit or ceiling on income and allowable personal assets based on a percentage of the federal poverty level (e.g., 100% of the poverty level, 50%, and so on). If the federal poverty level for a family of four is $14,350, a state with a ceiling of 50% of the poverty level would provide benefits to a family if the family's income is $7175 or less per year; if their income is $7200, they would be ineligible in that state. However, the same family might very well be covered in other states with higher ceilings. Figure 5–11 shows how one family might be affected by different state ceilings. It is estimated that Medicaid benefits do not reach one third to one half of the population below the poverty level because of variations in state eligibility rules (Pepper Commission, 1990; Feldstein, 1993).

The primary method under discussion for solving this type of inequity requires federal action. The solution, critics argue, is to mandate uniform federal standards for eligibility and service. Thus, each state would be expected to provide the same services to all who meet the federal standard of income need. Much debate on this issue can be expected in the near future. One of the main difficulties in enacting such requirements is that the federal government

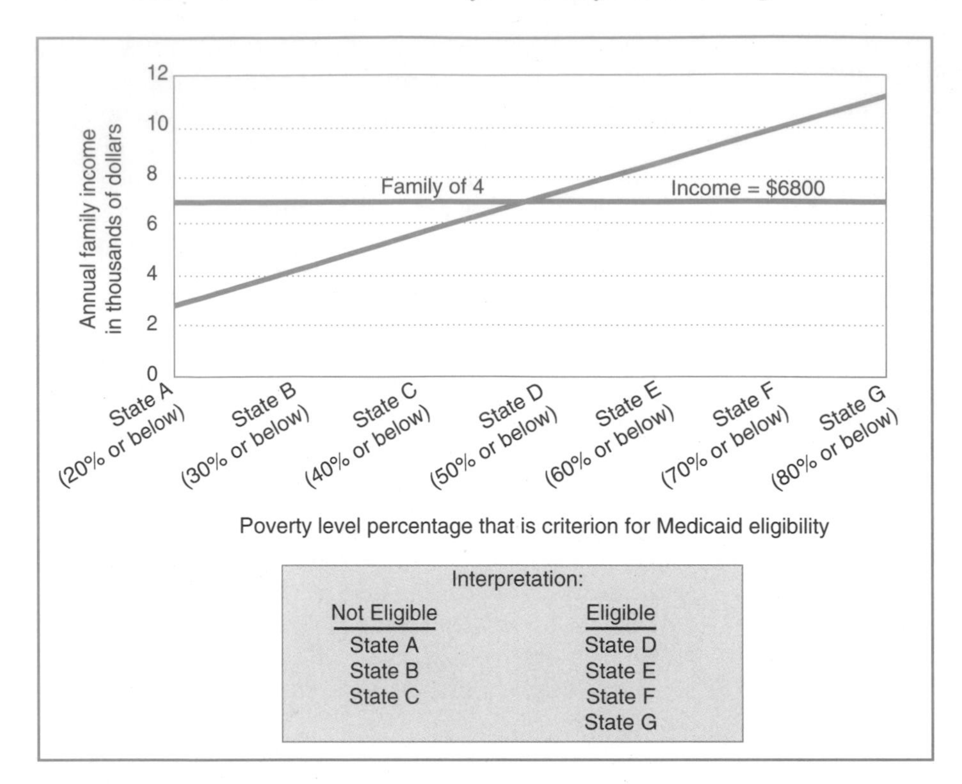

Figure 5–11 ● Income as percentage of poverty level as criterion for Medicaid eligibility in selected states. In states A, B, and C, hypothetical family is not eligible; in states D, E, F, and G, it is eligible.

would effectively dictate service populations and mandatory services without necessarily increasing its share of each state's Medicaid budgets. The net result would be an even greater burden on state budgets than is presently the case.

Financial Factors and Health Status

Financial resources play a major role in determining the quality of care available to people. Rationing of care by ability to pay is an obvious element of the current health care system (Hodges, 1991). Those who can least afford health care are at the greatest risk of poor health. The lower a person's income, the more likely it is that he or she will become ill or experience a chronic illness (Haan and Kaplan, 1985). The relationship among health status, access, availability, and quality of health care is undeniable.

RELATIVE MAGNITUDE OF THE POOR

When we think of the poor, we think of people living in poverty. What does that mean? How do we measure the scope of poverty in existence? Poverty is a relative term, meaning that in any country, some people are less well off than most of the population. However, the United States has chosen to use the term in an absolute sense and has set a living standard it considers "adequate." Persons who fall below this income are considered poor. The standard used in the United States is called the *poverty index.*

The poverty index is derived by determining the costs of purchasing specific goods and services. It incorporates the cost of food for a minimum adequate diet (called the *Economy Food Plan*) and multiplies that cost by a factor of three to arrive at a *basic subsistence standard.* Adjustments are made to that figure for family size, age of household members, and rural or urban residence (Schultz, 1985). In 1993, the poverty index for a family of four was $14,350. Any family of four whose income falls below this figure is considered to be poor, and any family above this level is not considered to be poor. However, the income standards used to set the poverty index are in dispute; criticism centers around conceptual and measurement issues.

Criticisms of the Poverty Index

There are two specific concerns with the criteria used to determine the poverty index: Both the diet plan and the subsistence indicator are considered flawed (Table 5–6).

In 1975, the Department of Agriculture proposed to replace the Economy Food Plan with a more nutritionally sound plan called the *Thrift Food Plan.* The Thrift Food Plan would have dramatically increased the number of persons below the poverty index. One study indicated that using the newer food plan as a calculation base would raise the poverty level by as much as 40% and would double the number of persons 65 years and older who were below the

TABLE 5–6

Criticisms of the Poverty Index

Diet Plan Measurements

The Economy Food Plan for determining poverty level is a minimally adequate diet intended to avoid serious immediate malnutrition. It is potentially detrimental to health if used over long periods of time. The Thrift Food Plan developed by the Department of Agriculture in 1975 has higher minimum nutritional standards and greater choice but has never been adopted (Yanochik-Owen & White, 1977).

Subsistence Factor Measure

People need a factor of more than three times the food plan as a subsistence measure. A factor of 3.4 to 5 times the cost of food is more realistic (Schultz, 1985; U.S. Dept. of Health, Education, and Welfare Poverty Studies Task Force, 1976). For example, if an adequate food budget was $300/mo, the 3x measure indicates that $900/month would be needed to live. A more realistic estimate of family expenses would be $1020 (3.4x) to $1500 (5x)/month.

Inflation Adjustment Measure

Periodic review is necessary to adjust for inflation in food prices. The poverty index has had only minor adjustments since 1980 (*Current Population Reports,* 1990). During the 1980s significant inflation reduced purchasing power. Without adequate annual adjustments, fewer people are counted below the poverty level. For example, after 4 years of 10% inflation, it would take $439 to purchase the same food bought for $300 4 years earlier. For example:

$300 × 3x factor = $900/month to qualify for poverty level

	Year 1	*Year 2*	*Year 3*	*Year 4*
10% inflation	$330	$363	$399	$439

At the end of year 4 $1217/mo would be needed to meet the same expenses that $900 would have purchased 4 years before, but $900 is still the qualifier for the poverty level.

poverty index (Sorkin, 1986). However, the Thrift Food Plan was never adopted.

The major criticism of the current poverty index is that it is an inadequate measure of poverty. Members of the Social Security Administration reported in testimony to the U.S. House of Representatives as early as 1967 that the living standard implied by the poverty index was inadequate. They recommended use of a broader measure, the low-income index. Despite recommendation, the low-income index has rarely been used in determining the numbers of people in economic hardship.

The poverty index is still the measure commonly used as a determinant of poverty status, and federal census data are reported using this criterion. Current figures indicate that 12.8% of all persons in the United States fall below the poverty level (U.S. Bureau of the Census, 1990). This translates into 31.5 million people, a very substantial number.

The poverty level has remained relatively stable since the mid-1970s. However, since then this country has experienced at least one period of high inflation, two episodes of substantial economic recession, and high unemployment, which have pushed a large number of families closer to the poverty index ceiling.

Proponents of changing the poverty measures believe the government's reluctance to revise the poverty index measures is tied to the political implications of such a move. If the newer measures were adopted or inflation adjustments were done yearly, a substantial number of people would be added to the poverty rolls. No one in government wants to be held responsible for increases in the poverty population.

Homelessness: A Poverty Measure

The incidence of homelessness is another indicator of the poverty problem. Homelessness is increasing, with the greatest increase occurring in the area of homeless families (see Chapter 23). There is a correlation between the lack of government support for programs that aid poor families and the increased rate of homelessness in this country. Government subsidies for renovation and construction of low-income housing programs have decreased by almost 90% (Bowman, 1992). The Department of Housing and Urban Development reduced the number of families involved in the federal rental assistance program by 74% between 1980 and 1992. During that same period, federal aid for urban programs was cut by 66% (Honey, 1993). These cuts have had their biggest impact on families on the edge of economic hardship.

Shrinking Middle Class at Risk of Poverty

The gap between rich and poor is widening, leaving the poor relatively poorer in general terms. The middle class is shrinking, and some middle-class families have lost ground and slipped into the lower economic level. While the majority of Americans are not in poverty, the trend toward increasing numbers is a point of concern. Americans who are relatively well off (median family income > $30,000) have become uneasy about their future status. The nation's experience with economic slumps or recessions and the growing government budget deficit serve as uneasy reminders that more of us could easily suffer economic reverses and join the poor.

EFFECTS OF SOCIOECONOMIC STATUS ON HEALTH

Socioeconomic status influences health status in many different ways. It is not sufficient to only consider access to health care; the general standard of living is also an important influence on a person's level of health. Diet, living conditions, and occupational hazards, as well as access to health care and the time frame in which medical care is sought, are all affected by income and in turn affect an individual's health. Public health care practitioners must be aware of all the risks associated with poverty if they want to improve health status in poor populations.

Mortality, Morbidity, and Poverty

Mortality figures are generally used as one means of measuring health status. The effects of income on mortality are measured directly and indirectly. Najman (1993) shows a direct link between low income and early death. Other studies suggest a similar link between very poor economic status and early death.

Two important indirect measures of the influence of income on health are (1) comparison of mortality rates for white and minority populations in the United States and (2) examination of the total mortality rates from illnesses that affect the poor to a greater degree than other income groups. Examining the differences between whites and minorities is an appropriate indirect measure of the effect of income on health, because minorities are at greater risk of poverty. Approximately 12.8% of the population is classified as poor, but if this group is broken down by racial composition, only 10% of white Americans are poor, while 30.7% of blacks and 26.2% of Hispanics are considered poor (*Current Population Reports,* 1990).

The mortality rate for blacks is about 50% higher than that for whites. In 1989, the death rate was 7.6 per 1000 persons for blacks and 5 per 1000 for whites (National Center for Health Statistics, 1990). Mortality rates for the three leading causes of death show the same trend in racial disparity. Heart disease, stroke, and cancer are all higher in blacks than in whites. The severity of illness is also different. Blacks have a greater chance of high health care expenditures, a measure of more severe illness (Berk & Monhert, 1992). Infant death rates are also higher for blacks (i.e., approximately double those for whites) (Nickens, 1990). In 1991, the black infant mortality rate was 17.9 per 1000 live births, which is double the national rate. The infant mortality rate for all other minorities was 35% higher than the national rate (Children's Defense Fund, 1991).

Certain illnesses have been identified as being more common among people living in poverty than in middle-income and high-income groups. These include anemia, arthritis, asthma, diabetes, hearing impairments, influenza, pneumonia, tuberculosis, and certain eye abnormalities (National Center for Health Statistics, 1981a, b; Andersen et al., 1987; Martin, 1992; Halfon and Newacheck, 1993). The mortality rates for these illnesses have dropped steeply since the introduction of Medicaid: 53% for influenza and pneumonia, 52% for tuberculosis not associated with human immunodeficiency virus infection, and 31% for diabetes. Califano (1986) argues that decreases in these illnesses and in mortality rates are a measure of the effect of increased access to health care for poor persons.

Personal Perceptions of Individual Health

Health interview surveys are frequently used to measure an individual's perception of health status. Lower income persons consistently report greater disability in terms of impairment of activities or confinement to bed, more worry and discomfort from illness, and higher dissatisfaction with health status (Haan and Kaplan, 1985; Andersen et al., 1987).

Diet, Health, and Socioeconomic Status

Income and nutritional status are positively correlated. Studies indicate that American Indians, Alaska Natives, Mexican Americans, and blacks—all populations with greater levels of poverty than whites—have a significantly greater risk of nutritionally related diseases. While some dietary choices are the result of cultural influences, income restrictions on diet choices play a greater role in nutritional deficiencies in minority groups.

In studies of minority children, vitamin and mineral deficiencies are relatively commonplace. In American Indian and Hispanic children there is an increased incidence of linear growth stunting (Trowbridge, 1984). Diet and weight relationships in minority children indicate greater deviation from average weights, either above or below the norm. Classic studies of minority populations in America found many more children either underweight or overweight with imbalanced diets (Carlile et al., 1969; Jacob et al., 1976; Yanochik-Owen and White, 1977).

Anemia is a frequent health problem in low-income persons. Studies have found anemia to be especially prevalent in blacks, American Indians, and Hispanics. The incidence in Indians has been reported to be triple the national rate (Calrendo, 1981). Anemia and concomitant low weight gain in pregnancy are also more prevalent in minorities (Schneck et al, 1990). One study reported that 40% of all pregnant black women have a hemoglobin level below 10 gm/dl (Trowbridge, 1984).

Many studies demonstrate a correlation among income, diet, and health during pregnancy (Schlesinger and Kronebusch, 1990; Coburn and McDonald, 1992; Wilson et al., 1992). Several government programs have been designed specifically to support the health and diet needs of poor pregnant women and their children (see Chapter 22).

WELFARE ASSISTANCE: SELECTIVE IMPACT ON HEALTH STATUS

Public health care practitioners seek to strengthen the basic standard of living for the American population in order to improve health status. In the United States, welfare assistance has been developed to help selected individuals improve their basic standard of living. A knowledge of the primary assistance programs, their benefits, and their scope of coverage is important to community health nursing. Nurses need this information so that they can refer and assist families in applying for the benefits for which they are eligible. Welfare assistance programs provide medical treatment and funds for basic needs for *some* families.

These programs may modify, but do not eliminate, all the risk imposed by poverty on a family's level of health.

The two primary government assistance programs for poor people are AFDC and Supplemental Security Income (SSI). Both provide monthly cash payments to eligible individuals. As previously mentioned, AFDC assists limited-income families with dependent children. The SSI program reaches similarly disadvantaged individuals who are aged, blind, or disabled. Both programs have stringent eligibility criteria. Not everyone below the poverty level is eligible for welfare assistance. In 1989, 11 million persons received AFDC, and the budget was $18.9 billion; SSI covered 4.3 million persons at a cost of $14.6 billion dollars (Library of Congress, October 1989). Both programs combined covered approximately 15.3 million persons, well below the 31.5 million persons in poverty that year.

To receive assistance under either program, an extensive application process is required. Financial status is the key determinant of eligibility, although states vary in the standards used to determine financial eligibility. Often, assets as well as income are considered. Assets may consist of personal property or the value of other types of assistance an individual receives. Dollar values are attached to personal assets, and this amount is added to income in gauging financial status. Some assets may be exempt from this formula; commonly a person's home and automobile are exempt up to a limited value. For example, according to the Maryland Department of Human Resources, in Maryland the value of a person's home may not exceed $25,000, and the automobile may not be valued at more than $4500. If a person sells property, the cash income from the sale is considered in determining eligibility.

Income provided by AFDC and SSI is minimal and does not reach the poverty level. In 1990, the average monthly income for an AFDC family was $392, or $4704 per year (U.S. Administration for Children and Families, 1991). Families who receive AFDC are usually eligible to receive food stamps, which are used to purchase food staples at grocery stores. The value of food stamps issued is dependent on the size of the household. A median AFDC household will receive $168 per month in food stamps, or an annual amount of $2016. This means that the average AFDC family receives a total of $6720 in assistance per year, well below the poverty level of $14,350. Participants in the SSI program receive similar benefits and medical assistance. Although the income benefits are reviewed and changed periodically, the disparity between stipend and need is constant.

Persons on these programs must undergo periodic review to renew their eligibility. If their financial situation has changed, there is always the possibility that payments will not continue.

It is difficult for families receiving assistance to budget appropriately in order to meet food, clothing, and shelter requirements. For example, consider your family's current budget. List what you pay for food, clothing, rent or mortgage, telephone, water, and electricity and/or gas. Then think of the "extras" you may need, such as an automobile, automobile insurance, gasoline or other transportation-related items, school supplies, and other household expenses. Now try to purchase these items or services on a total of $560 per month ($168 in food stamps and $392 in AFDC funds). Consider poverty from another perspective: on an average starting salary of $25,000, a nurse could support seven other people and would still exceed the salary ceiling for the poverty level (*Current Population Reports,* 1992).

These difficult budgeting choices confront millions of persons receiving government funding, as well as some 20 million individuals whose incomes fall just below or just above the poverty level. Health care services are only one of many needs that must be purchased on a severely limited budget. These individuals may have to choose between food, heat, or a physician office visit on an almost daily basis.

Trends in Reimbursement

Cost concerns have stimulated changes in the reimbursement structure and delivery of services. These changes are expected to continue and evolve in the future as efforts at cost containment intensify. Reimbursement mechanisms have significant implications for community nursing, as they affect the types of services nurses may provide and have a direct influence on the scope of independent practice.

THE CONCEPT OF MANAGED CARE

The most recent concept in cost containment is managed care. Managed care encompasses a wide variety of oversight techniques intended to deliver health care services while minimizing costs to the health care provider or third-party payer. Oversight may be minimal or intensive. Utilization review is an example of the more superficial form of managed care. HMOs and Medicare's diagnosis-related group (DRG) system are examples of the more intensive type. Reimbursement for managed care can be either retrospective or prospective depending on the nature of the contract and the organization or provider of care.

Prospective and Retrospective Reimbursement

The two payment systems for health care services are retrospective and prospective. In retrospective payment, which is the most common, service is provided and then paid for after the fact. A patient goes to his or her physician for a sore throat, for example, is seen and treated, and then is billed for the service. Retrospective payment is a cost-based reimbursement system. The total price charged for the service reflects the cost of service plus an overhead cost or profit margin. Retrospective payment essentially allows individuals and institutions to recover all costs of care. Some of the concerns with this type of payment system were discussed earlier relative to the rationale for implementing the DRG system in the Medicare program.

Retrospective payment is inflationary and provides no incentive for efficient management of health services. Costs are paid for regardless of whether a more economical method or alternative service would have been as effective and less costly. With retrospective payment the patient or third-party payer assumes all the risk of higher costs. The hospital, physician, or other providers of service bear no financial risks (Feldstein, 1993).

Prospective payment compensates the provider on a case basis for health services. The facility or provider can expect only a predetermined amount, regardless of the amount of time, energy, and service involved in providing care. Such a payment structure encourages efficiency; there is an incentive to provide care in an effective and cost-efficient manner.

Prospective payment is seen as a means of placing limits on the increasing costs of medical services and encouraging efficient management techniques. Any provider who reduces the cost of supplying service below the reimbursement price cuts operating losses and/or makes a profit. As an extra incentive, the provider is allowed to keep all monies paid even if the costs for that service are less than the reimbursement schedule.

The DRG system is the major prospective payment system currently in use. DRGs were initiated by the federal Medicare program and only affect hospitals. Other types of prospective systems are in operation and have become more popular as the cost of health care services has escalated.

Two examples of prospective payment systems are HMOs and preferred provider organizations (PPOs). An HMO provides all inpatient and outpatient care for an individual for a predetermined premium or price. Except in an emergency, the individual may not seek care outside of the HMO because that care will not be reimbursed.

A PPO has a looser organizational structure, with a variety of providers who are paid a fixed price or premium. Individuals may receive care at no additional charge or for a small fee for each service. If they seek care outside the PPO, they will be reimbursed for a predetermined amount; additional costs are the responsibility of the individual. An ophthalmologist examination, for example, might cost the consumer $5 for a visit with a PPO provider. If the consumer preferred an appointment with an ophthalmologist outside the PPO, she or he might be reimbursed for $20 of the cost and then will bear the responsibility for the remainder of the cost. The PPOs usually offer individuals more freedom of choice in providers than HMOs, especially when the PPO network has a large membership of physicians.

The cost of service for HMOs and PPOs is predetermined, thus supplying an incentive for the organization to provide or structure service in such a way that cost is low. The more expensive forms of services, such as hospitalization, are avoided whenever possible. Hospitalization is used as a last resort when other types of service are not available or are not appropriate. It has been suggested that efforts at cost containment in prospective payment systems could affect the quality of care provided; studies have both supported and disputed this claim (Reis, 1990; Faherty, 1991; Graveley and Littlefield, 1992; Krieger et al., 1992). Investigation of quality care issues continues.

Because both HMOs and PPOs have proven to be cost effective in delivery of care, they are expected to increase in popularity. Many employers have expanded their health benefits to include both, and federal and most state employees have these options. Some employers have limited employee options and provide only HMO or PPO choices. The Medicare and Medicaid programs are increasing their reliance on HMO/PPO systems.

While the DRG system affects only hospitals at the present time, consideration is being given to expanding this or a similar program to other service areas. Physician services, ambulatory clinics, dentists, and nursing homes are some of the service areas that could be affected. As long as the interest in reducing the cost of service persists, expansion of a DRG system is a very real possibility.

Reimbursement for Community Health Nursing Services. In the near future, the role of nursing in community settings can be expected to expand in all three areas: primary, secondary, and tertiary prevention. At the present time trends are heavily weighted toward expanded reimbursement for secondary and tertiary community nursing services. Although the majority of nurses will still be employed in hospital settings, the number of nurses involved in providing care for the ill and disabled in the community will increase. The overriding reason for these expanding opportunities is cost. The strategies for cost containment already mentioned, coupled with a number of other factors, are responsible for the growth in community-based services. Some of these factors are as follows:

- The DRG system has resulted in a reduction in the average length of hospital stay. As a result, patients are discharged earlier and more frequently require nursing service in the home (Morrisey et al., 1988).
- The financial cost of institutional care is greater than the cost of providing support services in the home and community. As a result, the government and insurance payers are expanding their coverage of community support services as a substitute for or as a means of delaying institutional care (Kane et al., 1991).
- The aging of the United States population makes it probable that there will be a larger population of

chronically ill elderly who require care, thus expanding the market for community services.

- The search for less costly labor substitutes will enhance the use of nursing services to provide additional care in the community (Feldstein, 1993).
- Care provided by nurses in independent practice settings demonstrates high quality and patient satisfaction (Etheridge, 1991; Pulliam, 1991).

The last factor has not come about without conflict, and competition among health professionals is projected to increase. There will be some struggle between nursing and medicine as nursing seeks to expand independent practice. Traditionally, physicians and the American Medical Association (AMA) have resisted direct third-party payment for nursing services. The American Nurses' Association believes that nurses should have the opportunity to be compensated for care by third-party insurers (Sullivan, 1992). Every effort to expand third-party reimbursement for nursing services has met with resistance.

Such a restriction on nursing's ability to receive reimbursement has resulted in restricted practice areas for nursing. While nothing prevents nurses from providing service for a fee in the community, the market for such services will remain constricted as long as consumers must personally bear the cost of such service. Allowing third-party reimbursement for independent nursing services will dramatically increase the demand for such services. Twenty-five states have passed legislation authorizing reimbursement to nurse practitioners from private and commercial insurers. The key to passage of such legislation lies in obtaining the support of third-party payers and prominent community leaders. As cost-cutting measures become more prevalent, the possibility of such support becomes more likely.

Federal and state governments have played a major role in expanding third-party reimbursement for nurses, especially in government-financed health programs. Federal employee insurance plans are authorized to make direct payment to nurse practitioners and clinical nurse specialists (Sullivan, 1992). The federal government supports projects aimed at increasing independent nursing practice in the community. These projects are geared toward providing service to geriatric populations and to rural and urban underserved populations (DeLeon, 1992). If they are shown to enhance health, prevent or delay more intensive care, and be more cost effective, they are expected to expand nationally. Community Nursing Centers are receiving direct payment for nursing services; currently there are 98 such centers. Some are funded by the Department of Health and Human Services; others, by a variety of state, local, and private sources. This type of service center is expected to increased in popularity and funding opportunities (*American Journal of Nursing News,* 1992).

Nurses' Role in Health Care Financing

Nurses are not accustomed to considering themselves part of the decision process involved in financing and reimbursement for health care services. Nursing practice has only relatively recently begun to emphasize this aspect of delivering care. Nurses generally become aware of the impact of finances through their own personal or professional experiences. However, it is possible to be completely insulated from issues of finance in some areas of practice; if your area of practice is one of these, then only personal experiences may direct you toward exploring this issue. In community health practice it is more likely that nurses will become aware of the financial concerns related to delivery of care, as their practice usually encompasses longer involvement with patients and emphasis on the psychosocial and family issues related to care.

There are a number of ways nurses may act to initiate or facilitate care for clients in the community setting; only a few are discussed here. Once they are sensitive to the link between finances and acquisition of services, nurses will be able to devise additional strategies.

REFERRING CLIENTS FOR BENEFITS AND SERVICES

Client referral is the simplest of nursing actions and one that can provide great benefit and financial relief to clients. Often it is just a matter of matching clients to existing programs for which they qualify. However, to do so, nurses will need baseline data on their local community services (i.e., local, state, and federal benefit programs) and on the insurance coverage of respective clients. This does not mean that nurses must become experts in program criteria, application processes, and benefit packages, but they should become aware of existing programs, the types of clients who are generally served by those programs, and the name and phone number of the initial contact for such programs.

Some of the major state and federal benefit programs have been discussed in this chapter, along with some general criteria for eligibility. This information will allow you to screen potential program–client matches. Remember that the selection criteria change from time to time, so your actions should not be directed toward narrowly applying selection criteria. Your role is to identify potential client–program matches, interpreting eligibility criteria broadly and leaving the reimbursing agency to investigate more stringently and examine client information against the agency's program criteria.

There are many community programs and resources that have not been listed or examined in this chapter. Each community health nurse will, in the course of her or his practice, devise her or his own community resources list and become familiar with the services that such resources can provide. It takes 3 to 6 months for a community health nurse to devise a basic list of community resources that include both widely known programs and those that are unique to the individual community. As the community health nurse becomes more proficient in her or his practice, the list of references and resources will grow. The information a nurse supplies to clients can reduce or eliminate some of the financial burdens imposed by illness, as well as secure access for primary care, health promotion, and health protection (e.g., immunizations).

ADVOCATING FOR CLIENTS IN APPEAL PROCESSES

Clients may apply for help and find that they have been denied service. Although most agencies should take time to inform clients, many clients may be confused about their rights of appeal and the reason for denial. There are a number of ways nurses can advocate for their clients in the appeal process.

First, ascertain the reason for denial of the claim. Frequently, inadequate information was supplied to the agencies. If this is the case, helping the client to complete the application correctly may be all the action needed. Other ways nurses can be an advocate include exploring the appeals method, personally contacting personnel within the agency to verify information or provide additional data, and enlisting the services of other experts who might assist them in the process.

IDENTIFYING ALTERNATIVE SOURCES OF PAYMENT

There are a variety of service sources available, especially within urban communities. If one program or agency has denied benefits to the client, seek other sources. As a nurse becomes proficient in identifying possible resources, he or she will become more expert at locating other potential service resources.

PROVIDING DOCUMENTATION TO ENSURE REIMBURSEMENT

Agencies and programs have become increasingly insistent on adequate documentation of services. Programs continually monitor claims for benefits to ensure that they meet selected standards. When documentation is not in a format acceptable to the agency, there is a risk that nursing services will not be covered. Even if the provided nursing services are considered reimbursable by the program, nurses should note in a way that is clear to the agency that the specified service has indeed been provided.

Inadequate or incomplete documentation of provided services has implications for both employers and clients. A nurse's agency will not be able to function effectively if it cannot recoup its costs for services. Similarly, a nurse's client may incur unexpected out-of-pocket expenses because he or she has to pay for covered services that should have been reimbursed by the insurance company. Complete and accurate nursing records reduce these risks.

COLLECTING DATA TO EVALUATE THE IMPACT OF REIMBURSEMENT MECHANISMS

As noted earlier, there are consequences of the reimbursement structure. Some of these are intended; others are unintentional. The rationale for Medicare implementation of a prospective payment method has also been discussed. The intent of this program change was to encourage hospitals to operate more effectively and to slow the rate of growth of hospital expenditures for the Medicare program. Both of those objectives have been accomplished; however, health care professionals are concerned that there may be additional unintended consequences of the DRG system.

The DRG system encourages hospitals to reduce a patient's length of stay. The longer the patient stays, the greater the cost of care. Longer stays are not profitable for hospitals because hospitals receive a set payment for each diagnosis. Health professionals are concerned that patients are being discharged in a sicker state and in need of more skilled community services than was previously the case (Kenney, 1991). There is an ongoing debate with respect to whether early discharge translates into poorer outcomes in the long run.

Community nurses providing care to the elderly and other patients after hospital discharge are an invaluable source of data to assist with risk assessment of early discharges. As this and other reimbursement mechanisms change and service practices are altered, nurses have a unique opportunity to collect data regarding the implications of such mechanisms and practices for health and health care delivery practice in the community.

LOBBYING FOR LEGISLATIVE AND ADMINISTRATIVE CHANGES

One of the most effective ways to affect health care delivery and reimbursement is through political action, an avenue on which the nursing profession continues to concentrate more attention.

One in every 10 women voters is a registered nurse; thus, the potential for political influence is enormous. Nurses can influence legislation in several ways. As individuals, they can become more involved in the process by identifying their state and federal representatives and contacting them on important health issues. Nurses can become active in their party affiliation or in campaigning for individuals who represent or support their views of health care needs. In these ways nurses can be an effective force in raising health care issues to the public agenda.

As a member of the nursing profession, you can support your representative organization's position on health care issues. You may want to become active in nursing organizations and help set the agenda of health concerns addressed by your profession. As nursing becomes more proficient at using the political process to address health goals, your support as an individual will become crucial to the success of such action.

Conclusion

It is imperative that nurses become involved in the decision-making processes related to delivery of health care services and reimbursement. Nursing practice is affected by such issues. Moreover, community health nurses and other public health professionals have always demonstrated concern for the social implications of health care delivery, particularly the issues of equity and accessibility of care.

The rising cost of health services, changes in the delivery of health care, and changes in the characteristics of the American population requiring service have forced those involved in the financing of the health care system to look at cost-cutting measures. With rising costs, hard choices will have to be made about the character and quality of services to be supplied and the structure in which they will be supplied. Nursing as a profession, and community health nurses as individual professionals, are in a position to provide valuable contributions to the decision-making process. It is crucial that we do so, for if we do not, the structure of health care financing and services will be redefined without our input into the process. We bear a professional responsibility to see that this does not happen. Community health nurses need to ensure that any changes in the system are designed to meet the basic health needs of all citizens without exception.

KEY IDEAS

1. The practice of nursing in community and hospital settings can be limited or directed by the cost of delivering health care services.
2. Nurses need to know about the financing system to understand its impact on individual clients and their health status.
3. Health care in the United States is costly and is rationed by the ability to pay.
4. Certain groups are at greater risk of limited access to health care services because of cost. The three groups at greatest risk are the elderly, the medically indigent, and poor children.
5. The health care market does not operate efficiently in the area of cost containment because consumer information and competition is limited and because providers often have dual interests in the welfare of their patients and in the profits from their medical investments.
6. Health care is financed by a variety of options (i.e., self-payment; health insurance, and health assistance). Medicare is a government-operated health insurance program. Medicaid is a government-operated health assistance program.
7. Employers have attempted to curb their costs by placing restrictions on the types of services covered under their health insurance plans, by limiting their employees' options of plans, by negotiating with health care providers for reduced fees, and by increasing the employees' share of health insurance premiums.
8. Medicare and Medicaid costs are a growing problem in government budgets and provide limited health care services to certain populations. Medicaid provides health care services to less than half the population below the poverty level.
9. Poverty is linked to poor health, limited access, and delay in seeking health care services. Cost containment measures that result in less access are not cost productive. Acute and delayed care are ultimately more costly than preventive services and immediate treatment.

GUIDELINES FOR LEARNING

1. Develop your ideas for the "ideal" method to finance health care delivery in this country. How close or different is your method to the present system for financing health care?
2. Identify groups that are affected by the way health care is delivered and paid for in this country. How might each of these vested interests be affected by your "ideal" method of financing health care? For those who would be affected by the change (if any), consider how you might present your position to convince them to support your proposal.
3. Interview a senior citizen. What kind of experiences have they had with health care services? Do they have any chronic conditions that require sustained medical care? Discover how much and what kinds of their medical bills Medicare pays. Ask if they would be willing to tell you their out-of-pocket expenses for medical care, including deductibles and co-payments under Medicare. Consider how these expenses might affect their ability to purchase other necessities such as food, shelter, and clothing, and how much is left to purchase incidentals and leisure treats.

④ Discover your state's cap for Medicaid eligibility for a family of three. What percentage of the current poverty level is your state's eligibility cap—30%, 50%, 70%, or some other percentage? Plan a 1-month budget for a family of three for minimally adequate food, clothing, and safe shelter. Include the cost of a telephone, electricity, and fuel. Compare your state Medicaid cap for this fictional family with your monthly budget. Is the capped income more or less than your expected monthly costs? If less, consider what you might be willing to forgo paying for or purchasing. What if you had additional expenses, including medical costs? How would you restructure your budget to meet these unexpected expenses? Is it achievable?

REFERENCES

Advocates for Senior Alert. (1990). The Medigap mess. Washington, DC: Author.

American Academy of Pediatrics. (1990). State access initiatives. *Child Health Financing, 7*(2), 2–3.

American Hospital Association. (1990). Uncompensated care fact sheet. Chicago: Author.

American Journal of Nursing News. (1992). Community nursing centers gain ground as solution to health issues. *American Journal of Nursing, 92*(7), 70–71.

American Nurses' Association. (1991). *Nursing's agenda for health care reform* (PR–12–91). Kansas City, MO: Author.

Andersen, R., Chen, M., Aday, L. A., & Cornelius, L. (1987). Health status and medical care utilization. *Health Affairs, 6*(1), 136–156.

Battistella, R. M., & Begun, J. W. (1984). The political economy of health services: A review of major ideological influences. In T.J. Litman & L.S. Robins (Eds.), *Health politics and policy.* New York: John Wiley & Sons.

Berk, M. L., & Monhert, A. C. (1992). The concentration of health expenditures: An update. *Health Affairs, 11*(4), 145–149.

Bowman, T. (1992, November 25). Rent is found to take food money from the poor. *Baltimore Sun,* p. 10D.

Brown, D. (1992, December 6). When healing, investing overlap: Physician self-referral divides medical community. *Washington Post,* pp. A1, A25–A26.

Burke, M. (1991). Medicaid expansion creates new dilemmas for state programs. *Hospitals, 65*(3), 34–36.

Burwell, B. O., & Rymer, M. P. (1987). Trends in Medicaid eligibility 1975–1985. *Health Affairs, 6*(4), 30–45.

Califano, J. A., Jr. (1986). *America's health care revolution: Who lives? Who dies? Who pays?* New York: Random House.

Calrendo, M. A. (1981). *Nutrition and preventive health care.* New York: Macmillan.

Capilouto, E., Thorpe, K. Z., & Dailey, T. E. (1992). How restrictive are Medicaid categorical eligibility requirements—a look at 9 southern states. *Inquiry—The Journal of Health Care Organization, Provision, and Financing, 29*(1), 451–456.

Carlile, W. D., Olson, H. G., Gorman, J., McCraken, C., Vanderwagen, R., & Connor, H. (1969). Contemporary nutritional status of North American Indian children. In *Nutrition, growth, and development of North American Indians* (NIH pub. no. 72-26). Washington, DC: U.S. Government Printing Office.

Childrens' Defense Fund. (1991) *The health of America's children.* Washington DC: Author.

Chisman, F., & Pifer, A. (1987). *Government for the people. The federal social role: What it is, what it should be.* New York: Norton.

Coburn, A. F., & McDonald, T. P. (1992). The effects of variations in AFDC and Medicaid eligibility on prenatal care use. *Social Science and Medicine, 35*(8), 1055–1063.

Cohen, M. A., Kumar, N., & Wallock, S. S. (1992). Who buys long term care insurance. *Health Affairs, 11*(1), 208–223.

Congressional Budget Office. (May 1992). *Staff memorandum: Factors contributing to the growth of the Medicare program.* Washington, DC: U.S. Government Printing Office.

Congressional Budget Office. (October 1992). Economic implications of rising health care costs. Washington, DC: U.S. Government Printing Office.

Creighton, H. (1986). *Law every nurse should know* (5th ed.). Philadelphia: W. B. Saunders.

Crenshaw, A. B., & Heath, T., (1992, November 29). Six blues said to be in trouble. *Washington Post,* pp. A1, A26.

DeLeon, P. H. (1992). Nursing: Policy agenda for the future. *Nursing Economics, 10*(2), 137–139.

Etheridge, P. (1991). A nursing HMO: Carondelet St. Mary's experience. *Nursing Management, 22*(7), 22–27.

Faherty, V. (1991). Home health care post-PPS: Some California data. *Home Health Care Services Quarterly, 12*(2), 35–52.

Feldstein, P. J. (1993). *Health care economics* (4th ed.). West Albany, NY: Delmar Publishers.

Freeland, M. S., & Schendler, C. E. (1984). Health spending in the 1980's: Integration of clinical practice patterns with management. *Health Care Financing Review, 5*(3), 1–68.

Freeman, H. C., Blendon, R. J., Aiken, L. H., Sudmans, S., Mullinix, C. F., & Corey, C. R. (1987). Americans report on their access to health care. *Health Affairs, 6*(1), 6–18.

Fuschs, V. R. (1991). National health insurance revisited. *Health Affairs, 10*(4), 7–17.

Ginsburg, J. A., & Prout D. M. (1990). Access to health care. *Annals of Internal Medicine, 112,* 641–661.

Gravely, E. A., & Littlefield, J. H. (1992). A cost-effectiveness analysis of three staffing models for the delivery of low-risk prenatal care. *American Journal of Public Health, 82*(2), 180–184.

Haan, M. N., & Kaplan, G. A. (August 1985). The contribution of socioeconomic position to minority health. In *Report of the Secretary's Task Force on Black and Minority Health* (Vol. 2). Washington, DC: Department of Health and Human Services, U.S. Government Printing Office.

Halfon, N., & Newacheck, P. W. (1993). Childhood asthma and poverty—differential impact and utilization of health services. *Pediatrics, 9*(1), 55–61.

Hodges, M. H. (1991). New perspectives on our national health care dilemma. *Health Care Management Review, 16*(3), 67–71.

Honey, P. (1993, January 17). Bill Clinton's ten biggest problems. *Washington Post,* p. A21.

Inglehart, J. (1983). Medicaid turns to prepaid managed care. *New England Journal of Medicine, 308*(16), 976–980.

Institute of Medicine (April 1986). *A study plan: Toward a national strategy for a long term care of the elderly* (IOM-85-05). Washington, DC: Author.

Jacob, J., Hunt, I. F., Dirige, O., & Swendseid, M. E. (1976). Biochemical assessment of the nutritional status of low income pregnant females of Mexican descent. *American Journal of Clinical Nutrition, 29,* 650–660.

Jacobs, P. (1991). *The economics of health and medical care* (3rd ed.). Gaithersburg, MD: Aspen.

Kaiser Family Foundation. (1993). *The Medicaid cost explosion: Causes and consequences.* Baltimore, MD: Henry J. Kaiser Family Foundation.

Kane, R. A., Kane, R. L., Illston, L. H., Nyman, J. A., & Finch, M. D. (1991). Adult foster care for the elderly in Oregon: A mainstream alternative to nursing homes? *American Journal of Public Health, 81*(9), 1113–1120.

Kenney, G. M. (1991). Understanding the effects of PPS on Medicare home health use. *Inquiry, 28*(2), 129–139.

Kliegman, R. B. (1992). Perpetual poverty—child health and the underclass. *Pediatrics, 89*(1), 710–713.

Knox, R. (1989, April 17). Is a solution in sight for 1990? *Boston Globe,* pp. A11, A14.

Krieger, J. W., Connel, F. A., & LoGerfo, J. P. (1992). Medicaid prenatal care: A comparison of use and outcomes in fee-for-service and managed care. *American Journal of Public Health 82*(2), 185–190.

Letsch, S. W., Lazenby, H. C., Levit, K. R., & Cowan, C. A. (1992). National health care expenditures 1991. *Health Care Financing Review, 14*(2), 1–30.

Levit, K. R., Lazenby, C. A., & Letsch, S. W. (1991). National health care expenditures 1990. *Health Care Financing Review, 13*(1), 29–54.

Library of Congress, Congressional Research Service. (October 1989). *Cash and noncash benefits for persons with limited income: Eligibility rules and expenditures data FY 1986–88* (Report no. 89-595).

Lurie, N., Ward, N., Shapiro, M., & Brook, R. (1984). Termination from Medi-Cal—Does it affect health? *New England Journal of Medicine, 311*(7), 480–483.

Martin D. A. (1992). Children in peril: A mandate for change in health care policies for low-income children. *Family and Child Health, 15*(1), 75–90.

Morrisey, M. A., Sloan, F. A., & Valvona, J. (1988). Shifting Medicare patients out of the hospital. *Health Affairs, 7*(5), 52–64.

Najman, J. M. (1993). Health and poverty—past, present, and prospects for the future. *Social Science and Medicine, 35*(2), 157–166.

National Center for Health Statistics. (1981a). *Hypertension in adults 25–74 years of age: United States 1971–1975.* (DHHS pub. no. 81-1671, series II, no. 221). Washington, DC: U.S. Government Printing Office.

National Center for Health Statistics. Series 11, no. 228. (1981b). *Eye conditions and related need for medical care among persons 1–74 years of age: United States 1971–72* (DHHS pub. no. 83-1678, series 11, no. 228). Washington, DC: U.S. Government Printing Office.

National Center for Health Statistics. (1990). *Annual 1989.* Washington, DC: U.S. Government Printing Office.

Newhouse, J. P., Manning, W. G., Morris, C. N., et al. (1981). Some interim results from a controlled trial of cost sharing in health insurance. *New England Journal of Medicine, 305*(25), 1501–1507.

Nickens, H. A. (1990). Health promotion and disease prevention among minorities. *Health Affairs, 9*(2), 133–142.

Pepper Commission (1990). *A call for action: Final report of the Pepper Commission.* Washington, DC: U.S. Government Printing Office.

Pulliam, L. (1991). Client satisfaction with a nurse managed clinic. *Journal of Community Health Nursing, 8*(2), 97–112.

Quinn, J. B. (1992, December 6). Will free market approach really curb Medical costs? *Washington Post,* p. H3.

Raffel, M. W., & Raffel, N. K. (1989). *The United States health care system: Origins and functions* (3rd ed.). New York: John Wiley & Sons.

Reinhardt, U. E. (1973). Proposed changes in the organization of health care delivery: An overview and critique. *Milbank Memorial Fund Quarterly, 51*(Spring), 169–222.

Reis, J. (1990). Medicaid maternal and child health care: Prepaid plans vs private fee-for-service. *Research in Nursing and Health, 13*(3), 163–171.

Rice, T., Desmond, K., & Gobel, J. (1990). Medicare catastrophic coverage act: A post mortem. *Health Affairs, 9*(3), 75–87.

Rice, T., & Thomas, K. (1992). Evaluating the new Medigap standardization regulations. *Health Affairs, 11*(1), 198–207.

Schlesinger, M., & Kronebusch, K. (1990). The failure of prenatal care policy for the poor. *Health Affairs, 9*(4), 91–111.

Schneck, M. E., Sideras, K. A., Fox, R. A., & Dupuis, L. (1990). Low-income pregnant adolescents and their infants: Dietary findings and health outcomes. *Journal of the American Dietetic Association, 90*(4):555–558.

Schultz, J. H. (1985). *The economics of aging* (3rd ed.). Belmont, CA: Wadsworth Publishing.

Scitovsky, A. A., & Snyder, N. M. (1972). Effects of co-insurance on use of physicians' services. *Social Security Bulletin, 35*(6), 3–19.

Segal, E. A. (1991). The unvenalization of poverty in the 1980s. *Social Work, 36*(5), 454–457.

Sidel, V. W. (1991). *Health care for a nation in need.* New York: Institute for Democratic Socialism.

Sloan, F., Mitchell, J., & Cromwell, J. (1978). Physician participation in state Medicaid programs. *Journal of Human Resources, 13*(supplement), 211–245.

Snyder, A. A., & McCall, N. (1977). Co-insurance and the demand for physician services: Four years later. *Social Security Bulletin, 40*(5), 19–27.

Sorkin, A. L. (1986). *Health care and the changing economic environment.* Lexington, MA: Lexington Books.

Sorkin, A. L. (1992). *Health economics: An introduction* (3rd ed.). New York: Lexington Books.

Statistical Abstract of the United States. (1992). Washington, DC: U.S. Government Printing Office.

Sullivan, C. B., Miller, M., Feldman, R., & Dowd, B. (1992). Employer sponsored health insurance in 1991. *Health Affairs, 11*(4), 172–185.

Sullivan, E. M. (1992). Nurse practitioners and reimbursement: Case analyses. *Nursing and Health Care, 13*(5), 236–241.

Trowbridge, F. L. (1984). Malnutrition in industrialized North America. In P.L. White & N. Selvey (Eds.). *Malnutrition determinants and consequences.* New York: Allen R. Liss.

U.S. Administration for Children and Families. (1991). *Public Assistance and Statistics Annual.* Washington, DC: U.S. Government Printing Office.

U.S. Bureau of the Census. (1990). *Current Population Reports* (Series P60, No. 169 RD). Washington, DC: U.S. Government Printing Office.

U.S. Bureau of the Census. (1991). *Current Population Reports* (Series P–25, No. 1045.). Washington, DC: U.S. Government Printing Office.

U.S. Bureau of the Census. (1992). *Current Population Reports* (Series P60, No. 175.). Washington, DC: U.S. Government Printing Office.

Wilensky, G. R. (1987). Viable strategies for dealing with the uninsured. *Health Affairs, 6*(1), 33–46.

Wilson, A. L., Murson, D. P., Schubat, D. B., Leonardson, G., & Stevens, D. C. (1992). Does prenatal care lower the incidence and cost of neonatal intensive care admissions? *American Journal of Perinatology, 9*(4), 281–284.

Yanochik-Owen, A., & White M. (1977). Nutrition surveillance in Arizona: Selected anthropometric and laboratory observations among Mexican children. *American Journal of Public Health, 67,* 151–154.

Yudkowsky, B., Cartland, J., & Flint, S. (1990). Pediatrician participation in Medicaid: 1978–1989. *Pediatrics, 89,* 567–577.

BIBLIOGRAPHY

Callahan, D. (1990). *What kind of life: The limits of medical progress.* New York: Simon & Schuster.

Clinton's big test: The fate of the budget, the economy and his first term rests on containing medical costs (1992). *U.S. News and World Report, 113*(20), 88–95.

Etzioni, A. (1991). Health care rationing: A critical evaluation. *Health Affairs, 10*(2), 88–95.

Feldstein, P. J. (1988). *The politics of health legislation: An economic perspective.* Ann Arbor, MI: Health Administration Press.

Fuschs, V. R. (1991). National health insurance revisited. *Health Affairs, 10*(4), 7–17.

Ginzberg, E. (1990). *The medical triangle: Physicians, politicians, and the public.* Cambridge, MA: Harvard University Press.

Goldwater, M. (1991). Impact of federalism on the state legislature. *Maryland Nurse, 10*(6), 2–3.

Inglehart, J. K. (1992). The American health care system: Private insurance. *New England Journal of Medicine, 326*(25), 1715–1720.

Inglehart, J. K. (1992). The American health care system: Managed care. *New England Journal of Medicine, 327*(10), 742–747.

Inglehart, J. K. (1992). The American health care system: Medicare. *New England Journal of Medicine, 327*(20), 1467–1472.

Mechanic, D. (1983). *From advocacy to allocation: The evolving American health care system.* New York: Free Press.

Reinhardt, U. E. (1991). Breaking America's health policy gridlock. *Health Affairs, 10*(2), 96–103.

Waldo, D. R., Sonnefeld, S. T., Lemieux, J. A., & McKusick, D.R. (1991). Health spending through 2030: 3 scenarios. *Health Affairs, 10*(4), 231–242.

Why the prognosis for reform is poor: A look at hospitals and communities shows how tough it will be to control medical costs. (1992) *U.S. News and World Report, 113*(20), 30–39.

SUGGESTED READINGS

Health care in crisis: A three part series. (1992). *Consumers Reports,* July, 435–448; August, 519–529; September, 579–592.

Ingelhart, J. K. (1992). The American health care system; Introduction. *New England Journal of Medicine, 326*(14), 962–967.

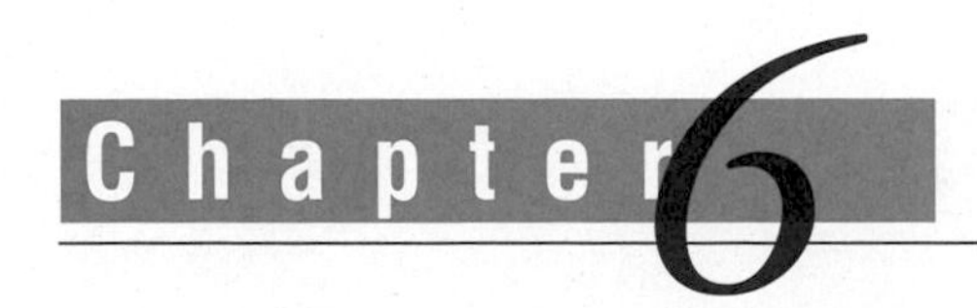

The Relevance of Culture and Values for Community Health Nursing

Judith Strasser, Frances A. Maurer, and Kathryn Hopkins Kavanagh

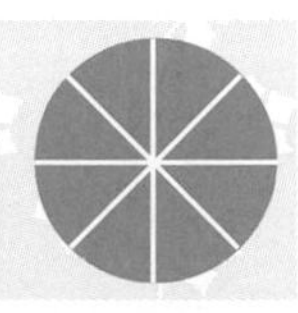

Continued

Focus Questions

PART ONE

What is culture, enculturation, and cultural diversity?

What is the relation of culture to health and health behaviors?

Why should community health nurses be concerned with culture?

What is liminality, and how does it relate to culture and health behaviors?

What type of nurse characteristics and nursing interventions are most effective when working with contrastive cultural groups?

What core categories should community health nurses explore when assessing culture?

PART TWO

What are the largest racial/ethnic minority groups in the United States?

What is the expected racial/ethnic mix of the population by the year 2025?

Continued

Focus Questions

Continued

What is the degree of cultural diversity within a racial/ethnic group?

What is the impact of race/ethnicity on health status?

What is the impact of poverty on health status?

What are some of the cultural norms of minority populations in the United States?

PART THREE

How do values influence attitudes, beliefs, and behaviors related to health and illness?

What role do nurses' value orientations play in the care clients receive?

What happens when community health nurses and clients have different value systems?

How can community health nurses understand their clients' value orientations?

How are community health nurses' and clients' value orientations involved in health care decision making?

What are nursing's values, and how do they relate to society's values?

Part 1: The Cultural Context for Community Health Nursing*

Judith Strasser

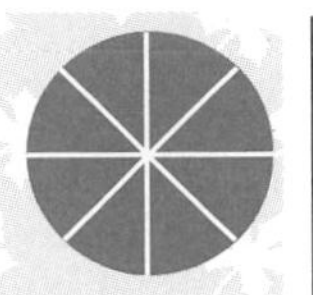

To understand individuals, families, and populations, we must explore their beliefs, values, and customs. Culture and other influences form an individual's value system, and people's view of health and the health services they seek are guided by their value system. Community health nurses can provide the best possible health care when they have some understanding of the cultural and values framework from which they and other people operate.

Culture

Culture can be viewed as learned, shared behavior and understanding that form an interrelated whole. Trotter (1988) calls culture "the social glue that holds relationships together and the mechanism by which we share our understanding with one another and understand other people. Culture is a behavioral map and a perceptual filter" (p. 3). People with a common culture may speak the same language or live in the same country or geographic area.

Ethnicity and Race

Ethnicity and race are overlapping concepts (Centers for Disease Control and Prevention, 1993). *Race* usually refers to a group of individuals who share common biological features. *Ethnicity* sometimes has a similar meaning but also may refer to a shared culture rather than shared biological characteristics. From this perspective, individuals who share a common culture may or may not have similar biological characteristics.

Ethnicity has been defined as classification of humans based on some commonality or affiliation. *Ethnic group* refers to designated or basic divisions or groups of humankind as distinguished by customs, characteristics, or language. In short, ethnicity is a difficult concept rooted in the designator's own cultural beliefs about what is different or distinguishable. Culture, ethnicity, and race are often used interchangeably, making the concepts difficult to understand.

Enculturation

The process of becoming a member of a cultural group is called *enculturation* and profoundly influences one's *world view.* A person's world view is just that—the way that individual sees the world. It is the frame of reference out of which all of us function with relation to all aspects of the environment and each other. Each person's world view is learned in the context of a specific culture. A person may be blind to his or her own culture, not recognizing that his culture is one of many. Those people who do not know or appreciate differences in world views are *culture bound.* For example, in an isolated village in Peru, visitors were thought to be crazy, defective, or stupid if they could not speak the language of the village. These villagers were culture bound and did not know there was any language other than their own.

Nurses, too, can be culture bound. For example a nurse taught a patient how to prepare a medicated solution for leg soaks. However, the patient had only taken medicines by mouth, so he drank the potassium permanganate solution. Luckily he survived to report to a physician that his lips were turning purple. In this case both the nurse and the patient were culture bound; neither knew the perspective of the other. More responsibility rests with the nurse, whose job it is to be sure the patient knows how to prepare *and* how to use the medication. The patient was able to demonstrate how to mix the solution, but he was never asked to demonstrate how to use it.

Many people are intimately familiar with more than one culture. People often blend aspects of several cultures or

*See focus questions on p. 139.

world views in their daily lives. Even in today's scientific and technological age, people may choose not to walk under ladders or step on cracks. Old adages such as "feed a cold, starve a fever" are often used in time of illness. A Hispanic patient, for instance, may go to a Western emergency department for treatment but may also obtain remedies from the local Hispanic healer (curandero). This practice of blending cultures is called *syncretism.*

Local remedies may be harmless or harmful. For example, a homeless woman eats a grapefruit each night to clean her teeth (Strasser, 1978). This practice does not clean teeth, but it does no harm. Other remedies may be beneficial in themselves, but become harmful when combined with modern treatments. For example, a woman might receive a prescription for digitalis from the emergency department and foxglove tea from the curandero (Trotter, 1988). This combination could be lethal. Health care personnel who understand and can work with both the patient and the curandero may find a mutually acceptable compromise.

Cultural Diversity

In heterogeneous cultures individuals are exposed to multiple world views, and new arrivals must adapt or adjust to a different cultural perspective. In the United States there are cultural differences based on geography (north or south; urban or rural) as well as ethnicity or national origin. New in-migrants or immigrants have a major adjustment to make. International communication (e.g., television) also exposes individuals to different cultures.

Migration

People migrate both across national borders and within them, doing so in official (legal) and unofficial ways and for a wide variety of reasons. Migration involves "hellos" and "good-byes," and if one migrates alone to a sharply contrastive culture, severe *culture shock* may occur. Culture shock is associated with feelings of panic, anger, denial, and depression and a sense of separation from others and even one's own self-identity. This experience can have serious health consequences. Culture shock can lead to acts of aggression toward self or others, a loss of appetite and/or sleep, and general malaise that can lead to death.

People who cross national borders are often referred to as *immigrants.* The more nationalistic a country, the more immigration is controlled. Multiple problems occur when large numbers of people cross a national border for an extended period of time. Countries may be poorly equipped to handle a large number of new residents. The established citizenry may resent or view the new inhabitants as rivals for precious resources such as food, shelter, or jobs. Countries develop rules to determine residency and citizenship status; access to employment; admission and employment of family members; time limits on length of stay; payment for work, sickness, maternity, invalidism, or old age; and employment and eligibility for education and health services, unemployment, or welfare subsidy.

Mass migration occurs when large numbers of people leave their homes and migrate to a new location. Political or religious upheaval, war, or some environmental or economic disaster usually precedes mass migration. *Chain, or social, migration* involves one or more people leaving their homeland, investigating the new location, acquiring resources, and then informing those at home that the new location is good or at least better in some way than the old. Thus, more immigrants come and are supported by relatives or friends. In this way, each new arrival encourages more to follow. Those who have arrived first provide emotional and financial cushions against culture shock.

Host countries have various ways of controlling both in- and out-migration. In the United States, in-migration is limited by a quota system and by visa requirements but many people enter illegally without following the prescribed procedures. In 1991 approximately 740,000 people came to the United States (Hollmann, 1993). Illegal in-migration is difficult to measure, but may be as high as one million people each year. In-migrants from different countries cluster together in different regions of the United States. For example, Jamaicans tend to locate in New York or Miami, Cubans in Florida, and Mexicans in California, Arizona, and Texas.

In-migrants are most successful when the host community is prepared for and welcomes their arrival. All migrants experience a sense of loss and the stresses of adaptation.

Liminality

Newcomers to any country experience a "push–pull" phenomenon—a seesaw of emotions from the old to the new and back again. This is known as *liminality,* or a state of transition (Turner, 1969). There are many kinds of transitions. Transitions occur, for example, when advancing in age from one group to another (such as from preadolescent to teenager, or from teenager to adult); when moving from one place to another; or when changing status, such as from wife to widow or from employee to retiree.

Being in a state of liminality is a precarious time in one's life. People in times of transition and change are more vulnerable to illness and injury. Their vulnerability lessens as they accept and are accepted into the new setting and let go of the old one.

Community health nurses caring for immigrant populations can anticipate that some individuals will experience difficulty with liminality. For new immigrants, transition generally is smoother when they are supported by others who have already been through the experience. Nurses can assist new immigrants to adjust to their new living conditions and a different health care delivery system. Helping newcomers to find others with whom they share cultural and life experiences is a very supportive strategy. Community nurses who do thorough assessments are sensitive to a community's changing population (both newcomers and departers) and are able to anticipate their needs.

A Cultural Perspective Regarding Care Concepts

Different cultures have different views and perspectives on everyday concepts and normal behavior. Recognition of the different meanings of some of these key concepts is very useful for nurses who practice in multicultural health care settings.

TIME AND SPACE

How people perceive and use both time and space are important considerations for community health nurses when assessing culture. Two central ways of viewing time are linear and circular. A *linear view* of time sees time as a straight line that can be divided into parts with a beginning and an end. A *circular view* of time sees time as a never-ending unity that repeats itself and is part of a continuous whole. Most often Western health care providers see time in a linear way, with segments marked off specifically into minutes, hours, days, weeks, and so on. We wear watches to alert us to the correct time, and presumably our watches are synchronous with others. Our work day begins and ends at a specific time, and we are where we are supposed to be at, or near, the appointed time. Time is seen as a precious commodity to be used or spent, and only with guilty trepidation is it wasted or "killed." Because time is money and is in limited supply, we are urged to both work and play fast, accurately, and smart. We spend our days trying to "catch up" with time and admire people who make good use of their time and control their time well.

Many people are enculturated with a very different way of perceiving time. Time may be seen as cyclical (continuous and never ending). It may also be seen as an omnipresent gift to be enjoyed, rather than a limited commodity to be used. People who are enculturated with this view of time may not have or use a watch, may not be at all concerned with punctuality, and may think that "if it doesn't get done today, maybe it will get done tomorrow or some other time." Also, if time is considered a gift to be enjoyed, practically anything may take precedence over a clinic appointment, a nurse's visit, or a day at school or work. Community health nurses and other health care professionals should be patient with individuals whose perspective of time is different from their own.

How human beings view and structure space differs among cultures in ways that are as profound and important as how they view and structure time. Space is linked with issues of territoriality, living, work and health care arrangements, touch, sound, and smell. Hall (1973) addresses the concept of space as physical boundary and territory: just as animals protect their territory, so do humans.

Culture determines the amount of personal space an individual requires. Some cultures are used to very little distance between people; others are more comfortable with a separation of several feet. When individuals from different cultures interact, there is a chance that one will violate the other's "personal space." Standing too close to another person can precipitate feelings of anger or fear in the person whose space is invaded.

Some cultural groups own land and mark their plots or acreage with fences to separate it from that of their neighbors. Some cultures perceive land as belonging to everyone and to no one in particular, and would not think of putting up fences. Some cultures value uniformity, and others, diversity. Although the United States places great emphasis on individual freedom and creativity, many U.S. towns have covenants that restrict the individual's right to alter his or her property in any unacceptable visible way.

How people construct and use public space is an important consideration when nurses conduct community meetings. Various cultural groups perceive space as more or less formal, and this can create problems among them. In one nursing home, Americans of African descent used the shared lobby on each floor as formal public space and dressed accordingly. Americans of European descent, on the other hand, used the shared space informally, wearing slippers, robes, and even hair curlers.

While in patients' homes, nurses are guests, and although the nurse is a professional guest, she or he must be aware of how space is structured and used. Certain chairs may be reserved for an authority figure, and the nurse should not sit in these chairs unless invited. Some rooms in the house may be "off limits" to outsiders, and nurses must be aware of cues regarding public and private space. Moreover, in working with people from a culture that contrasts with the nurse's culture of origin, the nurse *must* read the literature to explore how, in general, the patient's cultural group perceives and uses space and how limit-setting cues might be sent. The old saying, "When in Rome, do as the Romans do," does not always hold in home visiting, but the nurse has the responsibility to find out what the Romans do, to respect what the Romans do, and to work with the cultural system rules and values when possible.

RITES AND RITUALS

Rites and rituals are markers of important events within a culture. A *rite* is an event that marks a change in status from a lower to a higher level (Van Gennep, 1960). A *ritual* is a prescribed manner or process closely related to a culture's ideology (Herberg, 1989). Rites concern both critical and calendrical life events. Critical events include marriage, birth, death, or graduation. Examples of calendrical events include Thanksgiving (a religious and patriotic event), Christmas (a religious and social holiday), and Halloween (a religious and social festival). Types of events that are ritualized are events of separation, intensification, incorporation, and passage.

A rite of separation could formally mark a death, induction into the military, or a divorce. A rite of intensification could be the reenactment of a wedding after 25 years or some formal affirmation of group solidarity. A rite of incorporation could be formal acceptance into a group, club, or school, while a rite of passage marks growth from one state to another, such as from a girl to a woman or from a boy to a man.

Rites and rituals can indicate health and life in a community. Towns that have a carnival for a patron saint or a 4th of July parade every year are celebrating a calendrical rite of intensification. They are saying, "This is who we are, we rejoice in it, we mark it." Families who have ritual celebrations of Christmas or Hanukkah are celebrating both the holiday and themselves. Youths who go through a confirmation or bar mitzvah mark their rite of passage to a new time of greater maturity.

Culture's Relationship to Health

Culture is related to health in that culture teaches us the meaning of health and illness and the appropriate practices related to our beliefs. In many cultures, concepts such as cause and effect may not be relevant. Many cultural groups who adhere to the great traditions of Buddhism, Confucianism, and Taoism accept the fate of an illness and may not necessarily seek to discover the cause or cure. Many people may allow Fate to guide their lives and try to live in simplicity and harmony with nature.

It is important to know that many cultures do not accept the germ theory. Murdock (1980) describes 186 different cultural groups, only 31 of which have expressed theories concerning infection. In fact many cultural groups do not believe in natural causation (e.g., germs), but instead hold theories of supernatural causation. Natural causation theories concern infection, stress, organic deterioration, accidents, and human aggression. Murdock has identified three supernatural causation theories (Table 6–1): mystical, animistic, and magical.

Theories of causation are important because they help to define illness or disease in terms of etiology. Once the existence of ill health has been identified, people then find ways to interpret symptoms and, when appropriate, present themselves to the modern health care provider, folk healer, or some combination of providers, caregivers, and healers.

TABLE 6–1

Theories of Supernatural Causation of Illness

Theory	Type	Definition
Mystical causation (puzzling or mysterious cause)	Fate	Bad luck
	Ominous sensations	Sights, sounds, dreams thought to cause illness
	Contagion	Contact with polluting object, substance person
	Mystical retribution	Taboo violated: supernatural being punishes
Animistic causation (caused by personalized supernatural entity)	Soul loss	Departure of victim's soul from body
	Spirit aggression	Caused by malevolent or affronted supernatural being
Magical causation (ritual invocation of supernatural agencies)	Sorcery	Aggressive use of magical techniques by a human being independently or with a specialized magician or shaman (witchcraft); aggressive action by human being with special power

From Murdock, G. (1980). *Theories of illness—a world survey.* Pittsburgh: University of Pittsburgh Press.

SEEKING MEDICAL CARE

Decisions about presenting oneself to a health care provider are made in the context of the family, the community, and the culture. Typical patterns of behavior, such as when, where, why, and how to seek care, are learned from parents, neighbors, religion, and the health care system. The critical point in seeking an official health care practitioner also depends on the availability, acceptability of care, and the ability to reciprocate or pay in some way for the care given. In some countries and U.S. communities, goods or services are exchanged in lieu of money or health insurers' reimbursement.

What people do before requesting aid from the health care provider is also important to discover. "Starving a fever" and "feeding a cold" may have been tried without good results. Seeking to discover what else has been tried in a nonjudgmental way is essential to providing good care.

Because humoral medicine is practiced in many parts of the world, nurses need to have some awareness of what it is all about. Humoral medicine has its origins in ancient China and Greece (Landy, 1977) and involves the use of prescribed foods or elements which are hot or cold, wet or dry. The goal of humoral medicine is to promote and maintain health and to treat illness by achieving the natural and beneficial balance or equilibrium of hot and cold, wet and dry. The four humors and their properties are illustrated in Table 6–2. Some Spanish speaking, Asian, and other cultures may use humoral practices as well as Western treatments.

M. H. Logan (cited in Landy, 1977) describes the four humors as "the constitutional essence or innate character of a given item or personal state of being" (p. 489). Hot and cold do not mean physical temperature in terms of Centigrade or Fahrenheit, and wet and dry do not refer to actual water content. Some illnesses may be attributed to a problem with blood (e.g., hot and wet) and would require a cold and dry treatment to reestablish and maintain equilibrium. The labeling of treatments and illnesses as hot, cold, wet, or dry may vary from one region to another and may require knowledge of a specific cultural group's system of classifying illnesses and treatments.

TABLE 6–2

The Four Humors and Related Qualities

Humor	Quality
Blood	Hot and wet
Black bile	Cold and dry
Yellow bile	Hot and dry
Phlegm	Cold and wet

FOLK MEDICINES AND FOLK HEALERS

Folk healers and their remedies and recommendations are indigenous to a culture. Types of healers include curers, bone setters, herbalists, lay midwives, and spiritualists. Folk healers are practitioners of a lay medicine who work in face-to-face family and community contexts. According to Graham (1976), folk healers usually adhere to a well-organized and consistent theory of medicine. Because folk healers are present in both rural and urban communities, migrants to a different or new locale can often find a healer from their own cultural group who helps to link their new life with their former life and ties.

In addition to traditional folk healers, there are many "new age" health care providers and promoters. New age practitioners can be lay people with training in a specific technique, or licensed health care providers who add new age strategies to their repertoire of interventions. New age practitioners are usually well-educated, middle- or upper-class people who are humanistic in their approach to care. Skills used by these providers include therapeutic touch as described by Kreiger (1987); massage; reflexology; rolfing (deep massage); rebirthing (re-experiencing the birth process); mind control; regression hypnosis; health foods, tonics, and vitamins; mineral baths; acupressure; and the use of astrology, gemology, and modern witchcraft techniques. The preceding list is not inclusive, but illustrates the kinds of alternative care patients may be receiving.

There is much that is useful in folk medicine. As we move toward the 21st century, there is a renewed interest in incorporating folk practices into a healthy regimen. Holistic health care practitioners emphasize the quality and fullness of life, recognizing that empirical science and technology do not necessarily have the answers to every health concern.

RELIGION

Religion and spirituality are linked strongly to our identity as humans. An understanding of a wide range of religious beliefs and practices is important for the nurse, as health care must fit into a client's belief system for advice and prescribed treatments to be followed. If clients do not believe that treatments are justified or morally acceptable then it is not likely that they will comply with prescribed regimens.

To understand another religion, one must read the central literature of the faith. Examples of central literature are the Bible (Judaism and Christianity), the Koran (Islam), the Bhagavad-Gita (Hinduism), and the Talmud (Judaism). Some religions have no core book of belief but books that describe the religion. In some cultures religious beliefs and practices are handed down through oral tradition.

One question of critical importance for community health nurses is how religion influences dietary practices and other health behaviors. Some religious groups fast or feast or have specific food or drink regulations. Some religious ceremonies use alcohol or drugs as an integral part of the ceremony. Religious beliefs may influence the use of faith healers or the decision to participate in the medical system. Religion may also influence a person's willingness to participate in immunization, screening, and medical or nursing treatment.

THE MEANING OF SUFFERING

Pain and suffering (how we endure pain) are part of the human experience. Both pain and suffering are cultural as well as physical in nature. Pain—whether physical, mental, or spiritual—is experienced, influenced, and handled by individuals and groups in the context of their culture. How pain is interpreted and expressed varies across cultures. Some cultural groups minimize or emphasize pain and the expressions of pain. For example, some people see the suffering associated with pain as redemptive, while others differ and view suffering as punishment (just or unjust), as a fate to be accepted, or as plain bad luck.

When patients and families minimize or emphasize pain, unknowledgeable health care providers can misinterpret what is going on. Patients who minimize pain can be viewed as resting quietly and without pain, while those who emphasize pain can be viewed as nuisances, hypochondriacs, or malingerers. Any of these inaccurate assessments can impede appropriate diagnosis, referral, and treatment.

FOOD

Food habits are inextricably linked with culture. The perceptions and practices surrounding what, how, and with whom food is eaten provide important information about a cultural group and are so deeply rooted that they may be very difficult to change. Moreover, food customs require the thoughtful investigation of the health care provider. Landy (1977) states that, "Health workers should have an intimate detailed knowledge of the people's beliefs, attitudes, knowledge and behavior before attempting to introduce any innovation into an area" (p. 241).

Much about what people eat has to do with what foods are available and how people are enculturated with regard to food. Other factors such as biology and adaptation enter into the equation. Acceptable and prohibited foods may differ during a person's life span. Liminal periods such as pregnancy, nursing, weaning, and growth spurts may all require specific food practices in the context of culture. Certain foods in various cultures are thought to make people strong, virile, intelligent, or beautiful. Food taboos are often linked to religious belief systems rooted in the history and culture of people.

Food customs can be so ingrained in the past that people do not always know their origin. For example, pork prohibitions are thought to have originated because of health reasons such as fear of trichinosis. Farb and Armelagos (1980) disagree. They see the prohibition in Genesis 9:3 as a reaction of the Israelites to their Egyptian captor's worship of swine, rather than a safeguard against illness. Food customs are so deeply rooted within members of any cultural group that a kind of cultural revulsion can occur when they are presented with foods of other cultures. For example, what would a native-born American think of eating fish soup for breakfast, or rats, cats, worms, or dogs for dinner?

The sharing of food often involves symbolism (something that points to something beyond itself) and meaning. Wine, bread, or cake are used in Christian and Pagan services and can stand for blood and body, life supported by food and drink, the work involved in transforming grapes and grain, or the unity of sharing. An understanding of the meaning of food for peoples and the contexts and manner in which food is shared (or not shared) can be an important one for community health nurses who work with clients belonging to contrastive cultural groups.

RECIPROCITY AND EXCHANGE

Reciprocity implies a balance and equality in daily interactions. It includes the exchange of services and goods in the marketplace, as well as the exchange of gifts among friends, kin, and family. The concept is important for nurses when patients "tip" or give gifts as a reward for nursing services rendered or provide food (as a gift) or presents in the context of a home visit. Nurses also may give material gifts to patients.

Mauss (1966) describes three basic obligations of gift exchange: to give, to receive, and to reciprocate. Giving may occur to create a balance in a relationship by evening the scale or to create an imbalance in the relationship that helps to keep it going. Reciprocity is a cultural norm that appears to be universal and necessary for social life. Reciprocity in the giving of gifts is symbolic in that gifts stand for something beyond themselves. Gifts can stand for love, power, concern, the status of a relationship, or the promise of future interactions (Poe, 1977).

Little in the nursing literature provides guidance for nurses or clients in carrying out this important human process of exchange and reciprocity in the health care context. For nurses working with clients, the topic of gifts often evokes strong responses. There is a degree of awkwardness involved in deciding between refusing or accepting a gift. Some of the difficulties stem from administrative directives not to accept gifts while working as a professional. Other difficulties stem from the development of a caring and personal relationship with clients—a natural outgrowth of nursing, as it is often the reason people enter nursing in the first place. Personal relationships are an outgrowth and a natural evolution of professional relationships, which involve intimate, personal interactions; personal relationships also involve giving gifts. In deciding whether to refuse or accept a gift, nurses should consider the meaning of the gift to the client and how their decision will affect the gift giver.

FAMILY AND KINSHIP

Community health nurses provide care to individuals, families, and communities. Even when the focus of care is the individual, community health nurses look to the family as important caregivers, in addition to professional nursing and health aide services. Families provide and coordinate much of the care in the home and are sources of information with regard to the progress and care of the client.

To work with families, nurses need to identify family members. Nurses often define the family as the next of kin, or the people living in the same household. However, too often, this is not the way an individual or a family perceives itself. A family has many different forms and structures, depending on individual and family selection and culture.

In one study of a rural family, the family consisted of five fluid households, with meals, sleeping, play, and child care provided in different households on different days (Strasser, 1989). Family members were family by blood, marriage, or consensual union. Additional members included children who were "given" to an individual or couple to be raised and other individuals who, although not related by blood, were considered family members.

Sometimes how a family defines itself and its members may be different from the definition of their family unit imposed by outsiders. People who are "given" children to raise may have no legal right to sign for hospitalization or surgical procedures. Complications in providing nursing care can and do occur when the family defines itself one way, and the nurse and health care system, another. Efforts must be made by both sides to achieve a workable definition of the family that will best serve the family and take into account the family's view, however culturally different from the nurse's view. How families define themselves is a cultural construct that has endured and evolved over many generations.

SEXUALITY

Gender is more than a biological fact of life. It is also a cultural construct with expectations about behavior associated with being a boy or a girl, a man or a woman. Sexual orientation involves beliefs and practices about sexual behavior, as well as the social roles one assumes as a straight, gay, lesbian, bisexual, or transsexual. Culture also determines how people define a sex-related health problem. For example, if a culture sees teenage pregnancy as normal and expected, it will be difficult for health care professionals to reduce the number of teenage mothers.

Sexual beliefs and practices are emotionally charged issues in many cultures and serve as an arena for the airing of political, religious, and scientific differences. Some areas for exploration by community health nurses include how people learn about sexuality and how they are socialized into their sex roles. Issues surrounding circumcision, menstruation, mate selection, sexual intercourse, conception and birth, contraception, menopause or climacteric, sexual taboos, and sexual deviations from the norm are all areas for nonjudgmental assessment, literature review, and verification.

All cultures differentiate males from females, although the definitions of male and female behavior vary among cultures. In some cultures men carry purses, hold hands with other men, and publicly express affection in other ways; this is considered normative behavior for men in that culture. Often, when a behavior is considered normative for one sex, it is dropped by the other sex.

Among many Hispanics, sexual activity is expected to occur if a boy and girl are left alone. Males are believed to be unable to stifle sexual urges, and females are thought to be unable to resist. Other people are expected to prevent an unwed couple from being placed in such a situation. If a boy and girl are left alone, then sexual intercourse is presumed to have occurred. Knowing this will help community health nurses to understand the strict supervision placed on young Hispanic girls.

Community Health Nurse's Role in a Culturally Diverse Population

Community health nurses need to be aware of their own cultural orientation and to be sensitive to cultural differences between nurses and clients. A *nonjudgmental* and generally *tolerant* attitude is a must. Nurses in the community need to be *curious seekers* of *knowledge* about the lives and beliefs of people they care for. They need to be *optimists* who are secure in their ability to work with individuals, families, and communities to change things for the better. They need to be *creative* and *willing to take risks*. Community health nurses need to be *alert, skilled professionals* who are open to the world around them, willing to accept divergent views, and to listen and learn from clients.

Clinical nursing practice in community health is currently conducted from two complementary perspectives. The first concerns the care of individuals in their home setting. There, the family, neighborhood, and community are encountered as supports and adjuncts to the care of the individual. The second is a transindividual perspective—that is, looking across individuals as units of care and focusing on the family, neighborhood, group, or community as, themselves, "patients or unit of care."

Whether community health nurses focus on an individual, group, or community as the unit of care, the concept of culture is a critical variable that must be explored to have the best possible understanding of the people for whom they provide nursing care. If community health nurses do not know what people believe about health—what it is, and how and if it can (or should) be improved—then how can they change anything for the better with regard to groups or individual members of society? Several organizations that can help nurses learn about culture, health, and culturally sensitive nursing care are listed in Table 6–3. Culture and the values learned within a cultural group are critical for knowing how people perceive health, health care, and nursing care providers.

RESPONSIBILITIES OF THE COMMUNITY HEALTH NURSE WORKING WITH CONTRASTIVE CULTURAL GROUPS

In working with cultural groups, the community health nurse must be able to assess people and their cultures. To do this, a framework for assessment is required.

TABLE 6–3

Organizations Related to Culture, Health, and Nursing

American Anthropological Association (AAA)
P.O. Box 91104
Washington, DC 20090-1104
(202) 232-8800

Society for Applied Anthropology
P.O. Box 24083
Oklahoma City, OK 73124-0083
or contact AAA

Council on Nursing and Anthropology
Contact AAA

Medical Anthropology Society
Contact AAA

International Nursing Center
c/o American Nurses' Association
American Nursing Foundation
600 Maryland Avenue, SW
Suite 100 W
Washington, DC 20024-2571
(202) 554-4444, ext. 325

Transcultural Nursing Society
Madonna University
Division of Nursing and Health
36600 Schoolcraft Road
Livonia, MI 48150
(313) 591-8320
(313) 591-0156 (Fax)

One such framework (Table 6–4) is designed to structure the assessment of families and communities within a cultural perspective. Answers are "discovered" from observing and participating with people in a caring context, as well as interviewing people about their culture, family history, and beliefs and practices related to the health of individuals and groups. Some general community assessment tools address culture. However, when health care providers recognize that they are working with a cultural group that contrasts sharply with the providers' own experience, a more extensive cultural assessment needs to be conducted using a tool such as the one presented here.

STRATEGIES FOR THE COMMUNITY HEALTH NURSE WORKING WITH CONTRASTIVE CULTURES

In retrieving information about a culture, the nurse needs to use two additional sources: the library and good cultural informants. Most nurses know how to conduct a literature search, but the criteria for selecting an informant may be new knowledge. Spradley (1979) has delineated the following four characteristics of a good informant:

- Thoroughly encultured
- Currently involved in the culture
- A nonanalytic reporter
- Willing to participate

One who is thoroughly enculturated has been a part of the group represented for a long time. Current involvement means present and active participation in the culture to be investigated. A nonanalytic reporter is able to describe things in local terms rather than the way the reporter (informant) thinks the nurse wants to hear it. Someone who is willing to participate should want to share her or his time and knowledge about her or his own cultural group. Informants should be historically and actively a part of the culture. A good informant should be able to talk about what is a typical belief or behavior of the cultural group in the language of the people. Through the use of good informants and the library, nurses can put together a thorough assessment for validation with more informants.

Nursing interventions in community and family contexts should be culturally appropriate. This means that nurses should understand the culture in question as fully as possible and gear their nursing interventions to be acceptable to the cultural groups in question. In some cultures it may be rude to wear shoes in the house, and although clients may accept that the nurse is from a different cultural group, they may appreciate the respect the nurse shows by leaving his or her shoes at the door.

A primary role of the community health nurse with regard to culture is that of *culture broker.* Tripp-Reimer and Brink (1985) discuss the nursing intervention of culture brokerage, which is defined as "an act of translation in which messages, instructions and belief systems are manipulated and processed from one group to another" (p. 352). Community health nurses are responsible for being the bridges or links between their clients and the orthodox health care system. However, they will be in a good position to explain and interpret the nuances of one cultural group to the other only if they recognize their professional responsibility and have a good understanding of Western health care delivery and the culture of the clients with whom they are working.

USE OF TRANSLATORS

When clients do not speak English, the need for translators arises. Many agencies have a pool of available translators who can be called on to help in a given situation. Family members of the client are often used to translate, but the client may not wish the family member to know the details of his or her illness. Sometimes the family member asked to translate is a child, because he or she is learning English in school, although he or she may not be the best person to serve as translator. Issues of status, age, sex, and privacy should all be considered when selecting a translator.

One way of assessing the translator is to observe the balance between the translator's reply to a health question

TABLE 6–4

Community and Family Cultural Assessment Guide

Cultural Category	Questions for Community Assessment	Questions for Family Assessment
Definition of self	How does the community view itself? What are its cultural groups? What are its calendrical events, and how are they ritualized? What is the history of the community? What is the community's view of its future?	How does the family view itself? Are there fictive kin? Does the family have more or fewer members than the household? What are its calendrical events, and how are they ritualized? What critical events have occurred in the family, and how are they marked? What is the history of the family? What stories are told about the family? What does the family see as its future? What does the family tree (genogram) look like?
Definition of others	Who are the helping agencies? Who are the key informal helpers?	Who are the helping people? Who would help in time of need? What kind of help could be requested?
Definitions of health/illness	What groups does the community identify as well, worried and well, early ill, or ill? How are well/ill groups identified? What are the potential health problems of specific age and cultural groups? Who are the health and illness care providers in the community?	How does the family describe its health as a unit and the health of individuals within it? How and who within the family determines when a member is sick, and how? What are home treatments and nutritional remedies? Who decides when to seek folk or traditional scientific help?
Beliefs about health and illness	How do cultural groups perceive health and illness in terms of accepting, adapting, and controlling? What are the prevailing illnesses? How does the community view the cause, diagnosis, and treatment?	Does the family accept fate or use health promotion and illness prevention strategies? What illnesses is the family susceptible to? How do they view cause, diagnosis, and treatment?
Life ways and meaning	What is the prevailing meaning of life? How is life lived? What do people do each day?	What is the meaning of life to the family? How does the family live? What do the family members do each day?
Time	How is time structured? Is time viewed as a gift to be appreciated, as a commodity to be used, or in some other way? Are people present, past, or future oriented?	How is time structured? Is time viewed as a gift, a commodity, or in some other way? Are schedules used? Are schedules valued? Is the family past, present, or future oriented?
Space	How is space structured in the community? Is there open space? Are public buildings welcoming? Where are churches, shops, restaurants, bars, food stores, malls, public buildings, and health providers located?	How does the family structure space? Is the yard fenced? Who makes most use of what space? Where do family members eat and sleep? How close do family members get? How is observable touch used?
Physical objects	What visible objects represent the community? What are buildings like in terms of condition, cleanliness, and access? How are public facilities equipped and used?	What possessions are displayed? Is there misplaced matter? Is the house cared for? Is clothing clean, stylish, and in good condition? Is there evidence of conspicuous consumption ("keeping up with the Joneses")?
Food customs	What kind of eateries are present in the community? How are eating places patronized and by whom? Is there some ethnic style of eating noted? How do people communicate during meals?	Does the family eat together? Do they eat at a set time? What kinds of food are eaten? Who prepares the food? What and when do family members drink? What foods are adult foods? What foods are children's foods? Are any foods or drinks taboo? Do family members talk during meals? To whom is food given and in what order?
Religion	How many churches, mosques, or synagogues are located in the community? What denominations are represented? Do the organized religious groups provide any health care services? Are there designated healers or "nurses" in the churches? Do the churches sponsor health fairs or screenings?	Do family members participate actively in one religion or more than one religion? Do, or could, religious beliefs or practices affect health? Does church, mosque, or synagogue membership provide social support for the family now or if needed?
Clubs	What kinds of clubs are active in the community? What political parties are active in the community? What resources do the clubs have available? What kinds of people participate in clubs? Are there separate groups for men, women, and children?	To what clubs do family members belong? Are there clubs to which the entire family belongs? How active are family members at the present time in the club? What actual or potential resources can the club provide?

Continued

TABLE 6–4

Community and Family Cultural Assessment Guide *Continued*

Cultural Category	Questions for Community Assessment	Questions for Family Assessment
Work	What occupations exist in the community? How many people in the community work outside the home? How many work inside the home? What work hazards exist in the major occupations? How many people cannot find work? What employment support resources exist? Do people know about them? Are they accessible? What is the value and meaning of work?	What family members work outside and inside the home? What potential or actual work hazards are encountered by family members? What kind of health insurance plans do family members have from their jobs? How do members prepare for and cope with retirement, layoffs, or a company closing? What are the work duties in the household? What is the value and meaning of work?
Education	What kinds of schools are located in the community? Who attends these schools? What is the absence rate in the school? Is health care provided in the schools? What kind of health care is provided? What is the rate of nursing with regard to school health? Does the school play an active part in the community?	Do the children in the family attend school regularly? Is the family generally satisfied with the schools the children are attending? Do the parents/grandparents attend school? Are family members active in school activities? Is school seen as a way to a good or better life? Does the family identify specific problems with the school?
Play	What leisure activities are available in the community for various age groups? Are recreation facilities utilized? What groups use what kinds of resources? What is the value and meaning of play?	How many hours do family members spend in leisure activities? What kinds of activities do they enjoy as individuals and as a family? What is the value and meaning of play?
Power	How is official (formal) power structured in the community? Can informal power groups be identified?	How is power structured in the family? Who makes health decisions for family members?
Environment	Does the community environment (physical and social) foster health in the community? How?	Does the family environment (physical and social) foster its own health and the health of other community members? How?
In- and out-migrants and in-and out-migration	Who are the groups coming and going? How are in-migrant groups socialized to the community? How is out-migration justified?	How does the family accept newcomers and the loss of family members? Is the family open or closed to new groups in the community?
Deviance	How is deviance handled in the community? Who are the individual deviants and the deviant groups?	Who are the deviants in the family? How does the family cope with deviance? Is the family itself a deviant group within the community?
Change	What major changes have occurred in the community? How did the changes occur? Were the changes planned, unplanned, valued, or disvalued? How did the community accept or attempt to control the changes?	What major changes (anticipated and unanticipated) have occurred in the family? How did the family accept or attempt to control the changes? How does the family view change?
Sick role	Are there ways of identifying sick, frail, chronically disabled, and mentally ill individuals and populations in the community? How are these groups described? What are the expectations for sick role behavior among various cultural groups?	How is a family member identified as being "sick"? What are the behavioral expectations for those in the sick role? What are the behavioral expectations for chronically ill family members? Who assumes the role of caregiver? Who makes decisions for entry into a health care system?
Death ways and meaning	How are deaths marked by the community? Are there variations concerning the meaning of death among different groups in the community?	How are deaths marked by the family? What is the meaning of death? What are the rituals enacted at the time of a death? What are the expectations for individual family members?
Sexuality and sex roles	How do schools and religious groups socialize children with regard to male and female roles? How, where, and when is formal sex education taught? What are the prevailing ideas in the community about sexual behavior? Who are the sexual deviants? How is sexual deviance handled?	What are the sex role expectations across the life span? How, when, and by whom is sexuality discussed in the family? Who is responsible for monitoring the sexual conduct of family members? What are the rules for sexual conduct? How are boys and men supposed to act? How are girls and women supposed to act? When and how does a boy become a man? When does a girl become a woman? What are the sexual taboos?

TABLE 6–4

Community and Family Cultural Assessment Guide ***Continued***

Cultural Category	Questions for Community Assessment	Questions for Family Assessment
Childbearing	What are the shared practices of the community with regard to pregnancy and childbirth? Who attends the mother during delivery? Is early nurturing and mother-child bonding encouraged? Are there purification rituals for the mother? Is male (or female) circumcision practiced? What are the prevalent childbearing myths?	How are family members involved in the birth prenatally and at delivery? What are the expected roles of family members surrounding the birth experience? Who cares for the infant immediately after delivery? How is a newborn assimilated into the family?
Child rearing	What are community expectations with regard to child rearing? Does the community play a part in disciplining children?	Who are the main child rearers and caretakers? What is the expected role of siblings, other relatives, and fictive kin with regard to child rearing? Who are the sex role models? What are the privileges and responsibilities of children? What are the rules for child behavior? What are the patterns of discipline?
Growth and development across the lifespan	How does the community provide resources for all age groups? What health, education, and recreational resources are available for the needs of each age group?	How does the family provide for the very old and the very young? What are the expectations for behavior of each age group? How are life milestones marked?
Reciprocity and exchange	What is the means of exchange in the community (e.g., money, goods, services)? How is debt perceived?	When are gifts shared? Who purchases gifts, pays bills or taxes, etc.? What is the meaning of money, debt, wealth, and poverty? When and how does one give and receive?
Customs and laws	What laws and customs are followed in the community? Who are the law and customs enforcers?	What are the implicit and explicit family rules? Who makes the rules? Who breaks the rules? What are the consequences of rule breaking?
Health care providers	Who are the health providers (traditional and folk) in the community? What is the perception concerning the various kinds of health providers? How do cultural groups differ in their perceptions of health care providers?	What health care providers does the family use? How does the family perceive health care providers? When (under what circumstances) does the family use a health care provider? What does the family know about the traditional health care delivery system, including health insurance?

and the client's reply. The translator's job is to translate accurately and convert the client's words into the correct grammatical context. If the client's reply lasts for 2 minutes and the translator's reply lasts for 20 seconds, the nurse can be fairly certain that the entire reply is not being repeated accurately. Such an observation necessitates clarification of the translator's role and the request for a detailed translation.

Community health nurses who routinely care for clients with English language difficulties should be prepared in the event that no translator is available. The best strategy is for the nurse to become proficient in the language, especially when one language is predominant in the community. Nurses who are just learning or are unfamiliar with a language can prepare a "word board" or carry index cards with essential words or phrases to show clients. Clients can be asked to point to a descriptive phrase on a word board or the nurse can shuffle her index card to locate a key sentence such as "Where is your pain?" or "When did it start?" Sometimes the community health nurse can convey the correct idea through the use of hand motions, pantomime, or simple touch, although speech in a common language remains the most accurate way to communicate.

Part 2: Cultural Pluralism in the United States*

Frances A. Maurer

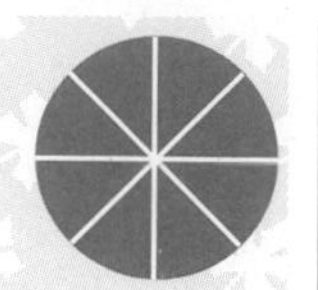

The United States is rich in racial and cultural diversity. At the present time there are approximately 254 million people living in the United States. The vast majority of these citizens are white, although many other racial and ethnic groups are represented in the population (Fig. 6–1). Population-based surveys by the federal government routinely collect data on blacks, Hispanics, Asians, Pacific Islanders, and Native Americans (American Indians, Eskimos, and Aleuts) as minorities, although small numbers of many other minorities live in the United States. Blacks and Hispanics make up the two largest minority groups.

Population experts predict that as the country moves toward the 21st century, it will continue to become more diverse. Whites, although still a majority, are expected to decrease in proportion to other segments of the population. Hispanics and Asians are the most rapidly growing minority groups. By the first quarter of the 21st century, Hispanics are projected to become the largest minority group (Fig. 6–2).

Immigration to the United States has become a significant contributor to population growth. Much of the growth in the Hispanic and Asian population is the result of immigration. In 1990 foreign-born individuals accounted for almost 8% of the total U.S. population, which is a larger percentage than at any time since World War II (Lapham, 1993).

For community health nurses, greater diversity means that nurses can expect to come into frequent contact with members of different ethnic and cultural groups. They must be careful to provide health care that respects and acknowledges these differences. Newer immigrants are most in need of special care. These families must cope with a bewildering array of new experiences, including the health care system. Many may have come from countries with different methods of health care delivery and different ways of interacting with health care providers. Many immigrant families over time adapt their health practices and lifestyles to accommodate to their

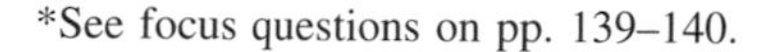

*See focus questions on pp. 139–140.

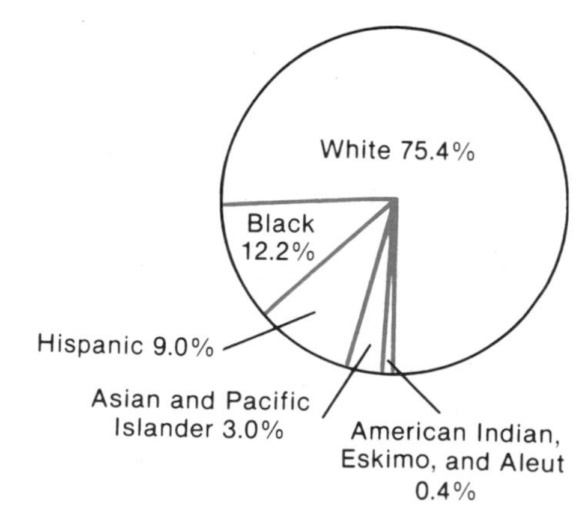

Figure 6–1 ● Population by race and Hispanic origin, 1990. (Data from U.S. Bureau of the Census. (1993). *Population profiles of the United States: 1993* (CPR, series p-23, No. 185). Washington, DC: Government Printing Office.)

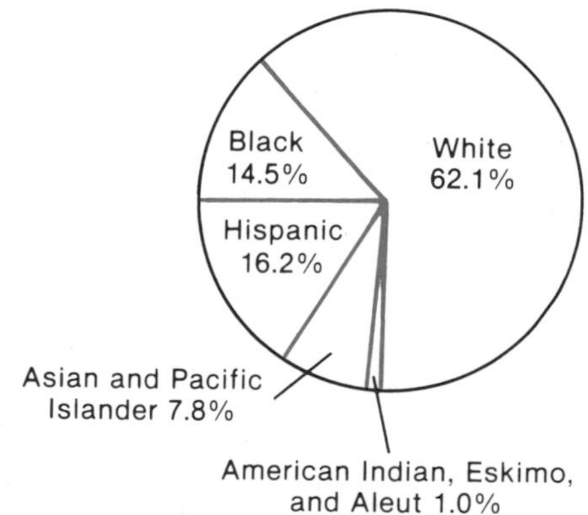

Figure 6–2 ● Population by race and Hispanic origin, 2025. (Data from U.S. Bureau of the Census. (1993). *Population profiles of the United States: 1993* (CPR, series p-23, No. 185). Washington, DC: Government Printing Office.)

TABLE 6–5

Definitions Related to Cultural Pluralism

Culture:	The sum total of ways of living built up by a group of human beings and transmitted from one generation to another.
Ethnic group:	A group of people who may or may not be of the same race, but who share a common and distinctive culture.
Race:	A group of people from an ethnic stock who share common biological features.

new country's patterns and practices, a process called acculturation.

Difficulty Determining the Racial/Ethnic Composition of the Population

Most federal data on racial differences were originally collected in two categories: black and white. These racial categories gradually expanded to include others. Collecting information according to racial composition poses a problem. The Bureau of the Census reports that several million people do not select a racial category on the census form (Rabin, 1993). In the United States, race is often blurred with ethnic origin, and children born of interracial unions are not easily placed in any one category (Table 6–5). People of the same ethnic background may have different racial characteristics. For example, some Hispanic Americans are black; others are white. To accommodate the racial diversity of Hispanics, the census categories currently blend race and ethnic origin. Hispanics (Cubans, Latin Americans, Mexicans, and Spaniards) of any race are counted as a single ethnic group. Black and white designations are limited to those who are not of Hispanic origin (e.g., white non–Hispanic or black non-Hispanic).

Cultural Diversity in Racial/Ethnic Group

Culture further expands the differences among people beyond race and ethnic origin. A racial or ethnic group may be very homogeneous, with a common culture and sharing many beliefs, health practices, and values (e.g., Japan). More often, however, a racial or ethnic group has greater cultural diversity. For instance, within the Asian/Pacific Islander cohort, there are actually more than 60 separate subgroups or cultures (Mass and Yay, 1992).

It is important for community health nurses to recognize the possibility of widespread differences in beliefs and practices among individuals even within the same group. For example, it would be a mistake to assume that all Hispanics share a completely similar culture. Because culture is not the sole source of behavior and values, individuals within a defined racial or ethnic group exhibit a wide range of behavior.

Impact of Race/Culture/Ethnicity on Health Status

Race or ethnic origin has a limited effect on the health status of individuals. There are diseases with a direct genetic link to race or ethnicity (e.g., sickle cell anemia [blacks] or Tay-Sachs disease [Jews]). Beyond such clear links, the health status of most individuals is influenced by a much broader spectrum of factors (Fig. 6–3).

Diseases are often the result of interactions between an individual's genetic inheritance and environmental forces (Bandaranyake, 1986). Even in the presence of a racial or ethnic susceptibility, disease will usually not develop unless the environment is suitably conducive. For example, persons who are genetically predisposed to allergies do not acquire them unless they are environmentally exposed to allergens. Rabin (1993) and others suggest that the root cause of observed racial/ethnic differences in health status actually consists of social factors such as lifestyle, behavior, attitudes, and socioeconomic status, not racial or ethnic influences. Of these, socioeconomic status is the single most important influence on health (Rabin, 1993; Williams, 1993). Poverty has an important negative impact on health status (see Chapters 5 and 11).

Poverty and Health Status

Poverty has a stronger influence on health status than does race (Centers for Disease Control, 1993). People of limited economic means have fewer resources to pay for food, clothing, and shelter and are frequently unable to

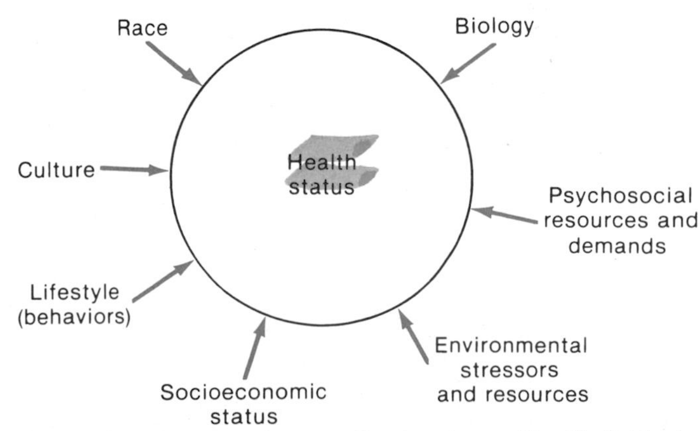

Figure 6–3 ● Selected factors affecting the health of individuals.

access or pay for health services and treatment. Many forgo medical care to purchase other necessities. Preventive care is a luxury few low-income people can afford. Poverty also brings other stressors that affect health: occupational and educational opportunities are limited, housing is often substandard and hazardous, and neighborhoods are not safe. These and other social stressors create a highly stressful environment that affects the health of individuals (Haan et al., 1987).

Minorities and Poverty

In the United States minorities are at greater risk of poverty and its associated problems: higher unemployment, lower educational levels, and shorter life expectancy (Table 6–6). Experts contend that many of the differences in health status are directly attributable to socioeconomic status rather than race/ethnicity (Centers for Disease Control, 1993). The health status of middle-class minority members more closely resembles that of other middle-class individuals than that of poor members of their own ethnic/racial minority. In other words, the health status of middle-class blacks is more similar to that of middle-class whites, than to that of poor blacks.

The epidemiological literature details particular health risks associated with selected minority populations. Much of the data do not consider economic status and other mitigating variables that affect health (Centers for Disease Control, 1993).

Community health nurses and other health professionals should be aware of minority-related health risks reported in research, but should exercise caution before generalizing to individual members of a minority population. The same warning holds true for using data about health risks in any population.

American Indians and Alaskan Natives

Native Americans (American Indians, Aleuts, and Eskimos) represent less than 1% of the U.S. population (CPR-P23-185, 1993). Although Native Americans live throughout the United States, the majority are concentrated in 33 states (Table 6–7). These 33 states are called *reservation states* because there are sufficient Native American populations to warrant health services provided by the Indian Health Service (IHS). The IHS is operated by the U.S. Public Health Service, which is authorized by the U.S. Congress to provide health care to select Native American populations. American Indians and Alaska Natives who reside outside the reservation states must find health services on their own. There is much available data on Native Americans because the IHS assumes the responsibility for collecting a broad base of information on Native Americans.

A common misperception is that almost all Native Americans live on reservations or in rural areas, but the majority (60%) live in urban areas. To meet some of their needs, the IHS operates 34 centers in large urban areas such as Phoenix, Arizona, and Portland, Oregon (Indian Health Service, 1991). Although the majority of Native Americans live in reservation states, about 40% reside in other areas of the country (Indian Health Service, 1991; *Statistical Abstract of the United States,* 1992).

Native Americans are poorer and have less education, higher unemployment, poorer health, and a shorter life expectancy than the general population. When compared with all other Americans, Native Americans have more than twice the unemployment and poverty rate; only about 55% graduate from high school and fewer than 8% are college graduates (Indian Health Service, 1991). The American Indian, Eskimo, and Aleut heritages place great importance

TABLE 6–6

Comparison of Education, Unemployment Rate, and Poverty Level Among Race/Ethnic Groups in the United States

Group	Percentage with High School Education	Unemployment Rate (%)	Percentage Below Poverty Level
Asians	80.4%	6.3%	13.8%
Blacks	66.7%	14.1%	33%
Hispanics	51.3%	7.8%	28.7%
Native Americans	55%	13.3%	28.2%
Whites	79.9%	6.4%	11%

Data from U.S. Bureau of the Census. *Hispanic Americans today* (CPR, series p-23, No. 183) 1993. *The black poulation in the United States* (CPR, series p-20 No. 471) (1992); *Population profiles of the United States* (CPR, series p-23 No. 185) (1993). Washington, DC: Government Printing Office.

TABLE 6–7

Reservation States

Alabama	Maine	North Dakota
Alaska	Massachusetts	Oklahoma
Arizona	Michigan	Oregon
California	Minnesota	Pennsylvania
Colorado	Mississippi	Rhode Island
Connecticut	Montana	South Dakota
Florida	Nebraska	Texas
Idaho	Nevada	Utah
Iowa	New Mexico	Washington
Kansas	New York	Wisconsin
Louisiana	North Carolina	Wyoming

From Indian Health Service. (1991). *Trends in Indian health.* Washington, DC: U.S. Dept. of Health and Human Services, Public Health Service, U.S. Government Printing Office.

on the wisdom of the elderly and incorporate a strong sense of community responsibility. Where that perspective continues, Native American clients may look to elders and leaders to help in their decision-making process. The strong sense of community ties may be reflected in individuals pitching in to help others in need. Extended family as well as neighbors will often help people with transportation, child care, and shelter needs.

Asians and Pacific Islanders

Although they make up only 3% of the total population, Asians and Pacific Islanders are a rapidly growing segment. Three fourths of the growth in this subgroup is the result of new immigrants. This is also perhaps the most diverse minority group, as there are many different cultures and languages, educational patterns and lifestyle habits, and immigration histories among Asians and Pacific Islanders (Takaki, 1993). The Japanese and Chinese are the oldest Asian immigrant groups; many families are now fifth- and sixth-generation Americans. The Vietnamese, Laotians, and Cambodians are relatively recent arrivals. The Hawaiian people are native to that state. Recognition of this diversity should sensitize community health nurses to the need to validate customs, health practices, and concerns on an individual basis.

Asians and Pacific Islanders are highly concentrated in the western states, Alaska, and Hawaii. Ninety-four percent of these people live in metropolitan areas, and they are about equally distributed between large cities and their suburbs (CPR-P20-459, 1992).

High school education levels meet or exceed those of the population as a whole. However, higher educational achievement varies greatly among subgroups of Asians and Pacific Islanders. Despite the widespread belief that all Asians do well in school and economically, they actually do no better than whites. The unemployment rate for Asians and Pacific Islanders is similar to that of the general population, and the poverty level is slightly higher than that of whites. The newer immigrant groups are more likely to live in poverty and to be less educated than older, well-established immigrant groups.

In the Asian culture filial piety and harmony are important (Mass and Yay, 1992). Elders and parents are respected and obeyed. There is a hierarchy of decision makers, with women generally having less status than men in this process. Harmony is valued, and individuals are encouraged to place group needs before individual needs to avoid confrontation and maintain peace. The family sense of obligation means that family members share responsibility for meeting the needs of other members, including health care, child care, and educational needs.

Blacks

Blacks are the largest minority group, representing one eighth (12%) of the U.S. population. Most blacks are native-born citizens. People from the Caribbean make up the largest black immigrant group but represent only a small proportion of all black citizens (Bennett, 1993). Slightly more than 50% of blacks live in large metropolitan areas, and a majority live in the southern states.

Consistent educational progress has resulted in about 70% of black citizens having at least a high school education. However, income has not kept pace with educational attainment. Black families still have three times greater the risk of poverty than do white families. During the 1980s, the number of blacks with very low incomes actually increased, and the rate of growth into middle-class status slowed (Swinton, 1990).

Black culture incorporates strong extended family bonds and shared child-rearing responsibilities (Prater, 1992). Because both parents in black families have long needed to work, in families with intact parents, both share the responsibilities for child care. In the past health care providers and social support agencies often viewed the resulting diverse child-rearing arrangements as chaotic and disruptive, rather than as a sign of flexibility. Community health nurses caring for black children should be careful to include extended family members in assessing how children's needs are being met.

Hispanics

Hispanics are the second largest minority group (9%) and are the fastest growing segment of the population (CPR-P23-183, 1993). Although most were born in the United States, Hispanics are the single largest new immigrant group. Most Hispanic immigrants come from Mexico and Latin America and represent many diverse cultures (Fig. 6–4). Because Hispanics are the largest immigrant group, Spanish is the most common second language spoken in the United States (Fig. 6–5). Community health nurses who care for Spanish populations can expect to come in contact with individuals who are not fluent in English. More than one third of Hispanics (8 million) do not speak English well or at all (CPR-P-23-183, 1993).

The vast majority of Hispanic Americans live in 10 states. California and Texas have the highest concentrations, followed by the northeastern states and Florida (Fig. 6–6). Immigrants tend to settle in areas with similar ethnic people, and therefore, Mexican Americans are concentrated in the southwestern region, Cubans in Florida, and Puerto Ricans in New York. Hispanic Americans are more likely

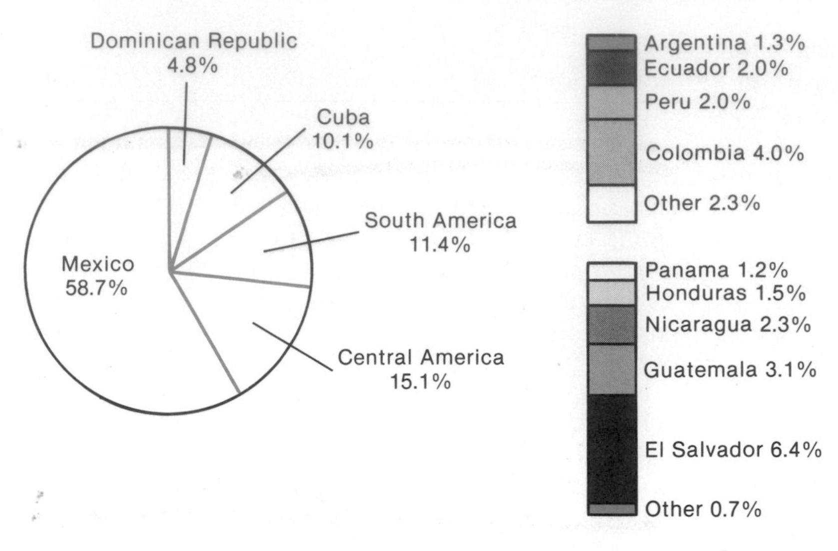

Figure 6–4 ● Foreign-born persons from Spanish-speaking Latin America, 1990 (percent distribution). (Redrawn from U.S. Bureau of the Census. (1993). *Hispanic Americans today.* (CPR, series p-23, No. 183). Washington, DC: Government Printing Office.)

to live in large cities and metropolitan areas; only about 10% live in rural areas and small towns (CPR-P23-183, 1993).

Hispanics are the second poorest minority group, and their health status reflects the influences of poverty. Hispanics actually have less access to health care than others, because more of them do not have any type of health insurance, either public or private, compared with rates in other racial/ethnic groups (Table 6–8).

The Hispanic culture places a deep importance on the family, and the family provides emotional and material support to its members. As in black families, there are strong extended family ties, although extended family members are less likely to live together (Delgado, 1992). As in Asian families, the father holds a position of authority, and Hispanics have a history of incorporating folk medicine and folk healers into their health care practices. Community health nurses need to assess family decision-making processes and scope of health practices when planning care. The use of folk medicine should not be opposed if it does not jeopardize the impact of medically prescribed treatment.

Generational Conflict

Conflict may arise within families as minorities assimilate and adapt to the general American culture. Families who traditionally shared responsibilities experience difficulty when younger members want to act independently. Families who have used a hierarchical and paternal decision-making process often have trouble when younger generations challenge those ideas. Community health nurses should be alert for the possibility of such tensions

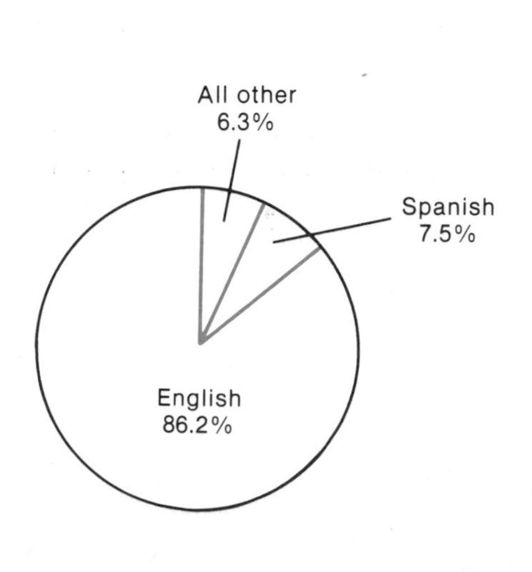

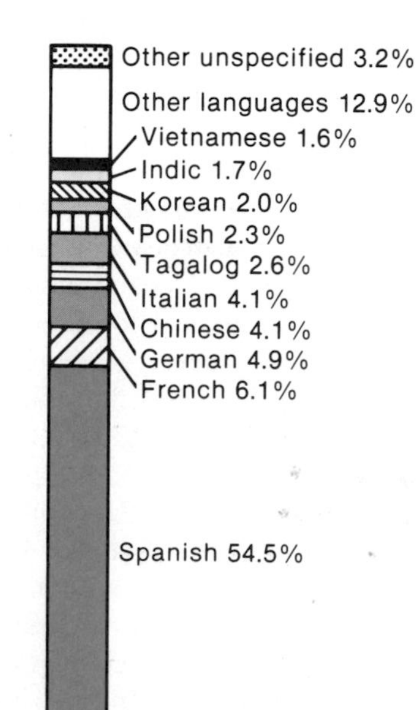

Figure 6–5 ● Language spoken at home, 1990 (percent distribution of persons 5 years and older). Bar graph on right indicates other and Spanish expanded to show specific languages spoken and frequency. (Redrawn from U.S. Bureau of the Census. (1993). *Hispanic Americans today.* (CPR, series p-23, No. 183). Washington, DC: Government Printing Office.)

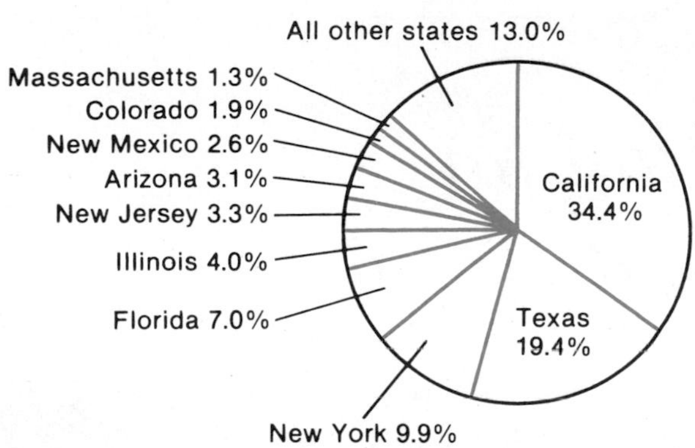

Figure 6–6 ● Hispanic population for selected states, 1990 (percent distribution). (From U.S. Bureau of the Census. (1993). *Hispanic Americans today* (CPR, series p-23, No. 183). Washington, DC: Government Printing Office.)

TABLE 6–8

Comparison of Health Insurance Coverage in Whites, Blacks, and Hispanics

	Percentage with Health Insurance
Whites	87.6%
Blacks	80.7%
Hispanics	73.0%

From *Statistical Abstract of the United States* (1992). Washington, DC: U.S. Bureau of the Census, U.S. Government Printing Office.

among family members and recognize that such tensions affect the entire family unit.

Role of Community Health Nurses in Culturally Diverse Populations

One of the rewards of community health nursing is the exposure to many different peoples and cultures. Caring and sensitive community health nurses have the opportunity to expand their knowledge and horizons while providing care to others. To ensure quality care, community health nurses should strive to incorporate all aspects of a client's usual habits and practices when planning care. For example, if a family is used to having the father make decisions, enrolling the father in the care process is likely to make treatment more successful. Any comprehensive assessment should include identification of values. Knowing and incorporating these into the nursing care plan goes a long way toward ensuring success.

Part 3: Values Clarification for Change and Empowerment*

Kathryn Hopkins Kavanagh

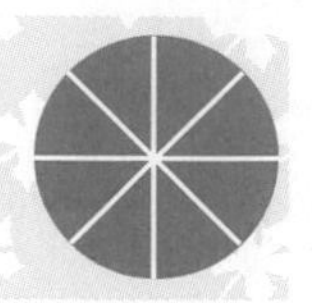

Values make us who we are. As nurses, our values reflect our personal and professional histories. We often pay little attention to values and may even be unaware of what they are or how our values differ from those of others. However, values are important in nursing, because they have the potential to create interactive barriers or positive communication and relationships. They influence every interpersonal interaction, every health care decision, and every caring behavior. When people interact, as nurses and clients do, their values interact.

As community health nursing moves toward a population-focused orientation, the need to clarify values becomes more obvious. Although values are important in one-to-one interactions, they are often assumed or overlooked. The goal of values clarification is to help make values more explicit—that is, less taken for granted—so that they can be used to work for better health at the individual, group, and community levels.

Values Affect Health Behavior

Values influence human behavior, including behavior related to health and illness (Table 6–9). We value what we view as worthwhile and important. Although each individual has values, the culture and society in which the individual lives or identifies usually strongly influences those values. Some primary values in American society include individualism, consumerism, competition, and mastery over nature. Certainly not everyone in the United States ascribes to these; indeed, entire subcultures may not. Nevertheless, these values influence our everyday life and the way the society functions. They influence the types of television programs that are popular and available, what is taught in schools, how the political system operates, attitudes toward disease and death, the advertisements that we are exposed to, and virtually every other aspect of societal life.

TABLE 6–9
Definitions Related to Values

Value: A preference or an ideal that gives direction to human life by influencing beliefs and behaviors. Values come in sets or systems that make up a specific view of the world. Culture, family, personality, and life experiences contribute to the formation of values.

Values conflict: A state of uncertainty in which two or more values are diametrically opposed and create a conflict. Values conflict may be intrinsic (i.e., within an individual) or extrinsic (i.e., between two or more persons with different values).

Value change: An exchange of one value for another or a reprioritization of values. May be gradual or sudden.

Values clarification: A strategy of discovery that brings into conscious awareness the values held by an individual or group.

Value Change

Values can and do change over time. Many of us live our lives within a single culture and might not notice the subtle influences that affect our values over time in a constantly changing society. We grow up and go to school, assuming adult and professional value orientations that we may never define as such, but they have a profound effect on us and on our interactions with others.

We were not born with the values we hold today. Nor are our values exactly like the values of those who raised us. Our values have changed and continue to do so. Values are constantly being shaped by our experiences in the world around us. Despite their ability to change, values change slowly. Whereas science causes modern societies and lifestyles to change rapidly (allowing mobility and

*See focus questions on p. 140.

changes in health care that were not even dreamed of in earlier times), people's values adapt only slowly. For example, the global problem of increasing population is in large part the result of innovations in modern technology. Improved sanitation and nutrition reduce death rates in any society, allowing more people to mature and reproduce. Traditional values, however, adjust slowly to the decline in infant mortality rates. Many people continuc to have large families (which were valued and adaptive in the past), so populations grow at rapid rates. Over time, people do adapt to lower mortality rates and produce smaller families.

Value Conflict

Although most people settle into fairly stable value orientations, it is not unusual at times to experience disharmony when values conflict. This disharmony can occur within an individual or between individuals. An example of a values conflict within an individual might be the problem associated with blending the roles of wife, mother, and career woman. Many women are torn between the competing demands of building a career and the more traditional role of family caretaker.

Value conflicts also surface on the interpersonal level, and it is these conflicts community health nurses most often face. Here the diversity of society comes to the forefront. Diversity exists everywhere there is not sameness; it is not limited to ethnicity or overt cultural, ethnic, or racial distinction. Differences are also rooted in age, health status, economic status, occupational and educational orientation, gender, sexual orientation, and life experiences. Sometimes we perceive significant differences, for example, in race, when only the social meaning of differences has impact. Genetically there is almost an inconsequential distinction between races, but socially there may be a profound effect on experience, especially in a society as stratified as that in the United States. Value conflict related to racial differences is not based on biology or genetics but is rooted in the high values placed on status and power.

Values Orientation and Culture

It has long been recognized that in every culture or society, there are basic values. These values emphasize shared ideas about time, activities, and relationships. Some of these shared ideas were previously identified in part 1 of this chapter. Basic values include nature (including the supernatural), time, activity, relationships with other people, and the nature of humankind (Kluckhohn, 1971; Kavanagh, 1991a).

Cultures that believe the relationships between people and nature are predetermined (by God, fate, or genetics) are more likely to believe that nature controls people. Cultures that believe that relationships can be altered are more likely to believe people can control nature.

People tend to be oriented toward the past, the present, or the future. People with a past orientation believe history may be emulated and the past reclaimed. They may even believe in ancestral spirits. People with a present orientation make the most of the moment and have little concern for the future (i.e., "Don't worry, be happy!"). People who have a future orientation are more likely to save money, to go to school to get credentials that will increase opportunities, and to set other long-range goals such as preventing diseases that might not occur for years, if ever.

Attitudes toward activity are also varied. For some people it is enough to just exist, to be; it is not necessary to accomplish great things to feel worthwhile. For others there is a sense of needing to develop the self, which is its own reward, with no outside recognition necessary. For still others, however, there is a belief that hard work will pay off visibly as well as psychologically. These orientations to life encourage people to be relatively passive or very energetic.

Values concerning social relationships and the nature of humans are equally diverse. Some cultures believe the welfare of the group is paramount, while others are more oriented toward individual rights and self-direction. Americans generally tend to value individualism very highly; only secondarily are they members of families or communities. Some people believe people are born to either lead or follow. These people do not expect "followers" to assume great responsibility for themselves or for decision making. Some cultures are more oriented toward believing all people are good and trustworthy, while others hold that humans are intrinsically evil and not worthy of trust.

VARIABILITY ACROSS AND WITHIN CULTURES

As previously noted, there are differences in values and customs, including health care beliefs and practices, among cultures. While members of a particular culture tend to share many ideas and values, there is also great diversity within that culture as well.

There is a sizable body of knowledge, called *transcultural nursing,* that focuses on the differences and similarities among people in terms of their values related to care (Leininger, 1978, 1988, 1991). This orientation is useful, because it provides a framework for understanding values and their importance in all aspects of nursing, whether the differences are overt (as when languages and cultures significantly differ) or covert (as when two individuals of the same culture view the same phenomenon in different ways).

The United States is probably the most diverse society to ever exist. As previously mentioned, it contains people from many different ethnic and cultural origins, as well as people from all classes or socioeconomic statuses.

Although most nurses are aware of cultural variations, class differences are less often acknowledged. Persons of different classes may share the same cultural, ethnic, religious, and political orientations, yet exhibit variability in time orientation.

A general pattern among the economically disadvantaged is to be oriented to the present, while the middle and upper classes tend to be oriented toward the future. Promoting disease prevention among poor people takes special strategies, because their priorities are more immediate (e.g., having shelter and food or enough money to get by). For example, the threat of heart disease years in the future may not seem real or important to anyone who thinks in terms of the present. They may not see the value in making changes in exercise and eating patterns in the present to postpone or avoid illness 10 or 20 years in the future. A future-oriented individual would be more likely to see value in such efforts.

DOMINANT AMERICAN CULTURAL AND HEALTH VALUES

Despite the wide variability in values held by people, there are some strong patterns of interrelated values that can be used to characterize society in general. Individualism and mastery over nature are dominant American values that permeate many aspects of health care. We increasingly hold individuals responsible for seeking and cooperating with health care and for promoting their own health and preventing illness. Medicine attempts to control disease and distress, using such aggressive terms as "conquering" cancer and "fighting" tuberculosis. Scientific knowledge, which was founded on a conviction that nature can be controlled and used, is applied through technology and technique in nearly every facet of health. There is little fatalistic submission to illness among health care providers as a result of the sophisticated armamentarium they use. Providers measure and control not only such aspects as room temperature and fluid intake, but also delicate blood gas levels, electrolyte balances, and other physiological phenomena. Such activities denote a belief in intervention and in a potential for mastery over whatever problem comes along.

Materialism is as apparent in the health care arena as in American society at large. Americans value money because of its potential to be turned into goods and services. Advertisements and media encourage consumerism, and status is often symbolized by the acquisition of material goods. Americans learn to want a vast array of things and services, often confusing standard of living (which is the ability to meet needs through access to consumer products) with quality of life and with more abstract values such as meaningful relationships, contentment, or a sense of fulfillment.

Individualism, personal achievement, materialism, and mastery over nature are reflected in individuals' choice of health care systems. The emphasis on mastery over nature has resulted in an emphasis on "cure" rather than caring and on prevention and promoting behaviors. An orientation toward the individual rather than the common good has resulted in a collage of health care structures and providers built on the free enterprise system. Health care in the United States has been a privilege to be earned or achieved; it has not been a right. As a result, millions of Americans do not have access to health care, and many more do not have adequate health care insurance coverage (see Chapter 3). This situation mirrors American society's predominant values: If an individual would just try hard enough, he or she would be able to afford health care or health care insurance.

Two additional values that affect health care are time and activity. Society is youth oriented; we try to deny and control the natural processes of aging and dying. We value opportunities that promise better futures and better lives. In lieu of appreciating the here and now, we yearn for something different or something more. At times this cultural trait is expressed in terms of valuing health and fitness, although this requires an orientation to the future and is more often observed among middle- and upper-class than lower socioeconomic class individuals and groups.

Our relationship with time is in large part measured in terms of efficiency and productivity. This is a problem for nursing, which tends to be time intensive. Efficiency requires streamlining and mass production of care, yet there is increasing evidence that quality care must be designed and provided according to the value-oriented requirements and expectations of divergent clients. Acceptable care is more effective than care that does not fit clients' needs, and effective care saves time. However, nurses often contend with situations in which they have too little time to provide quality care and are expected to focus on the technical aspects of nursing.

The familiar demand that one will be highly productive relates directly to the value of activity. The moral and ethical foundations of contemporary American values and beliefs denounced idleness and promoted hard work. Work is so important to us that our occupations often form the source of our personal as well as public identities. Occupations and employment serve as mechanisms for the distribution of status, power, and wealth. Work implies activity, and American society is oriented toward action and change. Health care reflects those values. It is often assumed (sometimes with little consideration of alternatives or consequences) that vigorous medical or nursing intervention will be beneficial and that immediate action is better than waiting.

Values Clarification

No values are implicitly right or wrong; they simply shape ideas and responses. Any assumption by health care providers that a given orientation is shared by all clients can be dangerously misleading. The most prominent values in the United States are reflected in its health care, but those values tend to represent the dominant cultural group (European American, middle-class, Christian males) and not the many subgroups within the country. The dominant culture's set of values is oriented toward individuals. Individuals, rather than groups, are viewed as responsible for making health-related decisions and their own health status. Privacy rights and personal freedom are based on the value of individualism. However, in many of the subcultures in the United States and around the world, individualism is not a primary value. Instead, belonging to family and community is most important.

Perhaps as you read the descriptions of different value orientations you recognized values that fit either you as an individual or the part of society with which you identify. If you did not, please re-read them and think about it. Ask yourself where your sense of personal identity came from and how it was formed, and where your values came from and how they were learned and shaped. Are they rooted in a particular ethnic, class, gender, or religious orientation? How are your values changing as you mature and age and experience different aspects of life? How do you want them to change? As you do this, be sure to question what your values really are, rather than what you would like them to be—that is, work toward understanding what you truly value; ignore what you think you should value. There is usually a difference between the real and the ideal, and pretending (even to yourself) will not make you a better nurse.

Values clarification involves bringing influences on behavior to conscious awareness. Values clarification is essential to providing quality care, and communication is the key to values clarification and understanding in nursing. To guide relationships that clients perceive as caring and helpful, nurses must communicate positively, and to do that, they must know both themselves and the client well. However it is not as easy to know oneself as it might seem. The community health nurse may take for granted much about himself or herself and may base ideas about clients on stereotypes. In both cases, values must be made explicit and must be acknowledged if communication is to be meaningful and effective. Take, for instance, the situation in which a nurse's values are influenced by a religion that views abortion as immoral. It is essential that the nurse recognize the impact such views will have on relationships with persons seeking to terminate a pregnancy. However, more subtle values also influence nurses' responses to clients. A high level of self-awareness is required to prevent imposing on others our own personal moral assessments or behavioral expectations that we may consider "normal," but are really based on a lack of knowledge about what others may consider normal.

The object of nursing is to provide quality care. To be viewed as valuable, care must be considered appropriate by the recipient. Because what the client considers to be good care is based on his or her value orientation, care that does not take values into account is little more than a hit-or-miss proposition. Nonetheless, much of the care providers give is based on nurses' and other providers' values, rather than on clients' values.

Reasons for Values Clarification

A community health nurse (or anyone else) cannot accurately and completely understand someone else's values, but nurses can be conscious of the possibility of diverse value sets among their clients, avoid stereotyping individuals and cultural groups, remain open minded, and seek to clarify others' values (especially health-related values) in planning nursing care. However, values conflicts will continue to exist.

CONFLICTING VALUES WITHIN HEALTH CARE

The fact that there are meaningful differences among people's values orientations poses both opportunities and challenges for community health nursing. Nurses and clients both have value orientations, and whether the nurse and client interact in a clinic or a home setting, their values interact. The fact that values shape expectations for giving care and for being cared for is the fundamental reason for value clarification. Failure to identify and consider values invites their interference, rather than support, in care. Where values differ, effective communication requires more flexibility and attention. Most Americans have learned to try to ignore differences; sometimes they avoid confronting differences because they have been taught that acknowledging them is risky; it might make them uncomfortable or "hurt someone's feelings." However, avoidance implies that the differences are not worth attention, which often leads to anger, frustration, rejection, humiliation, and even negative physiological consequences (Kavanagh and Kennedy, 1992). Avoidance of diversity communicates a message akin to, "It really does not matter what you think or how you feel; this is how we are going to do things." Avoidance frustrates good nurse–client relations and inhibits encounters that could be positive, respectful, and mutual.

Ideally communication is open and provides everyone involved with a sense of respect and integrity. This does not rule out conflicting encounters, as confrontation and conflict are not inherently offensive. Avoidance, in contrast, is harmful, because it ignores the issue (or part of the issue) and prevents it from being dealt with. If you have ever been ignored or made to feel unimportant, you know how it hurts. When ignored, people withdraw, get defensive or confrontational, resist, or just give in and comply. Too often that is what happens in health care; patients are cajoled (or coerced) into complying or blamed for not complying. Neither situation preserves the client's self-respect. Ideally communication should allow clients to make informed and independent decisions that maintain their respect and integrity. Both coercion and avoidance indicate failure to communicate effectively (Kavanagh and Kennedy, 1992).

CROSS-CULTURAL INTERACTIONS

Much of health care involves cross-cultural communication, even if that is only across the gap between professional providers (who represent the subcultural values of their disciplines) and lay clients. American society is so diverse that some cultural differences are obvious, yet nurses often are taught little about effective negotiation of those differences and how to use them to facilitate good care.

ACCOUNTABILITY AND SELF-RESPONSIBILITY IN NURSING

Nursing's code for ethics holds that all persons deserve respect and to be treated with dignity (American Nurses' Association, 1985). Community health nurses should be very sensitive to how their actions are delivered and perceived. Several studies have shown that clients who do not return for services after the first clinic visit often have values that differ significantly from those of the clinic's providers (Pedersen, 1981; Zola, 1981). Community health nurses have, both individually and collectively, a professional responsibility for developing the ability to understand their roles in communicating ideas. Many nurses inadvertently contribute to social distancing and discriminatory situations because they avoid the mutual communication that allows values to be clarified. They may not realize how others interpret their behavior, but by not recognizing that their ideas and behaviors conflict with the values and norms of others, they create social barriers and negate the worth of others (Hamill, 1988).

PROMOTING CLIENT PARTICIPATION AND FOLLOW-THROUGH

"Compliance is the extent to which a person's behavior coincides with health practitioners' advice" (Kozier et al., 1992, p. 239). Although innocuous enough by that definition, the concept of compliance has been exploited in health care to imply an "us-against-them" relationship between practitioners and clients. Too often the "noncompliant" client—that is, the client who did not conform to the expectations of the nurse or other provider—has been blamed for his or her failure to cooperate without attention to the reasons why alternative decisions or behaviors were chosen. Usually these reasons can be traced to differences in values, priorities, or resources that lead to differences in expectations and priorities. Clients are more likely to integrate health-related behaviors into their life when the suggested plan of care is consistent with their own values.

STRENGTHENING CLIENT SELF-EFFICACY

Self-efficacy is what one perceives and believes about his or her ability to change behavior (Pruitt, 1991). It has long been known that belief can strongly influence actual outcome. Understanding a client's values supports formulation of goals and plans that are both acceptable to the client and workable, which in turn strengthens a client's belief that he or she can successfully change behavior.

There is a shift toward collaborative and participatory relationships between clients and their health statuses (Lowenberg, 1989). Using a collaborative framework for intervention allows the client to participate in what happens to him or her (which is likely to motivate ongoing interest and cooperation in the process) and to feel acknowledged and respected. For example, the use of a collaborative model that encourages intravenous drug users to help prevent the human immunodeficiency virus (HIV) and the acquired immunodeficiency syndrome (AIDS) in their community has been acceptable and motivating for participants (Kavanagh et al., 1992).

When to Use Values Clarification

The community health nurse and the client, with their respective value systems, interact. Most nurses learn basic communication skills to facilitate interaction, but they may remain unaware of the impact that differences in values make. Values clarification can help community health nurses facilitate an effective relationship with clients by identifying factors that may affect the nurse's relationships with clients. There are many circumstances in which values clarification can be helpful; several of these will be discussed in more detail.

To Avoid Cultural Imposition. Culture is so much a part of everyday life that it is taken for granted. It leads us to assume that our own perspective is shared by others, including those for whom we care. It might be assumed, for example, that the client believes in professional health care and does not use folk remedies. It is often assumed that nursing care is value free and does not impose values on others. This, alas, is a myth. Nursing as it is currently practiced in the United States did not develop in a void. Like medicine, it reflects the dominant American culture. These values, like other values, are neither right nor wrong; they simply are. However, not everyone shares them.

When community health nurses practice with the idea that nursing's values and their values will be appropriate to the client, they are making huge assumptions and risk grave misunderstandings. This imposition of cultural values on others suggests a narrowness of view that inhibits an understanding of the client's beliefs, values, lifestyle, needs, and expectations. The key to developing and using awareness, sensitivity, and skills cross-culturally is flexibility (Pedersen, 1988). In our multicultural world there is a need to make care specific to individual and cultural needs and expectations, rather than imposing it on clients (Leininger, 1978, 1988, 1991). Values clarification skills are part of that. Do not be afraid of differences; learn to acknowledge them, use them, and enjoy them.

To Increase Control over Anxiety and Emotional Reactivity. Communication is sometimes associated with risk, as when there is uncertainty about how one will be received or whether one is doing the right thing. When situations are uneasy, it is common for anger, hurt, defensiveness, and resistance to occur. Defensiveness is a response to a perception of threat, while resistance involves barriers to trust or opposition to the goal of mutual communication.

The key to reducing defensiveness and resistance is recognizing these processes. When they are understood in specific terms, they can be managed. However, if they remain nonspecific (e.g., "But they never realize what I can do for them" or "He always makes me feel that way"), they are not controllable and are likely to perpetuate anger and negativity. Several strategies for identifying and reducing defensiveness and resistance are listed in Table 6–10.

To Handle Conflicts. Conflict arises when health care providers and clients disagree on how to handle a situation. Many times the conflict is the result of a different value orientation. When the relationship is mutual and communication open, it becomes easier to address the conflict. Defensiveness and resistance on the part of the nurse obstruct productive relationships. The community health nurse may conclude that a client's approach is totally wrong and requires radical overhauling, but sometimes this conclusion is based more on a lack of understanding of the client's stance than on necessity. Careful analysis by a flexible, sensitive, knowledgeable, and skillful nurse usually results in a desire to preserve the integrity of the client's view as much as possible, if for no other reason than that it is likely to promote the client's cooperation. However, occasionally perspectives conflict and the provider must take a stand for substantive change, as in cases of illegal or injurious behavior (e.g., child abuse).

To Help Clients and Nurses Solve Ethical/Moral Issues and Dilemmas. Values clarification is essential for clients to make informed and considered choices and as a guide for nursing intervention. Clients, like nurses, confront difficult decisions and often require help in knowing how to handle these decisions, (e.g., how to advise their teenagers to deal

TABLE 6–10

Strategies to Identify and Reduce Defensiveness and Resistance

1. State the obvious. "What you just said made me uncomfortable. Can we talk about it some more?" Acknowledging your responses attests to your integrity, honesty, and interest. There is no need to apologize for feelings.
2. Use humor, including humor that is self-directed. "Yes, I know I am late. I am sorry to keep you waiting. It seems I was born late, and I've been running to catch up ever since!"
3. Disclose selected, appropriate information to promote sharing and a sense of acceptance. "I know it's hard. My own baby never wanted me to do that to him either, but here's what I found worked for me. . . ."
4. Acknowledge and describe your own beliefs, behaviors, and responses in nonjudgmental ways. "I personally have never believed in spanking children, but I know people have different ideas about raising them."
5. Get help from others; you do not have to do everything alone. "I don't know very much about your mother's values and beliefs. Could you tell me about them so that I can provide the kind of care she expects and will find appropriate?"
6. Accept responsibility for interactive or behavioral errors by acknowledging them and apologizing to reinforce positive expectations for the relationship. "I am sorry that I did not know today is a religious holiday for you. Will you tell me about it?"
7. Be flexible; it prevents frustration. Plans are necessary for meeting goals, but flexibility is needed to realistically meet clients' needs and expectations. "I was hoping that you might be able to take him to see the doctor Monday, but will it be all right if I arrange it for Thursday?"
8. Show acceptance and understanding by clearly identifying the client's concern or understanding of the problem. "I understand that you think rubbing horse liniment on your knee will help the arthritis, but I wonder if you would also like to try this other medication."
9. Assess coping response patterns (including your own) to problematic and stressful situations. Such assessment promotes recognition of resistant or defensive responses.
10. Ask questions. Different cultural groups expect questions to be asked in different ways (perhaps indirectly or after considerable small talk), but nurses need information. "What would you like me to do for you?"
11. Recommend interventions that are not likely to meet with resistance or defensiveness. "I understand that your ethnic foods are very important to you. Will you help me figure out which ones will fit into this diet that the doctor wants you to be on?"
12. Openly acknowledge discrepancies between your views and the client's. "I know you do not like to drive in the snow, but I am concerned about Sara missing her physical therapy sessions."
13. To let it be known you understand them, accurately reflect, clarify, and interpret the client's behaviors, concerns, or ideas. "I think I heard you say that Juan's illness is because of the evil eye. Would you tell me more about that?"
14. Reflect and adjust your voice, body position, and other aspects of communication to synchronize with those of the client.
15. Get to know the client's informal system of social support. The client is part of a network and usually does not make decisions or act entirely without support from others. "Is there someone from your church who might stay with the children while you have that examination at the clinic?"

Adapted from Pederson, P. (1988). *A handbook for developing multicultural awareness.* Alexandria, VA: American Association for Counseling and Development; and Kavanagh, K. H., & Kennedy, P. H. (1992). *Promoting cultural diversity: Strategies for health care professionals.* Newbury Park, CA: Sage.

with their sexuality or whether, for the sake of possibly prolonged life, to significantly alter the diet of an aging family member who resists that change). Ethical concerns such as abortion, the right to die, and suicide strongly affect clients' lives. Frequently clients turn to nurses for support and direction. Working with clients to clarify their values, and with themselves to clarify their own, is essential for nurses to resolve value conflicts and moral or ethical problems.

Moral dilemmas involve personal options for choice that seem to be without satisfactory solution. The single mother who needs to work but also wants to be a conscientious parent may find herself morally torn by the situation. The strain of trying to perform both roles may interfere with each or even create a dangerous situation. For example, the mother tells the school nurse she leaves her 10-year-old child unattended during the night so that she can work the night shift and make more money. She and her daughter have established an elaborate safety routine because she cannot afford to hire someone to stay during the night. Aside from the obvious nursing responsibility to provide for the child's immediate safety, the nurse needs to help the mother sort out her priorities from the perspective of her values.

People have reasons for acting the way they do. Others may not understand or agree with those reasons, but generally people do the best they can in making decisions, given the options they perceive at the time. In many situations all alternatives are not realized, and priorities sometimes do not promote health, so nursing input is essential. An alternative search is one method nurses can use to help clients in the decision-making process (Table 6–11).

The development of sophisticated technology has led to increased numbers of moral and ethical problems. These can be painful and unsettling experiences; it is not easy to make the decision to "pull the plug," or even to know how best to set limits for a loved one. One cannot stand on one's values without first knowing them, and priorities cannot be intelligently set without consideration of the variables and alternatives. The clarification of values supports the making of decisions that promise to be the best for all involved.

TABLE 6–11

Alternative Search Form for Clients

Alternative	I'll Try It.	I'll Consider It.	I Won't Try It.
1.			
2.			
3.			
4.			
5.			
6.			
etc.			

From Simon, S., Howe, L., & Kirschenbaum, H. (1972). *Values clarification: A handbook of practical strategies for teachers and students.* New York: Heart Publishing Company.

To Facilitate Change in Behavior. Nursing care that fits clients' needs and value orientations is referred to as *congruent* because it works with clients and does not manipulate them. Culturally and personally congruent intervention is more effective in promoting healthy behavior than is the imposition of ideas and expectations that the client does not relate to (or that may contradict those the client does relate to).

The first step is identifying the client's values and perspective in terms of health and the specific situation at hand. Nearly always those values can be preserved or at least partly maintained, while at the same time improving health-related behaviors. It is important for the nurse to understand that deep-seated values are not easily changed, especially at someone else's direction. Overt attempts to modify client values may lead to superficial rather than intrinsic modification. A client would be very likely to perform some agreed-on health behavior in the nurse's presence, yet discontinue it when the nurse is not around or has completed home visiting.

To Validate (Un)Readiness to Change Behavior. The identification and prioritization of values validates unreadiness (or readiness) to change behavior. This clarification helps the nurse discern when people are willing to negotiate and when they are adamant in their positions. Most of the time, clarifying and understanding values opens the door for negotiation that results in mutually acceptable choices and outcomes. However, sometimes there is no room for negotiation. For example, a community health nurse became very upset when a family with whom she was working elected against corrective surgery for an infant with severe congenital anomalies. The surgery would be expensive, and even if it went well, there were few chances that the child would ever function as a productive adult. The nurse understood the financial, emotional and logistical costs involved, but she rejected the decision because, according to her values, individuals come first and should be given every opportunity for survival and success. To this large and extended family, however, the group came first, and decisions were based on that value. Both perspectives are legal and acceptable; they simply represent different priorities. It was unproductive and inappropriate to label the family as irresponsible or uncaring; they were neither. Yet this is what the nurse felt until she understood the intrinsic, value-rooted reasons for their decision. After some discussion with her peers, the community health nurse was able to accept the situation from the clients' perspective. Although she did not agree with their choice, she continued to work with the family and established adequate rapport to influence the child's care within the framework of the family's needs and expectations.

To Help Clients Handle the Impact of Emotions on Behavior Change. Knowledge alone does not change behavior and does not provide plausible options when it conflicts with established values, beliefs, or lifestyles. Believing that something "should" happen does not mean it will happen. The gap between intellectual decisions about behavior and actual behavior itself is fraught with poorly understood emotional barriers. No matter how much logical sense it makes, it is hard to motivate change that does not "feel right" or is not wanted because of conflict with taken-for-granted, implicit, and unspoken values. For example, a woman who wants a healthy infant may continue to occasionally drink alcohol. She might "know better," but her actions show she values other needs that result in health risks. Clients benefit from nonjudgmental assistance with clarifying their motivations for actions and identifying conflicting values that provide emotional interference with goals. When helping clients take control over those aspects of their lives that can lead to improved health, collaboration and sustained encouragement are frequently more effective than imposition or cajoling. The success of collaboration is based on use of and respect for the client's input and a recognition that change is not easy. The client is not forced into the nurse's way of thinking and doing things (i.e., forced to work with the nurse's values) (Kavanagh et al., 1992).

To Empower Clients to Work toward Their Visions and Goals. Since the earliest days of trying to develop, stabilize, and rehabilitate communities, it has been apparent that effective social actions are largely synonymous with empowerment from within. Although telling people what or how to change often generates defensiveness and resistance, helping them identify their problems and how they want to resolve them enables positive action. This is what empowerment is about.

Empowering people involves teaching them or helping them recognize tools that will allow them to accomplish their goals. The same values that help formulate those goals can help them to be reached, but the values must first be made explicit and clear. Choices cannot be made freely if there are unspoken value conflicts hindering the view of the options. The process of making choices and acting on them can also be affected by attitudes based on cultural values related to human nature, relationships between and among people, relationships between individuals and the cosmos or the supernatural, time, and activity (Kluckhohn, 1971; Kavanagh, 1991a). A nurse's understanding of the influence of such value orientations can vastly increase his or her effectiveness. Furthermore, helping the client to understand the relationship between values and behavior fosters potential for reasonable goals and satisfying, useful actions.

Values Clarification Throughout the Nursing Process

Because they are so often taken for granted as a part of everyday life, identifying the values of either the client or the nurse can be challenging. The most effective strategy to facilitate this important process is the most obvious: ask and listen. Sometimes nurse–client conversations may lead beyond the discussion of an immediate health issue. Clients may wonder why the nurse is asking such questions. A brief explanation of the connection between getting to know what is meaningful to the client and the health care that the nurse provides helps to ensure the client's cooperation. Some suggestions for approaching clients are presented in Table 6–12.

COMMUNICATION AND ARTICULATION OF THE SITUATION

Values clarification is grounded in meaningful interpersonal communication. The first step of this process involves

TABLE 6–12

Approaches to Clients

There are several additional recommendations to help set the stage for effective communication and values clarification:

1. Present yourself with confidence (not arrogance). Introduce yourself, and be open about the reason for your presence and what you intend to do. Shake hands if it is appropriate.
2. Strive to gain your client's trust, but do not resent it if you do not succeed. It is likely that the outcome is rooted in your client's personal history, not you.
3. Understand how the client perceives your relationship with authority.
4. Understand your client's desire to please.
5. Avoid assumptions about where people come from. Let the client tell you.
6. Emphasize the positive aspects of your client's beliefs and practices related to health care.
7. Show respect, especially for males, even if it is women or children you are interested in. Males are often the decision makers about follow-up.
8. Be prepared for the fact that children go everywhere in some cultural groups, as well as in poorer families who may have few options. Include them.
9. Be familiar with but do not discredit the traditional health-related practices you encounter unless you know for certain they are harmful.
10. Know the folk illnesses and remedies common to the people you work with.
11. Whenever possible, involve the leaders of local groups. Confidentiality is important, but the leaders know the problems and can often suggest acceptable interventions.
12. Learn to view the richness of diversity as an asset rather than a liability in your work.

From Kavanagh, K. (1991). *Values and beliefs.* In J. Creasia and B. Parker (Eds.), *Conceptual foundation of professional nursing practice* (pp. 187–210). St. Louis: Mosby-Year Book.

clarifying the issue and identifying the situation from the client's point of view. Only then can the nurse be actively involved in the client's relationship with his or her health. This approach is based on Pedersen's (1981, 1988) model for conceptualizing relationships, which are often a triad involving the client, the problem or health concern, and the health care provider. According to this model (Kavanagh, 1991b, p. 178):

1. The client has a relationship with the health issue as he or she sees it.
2. Effective intervention requires the ability to understand the health issue from both the insider's (client's) and outsider's (nurse's) point of view.
3. The influence of the nurse is less than that of the health issue, unless the nurse's influence can be combined with that of the client to form a partnership.
4. When the client and the nurse form a partnership, they can work together toward improving health. Nurses must ensure that their communications are a dialogue with give and take, rather than a nurse-dominated interview.

The alternative is being a powerless observer outside the client's relationship with the health issue.

RECOGNIZING AND REDUCING DEFENSIVENESS AND RESISTANCE

Numerous strategies have been described to facilitate the identification and reduction of defensiveness and resistance which are primary obstacles to effective communication, values clarification, and problem solving. It is important to understand defensiveness and resistance in specific terms, as nonspecific generalizations prohibit control over them.

RECOVERY SKILLS

Ventures into unfamiliar areas can be rewarding. They can also be frightening because of fear that mistakes might occur. When no communication mistakes are made, this implies that no communication is taking place; it is a "no risk, no gain" situation. Nurses should allow themselves to be honest and open communicators, to be adventurous (for there is no other way they can really get to know their clients), and even to risk an occasional mistake. To become confident and competent communicators, nurses can practice recovery skills (Kavanagh and Kennedy, 1992).

The most frequently used recovery skills are refocusing on the topic of discussion, changing the topic, using silence, reversing roles with the client (either mentally or interactively), role playing, negotiating or arbitrating, repositioning (i.e., changing stance on an issue), providing feedback, apologizing, and, if necessary, referring the client to another provider (Pedersen, 1988). Table 6–13 provides some examples of these techniques.

Perfect communication is an unrealistic goal; no one communicates flawlessly. It is not possible to know all of the interactive rules appropriate to more than 5 billion people representing thousands of cultures and subcultures and innumerable individual expectations. Because avoiding communication only makes things worse (often by communicating disinterest or rejection) and communication is essential to values clarification, nurses must learn to be sensitive, knowledgeable, and skillful communicators. That requires practice.

TABLE 6–13

Recovery Skills

Refocus:	"We were talking about your stomach problem. . . ."
Change the topic:	"Can you give me an example of your usual daily diet?"
Reverse roles:	"I know I would have some trouble juggling all your family's needs if I were in your shoes!"
Role play:	"I know you are having some difficulty talking to your mother about starting birth control. Suppose you pretend to be your mother and I will be you, and we can practice to see what approach you might be most comfortable with."
Negotiate:	"So, Mr. Jones, you are saying you cannot walk for 10 minutes at a time. How about trying two 5-minute walks about one-half hour apart to see how that goes?"
Give positive feedback:	"Well, it certainly looks as if you were able to make the diet changes we agreed on last week. I am glad you were able to help me make sure we stuck to the kosher requirements you always follow."

PROBLEM SOLVING

Problem solving involves decision making, which is a process of choosing specific responses and actions to pursue a desired goal (Kozier et al., 1992). Making decisions requires reasoning. Reasoning may progress from having bits and pieces of information to seeing the "big picture" on which the decision is based (i.e., inductive reasoning). Reasoning may also progress from the big picture—in this case, the situation or problem—to breaking the problem down into more manageable pieces (i.e., deductive reasoning). Both processes are appropriate and can lead to the deliberation necessary for making choices. Values clarification is an integral part of the problem-solving process. Effective problem solving requires the ability to determine options, predict the consequences of alternatives, examine motivating factors and barriers that influence choice, select alternatives and action plans and carry them out, and evaluate the intervention. Values can and do influence each part of this process. The clearer they are, the less the risk of value conflict and the greater the chances of appropriate problem resolution.

Summary

Examining others' values forces us to explore our own. As you help to clarify clients' values, ask yourself what you have learned about them, about communication styles, and about interviewing. How is this information meaningful and important in formulating relevant, acceptable, and potentially useful goals and nursing interventions? What did you learn about yourself and your own value orientation in the process? How did your values and world view affect the process and outcome of the values clarification? What would you do differently in the future?

It will take time and practice to make values clarification an effective tool in your own repertoire of skills. However, the investment will be well worth it as you become a more sensitive, knowledgeable, and skillful nurse in community health.

KEY IDEAS

1. Community health nurses need to be sensitive to the diversity of others. Diversity exists wherever there are differences (cultural, ethnic, racial, age, health status, economic status, occupational and education orientation, gender, sexual orientation, and life experience).
2. Nurses should seek to avoid labeling or stereotyping and assuming that all members of a culture are alike. Persons within a specific culture will demonstrate variations in their beliefs and behaviors.
3. Exploration of family and community culture and values is essential for providing appropriate, effective community health nursing.
4. Because nurses teach about health, illness, health promotion, disease prevention, care of the ill, and sexuality, nurses are agents of enculturation.
5. Nurses need to explore the use of Western, formal medical practices and other formal and informal health practices so that potential harms, conflicts, and interactions can be identified.
6. Culturally sensitive nurses can serve as translators between cultures, explaining and exploring with health professionals and clients such topics as Western medicine and other optional care strategies; differences in perceptions of time and the potential impact on keeping appointments and taking medicine; variations in child care and child discipline practices; and the differences in organization, delivery, and economics between the U.S. health care system and that from which clients have come.
7. Nurses need to recognize that persons undergoing cultural transitions may be stressed.
8. The United States is becoming more culturally diverse. Nurses, especially community health nurses, can expect to provide health care services for clients with many different cultural and values orientations.
9. All nursing interventions should be as appropriate as possible (i.e., not conflicting) with clients' culture and values.
10. To provide quality nursing care, nurses need to be aware of the values that influence human behavior in health and illness.
11. Values clarification is an important tool to assist nurses who are attempting to identify client and self values that may impinge on good nursing care.
12. Communication is the key to clarifying values. Coercion and avoidance indicate failure to communicate.
13. Community health nurses can seek to enter partnerships with clients to explore their health issues.

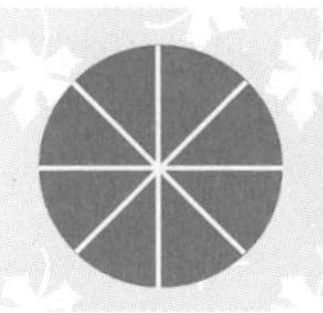

CASE STUDY

Cultural Assessment

Read each of the following scenarios. Review the suggested assessment areas in Table 6–4, and try to identify areas to assess.

Scenario 1

You are an Irish-American nurse who grew up in a large city. When making the first home visit to a 6-week postpartum African American rural family, you observe the grandmother chewing cooked ground beef and sharing the beef juice mouth-to-mouth with the infant. This is something you have never observed before.

What cultural categories would you address when assessing this family?

Cultural Category to Assess	Questions to Rephrase and Ask*
1. Food customs	• What kinds of food are eaten? • What foods are childrens' (infants') foods? • Who prepares the food? • Who in the family feeds infants, and how are infants fed?
2. Beliefs about health and illness	• What beliefs about health and illness are associated with the prechewed meat juice for this infant?
3. Child rearing	• Who are the caretakers and child rearers in this family?

*Questions should be asked in as nonthreatening a manner as possible. Why, who, what, when, where questions should be rephrased to avoid introducing your question with such words. An example is: "Can you tell me about what foods your family thinks are good for infants?"

Discussion

What if your findings reveal that prechewing meat and giving the juice to a newborn by mouth is seen as vital in contributing to the growth of a strong infant? You note also that the grandmother has raised 14 grandchildren the same way and that she is the primary caretaker and health care decision maker for the infant.

How would you intervene or not intervene? If you are not sure, where would you go for help?

Scenario 2

You are a black nurse visiting a Hispanic family to check five to eight children for immunization status. While there, you touch a toddler who feels hot and seems lethargic. The mother states that the child has not been feeling well and agrees with your request to take a rectal temperature. While examining the child, you notice several round, quarter sized marks that look like burns.

Cultural Category to Assess	Questions to Rephrase and Ask*
1. Definitions of illness	• Has anyone in the family determined that the toddler is ill? • What, if any, treatments have been used to help the toddler?
2. Beliefs about illness	• How does the family view cause, diagnosis, and treatment?
3. Definition of others	• Who helps when a child is sick?

*See footnote to table in Scenario 1.

Discussion

You find that the mother is breast-feeding the toddler and first noticed that the child felt hot. When the mother noticed this, she called her neighbor, who is known to be a curandero or healer. The curandero recommended that the mother burn lemon slices and apply them while hot to the child's abdomen. This practice is expected to "draw out" the fever.

How would you intervene or not intervene? If you are not sure, where would you go for help?

Scenario 3

You are a U.S.-born nurse, but your parents were born and grew up in Russia. You are working in the clinic when a man who recently migrated from Russia is welcomed by his primary nurse, who is wearing casual street clothes. The primary nurse's greeting is very informal. You know that the Russian client is shocked and displeased by the informality and will have a hard time relating to his primary nurse.

Cultural Category to Assess	Questions to Rephrase and Ask*
1. Definition of self	• Are your perceptions accurate? • Does the patient feel insulted by the nurse's attire and greeting?
2. Definition of others	• How does the client view the nurse's role, and what behavior does he expect of his primary health care provider?

*See footnote to table in Scenario 1.

Discussion

If you validate that the patient is offended by the informal dress and behavior of the nurse, what will you do? If you don't know what to do, where will you go for help?

Scenario 4

You are working with a community of native Ojibwa people from a clinic on the shore of Lake Manitoba. Hypertension is a problem in the community. A patient comes to you stating that his blood pressure is up and he has come to the clinic to have it checked. You checked the patient's blood pressure 2 days previously, and it was within normal limits. You know that among the Ojibwa people, many view hypertension as making them more susceptible to imbalances. Native healers strive to eliminate imbalance in the body, which may be related to a pathogen, deficiency, or curse.

Cultural Category to Assess	Questions to Rephrase and Ask*
1. Definitions of health and illness	• How did this patient determine that his blood pressure was up?
2. Beliefs about health and illness	• What does high blood pressure mean to this patient? • If his blood pressure is, in fact, high, what action will the patient take? • If the patient's blood pressure is high, what action does the patient expect of you?

*See footnote to table in Scenario 1.

Discussion

How might the diagnosis and treatment methods at your clinic fit with the native healer's efforts to achieve balance and harmony?

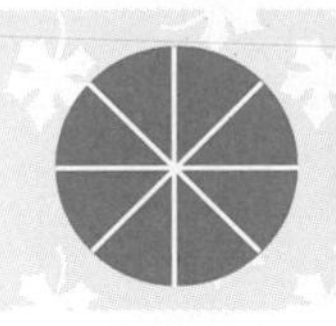

CASE STUDY

Values Clarification

Scenario

Megan: "Hello, Grandma, how are you?"

Juliane: "Why, hello, Megan. How nice to hear from you! I'm fine. How are you?"

Megan: "We're terrific, Grandma. I want to give you some great news!"

Juliane: "How nice, dear. What is it?"

Megan: "It's the baby, Gram. He finally came. Tom and I are adopting a beautiful baby. His name is Daniel. You have a new grandson, Grandma!"

Juliane: "Well, isn't that nice, dear! Is he colored?"

Megan: "He's beautiful and brown, Grandma. No one says "colored" anymore. Actually he is black, white, and American Indian. His hair and eyes are dark, his skin is coppery medium brown. He really is wonderful! You should see him!"

Juliane: "I think it's lovely, dear. I'm glad for you. Now you'll have help."

Megan: "Oh, Grandma! Daniel's not *help!* He's our son. And he's only 11 days old!"

Discussion

The preceding telephone conversation actually occurred. It illustrates profound value differences between two people in the same family. They love and respect each other, but disagree on the significance of race and its implications for social status. The depth of Juliane's convictions lies in her need to conceptualize both this event and Daniel, brought into her life by her only granddaughter, within the framework with which she is comfortable: she knows blacks only as service providers and cannot imagine one as a family member. However, she does not want to reject her granddaughter or her "young foolishness," for she has always supported Megan's whims, accepting them even when she did not understand them. Juliane avoids what she considers negative remarks.

Before analyzing the scenario, consider your initial response to reading it. What was your first reaction, and what values of yours did it reflect? Using what you know about values, list the values expressed by Megan and by Juliane in this scenario. (Pay special attention to the values related to relationships between and among people, the nature of humankind, and activity.) How different and how similar do you expect Juliane's and Megan's values orientations to be, based on this brief scenario? What do you need to know about each of the women to make sense of and understand (which does not imply acceptance of) their orientations and choices? What does knowing that Grandma Juliane is an affluent 70-year-old member of the Daughters of the American Revolution (as well as an old colonial family) suggest about her approach to the situation? What does knowing that Megan is a 25-year old college student in another state who corresponds with or phones her grandmother nearly every week suggest about her value orientation? How might these characterizations of Juliane and Megan contribute to the perpetuation of negative stereotypes if generalized beyond the context of the given situation?

Given what you know about defensiveness and resistance and the impact of these processes on communication and relationships, what difference might it make if Megan's final response to her grandmother in this conversation had a tone of anger rather than a chiding humor? As a community health nurse working with Megan before Daniel's adoption, how would you assist her with the values clarification appropriate to her decision making? As a community health nurse concerned with family process, parenting, and child development, how would you structure your assessment of this family?

GUIDELINES FOR LEARNING

1. Discuss your own cultural background with fellow students and faculty.
2. Describe cultural groups different from your own that you have encountered.
3. Identify a culturally sensitive person from your own culture. Discuss what he or she is like.
4. Identify a culturally sensitive person from another culture. Discuss what he or she is like.
5. Discuss how culture is related to health.
6. Discuss how culture is related to health and nursing care.
7. Discuss the health outcomes that you might expect when you assess and work with people from a variety of diverse cultural backgrounds.
8. Read about a culture in which you are interested but know little about. Discuss it with your classmates.
9. Observe a television program with the specific purpose of analyzing it for the values it expresses. A program with a health-related theme is particularly

useful for this exercise, but any production will do. If possible, videotape the show so that you can watch it more than once; what is immediately apparent may be only superficial when it comes to values. What values are expressed by the characters in the program, and how? What values are expressed by the theme or plot, and how? How do those values fit with the general pattern of American values? How was your response to the program influenced by your own value orientation? To what extent might you be willing to change your orientation or your behavior to fit ideas expressed by the television program? What is your motivation to change or not to change?

10. In school or at work, observe an interaction between two people. Analyze it for similarities and differences related to gender, ethnicity, age, job or position, role or relationship, education, socioeconomic status, and language. Identify any other factors that may influence the interaction. What impact do similarities or differences appear to have on the interaction? What values were expressed, and how were they responded to?

11. Observe a second interaction, but choose it according to the first. If the first observation was of persons who seemed more similar than different, choose a second interaction that is between two persons more different than similar; or vice versa. Analyze the second interaction in the same way. Then compare and contrast the two and your own responses to them.

12. Have a colleague describe an interaction with a client who differed from them ethnically, racially, or culturally. Analyze the information you receive about the client's view of the difference and about your colleague's view. Ask your colleague what each considered the main difference. How similar to or different from your own assessment is your colleague's assessment? What values are the answers based on? Discuss with your colleague how he or she would or did handle the differences. How would you deal with them? What are their implications for effective health care intervention?

13. There are far more nurses who are women than men in the United States. Analyze that situation for the values it reflects. Using the value systems that predominate in the United States and in nursing as a guide for your analysis, consider why more men do not become nurses. What values are related to the stereotypes, assumptions, and myths that are commonly used to describe male and female nurses? Discuss with a male nurse whether his values orientation has been respected, threatened, maintained, or changed as a nurse. The same exercise is effective with persons of ethnic backgrounds different from your own.

14. Using a tape recorder, tell yourself a story involving a client whom you considered difficult to work with. (Some people like to do this exercise in front of a mirror so that it seems more like talking with someone else.) When you are finished with the story, listen to your narrative. Using two columns on a sheet of paper, list your goals in the relationship in one column and your client's goals in the other. Be specific; do not generalize or stereotype. If you do not know exactly what the client's goals were, speculate on them as objectively as you can. Then, beside each of those goals, write the values reflected in these goals. What was difficult about your relationship with this client? What might have changed that?

15. Keep a journal for 2 weeks. In it record your observations pertaining to values and values clarification as they relate to health care and nursing. Focus on listening and observing in your dialogue with people, both in your clinical work and in your daily life. (A client aptly addressed a common communication problem when she reported, "I know to understand somebody I got to take the cotton out my ears and put it in my mouth.")

REFERENCES

PART 1: THE CULTURAL CONTEXT FOR COMMUNITY HEALTH NURSING

Centers for Disease Control and Prevention. (1993). Use of race and ethnicity in public health surveillance. *Morbidity and Mortality Weekly Report, 24*(RR-10), 1–17.

Farb, P., & Armelagos, G. (1980). *The anthropology of eating.* Boston: Houghton Mifflin.

Graham, J. S. (1976). The role of the curanderos in the Mexican American folk medicine system in West Texas. In W.D. Hand (Ed.), *American folk medicine: A symposium* (pp. 175–189). Berkeley, CA: University of California Press.

Hall, E. (1973). *The silent language.* Garden City, NY: Anchor Press/Doubleday.

Herberg, P. (1989). Theoretical foundation of transcultural nursing. In J.S. Boyle and M.M. Andrews (Eds.), *Transcultural concepts in nursing care.* Glenview, IL: Scott, Foresman.

Hollmann, F. W. (1993). National population trends. In *Population profiles of the United States (1993).* CPR-P23-185. Washington, DC: Bureau of the Census, U.S. Government Printing Office.

Kreiger, D. (1987). *Living the therapeutic touch: Healing as a lifestyle.* New York: Dodd, Mead and Co.

Landy, D. (Ed.). (1977). *Culture, disease and health,* New York: MacMillan.

Mauss, M. (1966). *The gift: Forms and functions of exchange in archaic societies.* London: Cohen and West.

Murdock, G. (1980). *Theories of illness—a world survey.* Pittsburgh: University of Pittsburgh Press.

Poe, D. (1977). The giving of gifts: Anthropological data in social psychological theory. *Cornell Journal of Social Relations, 12*(1), 47–63.

Spradley, J. (1979). *The ethnographic interview.* New York: Holt, Rinehart & Winston.
Strasser, J. (1978). Urban transient women, *American Journal of Nursing, 12,* 2076–2079.
Strasser, J. (1989). Qualitative clinical nursing research when a community is the client. In J. Morse (Ed.), *Qualitative Nursing Research.* Rockville, MD: Aspen.
Tripp-Reimer, T., & Brink, P. (1985). Cultural brokerage. In Bulechek, G., & J. McCloskey, (Eds.) *Nursing interventions and treatments for nursing diagnosis.* Philadelphia: WB Saunders.
Trotter, R. (1988). *Orientation to multicultural health care in migrant health programs.* Austin, TX: National Migrant Referral Project, Inc.
Turner, V. (1969). *The ritual process.* Ithaca, NY: Cornell University Press.
Van Gennep, A. (1960). *The rites of passage* (M.B. Vizedom and G.L. Coffee, translators). Chicago: University of Chicago Press.

PART 2: CULTURAL PLURALISM IN THE UNITED STATES

Bandaranyake, R. (1986). Ethnic differences in disease: An epidemiological perspective. In T. Rathwell and D. Phillips (Eds.), *Health, race and ethnicity.* London: Croom Helm.
Bennett, C. E. (1993). The black population. In *Population Profiles of the United States.* CPR-P23-185. Washington, DC: Bureau of the Census, U.S. Government Printing Office.
Centers for Disease Control. (1993). Use of race and ethnicity in public health surveillance. *Morbidity and Mortality Weekly Report, 42*(RR-10), 1–17.
Delgado, R. (1992). Generalist child welfare and Hispanic families. In N.A. Cohen (Ed.), *Child welfare: A multicultural focus.* Boston: Allyn & Bacon.
Haan, M., Kaplan, G., & Camacho, T. (1987). Poverty and health: Prospective evidence from the Alameda County study. *American Journal of Epidemiology, 125*(6), 989–998.
Indian Health Service (1991). *Trends in Indian health.* Washington, DC: U.S. Department of Health and Human Services, Public Health Service, U.S. Government Printing Office.
Lapham, S.J. (1993). The foreign-born population. In *Population profiles of the United States 1993.* CPR-P23-185. Washington, DC: Bureau of the Census. U.S. Government Printing Office.
Mass, A.I., & Yay, J. (1992). Child welfare: Asian and Pacific Islander families. In N.A. Cohen (Ed.), *Child welfare: A Multicultural Focus.* Boston: Allyn & Bacon.
Prater, G.S. (1992). Child welfare and African-American families. In N.A. Cohen (Ed.), *Child welfare: A multicultural focus.* Boston: Allyn & Bacon.
Rabin, S.A. (1993). A private sector view of health surveillance and communities of color. *Morbidity and Mortality Weekly Report, 42* (RR-10), 1–17.
Statistical Abstract of the United States. (1992). Washington, DC: United States Bureau of the Census, U.S. Government Printing Office.
Swinton D, (1990). The economic status of blacks, 1987. In J. DeWart, (Ed.), *The state of black America 1987.* New York: National Urban League.
Takaki, R. (1993). *A different mirror: A history of multicultural America.* Boston: Little, Brown.
U.S. Bureau of the Census. (1992). *The Asian and Philippine population in the United States: March 1991 and 1990* (CPR, series p-20, No. 459). Washington, DC: U.S. Government Printing Office.
U.S. Bureau of the Census. (1992). *The black population in the United States* (CPR, series p-20, No. 471). Washington, DC: U.S. Government Printing Office.
U.S. Bureau of the Census. (1993). *Hispanic Americans today* (CPR, series p-23, No. 183). Washington, DC: U.S. Government Printing Office.
U.S. Bureau of the Census. (1993). *Population profiles of the United States 1993* (CPR, series p-23, No. 185). Washington, DC: U.S. Government Printing Office.
Williams, D.R. (1993). Race in the health of America: Problems, issues and directions. *Morbidity and Mortality Weekly Report, 42*(RR-10), 1–17.

PART 3: VALUES CLARIFICATION FOR CHANGE AND EMPOWERMENT

American Nurses' Association. (1985). *Code for nurses with interpretive statements.* Kansas City, MO: Author.
Hamill, P. (1988, March). Breaking the silence: A letter to a black friend. *Esquire,* pp. 91–94, 96, 98, 100, 102.
Kavanagh, K. H. (1991a). Social and cultural influences. In J. L. Creasia and B. Parker (Eds.), *Conceptual foundations of professional nursing practice* (pp. 167–186). St. Louis: Mosby-Year Book.
Kavanagh, K. H. (1991b). Values and beliefs. In J. L. Creasia and B. Parker (Eds.), *Conceptual foundations of professional nursing practice* (pp. 187–210). St. Louis: Mosby-Year Book.
Kavanagh, K. H., Harris, R. M., Hetherington, S. E., & Scott, D. E. (1992). Collaboration as a strategy for acquired immunodeficiency syndrome prevention. *Archives of Psychiatric Nursing, VI*(6), 331–339.
Kavanagh, K. H., & Kennedy, P. H. (1992). *Promoting cultural diversity: Strategies for health care professionals.* Newbury Park, CA: Sage.
Kluckhohn, F. R. (1971). Dominant and variant value orientations. In C. Kluckhohn and H. A. Murray (Eds.), *Personality in nature, society, and culture* (pp. 342–357). New York: Alfred A. Knopf.
Kozier, B., Erb, G., & Blais, K. (1992). *Concepts and issues in nursing practice.* Redwood City, CA: Addison-Wesley.
Leininger, M. M. (1978). *Transcultural nursing: concepts, theories, and practices.* New York: John Wiley & Sons.
Leininger, M. M. (1988). Leininger's theory of nursing: Cultural care diversity and universality. *Nursing Science Quarterly, 1*(4), 152–160.
Leininger, M. M. (1991, April-May). Transcultural nursing: The study and practice field. *National Student Nurses Association/Imprint, 38*(April-May), pp. 55–56.
Lowenberg, J. S. (1989). *Caring and responsibility: The crossroads between holistic practice and traditional medicine.* Philadelphia: University of Pennsylvania Press.
Pedersen, P. (1981). The cultural inclusiveness of counseling. In P. Pedersen, J. Draguns, W. Lonner, & J. Trimble (Eds.), *Counseling across cultures* (pp. 22–58). Honolulu: University of Hawaii Press.
Pedersen, P. (1988). *A handbook for developing multicultural awareness.* Alexandria, VA: American Association for Counseling and Development.
Pruitt, R. H. (1991). Health promotion and wellness. In J. L. Creasia & B. Parker (Eds.). *Conceptual foundations of professional nursing practice* (pp. 211–223). St. Louis: Mosby-Year Book.
Zola, I. K. (1981). Structural constraints in the doctor-patient relationship: The case of non-compliance. In L. Eisenberg & A. Kleinman (Eds.), *The relevance of social science for medicine* (pp. 241–252). Dordrecht, The Netherlands: D. Reidel.

BIBLIOGRAPHY

PART 1: THE CULTURAL CONTEXT FOR COMMUNITY HEALTH NURSING

Aeschliman, D. (1973). Project Hope: Guidelines for cross-cultural health programs. *Nursing Outlook, 21*(10): 660–663.
Anderson J. (1990). Health care across cultures. *Nursing Outlook. 38*(3):136–139.
Antonovsky, A. (1979). *Health, stress and coping.* San Francisco: Jossey Bass.
Atkinson, D., Morten, G., & Wing S. D., (1989). *Counseling American minorities.* Dubuque, IA: William C. Brown Publishers.

Bates, D., & Lees, S. (1981). *Contemporary anthropology.* New York: Knopf.
Boyle, J., & Andrews, M. (1989). *Transcultural concepts in nursing care.* Glenview, IL: Scott, Foresman/Little, Brown College Division.
Brink, P. (1976). *Transcultural nursing.* Englewood Cliffs, NJ: Prentice Hall.
Brink, P. (1984). Key issues in nursing and anthropology. *Advances in Medical Social Sciences, 2,* 107–146.
Brownlee, A. T. (1978). *Community, culture and care.* St. Louis: Mosby.
Davitz, L., Davitz, J., & Higuehi, Y. (1977). Cross-cultural influences of physical pain and psychological distress. *Nursing Times, 73,* 556–558.
Ellen, F. R. (1984). *Ethnographic research: A guide to general conduct.* New York: Academic Press.
Ellis, C. (1986). *Fisher folk: Two communities on Chesapeake Bay.* Lexington: The University Press of Kentucky.
Geertz, H., & Geertz, C. (1975). *Kinship in Bali.* Chicago: University of Chicago Press.
Giger, J., & Davidhizer, R. (1991). *Transcultural nursing.* St. Louis: Mosby-Year Book.
Goffman, E. (1963). *Stigma.* Englewood Cliffs, NJ: Prentice Hall.
Green, J. (1982). *Cultural awareness in the human services.* Englewood Cliffs, NJ: Prentice-Hall.
Harrington, M. (1984). *The new American poverty.* New York: Holt, Rinehart & Winston.
Harwood, A. (Ed.). (1981). *Ethnicity and medical care.* Cambridge, MA: Harvard University Press.
Hatton, D. (1992). Information transmission on bilingual bicultural contexts. *Journal of Community Health Nursing. 9*(1), 53–59.
Hayfield, M. (1990). An exchange of gifts: The international language of friendship. *Nursing, 20*(5), 135.
Henderson, G., & Primeaux, M. (1981). *Transcultural health care.* Menlo Park, CA: Addison-Wesley.
Holmes, T. H., & Rahe, R. H. (1967). The social readjustment rating scale. *Journal of Psychosomatic Medicine, 11,* 203–218.
Howard, M. C., & McKim, P. C. (1983). *Contemporary anthropology.* Boston: Little, Brown.
Jeweski, M. (1993). Culture brokering. *Nursing and Health Care, 14,* 78–85.
Kelleher, K. (1989). *Nurse healers: A subculture of nurses.* Unpublished seminar paper, University of Maryland, Baltimore, MD.
Kitano, H., & Daniels, R. (1988). *Asian Americans, emerging minorities.* Englewood Cliffs, NJ: Prentice Hall.
Kleinman, A. (1980). *Patients and healers in the context of culture.* Berkeley: University of California Press.
Kreiger, D. (1979). *The therapeutic touch: How to use your hands to help or heal.* Englewood Cliffs, NJ: Prentice Hall.
LaFargue, J. (1985). Mediating between two views of illness. *Topics in Clinical Nursing, 7*(3), 70–77.
Lefley, H. (1979). Prevalence of potential falling-out cases among Black, Latin and non-Latin white populations of the city of Miami. *Social Science and Medicine, 13*B, 113–114.
Lefley, H. (1979). Female cases of falling-out: A psychological evaluation of a small sample. *Social Science and Medicine, 13*B, 115–116.
Leininger, M. (1978). *Transcultural nursing.* New York: John Wiley & Sons.
Leininger, M. (1985). Transcultural nursing: An essential knowledge and practice field for today. *Canadian Nurse, 80*(11), 41–45.
Lewis, O. (1970). *Anthropological essays.* New York: Random House.
Lichtman, A., & Challinor, J. (Eds.). (1979). *Kin and communities: Families in America.* Washington, DC: Smithsonian Institution Press.
Logan, M.H. (1977). Humoral medicine in Guatemala and peasant acceptance of modern medicine. In D. Landy (Ed)., *Culture, disease and healing.* New York: Macmillan.
Logan, M., & Hunt, E. (1978). *Health and the human condition.* Scituate, MA: Duxbury Press.
National League for Nursing (1976). *Ethnicity and health care.* Publ. no. 14-1625. New York: Author.
Neibel, B. (1990). *Transcultural health care: A nursing challenge for the 90's.* Covina, CA: Nursing Education of America.
Orgue, M., Bloch, B., & Monrroy, L. (1983). *Ethnic nursing care.* St. Louis: Mosby.
Rempusheski, V. (1989). The role of ethnicity in elder care. *Nursing Clinics of North America. 24*(3), 717–724.
Rubin, J. (1979). Falling-out: A clinical study, *Social Science and Medicine. 13*B, 117–127.
Rubington, E., & Weinberg, K. (1978). *Deviance: The interactionist perspective.* New York: Macmillan.
Salter, M. (Ed.). (1977). *Play: Anthropological perspectives.* West Point, NY: Leisure Press.
Schusky, E. L., & Culberot, T. P. (1987). *Introducing culture.* Englewood Cliffs, NJ: Prentice-Hall.
Shomaker, D. (1989). Age disorientation, liminality and reality: The care of the Alzheimer's patient. *Medical Anthropology, 12*(5), 313–323.
Smart, N. (1976). *The religious experience of mankind.* New York: Charles Scribner's Sons.
Spradley, J. (1970). *You owe yourself a drunk.* Boston: Little, Brown.
Spradley, B. (Ed.). (1991). *Readings in community health nursing* (4th ed.). Philadelphia: J. B. Lippincott.
Weidman, H. (1979). Falling-out: A diagnostic and treatment problem viewed from a transcultural perspective. *Social Science and Medicine, 13*B, 95–112.
Wenger, A. (1991). Culture specific care and the old order Amish. *Imprint. 38*(2), 80–82.
Wheeler, M. (1991). Nursing in a migrant setting. *Imprint. 38*(3): 70, 72, 127.

Readings About Culture, Health, and Health Care

Althen, G. (1981). *American ways.* Yarmouth, ME: Intercultural Press.
Galanti, G. (1991). *Caring for patients from different cultures.* Philadelphia: University of Pennsylvania Press.
Kleinman, A. (1981). *Patients and healers in the context of culture.* Berkeley: University of California Press.
Logan, M., & Hunt, E. (1978). *Health and the human condition.* North Scituate, MA: Duxbury Press.
Samova, L., & Porter, R. (1982). *Intercultural communication: A reader.* Belmont, CA: Wadsworth.
Sowell, T. (1981). *Ethnic America.* New York: Basic Books.
Spector, R. E. (1979). *Cultural diversity in health and illness.* East Norwalk, CT: Appleton-Century-Crofts.
Zborowski, M. (1969). *People in pain.* San Francisco: Jossey-Bass.

Readings About Haitian People

Dempsey, P. A., & Geese, T. (1983). The childbearing Haitian refugee: Cultural applications to clinical nursing. *Public Health Reports, 98*(3), 261–267.
Harris, K. (1987). Beliefs and practices among Haitian American women in relation to childbearing. *Journal of Nurse-Midwifery, 32*(3), 149–155.
Herskovits, M. J. (1971). *Life in a Haitian valley.* New York: Doubleday.
Laguerre, M. (1981). Haitian Americans. In A. Harwood (Ed.), *Ethnicity and medical care.* Cambridge, MA: Harvard University Press.
Leyburn, J. G. (1955). *The Haitian people.* New Haven, CT: Yale University Press.
Logan, M. (1975). Selected references on the hot-cold theory of disease. *Medical Anthropology Newsletter, 6*(2), 8–11.
Moskowitz, L., Kory, P., Chan, J., Haverkos, H., Conley, F., & Hensley, G. (1983). Unusual causes of deaths in Haitians residing in Miami. *Journal of the American Medical Association, 250*(9), 1187–1191.

Philippe, J., & Romain, J. (1979). Indisposition in Haiti. *Social Science and Medicine, 13*B, 128–133.
Rey, R. H. (1970). *The Haitian family.* New York: Community Service Society.
Scott, C. (1978). Health and healing practices among five ethnic groups in Miami, Florida. *Public Health Reports, 55,* 524–532.
Seligman, L. (1977). Haitians: A neglected minority. *Personnel and Guidance Journal, 2,* 409–411.
Snow, L. F. (1981). Folk medical beliefs and their implications for the care of patients: A review based on studies among Black Americans. In G. Henderson & M. Primeaux (Eds.), *Transcultural Health Care.* Reading, MA: Addison-Wesley.
Verdet, P. (1985). Trying times: Haitian youth in an inner city high school. *Social Work in Health Care,* pp. 228–233.
Wiese, J. (1976). Maternal nutrition and traditional food behavior in Haiti. *Human Organization, 35*(2), 193–200.
Wilk, R. (1986). The Haitian refugee: Concern for health care providers. *Social Work in Health Care, 11,* 61–74.
Williams, S., Murthy, N., & Berggren, G. (1975). Conjugal unions among rural Haitian women. *Journal of Marriage and the Family, 3*(4), 1022–1031.

Readings About Southeast Asian People

Cook, K., & Timberlake, E. (1984). Working with Vietnamese refugees. *Social Work, 29*(2), 108–113.
Crystal, D. (1989). Asian Americans and the myth of the model minority. *Social Casework, 70*(7), 405–413.
Eyton, J., & Neuwirth, G. (1984). Cross-cultural validity: Ethnocentrism in health studies with special reference to the Vietnamese. *Social Service and Medicine, 18*(5), 447–453.
Frye, B. (1990). The Cambodian refugee patient: Providing culturally sensitive rehabilitation nursing care. *Rehabilitation Nursing, 15*(3), 156–158.
Hoang, G., & Erickson, R. (1982). Guidelines for providing medical care for Southeast Asian refugees. *Journal of the American Medical Association, 248*(6), 710–714.
Huynh, T. D. (1987). *Introduction to Vietnamese culture.* San Diego, CA: Multi-functional Resource Center, San Diego State University.
Pickwell, S. (1989). The incorporation of family primary care for Southeast Asian refugees in a community-based mental health facility. *Archives of Psychiatric Nursing, 3*(3), 173–177.
Rosenblat, H., & Hong, P. (1989). Coin rubbing misdiagnosed as child abuse. *Canadian Medical Association Journal, 140*(4), 417.
Strand, P., & Jones, W. (1983). Health service utilization by Indochinese refugees. *Medical Care, 2*(11), 1089–1098.
Tien, J. L. (1984). Do Asians need less medication? Issues in clinical assessment and psychopharmacology. *Journal of Psychosocial Nursing and psychopharmacology. Journal of Psychosocial Nursing and Mental Health Services, 22,* 19–22.
Tripp-Reimer, T., & Thieman, K. (1981). Traditional health beliefs/practices of Vietnamese refugees. *Journal of Iowa Medical Society, 71*(12), 533–535.
Westermeyer, J., & Winthrop, R. (1979). Folk criteria for the diagnosis of mental illness in rural Laos. *American Journal of Psychiatry, 136,* 136–161.

Readings About Jewish American People

Bash, D. D. (1980). Jewish religious practices related to childbearing. *Journal of Nurse-Midwifery, 25,* 5.
Heller, Z. (1975). The Jewish view of death: Guidelines for dying. In E. Kubler-Ross (Ed.). *Death: The final stage of growth.* Englewood Cliffs, NJ: Prentice Hall.
Janowsky, O. (1964). *The American Jew: A reappraisal.* Philadelphia: Jewish Publication Society.
Rothchild, H. (1981). *Bio-cultural aspects of disease.* New York: Academic Press.
Schlesinger, B. (1971). *The Jewish family: A survey and annotated bibliography.* Toronto, Canada: University of Toronto Press.
Sperling, A. (1968). *Reasons for Jewish customs and traditions.* New York: Bloch.
Trepp, L. (1980). *The complete book of Jewish observances.* New York: Behman House.

Readings About Black/African American People

Bell, C., & Mehta, H. (1981). The misdiagnosis of black patients with manic depressive illness. *Journal of the National Medical Association, 73,* 101–107.
Bloch, B. (1976). Nursing intervention in black patient care. In D. Luckraft (Ed.). *Black awareness: Implications for black patient care* (pp. 27–35). New York: American Journal of Nursing Company.
Bloch, B. (1981). Black Americans and cross-cultural counseling experiences. In A.J. Marsella & P.B. Pedersen (Eds.). *Cross-cultural Counseling and Psychotherapy.* New York: Pergamon Press.
Dillard, J. L. (1972). *Who speaks black English: Its history and usage in the United States.* New York: Random House.
Giger, S., & Davidhizar, R. (1990). Developing communication skills for use with black patients. *The Association of Black Nursing Faculty in Higher Education Journal, 1*(2), 33–35.
Jacques, G. (1976). Cultural health traditions: A black perspective. In M.F. Branch & P.P. Paxton (Eds.). *Providing safe nursing care for ethnic people of color.* East Norwalk, CT: Appleton-Century-Crofts.
Knox, D. H. (1986). Spirituality: A tool in the assessment and treatment of black alcoholics and their families. *Alcoholism Treatment Quarterly, 2*(3–4), 313–343.
Poussaint, A., & Atkinson, C. (1970). Black youth and motivation. *Black Scholar, 1,* 43–51.
Remington, G., & DaCosta, G. (1989). Ethnocultural factors in resident supervision: Black and white supervisors. *American Journal of Psychotherapy, 43*(3), 343–355.
Smith, J. A. (1976). The role of the black clergy as allied health care professionals in working with black patients. In D. Luckraft (Ed.). *Black awareness: Implications for black care* (pp. 12–15). New York: The American Journal of Nursing Company.
Snow, L. E. (1977). Folk medical beliefs and their implications for care of patients. A review based on studies among black Americans. *Annals of Internal Medicine, 81,* 82–96.
White, E. H. (1977). Giving health care to minority patients. *Nursing Clinics of North America, 12,* 27–40.
Wintrob, R. (1973). The influences of others: Witchcraft and rootwork as explanations of behavior disturbances. *Journal of Nervous and Mental Disorders, 156,* 318.

Readings About Native Americans

Garro, L. (1988). The response to chronic disease: Changing models of illness in an Ojibwa community. In D. E. Young (Ed.). *Health care issues in the Canadian North,* University of Alberta. Boreal Institute for Northern Studies, Edmonton, Alberta.
Gottschalk, J. (1991). Said another way: Seeing the world through different lenses. *Nursing Forum, 26*(2), 30–35.
Hamilton, C. (1991). Nursing on the Navajo reservation. *Imprint, 38*(2), 174.
Phillips, S., & Lobar, S. (1990). Literature summary of some Navajo child health beliefs and rearing practice within a transcultural nursing framework. *Journal of Transcultural Nursing, 1*(2), 13–20.

Rose, V. (1991). Indian summer: The health of the Navajo. *Health Visitor, 11*(1), 40–42.

Readings About Arab Americans

Luna, L. (1989). Transcultural nursing care of Arab Muslims. *Journal of Transcultural Nursing, 1*(1), 22–26.

Martin, R. (1982). *Islam* Englewood Cliffs, N.J.: Prentice-Hall, Inc.

PART 2: PLURALISM IN AMERICA

Braithwaite, R., & Taylor, S. (Eds.). (1992). *Health issues in the black community.* San Francisco: Jossey-Bass.

Chavez, E., & Swaim, R. (1992). An epidemiological comparison of Mexican-American and white non-Hispanic 8th and 12th grade students' substance use. *American Journal of Public Health, 82*(3), 445–447.

Helsel, D., Petitti, D., & Kunstadter, P. (1992). Pregnancy among the Hmong: Birthweight, age, and parity. *American Journal of Public Health, 82*(10), 1361–1364.

Hingson, R., Strunin, L., Grady, M., Strunk, N., Carr, R., Berlin, B., & Craven, D. (1991). Knowledge about HIV and behavioral risks of foreign-born Boston public school students. *American Journal of Public Health, 81*(12), 1638–1641.

Magnus, M. (1991). Cardiovascular health among African-Americans: A review of the health status, risk reduction, and intervention strategies. *American Journal of Health Promotion, 5*(4), 782–790.

Stroup-Benham, C., & Trevino, F. (1991). Reproductive characteristics of Mexican-American, mainland Puerto Rican, and Cuban-American women: Data from the Hispanic Health and Nutrition Examination Survey. *Journal of the American Medical Association, 265*(2), 222–226.

PART 3: VALUES CLARIFICATION FOR CHANGE AND EMPOWERMENT

Althen, G. (1988). *American ways.* Yarmouth, ME: Intercultural Press.

American Nurses' Association (ANA). (1986). *Cultural diversity in the nursing curriculum: A guide for implementation.* Kansas City, MO: Author.

ANA. (1991). *Nursing's agenda for health care reform.* Kansas City, MO: Author.

Aroskar, M. A. (1982). Are nurse's mind-sets compatible with ethical nursing practice? *Topics in Clinical Nursing, 4*(April), 17–26.

Benner, P. (1984). *From novice to expert: Excellence and power in clinical nursing practice.* Menlo Park, CA: Addison-Wesley.

Blau, J. R. (1992). *The shape of culture: A study of contemporary cultural patterns in the United States.* New York: Cambridge University Press.

Bowser, B. P., & Hunt, R. G. (Eds.). (1981). *Impacts of racism on white Americans.* Beverly Hills, CA: Sage.

Brownlee, A. T. (1978). *Community, culture, and care: A cross-cultural guide for health workers.* St. Louis: C. V. Mosby.

Butterfield, P. G. (1990). Thinking upstream: Nurturing a conceptual understanding of the societal context of health behavior. *Advances in Nursing Science, 12*(2), 1–8.

Corcoran, S. (1988). Toward operationalizing an advocacy role. *Journal of Professional Nursing, 4*(4), 242–248.

Cortese, A. J. (1990). *Ethnic ethics: The restructuring of moral theory.* Albany, NY: State University of New York Press.

De Vita, P. R., & Armstrong, J. D. (1993). *Distant mirrors: America as a foreign culture.* Belmont, CA: Wadsworth.

De Waal Malefut, A. (1974). *Images of man: A history of anthropological thought.* New York: Alfred A. Knopf.

Donald, J., & Rattansi, A. (1992). *"Race," culture and difference.* Beverly Hills, CA: Sage, in association with the Open University.

Drucker, D. (1991). The new productivity challenge. *Harvard Business Review, 69*(6), 69–79.

Fry, S. T. (1987). Autonomy, advocacy, and accountability: Ethics at the bedside. In M. D. Fowler & J. Levine-Ariff (Eds.), *Ethics at the bedside* (pp. 39–49). Philadelphia: J.B. Lippincott.

Fry, S. T. (1991). Ethics in health care delivery. In J. L. Creasia and B. Parker (Eds.). *Conceptual foundations of professional nursing practice* (pp. 167–164). St. Louis: Mosby-Year Book.

Gadow, S. A. (1980). Existential advocacy: Philosophical foundation of nursing. In S. F. Spicker & S. Gadow (Eds.): *Nursing: Images and ideals—opening dialogue with the humanities* (pp. 79–101). New York: Springer.

Gadow, S. A. (1985). Nurse and patient: The caring relationship. In A. H. Bishop & J. R. Scudder (Eds.), *Caring, curing, coping* (pp. 31–43). Birmingham: University of Alabama Press.

Gadow, S. A. (1989). Clinical subjectivity: Advocacy with silent patients. *Nursing Clinics of North America, 24,* 535–541.

Galanti, G.-A. (1991). *Caring for patients from different cultures: case studies from American hospitals.* Philadelphia: University of Pennsylvania Press.

Gaut, D. A., & Leininger, M. M. (1991). *Caring: the compassionate healer.* Publ. no. 15-2401. New York: National League for Nursing Press.

Gilligan, C. (1982). *In a different voice: psychological theory and women's development.* Cambridge, MA: Harvard University Press.

Hunter, J. D. (1990). *Culture wars—the struggle to define America: Making sense of the battles over the family, art, education, law, and politics.* New York: Basic Books.

Kleinman, A. M. (1980). *Patients and healers in the context of culture.* Los Angeles: University of California Press.

Kochman, T. (1981). *Black and white: Styles in conflict.* Chicago: University of Chicago Press.

Kohnke, M. F. (1982). *Advocacy, risk and reality.* St. Louis: Mosby.

Lefley, H. P. (1984). Delivering mental health services across cultures. In P. Pedersen, N. Sartorius, & A. Marsella (Eds.). *Mental health services: The cross-cultural context* (pp. 135–171). Beverly Hills, CA: Sage.

Leininger, M. M. (1967). The culture concept and its relevance to nursing. *Journal of Nursing Education, 6*(2), 27–37.

Leininger, M. M. (1984). *Care: The essence of nursing and health.* Thorofare, NJ: Charles B. Slack.

Leininger, M. M. (Ed.). (1988). *Care: Discovery and uses in clinical and community nursing.* Detroit: Wayne State University Press.

Leininger, M. M. (Ed.). (1988). *Caring: An essential human need.* Detroit: Wayne State University Press.

Leininger, M. M. (Ed.). (1991). *Culture care diversity and universality: A theory of nursing.* Publ. no. 15-2402. New York: National League for Nursing Press.

Leininger, M., & Watson, J. (Eds.). (1990). *The caring imperative in education.* Publ. no. 41-2308. New York: National League for Nursing Press.

Nelson, M. (1988). Advocacy in nursing: A concept in evolution. *Nursing Outlook, 36*(3), 136–141.

Parrillo, V. N. (1990). *Strangers to these shores: Race and ethnic relations in the United States.* New York: Macmillan.

Shugars, D. A., O'Neill, E. H., & Bader, J. D. (Eds.). (1991). *Health America: Practitioners for 2005 (an agenda for action for U.S. health professional schools).* Durham, NC: The Pew Health Professions Commission.

Thomas, R. R. (1990) From Affirmative Action to affirming diversity. *Harvard Business Review, March–April,* 107–117.

Wali, A. (1992). Multiculturalism: An anthropological perspective. *Report from the Institute for Philosophy and Public Policy, 12*(1), 6–8.

Watson, J. (1979). *The philosophy and science of caring.* Boston: Little, Brown.

Winslow, G. R. (1984). From loyalty to advocacy: A new metaphor for nursing. *Hastings Center Report, 14*(3), 32–40.

Wuthnow, R. (1991). *Acts of compassion: Caring for others and helping ourselves.* Princeton, NJ: Princeton University Press.

SUGGESTED READINGS

Ailinger, R. (1988). Folk beliefs about high blood pressure in Hispanic immigrants. *Western Journal of Nursing Research, 10*(5), 629–636.

Arruda, E., Larson, P., & Meleis, A. (1992). Comfort: Immigrant Hispanic cancer patients' views. *Cancer Nursing, 15*(6), 387–394.

Blau, J. R. (1992). *The shape of culture: A study of contemporary cultural patterns in the United States.* New York: Cambridge University Press.

Clabots, R., & Dolphin, D. (1992). The multilingual videotape project: Community involvement in a unique health education program. *Public Health Reports, 107*(1), 75–80.

Clark, S., & Kelley, S. (1992). Traditional Native American values: Conflict or concordance in rehabilitation. *Journal of Rehabilitation, 58*(2), 23–28.

DeSantis, L., & Thomas, J. (1992). Health education and the immigrant Haitian mother: Cultural insights for community health nurses. *Public Health Nursing, 9*(2), 87–96.

Edwards, N., Ciliska, D., Halbert, T., & Pond, M. (1992). Health promotion and health advocacy for and by immigrants enrolled in English as a Second Language class. *Canadian Journal of Public Health, 83*(2), 159–162.

Hatton, D. (1992). Information transmission in bilingual, bicultural contexts. *Journal of Community Health Nursing, 9*(1), 53–59.

Henderson, S., & Brown, J. (1987). Infant feeding practices of Vietnamese immigrants to the Northwest United States. *Scholarly Inquiry for Nursing Practice, 1*(2), 171–174.

Jezewski, M. (1993). Culture brokering as a model for advocacy. *Nursing and Health Care, 14*(2), 78–85.

Lenart, J., St. Clair, P., & Bell, M. (1991). Childrearing knowledge, beliefs, and practices of Cambodian refugees. *Journal of Pediatric Health Care, 5*(6), 299–305.

Longman, A., Saint Germain, M., & Modiano, M. (1992). Use of breast cancer screening by older Hispanic women. *Public Health Nursing, 9*(2), 118–124.

Mall, P., McKay, R., & Katz, M. (1989). Expanding practice horizons: Learning from American Indian patients: Patient education for special populations. *Patient Education and Counseling, 13*(2), 91–102.

May, K. (1992). Middle-Eastern immigrant parents' social networks and help-seeking for child health care. *Journal of Advanced Nursing, 17*(8), 905–912.

Meister, J., Warrick, L., deZapien, J., & Wood, A. (1992). Using lay health workers: Case study of a community-based prenatal intervention. *Journal of Community Health. 17*(1): 37–51.

Meleis, A., Lipson, J., & Paul, S. (1992). Ethnicity and health among five Middle Eastern immigrant groups. *Nursing Research, 41*(2), 98–103.

Roberson, M. (1992). The meaning of compliance: Patient perspectives. *Qualitative Health Research, 2*(1), 7–26.

Simon, S., Howe, L., & Kirschenbaum, H. (1972). *Values clarification: A handbook of practical strategies for teachers and students.* New York: Hart Publishing Company.

Smith, L., & Gentry, D. (1987). Migrant farm workers' perceptions of support persons in a descriptive community survey. *Public Health Nursing, 4*(1), 21–28.

Stevens, P., Hall, J., & Meleis, A. (1992). Examining vulnerability of women clerical workers from five ethnic/racial groups. *Western Journal of Nursing Research, 14*(6), 754–774.

Toohey, J., & Valenzuela, G. (1983). Values clarification as a technique for family planning education. *Journal of School Health, 53*(2), 121–124.

Tripp-Reimer, T., Brink, P., & Saunders, J. (1984). Cultural assessment: Content and process. *Nursing Outlook, 32*(2), 78–82.

Weitzman, B., & Berry, C. (1992). Health status and health care utilization among New York City home attendants: An illustration of the needs of working, poor, immigrant women. *Women and Health, 19*(2–3), 87–105.

Unit II

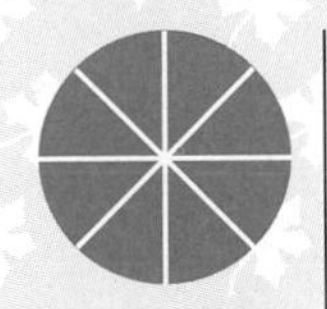

Family As Client

Chapter 7

The Home Visit: Opening Doors for Family Health

Claudia M. Smith 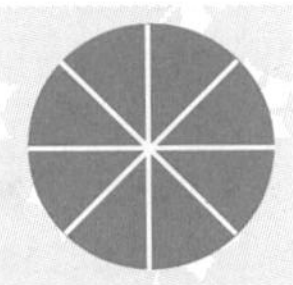

Continued

Focus Questions

Why are home visits conducted?

What are advantages and disadvantages of home visits?

How is the nurse-client relationship in a home similar to and different from nurse-client relationships in inpatient settings?

How can a nurse's family focus be maximized during a typical home visit?

What promotes safety for community health nurses?

What happens during a typical home visit?

How can client participation be promoted?

Nurses who work in all specialties and with all age groups can practice with a *family focus:* that is, thinking of the health of each family member and of the entire family per se, and considering the effects of the interrelatedness of the family members on health. Because being family-focused is a philosophy, it can be practiced in any setting. However, a family's residence provides a special place for family-focused care.

Community health nurses have historically sought to promote well-being of families in the home setting (Zerwekh, 1990.) Community health nurses seek to prevent specific illnesses, injuries, and premature death and to reduce human suffering. Through home visits, community health nurses provide opportunities for families to become aware of potential health problems, to receive anticipatory education, and to learn to mobilize resources for health promotion and primary prevention (Kristjanson and Chalmers, 1991; Raatikainen, 1991). In clients' homes, care can be personalized to a family's coping strategies, problem-solving skills, and environmental resources (see Chapter 9).

During home visits, community health nurses can uncover threats to health that are not evident when family members visit a physician's office, health clinic, or emergency room (Zerwekh, 1991). For example, during a visit in the home of a young mother, a nursing student observed a toddler playing with a paper cup full of tacks and putting them in his mouth. The student used the opportunity to discuss safety with the mother and persuaded her to keep the tacks on a high shelf. The quality of the home environment predicts the cognitive and social development of an infant (Engelke and Engelke, 1992). Community health nurses successfully assist parents in improving relations with their children and in providing safe, stimulating physical environments.

All levels of prevention can be addressed during home visits. Research has demonstrated that home visits by nurses during the prenatal and infancy periods prevent developmental and health problems (Olds et al., 1986). Families who received visits had fewer instances of child abuse and neglect, emergency room visits, accidents, and poisonings during the child's first 2 years of life. These results were true for families of all socioeconomic levels. The health outcomes for families who received home visits were better than those of families who received care only in clinics or from private physicians. Other research shows that home visits by nurses can reduce the incidence of drug-resistant tuberculosis and decrease preventable deaths among infected individuals (Lewis and Chaisson, 1993). This is achieved through directly observing medication therapy in the individual's home, workplace, or school on a daily basis or several times a week.

Several factors have converged to expand opportunities for nursing care to ill and disabled adults and children in their homes. The American population has aged; chronic diseases are now the major illnesses among elderly persons; and there are attempts to limit the rising hospital costs. As the average length of stay in hospitals has decreased since the early 1980s, families have had to care for more acutely ill adults and children in their homes. This increased demand for home health care has resulted in more agencies and nurses providing home care to ill persons and teaching family members to perform the care (see Chapter 29).

The degree to which families cope with a chronically ill or disabled member significantly affects both the individual's health status and the quality of life for the entire family (Burns and Gianutsos, 1987; Whyte, 1992). Family members may be called on to support an individual family member's adjustment to a chronic illness as well as take on tasks and roles previously performed by the ill member. This adjustment occurs over time and often takes place in the home. Community health nurses can assist families in making these adjustments.

Since the late 1960s deinstitutionalization of mentally ill patients has shifted them from inpatient psychiatric settings to their own homes, group homes, and the streets. Nurses in the fields of community mental health and psychiatry began to include the relatives and surrogate family members in the provision of critical support to enable the person with a psychiatric diagnosis to live at home.

The hospice movement also recognizes the importance of a family focus during the process of a family member's dying (American Nurses' Association, 1987). Care at home or in a home-like setting is cost-effective under many circumstances. As the prevalence of acquired immunodeficiency syndrome (AIDS) and the numbers of elderly continue to increase, providing care in a cost-effective manner is both an ethical and an economic necessity.

Nurses in any specialty can practice with a family focus. However, the specific goals and time constraints in each health care service setting affect the degree to which a family focus can be used. A home visit is one type of nurse-client encounter that facilitates a family focus. Home visiting does *not* guarantee a family focus. Rather the setting itself and the structure of the encounter provide an opportunity for the nurse to practice with a family focus.

Nurses who graduate from a baccalaureate nursing program are expected to have educational experiences that prepare them for beginning practice in community health nursing. Family-focused care is an essential element of community health nursing.

Most community health services are rendered in non–inpatient settings, including clinics, schools, worksites, homes, and other community-based residences.

Home visits may be made to any residence: apartments for the elderly, group homes, boarding homes, dormitories, domiciliary care facilities, and shelters for the homeless, among others. In such residences, the family may not be related by blood but rather they may be "significant others": neighbors, friends, acquaintances, or paid caretakers.

Nurses who are educated at the baccalaureate level are one of a few professional and service workers who are formally taught about making home visits. Some social work students, especially those interested in the fields of home health and protective services, also receive similar education. Training programs for homemakers and home health aides have been developed by the American Red Cross and the National Home Caring Council; not all aides have received such extensive training, however. Agricultural and home economic extension workers in the United States and abroad also may make home visits (Murray, 1968; World Health Organization, 1987).

TABLE 7–1

Family Health-Related Problems and Goals

Problem*	Goal
Lifestyle and Resources	Promote support systems and use of health-related resources
Health status deviations	Promote adequate, effective family care of an ill or disabled member
Patterns and knowledge of health maintenance	Encourage growth and development of family members; health promotion and prevention
	Promote healthful environment
Family dynamics and structure	Strengthen family functioning and relatedness

*Problems from Simmons, D. (1980). *A classification scheme for client problems in community health nursing.* (DHHS Publication No. HRA 80–16). Hyattsville, MD: U.S. Department of Health and Human Services.

The Home Visit

DEFINITION

A *home visit* is a purposeful interaction in a home (or residence) directed at promoting and maintaining the health of individuals and the family (or significant others). It may include supporting a family during a member's death. Just as a client's visit to a clinic or outpatient service can be viewed as an encounter between health care professionals and the client, so can a home visit. A major distinction of a home visit is that the health professional goes to the client rather than the client coming to the health professional.

PURPOSE

Almost any health service can be accomplished on a home visit. An assumption is that—except in an emergency—the client or family is sufficiently healthy to remain in the community and to manage health care after the nurse leaves the home.

The foci of community health nursing practice in the home can be categorized under five basic goals:

1. Promoting support systems that are adequate and effective and encouraging use of health-related resources
2. Promoting adequate, effective care of a family member who has a specific problem related to illness or disability
3. Encouraging normal growth and development of family members and the family, and educating the family about health promotion and prevention
4. Strengthening family functioning and relatedness
5. Promoting a healthful environment

The five basic goals of community health nursing practice with families can be linked to categories of family problems (Table 7–1). A pilot study to identify problems

TABLE 7–2

Advantages and Disadvantages of Home Visiting

Advantages	Disadvantages
Home setting provides more opportunity for individualized care	Travel time is costly
Most people prefer to be cared for at home	Less efficient for nurse than working with groups or seeing many clients in an ambulatory site
Environmental factors impinging on health, such as housing condition and finances, may be observed and considered more readily	Distractions such as television and noisy children may be more difficult to control
Information collection and understanding lifestyle values are easier in families' own environment	Clients may be resistant or fearful of the intimacy of home visits
Participation of family members is facilitated	Nurse safety can be an issue
Individuals and family members may be more receptive to learning because they are less anxious in their own environment and because the immediacy of "needing to know" a particular fact or skill becomes more apparent	
Care to ill family members in the home can reduce overall costs by preventing hospitalizations and shortening the length of time spent in hospitals or other institutions	
A family focus is facilitated	

common in community health nursing practice settings revealed that problems clustered into four categories: (1) lifestyle and living resources; (2) current health status and deviations; (3) patterns and knowledge of health maintenance; and (4) family dynamics and structure (Simmons, 1980). Home visits are one means by which community health nurses can address these problems and achieve goals for family health.

ADVANTAGES AND DISADVANTAGES

Advantages of home visits by nurses are numerous. Most of the disadvantages relate to expense and concerns about unpredictable environments (Table 7–2).

Nurse-Family Relationships

How nurses are assigned to make home visits is both a philosophical and a management issue. Some community health nurses are assigned by geographic area or "district." This generally was the case in the United States before the 1970s. Home visiting by geographic area exists today primarily in England, Canada, and the rural United States. With such assignments, the nurse has the potential to work with the entire population in a district and to handle a broad range of health concerns; the nurse can also become well acquainted with the community's health and social resources. The potential for a family-focused approach is strengthened because the nurse's concerns consist of all health issues identified with a specific family or group of families. The nurse remains a clinical generalist, working with people of all ages.

The size of the geographic area for home visits varies with the population density. In a densely populated urban area a nurse might visit in one neighborhood; in a less densely populated area the nurse might be assigned to visit in an entire county.

Other community health nurses are assigned to work with a population aggregate in one or more geopolitical communities. For example, a nurse may work for a "categorical" program that addresses family planning or adolescent pregnancy, in which case the nurse would visit only families to which the category applies. This type of assignment allows a nurse to work predominantly with a specific interest area (family planning and pregnancy) or with a specific aggregate (families with fertile women).

PRINCIPLES OF NURSE-CLIENT RELATIONSHIP WITH FAMILY

Regardless of whether the community health nurse is assigned to work with an aggregate or the entire population, several principles strengthen the clarity of purpose.

- By definition, the nurse focuses on the family.
- The health focus can be on the entire spectrum of health needs and all three levels of prevention.
- The family retains autonomy in health-related decisions.
- The nurse is a guest in the family's home.

To relate to the family the community health nurse does not have to personally meet all members of the household, although varying the times of visits might allow the nurse to meet family members usually at work or school. To relate to the family requires that the nurse be concerned about the health of each member and about each person's contribution to the functioning of the family. One family member may be the primary informant; in such instances the nurse should realize that the information received is being "filtered" by the person's perceptions.

The community health nurse should take the time to introduce herself or himself to each person present and address each by name. The nurse should use the clients' surnames unless they introduce themselves in another way or give permission for the nurse to be less formal. It is important to interact with as many family members as possible. The nurse should ask for an introduction to pets and ask for permission before picking up infants and children, unless it is granted nonverbally.

Through assessment, the community health nurse attempts to identify what actual and potential problems exist with each individual and, thematically, within the family (see Chapter 9). Issues of health promotion (diet) and specific protection (immunization) may exist, as may undiagnosed medical problems for which referral is necessary for further diagnosis and treatment. Actual family problems in coping with illness or disability may require direct intervention. Prevention of sequelae and maximization of potential may be appropriate for families with a chronically ill member. Health-related problems may appear predominantly in one family member or among several members. A thematic family problem might be related to nutrition. For example, a mother may be anemic, a preschooler obese, and a father not following a low-fat diet for hypertension.

There are a few circumstances in our society in which the health of the community, or "public," is considered to have priority over the right of the individual person or family to do as they wish. In most states there are statutes (laws) that provide that health care workers, including community health nurses, have a right and an obligation to intervene in cases of family abuse and neglect, potential suicide or homicide, and existence of communicable diseases that pose a threat of infection to others. Except for these three basic categories, the family retains the ultimate authority for health-related decisions and actions.

In the home setting family members participate more in their own care rather than depend on the nurse for assistance in vital functioning and daily living. Nursing care in the home is intermittent, not 24 hours a day. When the visit ends, it is the family who takes responsibility for their own health, albeit with varying degrees of interest, commitment, knowledge, and skill. This is often difficult for beginning community health nurses to accept; learning to distinguish what the family is responsible for from what the nurse is responsible for involves experience and consideration of laws and ethics. Except in crises it is usually not appropriate to take over for the family in areas in which they have demonstrated capability.

For example, if family members typically call the pharmacy to renew medications and make their own medical appointments, it is not appropriate for the nurse to begin doing these things for them. Taking over undermines self-esteem, confidence, and success.

Being a guest as a community health nurse in a family's home does not mean that the relationship is social. The social graces for the community and culture of the family must be considered so that the family is at ease and is not offended. However, the relationship is intended to be therapeutic. For example, many elderly persons believe it is important to offer something to eat or drink as a sign that they are being courteous and hospitable. Your refusal to share in a glass of iced tea may be taken as an affront, but you certainly have the right to refuse, especially if infectious disease is a concern.

Validate with the client that the time of the visit is convenient. If the client fails to offer you a seat, you may ask whether there is a place that you and the family could sit to talk. That place may be any room of the house or even outside in good weather.

PHASES OF RELATIONSHIPS

Relatedness and communication between the nurse and the client are fundamental to all nursing care. A nurse-client relationship with a family (rather than an individual) is critical to community health nursing. The phases of the nurse-client relationship with a family are the same as with an individual. There are different schemes for naming phases of relationships. All schemes have (1) a preinitiation or preplanning phase, (2) an initiation or introductory phase, (3) a working phase, and (4) an ending (Arnold and Boggs, 1989). Some schemes distinguish a power and control or contractual phase that occurs before the working phase.

The initiation phase may take several visits. During this phase the nurse and the family get to know one another and how the family health problems are mutually defined. The more experience the nurse has, the more efficient she or he will become; initially it may take many community health nursing students four to six visits to feel comfortable and to clarify their role.

The nursing student should keep in mind that the relationship with the family usually involves many encounters over time—home visits, phone calls, or visits at other ambulatory sites, such as clinics. Several encounters may occur during each phase of the relationship (Fig. 7–1). Each encounter also has its own phases (Fig. 7–2). It is helpful to preplan each phone call and home visit.

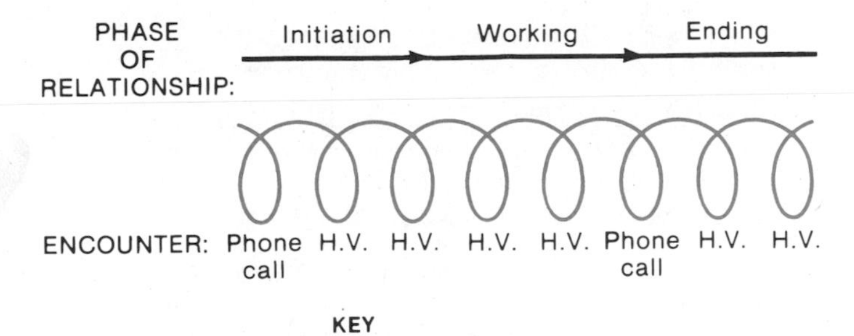

Figure 7–1 ● A series of encounters during a relationship. (Redrawn from Smith, C. (1980). *A series of encounters during a relationship.* Unpublished manuscript. Baltimore, MD: University of Maryland School of Nursing.)

Table 7–3 lists activities that community health nurses usually engage in before a home visit. The list can be used as a guide in helping novice community health nurses to organize previsit activities efficiently.

The visit begins with a reintroduction and a review of the plan for the day; the nurse must assess what has happened with the family since the last encounter. At this point the nurse may renegotiate the plan for the visit and implement it. The end of the visit consists of summarization, preparation for the next encounter, and leave-taking. Table 7–4 describes the community health nurse's typical activities during a home visit.

CHARACTERISTICS OF RELATIONSHIPS WITH FAMILIES

Some differences are worth discussing in nurses' relationships with families compared with those with individual clients in hospitals. The difference that usually seems most significant to the nurse who is learning to make home visits is the fact that the nurse has less control over the family's environment and health-related behavior. The relationship usually extends for a longer period. A more

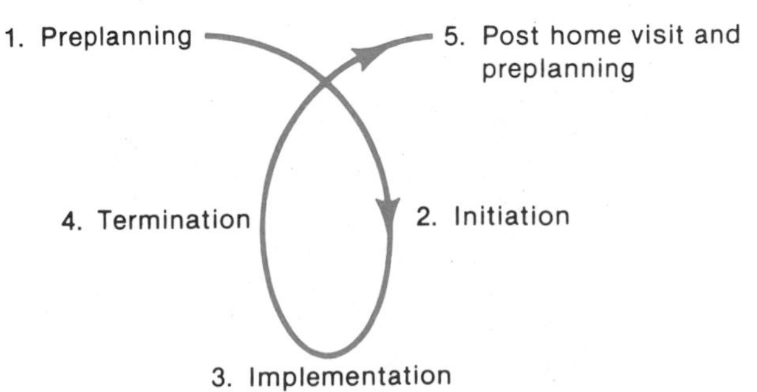

Figure 7–2 ● Phases of a home visit (h.v.). (Redrawn from Smith, C. (1980). *Phases of a home visit.* Unpublished manuscript. Baltimore, MD: University of Maryland School of Nursing.)

TABLE 7–3

Planning Before a Home Visit

1. Have name, address, and telephone number of family with directions and a map.
2. Have telephone number of agency where supervisor or faculty can be reached.
3. Have emergency telephone numbers for police, fire, and rescue personnel.
4. Clarify who has referred family to you and why.
5. Consider what is usually expected of a nurse in working with a family who has been referred for these health concerns (e.g., postpartum visit) and clarify the purposes of this home visit.
6. Consider whether any special safety precautions are required.
7. Have a plan of activities for the home visit time (see Table 7–4).
8. Have equipment needed for handwashing, physical assessment, and direct care interventions or verify that client has the equipment in the home.
9. Take any data assessment or permission forms that are needed.
10. Have information and teaching aids for health teaching as appropriate.
11. Have information about community resources as appropriate.
12. Have gas in your automobile or money for public transportation.
13. Leave an itinerary with the agency personnel or faculty.
14. Approach the visit with self-confidence and caring.

interdependent relationship develops between the community health nurse and the family throughout all steps of the nursing process.

Families Retain Much Control

The family can control the nurse's entry into the home by explicitly refusing assistance, establishing the time of the visit, or deciding whether to answer the door. Unlike hospitalized clients, family members can just walk away and not be home for the visit. Being rejected by the family is often a concern of nurses who are learning to conduct home visits. As with any relationship, anxiety can exist in relation to meeting new, unknown families. Families may actually have similar feelings about meeting the nurse and may wonder what the nurse will think of them, their lifestyle, and their health care behavior.

It will help you keep your perspective if the nurse remembers that *if the clients are home for the nurse's visit, they are at least ambivalent about the meeting!* If they are there to answer the door, they are willing to consider what the nurse has to offer.

Most families involved with home care of the ill have requested assistance. Because only a few circumstances exist (as previously discussed) in which nursing care can be forced on families, the home visit can be viewed by the nurse as an opportunity to explore voluntarily the possibility of engaging in relationships. The nurse is there to offer services and engage the family in a dialogue about health concerns, barriers, and goals. As with all nurse-client relationships, the nurse's commitment, authenticity, and caring constitute the art of nursing practice that can make a difference in the lives of families. Just as not all individuals in the hospital are ready or able to use all of the suggestions made to them, families have varying degrees of openness to change. When, after a discussion of the possibilities, the family declines either overtly or through its actions, the nurse has provided an opportunity for informed decision-making and has no further obligation.

TABLE 7–4

Nursing Activities During Three Phases of a Home Visit

Initiation Phase of Home Visit

1. Knock on door and stand where you can be observed if peephole or window exists.
2. Identify self as __(name)__, the nurse from __(name of agency)__.
3. Ask for the person to whom you were referred or the person with whom the appointment was made.
4. Observe environment as regards your own safety.
5. Introduce yourself to those present and acknowledge them.
6. Sit where family directs you to.
7. Discuss purpose of visit. On initial visits discuss services to be provided by agency.
8. Have permission forms signed to initiate services. This may be done later in the home visit if more explanation of services is needed for the family to understand what is being offered.

Implementation Phase of Home Visit

9. Complete health assessment database for the individual client.
10. On return visits assess for changes since the last encounter. Explore degree that family was able to follow up on plans from previous visit. Explore barriers if follow-up did not occur.
11. Wash hands before and after conducting any physical assessment and direct physical care.
12. Conduct physical assessment as appropriate and perform direct physical care.
13. Identify household members and their health needs, use of community resources, and environmental hazards.
14. Explore values, preferences, and clients' perceptions of needs and concern.
15. Conduct health teaching as appropriate and provide written instructions. Include any safety recommendations.
16. Discuss any referral, collaboration, or consultation that you recommend.
17. Provide comfort and counseling as needed.

Termination Phase of Home Visit

18. Summarize accomplishments of visit.
19. Clarify family's plan of care related to potential health emergency appropriate to health problems.
20. Discuss plan for next home visit and activities to be accomplished in the interim by the community health nurse, individual client, and family members.
21. Leave written identification of yourself and agency, with telephone numbers.

Goals of Nursing Care Are More Long Term

A second major difference in nurse relationships with families is that the goals are usually more long term than with individual clients in hospitals. Clients may be in hospice programs for 6 months. A family with a member who has a recent diagnosis of hypertension may take 6 weeks to adjust to medications, diet, and other lifestyle changes. A school-age child with a diagnosis of attention deficit disorder may take as long as half the school year to show improvement in behavior and learning; sometimes it can take as long as a year for appropriate classroom placement.

For some nurses, this time frame is judged to be slow and tedious. For others, the time frame is seen as an opportunity to know a family in more depth, share life experiences over time, and see results of modifications in nursing care. For nurses who like to know about a broad range of health and nursing issues, relationships with families stimulate that interest. It is helpful for nurses who work in inpatient settings to have had some experience in home visiting, which allows them to appreciate the scope and depth of practice of community health nurses who make home visits as a part of their regular practice. Such experiences can sensitize hospital nurses to the home environments of their clients and can result in better hospital discharge plans and referrals.

Because ultimate goals may take a long time to achieve, it is important that short-term objectives be developed to achieve long-term goals. For example, a family needs to be able to plan lower-calorie menus with sufficient nutrients before weight loss is possible; a parent may need to spend time with a child daily before unruly behavior improves.

Nursing interventions in a hospital setting become short-term objectives for client learning and mastery in the home setting. In an inpatient setting "giving medications as prescribed" is a nursing action. In the home "the spouse will give medications as prescribed" becomes a behavioral objective for the family; the related nursing action is teaching.

Human progress toward any goal usually does not occur at a steady pace. You may start out bicycling faithfully three times a week and give up abruptly. Likewise, clients may skip an insulin dose or an oral contraceptive. A family may assertively call appropriate community agencies, keep appointments, and stop abruptly. Families can be committed to their own health and well-being and yet not act on their commitment consistently. Recognizing that setbacks and discouragement are a part of life allows the community health nurse to be more accepting of reality and have the objectivity to renegotiate goals and plans with families. Table 7–5 includes ways to foster goal accomplishment.

Changes are sometimes subtle or small. Success breeds success, at least motivationally. It is important to make clear what short-term goals have been agreed on so that the nurse and the family members have a common basis for evaluation. Goals can be set in a logical sequence, in small steps, to increase the chance of success. In an inpatient setting it is the skilled nurse who notices the subtle changes in client behavior and health status that can warn of further disequilibrium or can signal improvement. Likewise, during a series of home visits it is the skilled nurse who is aware of slight variations in home management, personal care, and memory that may presage a deteriorating biological condition.

TABLE 7–5

Fostering Goal Accomplishment with Families
1. Share goals explicitly with family.
2. Divide goals into manageable steps.
3. Teach family to do for themselves.
4. Do not expect family to do something all of the time or perfectly.
5. Be satisfied with small, subtle changes.
6. Be flexible.

Nursing Care Is More Interdependent With Families

Because families have more control over their health in their own homes and because change is usually gradual, there must be greater emphasis on mutual goals if the nurse and family are to achieve long-term success.

Except in emergency situations, the client determines the priority of issues to be dealt with. A parent may be adamant that obtaining food is more important than obtaining their child's immunization. A child's school performance may be of greater concern to a mother than her own abnormal Papanicolaou (Pap) smear. Failure of the nurse to address the family's primary priority may result in the family perceiving that the nurse does not genuinely care. Even if the priority problem is not directly health-related, or if the solution to a health problem can be handled better by another agency or discipline, the empathic nurse can address the family's stress level, problem-solving ability, and support systems and make appropriate referrals. When the nurse takes time to validate and discuss the primary concern, the relationship is enhanced.

Flexibility is a key. Because visits occur over several days to months, other events (e.g., episodic illnesses, a neighbor's death, or community unemployment) can impinge on the original plan. Family members may be rehospitalized and receive totally new medical orders once they are discharged to home. The nurse's clarity of purpose is essential in the identification and negotiation of other health-related priorities after the first concern has been addressed.

Increasing Nurse-Family Relatedness

What promotes a successful home visit? What aspects of the nurse's presence promote relatedness? What structures provide direction and flexibility? The nursing process provides a general structure, and communication is a primary vehicle through which the nursing process is manifested. The foundation for both the nursing process and communication is relatedness.

FOSTERING A CARING PRESENCE

Nursing efforts are *not* always successful. However, by being concerned about the impact of home visits on the family and by asking questions regarding her or his own motivations, the nurse automatically increases the likelihood that home visits will be of benefit to the family. The nurse is acknowledging that the intention is for the relationship to be meaningful to both the nurse *and* the family.

The relatedness of nurses in community health *with* clients is important (Goldborough, 1969; Mayers, 1973).

> "Involvement, essentially, is caring deeply about what is happening and what might happen to a person, then doing something with and for that person. It is reaching out and touching and hearing the inner being of another. . . . For a nurse-patient relationship to become a moving force toward action, the nurse must go beyond obvious nursing needs and try to know the patient as a person and include him in planning his nursing care. This means sharing feelings, ideas, beliefs and values with the patient. . . . Without responsibility and commitment to oneself and others . . . [a person] only exists. It is through interaction and meaningful involvement with others that we move into being human (Goldsborough, 1969, pp. 66–68)."

Mayers observed 16 randomly selected nurses during home visits to 37 families and reported that "regardless of the specific interaction style [of each nurse], the patients of nurses who were patient-focused consistently tended to respond with interest, involvement and mutuality" (Mayers, 1973, p. 331). A client-focused nurse was observed as one who followed client cues, attempted to understand the client's view of the situation, and included the client in generating solutions. Being related is a contribution that the nurse can make to the family, independent of specific information and technical skills. It is a contribution that students often underestimate.

Although being related is necessary, it is inadequate in itself for high-quality nursing. A community health nurse must also be competent. Community health nursing also depends on assessment skills, judgment, teaching skills, safe technical skills, and the ability to provide accurate information. As a community health nurse's practice evolves, tension always exists between being related and doing the tasks. In each situation, there is an opportunity to ask, "How can I express my caring *and* do (perform direct care, teach, refer) what is needed?"

Barrett (1982) and Katzman and colleagues (1987) report on the differences that students actually make in the lives of families. Barrett demonstrated that postpartum home visits by nursing students reduced costly postpartum emergency room and hospital visits. Katzman and coworkers considered hundreds of visits per semester made by 80 students in a southwestern state to families with newborns, well children, pregnant women, and members with chronic illnesses. Case examples describe how student enthusiasm and involvement contributed to specific health results.

Everything a nurse has learned about relationships is important to recall and transfer to the experience of home visiting. Carl Rogers (1969) has identified three characteristics of a helping relationship: *positive regard, empathy,* and *genuineness.* These are relevant in all nurse-client relationships, and they are especially important when relationships are initiated and developed in the less-structured home setting.

How is it possible to accept a client who keeps a disheveled house, or who keeps such a clean house that you feel as if you are contaminating it? How is it possible to have positive feelings about an unmarried mother of three when you and your spouse have successfully abstained from pregnancy? Having positive regard for a family does not mean giving up your own values and behavior (see Chapter 6). Having positive regard for a family who lives differently than you does not mean you need to ignore your past experiences. The latter is impossible. Rather, having positive regard means having the ability to distinguish between the person and her or his behavior. Saying to yourself, "this is a person who keeps a messy house" is different from saying, "this person is a mess!" Positive regard involves recognizing the value of persons because they are human beings. Accept the family, not necessarily the family's behavior. All behavior is purposeful, and without further information you cannot determine the meaning of a particular family behavior. Positive regard involves looking for the common human experiences; for example, it is likely that both you and the family members experience awe in the behavior of a newborn and sadness in the face of loss.

Empathy is the ability to put yourself in someone else's shoes, to be able to walk in his or her footsteps so as to understand his or her journey. "Empathy requires sensitivity to another's experience . . . , including sensing, understanding, and sharing the feelings and needs of the other person, seeing things from the other's perspective" according to Rogers (cited in Gary and Kavanagh, 1991, p. 89). Empathy goes beyond self and identity to acknowledge the essence of all persons. It links a characteristic of a helping relationship with spirituality —"a sense of connection to life itself" (Haber, 1987, p. 78). Empathy is a necessary pathway for our relatedness.

But what does it mean to understand another's experience? More than emotions are involved. A person's experience includes the sense she or he makes of aspects of human existence (van Manen, 1990). Being understood means that one is no longer alone (Burgess, 1990). Being understood provides support in the face of stress, illness, disability, pain, grief, and suffering. A person's being understood in a nurse-client partnership (side-by-side relationship) contributes to an experience of being cared for (Beck, 1992).

To understand another's experience, you must be able to imagine being in another's place, recognize commonalities among persons, and have a secure sense of yourself (Davis, 1990). Being aware of your own values and boundaries is helpful in retaining your identity in interaction with others. To understand another's experience, you must also be willing to engage in conversation to negotiate mutual definitions of the situation. For example, if you are excited that an elderly person is recovering function after a stroke, but the person's spouse sees only the loss of an active travel companion, a mutual definition of the situation does not exist. Empathy will not occur unless you can also understand the spouse's perspective.

Each of us likes to perceive that we have some control in our environment, some choice. We avoid being dominated and conned. The nurse's *genuineness* facilitates honesty and disclosure, reduces the likelihood that the family will feel betrayed or coerced, and enhances the relationship. Genuineness does not mean that you speak everything that you think. Genuineness means that what you say and do is consistent with your understanding of the situation.

Self-expression by others can be promoted by your creating an atmosphere of trust, accepting that each person has a right to self-expression, "actively seeking to understand" the others, and assisting them to become aware of and understand themselves (Goldsborough, 1969, p. 66).

The reciprocal side of genuineness is being willing to undertake a journey of self-expression, self-understanding, and growth. A recent nursing graduate wrote about her growing self-responsibility:

> "Although I felt out of control, I felt very responsible. I took pride in knowing that these families were my families and I was responsible for their care. I was responsible for their health teaching. This was the first semester where there was not a faculty member around all day long. I feel that this will help me so much as I begin my nursing career. . . . I have truly felt independent and completely responsible for my actions in this clinical experience."

This student, who preferred predictable environments, was able to confront her anxiety and anger in environments where much was beyond her control. A mother was not interested in the student's priorities. A family abruptly moved out of state in the middle of the semester. Yet the student was able to respond in such circumstances. She became more responsible and she was able to temper her judgment and work with the mother's concern. When the family moved, the student experienced frustration and anger that she would not see the "fruits of her labor" and that she would "have to start over" with another family. However, her ability to respond increased because of her commitment to her own growth, relatedness with families, and desire to contribute to the health and well-being of others.

In a context of relating *with* and advocating *for* the family, the relationship becomes an opportunity for growth in both the nurse's and the family's lives (Glugover, 1987). Imagine standing side by side *with* the family, being concerned *for* their well-being and growth. Now imagine talking *at* a family face to face, attempting to have them do things your way. The first image is a more caring and empathic one.

CREATING AGREEMENTS FOR RELATEDNESS

How can communications be structured to increase the participation of family members? Without the family's engagement, the community health nurse will have few positive effects on the health behavior and health status of the family and its members.

Nurses are expert in caring for the ill; in knowing about ways to cope with illness, to promote health, and to protect against specific diseases; and in teaching and supporting family members. *Family members are experts in their own health.* They know the family health history, they experience their health states, and they are aware of their health-related concerns.

Through the nurse-family relationship there is a fluid process of matching the family's perceived needs with the nurse's perceptions and professional judgments about the family's needs. Paradoxically the more skilled the nurse is in forgetting his or her own anxiety about being the "good nurse," the more likely the nurse is to listen to the family members, validate "their reality," and negotiate an adequate, effective plan of care.

One study of home visits revealed that more than half of the goals stated by public health nurses to the researcher could not be detected, even implicitly, during observations of the home visits. Therefore, half of the goals were known only to the nurse and were therefore not mutual. The more specifically and concretely that the goals were stated by the nurse to the researcher, the greater the likelihood that the clients understood the nurse's purposes (Mayers, 1973). To negotiate mutual goals, the client needs to understand the nurse's purposes.

The initial letter, telephone call, or home visit is the time to share your ideas with the family about why you are contacting them. During the first interpersonal encounter by telephone or home visit, explore the family members' ideas about the purpose of your visits. This is essential to establishing a mutually agreed on basis for a series of encounters.

Family members may have had previous relationships with community health nurses and students. Family members may be able to share such information as what they found to be most helpful, why they are willing to work with a nurse or student again, and what goals they have in mind. Other families who have had no prior experience with community health nurses may not have specific expectations. It is important to ask.

A contract is a specific, structured *agreement* regarding the process and conditions by which a health-related goal will be sought. In the beginning of most student learning experiences, the agreement usually entails one or more family members continuing to meet with the nursing student for a specific number of visits and/or weeks. Initially specific goals and the nurse's role regarding health promotion and prevention may be unclear. (If this were already clear it would not be necessary to undergo a period of study and orientation.)

Initially the agreement may be as simple as "we will meet here at your house next Tuesday at 11:00 until around noon to continue to discuss what I can offer related to your family's health and what you'd like. We can get to know each other better. We can talk more about how the week has gone for you and your family with your new baby." This is the nurse's oral offer to meet under specific conditions of time and place. The process of mutual discussion is mentioned. The goals remain general and implicit: fostering the family's developmental task of incorporating an infant and fostering family-nurse relatedness. For the next week's contract to be complete the family member or members would have to agree. The most important element initially is whether agreement about being present at a specific time and place can be reached. If 11:00 is not workable for the family, is there another time during the day when you both are available that is mutually agreeable? For families who do not focus as much on the future, a community health nurse needs to be more flexible in scheduling the time of each visit.

The word *contract* often implies legally binding agreements. This is not true of nurse-client contracts. Nurses are legally and ethically bound to keep their word in relation to nursing care; clients are *not* legally bound to keep their agreements. However, establishing a mutual agreement for relating increases the clarity of who will do what, when, where, for what purposes, and under what conditions. Because of some people's negative response to the word *contract, agreement* may be better.

Agreements may be oral or written. For some families, written agreements, especially early in the relationship, may be a threat. For example, a family who has been conned by a household repair scheme may be very suspicious of written agreements. Families who are not legal citizens may not want to sign an agreement, for fear that if it is not kept they will be punished. Do not push for a written agreement if the family is uncomfortable. And if you do notice such discomfort, this may be a good opportunity to explore their fears.

Helgeson and Berg (1985) described factors affecting the contracting process by studying a small convenience sample of 15 community health nursing students and 12 client responses. Of the 11 students who introduced the idea of a contract to clients, all did so between the second and the fourth visits of a 16-week series of visits; 9 did so orally rather than in writing. There was *not* "one specific time that was best." Eight clients were very receptive to the idea because they "liked the idea of establishing goals to work toward and felt the contract would serve as a reminder of their responsibility." The very process of developing a draft agreement to present to families provides the novice practitioner with an increased focus of care, clarity of nurse and family responsibilities and activities, and a basis from which to negotiate modifications in client behaviors (Helgeson and Berg, 1985; Sheridan and Smith, 1975).

Figure 7–3 lists nurse behavior that is appropriate for home visits, especially initial home visits and those early in a series of home visits. This list may be used as a preplanning tool by nurses to assist them in identifying their readiness to conduct a specific home visit. The tool has also been used by students and community health nurses to evaluate initial home visits and identify their behaviors that were omitted and needed to be included on the second home visits. It has also been used jointly as an evaluation tool by nurses and supervisors and students and faculty.

INCREASING UNDERSTANDING THROUGH COMMUNICATION SKILLS

It is the nurse's ability to *be* with family members that determines the success of the nurse-family relationship. A nurse can employ techniques of speaking and listening appropriately and still not have a working relationship because caring is not there. Mayers (1973) reported that each of the community health nurses studied had their own interactional style: some were nondirective listeners, calm and relatively quiet; others were more verbally active and directive. Most did not demonstrate a balanced use of communication techniques, yet those who could *be* with the families had a successful relationship in spite of their imperfect technique.

Communication techniques do have their place as skills for community health nurses. It is through communication that the nurse discovers the meanings of particular things to families and validates those meanings. It is through communication that the nurse comes to understand the family and their circumstances, goals, and preferences.

Leitch and Tinker (1978) discuss clusters of communication skills and their purposes and guidelines for use. Listening, leading, reflecting, and summarizing are important communication skills. Listening skills assist nurses in clarifying and validating messages. "Leading" skills

HOME VISITING EVALUATION TOOL

This Home Visiting Evaluation Tool is built upon behaviors of initiation, implementation, and termination within each visit.

Directions: Place a check in the appropriate box below:

Family name	Date and time of home visit					
Nursing Activities	Present	Absent	N/A	Present	Absent	N/A
1. Determines name, etc., of client						
2. Has planned the visit						
3. Introduces self						
4. Links self with others						
5. Accepts client non-judgmentally						
6. Identifies household members						
7. Assesses client's capacity to comprehend						
8. States with whom you will communicate						
9. Initiates contract						
a. Time						
b. Day						
c. Beginning week						
d. Ending week						
e. Attendance						

Figure 7–3 ● Home visiting evaluation tool. (From Chichester, M., & Smith, C. (1980). *Home visiting evaluation tool.* Unpublished manuscript. Baltimore, MD: University of Maryland School of Nursing.)

Illustration continued on following page

assist nurses in focusing and questioning for the purposes of expanding the scope and depth of factual and emotional messages and reducing confusion. These skills are basic to all nursing relationships, and they are especially important to community health nurses because the nurse is probably the sole collector of information. Time passes between home visits during which events occur in the family's life. Unlike in a hospital setting where records or reports are given from nurses on previous shifts, on home visits the nurse must update the assessment, based mainly on what the family says. Reflecting skills allow community health nurses to understand the family's frame of reference and the meaning of its concerns. Reflecting also allows the family members to know that they have been understood.

In working with families and individuals over time, the opportunity to identify themes of communication emerges. Analytical skills can be of assistance. When themes become clearer the family and nurse can work on more basic issues, rather than on piecemeal episodes. For example, during week 2 of a series of home visits, a young mother had missed a well-child appointment; during week 4 she missed her own appointments to a general practitioner to monitor the blood levels of her antiseizure medications and to the dentist to treat her related gum problems. By week 6 she had not made any new appointments. The student was able to recognize a theme of unkept appointments and summarize the past weeks with the mother.

When she confronted her own feelings, the student realized she was frustrated and angry that the mother had not kept her word and had not made progress toward what the student believed had been mutual goals. The student expressed the intensity of her own feelings to faculty and peers rather than directly with the client. The student wanted neither to blame nor to attack the mother with her own anger. Rather, the student expressed herself calmly to the mother by describing the pattern of making, and missing, and not making appointments.

When the student asked the mother to explain, the mother agreed that the infant's shots were important, that she had been "worried about her living arrangements and felt tired," and that she would make and keep the infant's future appointments. She explained that since she had had

Family name	Date and time of visit					
f. Cancellations						
g. Purpose						
h. What you will offer						
i. Your constraints						
j. Exploration of expectations						
k. What client may offer						
10. Negotiates mutually acceptable contract						
11. Reduces distraction						
12. Listens actively						
13. Allows and supports distance						
14. Explores client's ideas						
15. Relates own understanding of what has been said						
16. Seeks shared meanings of words						
17. Explores ambivalence						
18. Tolerates silence						
19. Has verbal/nonverbal communications that are congruent						
20. Focuses discussion appropriately						
21. Completes a relevant tangible intervention						
22. Reinforces positive behaviors						
23. Avoids giving disapproval						
24. Avoids defending others						
25. Avoids "talking down" to client						
26. Avoids cliches/stereotyping						
27. Avoids prolonging the contact						
28. Gives client in writing						
a. Your name						
b. Agency phone number						
c. Other significant information						
29. Summarizes agreed upon points						
30. Leaves promptly						

Figure 7–3 ● Continued

seizures for so long she knew to go to the physician when she was seriously ill but would not go routinely. Although the student did not like the mother's response about her own health, the student did accept it as the mother's own frame of reference. The student pointed out that more frequent medical appointments might help to prevent seizures. The mother still said she would not go.

The student returned from the home visit no longer angry. She expected that the mother would have her son immunized before the end of the semester (12th visit) and that she would not obtain medical care for herself at this time. Her expectations were fulfilled.

The efficiency of identifying themes usually increases with the nurse's experience. Discussing families with your peer group and faculty or supervisor allows you to identify others' perceptions of family themes. Expanding possible meanings provides you more flexibility and depth of interpretations. You have an opportunity to return to the family with renewed ability to validate the meaning of behavior with the family. This process may result in the family having a clearer understanding or interpretation of their own behavior.

Reducing Potential Conflicts

Acknowledging that uneasiness can arise in the nurse owing to reduced control during home visits, how is mutuality facilitated? As coercion has little place in public health and nursing, how can a nurse have influence over the health of family members?

The truth is that the one person you *can* change is yourself. This is under your direct control. Through changes in *yourself,* you *may* be able to affect your relationship with a client so that there may be a shift in his or her being and behavior. A paradox of relationships is that the more you focus on changing, fixing-up, or making another person "better," the more likely that person is to feel dominated and to resist change. Through managing your own anxiety and your degree of self-attention, you may shift your being and behavior sufficiently to provide the family members with openness and self-expression. By attuning to their perception of reality, you have a basis for dialogue, therapeutic relationship, and practical problem-solving.

How does a nurse manage his or her own anxiety or self-absorption in a home that is likely very different from the nurse's own home? Expectations, role insecurity, value interference, and the client's reaction to the nurse are potential sources of conflict (Friedman, 1983).

MATCHING THE NURSE'S EXPECTATIONS WITH REALITY

Surprises often shock or unnerve and reduce a person's ability to feel in control. Have you ever attempted to use a new piece of medical equipment which you have never seen before? Did you wonder how to make it work? Did you feel anxious that you might do something foolish? Were you thinking that other people were watching you and thinking you were an incompetent nurse? If someone had described the machine to you ahead of time, talked you through the procedure, and warned you of the machine's idiosyncracies, might you have felt more prepared, more in control, and less anxious? For many of you, the answer is yes.

Similarly, learning about a neighborhood and a family prior to your home visit can allow you to anticipate what you will find, reduce surprises, and promote your feelings of calmness and self-control. In such a state, you are much more likely to be attentive in your relationship with family members.

Learning about the family before the home visit can be accomplished by gathering as much information as possible. These data may be obtained by calling the person who initiated the referral to you, by having the liaison nurse or discharge planner obtain the information from the hospitalized family member, by calling the family, and/or by looking at the family identification information if you are working in a health maintenance organization or health department.

1. Who is in the family? How old are they? Who is likely to be there during your home visit? If you know there are three preschoolers at home, you can be mentally prepared for relating with children and for the possible exuberance of their presence.
2. What are the related developmental tasks of the family members? Anticipating these tasks can suggest possible situations in the family that are timely topics for discussion. For example, if it is fall, is a child adjusting to kindergarten or first grade?
3. How receptive might this family be to your visit? Has the family initiated the request for service? If not, what have they been told about the referral to you? Has the family been visited previously by community health nurses or nursing students? What is the family's past or current relationship with the agency with which you are affiliated? Does the family usually keep outpatient office and clinical appointments? Nurses previously involved with the family may be able to describe the family's usual way of presenting themselves.
4. What other health and social service agencies and providers are the family involved with? Are all of the relationships voluntary or are some court-ordered? This information assists you to clarify part of the family's support system as well as to initiate discussion about persons already known to the family.
5. What will the environment be like? In some neighborhoods it is misleading to predict what the inside of a home looks like based on the exterior of the building.

A disadvantage of collecting information about the family prior to your initial home visit is that the information may bias your point of view about the family. Some nurses prefer to visit first and then validate their perceptions with data from other sources.

CLARIFYING NURSING RESPONSIBILITIES

The purpose of the visit constitutes another category of data to be collected in the preinitiation phase of the relationship before the home visit. What has the family been told about the purpose of your visit and what are the family's expectations? If the family initiated the request for services, what specifically do they want? What is the goal of the agency or program for whom you are working? What is the job description for you and your peers?

Uncertainty and ambivalence are common responses of nurses who have little experience in home visiting. Talk about your anxieties with faculty, supervisors, or more experienced nurses.

For registered nurses who are skilled at providing nursing practice in inpatient settings, home visiting adds complexity. The reduced control, increased focus on family, expanded teaching, adaptation of care to the home, and increased primary prevention add complexity to the already-established role (see Chapter 1).

Once you have contacted the family by phone or at their home, listen actively to the specifics and themes of what is communicated. What is not talked about may be as important as what is mentioned. Following up on cues can provide important information for you. For example, when reviewing the health of household members with the nurse during a home visit, a mother spoke positively about all of her children except Patti. When the mother did not even mention Patti, the nurse specifically commented, "We haven't talked about Patti yet." The mother hesitantly said they did not get along and changed the subject. The nurse now knew more about the meaning of the mother's omission.

The desire to have families be appreciative and cooperative can backfire. Families may test what the nurse is willing to do, or they may be so overwhelmed and looking for help that they make inappropriate or unrealistic demands. Sometimes families ask for time, money, rides, or assistance with tasks that they can accomplish themselves. Other families are so emotionally distraught that they seek relief from their uncomfortable feelings by placing unrealistic hopes on the nurse. The nurse tries to develop a relationship with a family that inspires their trust. Limit-setting on the part of the nurse helps to establish trust. For example, if a client asks for a loan to pay the rent, you might reply, "I will not loan you money, but I will help you think about other plans for paying your bills." Agreeing to demands that are unrealistic or uncomfortable for the nurse will eventually erode the relationship. The nurse needs to learn to be comfortable identifying and stating limits to the family starting at the very first visit.

You would not have come this far in your nursing education and practice were you not committed to being a successful nurse and contributing to the well being of other persons. Rather than worry about your success in a new environment, attempt to experience your home visits as the next step in your nursing journey.

MANAGING THE NURSE'S EMOTIONS

As with all relationships in nursing, our emotions can get in the way of our providing client-centered care. Anxiety has already been mentioned; sadness, disgust, anger, joy, and fear can also be evoked. Our emotions are linked through associations to events and situations in our lives. Although our emotional responses are often automatic and certainly color our perceptions, they are usually not rational. What seems to be *the* only feeling possible at the moment is really one of many. Another person may associate the environmental cue with an entirely different meaning and thereby have an entirely different emotional response.

Although community health nurses are confronted with a variety of home settings, lifestyles, family types, and cultures, and strong emotions may be triggered, family members may end the relationship if nurses are judgmental. One goal in therapeutic nursing relationships is to be open to possible interpretations of the situation other than your initial, automatic one. For example if on an initial home visit a mother does not maintain eye contact with the nurse and the preschoolers shelter themselves behind her, the nurse might automatically conclude that she or he is not wanted and act accordingly, by leaving the visit prematurely. Perhaps the mother has low self-esteem or is relatively shy with strangers. Not making eye contact may also be a respectful gesture, especially to authority figures. To consider these possible meanings of the family's reaction to the home visit will at least remind the nurse that the meaning of the mother's behavior is not known. "Not knowing" provides an opportunity for further discussion of the purpose of the visit and of the mother's perception of that purpose, as well as of her concerns and possible ambivalence.

MAINTAINING FLEXIBILITY IN RESPONSE TO CLIENT REACTIONS

The nurse should not assume that a client's behavior is a reaction rationally linked to the nurse's behavior. The way a particular individual behaves at a given moment is influenced by his or her culture, family values, and personal experience. In the example given previously, the mother may rarely maintain eye contact with anyone except a close friend or sister. Also because the nurse-family relationship is in the initiation stage, some testing behavior may automatically occur regardless of the nurse's behavior. The client may unconsciously ask, "Is the nurse sufficiently interested to continue caring for *me?*"

Conversely do not assume that your behavior has no effect on the client's responses and behavior during the home visit. By definition, communication is interactive. How you present yourself with family members makes a difference with them.

CLARIFYING CONFIDENTIALITY OF DATA

If both the nurse and the family members are clear about who is working with the family and what information is being shared, there will be far less potential for conflict.

The nurse and family expectations about shared information will be aligned.

Clients have a right to know what information is being entered in the legal health record and with whom the nurse is sharing that information. Remember that individual clients have the right to read their own health records and the records of their children and of those under their guardianship. Keep this in mind when recording; objective data, not inferences or generalizations, should be recorded. Describe client behaviors but do not attribute motivation. For example, note that the "client spoke rapidly, 'they can't make me give my child medicine.'" Do not record that the "client doesn't like health providers," which is an unvalidated, overgeneralized conclusion.

Other health care providers employed by your health care agency may have access to the legal record if they are involved in providing direct care, consulting with you, or supervising your care. It is honest and fair to identify with the client those health care providers with whom you will share information routinely. For example, "I will share this information about your child with my supervisor, the nurses who work in the clinic and the physician(s) there. Sometimes I may speak with Dr. X, your pediatrician."

Written permission of the client or of the parent or guardian of a minor is required to obtain or release written information from other agencies or disciplines in private practice (see Chapter 4). With the client's knowledge you can share and seek information orally to collaborate in providing care. As discussed earlier, there are some situations in which the nurse is required by law to share information without client consent. Even when you are initiating a referral for suspected abuse or neglect, it is appropriate to discuss your problem-solving with the available family members. Though they may be unhappy or angry, you have acknowledged them by providing information. Remember that the right of minors to sign for permission for their own treatment varies from state to state.

Prior to the home visit, clarify your state's laws that govern consent of minors and mandatory reporting of selected circumstances (such as child abuse) by health providers. With your supervisor or faculty, identify the usual and customary people within the agency with whom you will be sharing information.

Promoting Nurse Safety

The safety of the community health nurses is critical. The purpose of the home visit is to offer or provide nursing services that make a contribution to the family's health *and* to do so while maintaining the nurse's safety. The purpose of a home visit is not to provide care "at all costs." Assertiveness, not abandonment of one's own needs, is required. This is especially true when you are learning to be a community health nurse and testing yourself and the boundaries of your professional role.

CLARIFYING THE NURSE'S SELF-RESPONSIBILITY

Nurses will encounter some clients who are hostile, angry, volatile, or potentially violent. This is true of individuals in an acute inpatient setting and in their homes (e.g., a person with dementia who is combative). Therefore, why do many nurses beginning home visits (as well as their families) express anxiety and fear? The reason is largely because the nurse has less control over the environment on a home visit.

The experience of home visiting is new and unknown. There are no hospital or agency walls within which to practice, no backup personnel immediately available, no receptionist, and, often, no security guards. The community health nurse often visits alone.

Community health nurses visit in every type of household and neighborhood. Each nurse has grown up in a specific family constellation and neighborhoods with particular socioeconomic, ethnic, religious, and racial compositions. We are more comfortable with people like ourselves and with environments similar to those we are most accustomed to. Practicing as a community health nurse probably will expand those boundaries.

As the incidence of violence in our society has increased, concerns about safety in general have grown. This has become especially true in neighborhoods in which drug trafficking, gang activity, and violent crimes occur. Having acknowledged all this as being so, it is necessary to put the potential threats in perspective. Community health nurses are generally known in communities and acknowledged as having special skills and relationships that contribute to the residents' well-being. Community health nurses collectively have been seen as caring, helpful, constructive persons throughout their history. As a visitor who represents nursing, you have the protection of this general community attitude.

Also community health nurses usually are perceived differently in a community than are police and social workers because nurses' roles are perceived to have less "threat of law." As discussed elsewhere, community health nurses are usually invited in, or families at least have the opportunity to decline nursing services. Consequently, nurses are seen as being helpful rather than threatening.

What is done to promote the safety of community health nurses? In very high-risk neighborhoods, some nurses are accompanied by police, neighborhood volunteers, or paid security escorts (Nadwairski, 1992) (Table 7–6). Almost universally, nurses may request that another nurse or their supervisor accompany them on visits to neighborhoods and homes in which they are uncomfortable. In some agencies, the ethical decision has been made to forbid nursing visits to selected neighborhoods, apartment developments, or families for the nurse's protection. Family members can be invited to more neutral territory, such as a school, clinic, or library, for an interaction. Phone visits may at times be substituted for some home visits.

TABLE 7–6
Safety and Home Visiting

1. If possible, obtain the family's permission to work with them by telephone prior to home visiting. Ask for directions to their road, driveway, building, or apartment.
2. Always have an itinerary with the agency for each clinical day that includes the name of the family to be visited, their address and telephone number, and the license tag number and make of the automobile you're driving.
3. Do not carry purses or wear jewelry other than engagement or wedding rings. Do not wear rings with large gems.
4. Wear the appropriate dress (uniform or street clothes) determined by the agency.
5. Carry coins for telephone calls and a small amount of money for emergencies.
6. Carry an identification badge and wear a name pin.
7. Avoid secluded areas such as stairwells, alleys, basements, and empty buildings or obtain an escort.
8. Avoid areas where persons are loitering or obtain an escort.
9. Use discretion about visiting a family. If you feel unsafe—*do not visit.*
10. If approached on the street by someone requesting a home visit, refer them to the office of the public health or home health agency.
11. Consider whether an escort is needed to avoid visiting a lone male if you are female or visiting a lone female if you are male.
12. Request a nurse partner or escort to a home visit if needed.
13. Avoid entering a home in which fights, drug use, or drug sales are in progress.
14. Always report back to the agency in person or by telephone at the end of the clinical day.
15. Visit only during your scheduled work hours. If you must make an exception to this, permission from your supervisor must be obtained.

PROMOTING SAFE TRAVEL

All community health nurses can benefit from basic crime prevention courses provided by local or state police regarding safety on the street and in automobiles. It is especially helpful for a community health nurse to know that he or she is incorporating basic self-protection behaviors. For nurses driving in remote areas, cellular phones, citizens band radios, and knowing what to carry for weather emergencies are especially important.

HANDLING THREATS DURING HOME VISITS

Actual and potential threats can occur during home visits. What should a community health nurse do if the family is engaged in an altercation or fight when the nurse arrives? What if family members appear to be intoxicated or under the influence of drugs? What if someone in the family displays a weapon? There is no one absolutely correct response, but there are some guiding principles. The first rule is to protect your own safety because you are of no assistance if you become entangled in an altercation or are harmed. If you are feeling sufficiently fearful or anxious that your functioning is compromised, or if you perceive that your presence is further aggravating the circumstances, then either do not enter the home or leave the home if you have already entered.

You can ask the family whether another time to visit would be better; or you can announce that you will not stay and that you will call or come at another time. Sometimes by having their focus shifted by the presence of an outsider, the situation is temporarily defused. Always notify your supervisor or faculty as soon as possible. Remember, though, as a beginning community health nurse you may feel less confident than someone with more experience. It is acceptable to err on the side of being "too cautious" as regards your own safety. If, however, you are finding that most home visits seem threatening, you must speak with your faculty, preceptor, or supervisor to help identify the source of perceived threats and ways to relieve them.

PROTECTING THE SAFETY OF FAMILY MEMBERS

The second principle is to protect the safety of each family member. How can you do this if you are no longer in their house? If you believe someone is in imminent physical danger or is being injured, you need to call the policing authority that responds to domestic violence. If someone has been injured, you should call for both police and rescue workers. If you believe that dependent children or adults are being neglected or abused, you need to contact your faculty or supervisor and follow your school's or agency's policies and procedures. Short of these priorities, the community health nurse is not legally bound to respond.

After you have gained experience with a specific family or are more experienced in dealing with family anger in general, you can use communication and crisis intervention to alter the family's self-expression. All of your knowledge and experience in psychiatric–mental health nursing is of value in such circumstances. In some agencies psychiatric nursing consultants are available to coach you in responding to families who exhibit anger. Psychiatric emergency teams are available for home visits in some communities.

Generally families present a more reserved, social self to nurses, especially at first. Consequently illegal behavior is often hidden from the nurse. As a beginner do not probe your speculations about illegal behavior. For example if several different people are coming in and out of a house during each of your visits, you might suspect that drug sales are taking place. However, you usually would not ask, "Is someone here dealing drugs?" Seek consultation from your faculty or supervisor instead. In some households, members may be intoxicated from alcohol consumption or may be using illicit drugs during the visit. Such individuals are likely to be cognitively impaired and will not benefit from your visit. You should indicate that you will return at another time and leave the home. If other family members who are at risk of harm (such as an infant who is not being supervised) are being cared for by the intoxicated person, you should follow the policies and procedures for notifying the appropriate authorities.

If clients have weapons that are unsafely displayed in the home, it is your right to request that weapons be put away during or prior to your visits. For example, an elderly man kept a loaded pistol with him for protection in his efficiency apartment. The nurse requested that, since he knew when she was coming, he put his gun away before he answered the door for her. When he refused he was given a choice between keeping his gun out and having nursing visits. After some discussion he chose to store his gun when the nurse visited.

Ethically you need to encourage family safety related to proper storage of weapons, especially when there are children or adults with compromised cognition or proneness to violence. Some states have legislation governing safe gun storage in homes.

Managing Time and Equipment

The community health nurse's effectiveness depends on planning the day for the efficient use of time and other resources. Physical resources are often limited to equipment carried by the nurse and/or provided by the family at the home. Consequently, "making do" with what is at hand and doing this consistent with basic principles of safety and infection control are the hallmarks of a skilled community health nurse, although more specialized equipment is being used in the home to care for sicker individuals (see Chapter 29). Table 7–3 discusses activities for planning a home visit that will increase efficiency.

STRUCTURING TIME

The time devoted to a home visit may vary; an hour is often used as a basis for planning. As many as seven visits per day may be expected of nurses in some agencies. Geographic location, travel time, and client priorities help establish the order of visits. Visits to persons with infected wounds should be scheduled after home visits to healthy or immunosuppressed individuals.

Some visits may last only the few minutes it takes to determine that a family either is absent from the home or is engaged in other activities that make home visiting inappropriate at that time. Other visits may approach 2 hours in length, especially an initial visit to a family with a member who is being admitted to services of a home health agency. In such a case consent forms must be signed, assessments must be performed, environmental evaluations must be done to determine equipment needs, and direct care techniques must be demonstrated to family members. An hour for novices usually proves sufficient time to accommodate some inefficiencies in interviewing, relating, and performing nursing care. If family members are especially anxious or upset, visits may take a longer time. If equipment must be improvised or modified or if there is a health-related emergency, more time will probably be needed.

Conversely visits may need to be shortened when the stamina of the family members is compromised. An interview with a person with shortness of breath, for example, needs to be paced so that the person does not become tired. Some family members think concretely rather than abstractly, so short, frequent visits allow the nurse to focus on one or two items at a time. Shorter visits result in greater clarity and timely correction and/or reinforcement of the family's health-related behaviors.

HANDLING EMERGENCIES

Emergencies in the family may extend the length of the home visit and are *always* to be handled before the nurse leaves unless the safety of the nurse is threatened. It is true that if the nurse were *not* making the home visit the family would probably deal with the emergency without the nurse, unless the nurse were one of the resources contacted by the family. More likely the family would contact other family members, their private physician, the emergency room of a hospital, an ambulatory emergency center, or the rescue system. However, once the nurse is made aware that an emergency exists, it is the nurse's professional and legal responsibility to address the emergency within the scope of nursing and to support the family to obtain appropriate resources.

Responding to a medical emergency in the home is similar to responding to a patient's emergency in the hospital, in that in both circumstances the nurse has knowledge of basic assessment skills, cardiopulmonary resuscitation (CPR), asepsis, and nursing interventions to reduce client anxiety, conserve client energy, promote comfort, and prevent further dysfunction. However, the nurse in the home does not have the equipment and team members that are available to the hospital nurse. Equipment in the home is probably limited to what the nurse brings—soap, clean gloves, a sphygmomanometer, a stethoscope, thermometers, and clean dressings. The only medication available is that of the respective family members. The medical orders are those of the family member's physician or nurse practitioner, which may be known to the nurse from written medical orders to the nurse or written and oral instructions to family members. Many agencies also have written policies and procedures for handling a variety of emergencies. Knowledge of basic and advanced first aid is appropriate for any nurse making home visits. In addition to knowing what family members are taught to do in emergencies, a nurse who starts with first aid skills and incorporates basic nursing practice and agency policy will be functioning on a firm foundation.

As presented in CPR classes, the priorities in physiological emergencies are the ABC's—Airway, Breathing, Circulation. In these three emergencies, appropriate use of

CPR is required, which includes activating the emergency rescue system.

Poisoning is usually considered the fourth life-threatening priority. Nurses should always carry their state's poison control telephone number; nurses are to call this number to verify the importance of any suspected poisoning and to ascertain the need for any immediate treatment prior to medical treatment.

Other physical emergencies include acute deficits in hydration or nutrition and environmental safety hazards that may be life threatening. Of similar magnitude are the psychological emergencies of potential suicide, homicide, and abuse, which have been discussed previously.

Community health nurses often encounter family members who exhibit signs or symptoms that have not yet been diagnosed by a physician or nurse practitioner. Are these signals of normal variations that bother the family member? Is a referral for medical diagnosis appropriate? Are these signals of an unstable condition or an impending emergency that requires immediate referral? These are distinctions that community health nurses assist families to make.

Families also have emergencies. Unexpected situations requiring immediate action do constitute emergencies for families. Often emergencies relate to an unhealthy environment, such as loss of heat, potable water, or refrigeration for food. Families may have insufficient funds to pay heat bills or repair a refrigerator. Or community disasters, such as storms or fires, may have interrupted utilities. A family may be experiencing an impending or actual eviction. Food, water, clothing, shelter, and safety are basic for survival, and their loss usually constitutes an emergency.

Families may also experience crises in which the stressors exceed their coping skills. A birth, death, unemployment, or chronic illness may tax their coping. Stress may manifest as acute physical or psychiatric illness in one or more family members.

How does a community health nurse relate to such emergencies? What does the nurse do? Referrals are appropriate for emergency food, clothing, and shelter. The local or state department of social services has some resources for emergency food stamps and shelter. Agencies such as the Salvation Army and Red Cross, as well as religious and civic organizations, supply emergency provisions. Members of the extended family, neighbors, or volunteers may be mobilized to stay with the family for support during the crisis.

PROMOTING ASEPSIS IN THE HOME

The goals of infection control in the home are to prevent the spread of communicable organisms from one family member to another and from one household to another, to protect individual family members who are especially susceptible to infection, and to protect the nurse from infection. The Centers for Disease Control and Prevention publishes infection control standards for the hospital and other settings (CDC, 1985). The community health nurse adapts these standards to the circumstances of each household and the specific needs of the family.

Some visits will be entirely "talking" visits and involve no direct physical care. For example, you might be making a home visit to a mother of school-age children when they are in school. If your initial purposes are to introduce yourself, obtain the mother's agreement to work together, and collect identifying information and health history for the record, there may be no direct physical contact. Unless the mother herself is ill and requires some physical assessment or she exhibits risk factors that indicate the need for screening (such as high blood pressure), there is no need to wash your hands and use equipment from the nursing bag. Your hands are clean from having washed them prior to leaving the agency or the previous home visit.

Airborne organisms can be transmitted to and from you and among family members, even without direct contact. Noticing respiratory symptoms among family members offers an opportunity to teach family members about managing coughs and sneezes and performing handwashing and other infection control measures. If you are ill yourself, you need to identify the likely degree of communicability; as in the hospital, nurses need to distinguish their allergies from colds, manage their symptoms, and avoid patients with compromised immunity. In community health nursing, the nurse may wear a mask and be fastidious about handwashing, postpone the visit until another day, or have another nurse act as a substitute.

Lice and scabies can be transmitted from clothing, bedding, and upholstered furniture. In some households the furniture is multipurpose—used for sleeping and for sitting. Where this is so it is best to sit in unupholstered furniture, if available, such as a wood or plastic chair. Routinely avoid sitting on beds, both as a protection to yourself and so as not to transmit any organisms from your clothing to the bedding. When you remove your coat, either continue to sit on it or remove it completely and fold it with the outside out; it is the outside that is considered less clean to you. Washing uniforms in hot water (60°C for 20 minutes) or dry cleaning promotes infection control (Benenson, 1990).

Direct physical contact and the use of equipment introduce the necessity for medical asepsis or clean technique by the community health nurse. Take as little equipment into the home as you anticipate you will need; do not carry purses, knapsacks, extra records, or books. If you travel by car, you can stock extra equipment and resources there. It is usually sufficient to take pen, paper, permission forms to be signed, health records to be completed, emergency telephone numbers, educational materials, and a nursing bag (with handwashing equipment and basic physical assessment equipment) into the home. Some agencies also provide small policy and procedure handbooks.

Handwashing is an essential component of infection control in homes as it is in all other settings of practice. In the hospital, nursing home, or clinic, the sink with water, soap, and paper towels is an expected part of the environment. Running water will not always be available in homes. The water may be temporarily shut off while the pipes or hot water heater are being fixed. In one instance a family owned its own condominium and had faucets that leaked excessively; rather than pay for a plumbing bill, the family turned the water off under each sink until it was needed. Some homes have well or cistern water that must be carried in from outside, sometimes over a great distance.

All sinks in homes are considered to be dirty. This is not meant as a judgment of the family's house-cleaning skills, rather, it is a basic principle of medical asepsis. The community health nurse does not know what else has touched the sink or how the sink has been used.

Some homes will have sinks, running water, liquid soap, and separate hand towels for guests. Unless there is a known infection in the home, the nurse may use these family supplies for handwashing.

Other homes will have sinks and running water, but will have a bar of soap and towel used by everyone in the household. In this case neither the soap nor the towel is clean enough for the community health nurse to use. Sometimes there will be no waste receptacle. Consequently, the community health nurse must always include soap, paper towels, and bags for waste as a part of the standard equipment for home visiting (Table 7–7.)

Proper handling of equipment prevents spread of communicable organisms. Each agency usually specifies standard equipment each nurse is to have on a home visit; minimally, equipment for physical assessments is included. When sterile equipment is needed it is usually obtained by the family from a supply company. Cleansing equipment in the home is sometimes needed to prevent contamination of the nursing bag and subsequent transmittal of organisms to other households and individuals (Table 7–8).

The CDC has recommended that *all* individuals be cared

TABLE 7–7

Handwashing Procedures

Handwashing Procedure with Running Water

Equipment

1. Liquid soap containing a germicide in squeeze bottle
2. Paper towels
3. Trash receptable (paper or plastic bags)

Procedure

1. Remove soap and paper towels from nursing bag.
2. Place one paper towel down as a clean field.
3. Squeeze soap into the palm of one hand, and place the soap container on the clean field.
4. Carry the remaining paper towels to the sink area. Place paper towels under one arm and hold them against your side. This prevents them from getting wet or being placed on the dirty sink.
5. Turn on the water, adjust temperature to warm, wash and rinse hands.
6. Dry hands with paper towels.
7. Turn off water with paper towels.
8. Dispose of paper towels in household receptacle or return to nursing bag and use the receptacles provided.

A major advantage of this procedure is that the equipment does not have to be taken to the dirty sink where it can get wet and contaminated. The disadvantage is that the soap may be left out of sight of the nurse; this could be a poisoning hazard to a confused family member or a child. If you have any doubts, take the soap with you, replace it in the bag before going to the sink, or assign a responsible person to guard the equipment. There are other procedures that involve taking the soap to the bathroom.

Handwashing Procedure with Poured Water

Substitute step 5 above with the following:

5. Have another person pour a small amount of water from a clean pitcher, glass, jar, or other utensil over your hands. (To warm water, water may be heated in a small saucepan on a stove, burner, or fire, then cooled with additional water as needed.)

Handwashing Procedure without Water

Germicide liquids and aerosols are commercially available from hospitals and medical supply companies for handwashing without water and can be carried in the nursing bag.

Equipment

1. Bottle or can of handwashing germicide.

Procedure

1. Squeeze or spray small amount onto hand.
2. Rub germicide onto all surfaces of hands, fingers, and fingernails for 30 seconds. The germicide evaporates and no towel is needed (Trotter, 1992).
3. Handwashing with germicide is only effective for four cleansings. Water must be used for the fifth washing.

TABLE 7–8

Cleaning Equipment in the Home

Remember, the rule of thumb is to bring as little equipment in and out of the home as possible to decrease the possibility of cross-contamination.

Equipment

Article to be washed
Soap
Running water
Paper towels
Plastic bags
Disposable gloves

Procedure

1. Don disposable gloves when working with equipment contaminated with any body fluids or blood.
2. Rinse article with *cold* running water. (Rationale: Cold water releases organic material from the equipment whereas warm or hot water will make the material adhere.)
3. Wash with warm, soapy water using friction.
4. Rinse well with clear water.
5. Dry thoroughly.
6. Remove disposable gloves.
7. Dispose of gloves (inside out) into plastic trash bag using blood and body fluid precautions.
8. Disinfect equipment or article as indicated.
9. Dry article thoroughly or store as agency procedure indicates.
10. Wash hands.

From Trotter, J. (1992). Home care. In S. Smith and D. Duell (Eds.). *Clinical nursing skills* (3rd ed.). Norwalk, CT: Appleton & Lange.

for as though they are potentially positive for human immunodeficiency virus (HIV) and other blood-borne infections. All health agencies adopt universal precautions when handling blood and body fluids, needles, and other materials (see Chapter 29). Infection control guidelines for people living with AIDS in the community also are included.

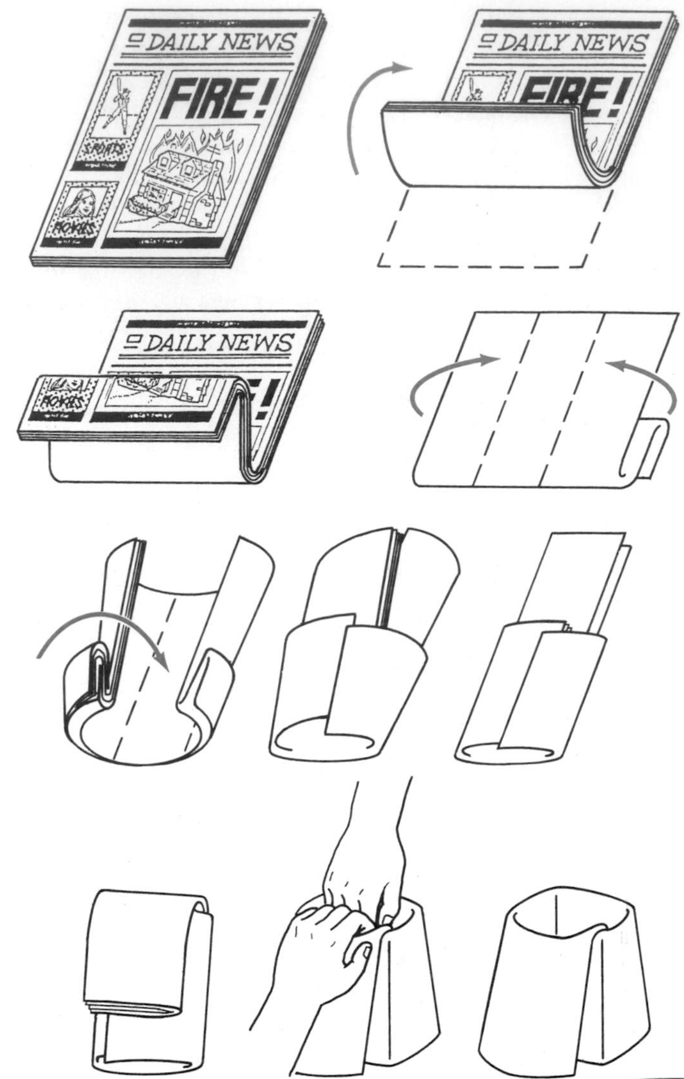

Figure 7–4 ● Step-by-step illustration of how to fold a newspaper to make a waste disposal bag. (Redrawn from American Red Cross. (1979). *Family health and home nursing* (p. 520). Garden City, NJ: Doubleday.)

MODIFYING EQUIPMENT AND PROCEDURES IN THE HOME

From its inception district nursing involved teaching families in the home about the care of the ill and preventive hygiene practices. The nurse assisted the family in using available equipment, in modifying household items for health-related purposes, and in making equipment. How can a family make bed tables and bed rails? How can a drawer become an infant bed? Between 1913 and 1979, the American Red Cross published eight editions of a book for family caretakers that addressed hygiene and home care of the sick. Olson's (1947) handbooks taught nurses about improvising equipment in the home to care for the sick.

The need to modify home equipment has been reduced by the availability of durable medical equipment for purchase and rent (such as hospital beds and commodes) and disposable equipment (such as dressing trays). Medicare and some other health insurance and assistance plans often pay for such equipment. However, many are not eligible for reimbursement because they are not eligible for skilled home health care (see Chapter 29). Therefore, improvised equipment is a cost-effective means of assisting families to care for such individuals. Books for families (Parker and Dietz, 1980) and for nurses (Humphrey, 1986) discuss equipment modifications.

As previously discussed, the community health nursing bag usually contains only the necessary equipment for basic medical asepsis, physical assessment, and disposal of wastes. Newspaper can be folded to make small waste disposal bags for noninfectious waste that are both inexpensive and biodegradable (see Figure 7–4).

En route to homes, the nursing bag is to be kept clean and safe from theft. Always keep the bag in sight or have it locked in the vehicle's trunk or covered hatch or in a covered box. For example, do not drive to a restaurant for lunch, open the trunk, and place the bag in the trunk. Rather, immediately before leaving a home, put the bag in the trunk, then drive away. The bag is safe and out of sight until it is needed at another home visit.

Just as the floor in a hospital is considered dirty, so too are streets, sidewalks, the ground, vehicle floors, and floors in homes. Do not place a nursing bag on any of these surfaces. Newspapers are considered clean and provide a field on which to place your nursing bag.

Modifications in the use of assessment equipment may also be needed. For example, infant scales are not always available. An alternative procedure is to weigh a parent on the bathroom scale, weigh the parent again with the infant, and subtract the first value. Although the parent should be dressed similarly at each visit to reduce variation, this procedure provides a gross estimate of infant weight.

Teaching family members to assess their own health status is often a responsibility of community health nurses. By using the family's equipment, the procedures can be tailored to specific circumstances. For example it may be more appropriate to use the thermometer available in the home and assist the family members in effective, safe, clean use. Cool water can be used as a lubricant for rectal temperature-taking if clean petroleum jelly is not available. Family members can be taught that it is unhygienic to insert thermometers into a jar of petroleum jelly that is also used for chapped hands and lips.

When families give medications, especially liquids, it is important to validate the type and size of spoons and droppers used to ensure that the doses given match the doses prescribed. Alarm clocks can be used to assist families to remember medication schedules.

Postvisit Activities

You have prepared yourself for a home visit, considered your own safety, and conducted a home visit. You have considered your relatedness with the family and management of time and equipment. You have a right to feel successful and pleased with yourself. What comes next?

Postvisit activities provide a time for your evaluation and work on behalf of the family: collaboration, referral, and recording. This conclusion of one visit becomes the beginning or preinitiation for the next encounter. A plan of care is derived from the information you have assessed. The initial home visit, the first of few or many visits in your nurse-family relationship, is complete.

EVALUATING AND PLANNING THE NEXT HOME VISIT

How does a community health nurse determine whether the home visit has been successful? What criteria are used to determine the success of any nurse-client encounter? Usually the nurse looks at the scope and specificity of the nursing process, the degree of client satisfaction, the quality of the nurse-client relationship, and the health behavior and status of the client.

How can these criteria be applied to the evaluation of a specific home visit? Table 7–9 lists questions that were derived from the criteria; you may wish to develop more.

TABLE 7–9

Determining the Success of Your Home Visit

Preinitiation

Was your preplanning adequate in scope to assist you in anticipating the needs of the family?

How did a review of nursing literature before the home visit strengthen your knowledge base and foster your role security?

Home Visit

To what degree were you able to express your purpose for the home visit and to elicit the perception of family members?

How were you able to address the purpose?

Did any major issues arise for which you were not prepared? If so, how did you handle them?

What data do you have to support your inferences about the family's satisfaction with the home visit? To what degree did you validate the accuracy of your inferences with the family members?

How satisfied were you with your visit? What contributed to your satisfaction?

What cues indicate that you and the family are engaged in the relationship?

What cues indicate that the interactions were appropriate to the phase of the relationships?

What health care behaviors did one or more family members agree to initiate or modify? Or what information did they indicate they were clearer about?

Can you identify any changes in the health status of one or more family members?

Postvisit Activities

How complete were your legal records? Were gaps in your data-base revealed? If so, what plans are necessary for collecting the missing data?

What activities are necessary to complete any referrals?

What consultation with your faculty, supervisor, and/or other members of the health care team would be helpful?

What plans are evolving for your next home visit in the areas of data collection, teaching, other direct care, and referral?

What changes, if any, in equipment, asepsis, or safety require planning prior to the next home visit?

Adapted from Smith C. (1987). *Determining the success of your home visit.* Unpublished manuscript. Baltimore, MD: University of Maryland School of Nursing. Used with permission.

CONSULTING/COLLABORATING WITH THE TEAM

Consultation is seeking the advice or opinion of an expert. Community health nurses may consult with an array of practitioners in other disciplines, such as medicine, physical therapy, and environmental hygiene. Nurses with specialties are also available. For example, psychiatric nurses can assist in formulating a plan of care for an interpersonally intense family situation; pediatric nurses in regional neonatal intensive care units can demonstrate the use of monitoring equipment to you and the parents before an infant at risk for sudden infant death syndrome is discharged to home. Your supervisor and peers are also available to share opinions about family care in formal and informal conferences.

Even if you are just beginning community health nursing practice, you are the individual who has made the home visit and experienced meeting the family in their environment. You are therefore in a position to collaborate with nursing and multidisciplinary teams. You are in a position to share assessment information, what it means to the family, and what nursing inferences you have derived. You are also able to contribute ideas for realistic goals and time frames. Development of a plan agreed on by the entire team helps to prevent duplication and gaps in care. For example, will home visits be made jointly by disciplines to prevent family confusion or will home visits be made separately to promote intermittent reinforcement?

Consultation and collaboration may occur via phone, by mail, or in person, depending on the complexity and urgency of the situation. Emergencies are best handled with telephone calls followed by written communications. Complex situations are best handled by face-to-face conferences, in which all disciplines can hear the same information simultaneously. One participant can be designated to write and circulate a meeting summary.

As a beginner it is safest to always report to your supervisor about changes in family health status and functioning, emergencies, threats to your safety, and situations that you do not understand clearly. This is considered necessary for sound legal practice.

MAKING REFERRALS

Referral is the act or instance of sending or directing someone for treatment, aid, information, or a decision. If the family members have needs that cannot be satisfied with available resources and the problem is not within the scope of your responsibility and capability (or that of your team), making a referral may be necessary.

Referrals may be indicated for the following reasons: screening procedures; medical diagnostic consultations, laboratory tests, or procedures; emergency services; nursing home placement; educational, vocational, and social services; or consultations with medical, nursing, and other disciplines regarding the treatment and care regimen (Smith, 1972).

Referral always consists of communication among three individuals: the client, the person making the referral, and the person or persons to whom the client has been referred. The most short-term goal is that the family member or members and the person to whom they are referred make contact. The intermediate goal is that the family receive the desired treatment, aid, or information. The ultimate goal is that the family's needs will be met because of the relationship with the third person. It is ideal for the nurse to stay involved with the family until connections have been made between the family and the third person. The nurse can evaluate the degree to which the family and agency are satisfied with the referral. At times the original referral proves to be inappropriate for family needs and additional referrals are necessary.

The nurse initiating the referral must have prior knowledge of *both* the family and the agency or specialist to whom the family is being referred. The nurse must then decide what information about the family needs to be shared with the agency and what information the family needs to be given about the agency. It often takes up to 6 months for a community health nurse to learn the details about health and social agencies and private practitioners in the specific geographic area of practice. Since personnel and policies frequently change, keeping up to date is a continual process (see Chapter 17).

LEGAL RECORDING

All home visits are to be documented on the legal record. Telephone calls from and to the family and with other disciplines involved are also to be recorded. Ineffective telephone calls and home visits are recorded to show effort and timeliness of nursing attempts to provide care.

Most community health agencies use some version of the problem-oriented recording (POR) system, which consists of forms for databases, including identifying information; problem lists; selected flow sheets; progress notes; and discharge summaries. In agencies that do not use POR, narrative progress notes and flow sheets are used.

KEY IDEAS

1. Home visiting is a traditional activity of community health nurses for providing health promotion and all levels of prevention to individuals and families.
2. Home visits provide opportunities for family-focused care, for personalizing care within the environment in which the care will actually be implemented, and for modifying care to family preferences. Home visits also provide an opportunity for detecting health threats of which the family may be unaware.
3. Despite budget cuts during the 1980s for home visiting by health departments, home visiting for care of the ill and disabled persons is the fastest growing segment of community health nursing. Home visiting for care of the ill and disabled has proved to be cost-effective when compared with providing care in hospitals and nursing homes.
4. Practice and research indicate that positive preventive health outcomes result from home visits by community health nurses. Although the health results obtained from home visits can exceed those obtained by visits to clinics and private physicians, political debate continues regarding the cost-effectiveness of home visiting for health promotion and primary prevention.
5. Home visiting involves a process of initiating relationships with family members, negotiating and implementing a family-focused plan of care, and evaluating health outcomes and family satisfaction.
6. Each home visit involves several phases or steps: preplanning the visit, traveling to the home and initiating the visit, accomplishing the interventions, evaluating and summarizing the visit with the family, ending the visit and leaving the home, and conducting postvisit activities.
7. Relationships with families within their homes are different from nurse-client relationships in inpatient settings. Families retain more control over the environment; the relationship may extend over weeks, months, or years; and goal achievement depends more on an interdependent partnership between the nurse and the family.

8. Nurses can reduce potential conflicts in their relationships with families by clarifying the purpose of the visits, carefully negotiating contracts with family members, being aware of their own feelings and values, and honoring confidentiality.
9. Maintaining nurse and family safety and appropriately handling emergencies are important responsibilities when making home visits.
10. Efficiency is increased when community health nurses wisely manage their time and equipment. Promoting personal hygiene and a clean home environment reduces the likelihood of the transmission of communicable diseases among family members and between households.
11. Postvisit activities include evaluating the visit and the plan of care, collaborating with other team members, conducting referrals, making an entry in the legal health record, and planning for future contacts with the family.
12. Community health nurses need to continue to demonstrate the cost-effectiveness of home visits with various aggregates. Community health nurses are exploring creative models of nursing care that reintegrate care of the sick with health promotion and primary prevention within families.

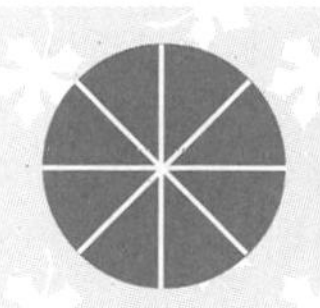

CASE STUDY

Home Visiting

A community health nurse employed by a suburban county health department in a maternal child health program received a referral from the local hospital for a young mother and her newborn daughter. The referral was initiated by a nurse who was employed by the health department and the hospital for the express purpose of interviewing and identifying families at risk for child health problems.

Planning for the Home Visit

The community health nurse reviewed the referral for identifying information, information about the family, and the purpose of the referral. The referral included the parents' and infant's names, address, and telephone number; a brief delivery history (normal, 5 lb. 7 oz. female infant born of vaginal delivery); the results of screening tests for illicit drugs and sexually transmitted diseases (negative); the method of infant feeding (breast-feeding); and a description of mother-infant interactions (anxiety regarding breast-feeding and living arrangements) observed by the hospital nurse. The mother had agreed to being contacted by a community health nurse for home visits.

The referral further stated that the mother had moved to the county 2 months ago, interrupting her prenatal care. She was staying with her cousin while her husband traveled to a neighboring state in search of employment. Therefore the community health nurse inferred that it would be especially important to further assess the mother's support systems, knowledge of health care resources, and finances.

When the community health nurse telephoned the home to make an appointment for a home visit she could hear the voices of children in the background; their volume made it difficult to hear the mother. The community health nurse introduced herself by name, stated that she worked for the health department, and indicated that she had been notified by the hospital that the mother had delivered a baby girl. The nurse asked how the mother and infant were doing. The mother replied that she was very tired and was not sure that her infant was getting enough to eat; she was giving her infant formula from a bottle and trying to breast-feed at alternate feedings. Yes, she was eager to have the nurse visit in her cousin's home. The nurse arranged a visit for the next day at a time when the infant usually was being fed.

The nurse determined that the family lived in a trailer behind an old farmhouse near a new housing subdivision. The nurse found the address on her county map and decided that she felt the area was adequately safe to visit alone.

After completing the telephone call, she reflected that the purpose of the maternal child health program was to promote the well-being of families with infants, to prevent problems such as infant "failure to thrive" and injuries, to ensure that family members received appropriate immunizations and health care, and to promote positive parent-child relationships and child development. Her focus would be on the infant, the mother, and other household members.

In preparation for the visit the community health nurse obtained the appropriate agency forms for recording postpartum and newborn care in the home and obtaining the mother's written permission for services. She restocked her nurse's bag with soap, towels, disposable tape (used to measure infant head circumference), thermometers, sphygmomanometer, and stethoscope. She obtained an infant scale. To be prepared for teaching the mother, the nurse collected pamphlets on postpartum care, care of a newborn, breast-feeding, infant safety, and community resources. Before leaving the office she left an itinerary of her visits for the next day; she would go directly from her home to her first visit.

Initiating the Home Visit

As she drove to the home, she noticed that there was a "for sale" sign on the farm property and that tall grass and weeds grew in the field. A relatively new trailer sat next to a farmhouse, which was in disrepair. The yard around the trailer was mowed and contained a plastic swimming pool and several children's bikes. No animals appeared.

As she parked her car and approached the trailer a woman appeared at the trailer door and called, "Are you the nurse?" The nurse replied that she was and introduced herself by name. The woman introduced herself, stated that her cousin and the cousin's infant were inside, and motioned for the nurse to come in.

The nurse noticed three preschoolers playing on the floor and a young woman sitting with an infant on a sheet-covered sofa. The nurse introduced herself and so did the mother. The nurse said hello to the children as well. The chairs were piled with clothes and there was nowhere in the room to sit. The nurse noticed the dinette chairs and asked if she could move one to the living room to sit down; the cousin agreed.

The nurse repeated that she was from the health department and was there to be of assistance to the mother and her newborn. The nurse sat quietly, looking at the mother and newborn, waiting for the mother to speak. The mother smiled faintly and asked if the nurse would like to hold her infant. The mother was dressed in nightclothes; her hair was uncombed and she had dark circles under her eyes. The nurse stated she would be delighted to hold the infant but that she would like to wash her hands first.

Implementation of the Home Visit

After washing her hands, the nurse held the infant, looked into her face, and spoke softly about how alert she was. She asked the infant's name. The nurse noticed that the infant's respirations were regular and her color was good; her fontanelles were not depressed or bulging and her mucous membranes were moist; her umbilical cord was drying without exudate; she did not appear to be in any distress. Therefore, the nurse focused on the mother.

The mother offered that she was tired because the infant did not yet sleep through the night. She was sleeping on the couch and the infant slept in an infant car seat that belonged to her cousin. She was disappointed that her husband had not yet come to see his daughter. He had telephoned about his job interviews and had wired her some money from his unemployment check. Yes, she was able to purchase some diapers and had a few bottles. Her cousin had loaned her some infant clothes.

When asked specific questions about her postpartum status she replied that her vaginal bleeding was getting lighter and did not contain any clots. She did not have any bothersome pains in her abdomen or her legs. Her blood pressure was 130/76 mm Hg. She was eating two meals a day, but wondered what to eat to "help make my milk." Her breasts were engorged and she reported difficulty getting the infant to latch onto her nipples.

The infant began to fret and root as if she were hungry. The mother noticed the infant's behavior and stated it was time for her to eat. The nurse stated she would like to observe the breast-feeding so she could make suggestions; the mother eagerly agreed. The nurse used the opportunity to demonstrate several positions for holding the infant during breast-feeding and how to use the rooting reflex and position her nipples to assist her daughter. The nurse explained that the more the infant sucked and emptied the breasts, the more milk would be produced. The nurse suggested the mother empty one breast before going to the second. The nurse affirmed what the mother was doing correctly and worked with the mother to improve her technique.

As the infant fell asleep, the nurse had the mother sign the permission form for home visiting services. Most of the visit was devoted to teaching related to breast-feeding because this was the immediate concern of the mother and was also essential for the hydration and nutrition of the infant. The nurse assessed that the mother had completed high school and had worked in an office for a while. The nurse reviewed the written pamphlets on breast-feeding, postpartum changes in mothers, safety for newborns, and medical emergencies. She gave the mother the telephone numbers of a local church, which supplies infant clothes and equipment, and the local La Leche League group, which provides information and support for breast-feeding women.

The nurse further assessed the mother's living arrangements, financial circumstances, and plans for obtaining a postpartum examination for herself and well-child care for the infant. She had no health insurance but had initiated application for medical assistance while in the hospital. She had applied for Women, Infants, and Children (WIC) vouchers to help obtain nutrition for herself while she breast-fed. She would return to the hospital for a postpartum visit, but she did not know where to obtain care for her infant. The nurse provided a list of pediatricians who accepted medical assistance payments and the health department's well-child clinics.

The cousin and the mother both confirmed that the mother planned to stay for a "couple of months," until her husband returned for her. Yes, it was crowded in their trailer, but "families need to help each other out and I know a lot about caring for babies," the cousin asserted.

Ending the Home Visit

The nurse stated it was almost time for her to leave. The mother volunteered that she felt much more confident with her breast-feeding and that she understood she did not have to feed both formula and breast milk. She would call the church for more infant clothes and call the La

Leche League. The nurse reinforced that she was doing well caring for her infant and had a plan for obtaining medical care when she needed it.

The nurse left her written name, agency address, and telephone number. The nurse stated that she would telephone the next day to see how the breast-feeding was working and whether the mother's breast engorgement had decreased. A second home visit was planned for the next week.

Postvisit Activities

During the evaluation of her home visit, the community health nurse was pleased that she had been able to establish a relationship with the mother and to offer information related to breast-feeding that was immediately helpful. No additional referrals or consulations were needed.

The community health nurse completed her legal recording on the client identification form, postpartum assessment form, newborn infant assessment form, and progress note. She identified the problems as altered breast-feeding; potential for growth related to care of firstborn; knowledge deficit related to community resources; and income deficit related to unemployment.

The family strengths included the father's motivation to seek employment, the mother's education and readiness to learn, the mother's attentiveness to her newborn, and the support from her extended family. The nurse concluded that she needed more information about the social situation before she could predict how long she would need to continue the home visits. Her assessment priorities for the next home visit included information about the spousal relationship and the mother's coping skills, more about the cousin's family and their health needs, a home safety assessment, and a developmental assessment of the infant.

The community health nurse would start her next home visit by inquiring about how the week had gone, how the mother was feeling, and whether breast-feeding had improved. She would also evaluate whether the mother had contacted the church and La Leche League and the degree to which these resources had been helpful.

GUIDELINES FOR LEARNING

1. Describe experiences you have had with home visits to households in which you did not know anyone (e.g., selling newspapers or collecting money for charities). Recall your feelings. What did you do that was usually effective? Share your ideas with others.
2. Describe your own home and compare it with another home that is much different. Notice what categories you use for comparison: (a) What are the themes in your comparison (e.g., did you compare the level of activity in the home or did you compare the amount and type of furniture)? (b) Which of your senses are represented in your comparison, in addition to sight?
3. After an initial home visit to a family, describe the physical features of the home without including value judgments or generalized conclusions such as "the furniture was in good shape." Have another person critique how successful you were. Notice which of your values or biases were revealed.
4. After a home visit to a family, describe several behaviors of family member(s) that you believe to have been in response to your interactions. Speculate on at least three possible meanings of the behaviors. Create a plan to validate which of the meanings is most accurate.
5. Write an agreement that you desire to negotiate with a family on the first home visit. Role play how this might be expressed verbally to the family members; be certain to validate with the "clients" what they actually agree to.
6. Discuss how a family focus can be fostered during a home visit when there is only one household member present.
7. After an initial home visit, use the guide for Determining the Success of Your Home Visit (Table 7–9) or the Home Visiting Evaluation Tool (Figure 7–3) to help preplan for your second visit.
8. Create an artistic expression of what "relating with a family, being concerned for their well-being and growth" means to you. (You might work with drawing, painting, music, prose, dance, or poetry, for example.)

REFERENCES

American Nurses' Association. (1987). *Standards and scope of hospice nursing practice.* Washington, DC: Author.

American Red Cross. (1979). *Family health and home nursing.* Garden City, NJ: Doubleday.

Arnold, E., & Boggs, K. (1989). *Interpersonal relationships: Professional communication skills for nurses.* Philadelphia: W. B. Saunders.

Barrett, J. (1982). Postpartum home visits by maternity nursing students. *Journal of Obstetric, Gynecologic, and Neonatal Nursing, 11*(4), 238–240.

Beck, C. (1992). Caring among nursing students. *Nurse Educator, 17*(6), 22–27.

Benenson, A. S. (Ed.). (1990). *Control of communicable diseases in man* (15th ed.). Washington, D.C.: American Public Health Association.

Burgess, A. (1990). *Psychiatric nursing in the hospital and the community* (5th ed.). Norwalk, CT: Appleton & Lange.

Burns, P., & Gianutsos, R. (1987). Reentry of the head-injured survivor into the educational system: First steps. *Journal of Community Health Nursing, 4*(3), 145–152.

Centers for Disease Control (CDC). (1985). *Guidelines for prevention and control of nosocomial infections* (P.B. 86–133022LL). Springfield, VA: National Technical Information Service.

Davis, C. (1990). What is empathy, and can empathy be taught? *Physical Therapy, 70,* 707–711.

Engelke, M., & Engelke, S. (1992). Predictors of the home environment of high-risk infants. *Journal of Community Health Nursing, 9*(3), 171–181.

Friedman, M. (1983). *Manual for Effective Community Health Nursing Practice.* Monterey, CA: Wadsworth.

Gary, F., & Kavanagh, C. (1991). *Psychiatric mental health nursing.* Philadelphia: J. B. Lippincott.

Glugover, D. (1987). Community health nurses: Role models for change in our lives and in our client's lives. *Caring, 84,* 14–15.

Goldsborough, J. (1969). Involvement. *American Journal of Nursing, 69*(1), 66–68.

Haber, J., Hoskins, P., Leach, A., & Sideleau, B. (1987). Self-awareness. In J. Haber, A. Leach, & B. Sideleau (Eds.). *Comprehensive Psychiatric Nursing* (pp. 77–86). New York: McGraw-Hill.

Helgeson, D., & Berg, C. (1985). Contracting: A method of health promotion. *Journal of Community Health Nursing, 2*(4), 199–207.

Humphrey, C. (1986). *Home care nursing handbook.* Norwalk, CT: Appleton-Century-Crofts.

Katzman, E., Cohen, C., & Lukes, E. (1987). Students *do* make a difference. *Journal of Community Health Nursing, 4*(1), 49–56.

Kristjanson, L., & Chalmers, K. (1991). Preventive work with families: Issues facing public health nurses. *Journal of Advanced Nursing, 16,* 147–153.

Leitch, C., & Tinker, R. (1978). *Primary Care.* Philadelphia: F. A. Davis.

Lewis, J., & Chaisson, R. (1993, September). *Tuberculosis: The reemergence of an old foe.* Paper presented at the Baltimore City Health Department 200th Anniversary Celebration Conference, Baltimore, MD.

Mayers, M. (1973). Homevisit—Ritual or therapy? *Nursing Outlook, 21*(5), 328–331.

Monteiro, L. (1985). Florence Nightingale on public health nursing. *American Journal of Public Health, 75*(2), 181–186.

Murray, S. (1968). *Farm and home visits: A guide for extension workers in many countries.* Washington, DC: U.S. Department of Agriculture.

Nadwairski, J. (1992). Inner-city safety for home care providers. *Journal of Nursing Administration, 22*(9), 42–47.

Olds, D., Henderson, C., Chamberlin, R., & Tatelbaum, R. (1986). Preventing child abuse and neglect: A randomized trial of nurse home visitation. *Pediatrics, 7*(1), 65–78.

Olson, L. (1947). *Improvised equipment in the home care of the sick.* Philadelphia: W. B. Saunders.

Parker, P., & Dietz, D. (1980). *Nursing at home: A practical guide to the care of the sick and the invalid in the home plus self-help instructions for the patient.* New York: Crown.

Raatikainen, R. (1991). Self-activeness and the need for help in domiciliary care. *Journal of Advanced Nursing, 16,* 1150–1157.

Rogers, C. (1969). *Freedom to learn.* Columbus, OH: Charles E. Merrill.

Sheridan, A., & Smith, R. (1975). Family-student contracts. *Nursing Outlook, 23*(2), 114–117.

Simmons, D. (1980). *A classification scheme for client problems in community health nursing* (DHHS Publication No. HRA 80–16). Hyattsville, MD: U.S. Department of Health and Human Services.

Smith, C. (1972). *Referral as triadic communication.* Unpublished manuscript.

Spradley, B. (Ed.). (1991). *Readings in community health nursing* (4th ed.). Philadelphia: J. B. Lippincott.

Trotter, J. (1992). Home care. In S. Smith & D. Duell (Eds.). *Clinical Nursing Skills* (3rd ed.). Norwalk, CT: Appleton & Lange.

van Manen, M. (1990). *Researching lived experience: Human science for an action sensitive pedagogy.* London, Ontario: The State University of New York.

Whyte, D. (1992). A family nursing approach to the care of a child with a chronic illness. *Journal of Advanced Nursing, 17,* 317–327.

World Health Organization (1987). *The Community Health Worker.* Geneva: Author.

Zerwekh, J. (1990). Public health nursing legacy: Historical practical wisdom. *Nursing and Health Care, 13*(2), 84–91.

Zerwekh, J. (1991, October). Tales from public health nursing: True detectives. *American Journal of Nursing,* pp. 30–36.

SUGGESTED READINGS

American Red Cross. (1989). *Nurses Assistant Training.* Washington, DC: Author.

American Red Cross. (1992). *Responding to emergencies.* St. Louis: Mosby–Year Book.

Brofman, J. (1979, October). An evening home visiting program. *Nursing Outlook,* pp. 657–661.

Centers for Disease Control. (1989). Guidelines for prevention of transmission of human immunodeficiency virus and hepatitis B virus to health-care and public-safety workers (No. S–6). *Morbidity and Mortality Weekly Report, 38,* 1–37.

Helvie, C., Hill, A., & Bambino, C. (1968, August). The setting and nursing practice: Part I. *Nursing Outlook,* pp. 27–29.

Keeling, B. (1978, March). Making the most of the first home visit. *Nursing 78,* pp. 24–28.

Lentz, J., & Meyer, E. (1979, September). The dirty house. *Nursing Outlook,* pp. 290–293.

Nadwairski, J. (1992). Inner-city safety for home care providers. *Journal of Nursing Administration, 22*(9), 42–47.

Price, J., & Broden, C. (1978, September). The reality in home visits. *American Journal of Nursing,* pp. 1536–1538.

Pruitt, R., Keller, L., & Hale, S. (1987). Mastering distractions that mar home visits. *Nursing and Health Care, 8*(6), 345–347.

Sargis, N., Jennrich, J., & Murray, K. (1987). Housing and health: A crucial link. *Nursing and Health Care, 8*(6), 335–338.

Stulginsky, M. (1993). Nurses' home health experience—Part I: The practice setting. *Nursing and Health Care, 14*(8), 402–407.

Stulginsky, M. (1993). Nurses' home health experience—Part II: The unique demands of home visits. *Nursing and Health Care, 14*(9), 476–485.

Chapter 8

A Family Perspective in Community Health Nursing

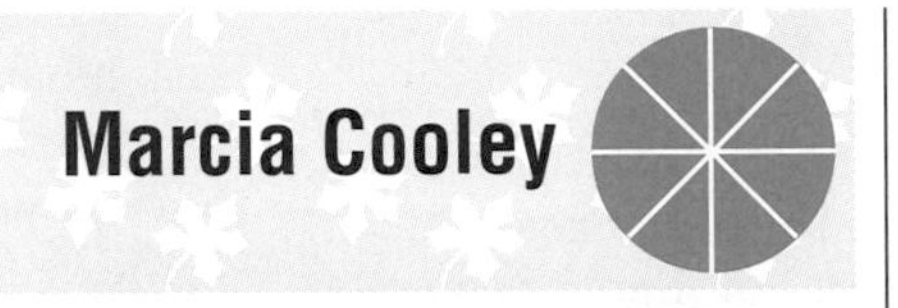
Marcia Cooley

Focus Questions

Why use a family perspective in community health nursing?

How do families differ? How are they the same?

What different family approaches have been proposed in the past?

How can these approaches be integrated?

What is family nursing?

How is the family perspective used within the practice of the community health nurse?

A Family Perspective

Family nursing can and should be practiced by all nurses. People are born, grow, live, and die within their families. Everyone has a family. Families have different structures and sizes, have different levels of connection and ways of operating with each other, and may be geographically close or distant. Families can offer support and love and can also bring their members disappointment and grief. People grow older, may move away, or may sometimes try to pretend they do not have a family, but ultimately the person one becomes is a reflection of the family from which he or she came.

THE FAMILY AS CLIENT

The family as a unit of care has been a focus in community health nursing since its beginning (Whall, 1986). Nurses and other workers in the community recognized that the family became a major source of support and influence in many situations. Whether the issue was an ill family member, a change in the family (e.g., a birth or a death), or disease prevention, the community health nurse learned to include the family in nursing care. People's lifestyles and, consequently, their health are intimately tied to the culture, values, beliefs, practices, and socioeconomic status they share with their families.

Appreciation of the family as a unit of care evolved naturally as community health nurses worked within the community. With this work came a recognition that not all families are able to provide all their members with what they need to reach optimum levels of health. Community health nurses have a unique position, because they are broadly educated and able to integrate different perspectives that make up an understanding of family functioning. Nurses also have a unique role within the community that offers them access to family situations. Focusing on the family is a helpful step to take in working toward a broader perspective of caring for the individual, the family, and the entire community.

Is there really a difference in using a family rather than an individual perspective? Consider the following example:

Michelle is a 13-year-old girl referred to the community health nurse by administrators at her middle school. Her attendance has been very poor, she is irritable and rebellious in class, her previously good grades are dropping, and she has recently gained so much weight the school nurse wonders if Michelle is pregnant. Depending on the professional's point of view, there are many different ideas of her "problem." The school system views her behavior as truant, the school psychologist wonders about depression, and her teacher views her as a behavior problem. Repeated attempts to involve her mother have had little success.

Suppose the community health nurse has been alerted to the need to visit and assess the family. During the visit, she realizes Michelle is staying home from school to watch her younger brother and sister on days her grandmother goes to work and has no other baby-sitter. Michelle is very unhappy about having to miss school but does not want anyone to know the situation at home. Her mother, who had been taking care of the children, is abusing drugs and is not a reliable person to care for the children. The younger children, age 6 and 8 years, have had repeated throat infections during the winter. No one has been able to take them to the clinic. Michelle is not pregnant, but has been so unhappy that she is overeating and gaining weight.

Thus, the opportunity to look at a bigger picture gives a very different perspective than the one presented when one takes an individual view of Michelle. It is difficult to view the situation as "Michelle's problem." The community health nurse may still choose to focus only on Michelle's difficulties, but realizes that these difficulties are connected to other issues and to the health of other people. Not only is Michelle's health a concern, but the health of the family is also at risk. The family could either be supportive of Michelle or block attempted interventions. Community health nursing recognizes the importance of the family and defines the entire family as the unit of treatment: Michelle will be involved, but the whole family will become the focus for nursing care.

There are many ways to look at a problem. In the past, science has often used a cause-and-effect way of thinking. "Germ A causes sickness B. Applying medicine C cures it." This is an example of cause-and-effect thinking, which became popular in the medical field after medications and inoculations proved to be successful in combatting specific infectious illnesses.

However, real life is more complex. Not every person exposed to a certain pathogen becomes ill. Becoming infected depends on such variables as general level of health, stress level at the time, previous antibody development, and genetic susceptibility. Many different events occur at the same time. When the organism experiencing these factors is in balance, health is usually maintained. When there is imbalance, illness or dysfunction may occur—not because of any one event, but because of a combination of factors. This recognition of the complexity and interconnectedness of a living organism is a systems, rather than a cause-and-effect, way of thinking.

Individuals in a family can be thought of as a "living" system. Each person is one of the elements that is interrelated with the others. A *boundary* or imaginary wall exists around the family, similar to the thin membrane of a cell wall. This boundary can vary. It can be rigid and impenetrable, or it can be a permeable membrane that allows exchange in and out of the system. Each member, although only a part of the system, has the potential to change the patterns and organization of the entire system. The individuals within the family make up something new that is different and greater than the simple sum of its members.

Living systems have parts that undergo growth and change. At any given point in time, the individuals in the family will be undergoing change themselves. The members are growing, developing, learning, and changing, usually on trajectories or paths that are recognizable as part of the life cycle. Thus, the family as a living system is constantly changing.

The boundaries of the system permit some exchange of information between the inside and outside. The family is one system; the community outside it is another. Bronfenbrenner (1979), while studying children in families, proposed the idea of different levels of systems: a mesosystem, a macrosystem, and an endosystem. The three levels constitute broader and broader environmental contexts in which the child will grow. Scheflen (1981) takes a similar approach in explaining different perspectives of schizophrenia. He describes how this one phenomenon can be viewed from genetic, biochemical, individual, family, community, and societal perspectives. Figure 8–1 depicts some different levels of analysis that could be used when thinking about family nursing care. Notice that family is not the only perspective, but one piece in an ever-broader context of conceptualizing the appropriate target of intervention.

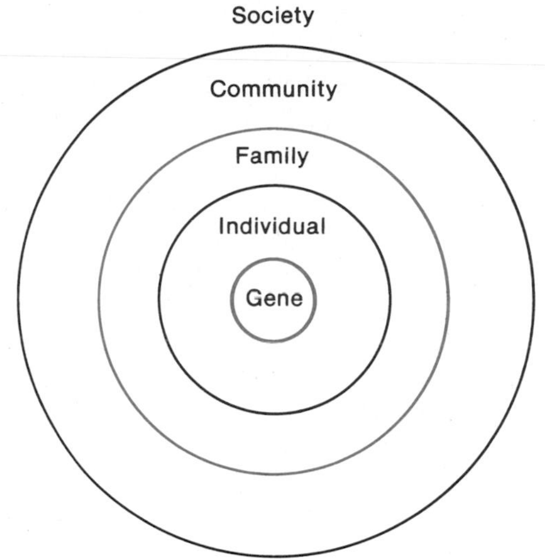

Figure 8–1 ● Levels of systems. (See text for explanation.)

WHY CHOOSE A FAMILY PERSPECTIVE?

Family Thinking Gives a Broader Picture. Viewing an individual in a smaller framework may narrow the information and understanding of the problem. It assumes that individuals act independently and in an isolated way when they are actually intimately connected with larger systems. When assessing a family member, the person may be able to be completely understood only if he or she is viewed within the context of the gestalt—the whole situation. Assessment using an individual perspective may miss important interrelated aspects of the problem or resources that can be used to promote health and alleviate distress.

The Family Is a Unit of Care. People often live in households as families. Families are organized in a structure with identified roles and leadership, and society expects families to assume some responsibility for each of their members. Economic resources are divided up by family. Family members also have emotional ties to each other. Even though society is assuming more and more of the family's functions, the family remains a workable unit.

The Family Assumes a Crucial Role in Maintaining Health. There is such a strong relationship between the family and health care that the role of the family becomes paramount in maintaining health. The family is a critical resource in the delivery of health care to people. Accessibility to health resources, making decisions about when to seek care, how health care is paid for, and how the recommended treatment regimens are carried out are all enacted within the family. Sometimes the family is the primary care provider for its ill and dependent members. Changes in lifestyle are often required for the whole family if the level of wellness for one of the members is affected.

Dysfunction in One Member May Be Related to Disturbance in the Whole Family. Because a family operates as a system, a symptom in one member may be a signal that something is happening in the family as a whole. Sometimes the family will work very hard on one health problem with some good results, only to have another health problem present in a second family member. A familiar example of this is an alcoholic family in which one spouse stops drinking, only to have the marriage break up or the "healthy" spouse become ill. Physical, emotional, and social problems are thought to be related to the degree of anxiety and emotional immaturity present and shared among family members in the entire system.

Dysfunction in One Member May Lead to Added Stress and Depletion of Resources for a Family. Some believe that any family member who is dysfunctional will ultimately affect the health of the entire system. Caring for an ill or dependent member can deplete financial resources, physical energy, and other sources of family support. Sometimes the health of other members is disturbed. Often the ability of the family to fulfill its maintenance functions for its members (such as giving time and attention to young children or sharing recreational activities) is affected by illness in a member.

Family and Intimate Relationships Are Important for Tracking the Occurrence and Incidence of Disease. To community health nurses attempting to prevent, track, and record disease processes, the relationships within families and other intimate partners are clearly significant. Family information is used in assessing needs, determining health care priorities, case finding, tracking and preventing the spread of communicable diseases, educating for preventive purposes, and organizing the delivery of care to special and large populations. The family is an essential piece of these epidemiological health care functions.

The Unique Goals of Family Nursing: Individual Health, Supportive Interpersonal Relationships, and an Effective Family Unit Can Be Achieved Only by Using a Family Perspective. Family nursing is a movement in nursing that is coming into its own identity. By definition, all nursing practice is oriented toward achievement of goals that are beneficial to the health and well-being of individuals within society. Nursing practice must be expanded to include all the above goals. The goals that are put forth in family nursing—goals for individuals, relationships, and the family unit—can be addressed only by using a family perspective.

What Is a Family?

DEFINITION OF FAMILY

Thus far this text has talked about families as if all families are alike and everyone understands what is meant when the word *family* is used. However, in the United States there are actually many different kinds of families. Community health nurses need a definition broad enough to encompass the many ways they will be interacting with families (Table 8–1). This definition must not ignore the atypical or nontraditional family forms that will often be encountered in current communities. The definition should also provide some structure to the way nurses think about families to establish a framework for intervention. The definition adopted by this text is as follows:

> A family is an open and developing system of interacting personalities with a structure and process enacted in relationships among the individual members, regulated by resources and stressors, and existing within the larger community.

TABLE 8–1

Definitions of Family

A married couple or other group of adult kinfolk who cooperate economically and in the upbringing of children, all or most of whom share a common dwelling (Gough, 1986).
The family is a haven in a heartless world (Lasch, 1986).
A family is a unity of interacting personalities (Burgess, 1926).
The basic unit of society and the social institution that has the most marked effect on its members (Friedman, 1986).
An open system that functions in relation to its broader sociocultural context and that evolves over the life cycle (Walsh, 1982).
A human social system with distinct characteristics that is composed of individuals whose characteristics are equally distinct (Friedemann, 1989).

HOW ARE FAMILIES ALIKE AND DIFFERENT?

All living systems need some sort of organization and pattern to function. Families also have this organization. Many people use a framework of structure, process, and function to describe the complex nature of families.

Structure. *Structure* refers to the elements in and organization of those elements within the family. Over the life of a family, structure does not remain exactly the same, but a certain continuity of structure is maintained. Structure is defined in several ways. Some define it anthropologically, using family types defined according to lineage and power. For example, families may be matriarchal or patriarchal. Others look at the arrangement of members within the system in terms of subsystems, coalitions, and other structures that have hierarchies and boundaries; this is explored in more depth in the structural-functional approach discussed later in this chapter. Still others believe structure means the diversity of family forms.

Family Forms. Some type of family exists in all societies, although there are a wide diversity of forms and even variations among classes within the same society. In Greece and America, for example, slaves were prevented by law from forming legal families. Even so, the family in some form (although not necessarily the traditional nuclear family) is an ideal that most people try to attain.

Family structures have changed across societies and over time. Our idea of the traditional American family living in a household with extended family members such as grandparents is actually a myth that has been popularized through the years (Hareven, 1982). The National Council of Family Relations suggests that current family types are varied and changing (Olson and Hanson, 1990). Table 8–2 presents some different family forms.

Process. A *process* is a phenomenon that occurs over a period of time. Families, individuals, and society go through processes of growth, development, and change. The term implies change, but within every change there is often some pattern and connectedness with previous and future patterns.

Family process can be defined as predictable and repetitive interaction patterns within families. For example, Mom always watches Johnnie's behavior very closely. Johnnie gets upset with her attention and complains to Dad. Dad goes to Mom and complains that she is too harsh with Johnnie. Mom backs off for a while but soon resumes her attention. Such interaction can be observed in dyads, or two-person groups, or in interconnecting "triangles" (three-person groups) within the family.

Families also seem to have a characteristic way of interacting as a unit in relation to the outside world; this process is open or closed, separate or connected. Families may allow information from the environment to help them

TABLE 8–2

Family Forms

Nuclear: A father, mother, and child living together but apart from both sets of their parents.
Extended: Three generations, including married brothers and sisters and their families.
Three-generational: Any combination of first-, second-, and third-generation members living within a household.
Dyad: Husband and wife or other couple living alone without children.
Single-parent: Divorced, never married, separated, or widowed male or female and at least one child. Most single-parent families are headed by women.
Step-parent: One or both spouses have been divorced or widowed and have remarried into a family with at least one child.
Blended or reconstituted: A combination of two families with children from one or both families and sometimes children of the newly married couple.
Single adult living alone: An increasingly common occurrence for the never married, divorced, or widowed.
Cohabiting: An unmarried couple living together.
No-kin: A group of at least two people sharing a relationship and exchanging support who have no legalized or blood tie to each other.
Compound: One man (or woman) with several spouses.
Gay: A homosexual couple living together with or without children. Children may be adopted, from previous relationships, or artificially conceived.
Commune: More than one monogamous couple sharing resources.
Group marriage: All individuals are married to each other and are considered parents of all the children.

problem-solve or close themselves off from outside influence. Families may act together in a cohesive manner, withdraw from each other, or even split apart. Their behavior may be random and chaotic or very rigid and predictable.

Function. Family functioning is used in this context to describe results for families. Does this family operate in a way that successfully provides for the needs of its members? Successful functioning means a measure of normality or health. How well individual family members care for self and others is a way of assessing that family's level of health. Unhealthy families are called *dysfunctional.*

Family functioning is best viewed as a continuum. When using the words *functional* or *dysfunctional,* one can get caught in thinking of family functioning as "good" or "bad." There is no such thing as a good or a bad family. All families fall somewhere on a continuum of optimal functioning in which all members benefit. There are many different ways to assess families according to different views of optimal family functioning. Bowen (1978) describes families as more or less healthy according to (1) their ability to separate thinking from feeling and (2) the amount of anxiety that is present in the family. Tapia (1982) defines levels of family functioning from chaotic to adult according to the family's degree of emotional maturity. Olson et al. (1982) suggest families should have moderate degrees of cohesion, coordination, and adaptability for healthy family function.

The important thing to remember is that for optimal family functioning, the structure and process must combine in a way that allows the family to function. To truly understand the functioning of a particular family, one must know about the particular stresses and history that have shaped this family's current way of operating. Conversely, the typical level of functioning of a family may determine the processes it develops and the decisions and events that alter family structure (e.g., divorce, single parenthood, the arrangement of subsystems). Structure, process, and function are interrelated, and all must be considered when assessing a family. However, no one structure, process, or type of function is proposed here as the "right" one. There are many variations within these dimensions that can lead to healthy families.

Historical Frameworks

The study of family does not fit neatly into any one field, be it genetics, physiology, anthropology, sociology, or psychology; many disciplines have contributed to the understanding of family functioning. The study of family is interdisciplinary, and theories of family have been broadly adapted and used. However, most frameworks in family have been drawn from family sociology or family therapy.

Sociologists have studied families since the earliest origins of that science in the United States. Developments during the 19th and early 20th century sprang from the need to solve emerging social problems. The 1950s saw an emergence of conceptual frameworks in family theory. About that time, interest in the family as a unit of treatment emerged in the psychiatric field. Family therapists began focusing on pathology within families. Relatively recent trends have included family theories attempting to describe the characteristics of healthy families, theories of family coping with stressful situations, and the emergence of frameworks for family nursing.

Family approaches can be separated into several areas that provide different viewpoints describing the complexity of the family. Families develop, interact, and communicate; have structures; cope with stress; develop identity; and operate as systems. The following pages describe these in more detail.

FAMILY DEVELOPMENT

The family development approach attempts to track change over time in a family. Families and individuals are engaged in a developmental process of growth, aging, and change over their life span. In this approach, a longitudinal view of the family classifies and predicts differences in families as they develop. It assumes that both individuals in the family and the family as a whole need to accomplish certain tasks at specific times in their life cycles. As the family confronts various *stages* of the life cycle, *developmental tasks* must be achieved if the stage is to be negotiated successfully. These tasks carry certain role expectations. If the tasks are not achieved at specific times as a result of stress, crises, lack of resources, or unhealthy family structure and process, they may never be completely achieved. The better equipped a family is to help each member meet his or her developmental tasks and the family meet its group tasks, the more successful the development of the family. The theory assumes there are commonalities to these changes and attempts to predict what will happen for all families.

Duvall (1957) adapted this approach from the theory of individual developmental tasks proposed by Havighurst. Duvall defined nine ever-changing family developmental tasks that span the family life cycle (Table 8–3) and outlined eight stages of the family life cycle and specific tasks for each stage. Family stages are defined by the age of the oldest child. For example, a family that has two children, aged 7 and 2, would be considered a school-age family rather than a preschool family.

In the cycle of family development, the *transition* from one stage to the next is the critical period. The ease with which a family progresses through these critical phases is determined to some extent by the completion of earlier tasks. For example, a family in the launching stage typically has a young adult who is preparing to leave home. The family in this stage must successfully release the young adult, maintain a supportive home base, and reestablish the relationships and structure within the family to adjust to the missing member. The transition is easier if the family has completed earlier transitions successfully. For example, what if a family is trying to launch a young adult but has never worked out a way to share the responsibilities involved with day-to-day life? The member who is about to be launched might be unprepared to accept adult responsibilities.

Duvall's ideas provide a structured and logical way of looking at family life. However, this framework tends to view all families as nuclear (i.e., mother-father-children).

TABLE 8–3

Stages of the Family Life Cycle

A married couple: Newly established, without children.
Childbearing: Oldest child, birth to 2½ years.
Preschool-age: Oldest child, 2½ to 6 years.
School-age: Oldest child, 6 to 13 years.
Teenage: Oldest child, 13 to 20 years.
Launching: Period from departure of the oldest child to departure of the youngest (empty nest).
Middle-aged: Empty nest to retirement.
Aging: Period from retirement to death of both spouses.

From Duvall, E.M. (1957). *Family development.* Chicago: J.B. Lippincott.

The organization of the developmental stages is based on the assumption that every family will experience the birth and eventual release of children. This portrait of family life does not represent modern families.

Others have expanded Duvall's ideas to include categories of family life that also take into account the position of the younger siblings. McGoldrick and Carter (1982) have recognized that families take different forms and are often three-generational in nature. In their model, the family life cycle is more than one generation, and families react to both the past and the future. For many families, for example, when the youngest child leaves home, increased responsibilities for elderly parents often arise.

A community health nurse who is aware of developmental family theory will attempt to determine the family's stage in the life cycle and to assess the family's knowledge of current developmental demands, the strategies they are using to meet these demands, and their success at accomplishing them. Some families need information about the "usual" course that can be expected. Others may benefit from interventions that help them arrange some balance between the developmental demands and other demands such as illness, losing a job, or scarce family resources. Sometimes in families with an ill member, the needs of a healthy child will get lost in the shuffle. The goal is to enable the family to accomplish its function for all its members, not just the ones who are ill or otherwise in the forefront.

THE FAMILY AS A SYSTEM

Thinking about the family as a system is so common that many other approaches actually combine their way of thinking about families with a systems perspective. The systems perspective views the family as a unit and was first proposed by von Bertalanffy (1968) as the *general systems theory.* He described certain principles applicable to all systems; some are as follows:

1. A system is a unit where the *whole* is greater than the sum of its parts.
2. There are certain *rules* that govern the operation of such systems.
3. Every system has a *boundary* that is somewhat open or closed.
4. Boundaries allow exchange of information and resources into *(inputs)* and outside *(outputs)* the system.
5. *Communication* and feedback mechanisms between parts of the system are important in the function of the system.
6. *Circular causality* helps to explain what is happening better than linear causality. A change in one part of the system leads to change in the whole system.
7. Systems operate on the principle of *equifinality.* The same end point can be reached from a number of starting points or in different ways.

8. Systems appear to have a purpose. This purpose is often the avoidance of *entropy,* or complete randomness and disorganization.
9. Systems are made up of *subsystems* and are themselves part of *suprasystems.*

Family therapists were the first to apply systems theory to families. Approaches such as Minuchin and Fishman's (1981) and Satir's (1972), described later in this chapter, are based on the idea of the family as a system in which the whole is different and greater than the individual members. A family system perspective recognizes that change in one part of the system will affect the entire family. Because the system has the tendency to want to stay the same *(morphostasis),* the family will usually attempt to resist the change even if it is a helpful one. Nurses who are planning interventions with families must take into account this resistance and the implications for the entire system.

Suppose a family with a disabled child is not complying with daily treatments. Planning an intervention that encourages the mother to spend more time on these treatments may help the disabled child, but may take the mother away from tasks that need to be accomplished for her other children. The goal of viewing families as an interconnected system makes nursing care more difficult to plan and perform but is a more accurate way to think about families.

Families tend to have boundaries that have different permeabilities. Some are more open or closed to the environment. Some will allow information and resources to pass back and forth freely, while others shut off this exchange. Families are exposed to stress over time. When stress is present in an open system, it can result in adaptation and growth in the individuals. When stress is present in a more closed family system, it results in maladaptation; distorted perceptions, thoughts, and feelings; and less capable individuals. Community health nurses interacting with families need to be aware of the character of a particular family's boundaries. Helping a family become aware of its tendencies to use resources from the environment often promotes family health.

Family systems tend to want to reach relatively steady states, but change can occur. Change occurs most often when at least one member of the system, often the one who is the most flexible or free of constraints and has some power in the family, makes a change in his or her way of functioning within the family. In this way of thinking, interventions for families are not directed at the member who is ill, injured, or at risk, but at the members who are strongest and most able to change. This means the nurse will plan and target interventions with the members in the system who have some freedom and strength to carry out the interventions. A nurse who is working with a family caring for an aging mother may choose to spend more of her time with a daughter-in-law who has indicated a willingness to help, rather than with the aging mother or her ill spouse, who is having difficulty himself. Family interventions include the entire family, building on its strengths rather than focusing on its weaknesses.

BOWEN'S FAMILY SYSTEMS THEORY

Murray Bowen is the founder of a school of family therapy that developed the family systems approach in more specific ways. Bowen's thinking about families was stimulated during his work at the National Institute of Mental Health, where he began observing families of schizophrenics. He and his staff had the opportunity to observe family interaction on a psychiatric inpatient research unit. His observations of first the mother, then the nuclear family, and eventually other generations of the family have been articulated in Bowen's family systems theory (Bowen, 1978).

A key concept involves the *level of differentiation,* or a person's ability to separate his or her emotions and thoughts. People exist on a continuum that ranges from being able to separate decisions and emotional reactions to being totally driven by automatic emotional responses. When one is operating in a high feeling state, the need to be approved of or close to other people is paramount; operating in an autonomous or self-directed way becomes very difficult. A person's level of differentiation will relate to his or her ability to operate successfully in the many spheres of life, including job, parenting, managing money, and health habits. A person's physical, emotional, and social functioning is related to his or her level of differentiation and the amount of anxiety present in the family system.

The *triangle* is another concept that is helpful in understanding family operations (Fig. 8–2). Any two-person system is unstable. Within a short period of time, tension develops between the two people and results in the automatic "triangling in" of a third person. Each triangle has three sides: a close one where two people are allied, a conflictual one where two people are in disagreement, and a distant one where two people are emotionally separated (Triangle A). In periods of calm, the distant position is uncomfortable. The distant person (person 2) will usually try to move into a closer position (Triangle B). In periods of anxiety, the distant position is preferred. People try to maneuver that position to escape the tension. Triangles are usually dynamic (i.e., constantly changing), although in families they often have predictable and rigid forms.

A community health nurse interacting with a family can use this knowledge of triangles. Remembering that he or she will automatically become a member of one or several triangles when interacting with a family, the nurse can monitor his or her behavior and be aware of the pull toward automatic behaviors. For instance, a nurse interacting with two brothers trying to make plans about moving their mother into a nursing home may find herself taking sides with the brother who first contacted her. Being able to

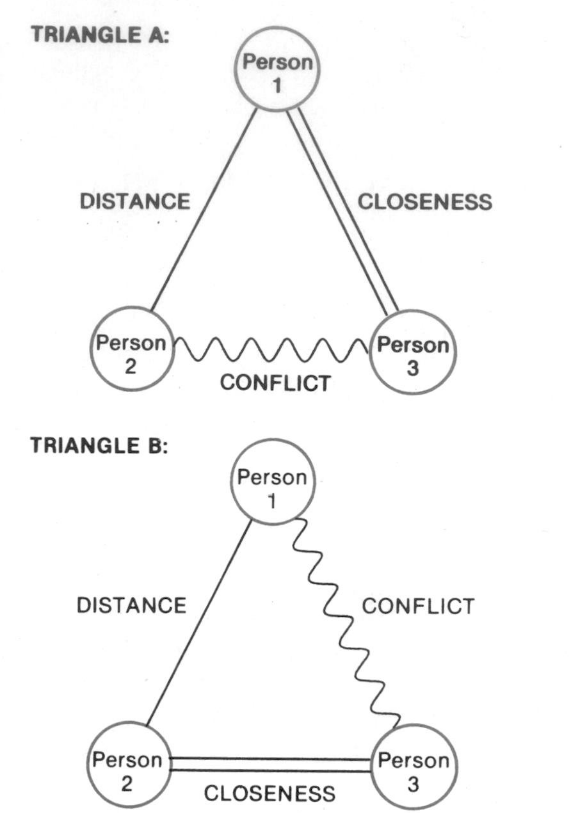

Figure 8–2 ● Triangles are dynamic. (See text for explanation.)

operate in somewhat neutral ways and maintain contact with all is likely to be more helpful than taking sides with one of the family members. Nurses cannot avoid triangles, but they can be aware of the behaviors within them.

Anxiety is another concept that is important in this theory. The more anxiety that is present, the more likely it is that people will react with automatic rather than thoughtful actions. These automatic reactions tend to escalate triangles and patterns of interactions within the system that have developed over time in attempts to manage tension. Nurses who can become aware of their own anxiety and how their way of operating in a particular system may have an escalating or calming effect on the system can be more valuable and effective. If a nurse can enter an anxious system and retain a somewhat calm presence in the midst of great tension, others in the system may be able to do this also. A nurse cannot change the functioning of the system, but she or he can change the ways she or he is operating within it.

Bowen's work with families led him to think more and more broadly about individuals and families within the larger contexts of society and evolutionary time. An understanding of a family at one point in time is helped by gaining more information about its history. Perhaps even larger groups such as work systems, communities, and society share the patterns first observed in families.

Bowen (1978) emphasized theory rather than technique in his work with family therapists in training. A community health nurse using family systems ideas with families realizes that monitoring self-functioning is the prerequisite to any intervention. A person who is anxious and not thinking clearly will take that anxiety into the family. Being in contact with a family without being anxious, overresponsible, or taking sides is sometimes difficult. The nurse who can do this and continue to relate to the family in a way that enables her or him to calmly see the "problem" in a broad and thoughtful way is believed to be more helpful to a family system than a nurse who is determined to find a way to "fix" the family.

FAMILY STRUCTURE AND FUNCTION

In a structural-functional approach, the family is viewed as an organization arranged in a *structure,* or hierarchy, that enables it to assume certain *functions.* The family is arranged in smaller parts, or *subsystems.* Some of the important concepts within this framework include *values, boundaries, roles, status, power,* and *interactional patterns.*

Structural-functional theory originated in family sociology and was at its peak during the 1960s. This theory has an outcome orientation: "What does the family do in relation to society at large?" Three major areas of function were emphasized by family sociologists: the functions of the family *for society,* the functions of subsystems within the family *for the family,* and the functions of the family *for individual members* (Nye and Berardo, 1981). Examples of functions of family that are frequently mentioned include socialization of new members into society, reproduction, maintenance (of the family as an organization), and affective (stabilization of adult personalities) and economic (providing for members' food, clothing, and shelter) functions.

Structural-functional concepts also emerged in family therapy. According to Salvatore Minuchin (1981), a structural family therapist, symptoms of family members can be resolved through appropriate family organization. The concept of boundaries between subsystems is emphasized in his approach. Boundaries are rules that define participants in a subsystem and regulate their behavior. Families with clear and age-appropriate boundaries are believed to function better than families with rigid or ill-defined boundaries. Subsystems enable the family to perform its functions. Each subsystem has different territories and makes certain demands on its members. Commonly discussed family subsystems include *spousal, parental,* and *sibling* subsystems.

Interactional styles describe the way family members relate to each other. Sometimes families develop repetitive patterns of interaction that prescribe their behavior. A family therapist observing a family would ask, "Do certain patterns reappear that seem to be regulated by the structure and past behaviors within the family? Are these patterns functional in that they help the family achieve its goals? Do they function to keep things the same, or do they seek change?"

How is the family organized in general? Is it *enmeshed,* with boundaries blurred and a strong feeling of overinvolvement? Are family members *disengaged,* with members barely connecting with each other? Are they somewhere in between? Are boundaries so rigid that no growth or adaptation is possible? Structural family therapists often use a tool called a *family map* to diagram the spatial and relationship qualities within a family system. This is discussed in more detail in Chapter 9.

FAMILY INTERACTION AND COMMUNICATION

Burgess (1926) described the family as "a unit of interacting personalities." Family sociologists began using the term *symbolic interaction* to describe the way family members interact with each other. *Interaction* is defined as a set of processes taking place among individuals that cannot be separated into isolated parts. Behaviors of one person are both the cause and effect of behaviors in another. A *symbolic environment* is an environment that has significant symbols attached to it. Learned meanings and values define the situation and shape the ways a person acts within it. A representation of self is also learned through values and symbols communicated to the actor by other people.

Symbolic interaction is perhaps most clearly demonstrated when we think about the process of child development—how a child learns about himself or herself and his or her position and status within the world. This concept is appropriate for all family interactions. For example, in every marriage many actions become regulated through symbols and shared meanings that define the situation and each spouse's relationship to the other. For example, playing a part (e.g., the "competent husband" or the "comforting wife") may typify many of the interactions in a marriage.

Communications theory, which is based on systems theory, developed from family therapists. This theory, in which communication is the primary tool for looking at and working with families, developed from work done in California by Watzlawick, Beavin, and Jackson (1967) and by Satir (1972). An example is double-bind communication in schizophrenic families. A *double-bind communication* sends two conflicting messages. For example, a mother may say, "Come here, I love you" to a child, yet remain rigid and cold when the child approaches. Not only is the child in a double bind by being unable to respond to both messages, but the communication also usually includes the unspoken message, "Don't comment on how incongruent this communication is."

Early observations of communication and interaction among people led to several components of communication theory:

1. It is impossible not to communicate, because every verbal or nonverbal behavior includes a message. Even silence is communication.
2. Communication has several levels. On one level, the content or literal meaning of the message is communicated: "I want you to go to the store." On another level, information about intimacy, power, or conflict is transmitted. This is known as *metacommunication.* "I want you to go to the store," can be said in many different ways intending to communicate power, helplessness, intimacy, conflict, or many other messages about the relationship between the communicators.
3. Communication implies an exchange of information. Within a family these interactions become *patterns* that are predictable and repeated. For example, in one family the only way to complain about something may be for the mother to talk to the son, who will then talk to the father. This communication may always occur in a derogatory way so that the father is blamed for what is happening. Because families have a long history of repeated contacts with each other, these patterns tend to repeat themselves in somewhat predictable ways.
4. In functional families, communication is usually one of the following:
   a. A tool to help children learn about the environment.
   b. A way to communicate *rules* about how people in the family should think and act.
   c. A tool for *conflict resolution.*
   d. A nurturing method that leads to the development of *self-esteem.*
5. Healthy communication is open, honest, direct, and congruent with internal feelings.
6. Family members assume certain *roles* relating to family communication.

Virginia Satir (1972) is a communication theorist who emphasizes the messages about self-esteem communicated within families. Her book, *Peoplemaking,* provides interesting exercises and reading for those who want to learn more about family communication.

The community health nurse using communications principles with families would first assess the family's style of communication. Families will have certain rules that govern the way they communicate. Their patterns of interaction will repeat themselves and can be used as a source of information about the family's communication and members' relationships with each other. The nurse will want to observe what kinds of messages family members receive about themselves as people and about the problem at hand. Ideally communication will be open (members discuss events with each other rather than engage in circuitous ways of transmitting the information), honest (members feel free to say what they think and feel), direct (members go directly to the person involved rather than communicate through another), and congruent (verbal messages match internal feelings); however, the family may not be able to communicate in these ways. On some occasions it may be appropriate to help family members alter their communication; in other circumstances the nurse may choose to alter interventions to match the family communication. For example, if a family has a rule that all communication goes through the father, the nurse may choose to communicate with the family in their preferred way.

Even if the situation is not conducive to changing family communication, the community health nurse can influence the family situation by being careful of her or his own communication. Taking steps to ensure that communication is open, honest, direct, and congruent accurately sends information to the family and increases the chance that the family will perceive it accurately. The nurse may sometimes intervene most effectively simply by being a role model of an effective communicator. Sometimes the nurse's "meta" position—the ability to be outside the family and observe more accurately what goes on—enables her or him to communicate information about family communication patterns that the family cannot observe. All family members in the family deserve communication from the health care system that recognizes their importance and worth as individuals in the family. *How* the nurse communicates to each member may be as important as *what* is said.

DISTINCTIVE CHARACTERISTICS OF FAMILIES

Other family scholars have attempted to describe families by identifying their distinctive characteristics. How do families differ from each other? Are there "types" of families? Many of these models focus on healthy or "normal" families in contrast to the earlier theories which focused on family problems.

Beavers (1982) studied healthy families and developed a model that describes levels of family functioning that range from "healthy" to "midrange" to "severely dysfunctional." He used two dimensions—family *competence* and family *style*—to describe families. Style is *centripetal* or *centrifugal,* meaning families tend to look for gratification within the family or outside of it, respectively. Family styles tend to vary along developmental lines. For example, the family that is newly formed will often be centripetal, while a middle-age family is often centrifugal.

Riess and Olivieri (1980) describe families according to their styles of perceiving the social environment. The ways a family perceives the social situation and its place within it—the *family paradigm*—seems to shape the family's typical way of interacting with the environment and to have an effect on day-to-day living. There are three dimensions along which the family paradigm varies: configuration,

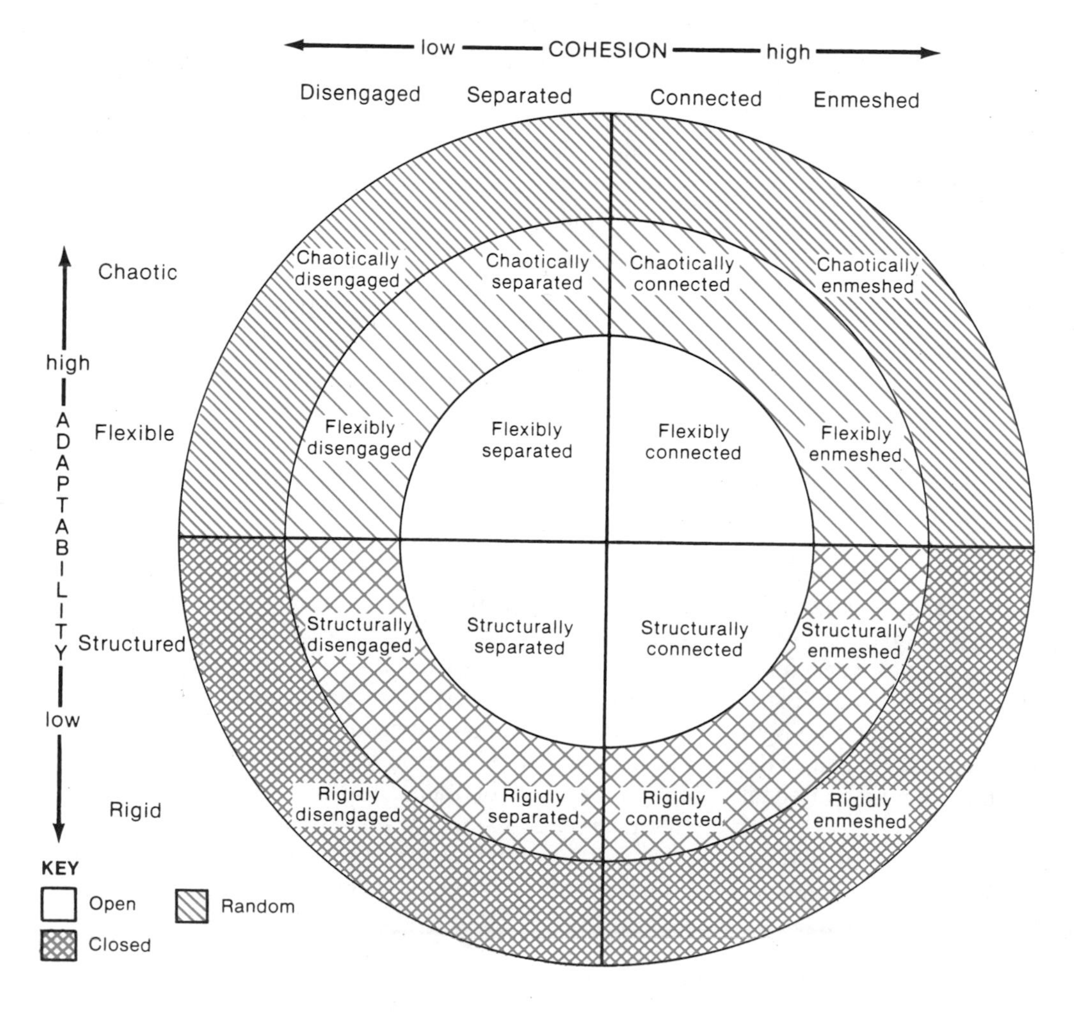

Figure 8–3 ● The Circumplex Model of family systems. (Redrawn from Olson D. H., & McCubbin H. I.: Circumplex model of marital and family systems: V. Applicaton to family stress and crisis intervention. In H. I. McCubbin, A. E. Cauble, & Patterson, J. M. (Eds.). *Family stress, coping, and social support.* Springfield, IL, Charles C Thomas, 1982, p 54.)

coordination, and closure. *Configuration* refers to the family belief that the social world has order, is understandable, and is able to be mastered by the family. *Coordination* refers to the family's belief that the environment has a uniform impact on all family members, and to their subsequent tendency to act as a unit. *Closure* refers to family perceptions of the social world as consistently familiar, or as fresh, new, and demanding different responses. The family's ability to problem-solve and to manage demands imposed by the outside world is believed to be shaped by these dimensions.

Olson et al. (1982) has advanced a circumplex model of families based on the family dimensions of cohesion and adaptability. *Cohesion* is the tendency of the family to interact as a unit and can vary from open to closed. *Adaptability* or *flexibility* refers to the family ability to adopt new ways of operating. Families vary from rigid to extremely flexible; 16 different types are possible. The model suggests that a balanced level of cohesion and adaptability is most functional, but no one family type is believed to be the "best" (Fig. 8–3).

These different models suggest that there are many variations in the ways families can operate and still be "healthy." When working with families, the community health nurse would want to assess different family styles to gain an understanding of how the family operates. Knowing the family style will help the nurse plan the best way to proceed to fit into the family's usual way of dealing with the world. For example, a family that is operating in a disconnected way may not be able to present all its members together at a prearranged conference. However, the nurse may be able to see different family members at different times and discuss issues with individuals. Families that prove to be at either extreme of the continuum may find themselves in trouble if their conventional way of operating is not working for the current situation. Some families might be receptive to suggestions about alternative ways to do things, and others might not. The goal for the nurse is to maximize what can be done within the family style.

FAMILY COPING WITH STRESS

Interest in how families cope with stress has been growing, and the emphasis in family theories has changed from concentrating on the pathology within families to focusing on family strengths, resources, and adaptability. This switch in focus results in attempts to maximize families' abilities to cope with expected and unexpected stressors in their lives.

As early as 1949, Hill proposed a model that describes family reaction to stress as a process in which the family experiences several phases or changes (Fig. 8–4). In the ABCX (crisis) Model of family coping, *a* (the event) interacts with *b* (resources), which interacts with *c* (the definition the family makes of the event) to produce *x* (the crisis). The family is thought to experience a roller coaster course of adjustment, a process involving disorganization, recovery, and a subsequent level of reorganization. Burr (1973) added the concepts of *vulnerability* and *regenerative power* to Hill's framework, stressing that families vary in their internal resources or abilities to respond to crisis.

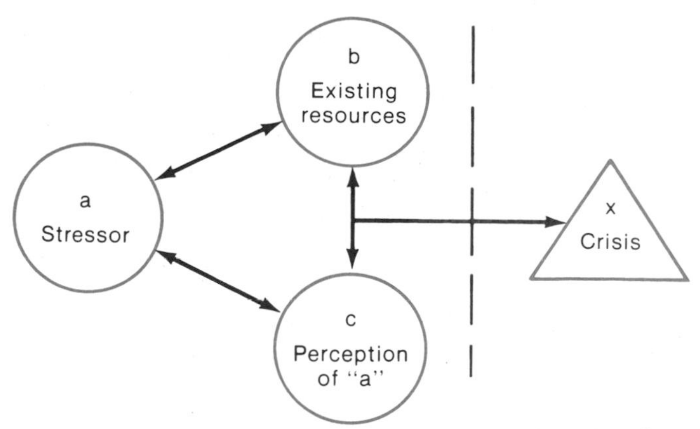

Figure 8–4 ● Hill's ABCX Model of family coping. (Redrawn from McCubbin, H. I., & Patterson, J. M.: Family adaptation to crisis. In H. I. McCubbin, A. E. Cauble, & J. M. Patterson (Eds.). *Family stress, coping, and social support.* Springfield, IL, Charles C Thomas, 1982, p 46.)

McCubbin et al. (1982) proposed the Double ABCX Model of family stress and adaptation. This model adds the concepts of *pileup of demands, family system resources,* and *postcrisis behavior.* How a family responds to crisis will in part depend on its response to previous crises. When crises pile up, the family is more at risk for being unable to maintain sufficient resources and healthy coping behaviors (Fig. 8–5).

Consider the case of a family who experiences the birth of a child with a disability. Their coping will be related to their internal resources (money, internal strengths, emotional health), social support (availability of baby-sitters, access to health care, the educational system within the community), and beliefs about the disability. They will probably experience a period of disorganization at first, and at some point they will begin to work through their feelings and make changes that will help them care for the child. Eventually the family will stabilize in ways that are different from how they were before the birth.

Suppose, however, that shortly before the birth of the child the father had taken a new job; the family had moved to a new community; and that Grandma, who had helped when the older children were young, had fallen and needed some help herself. The pileup of demands for this family might exhaust their resources and drive them into less effective coping behaviors. Their behavior after the earlier stresses will affect the way they manage the latest crisis.

The outcome for this family must be considered in terms of the effect on the individual members and the family as a whole. It is possible that resources could be very effectively mobilized to provide safe care for the child, but the marriage of the parents might end in divorce. This requirement of simultaneous balancing of individuals and

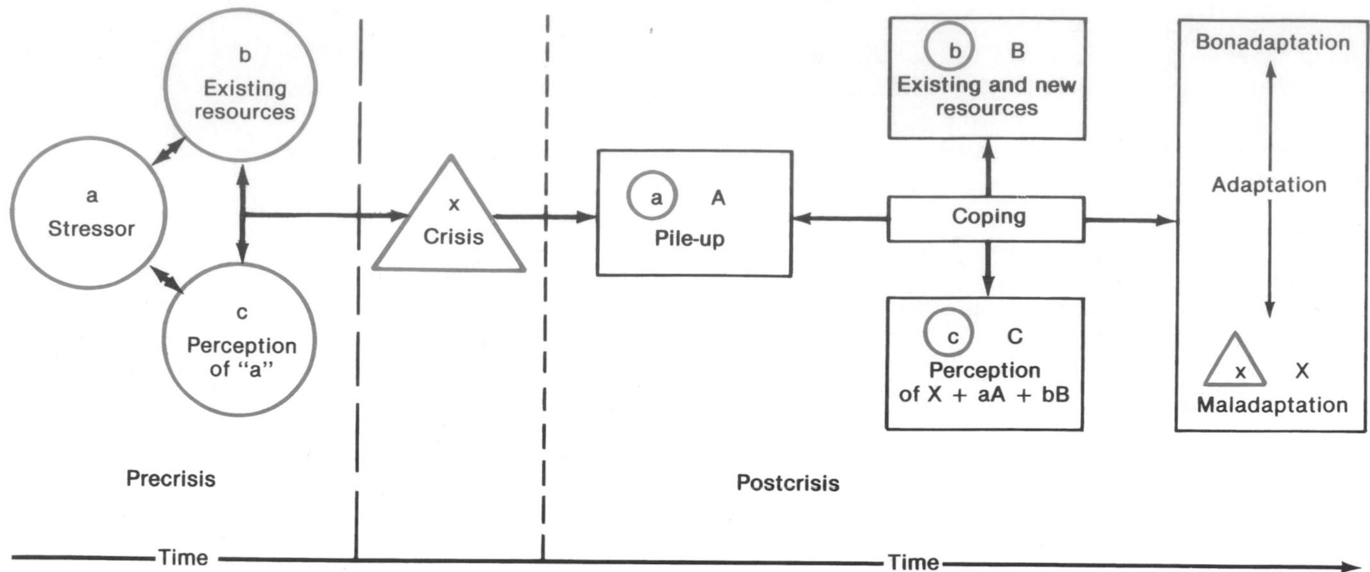

Figure 8–5 ● The Double ABCX Model of family stress and adaptation. (Redrawn from McCubbin, H. I., & Patterson, J. M.: Family adaptation to crisis. In H. I. McCubbin, A. E. Cauble, & J. M. Patterson (Eds.). *Family stress, coping, and social support.* Springfield, IL, Charles C Thomas, 1982, p 46.)

the family needs should be understood by anyone who works with families.

How Can These Approaches Be Integrated?

It is evident from the material presented here that understanding the family is not a simple task. The models and theories provide a wide array of ideas about how families work. Some concepts, however, seem to be universal or to occur over and over throughout the theories. A summary of these concepts is presented in Table 8–4. Understanding the concepts and how they relate to a functional family will help the beginning nurse in early family nursing practice.

Family Perspectives in Nursing

The practice of nursing involves the use of theoretical frameworks from a variety of sources. Traditionally nursing has borrowed theory and knowledge from other disciplines and has used the parameters presented within the frameworks to guide assessment, to design appropriate interventions, and to evaluate outcomes against parameters of normal identified within the frameworks. Nurses have proved that they are able to synthesize large amounts of information and organize it in a useful way. However, when a theory is designed for a different purpose, problems can arise in the adaptation of it to another setting. For example, a theory developed to guide a scientist researching broad social problems is not specific enough to guide day-to-day interactions with a client. Therefore, these concepts and principles from family theories must be used within a framework that considers the role of the nurse and the relationship between the nurse and the client.

Some nursing theorists have included the idea of family in their theories. King (1981) identified the family as a social system as one of her major concepts; her theory treats the family as a unit of care. Other theorists did not include family in their early work but added the component later (Newman, 1979; Orem, 1971: Rogers, 1970). All discuss the family as a unit that can be the focus of care (Newman, 1983; Orem, 1980; Rogers, 1983). However, none of these nursing theories describes the family or interventions for the family in enough detail to direct family–nurse interactions.

Other theorists are beginning to formulate frameworks specifically for family nursing. Gillis (1983) described families and their relationship to health and illness. Wright and Leahey (1984) have developed a framework for family nursing adapted from Tomm's Calgary model. In this framework the family is viewed as a system with three categories to be assessed: structure, development, and function. The principles directing family intervention are related to change, and family care cannot be separated into care for individuals or care for the family as a unit. Emphasis is placed on the interaction between these levels. Zerwekh (1991) developed her framework from interpretations of home visiting nurses' experiences. She identifies three family caregiving competencies: locating the family, building trust, and building strength. Anderson and Tomlinson (1992) identified five realms of family experience to direct nursing practice: interactive processes, developmental processes, coping processes, integrity processes, and health processes.

TABLE 8–4

Characteristics of Functional Families

Developmental stages and tasks: A family goes through predictable stages according to the age and development of its members. Tasks must be achieved at the stage-appropriate time or they may never be achieved. Maturational crises are predictable. Some crises are unpredictable and interfere with achievement of tasks.

Roles: Define certain patterns of expected behavior. Often are male/female linked. Need to be appropriate for age and sex. Also need to be flexible, not rigid, and able to support family functioning.

Boundaries: Exist around the system to handle exchange between the family and the environment. Also exist between subsystems to differentiate members belonging to each subsystem. Need to be permeable to allow information and resources in and out. Boundaries between subsystems should have clear generational lines and support a strong parental coalition. Should be neither too rigid nor diffuse.

Subsystems: Each member of the family belongs to several simultaneously: spouse, parental/child, sibling, grandparents. Subsystems should include all (and only) age-appropriate members.

Patterns of interaction: Repeat themselves. Are healthier when one member does not end up blamed, left out, or put down in the interaction. Should be somewhere in between enmeshed and disengaged. Communication theorists describe how people communicate (e.g., placator, blamer, superresponsible one). Bowen talks about four ways of handling fusion: distance, conflict, projection, dysfunction.

Power: Results from clear role definition and appropriate rules. Should be somewhat shared, appropriate to age, and within the parental subsystem until the children are independent.

External stressors: Usually present at some point. If they vary, are not very intense, and are spread out over time, the family has a chance to adapt. Illness brings its own set of demands to the family.

Open/Closed system: As the system closes, all variables and patterns become fixed and less adaptable. Energy is used in dysfunctional ways. Open systems can adapt and change as feedback is received from within and outside the system. This is related to permeability of boundaries.

Communication: Healthier when it is clear, honest, direct, congruent, and specific, and when the family is able to use it as a mechanism to resolve conflict.

Values: Related to cultural, socioeconomic groups. Provide some stability, rules, and guidelines. Need to be able to change with changing times.

Encouragement of autonomy/acceptance of difference: A balance needs to exist between autonomy of members and the need to be a cohesive group.

Level of anxiety: When the family is calm, people in the family can think and problem-solve better. The family tends to do better than in times of stress. Anxiety can be transitional or long-term. Long-term anxiety tends to wear down the ability of the family to function well.

Resources/social support: Available to most families from within and outside the family, but the family must be able to use them. Extended family is often used. Socioeconomic status and geographic location tend to influence these. All families have some strengths.

Meaning, perception, and paradigm: The way a family perceives a situation, the meaning it attaches to the events, and its typical way of relating to the outside environment influence the ways families react.

Adaptability: Flexibility, adaptability, and resilience are necessary for a family to be able to cope with changing demands. A family needs to maintain a certain degree of flexibility and yet a certain degree of cohesiveness and predictability.

WHAT IS FAMILY NURSING?

In the frameworks described earlier, family is viewed in nursing in two ways: family as client and family as context for the individual (Whall, 1986; Wright and Leahey, 1990). Some nurses believe that a nurse practicing with families as client should be a specialist with advanced preparation in family nursing. Others suggest that all nurses practice family-centered care.

Friedemann (1989) discusses this dilemma and makes several suggestions. Friedemann proposes a system-based conceptualization of family nursing, with family nursing practiced on three levels. The *individual level* is directed at the family as a composite of individuals. The *interpersonal level* is directed at dyads and other small groups of people within the family. The *family system level* is directed at the total system as it interacts with the environment. Friedemann believes that family nursing falls within the scope of all nurses; however, different amounts of expertise are brought to the family situation by different nurses. All nurses practice at the individual level, while interpersonal family nursing can be practiced only by a nurse who sits with more than one family member and guides the communication process through the appropriate channels. Community health nurses practice at the interpersonal level when they assist parents to communicate with their preschool children or assist family members to share their thoughts with a terminally ill member. A nurse practicing at the family system level should be prepared educationally to offer family therapy type interventions. Friedemann suggests that interventions at the interpersonal and family system levels require expertise beyond that of the novice nurse.

If this definition of family nursing is adopted, how can what we have discussed be brought together in a meaningful way to direct family nursing practice? At this point our model includes a conceptualization of different levels of systems; Friedemann has chosen to focus on three. This text adds a fourth level. Sometimes the environment itself may need to be addressed. Novice community health nurses can reduce environmental hazards, link families with resources, and develop resources external to families. Community health nurses are often involved at a level where they are addressing legislation, policies, and practices at a local, state, national, or even international level. The community or even the larger system of society are also appropriate levels of intervention. Thus, the four levels of intervention for the community health nurse are the

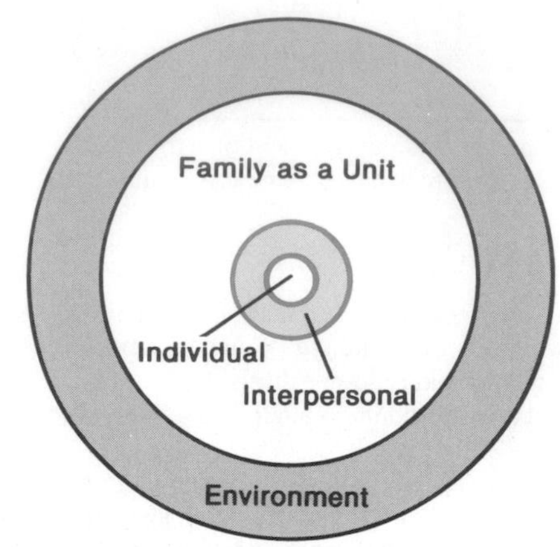

Figure 8–6 ● Levels of intervention in family nursing.

individual, the interpersonal, the family system, and the environmental levels (Fig. 8–6), all four of which are discussed more in Chapter 9.

The definition of family nursing proposed by this text is as follows:

> Family nursing is the practice of nursing directed toward maximizing the health and well-being of all individuals within a family system. It incorporates two views of family: family as the unit of care and family as context. Family nursing views the family as a system existing within a larger system. Levels of intervention are the individual, the interpersonal, the family system, and the environmental level. The goals of family nursing include optimal functioning for the individual and for the family as a unit.

The family as a unit of care means that the entire family is the recipient of the nursing intervention. This viewpoint recognizes the mandate in the American Nurses' Association (1986) *Standards of Community Health Nursing Practice* that identifies clients as individuals, families, and communities. In contrast, the family as context recognizes the impact the family has on an individual. This viewpoint underscores the need to understand the family environment in which the individual exists.

HOW IS FAMILY NURSING PRACTICED?

Family nursing practice, like any nursing practice, begins with the nursing process. By using this process, the nurse practicing with a family perspective is potentially able to effectively intervene at any of the levels. After an assessment of the individuals, dyads, family unit, and suprasystem, the nurse is ready to begin to identify areas of concern or need. Smith (1985) suggests that nurses working within the community will discover that *family needs* fall into one or several of five categories: families dealing with normal growth and development, families coping with illness or loss, families dealing with external stressors, families with inadequate resources or support, or families with disturbances in organization. In addition to their needs, the *family style,* or process, must be considered as the nurse works with the family. Finally, *family function* must be assessed to determine the realism of the goals. This framework for family nursing is based on these four assumptions:

1. Improvement in the functioning of an individual will elicit improvement in the functioning of the whole family.
2. Because of the systemic nature of family, interventions can be directed at any of several levels with a resultant change in family operation.
3. The nature of the nurse–client interaction is a crucial part of family nursing intervention.
4. Family nursing interventions need to be modified to match different family needs, family styles, and levels of family functioning.

To begin this transition to using a family perspective, it is suggested that the nurse guide her or his family practice with some questions about the nature of the contact:

- What have I learned during my assessment of family structure, process, and function that best explains the phenomena happening in this family?
- What does the family want from me? What are they expecting me to do?
- What does the larger system expect/require of me? What is a community health nurse's responsibility in this situation?
- What level of expertise and skill am I bringing to the situation? What do I have the skills to do?
- What have I learned from science and theory that seems to apply to this situation?
- What might I know or be able to offer to help the individuals and the family achieve a more optimal level of health? How do I present this as a choice to the system?
- At what level of the system (individual, interpersonal, family system, or environment) will I intervene?

The decisions and actions of a nurse with families are performed within the nursing process. How family nursing is actualized within each step of the process—assessment, planning, implementation, and evaluation—is discussed in more detail in the next chapter. Working toward family health is a goal that will support people today and strengthen our society as we enter the future. Family nursing is an essential basis of community health practice.

KEY IDEAS

1. Using a family perspective is necessary for the community health nurse.
2. The nature of the American family is changing, resulting in many different family forms.

3. There is no one type of healthy family. Families organize themselves in different ways that work for them.
4. Historical frameworks from social sciences and family therapy provide information about the nature of families.
5. Recent efforts in developing nursing frameworks identify the family as the context in which an individual lives or as the unit of care.
6. Community health nurses can intervene with families at any of several levels: individual, interpersonal, family system, or environmental.
7. Family nurses need to identify family needs, family styles, and family level of functioning.
8. Helping individuals maintain or restore their functioning will ultimately help strengthen the family.
9. Nurse–client interaction is the crucial part of family nursing and is adjusted for differing family situations.

GUIDELINES FOR LEARNING

1. Write a description of an ideal family. Take a moment to reflect on where these ideas came from. In what ways is your family alike and different from your ideal?
2. Compare the concepts applicable to functional families to those of a clinical family (see Table 8-4). In what ways does the family exhibit the ideal, and where is it weak? Can you see where some of the concepts begin to relate to each other? For example, are boundaries between subsystems related to communication patterns?
3. Observe a family in a public place such as a restaurant or shopping center. What does their interaction tell you about the family? Do you get a sense of the emotional tone and what the experience would be like to live within this family?
4. Mentally review the families living in your neighborhood. How many of these families are a traditional family? What other family forms do you recognize? From your knowledge of any of these families, do you think family form determines family health?
5. Watch a television show depicting family life. What form does this family represent? In your opinion, is it a healthy or not-so-healthy family? Where is the drama or comedy in the show coming from? Is the show making fun of the family, using it to explain the drama, or presenting it as the answer to the heroic dilemma in the plot?
6. Think about intervening at the individual, interpersonal, family, or environmental level. At what levels have your past interventions been? At what levels do you feel comfortable intervening now? What additional experience or skills would you eventually like to have to intervene at all these levels?
7. Write your family a plan for improving family health.

REFERENCES

American Nurses' Association. (1986). *Standards of community health nursing practice.* Washington, DC: Author.

Anderson, K. H., & Tomlinson, P. S. (1992). The family health system as an emerging paradigmatic view for nursing. *Image: Journal of Nursing Scholarship, 24*(1), 57–63.

Beavers, W. R. (1982). Healthy, midrange, and severely dysfunctional families. In F. Walsh (Ed.). *Normal family processes.* New York: The Guilford Press.

Bowen, M. (1978). *Family therapy in clinical practice.* New York: Jason Aronson.

Bronfenbrenner, U. (1979). *The ecology of human development.* Cambridge, MA: Harvard University Press.

Burgess, E. W. (1926). The family as a unit of interacting personalities. *Family, 7,* 3–9.

Burr, W. (1973). *Theory construction in the sociology of the family.* New York: John Wiley & Sons.

Burr, W. R., Hill, R., Nye, F. I., & Reiss, I. L. (1979). *Contemporary theories about the family.* New York: The Free Press.

Duvall, E. M. (1957). *Family development.* Chicago: Lippincott.

Friedemann, M. L. (1989). The concept of family nursing. *Journal of Advanced Nursing, 14,* 211–216.

Friedman, M. M. (1986). *Family nursing: Theory and assessment.* Norwalk, CT: Appleton-Century Crofts.

Gillis, C. L. (1983). The family as a unit of analysis: Strategies for the nurse researcher. *Advances in Nursing Science, 5*(3), 59–67.

Gough, K. (1986). The origin of the family. In A. Skolnick & J. Skolnick (Eds.). *Family in transition.* Boston: Little, Brown.

Hareven, T. K. (1982). American families in transition: Historical perspectives in change. In A. Skolnick & J. Skolnick (Eds.). *Family in transition.* Boston: Little, Brown.

Hill, R. (1949). *Families under stress.* New York: Harper & Row.

King, I. (1981). *A theory of nursing: Systems, concepts, process.* New York: John Wiley & Sons.

Lasch, C. (1986). The family as a haven in a heartless world. In A. Skolnick & J. Skolnick (Eds.). *Family in transition.* Boston: Little, Brown.

McCubbin, H. I., Cauble, A. E., & Patterson, J. M. (1982). *Family stress, coping, and social support.* Springfield, IL: Charles C Thomas.

McCubbin, H. I., & Patterson, J. M. (1982). Family adaptation to crisis. In H. I. McCubbin, A. E. Cauble, & J. M. Patterson (Eds.). *Family stress, coping, and social support* (p. 46). Springfield, IL: Charles C Thomas.

McGoldrick, M., & Carter, E. A. (1982). The family life cycle. In F. Walsh (Ed.). *Normal family processes.* New York: Guilford Press.

Minuchin, S., & Fishman, H. C. (1981). *Family therapy techniques.* Cambridge, MA: Harvard University Press.

Newman, M. (1979). *Theory development in nursing.* Philadelphia: F. A. Davis.

Newman, M. (1983). Newman's health theory. In I. Clements & F. Roberts (Eds.). *Family health: A theoretical approach to nursing care.* New York: John Wiley & Sons.

Nye, F. I., & Berardo, F. E. (1981). *Emerging conceptual frameworks in family analysis.* New York: Praeger.

Olson, D. H., & Hanson, M. H. (Eds.). (1990). *2001: Preparing families for the future.* NCFR Presidential Report. Minneapolis, MN: National Council of Family Relations.

Olson, D. H., & McCubbin, H. I. (1982). Circumplex model of marital and family systems: V. Family stress and crisis intervention. In H. I. McCubbin, A. E. Cauble, & J. M. Patterson (Eds.). *Family stress, coping, and social support* (p. 54). Springfield, IL: Charles C Thomas.

Olson, D., Sprenkle, D., & Russell, C. (1982). Circumplex model of marital and family systems. *Family Process, 18*(3), 3–27.

Orem, D. (1971). *Nursing: Concepts of practice.* New York: McGraw-Hill.

Orem, D. (1980). *Nursing: Concepts of practice* (2nd ed.). New York: McGraw-Hill.

Riess, D., & Oliviri, M. E. (1980). Family paradigm and family coping: A proposal for linking the family's intrinsic adaptive capacities to its responses to stress. *Family Relations, 29,* 431–444.

Rogers, M. (1970). *An introduction to the theoretical basis of nursing.* Philadelphia: F.A. Davis.

Rogers, M. (1983). Science of unitary beings: A paradigm for nursing. In I. Clements & F. Roberts (Eds.). *Family health: A theoretical approach to nursing care.* New York: John Wiley & Sons.

Satir, V. (1972). *Peoplemaking.* Palo Alto: CA: Science and Behavior Books.

Scheflen, A. E. (1981). *Levels of schizophrenia.* New York: Brunner/Mazel, Inc.

Smith, C. (1985). *Goals for community health nursing.* (Unpublished manuscript.) Baltimore, MD.

Tapia, J. A. (1982). The nursing process in community health. In B. W. Spradley (Ed.). *Readings in community health nursing* (2nd ed.). Boston: Little, Brown.

von Bertalanffy, L. (1968). *General systems theory.* New York: George Braziller.

Walsh, F. (1982). *Normal family processes.* New York: The Guilford Press.

Watzlawick, P., Beavin, J., & Jackson, D. (1967). *Pragmatics of human communication.* New York: W.W. Norton & Co.

Whall, A. (1986). The family as the unit of care in nursing: A historical review. *Journal of Advanced Nursing, 14,* 211–216.

Wright, L., & Leahey, M. (1984). *Nurses and families.* Philadelphia: F.A. Davis.

Wright, L. & Leahey, M. (1990). Trends in nursing of families. In J. Bell, W. Watson, & L. Wright (Eds.). *The cutting edge of family nursing.* Calgary, Alberta, Canada: University of Calgary.

Zerwekh, J. (1991). A family caregiving model for public health nursing. *Nursing Outlook, 39*(5), 213–217.

BIBLIOGRAPHY

Bell, N. W., & Vogel, E. F. (1968). *A modern introduction to the family.* New York: The Free Press.

Caplan, G. (1976). The family as a support system. In G. Caplan & M. Killiea (Eds.). *Support systems and mutual help.* New York: Grune & Stratton.

Combrinck-Graham, L. (1985). A developmental model for family systems. *Family Process. 24*(2), 139–150.

Duvall, E. M. (1977). *Family development* (5th ed.). Philadelphia: J. B. Lippincott.

Fine, M., Schwebel, A. I., & James-Myers, L. (1987). Family stability in black families. *Journal of Comparative Family Studies. 18*(1), 1–23.

Friedman, M. (1992). *Family nursing: Theory and assessment* (3rd ed.). Norwalk, CT: Appleton & Lange.

Garfinkel, I., & McLanahan, S. S. (1986). *Single mothers and their children: A new American dilemma.* Washington, DC: The Urban Institute Press.

Glick, P. C. (1988). Fifty years of family demography: A record of social change. *Journal of Marriage and the Family, 50,* 861–873.

Hall, J. E., & Weaver, B. R. (1974). *Nursing of families in crisis.* Philadelphia: J.B. Lippincott.

Hansen, D. A., & Hill, R. (1964). Families under stress. In H. T. Christensen (Ed.). *Handbook of marriage and the family.* Chicago: Rand McNally.

Hansen, D. A., & Johnson, V. A. (1979) Rethinking family stress theory: Definitional aspects. In W. Burr, R. Hill, E. Nye, & I. Reiss (Eds.). *Contemporary theories about the family.* New York: The Free Press.

Jacob, T. (1987). *Family interaction and psychopathology.* New York: Plenum Press.

Kantor, D., & Lehr, W. (1975). *Inside the family.* San Francisco: Jossey Bass.

McAdoo, H. P. (1978). Factors related to stability in upwardly mobile black families. *Journal of Marriage and the Family, 40*(4), 761–776.

McCall, G. J., & Simmons, J. L. (1978). *Identities and interactions.* New York: The Free Press.

McCubbin, H., Joy, C., Cauble, A., Comeau, J., Patterson, J., & Needle, R. (1980). Family stress and coping: A decade review. *Journal of Marriage and the Family, 10,* 855–871.

McCubbin, M. (1984). Nursing assessment of parental coping with cystic fibrosis. *Western Journal of Nursing Research, 6*(4), 407–421.

Miller, J. R., & Janosik, E. H. (1980). *Family-focused care.* New York: McGraw-Hill.

Miller, S. R., & Winstead-Fry, P. (1982). *Family systems theory in nursing practice.* Reston, VA: Reston Publishing Co.

Moos, R. H. (1977). *Coping with physical illness.* New York: Plenum Press.

Moos, R. H. (1984). *Coping with physical illness, 2: New perspectives.* New York: Plenum Press.

Nichols, M. (1987). *The self in the system.* New York: Brunner/Mazel.

Riess, D., Gonzalez, S., & Kramer, N. (1986). Family process, chronic illness, and death: On the weakness of strong bonds. *Archives of General Psychiatry, 43,* 795–804.

Riskin, J., & Faunce, E. E. (1972). An evaluative review of family interaction research. *Family Process, 11*(4), 365–411.

Rolland, J. (1987). Chronic illness and the life cycle: A conceptual framework. *Family Process, 26,* 203–221.

Skolnik, A. S., & Skolnick, J. H. (1986). *Family in transition.* Boston: Little, Brown.

Sussman, M., & Steinmetz, S. (1987). *Handbook of marriage and the family.* New York: Plenum Press.

Turner, J. G., & Chavigny, K. H. (1988). *Community health nursing: An epidemiological perspective through the nursing process.* Philadelphia: J.B. Lippincott.

Wright, L. and Leahey, M. (1994). *Nurses and families* (2nd ed.). Philadelphia: F. A. Davis.

Wynne, L. C. (Ed.). (1988). *The state of the art in family therapy research: Controversies and recommendations.* New York: Family Process Press.

Zinn, M. B., & Eitzen, D. S. (1987). *Diversity in American families.* New York: Harper & Row.

Chapter 9

The Nursing Process and Families

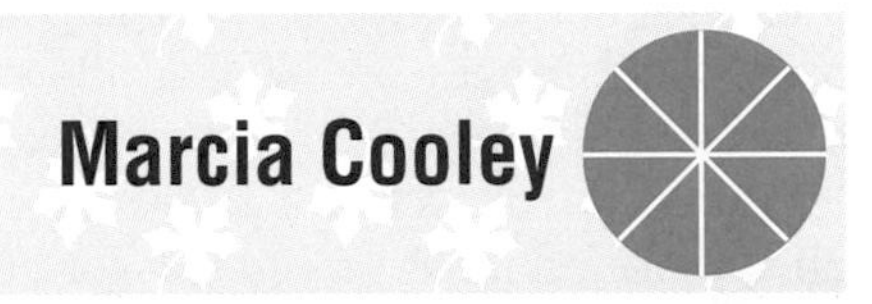

Focus Questions

What is the purpose of family assessment?

What methods and tools are used for assessing individuals? subsystems? the family unit? the family within the environment?

How does the nurse analyze family data?

What are family nursing diagnoses?

How are priorities determined in family nursing?

What principles will help the nurse and family develop an effective plan of care?

How do family functioning and family style influence care planning?

How do family–nurse interactions vary with different family needs?

What are the possible outcomes of the evaluation phase of the nursing process?

How does the nurse coordinate termination with a family in a way that will benefit the nurse and the family?

Family health nursing is the practice of nursing directed toward maximizing the health and well-being of all individuals within a family system. It incorporates two views of a family: family as the unit of care and family as context for individuals and subsystems. When working with families, the community health nurse's goal is to promote optimal health for each member of the family and for the family as a unit. Bringing a family perspective to the arena in which the nurse will meet with the family will change the way the nurse practices. The nurse begins to consider more complex needs and more complex interactions as care is offered. As with all nursing encounters, this practice builds on the foundation of the nursing process. Community health nurses assess, diagnose, plan, implement, and evaluate their nursing care for and with families.

For nurses dealing with families, extra challenges are posed in the complexity and skill that is sometimes required to deal with these larger and more intensely connected groups of people. The nurse's ability to establish a relationship that respects the family's rights and strengths becomes more important than any other task. Trust, open communication, and acceptance of diverse family values are essential. While the community health nurse has responsibilities to the community and wishes to affect the health of each family member and the family as a whole, he or she must always remember that the family is ultimately responsible for what it does. The nurse's role is limited to that of a facilitator, educator, or advocate except in the most extreme cases of personal safety or abuse. Success depends not on what the nurse does, but on his or her talent at empowering the family to act for itself.

Family Assessment

As with all assessment, the nurse uses as many possible sources of data as practical to help fill in a complete picture of the family and each member. Of course, before discussing a family or reviewing the family's records with a member of the health care team from another agency, the family's permission must be obtained. Sources of data can include, but should not be limited to, charts and written health records, collection of biological data such as blood pressures or specimens, telephone calls and conversations with other health care team members, information from social service agencies involved with the family, and environmental and community information. However, the most accurate and complete information can be obtained only by observing and interviewing the family itself.

Interviewing families can be more difficult than interviewing an individual client and, for a nurse not familiar with this situation, a little frightening. After all, the family has been together for a long time and has a history together that gives even the most dysfunctional family strength and a collective power. Interviewing families can also be a rich source of information and a path to establishing relationships that are fulfilling and meaningful for both the nurse and family members.

Families may first be seen in the hospital, clinic, community setting, or in their own home. Seeing families in their own environment is preferable, because the nurse can observe firsthand the physical and environmental conditions, as well as the way family members act with each other on their own turf. Preparing for a home visit is discussed in Chapter 7. Ideally, the nurse will plan the first meeting with the family keeping those principles in mind. Families can then be assessed on several levels: assessment of individuals within the family, assessment of interactions among subsystems, assessment of the family as a unit, and assessment of the family within the environment.

The goal of family assessment is to gather information that allows the nurse and family to identify family needs together and to plan care that will allow the family to work toward more optimal health for individual family members and for the family as a whole. Remember that family nursing can occur on multiple levels: individual, subsystems, family as a unit, and family interacting with the environment. A comprehensive family assessment should include information gathered about and from all these levels. Data that are essential to collect include household composition, health status and behaviors of all members, interaction among the family members, and the relationship of the family with its community.

ASSESSING INDIVIDUAL NEEDS

Typically, one member of the family is identified as the patient or client who is to be the recipient of nursing care. This client may have an identified health problem (e.g., a recent discharge from a hospital after a stroke), a chronic illness that needs continued monitoring (e.g., diabetes), or a potential problem (e.g., a new mother needing education about her infant). Adequate identification and collection of information about the client's response to these actual or potential health problems is the first priority in family assessment.

However, many families will have more than one member with actual or potential health problems. Because family members are interconnected, the health of all members is a concern to the nurse. Depending on the mission and guidelines of the agency and the nurse's role, all family members are potential targets of individual assessment. For example, suppose the identified client is a 55-year-old man who has developed a foot ulcer. He may eventually need assistance with moving and transferring. What if the only other member of the family, his wife, has chronic obstructive pulmonary disease and is unable to help? Family health is interconnected because members share their environment and depend on each other.

Individual assessment will vary with the age and particular health status of each person. It may include comprehensive health or physical assessment, assessment

TABLE 9–1

Examples of Individual Assessments

General Assessments
Physical assessment of the newborn
Pediatric physical assessment
Pediatric health history
Adult physical examination
Adult health history
Instrumental Activities of Daily Living (Lawton & Brody, 1969)
Growth measurements
Mortality Risk Appraisal (Pender, 1987)
Assessments with a Specific Focus
Barthel Rehabilitation Index (Hens, 1989)
Denver Eye Screening Test (Wong & Whaley, 1990)
Diet history
Dementia assessment (Kane et al., 1989a)
Incontinence assessment (Kane et al., 1989b)
Spiritual assessment (Zerwekh, 1989)
Mental status examination (Jernigan, 1986)
PULSES Profile of Well-Being (Hens, 1989)
Quadriplegia Index of Function (Hens, 1989)
Pain Assessment Tool (McCaffrey & Beebc, 1989)
Social Readjustment Rating Scale (Holmes & Rahe, 1967)

of developmental level, mental status assessment, focused information about specific health problems such as incontinence or decubiti, or assessment of coping and adaptation. Some specific individual assessments are outlined in Table 9–1.

ASSESSING FAMILY SUBSYSTEMS

Families interact in small interpersonal groups. Understanding the interactions and functioning of these dyads and triangles is important to understanding the functioning of the family and ascertaining available support. Subsystems such as the parent–child subsystem, the marital pair, and the sibling subsystem should always be assessed. Other, less obvious subsystems might be grandparent–grandchild, foster parent–child, or parents–young married couple. Tools that can be used include maps of social interaction, tools that assess the health of developmental bonds such as mother–child interaction, and tools that target problems in dyads, such as elder abuse screening tools. Examples of these assessments are presented in Table 9–2.

TABLE 9–2

Examples of Interpersonal Assessments
Brief Screening Inventory for Postpartum Adaptation (Affonso, 1987)
Elder Abuse Assessment Tool (Fulmer, 1984)
Lubben Social Network Scale (Lubben, 1988)
Mother/Infant Screening Tool (MIST) (Reiser, 1981)
Neonatal Perception Inventory (Broussard & Hartner, 1992)
Social Assessment of the Elderly (Kane et al., 1989)

TABLE 9–3

Examples of Family Assessments
Family APGAR of Family Functioning (Smilkstein, 1978)
Family Coping Index (Lowe & Freeman, 1981)
Family Inventory of Life Events and Changes (FILE) (McCubbin & Thompson, 1987)
Family Map (Minuchin, 1974)
Family Nutritional Assessment Tool (James, 1989)
Family Self-Care Patterns (Pender, 1987)
Genogram (McGoldrick & Gerson, 1985)
Family Strengths (Otto, 1973)

ASSESSING THE FAMILY AS A UNIT

While it is helpful to assess families in smaller segments, these assessments do not capture the nature of the family as a whole. Families have unique identities that cannot be understood when thinking about only the segments. Parameters that are often assessed include family processes, roles, communication, division of labor, decision-making, boundaries, styles of problem-solving, and coping abilities. Some specific tools are outlined in Table 9–3, while some of the more widely used family assessments are discussed in the sections that follow.

Family Maps. A family map is a tool that originated with structural/functional family therapists (Minuchin and Fishman, 1981). They began observing the structure and interaction of families in therapeutic situations and mapping families to understand their hierarchies, roles, and power. After an interview in which the family is observed in an interactive situation, a map is drawn that details the *subsystems,* the *boundaries* between subsystems, and interactive patterns such as *coalitions, conflict,* and *avoidance.*

A healthy family will demonstrate age-appropriate subsystems. Power will reside with parents, and children will have the nurturant guidance they need to grow. Spousal subsystems will have a clear identity. Boundaries between subsystems will be clear and permeable. Diffuse boundaries allow too much confusion, as members move back and forth without clear definition of roles. Rigid boundaries serve to shut off necessary interaction and discourage flexibility and adaptiveness. Interactive patterns tend to repeat themselves and provide information about who will communicate and what that communication may be like. Symbols for the maps are shown in Figure 9–1.

Genograms. A genogram is a format for drawing a family tree that records information about family members and their relationships for at least three generations (Cain, 1981). Genograms make it easier for a community health nurse to keep in mind the family members, patterns, and significant events that are important in the family's care. The picture of the family that is presented on the genogram helps the observer think about the family systemically and over time. Sometimes when a larger picture is presented,

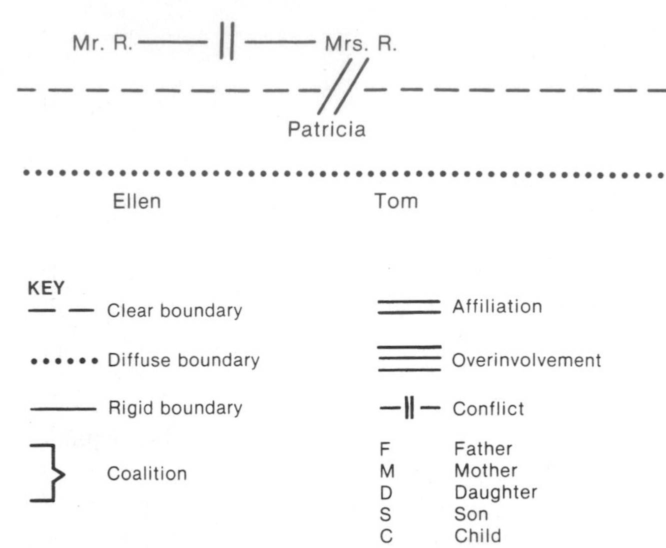

Figure 9–1 ● Family map using family example from chapter case study. (Adapted from Minuchin, S. (1974). *Families and family therapy.* Cambridge, MA: Harvard University Press, p. 53.)

connections between events and relationships become clearer and are viewed in a more objective way.

Genograms serve several other functions. The process of collecting and recording information for the construction of a genogram serves as a way for the interviewer and family to connect in a personal but emotionally safe way. It also provides the interviewer with information about how the members of the family think about family problems and interact with other members. Recording information on a genogram can serve to detoxify issues or reduce anxiety about the family problem. During the process, family members are required to think, organize, and present facts. The nurse helps the family normalize and reframe problems so that they are viewed in a larger context. This type of interaction can help family members step back and think about an issue in a calmer way.

Typically the genogram is constructed in the first or a very early session and revised as new information becomes available. There are three parts to genogram construction: mapping the family structure, recording family information, and delineating family relationships.

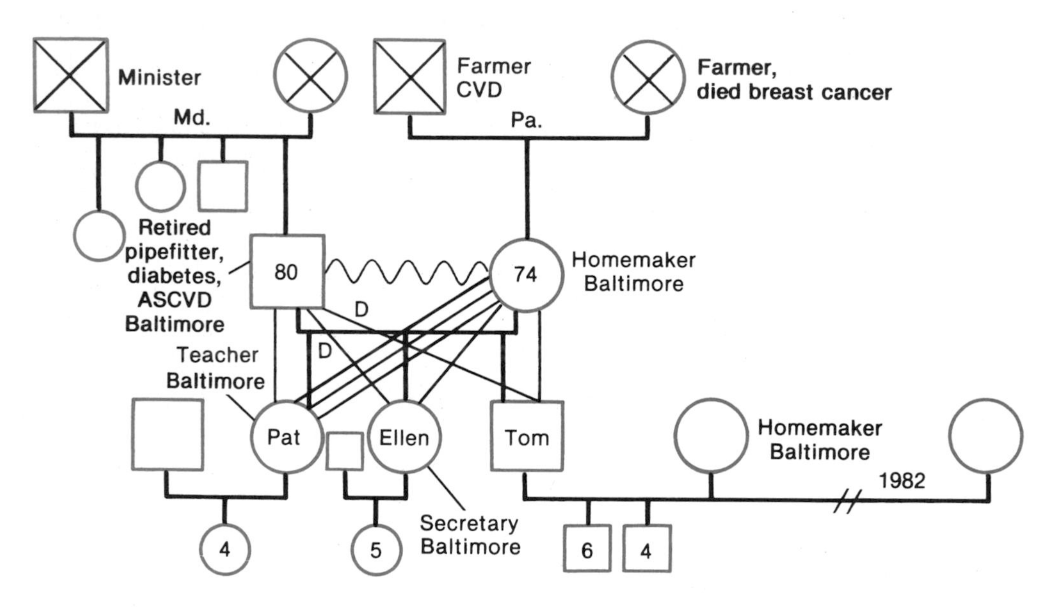

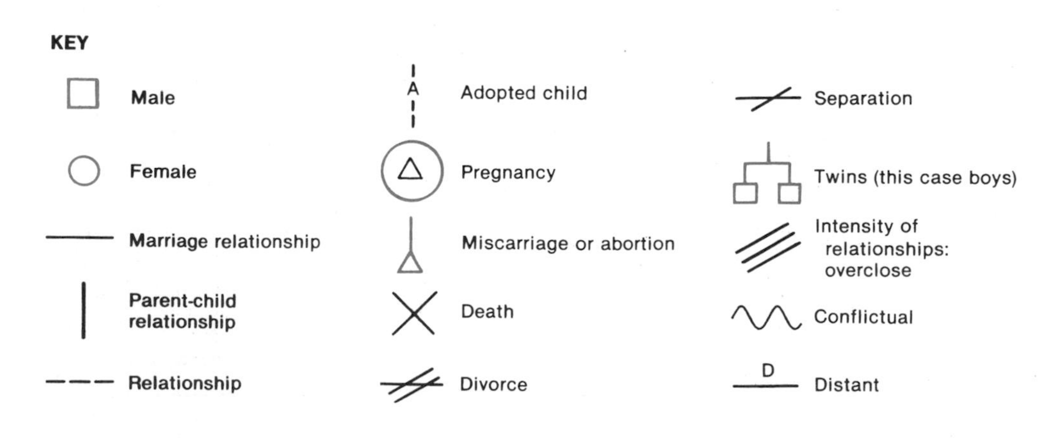

Figure 9–2 ● Genogram using family example from chapter case study. Adapted from Cain, A. (1981). Assessment of family structure. In J. Miller & E. Janosik (Eds.). *Family-focused care* (p. 117). New York: McGraw-Hill.)

TABLE 9–4

Examples of Environmental Assessments

Assessment of Immediate Living Environment (Skelley, 1990)
Building Accessibility Checklist (Mumma, 1987)
Eco-map (Hartman, 1978)
Home Observation for Measurement Environment (HOME) (Caldwell, 1976)
Occupational/Environmental Health History (Wiley, 1989)

A diagram of family members in each generation is drawn using horizontal and vertical lines. Symbols used to represent pregnancies, miscarriages, marriages, and deaths are presented in Figure 9–2. Males are placed on the left of the horizontal line; females on the right. Birth order is represented by placing the oldest sibling on the far left and progressing toward the right. In the case of multiple marriages, the earliest is placed on the left and the most recent on the right.

Family information that is usually helpful includes ages, dates of birth and death, geographic location, occupation, and educational level. Critical family events and transitions such as moves, marriages, divorces, losses, and successes are recorded. Family members' physical, emotional, or social problems or illnesses are identified. A chronology, or time line, of family events is often very useful to help people see relationships between events and behavior changes. Observing and describing family relationships is the stage that is the most crucial and often the most helpful to the family, but is often ignored. Relationship patterns can be quite complex and are inferred from observations and from family members' comments and analyses. Some symbols used to represent relationships are presented in Figure 9–2. Triangles are present in every family. Attempting to map the primary or most influential triangles in the family is a part of describing the family relationships (see Chapter 8).

The genogram is an assessment tool that can be useful throughout the contact with the family. At some point it may also be used as a therapeutic tool where information is interpreted and used to help individuals define the way they would like to operate within the group. While the nurse may fall into thinking he or she knows what the family should do, interpretations that come from family members themselves are usually more accurate and useful for change.

ASSESSING THE FAMILY WITHIN THE ENVIRONMENT

The family is a group of interacting people who also live within an external physical and interpersonal environment. Data about the family's physical environment, such as the presence of accident hazards, screens, plumbing, and cooking facilities, help the nurse (1) plan care that matches or supplements family resources and (2) identify potential health problems. Some physical conditions that should be assessed are presented in Table 9–4. Home Observation for Measurement Environment (HOME), an observation tool developed to assess the potential of the environment for development of children from birth to 6 years of age, is an example of a tool that can be used to collect data about the physical environment (Caldwell, 1976).

Community resources and facilities available to the family should also be noted. However, some families can live within a fairly resource-rich environment and not be able to maintain the connections that are needed to tap those resources. An eco-map (Hartman, 1978) is a tool that can be used to help the nurse and family discover the patterns of energy flow into and outside of the family. The family's relationships to significant community resources, activities, and agencies are diagrammed. Are these connections strong, tenuous, or stressful? The diagram illustrates the amount of energy used by a family to maintain its system and what support is available. After the nurse helps the family prepare the diagram, the eco-map helps family members visualize how relationships with external systems are affecting their state of well-being. An eco-map is presented in Figure 9–3.

Families also are affected by other aspects of the

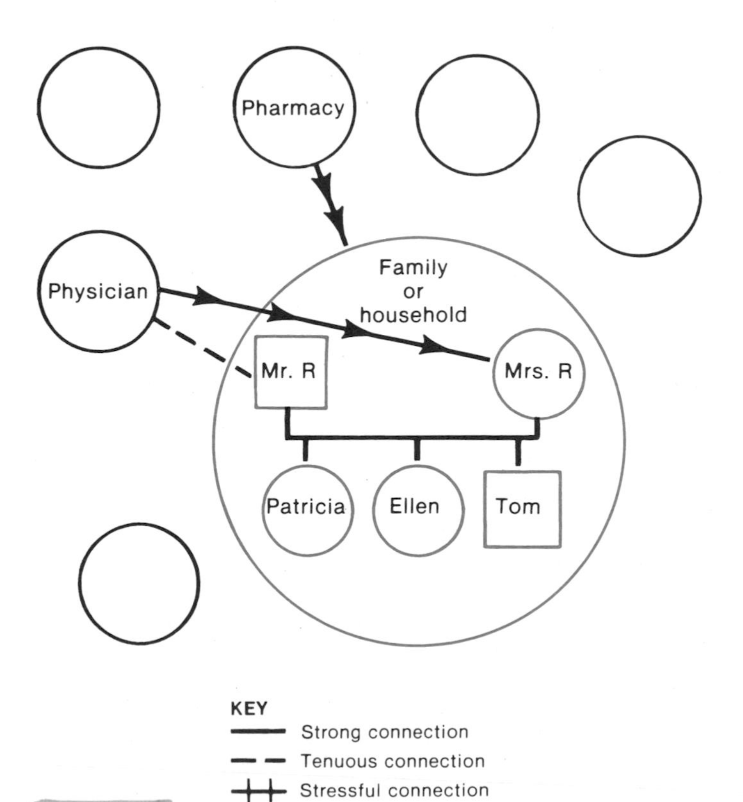

Figure 9–3 ● An eco-map using family example from chapter case study. Directions: Fill in connections where they exist. Indicate their nature by descriptive words or different lines. Draw arrows along lines to signify flow of energy and resources. Identify significant people. Fill in empty circles as needed. (Adapted from Hartman, S. (1978). Diagrammatic assessment of family relationships. *Social Casework, 59,* p 470.)

environment, such as hazards within the workplace, air quality, and exposure in neighborhoods with a high level of criminal activity. An example of a tool that provides an assessment of a family's occupational and environmental history is the Occupational/Environmental Health History (Wiley, 1989) in Table 9–5.

Analyzing Family Data

The different types of assessments just discussed provide a comprehensive assessment, but also a massive amount of data. Family assessments can be complex and confusing if

TABLE 9–5

Occupational/Environmental Health History

Identifying Data

Name: ________________

Address: ________________

Telephone: ________________

Social Security Number: ________________

Sex: ________

Age: ______ Date of Birth: ________________

Chief Complaint and Stressors Perceived by the Client: ________________

Key Questions:

1. Describe the health problem or injury you are currently experiencing. ________________
2. Are any other members of your family experiencing this problem: Any co-worker? Any acquaintance? ________________
3. Do you smoke? ______ Use chewing tobacco? ______ Consume alcohol? ______ Use any other drugs? ______ (Packs per day, quantity, frequency, years' duration) ________________
4. Do you smoke while on the job? ______ At home? ______ Do your co-workers smoke on the job? ______ Do family members smoke while you are in the room? ________________
5. Have you missed work within the past 6 weeks? ______ When did these symptoms begin? ______ Have you stayed in bed since this started? ______ Are you distressed by your disability now? ________________
6. Have you ever worked at a job or other activity that has caused you to have this problem before? ______ If so, describe the pattern of illness or difficulty. ________________
7. Have you ever found yourself short of breath, light-headed, dizzy, with a cough, or wheezing at work? ______ After work? ______ At the beginning of the work week? ______ At the end of the work week? ______ During the weekend? ________________
8. Have you ever changed jobs, homes, or hobbies because of a health problem? ________________
9. Have you ever experienced muscle or moving difficulties (back pain, fractures, sore muscles, decreased ability to move around, joint pain) related to work, home, or play? ________________
10. Name the chemicals and compounds you work with and the frequency of your contact with each. ________________
    Name the chemicals and compounds that your spouse or other family member works with. ________________
11. Does your skin ever come in contact with any chemicals or substances at work or play? ________________
12. Describe your neigborhood. ________________
    Map out the location of industrial areas, waste disposal sites, water sources, and waste disposal. ________________
13. Have any community environmental problems evolved recently? ________________
    Have there been any toxic spills, sewage breakage, smog changes, or OSHA investigations pertinent to the client's condition? ________________
14. What types of pesticides, cleaning solutions, glues, solvents, metals, or poisons are used in your home? ________________
15. What type of heating and cooling system is used in the home? ________________
    What is its impact on the illness pattern? ________________

Adapted from Wiley, O. (1989). Family environmental health. In P. Bomar (Ed.). *Nurses and family health promotion: Concepts, assessment, and interventions.* Baltimore: Williams & Wilkins.

these data are not sorted and analyzed in some way. What does this information mean, and in what way can it be used to help the nurse and family plan their work together? The information must be integrated and analyzed before decisions about the plan of care can be made. The following steps can be used to help organize these data:

- Determining family needs or areas of concern
- Determining family functioning
- Determining family style
- Determining targets of care
- Determining nursing's contribution
- Determining priorities of identified health needs

Determining Family Needs. What needs or concerns do the nurse and family want to work on? These needs are identified on multiple levels: needs of individual members, needs in family subgroups, needs of the family as a whole, and needs related to the family interacting with the environment. Nursing diagnoses can be developed that represent each of these areas. The North American Nursing Diagnosis Association (NANDA) has been identifying and listing diagnostic nomenclature since the early 1970s (North American Nursing Diagnosis Association, 1987). These diagnoses are formulated to help nurses choose and focus nursing interventions by concentrating on patient responses to actual or potential health problems rather than on the disease process. Each diagnosis consists of two parts: the unhealthy response and an indication of the factors contributing to the response. Problems can be existing (actual) or possible in the future (potential).

Individual nursing diagnoses are identified just as they are when an individual is the sole target of care. Diagnoses that represent responses to health problems are organized according to patterns or clusters of behaviors such as sleep/rest, elimination, activity/exercise (Cox et al., 1989).

Interpersonal nursing diagnoses may include needs that represent the interaction of more than one person, such as "breast-feeding, ineffective," or diagnoses that affect more than one person, such as "social interaction, impaired." Examples of individual and interpersonal nursing diagnoses are presented in Table 9–6.

Family nursing diagnoses have also been identified by NANDA. The nomenclature used includes "family processes, altered," "family coping, ineffective," and "family coping, potential for growth." The major defining characteristics that correspond to these diagnoses include most of the concepts discussed within the family chapters in this book and are presented in Table 9–7.

However, some find that the NANDA family nursing diagnoses are not sufficiently specific. Smith (1985) suggests that there are five major areas in community health nursing where families and nursing intersect (Table 9–8). This delineation may help the nurse identify more specific family needs. Families meeting normal growth and developmental challenges often benefit from preventive education or supportive contact as the family

TABLE 9–6

Interpersonal Nursing Diagnoses
Adjustment, impaired
Breast-feeding, ineffective
Home maintenance management, impaired
Individual coping, ineffective
Parenting, altered
Role performance, altered
Self-care deficit
Sexual dysfunction
Social interaction, impaired
Social isolation
Verbal communication, impaired
Violence, potential for

From North American Nursing Diagnosis Association. (1987). *Taxonomy I with complete diagnosis.* St. Louis: Author.

masters behaviors appropriate for their new stage of life. Families coping with illness or loss need not only emotional support, but also concrete help such as direct care, education, and connection to services. Families dealing with external stressors such as natural disasters, unemployment, or societal violence benefit from emotional and physical support. During this time of crisis the family may be strained and not as functional. However, it may also be a time for the family to grow and discover strength under stress.

Inadequate resources or support can be temporary or long-term. For example, a family with several events happening at once (e.g., children in college, an illness, and an aging parent) may find its usually sufficient resources inadequate. Other families deal with the chronic problem of poverty, lack of access to resources, and inadequate energy to maintain self-esteem and meet others' emotional needs.

Families with disturbances in organization create stress from within. The unhealthy way in which they operate tends to add to rather than mediate their stress. Of course, families can have combinations of these problems, or some of the problems may potentiate others. However, this framework covers most of the needs families will present in the community health setting.

Environmental problems for families are described in the Omaha System problem classification scheme (Martin and Scheet, 1992). Problems with material resources and physical surroundings include income, sanitation, residence, and neighborhood and workplace safety (Table 9–9). Family problems related to the social environment may occur in the areas of communication with community resources and social contacts (Table 9–10). For each problem there may be actual or potential impairments, or opportunities for health promotion.

Determining Family Functioning. What is the potential for change? How much energy is available for growth and change? To determine the level of family functioning the nurse may want to integrate information about family strengths, resources, and coping. Families with the most

TABLE 9–7

Major Defining Characteristics of Family Diagnoses

Family Processes, Altered

The state in which a family that normally functions effectively experiences a dysfunction.

In families with this diagnosis, the family system or family members have the following characteristics:

a. Unable to meet physical needs of members.
b. Unable to meet emotional needs of members.
c. Unable to meet spiritual needs of members.
d. Parents do not demonstrate respect for each other's views on child-rearing practices.
e. Family members unable to express or accept wide range of feelings.
f. Family members unable to express or accept feelings of other members.
g. Unable to meet security needs of its members
h. Unable to relate to each other for mutual growth and maturation.
i. Uninvolved in community activities.
j. Unable to accept or receive help appropriately.
k. Rigid in function and roles.
l. Do not demonstrate respect for individuality and autonomy of its members.
m. Unable to adapt to change or deal with traumatic experiences constructively.
n. Fail to accomplish current or past developmental tasks.
o. Unhealthy decision-making process.
p. Fail to send and receive clear messages.
q. Boundary maintenance is inappropriate.
r. Inappropriate or poorly communicated family rules, rituals, or symbols.
s. Unexamined family myths.
t. Family has inappropriate level and direction of energy.

Family Coping, Ineffective; Compromised and Disabling

Compromised: insufficient, ineffective, or compromised support, comfort, assistance, or encouragement, usually by a supportive primary person (i.e., family member or close friend). Client may need it to manage or master adaptive tasks related to his or her health challenge.

Disabling: behavior of a significant person (i.e., family member or other primary person) that disables his or her own capacities and the client's capacities to effectively address tasks essential to either person's adaptation to the health challenge.

1. Compromised
   a. Subjective
      (1) Client expresses or confirms a concern or complaint about significant other's responses to his or her health problem.
      (2) Significant person describes preoccupation with personal reactions (e.g., fear, guilt, anticipatory grief, anxiety) to client's illness, disability, or situational or developmental crisis.
      (3) Significant person describes or confirms inadequate understanding or knowledge base that interferes with effective assistive or supportive behavior.
   b. Objective
      (1) Significant person attempts assistive or supportive behavior with less than satisfactory results.
      (2) Significant person withdraws or enters into limited or temporary personal communication with the client at the time of need.
      (3) Significant person displays protective behavior disproportionate to the client's abilities or need for autonomy.
2. Disabling
   a. Neglectful care of the client in regard to basic human needs or illness treatment
   b. Distortion of reality regarding the client's health problem, including extreme denial
   c. Intolerance
   d. Rejection
   e. Abandonment
   f. Desertion
   g. Carrying out usual routines, disregarding client's needs
   h. Psychosomaticism
   i. Taking on illness signs of client
   j. Decisions and actions by family that are detrimental to economic or social well-being
   k. Agitation, depression, aggression, hostility
   l. Impaired restructuring of meaningful life for self, impaired individualization, prolonged overconcern for client
   m. Neglectful relationship with other family members
   n. Client development of helpless inactive dependence

Family Coping, Potential for Growth

Effective management of adaptive tasks by family member involved with the client's health challenge, who now is exhibiting desire and readiness for enhanced health and growth in regard to self and in relation to the client.

a. Family member attempting to describe growth impact of crisis on his or her own values, priorities, goals, or relationships.
b. Family member moving in direction of health-promoting and -enriching lifestyle.
c. Individual expressing interest in making contact with another person who has experienced a similar situation.

From North American Diagnosis Association. (1987). *Taxonomy I with complete diagnosis* (pp. 67, 74–76). St. Louis: Author.

TABLE 9–8

Determining Family Needs

1. **The Family Dealing with Normal Growth and Development**
   - Transitions such as births, divorces, and a child going to college are stressful for all families.
   - As children grow older, the family must adjust and learn new roles and ways of operating together.
   - Normal age-related behaviors may be unexpected or unfamiliar to the family.
2. **The Family Coping with Illness or Loss**
   - Illness may be acute or chronic but is almost always accompanied by demands such as financial strain or inability to perform family roles.
   - The family often needs to accomplish health care tasks such as special diets, exercises, or tracheostomy care.
   - It is a myth that all people should be encouraged to talk about their feelings. Individuals cope in different ways: humor, action, denial, intellectualizing, seeking support of others.
   - It is a myth that family coping requires simple, open communication. Families cope in different ways: pulling together, depending on one member, distancing, seeking help from the community.
3. **The Family Dealing with an External Stress**
   - Stress from the environment is usually unexpected and therefore more difficult to deal with.
   - The event may be positive or negative, but is still stressful because it requires the family to rearrange itself or to adjust emotionally.
   - The environment may be hazardous.
4. **The Family with Inadequate Resources and Support**
   - The family may lack equipment, money, tools, space, or other materials.
   - The family may lack emotional or social support.
   - The family may have never had the resources, may have depleted them, or may not know how to connect with available supports.
5. **The Family with Disturbances in Organization**
   - Internal dynamics lead to relationships that are problematic and ineffective.
   - Power and authority are not appropriately placed.
   - Organization may be chaotic and unpredictable or too rigid and inflexible.
   - Family members are not responsible for self: they either push things onto others or assume extra responsibility that should belong to another.
   - Unhealthy patterns are used, such as blaming, conflict, scapegoating, withdrawal, or sacrifice of one member.

Categories adapted from Smith, C. (1985). *Goals for community health nursing.* (Unpublished manuscript).

strengths and support and the widest ranges of coping behaviors are more able to manage multiple stresses and strains. A family with limited health may appear functional in times of calm but fall apart with relatively little stress. Conversely, a very healthy family may be able to function well in the presence of crushing adversity. A family with greater functional and adaptive ability will be able to progress more quickly and with less dependence on the nurse than a family with less ability.

TABLE 9–9

Nursing Diagnoses for Environmental Problems

Problem	Signs/Symptoms
Income	Low/no income; uninsured medical expenses; inadequate money management; able to buy only necessities; difficulty buying necessities; other
Sanitation	Soiled living area; inadequate food storage/disposal; insects/rodents; foul odor; inadequate water supply; inadequate sewage disposal; inadequate laundry facilities; allergens; infectious/contaminating agents; other
Residence	Structurally unsound; inadequate heating/cooling; steep stairs; inadequate/obstructed exits/entries; cluttered living space; unsafe storage of dangerous objects/substances; unsafe mats/throw rugs; inadequate safety devices; presence of lead-based paint; unsafe gas/electrical appliances; inadequate/crowded living space; homeless; other.
Neighborhood/workplace safety	High crime rate; high pollution level; uncontrolled animals; physical hazards; unsafe play areas; other

Adapted from Martin, K., & Scheet, N. (1992). *The Omaha System: Applications for community health nursing.* Philadelphia: W.B. Saunders.

Schema to measure functioning can be used. Tapia (1972) presents a classification system for family functioning that helps guide nurses' decisions. Families are classified according to their level of maturity and potential to function independently (Table 9–11).

Determining Family Style. What about the way the family typically acts will affect the way the nurse should plan and implement care with this family? In what ways does the family usually act to process information, solve problems, and open or close itself to the environment? Most families have characteristic styles that they use to meet challenges and deal with others. Identifying this style will help the nurse choose appropriate actions and ways of working with the family. Information gained from tools that assess the family's coping ability, patterns of interaction, and use of

TABLE 9–10

Nursing Diagnoses Related to the Use of Social Resources

Problem	Signs/Symptoms
Communication with community resources	Unfamiliarity with options/procedures for obtaining services; difficulty understanding roles/regulations of service providers; unable to communicate concerns to service provider; dissatisfaction with services; language barrier; inadequate/unavailable services; other
Social contact	Limited social contact; uses health care provider for social contact; minimal outside stimulation/leisure time activities; other

Adapted from Martin, K., & Scheet, N. (1992). *The Omaha System: Applications for community health nursing.* Philadelphia: W.B. Saunders.

TABLE 9–11

Criteria for Selection of Family Functioning

Characteristics	Nursing Goal
Level I: The Chaotic Family	
1. Disorganization in all areas of family life a. Barely meets needs for security and physical survival b. Members unable to secure adequate wages or housing c. Unable to budget money d. Unable to maintain adequate nutrition, clothing, heat, and cleanliness e. No future orientation 2. Inability to provide for healthy emotional and social functioning of its members (apparent alienation from community) a. Distrusts outsiders b. Unable to utilize community services and resources c. Become hostile and resistant to offers of help 3. Poor role identification a. Immature parents unable to assume responsible adult roles (child neglect or abuse often seen) b. Parents unable to act as mature role models for children 4. Family fails to provide support and growth for its individual members a. Exhibits depression and feelings of failure b. Insecurity of family members prevents change 5. Family sees the nurse as a "good parent" and will test her or him for consistency and try to be dependent	To establish a trusting relationship
Level II: The Intermediate Family	
1. Lesser degree of disorganization of family life than Level I family a. Slightly more able to meet their needs for security and physical survival b. Variation in economic level c. More hope for better way of life 2. Family unable to support and promote growth of members a. Members appear unable to change b. Defensive and fearful c. Lacks resources to gain a sense of accomplishment d. Does not seek help actively e. Requires much assistance to acknowledge problems realistically 3. Role identification a. Parents are immature; socially deviant behavior may occur b. Distortion and confusion of roles exists, but parents are more willing to work together for benefit of whole family c. Children not neglected to the extent that they must be removed from the home 4. The family will see the nurse as a sibling—that is, they will vacillate between dependence and independence, and compete for attention and control	To increase the ability of the family to understand themselves in their interaction as a group and grow to the point where they can work on solutions to some of their problems
Level III: The Adolescent Family	
1. Essentially normal but has more than the usual amount of conflicts and problems a. More capable of physical survival and providing security for its members (abilities may vary greatly) b. Variation in economic levels c. Future oriented, even though present may be painful 2. Increased ability to provide healthy emotional and social functioning of its members a. Greater trust in people b. Have knowledge and ability to utilize some community resources c. Less openly hostile to outsiders d. Increased ability to face some of its problems and look for solutions 3. Role identification a. Usually one parent appears more mature than other b. Children have less overall difficulty adjusting to changes in family, school, environment c. Difficulty in providing sexual differentiation and training of children d. Because one parent may appear quite immature, adult role model for one or more of the children may be lacking (physical care usually adequate, but emotional conflicts usually present) 4. Family members experience achievements and successes outside the family to replace missing satisfaction within family life 5. The nurse will be seen by the family as an adult helper with expertise in the solution of problems	To help them improve the ability to manage their roles and tasks as they proceed from one problem to another

TABLE 9–11

Criteria for Selection of Family Functioning (Continued)

Characteristics	Nursing Goal
Level IV: The Adult Family	
1. Normal organization in most areas of family life a. Capably provides for physical security and survival b. Steady adequate wage earner c. Enjoy present and plan for future 2. Capably provides for emotional and social functioning a. Family has ability to adapt and change in crisis situations b. Is able to handle most problems as they arise; however, may show anxiety over these problems c. Often refer themselves to outside services for help d. Individual and group needs and goals are usually brought into harmony by this family 3. Family confident in roles 4. Main problems center around stages of growth and developmental tasks 5. Family sees the nurse as an expert teacher and partner and is able to utilize this partnership	Preventive health teaching to enable family to maintain its health and to increase the members' self understanding and effectiveness in group functioning

Adapted from Tapia, J. (1972). The nursing process in family health. *Nursing Outlook, 20*(4), 267–270.

support from others can be integrated to complete this analysis. Table 9–12 presents a format for thinking about family style.

Determining Targets of Care. Who will be involved in the care, and at what level? Who is the most likely person in the family to be able to change his or her own behavior? Who is likely to communicate with or assert power over other members? What members are so burdened by problems that they need support rather than new challenges?

The family assessment may reveal many actual needs or potential problems. There may be too many to deal with at once, and some people may not wish to be involved in the care. Because families act as systems, an action applied to one member will influence the other members. The nurse may need to make predictions about how certain actions may affect individual members and the family as a whole. For instance, if a child who is afraid of school is successfully encouraged to return to school, another child in the family may begin to "act out." Of course, the most useful care plan will develop from the wishes of the family members who will be responsible for implementing it. Targeting some individuals as recipients of care without their cooperation will be less helpful than if the idea to participate comes from within.

Determining Nursing's Contribution. What can the nurse do for and with this family? The nurse needs to define a focus not only for the family, but also for self. The needs of the family may be beyond the scope of the nurse's competence or energy, and time and resources become a factor in making decisions about what a nurse can do. The role of the nurse is also dictated by the agency and reimbursement mechanisms. A successful community health nurse will be very aware of his or her strengths and preferences and try to use them whenever possible. Being able to say "no" or to give up responsibilities is helpful in the long run when potential nursing actions are not realistic. Friedemann's (1989) description of nursing roles is helpful here. The nurse, depending on the analysis of the family and the nurse's experience, chooses to focus on individuals, interpersonal interactions, the family as a whole, or the family's interface with its community.

Determining Priorities of Identified Needs. What is most crucial? What is the most essential or necessary? What is possible given current constraints? What is most likely to empower the family to act in healthy ways in behalf of itself in the future? Some people will use a framework such as that developed by Maslow (1972) to help them determine priorities. Usually anything that is life threatening or a threat to physical safety will be the top priority. Beyond that, certain decisions need to be made to help ensure that the care of the family will be effective. Dunst et al. (1988) suggest that the key to working with families is recognizing their need for empowerment. Helping the family discover or regain its sense of power and hope is the basis for the members to be able to continue to build adaptive behaviors and strengths. When working with families, the need that assumes top priority (after life-threatening emergenices) is the need the family itself identifies as most important. Sometimes this may conflict with the nurse's ordering of priorities. Dunst et al. urge the nurse to choose the family's identified need first, achieve some success and trust when a realistic and achievable goal is accomplished, and then go on to priorities suggested by the nurse.

Once the family and the nurse have identified the family needs and strengths and established priorities, plans for action can be made. Interventions with the family system

TABLE 9–12

Determining Family Style

A Receptive Family
- Opens up to suggestions.
- Is eager to work with the system.
- Will accept part of the responsibility for the problem and solution.

A Distancing Family
- Understands the problem but has difficulty making connections with resources.
- Is embarrassed or tries to deny the problem's existence.
- Has difficulty dealing with the emotions surrounding the contact.

A Resistive Family
- Denies or disagrees with institutional interpretation of the problem or the solutions.
- Feels powerless in the face of the larger system.
- May play along without really cooperating or following through on suggestions.

A Chaotic Family
- Is flexible and experiences frequent and quick changes.
- May be extremely adaptive or so disorganized or pressured that this problem is only one of many.
- May have difficulty cooperating with planning or solutions because family life is unpredictable and unstructured.

A Rigid Family
- Has a fixed way of dealing with things that cannot easily be changed to accommodate new demands or behaviors.
- May see itself as incapable of carrying out new routines, even if the family accepts the solutions.

A Lopsided Family
- Power or responsibility lies mostly with one adult member.
- Member may be too burdened to accomplish all that needs to be done.
- The "doer" may have to struggle with another adult to accomplish the changes.

An Ordered Family
- Hierarchy, roles, and lines of communication are clearly spelled out.
- The way the family usually works together results in success and accomplishments.

A Tight Family
- Family members depend on each other for physical assistance and emotional support.
- Talking to one member usually means the rest of the family will receive the information quickly.
- The family prefers to look to its own rather than to those outside.

are the most exciting and challenging part of the nurse's role in family nursing. However, the nurse who enters into this role without an appropriate understanding of some principles risks frustration and disappointment. Sometimes inexperienced nurses believe that they must change the internal dynamics of the family system if their nursing care is to be successful. However, a change to the family system can come only from within the family. Sometimes other goals (e.g., strengthening support systems and learning to cope with an illness) are helpful and more appropriate when working with families.

Developing a Plan

Planning family nursing care occurs after the family system is assessed and data are analyzed in a systematic way. Priorities are determined with the family. Remember that nursing interventions are primarily directed toward the five areas of needs that are identified through most family–nurse interactions: growth and development, coping with losses and illness, adapting to the demands of or modifying the environment, strengthening inadequate resources and support, and dealing with disturbances in internal dynamics. The target of the interventions may be an individual, a subsystem, the family unit, or the interaction with the environment. The level of family functioning will affect the type and extent to which goals can be achieved. For example, families with lower levels of functioning need goals that are short term, realistic, concrete, and compatible with their definitions of what is needed. Also, family style will determine the way the nurse applies interventions.

PRINCIPLES OF FAMILY CARE PLANNING

Mutuality. The biggest mistake a nurse can make is to forget that the care plan is supposed to benefit the family. If the family has identified the problem and some solutions that they are willing to work toward, their energy and attention will be directed toward a goal that both the nurse and family support. Dunst et al. (1988) remind us that "a need is an individual's judgement of the discrepancy between actual states or conditions and what is considered normative, desired or valued *from a help seeker's and not a help giver's perspective.*" Unless there is an indicated need on the part of the help seeker, there may not be a need, regardless of what the professional believes to be the case. Mutuality in family–nurse interactions must occur during identification of the family's needs, definition of goals, choices for nurse and family actions, and evaluation of effectiveness.

Individualization. Even though many families experience similar issues and have common health problems, each family care plan must be unique for that family. The family structure, style of operation, values, strengths, perception of the problem, resources, preferred goals, and level of functioning all will influence the way nursing care should be planned. Two families may have the same health problem and yet require a very different nursing intervention.

Realistic Goals. When a nurse first connects with a family, the tendency is to try to do everything at once. An outsider looking in on a family can often see many things that hinder the growth and happiness of some of the members. Just because they are identified as potential problems by the nurse, however, does not mean that these problems concern the family or that the family wants to change. Time and resources are also limited, and goals must be adjusted to the limitations determined by the nurse's employer or by funding. To some extent, family functional level will also determine the level of goal that can be achieved. According to Tapia (1972) a family that is operating on an adult level will be able to achieve goals that have to do with health prevention and minimization of potential problems. In contrast, a realistic goal for a chaotic family would be connecting the family to a resource that will perform some of the family maintenance functions and then coaching them to use the resource appropriately.

Values and Health Care Beliefs. Behavior begins with thoughts and feelings about the situation. The family's beliefs and values will direct their responses to any situation. A care plan that takes the family's values into account will have a greater chance of success than a plan that works against family values (see Chapter 6).

Coordination with the Health Care Team. Neither the nurse nor the family operates in isolation from other professionals and institutions within the community. The plan must be coordinated with all involved for it to be successful, avoid duplication, and maximize the use of resources. Nothing is more frustrating to a family than to be pulled or advised in two different directions by two agencies that are supposed to be helping them.

Defining Self. For the nurse who works within the community, the demands and needs that he or she sees will be great, and sometimes overwhelming. In a community where many people are operating with scarce resources, many people must do as much as they can. The nurse who wants to work in a community setting for any extended period of time will soon realize that choices must be made about how time and resources are spent. Being aware of her or his own beliefs and purpose within the setting will help the nurse to make these choices in ways that continue to be satisfying and do not overextend the capabilities of any one person. Sometimes the nurse will encounter a situation that is at odds with her or his personal beliefs. Being clear about one's operating principles helps one to respond in a thoughtful and ethical way rather than an automatic, emotional way.

A traditional care plan format is presented in Table 9–13.

Implementing the Plan

HELPING THE FAMILY COPE WITH ILLNESS OR LOSS

Nurses often view their role as one that supports a family's coping. Most nurses think this means the nurse is expected to provide emotional support for a family that is experiencing stress. This is often accomplished in conversations in which the nurse is available and empathetic to family concerns. However, many families actually need other, different types of interventions to support their coping.

Coping is a set of behaviors that emerge whenever a person or family is confronted with a stressor that requires some mobilization of energy. The stressor can be a positive or negative event, but it often demands some adaptation or change in behavior from a member or the family as a whole. Effective coping will result in an outcome that is positive not just for one family member, but for the whole family. Coping requires both *instrumental* and *affective* actions. *Instrumental actions* are coping behaviors that accomplish a task, such as changing a dressing, locating a source of oxygen supply, or making a clinic appointment. *Affective actions* are coping behaviors that help modify negative emotions that might arise during the stressful situation. Examples of affective coping include talking to others, putting the illness out of one's awareness, or using humor to diffuse tension.

Families and individuals within families already have a repertoire of coping behaviors that they use when stress arises. Sometimes these coping behaviors are effective, and sometimes they are not. When a stressful situation first arises, the nurse can be most helpful in assisting a family to think about the crisis. How a family perceives a crisis may greatly affect how they are able to deal with it. The same situation may be perceived by one family as an event from which there is no recovery, and by another family as an opportunity to forge new bonds. After the crisis is identified and an accurate perception of what is happening is shared, some family members may benefit from discussing their emotional reactions to the crisis, while some may be very uncomfortable with this strategy. In this early stage of the crisis, the nurse can help the family identify its typical coping behaviors and support or

TABLE 9–13

Components of a Care Plan

Nursing Diagnosis	Goals	Nurse-Family Actions	Rationale	Evaluation
Individual, interpersonal, family, and environmental diagnoses	Long- and short-term	Interventions to be performed	Scientific: derived from research or theory; individualized	Criteria are observable, measurable outcomes

encourage their use. A family in crisis should not try to change unless what it is doing is dysfunctional or not working.

There is no single right or wrong way to cope. For example, denying a problem or distancing oneself from it in some cases may be protective and necessary until the situation changes. Sometimes the coping that is chosen by the family does not work or does not work in a healthy way for the entire family. At this point, the nurse can help the family identify alternative coping behaviors. Coming up with a list of alternatives can be accomplished jointly with the nurse who may have more ideas or information than the family.

The nurse then helps the family select alternative coping behaviors that seem workable to them. As the family tries these new ways of coping, the nurse is available to offer feedback, reinforce new behaviors, and act as a sounding board as the family makes decisions about the next course of action.

Families who are dealing with illness and loss may encounter experiences where nothing that they do will make the situation better. When tragedy strikes, a loved one dies, or a family must confront an irreversible loss, there are no actions that will make the situation right again. In these situations, both the nurse and the family often resolve the situation by searching for some meaning within what has happened. Dass and Gorman (1986) ask "How can I help?" The nurse who can find meaning in what she or he does when she or he cannot "help" is very valuable to a family in this situation. Having a compassionate and thoughtful contact within the health care system is useful for almost any family dealing with a crisis.

TEACHING THE FAMILY EXPERIENCING DEVELOPMENTAL CHANGES

Every family deals with the experience of members who grow older and confront day-to-day life in new ways. Many families add or lose members as the family reproduces, the children grow to adulthood, and the family ages. The developmental stage of a family will indicate typical tasks that need to be completed. Even the most functional families are novices during the experience of growing into a new stage. Other families confronted with *situational* as well as *maturational* tasks may be more overwhelmed by dealing with many new things simultaneously. Families at lower functional levels may be poorly prepared to deal with any additional demands and may view new behaviors of developing members with anger or misunderstanding (see Chapter 10).

The nurse's role when dealing with families who are confronting developmental demands is primarily educational. Providing information about normal growth and development and the adaptations required by parents, children, and extended family members can prevent potential problems and help families manage current ones. The information that is provided may be new to the family, or it may be a reinforcement of what the family already knows but has not recognized as important. Families will differ in their ability to hear information presented by the nurse, especially if the timing competes with other demands that seem more pressing. To effectively teach families with developmental needs, the nurse must assess each member's current knowledge of the developmental issue and then gain agreement from family members that this is something they would like to learn more about. Teaching–learning interactions should be planned for maximum effectiveness, considering timing, the learner's ability, and the method of presentation. After each session, the nurse validates the family's understanding of the content. Finally, the nurse helps the family problem-solve solutions that will satisfy the current or potential developmental demands.

Through this entire process, the nurse is concerned with normalizing the situation for the family. In other words, the more family members can perceive this situation as something that all families go through, the more objective they may be about it. Even though a situation is normal, families may feel pressured or uncomfortable. Not all families will or should adapt to the situation in the same way. Helping the family use its knowledge of its strengths and values to choose operating principles that are compatible must be done on an individual basis for each family.

CONNECTING THE FAMILY TO NEEDED RESOURCES

Some families do not have the necessary resources; other families have difficulty accessing them. Resources are both internal and external—that is, both within the family and in the community. Resources can be tangible (e.g., money, clothing, transportation, or shelter) or intangible (e.g., strong values, emotional support, religious beliefs, or a sense of family solidarity). Resources for health promotion, prevention, and early detection of health probelms are especially important (see Chapters 16 and 17). One of the most obvious roles of the community health nurse is helping families identify and access resources. Families may not know their way around the community or the health care system as well as an effective community health nurse does. The ability to act as a provider of information, a liaison, or a coordinator of resources is essential for community health nurses.

The nurse who desires to help families access resources will thoroughly assess tangible and intangible resources that have the potential for being useful in the situation. Many families have a need for multiple resources; identifying the one or two that are most helpful to the need will target the nurse's and family's energies.

Sometimes resources that are not typically seen as helpful may be used creatively in certain situations. For example, the family may think there is no one to care for an ill member but be ignoring a family member who could, but typically does not, perform this role. Encouraging the family to open itself up to new ways of using internal resources is useful.

Families that are closed—that is, families with boundaries that are not very permeable—often like to try to deal with problems themselves. These families may have strong beliefs that they should manage troubles themselves. Helping them accept aid from extended family members, the community, or professionals may involve exploring their beliefs and offering help while acknowledging the family's preferred style. Other families may have had past experiences with resources that have turned out to be ineffectual or inadequate. Making sure that resources are reliable and that the family has realistic expectations of what the resource can provide are ways to prevent repeats of earlier experiences.

COACHING THE FAMILY TO CHANGE ITS INTERNAL DYNAMICS

The process of change within a family will occur naturally as the family grows and adapts to new and ever-changing environmental circumstances. Most families do not need help to change their way of operating in general; instead, they need help to adapt and cope with new developmental, situational, and environmental challenges. The nurse assists the family to change not because there is something wrong with the family, but because the family style and organization are not effectively meeting the current demands.

Sometimes, however, families do not effectively meet the needs of their members even in times that are relatively calm. These families with disturbances in internal dynamics are candidates for change in the family system.

The community health nurse who is informed about the dynamics of families and has some training in family coaching is in the perfect position to serve as a catalyst for change. Often family coaching is taught at the graduate level.

Principles of Change

1. Many families are resistant to change. Even when the change would probably be beneficial to the family, families may prefer to remain as they are. It is easier to remain in what is known than to exert energy to move into the unknown.
2. Sequencing/timing will affect the outcome. Families have difficulty changing during times of crisis or stress. However, this is often the best time to change, because the family sees the need for it then. Change is most likely to happen after perceptions of the situation begin to change. Working on the family's cognition or thinking about the problem is the first step in an intervention. Helping the family modify affect and behavior comes next.
3. Past patterns must be interrupted. Families tend to operate in patterns of interaction that repeat themselves. Triggers set up behaviors that all family members respond to automatically. It is difficult to break these patterns and start healthier behavioral sequences, but it can be done.
4. A change in one part of the system will affect the whole system. No person can change another, but any person can change himself or herself. What we do and the way we react has an impact on others. When any one person in a system changes, the system will automatically change.
5. The more important a family member is to the family's functioning, the more impact a change in that family member will have. Not all family members will change equally or have equal capacity to change. Identifying the family member who is most likely to be able to change is a good strategy for the nurse who desires to help the family modify its functioning.
6. Family strengths are as important as family problems. The perception of the family problem is often unhealthier than the problem. When one family member is blamed or held responsible for others, the shared nature of the family problem cannot be recognized. For example, at times Harry is lazy and irresponsible. Is it also possible that Harry adds humor and genuineness to a restricted family environment? Can the problem be reframed and seen as an asset?
7. A family's capacity to change is related to its level of functioning. The family has probably operated at a certain level of health for some time before the nurse appears on the scene. Having realistic ideas about what can be accomplished for each family is necessary. The nurse who can help the family think about issues in ways that lead to a small improvement in or maintenance of functioning will mean the family is in better shape than having no intervention at all.

Techniques that nurses use to help families change include contracting, tracking family process, increasing cognitive awareness, reframing, aligning or maintaining neutral connections to family members, exploring affect, restructuring, suggesting direct interventions, and offering paradoxical interventions (Minuchin and Fishman, 1981) (Table 9–14). Formulating a contract with the family at the beginning of the interaction, having a definite goal, and limiting the number of sessions helps keep the interaction focused. At different times during the sessions, the professional carefully chooses a position in relation to family members, such as aligning with a weak member or maintaining neutral but meaningful connections to all.

Reframing is a way to label negative as positive. Something that is perceived as negative can be explored and renamed in a positive way. This breaks up the family's typical way of thinking about the problem and helps them

TABLE 9–14

Strategies for Helping Families Change Internal Dynamics

Contracting
Exploring affect
Teaching–learning interactions
Problem-solving techniques
Exploring coping strategies
Offering feedback and emotional support
Referral
Role modeling
Family coaching
Reframing
Restructuring
Aligning
Detriangling
Paradoxes and reversals
Tracking family process

begin to think of alternatives. Cognitive perceptions and knowledge about family dynamics can be broadened. When this happens, objectivity about the family problem is increased and family members are able to act in less reactive ways.

During early sessions, the family process or patterns of interaction are tracked by the professional and brought into the awareness of the family. Seeing the repetitive nature of the behavior sequences and recognizing the behavioral triggers is the first step to being able to modify behavior. Affect or feelings that accompany behavioral sequences can be named and examined. Many times, if the behavioral sequence is changed, the emotion that accompanies it will also change.

Direct interventions are directions or activities suggested by the nurse to be carried out by the family. These include suggestions to do something or to stop doing something. Often this is given in the form of "homework" to be tried out over the next week. *Restructuring,* one type of direct intervention, is a suggestion by the nurse that helps to reorder the family power and subsystems in ways that are healthier and more age appropriate. For example, a father may be encouraged to discuss his intense work frustrations more with his wife than with his preteen daughter. This suggestion seeks to strengthen the spousal subsystem and keep the daughter within the parent–child subsystem.

Indirect interventions are interventions that are not clearly presented as orders. One example is a paradoxical intervention, which is an admonition by the professional to the family to do the opposite of what is expected, or an instruction not to do something. These interventions must be used skillfully, but they often have great impact because they are a surprise and an interruption to the family process.

Helping a family change its internal dynamics is not a goal to be attempted by every nurse, but with practice and training many nurses become effective family coaches.

HELPING THE FAMILY REMAIN HEALTHY WITHIN THE ENVIRONMENT

The world in which families live is resource rich, and our society performs many functions that used to be the responsibility of the family. Families and family members are healthier and have access to many more living aids than did families in the past. However, today's world is also a potential threat to health in many ways. Pollutants in our air, water, food, homes, schools, and occupational settings are threats to family health. Our social environment also exposes us to unsafe situations of crime, violence, drug abuse, and deteriorating interpersonal behavior. Many families make plans for their lives, only to have them affected by situations beyond their control, such as buy-outs and mergers of employers, changes in health and retirement benefits, and a changing economy.

The community health nurse interested in family health will consider family–environment interactions (see Chapter 24). Actual health problems may be related to or aggravated by environmental issues, and potential health problems related to environmental issues may be diverted. Surveillance, detection, and correction of environmental threats become a way to help families maintain their health. Education of families and communities is crucial to help the public become aware of potential health threats and strategies for dealing with them. Nurses also have the opportunity to intervene by providing data that influence health care decisions and by participating in legislative and executive processes that formulate health policy.

Evaluation

Evaluation is the final step of the nursing process, but it is also a step that starts at the beginning of the contact and occurs continuously as the contact progresses. The word *evaluate* means to determine the worth of something. There are many methods that can be used to evaluate nursing care, but the key to evaluation is to determine the correct criteria that demonstrate the value of the nursing contact. Criteria for evaluating client outcomes are derived from the objectives developed with the family. Because the outcomes of nursing interventions occurring during one visit may not be apparent until later, both long- and short-term evaluative criteria should be developed.

Methods. Two methods of evaluation are *formative* and *summative* evaluation. *Formative evaluation* is evaluation that occurs during the course of nurse–family interactions. It can be used to guide decisions about modification of goals, objectives, nursing actions, and priorities as the nursing encounters unfold. Data are collected once or multiple times during the home visiting process. Examples of formative evaluation methods include keeping daily records of blood glucose levels, holding monthly health care team meetings to discuss family progress, or asking the family for feedback at the end of each visit. Formative evaluation helps the nurse and family modify nursing care in a more effective way.

Summative evaluation occurs at the end of the family–nurse relationship and is used to summarize the value of the interaction to the family. A description of the extent of goal accomplishment and remaining family needs helps the family make choices about termination or referral. The family can review with the nurse the actions that it used to achieve its goals and can leave the relationship with a sense of accomplishment. Summative evaluation can also help inform the nurse about her or his effectiveness and provide feedback about specific nursing actions and suggestions for working with other families in the future. Examples of summative evaluation include an oral quiz about a client's knowledge of his or her medication, a discharge planning meeting with the health care team, or a conversation with a family about the series of visits.

Factors Influencing Evaluation. Many factors influence evaluation; an example is the availability of data. If data are easy to obtain and have been carefully collected, the evaluation is likely to be accurate and complete. The resources available to the nurse and health care team also influence the outcomes being judged during evaluation. In a community health situation that is resource rich, it is expected that many of the family's needs will be met. In a situation with fewer resources, outcomes are likely to be judged more leniently. Family expectations also influence evaluation. If the family began the encounter with a realistic expectation of what could be accomplished and under what circumstances the nurse would leave, the family is more likely to be satisfied with what has happened. Families who expect something the professionals are unlikely to be able to deliver will naturally leave the interaction disappointed. Also, the nature of the family–nurse–health care team interaction often influences the way people view the encounter. Relationships that have been pleasant and mutually satisfying are more likely to lead to perceptions that the nursing care has been effective than are relationships in which some or all of the parties have been dissatisfied or uncomfortable.

Finally, the nurse's attitudes will influence her or his judgment of success. Many new nurses enter community health situations with unrealistic expectations of their own power. Nurses cannot "fix" families, but they can help families maintain or improve their level of wellness within realistic limits.

What to Evaluate

Examination of Goals. At the beginning of the planning process, the nurse and family state the criteria for goal achievement. If these criteria are clearly stated and data are available, then it is a simple matter to determine goal achievement. Goals should be written in the form of outcomes so that the true impact of the nursing intervention can be determined. For example, knowing that a family member read a pamphlet about insulin administration is not the same as seeing the family member administer an injection.

Remember that there are both short-term and long-term objectives. During the evaluation process, examination of short-term objectives may make it evident that the long-term goal is not going to be achieved. Revision of either the long-term goal or the actions performed to accomplish the goal may be necessary.

Examination of Effect on the Ill Member. Many family nursing encounters are initiated because someone in the family has been identified as sick. The person who is the focus of care, especially one who has been identified by an agency or reimbursement mechanism, is the primary person to be evaluated. What effect have nursing actions had on the ill family member? Is his or her health status improved? Has his or her position and role within the family changed in any way? To what extent is this person satisfied with the nursing contact?

Examination of Effect on Individuals. Many times other individuals within the family have health needs of their own. Other members will be involved in offering care to the ill person or in coping with necessary changes. Family nursing interventions often upset the balance within a family. What is the impact on each member of the family? To what extent have individual health needs been met? To what extent is each person satisfied with the nursing contact?

Examination of Effect on Subsystems. A subsystem of the family may have been the target of care or may be particularly affected by the activities of the family. For example, the nurse may have been working with a single mother with regard to her parenting of a toddler. The sibling subsystem—two older children in the family—may feel left out or may have benefited by the mother's new skills. As families learn new behaviors, other groups of people within the family may be affected. Have the changes been beneficial and satisfying for all the members of the system? Do interventions need to be planned for another portion of the family to balance recent activity?

Examination of Effect on the Family Unit. A family is more than a collection of individuals; it is a unit that can stand on its own. How has the family as a whole benefited or responded to the nursing interventions? Is it able to function more effectively? Does the family operate more smoothly as a unit? What is the affective response to the interactions? Is the family more able to master situations and problem-solve for itself?

Examination of Interaction with the Environment. The family is not isolated, but lives within an environmental context. How has the family–environment interaction changed? Is this change beneficial to the family? Is it beneficial to the community? Is there reason to plan more or different actions directed toward the family's interaction with their context?

Examination of Nursing Performance. The nurse also will benefit from evaluating self. Was the nurse prepared for each nursing visit? What knowledge did the nurse bring to the visit? What new knowledge would have been helpful? How skillful was the nurse during the performance of his or her tasks? Are there other skills the nurse needs to acquire? How did the nurse's own values and attitudes influence the interactions? Did the nurse use feedback to modify performance? How much effort was put into communicating and coordinating care with other members of the health care team? To what extent is the nurse satisfied with the family interactions? These insights can be used to maintain the quality of the current family care and for the nurse's future family contacts.

Outcome of Evaluation. Sometimes people think of evaluation as the end of the nursing process. In many situations, however, it is just the beginning. If evaluation is used properly at several predetermined times during the nurse–family relationship, it should help the nurse refine the nursing care plan and improve its quality. There are three possible outcomes: modification, continuation, and resolution.

Modification. Modification or change may be necessary in any part of the nursing care plan, including identification of needs, establishment of priorities, selection of short- or long-term goals, or choice of nursing or family actions. The nurse and family may change their ideas about timing or which family member will perform certain tasks. Modification is a necessary step in a nursing care plan if it is to be a plan that the family really needs.

Continuation. The evaluation may show that the plans that have been made are working or are likely to work. Continuation of the plan is evidence of successful planning but does not imply that termination is imminent.

Resolution. Hopefully, some or all of the original needs will be resolved or no longer require nurse and family actions. A need is resolved when outcome criteria have been achieved or when the family no longer perceives it as a need. Resolution of some needs may allow the family to proceed to needs perceived as having less priority or to decide that terminating the nurse–family relationship is appropriate.

Terminating the Nurse–Family Relationship

Ending a meaningful relationship always elicits feelings for the family and for the nurse. In any relationship that has been defined as potentially therapeutic for the family, attention should be paid to the termination process. During termination everyone involved must deal with their personal feelings about separation. Many people have a preferred form of separation: they may distance themselves; attempt to prolong the contact; become angry, sad, or "act out"; or deny that the relationship has been important. The type of reaction depends to some extent on the way separations have happened in the past.

In the community health setting, the nurse frequently experiences termination. Clients may experience them all too often when community health nurses are transferred or cases are discharged without much notice. Careful planning, advance notice, and talking about the emotions and issues that arise are helpful for all involved. Often the nurse will bring up the issue of termination before the client is ready. Allowing clients to express reactions and helping families perceive themselves as able to master upcoming situations independently will help the family make the transition to independence and termination.

During the final visits, the nurse begins to prepare the family by reminding them that the time together is limited. A date or goal should be set that is understood as the marking point for termination. Goal accomplishment, satisfaction with the process, and plans for continuation of health maintenance should be discussed. If referrals or transfers are needed, they are arranged at this time. Criteria should be established for the family to know when to seek health care again; for example, reappearance of the signs and symptoms of a chronic mental illness would be a signal for the family to contact the clinic. Hopefully, the nurse will find a way to frame the outcomes of the visits in a way that indicates success for the family even if the original goals were not met. In almost every contact, there is something the nurse and family learned or some way that they grew that could be presented as a success.

KEY IDEAS

1. Family nursing takes place within the framework of the nursing process.
2. Families are assessed on several levels: individual, subsystem, family unit, and family–environment interaction.
3. The goal of family assessment is mutual identification of needs and care planning that includes both the nurse and the family.
4. A family map diagrams the structure and organization of the family and its subsystems.
5. A genogram identifies family facts and process, including multigenerational patterns of relationships.
6. An eco-map describes the energy exchanges between the family and the environment.
7. Analysis of family data helps the nurse determine family needs, family style, and family functioning.

8. Analysis of family data includes determination of the targets of care, nursing contribution, and the priorities of family needs.
9. NANDA has specified several nursing diagnoses related to families focusing on family process and family coping.
10. The Omaha System identifies family problems related to the use of social resources and the environment.
11. Family strengths are as important as family problems.
12. The success of family health care depends on setting realistic goals related to family functional level.
13. Different nursing strategies are used for each family need: developmental and health promotion needs, coping with illness or loss, inadequate support, coping with the environment, and disturbances in internal dynamics.
14. Families are resistant to change, but a time of crisis is often the best opportunity for change.
15. As the importance of the family member increases, the impact of a change in that member on the family increases.
16. Helping a family change its internal dynamics is not a goal for every community health nurse or every family.
17. The two kinds of evaluation are formative and summative.
18. Evaluation should include examination of goals and the effect of intervention on the ill family member, other individuals, family subsystems, the entire family, and the environment.
19. Evaluation should also include evaluation of the quality of nursing performance.
20. The outcome of evaluation may be modification of the plan, continuation of the plan, or resolution of the problem.

GUIDELINES FOR LEARNING

1. Choose one of the family assessment tools and apply it to a family you know. In what ways does the tool help you identify information to collect? Would you have considered this information important without the guidance of the tool? In what ways does the tool restrict your thinking about the family? What important information did not get included?
2. Trace the origins of one of the assessment tools back to the original theoretical concepts from which it evolved. Is the theory appropriate for thinking about this family? Would different concepts seem to fit better?
3. Draw a structural–functional map of an ideal family. Then draw a structural–functional map of a family you know from television programs such as "The Simpsons," "The Waltons," "Step by Step," or "Family Matters." In what ways does the television family match your ideal?
4. Try to complete a genogram of your own family for at least three generations. What was it like to ask family members questions about your family? Did you find out information that was not known to you before? How did family members respond to thinking about past generations? Can you figure out the relationships as well as the facts of the family? Where would you go to find out missing information?
5. What functional level would you assign to your family of origin? What data support your analysis?
6. Think about a patient you have known as an inpatient. Can you apply some of the family concepts to his or her situation? How might knowing more about the family have helped you with his or her care?
7. Think about the family you have in your community health clinical practicum. What categories of needs does this family have? Do the family needs fit into more than one category? Which category of needs do you feel most prepared to deal with as a nurse? Which are you the least informed about? What do you need to learn to prepare you to deal with these types of needs?
8. Assess your clinical family's environment. How does the environment affect your thinking about your care planning?
9. How many different dyads (two-person groups [e.g., mother–infant]) can you think of that might occur in a family? Where do health priorities and problems fit into these dyads?
10. In a student group, role play an initial encounter with a family. Introduce yourself, engage the family, do some initial assessment, and set up a contract for your repeated visits.
11. In a student group, role play a visit in which you and the family are planning mutual goals. Have an observer set up the situation so that the goals of the family and the goals of the nurse are slightly different. Can you negotiate and come to an agreement?
12. Think of three examples of summative evaluation and three examples of formative evaluation in your clinical area. What formative and summative evaluation methods would be appropriate for your clinical family?

⑬ Identify the family style of one family that you know. Try different interpersonal approaches with this family. Which ones seem to work best? Does the family give you any clues about how they would like you to interact with them?

⑭ Watch a movie that demonstrates family interaction (e.g., *Dad* or *A River Runs Through It*). Try to apply family assessment tools to the family. Can you make a care plan that addresses this family's needs, style, and level of functioning?

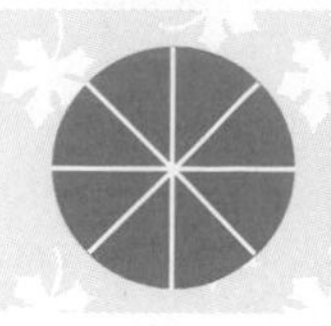

APPLYING THE NURSING PROCESS: *Formulating a Family Care Plan*

Mr. R is an 80-year-old retired pipe fitter who lives with his wife; he has had diabetes for 15 years. Although his diabetes has been moderately controlled with diet and daily insulin, some complications have occurred. He experiences arteriosclerotic cardiovascular disease (ASCVD) and peripheral neuropathy, and recently he spent 2 months in the hospital with circulatory problems in his left leg. The progressive deterioration of circulation resulted in an amputation below the knee. Although fitting him with a prosthesis would be possible, he currently refuses this and is wheelchair bound. Currently he is depending on someone else to help with transfers. He is cranky, irritable, and demanding to almost everyone. He has recently stopped following his diabetic regimen because he claims it just doesn't matter anymore.

Mr. R's wife, Doris, is a 74-year-old woman who has been a homemaker most of her life. She has always been the "watchdog" for Mr. R's health. It is mostly through her changes in food preparation and her lifestyle adjustments that Mr. R's diabetes has been cared for. She schedules his physician appointments, buys his medical supplies, and administers his insulin. He is now refusing to accept her help, and she is anxious and angry about his behavior. They frequently argue, after which Mrs. R retreats to her room.

Mr. and Mrs. R have three children and four grandchildren who live in the same city. The eldest daughter, Patricia, calls or stops by about once a week. The other children, Tom and Ellen, are busy with their families and see their parents mostly on holidays. They have very little communication with Patricia or their parents. When the children do come to visit, Doris tries to put on a happy expression and pretend everything is going well so she won't worry them. She is also embarrassed about Mr. R's behavior and doesn't want anyone from outside the family to see what is going on.

On her initial home visit to this family, the community health nurse noted that Mr. R appeared somewhat drowsy and unkempt. Mrs. R looked anxious and tired, her skin color was slightly ashen, and she had circles under her eyes. When the nurse asked them what they hoped to get out of the nursing visits, Mrs. R said, "Actually, you don't need to keep visiting. In a few weeks we'll be back to normal and doing fine."

Formulating a Care Plan

Based on a thorough assessment of the family, the community health nurse may begin to develop a mutually acceptable plan of care with the family.

Assessment

In the initial interview, the community health nurse completed a genogram and an eco-map with the family (see Figs. 9–2 and 9–3). After the second family interview, the nurse was also able to complete a family map that described members' interactions with each other (see Fig. 9–1). A family guide to help structure a family assessment is presented in Table 9–15.

Completing the genogram helped break the ice to get the family to talk about their situation. It provided a safe and thought-provoking way for Mrs. R to supply appropriate information about the situation. During this process, the nurse obtained information about other family members, their general level of functioning, and the possibility of acting as resources. She was able to identify family members' patterns of closeness and distance.

Continued on page 244

TABLE 9–15

Family Assessment Guide

I. Identifying Data

Name ______________________________

Address ______________________________

Phone ______________________________

Household members (relationship, sex, age, occupation) ______________________________

____

____

Financial data (sources of income, financial assistance, medical care plans, expenditures) ______________________________

____

____

Ethnicity ______________________________

Religion ______________________________

Identified patient(s) ______________________________

Source of referral and reason ______________________________

____

____

II. Genogram

Include household members, extended family, and significant others
Ages or date of birth, occupation, geographic location, illnesses, health problem, major events
Triangles and characteristics of relationships

III. Individual Health Needs

Identified health problems or concerns ______________________________

____

Medical diagnoses ______________________________

____

Recent surgery or hospitalizations ______________________________

Medications and immunizations ______________________________

____

Physical assessment data ______________________________

____

____

Emotional and cognitive functioning ______________________________

____

Coping ______________________________

Sources of medical and dental care ______________________________

Health screening practices ______________________________

Table continued on following page

TABLE 9–15

Family Assessment Guide (Continued)

IV. Interpersonal Needs

Identified subsystems and dyads ____________

Prenatal care needed ____________

Parent–child interaction ____________

Spousal relationships ____________

Sibling relationships ____________

Concerns about elders ____________

Caring for other dependent members ____________

Significant others ____________

V. Family Needs

A. Developmental

Children and ages ____________

Responsibilities for other members ____________

Recent additions or loss of members ____________

Other major normative transitions occurring now ____________

Transitions that are out of sequence or delayed ____________

Family proceeding at expected sequence ____________

Tasks that need to be accomplished ____________

Daily health promotional practices for nutrition, sleep, leisure, child care, hygiene, socialization, transmission of norms and values ____________

Family planning used ____________

B. Loss or Illness

Non-normative events or illnesses ____________

Reactions and perceptions of ability to cope ____________

Coping behaviors used by individuals and family unit ____________

Meaning to the family ____________

Adjustments family has made ____________

Roles and tasks being assumed by members ____________

Any one individual bearing most of responsibility ____________

TABLE 9–15

Family Assessment Guide (Continued)

Family idea of alternative behaviors available ______________________________

Level of anxiety now and usually ______________________________

C. Resources and Support

General level of resources and economic exchange with community ______________________________

External sources of instrumental support (money, home aides, transportation, medicines, etc.) ______________________________

Internal sources of instrumental support (available from family members) ______________________________

External sources of affective support (emotional and social support, help with problem-solving) ______________________________

Internal sources of affective support (who in family is most helpful to whom?) ______________________________

Family more open or closed to outside? ______________________________

Family willing to use external sources of support? ______________________________

D. Environment

Type of dwelling ______________________________

Number of rooms, bathrooms, stairs, refrigeration, cooking ______________________________

Water and sewage ______________________________

Sleeping arrangements ______________________________

Types of jobs held by members ______________________________

Exposure to hazardous conditions at job ______________________________

Level of safety in the neighborhood ______________________________

Level of safety in household ______________________________

Attitudes toward involvement in community ______________________________

Compliance with rules and laws of society ______________________________

How are values similar to and different from those of the immediate social environment? ______________________________

E. Internal Dynamics

Roles of family members clearly defined? ______________________________

Authority and decision-making rest where? ______________________________

Subsystems and members ______________________________

Hierarchies, coalitions, and boundaries ______________________________

Typical patterns of interaction ______________________________

Communication, including verbal and nonverbal ______________________________

Table continued on following page

TABLE 9–15

Family Assessment Guide (Continued)

Expression of affection, anger, anxiety, support, etc. ______

Problem-solving style ______

Degree of cohesiveness and loyalty to family members ______

Conflict management ______

VI. Analysis

Identification of family style ______

Identification of family functioning ______

What are needs identified by family? ______

What are needs identified by community health nurse? ______

The eco-map presented a picture to both the nurse and Mr. and Mrs. R of a family that was not very connected to outside resources. Little energy was coming in or going out of the immediate family system, with the exception of intervention by the health care system, which the family wanted to discontinue. When the community health nurse later completed a family map, she became aware of Mrs. R's tendency to act as a parent and Mr. R's tendency to act as a child. This blurring of boundaries had set up a behavior pattern in which Mr. R "gave away" responsibility for his own health. At the same time, however, the rigidity of these boundaries kept the children out of these interactions.

After assessing the family, the nurse tried to guide her practice with some questions. She asked herself about the family's needs, functioning, and style. She examined the family's priorities and the strengths and resources they were using or potentially able to use. She looked at her skills and abilities and attempted to define her responsibility to the family system. These questions helped her begin to analyze the family data. This analysis led to several determinations.

Family Health Needs. The family needs help coping with this illness and connecting with resources and sources of support. Some minor disturbances in organization are influencing the way the family is dealing with the problem. The nurse assigns the family the nursing diagnosis, "family coping, ineffective: compromised."

Family Style. This family is a distancing family that prefers to keep its problem-solving to itself. However, this limits family members' ability to support each other. The community health nurse must adjust her nurse interactions to accommodate this family's style of operating. The nurse should respect the family's need for distance, approach them cautiously, and observe for cues that indicate they are becoming anxious.

Family Functioning. Even though the family is currently stressed, long-term functioning is fairly healthy. No one member has consistently been a problem or has failed to fulfill his or her role. The adult children are not acting in their age-appropriate roles of support to parents. This seems to reflect the family style but could possibly be modified.

Targets of Care. The community health nurse believes several levels of this family—the individuals with health problems (both Mr. and Mrs. R), the couple, and the family as a unit—are potential targets for care. When she reviews who is the most likely person in the family to be able to change behavior, she looks for someone who seems willing to change. She decides this person is Mrs. R and potentially the children.

Nursing's Contribution. The community health nurse reviews her own caseload and her available time and attempts to make an accurate assessment of her skills. She is fairly comfortable in dealing with families and decides she will intervene on three levels: individual, subsystem, and family unit. Her contribution will be to offer information, counseling, and connection with other resources. She can visit one time per week and will try to schedule those visits when some of the children can be present.

Priorities. The family has several needs. What is most crucial? Anything life threatening must be top priority, but nothing will be accomplished without the family's agreement that this is their concern. After discussing these ideas with the family, the nurse and the family decide to first address individual health concerns. Mr. R's hyperglycemia is noted, and he admits it is making him feel bad. Mrs. R's cardiac status is to be assessed next week at an appointment with the family physician. While Mr. R seems agreeable to resuming his insulin injections, he has no desire to change his diet or learn how to walk with a prosthesis. The community health nurse shelves these problems for the time being and addresses Mrs. R. She wonders if Mrs. R would be interested in exploring her current care for herself? Mrs. R tentatively agrees. Pulling in additional resources to help Mr. R transfer is something that could be accomplished, but the family is still reluctant about it. This, too, is put off to a later time.

The community health nurse and the family together develop both long- and short-term goals.

Mr. R:

- Will monitor and record blood glucose levels every morning;
- Will accept administration of insulin by Mrs. R;
- Will begin range-of-motion and strengthening exercises to promote mobility for eventual transfer of self to chair;
- Will communicate to Mrs. R his ability to take care of any of his own needs as each opportunity arises; and
- Will demonstrate improved blood glucose levels within 1 month.

Mrs. R:

- Will have her cardiac status evaluated within 2 weeks;
- Will self-monitor her health and record her health status for 1 week;
- Will decide on one goal to take care of herself within 2 weeks;
- Will practice this behavior for 1 month; and
- Will allow Mr. R to care for himself when he desires.

Mr. and Mrs R together:

- Will experience decreased frequency of arguments within 1 month; and
- Will spend some relaxed time together every evening.

The Family:

- Will discuss new ways of coping with this situation as a group;
- Will try out two behaviors that use different family members within 2 weeks; and
- Will accept one resource to help within 1 month.

Implementation

The community health nurse is aware that the disturbances in the family's coping ability are fairly recent. The behaviors they have used in the past—self-reliance, appropriate action, distancing, and some denial of the problem—are not working in this situation. The first goal for nursing implementation addresses individual health needs. The second involves helping Mr. and Mrs. R think about the crisis and identify their present coping strategies. Because the nurse knows that the family style is distant, she will proceed slowly with this step, adjusting to suit the family's pace. She will initially keep the discussion focused on thoughts and facts rather than feelings. Mr. R perceives the situation as hopeless. Helping the family reframe this perception so that the current crisis is seen as being able to be modified is important. Subsequent plans with regard to family coping would include identifying alternate coping behaviors and practicing them. Because the family level of functioning is fairly high, the community health nurse would expect the family to be able to use information to appropriately problem-solve in this crisis. The family may also use the situation as a way of growing into new behaviors that foster family health.

Connecting the family with resources must be done in a way that allows this family to make the choice about outside care. Providing information about the extent to which other modern families use these resources may help them accept this intrusion into their world. Internal resources available to the family include the adult children, who may be able to offer instrumental or emotional support simply by being made aware of the extent of the need.

The internal dynamics of the family, in which the couple's roles are unbalanced as the wife has assumed more and more responsibility for the husband, are likely to be long-term patterns. Expecting a family at this stage of life to change a formerly effective pattern of relating to each other is unrealistic and ill advised. Instead, helping Mrs. R to focus on herself more to care for her needs and helping Mr. R to increase his awareness about his responsibility for his health and to his wife are more appropriate interventions.

Evaluation

The community health nurse reviewed the care plan periodically with the family and at the end of the contact. This evaluation included examination of goals. As the family crisis subsided, goals were quickly accomplished and revised weekly.

The family also examined the effect of the interaction on the ill member (Mr. R). His hyperglycemia was modified the first week and blood glucose levels dropped to a normal range within several weeks of contact. He accepted his insulin and even expressed interest in administering it himself. His stance about eating whatever he wanted also changed, and he began to follow his diet more closely. He continued to resist attempts to be fitted for a prosthesis, but eventually learned to assist with his transfers. As the community health nurse left this family, a goal still to be accomplished was his learning to use a walker.

Examination of the intervention's effect on individuals included looking at Mrs. R's health status and that of the adult children. Mrs. R's cardiovascular status had deteriorated. She began some cardiotonic medication and was urged to moderate her activity and stress level. All three of the adult children began sharing in the care of their father. Although they were busier than before, the impact on them was manageable.

Examination of the effects on the subsystem included effects on the interactions of the marital couple. Mr. and Mrs. R both began to assume more appropriate responsibility for themselves. The arguments and anger lessened, although their long-term way of relating to each other did not change very much.

The effect on the whole family was also examined. Bringing in additional resources led to decreased perception of crisis and increased calm in the family. As the members began to renew connections with each other, they discovered new sources of emotional support. Several months later, Mr. R died after experiencing pulmonary emboli. The children were able to support their mother during this time of loss.

In examining the family's interaction with the environment, it became apparent that the family members had become more aware of the community resources available to members. Members were still very private, but began to use available resources appropriately. Members' home environment was relatively safe.

As she was working with this family, the community health nurse continually sought feedback to evaluate her own performance. She carefully monitored the family's reaction to her interventions and her reactions to the family. She was frustrated at the need to proceed slowly with the family, but was satisfied with her choice when she saw that the strategy had worked. Her contact with the family led her to enroll in a course about noncompliance in clients. She learned to be patient during this experience and took those behaviors with her in her future contacts with families.

REFERENCES

Affonso, D. (1987). Assessment of maternal postpartum adaptation. *Public Health Nursing, 4*(1), 9-16.

Broussard, E., & Hartner, S. (1992). Neonatal perception inventory. In M. Stanhope & J. Lancaster (Eds.). *Community health nursing: Process and practice for promoting health* (pp. 953-954). St. Louis: Mosby-Year Book.

Cain, A. (1981). Assessment of family structure. In J. Miller & E. Janosik (Eds.). *Family-focused care* (pp. 115–131). New York: McGraw-Hill.

Caldwell, B. (1976). *Home observation measure of the environment.* Little Rock, AR: University of Arkansas Center for Child Development and Education.

Cox, H., Hinz, N., Lubno, M. A., Newfield, S., Ridenour, N., & Sridaromont, K. (1989). *Clinical applications of nursing diagnosis.* Baltimore: Williams & Wilkins.

Dass, R., & Gorman, P. (1986). *How can I help?* New York: Knopf.

Dunst, C., Trivette, C., & Deal, A. (1988). *Enabling and empowering families: Principles and guidelines for practice.* Cambridge, MA: Brookline Books.

Friedemann, M. L. (1989). The concept of family nursing. *Journal of Advanced Nursing, 14,* 211–216.

Fulmer, T. (1984). Elder abuse assessment tool. *Dimensions of Critical Care Nursing, 3*(4), 1984.

Hartman, A. (1978). Diagrammatic assessment of family relationships. *Social Casework, 59*(8), 465–476.

Hens, M. (1989). Functional evaluation. In S. Dittmar (Ed.). *Rehabilitation nursing.* St. Louis: Mosby-Year Book.

Holmes, T. H., & Rahe, R. H. (1967). The social readjustment rating scale. *Journal of Psychosomatic Research, 11*(2), 213-218.

James, K. (1989). Family nutrition and weight control. In P. Bomar (Ed.). *Nurses and family health promotion: Concepts, assessments, and interventions.* Baltimore: Williams & Wilkins.

Jernigan, D. (1986). Mental health assessment and intervention: An integral part of nursing service. *Caring, 5*(7), 4–10.

Kane, R., Ouslander, J., & Abrass, I. (1989a). Dementia assessment. In R. Kane (Ed.). *Essentials of clinical geriatrics.* New York: McGraw-Hill.

Kane, R., Ouslander, J., & Abrass, I. (1989b). Social assessment of the elderly. In R. Kane (Ed.). *Essentials of clinical geriatrics.* New York: McGraw-Hill.

Lawton, M., & Brody, E. (1969). Assessment of older people: Self-maintaining and instrumental activities of daily living. *The Gerontologist, 9*(3), 179–186.

Lowe, M., & Freeman, R. (1981). Family coping index. In R. Freeman & J. Heinrich (Eds.). *Community health nursing practice* (pp. 555–566). Philadelphia: W.B. Saunders.

Lubben, I. (1988). Assessing social networks among elderly populations. *Family and Community Health, 11*(3), 42–52.

Martin, K., and Scheet, N. (1992). *The Omaha System: Applications for community health nursing.* Philadelphia: W.B. Saunders.

Maslow, A. (1972). *Toward a psychology of being.* New York: Van Nostrand Reinhold.

McCaffrey, M., & Beebe, A. (1989). *Pain: A clinical manual for nursing practice.* St. Louis: Mosby-Year Book.

McCubbin, H., & Thompson, A. (1987). Family inventory of life events and changes. In H. McCubbin & A. Thompson (Eds.). *Family assessment inventories for research and practice.* Madison, WI: University of Wisconsin at Madison.

McGoldrick, M., & Gerson, R. (1985). *Genograms in family assessment.* New York: W.W. Norton.

Minuchin, S. (1974). *Families and family therapy.* Cambridge, MA: Harvard University Press.

Minuchin, S., & Fishman, H. C. (1981). *Family therapy techniques.* Cambridge, MA: Harvard University Press.

Mumma, C. M. (1987). Building accessibility checklist. In C. Mumma (Ed.). *Rehabilitation nursing, concepts and practice: A core curriculum.* Evanston, IL: Rehabilitation Nursing Foundation.

North American Nursing Diagnosis Association. (1987). *Taxonomy I with complete diagnosis.* St. Louis: Author.

Otto, H. (1973). A framework for assessing family strengths. In A. Reinhardt & M. Quinn (Eds.). *Family-centered community nursing* (pp. 87–93). St. Louis: C.V. Mosby.

Pender, N. J. (1987). *Health promotion in nursing practice.* Norwalk, CT: Appleton & Lange.

Reiser, S. L. (1981). A tool to facilitate mother-infant attachment. *Journal of Obstetrical and Gynecological Nursing, 10,* 297.

Skelley, A. (1990). Assessment of Immediate Living Environment. In B. Bullough & V. Bullough (Eds.). *Nursing in the community.* St. Louis: C. V. Mosby.

Smilkstein, G. (1978). The Family APGAR: A proposal for family function test and its use by physicians. *Journal of Family Practice, 6*(6), 1231–1239.

Smith, C. (1985). *Goals for community health nursing.* (Unpublished manuscript.)

Tapia, J. (1972). The nursing process in family health. *Nursing Outlook, 20*(4), 267–270.

Wiley, O. (1989). Family environmental health. In P. Bomar (Ed.). *Nurses and family health promotion: Concepts, assessment, and interventions.* Baltimore: Williams & Wilkins.

Wong, D., & Whaley, L. (1990). *Clinical manual of pediatric nursing.* St. Louis: Mosby-Year Book.

Zerwekh, J. (1989). Homecare of the dying. In I. Martinson & J. Widmer (Eds.). *Home health nursing care.* Philadelphia: W.B. Saunders.

BIBLIOGRAPHY

Barbarin, O., & Chesler, M. (1984). Coping as interpersonal strategy: Families with childhood cancer. *Family Systems Medicine, 2*(10), 279–289.

Danielson, C. B., Hamel-Bissell, B., & Winstead-Fry, P. (1993). *Families, health, and illness: Perspectives on coping.* St. Louis: Mosby-Year Book.

Donnelly, E. (1990). Health promotion, families, and the diagnostic process. *Family & Community Health, 12*(4), 12–20.

Folkman, S., & Lazarus, R. (1985). If it changes it must be a process: A study of emotion and coping during three stages of a college examination. *Journal of Personality and Social Psychology, 48*(1), 150–170.

Greenberg, L. S., & Johnson, S. M. (1988). *Emotionally focused therapy for couples.* New York: Guilford Press.

Jacob, S. (1991). Support for family caregivers in the community. *Family & Community Health, 14*(1), 16–21.

Karpel, M. (1986). *Family resources: The hidden partner in family therapy.* New York: The Guilford Press.

Kerr, M. E., & Bowen, M. (1988). *Family evaluation.* New York: W.W. Norton Co.

Kupferschmid, B., Briones, T., Dawson, C., & Drongowski, C. (1991). Families: A link or a liability? *Critical Care Nurse, 2*(2), 252–257.

Lazarus, R. S., & Folkman, S. (1984). Coping and adaptation. In W. Doyle (Ed.). *Handbook of behavioral medicine.* New York: Guilford Press.

Leahey, M. (1987). *Families and chronic illness.* Springhouse, PA: Springhouse.

McCubbin, M. (1984). Nursing assessment of parental coping with cystic fibrosis. *Western Journal of Nursing Research, 6*(4), 407–421.

McCubbin, H., Cauble, A., & Patterson, J. (1982). *Family stress, coping, social support.* Springfield, IL: Charles C Thomas.

McCubbin, H., Joy, C., Cauble, A., Comeau, J., Patterson, J., & Needle, R. (1980). Family stress and coping: A decade review. *Journal of Marriage and the Family, 10,* 855–871.

Miller, J. R., & Janosik, E. H. (1980). *Family-focused care.* New York: McGraw-Hill.

Miller, S. R., & Winstead-Fry, P. (1982). *Family systems theory in nursing practice.* Reston, VA: Reston Publishing Co.

Moos, R. H. (1984). *Coping with physical illness 2: New perspectives.* New York: Plenum Press.

Pendagast, E., and Sherman, C. (1979). A guide to the genogram. In E. Pendagast (Ed.). *The best of the family: 1973–1978.* New Rochelle, NY: Center for Family Learning.

Pender, N. J. (1986). Health promotion: Implementing strategies. In B. B. Logan & C. E. Dawkins (Eds.). *Family-centered nursing in the community.* Reading, MA: Addison-Wesley.

Pratt, L. (1976). *Family structure and effective health behavior: The energized family.* Boston: Houghton Mifflin.

Schilling, R., Schinke, S., & Kirkham, M. (1985). Coping with a handicapped child: Differences between mothers and fathers. *Social Science Medicine, 21*(8), 857–863.

Shapiro, J. (1986). Assessment of family coping with illness. *Psychosomatics, 27*(4), 262–271.

Terkelson, K. G. (1980). Toward a theory of the family life cycle. In E. A. Carter & M. McGoldrick (Eds.). *The family life cycle: A framework for family therapy* (pp. 21–52). New York: Gardner Press.

Wright, L., & Leahey, M. (1984). *Nurses and families: A guide to family assessment and intervention.* Philadelphia: F.A. Davis.

SUGGESTED READINGS

Fife, B. (1985). A model for predicting the adaptation of families to medical crisis: An analysis of role integration. *Image: Journal of Nursing Scholarship, 17*(4), 108–112.

Martin, A. C., & Starling, B. (1989). Managing common marital stresses. *Nurse Practitioner, 14*(10), 11–22.

McFarland, J. (1988). A nursing reformulation on Bowen's family systems theory. *Archives of Psychiatric Nursing, 2*(5), 319–324.

Phillips, L. (1989). Elder family caregiver relationships: Determining appropriate nursing interventions. *Nursing Clinics of North America, 24*(3), 795–807.

Pesnecker, B., & Zerwekh, J. (1989). The mutual-participation relationship: Key to facilitating self-care practices in clients and families. *Public Health Nursing, 6*(4), 197–203.

Zerwekh, J. (1991). A family caregiving model for public health nursing. *Nursing Outlook, 39*(5), 213–217.

Chapter 10

Multiproblem Families

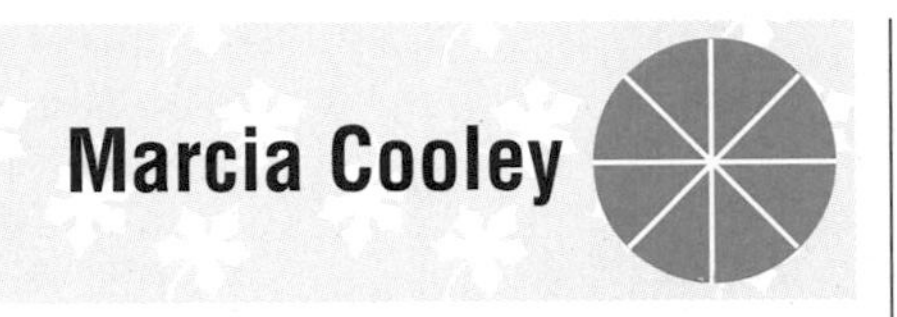

Marcia Cooley

Focus Questions

What characterizes a family in which members are unable to meet basic needs or maintain optimal levels of health?

What kinds of feelings are experienced by nurses who attempt to offer care for multiproblem families?

How do nurse and family values interact in these nurse–client relationships?

How does one work toward mutual goal setting with multiproblem families?

What guidelines can the nurse use in searching for strategies that are effective with multiproblem families?

How does a nurse transcend labeling, blame, and cutoff when a multiproblem family is encountered?

To what extent does clear definition of the nursing role play a part in moderating nursing frustration?

What are appropriate and achievable goals for multiproblem families?

Working with families is challenging, but the true challenge for a community health nurse is working with families who have problems in several areas simultaneously. Many of us as health professionals base our appraisal of the behavior of the family on our own "comfort zone" that defines what is normal. These preconceived ideas of healthy families need to be modified as one works with multiproblem families. Most of these families can be divided into two general types: families experiencing crisis and families with chronic problems.

Families Experiencing Crisis

Even the healthiest family encountering multiple stressors and stress of long duration can be pushed beyond its resources and begin to have multiple problems leading to crisis. Often these families can be supported through the crisis and can regain some measure of their previous level of health. What leads a family to crisis?

Family crisis is a continuous disruption, disorganization, or incapacitation in the family social system (Burr, 1973). Families in crisis have serious disturbances in family organization and require basic changes in family patterns of functioning to restore stability. Crises come in many forms. Revisiting the Family Stress and Coping Model of McCubbin (1982) reminds us that the *stressor* acting with the *resources* and the *appraisal* of the event combine to drive the family to adaptation or to crisis (See Figure 8–5 in Chapter 8). Part of the family's response is influenced by the characteristics of the stressor, including the extent, severity, duration, type of onset, predictability, and amount of stigma attached to the stressor (Danielson et al., 1993). Each dimension will have a different ability to affect the family. For example, an intense, unpredictable event such as a sudden death is more stressful than the expected loss of an elderly family member.

The appraisal the family makes of the situation is another factor. When presented with a stressor, the family makes a judgment about their overall capability in relation to the event. If family members judge themselves as inadequate to meet the demands, the tension increases.

Another factor is the family's resources, including inherent family strengths and specific coping abilities. Resources can include personal assets, such as innate intelligence or a sense of humor; family system resources, such as communication and problem-solving ability; and social support.

It is through the process of situational appraisal, including evaluation of the stressor, assessment of the family's capabilities and strengths, and consideration of alternative courses of action and coping strategies, that the family ultimately comes together as a unit to cope with stress. The successful family has a number of coping strategies that include internal and external mechanisms. Such a family knows how to use the coping mechanism most appropriate to the problem presented. However, families who have experienced a pileup of demands—that is, long-term accumulation of and exposure to multiple stressors—will sometimes exhaust their ability to be resilient. They are more vulnerable to stress when it is presented again. These families may find themselves in crisis.

Helping families cope with crisis is within the scope of the community health nurse's role. Interventions useful to this process are presented in Table 10–1.

TABLE 10–1

Helping Families Cope with Crisis

1. Start by recognizing sources of family resiliency and strength.
2. Offer hope.
3. Help the family identify and describe the nature of the stressors.
4. Explore the family's appraisal of the situation, including its meaning to them and their judgment of their ability to respond.
5. Provide information about the nature and demands of the stressor that may not be known to the family.
6. Help the family divide the tasks required by the stressor into manageable pieces.
7. Help the family explore current and alternative coping mechanisms.
8. Validate and emphasize the use of internal family resources including personal and family strengths.
9. Pull in external sources of social support.
10. Arrange for tangible sources of external support such as financial assistance, health care, home visitors, support groups, food assistance, and transportation.
11. Encourage a positive reappraisal of the situation as the family moves from adjustment to adaptation to their new state.

Families with Chronic Problems

Since nurses began visiting in the community, there have been families who have chronic problems and many barriers to gaining optimal health. Many of these families with chronic multiple problems have disturbances in their internal dynamics. The personal and family resources available to them, their range of coping behaviors, and their willingness and ability to utilize external sources of support all combine to keep them in a perpetual state of chronic problems. Experienced community health nurses recognize this situation and become aware of their own frustrations in dealing with families who seem unable or unwilling to change. The interface between multiproblem families and community health nurses will be the focus of the remainder of this chapter.

MULTIPROBLEM FAMILIES

A multiproblem family is one that has needs in several areas simultaneously: development, support, illness or other stress, internal functioning, or environment. Multiproblem families are families in which combinations of functional level, multiple stresses, multiple symptoms, and lack of support interact to prevent the family from meeting the physical, social, and emotional needs of its members. Several things predispose a family to having multiple problems. (See Applying the Nursing Process: Working with a Multiproblem Family in this chapter.)

VULNERABLE FAMILIES

Vulnerable families are families at special risk because of the intensity and clustering of stressors associated with a certain life event (Gillis, 1991). Examples of families at high risk for future health problems include families with members who are chronically ill or have Down's syndrome or alcoholism. Special events such as the loss of a child, teenage pregnancy, or sexual abuse can also predispose a family to subsequent physical, emotional, and social problems. The combination of intense stressors and depletion of resources can push the family beyond its capacity to cope.

FAMILIES WITH NEGATIVE CHOICES

Community health nurses assist families to cope with stress by helping them identify their previous coping style, their resources, and their alternatives for action. For some families, however, coping with stress remains a problem even after nursing intervention, because the choices for action are all negative (Wilson, 1989). Sometimes none of the available choices will modify the problem. Sometimes the consequences of the choices are all negative and create more problems. For example, suppose a family is dealing with a husband and father who has Alzheimer's disease. The wife, having assumed the caregiver role, is exhausted and needs to spend some time out of the house. However, her husband becomes anxious and more confused whenever any other person takes over his care. None of the choices available to this family solves or completely alleviates the problem. The wife must choose among "solutions" with negative implications.

Families who must cope when all the choices are undesirable are also a special risk group.

FAMILIES IN POVERTY

The impact of poverty and living in a resource-depleted or hostile environment is also a factor in family coping. The poor, as both individuals and a group, are continually faced with multiple and chronic stressors, including frustration over employment options, inadequate and unsafe housing conditions, repeated exposure to violence and crime, inadequate child care assistance, and insensitive attitudes and responses of health and social service agencies (Berne et al., 1990). As family coping abilities are strained by unpredictable and unrelenting stressors, mastery of the situation decreases. Feelings of helplessness and hopelessness increase, and self-esteem suffers. The spiral continues as people become anxious and depressed, feel powerless, and thus are less able to marshal energy to meet the next day's problems.

Poverty also brings its own set of health problems. Correlates of poverty include increased communicable diseases, especially tuberculosis and human immunodeficiency virus, more episodes of illness, less preventive care, higher rates of chronic disease and premature death, occupational hazards, and unsafe housing. Unfortunate correlates for children include delayed development, childhood depression and anxiety, and increased separation from families into foster care. Poor neighborhoods may also have greater environmental risks such as industrial sites, landfills, and toxic waste sites. Living within a poverty area may contribute to excess mortality, independent of an individual's own health behaviors (Haan et al., 1987). Poor individuals are also more likely to be homeless and to lack access to health care (Berne et al., 1990).

FAMILIES WITH DISTURBANCES IN INTERNAL DYNAMICS

Multiproblem families are often unable to provide for security, physical survival, emotional and social functioning, sexual differentiation, training of children, and promotion of growth of individual members (Tapia, 1972). These families are characterized by insufficient internal support, frequent or intense emotional conflict, inability to conform to societal expectations, and acting out of family members.

What makes a family adaptive or resilient? What are the characteristics of families that are able to bounce back from stress? Riess and Oliveri (1980) suggest that the family's openness, or lack thereof, toward accepting help will determine its response to crisis. The successful family will gather information, make clear decisions and implement them, and resolve conflict. The successful family will provide for the growth of individuals in the family, as well as try to maintain its wholeness. This type of family creates an emotional atmosphere that fosters trust, cooperation, and acceptance; it has a number of coping strategies, including internal and external ones. Internal coping strategies include rearranging roles and tasks of family members, offering each other emotional support, or communicating information. Examples of external coping strategies include seeking financial assistance or seeking information from an informed source. The successful family knows how to use the coping mechanism most appropriate for the problem presented. Finally, it engages in productive and adaptive activities for the family's own needs and to meet society's expectations.

Family systems theory provides some thoughts about how the level of health of a family might develop. Multigenerational patterns that are passed down from one generation to another can be adaptive or maladaptive. The tendency to repeat these patterns is great, especially when one considers that the family members have known no other family experience. Often doing what one knows, even if it brings unhappiness and failure, is easier than changing behavior to something unfamiliar and unknown.

TABLE 10–2

Families with Disturbances in Internal Dynamics

Developmental stages and tasks: The family has difficulty achieving tasks at the stage-appropriate time. Situational and maturational crises occur simultaneously. Tasks for the next stage are delayed or not accomplished.

Roles: Patterns of expected behavior are not appropriate to age and ability, are rigidly assigned, and are unable to support family functioning.

Boundaries: Boundaries are closed and impermeable or completely diffuse. They fail to allow appropriate exchange with the environment or fail to define the family unit. Boundaries between subsystems have no clear generational lines and do not support a strong parental coalition. Subsystem boundaries may be unclear, rigid, or diffuse.

Subsystems: As in most families, each member of the family belongs to several subsystems simultaneously: spouse, parent–child, sibling, grandparent. However, subsystems may include inappropriate members.

Patterns of interaction: Repetitive and fixed. Focus on one member who is blamed, left out, or put down in the interaction. Family cohesion is extremely enmeshed or disengaged. Communication patterns of placator, blamer, superresponsible one, and distractor are often used. Distance, conflict, projection, and overresponsibility/underresponsibility are common.

Power: No clarity of role definition and appropriate rules. Power is not shared, appropriate to age, or within the parental subsystem until the children are independent.

External stressors: Are very intense, numerous, and occur simultaneously. The family has little chance to adapt. Chronic illness adds to family stress.

Open/closed system: As the system closes, all variables and patterns become fixed and less able to adapt. Energy is used in dysfunctional ways.

Communication: Is unclear, not honest, and indirect; contains incongruency of feelings and words; and is nonspecific. The family is not able to use it as a mechanism to resolve conflict.

Values: Do not provide guidelines for behavior acceptable to society and culture. Unable to be modified to adapt to changing times.

Encouragement of autonomy/acceptance of difference: A balance does not exist between autonomy of members and the need to be a cohesive group. There are strong pressures to conform and to sacrifice individual needs for the purpose of the group.

Level of anxiety: Is extremely high. People in the family have difficulty thinking and problem-solving. Long-term anxiety tends to wear down the ability of the family to function well.

Resources/social support: Family has few internal and external sources of support. Those that are available are not used to their capacity or are overused. All families have some strengths, but the strengths may be different from those expected by society.

Meaning, perception, and paradigm: The family agrees to allow myths and secrets to structure the meaning of many situations. Life problems are viewed as unsolvable problems rather than challenges. The family views itself as powerless.

Adaptability: Resilience is necessary for a family to be able to cope with changing demands. These families are not able to be flexible or are so chaotic that cohesiveness and predictability are missing.

The level of differentiation of a family is a crucial variable in the appearance of symptoms (Kerr and Bowen, 1989). Families have varying levels of differentiation or ability to separate emotion from thought. Families on the low end of the continuum have greater difficulty living their lives in a thoughtful way, responding to situations automatically in attempts to manage their high levels of anxiety. At the opposite end of the continuum are families with the ability to distinguish thought from feeling. These families have members who are able to think of themselves as separate persons, as well as group members, and who can define life goals and pursue them in a thoughtful way. Families on the thoughtful end of this continuum have fewer life problems than families caught in automatic emotional reactivity. Most multiproblem families tend to fall on the more emotional side of differentiation of self. Family theory suggests that these levels are transmitted from generation to generation through the projection process, which is the amount of the child's relationship dependence or the degree to which each child is involved in maintaining the emotional lives of its parents. Some suggest that stressors and events that occur during the formation of early attachments predispose the parent–child relationship to problems. Premature infants separated from parents, prolonged hospitalizations or illness, unexpected crises such as homelessness or imprisonment, deaths, or emotional illnesses are examples of disruptions in family life that can interfere with parenting and early development. Tension or lack of nurturing during the child's earliest interactions influences the growth and development of the child and the child's subsequent ability to nurture his or her own children. Not only multigenerational patterns, but perhaps even basic emotional health is passed from generation to generation.

Chapter 8 contains a list of healthy family characteristics; a comparison list of characteristics of families with disturbed internal dynamics is outlined in Table 10–2. The multiproblem family may have disturbances in many of these characteristics, such as inadequate support, multiple stressors, high levels of anxiety, dysfunctional family boundaries, unhealthy communication patterns, dysfunctional expression of emotion, inadequate problem-solving, under- or rigid organization, unclear roles, and repetitive patterns of interaction that blame or shift responsibility.

Scapegoating, or identifying one family member as "the problem," is one pattern that may be used. Distancing and cutoff of family members can occur when the anxiety rises to such a point that family members can no longer tolerate contact with each other. In some areas, it is not unusual to see members of a family who live on the same street but have not spoken to each other in years. Repetitive patterns of emotional conflict occur in which the conflict seems to be resolved and then erupts again. These families often contain many active and interlocking triangles and may use this pattern with outsiders when tension rises. "Triangling-in" the social worker, police, or nurse helps relieve anxiety.

Responsibilities of the Community Health Nurse

Families defined as multiproblem are often the most challenging, most time consuming, and least rewarding families in a community health nurse's caseload (Fox, 1989). Nurses often need support to continue working in situations in which their efforts are frustrated. As experienced and educated health care workers, we expect ourselves to have the answers and that our expertise will be accepted and acted on. This assumption is in direct conflict with the family's perception of a health care worker who is unable to be trusted and whose advice does not seem to affect their quality of life. If one also assumes that families have the right to self-determination and know what is best for themselves, then there is a conflict between these two ways of viewing family care. Only after examining his or her own values and resolving this conflict can the community health nurse be effective with multiproblem families.

ASSESSMENT

Most of the time, multiproblem families operate at a low level of functioning, according to Tapia (1972). Families at level I (chaotic families) are characterized by disorganization in all areas of life. In these extremely immature families, adults may be unable to fulfill their roles and responsibilities. Children or others may be expected to assume these roles, which are inappropriate and interfere with normal growth and nurturing needs. Physical and emotional resources may be inadequate. Family members are often depressed, with a sense of hopelessness and powerlessness. They may have little self-esteem, a high sense of failure, and little reason to trust another health care worker who comes with promises that are most often unfulfilled.

Families at Tapia's level II (intermediate) are able to meet their basic survival needs but are immature and unable to meet many needs of family members. They are often defensive, unable to trust, and alienated from the community. However, these families retain some hope and have some capacity to change and improve their functioning.

Assessment of multiproblem families should pay special attention to the interaction of the family's many needs, style, functional level, coping patterns, resources and supports, strengths, and past experiences with health care workers (see Chapter 9). Special areas of focus should include the number and duration of stressors the family has experienced over time, the family's perception of the event, an estimation of the severity of any symptoms the family may be experiencing (e.g., depression, alcohol use, or physical abuse), and contacts with other health care resources. Tools such as the Holmes and Rahe (1967) Stressful Events Scale, the Family Coping Index (Lowe and Freeman, 1981), or an eco-map (Hartman, 1978) may be especially helpful.

PLANNING

After analyzing the data, the nurse will have a better understanding of realistic goals and expectations of what will happen in the family encounters. Perfection should not be sought. Goals should be concrete and realistic and mutually defined by family and nurse. Sometimes, in the presence of what seem to be overwhelming problems, it is difficult for a nurse to identify family strengths. Our values set up expectations that block our identification of strengths. As the community health nurse truly listens and asks the family to identify its strengths, they become more apparent. Otto (1973) was one of the first to emphasize family strengths; his schema is presented in Table 10–3. Karpel (1986) suggests that some personal strengths are often hidden, such as self-respect, protectiveness, caring in action, hope, tolerance, affection, humor, and playfulness. Relational strengths include respect, reciprocity, reliability, the ability to repair, flexibility, and family pride. He suggests that loops of family interaction repeat themselves to amplify resources, and that symptoms can be reframed to allow people to see the situation in a positive way. For example, suppose one family member loses her job. When her sisters and brothers become aware of this, the situation is redefined as one that allows her to spend more time with her young children. The sisters and brothers engage in a series of telephone calls and conversations in which all agree to offer a little financial help and a lot of emotional support until the situation changes. This family has maximized its resources.

TABLE 10–3

Family Strengths
Ability to provide for physical needs
Ability to provide for emotional needs
Ability to provide for spiritual needs
Respect for parental views and decisions on child rearing
Ability to communicate openly and indepth
Consensual decision-making
Poviding for security, support, and encouragement
Ability to relate to each other and to foster growth-producing relationships
Responsible community relationships
Growing with and through children
Ability to help itself and accept help when needed
Flexibility of family functions and roles
Mutual respect for individuality
Ability to see crisis as a means of growth
Family unity and loyalty and intrafamily cooperation
Flexibility of family strengths

From Otto, H. (1973). A framework for assessing family strengths. In A. Reinhardt & M. Quinn (Eds.). *Family-centered community nursing* (pp. 87–93). St. Louis: C.V. Mosby.

Alterations in the Nurse–Family Relationship. Sometimes the multiproblem family's past experience with health care workers has led the family to distrust other encounters. After hoping to have some of their needs met and then being left with problems that are unresolved, the family may pull away or be reluctant to engage with another health care worker. Especially when values are different, the family may "play along" with the nurse, feeding the nurse inaccurate information that the family believes she or he wants to hear. They may agree to make appointments and then not keep them, preferring to break the contact rather than be disappointed. The family may test the nurse while trying to determine her or his reliability and consistency. This may even feel to the nurse like manipulation. However, frequently this is a pattern the family has found helpful in the past to maintain some control. Zerwekh (1992) describes three responsibilities of the community health nurse in response to this pattern: locating families, building trust, and building strength.

When it is time for problems to be identified, the nurse may find that the family cannot agree on or clearly identify problems. The family's ability to sort through multiple priorities and clearly see the problem and what can be done may be weakened by their anxiety and their sense of being overwhelmed. The family members may have no previous experience with this style of thinking and so may resort to impulsive and automatic patterns as explanations for their distress.

For the family to continue to engage in care, some commitment and resources are necessary. Other needs may compete for priority. For instance, the usual time a nurse might meet with a family member is during the day. A mother who has to work at a 9-to-5 job may be unable to take the time off to keep up with nurse contacts, and a mother caring for a toddler with an earache may find herself at the pediatric clinic waiting to be seen and then spend several hours getting home on the bus. Families with fewer resources seem to have to work harder and deal with more obstacles to getting things done that others take for granted.

Mutual Goal Setting. A mutual goal is one that is shared by both the family and the community health nurse. This means the family and the nurse agree on the need for the goal and to work together toward meeting it. Carey (1989) identifies the process of mutual goal setting as the single most important skill to bring to multiproblem families. Individuals have a right to knowledge about themselves and to participate in decisions that influence their life and health. Health professionals have a responsibility to share information that helps individuals make informed decisions about their care. Sometimes our education and knowledge get in the way of family interactions. People tend to resist being told what to do and are therefore more likely to work toward goals they choose and support. Instead of "investing" herself in the outcome, the nurse should let go of the outcome and invest in respect and support of the client.

Determining the Level of Intervention. Potential levels of intervention include individual, interpersonal, the family as a unit, and the family within the environment. How does the community health nurse determine the appropriate level of intervention with multiproblem families? For some families, working with the family as a unit may not be possible because of access, time constraints, or disconnected relationships. For example, the community health nurse may be referred to work with a mother who has lost permission to see her children because of abuse. In multiproblem families, the nurse takes every opportunity to work with any part of the family, recognizing that more optimal ways may be unavailable.

Working on the individual level will include interventions directed at individual health problems as well as strengthening individual functioning. For example, the nurse who works to prepare the previously mentioned mother for the return of her children may be educating her about parenting skills, helping her find and maintain employment, and connecting her to resources in her community. The development of personal strengths is always beneficial to someone in the family.

Working on the interpersonal level is often a choice the community health nurse will make. Multiproblem families will frequently manifest problems in areas related to interpersonal relationships, such as inadequate prenatal care, unsafe parent–child interactions, marital conflict, or elder abuse. Helping subsystems within the family learn new ways of interacting and coping ultimately helps the whole family.

Some thoughts about working with the family as a unit are outlined later. For many family health nurses, this is the preferred strategy. Knowing that the family functions as a unit makes the experienced nurse wary of addressing it in segments.

It can be argued that the most appropriate role for a nurse is at the macro, or environmental, level. It is a fact that the realities of life for many multiproblem families are related to factors that are beyond their internal control. Coping with exposure to environmental hazards, health risks in air and water, violence in the street, deterioration of the neighborhood, inadequate education, limited access to health care, and unavailability of adequate employment would tax the resiliency of any person or family. Nurses who assume the role of advocate for families within a larger social context ultimately may make the most impact on family health.

ISSUES IN INTERVENTION

There are two basic approaches for nurses who offer care to families in the community. In the first, nurses approach families with the expectation that they will participate as equal members in the process of planning and implementing care. Families are asked what they want or need to work on. Clients identify their own problems and monitor their own progress. Nurses assist the family by clarifying ideas, breaking problems down into more manageable units, helping families set priorities, and giving feedback and positive support. When a goal is reached, the family may start working toward a new goal.

With less functional families, this nursing approach may not work. We have already discussed families who may not have the ability to identify their needs or ask for specific kinds of help. They may have difficulty engaging and continuing in the relationship. Impulsivity and competing demands may alter their ability to stick with the care plan. With these families the nurse must alter the approach. From the beginning the nurse must be consistent and reliable in her or his contact. A regular and continued physical presence that the family can count on is necessary to reassure the family that the relationship can be trusted.

If the family cannot identify its own goals, the nurse acts as an information giver, sharing the assessments and diagnoses. Visual or concrete portrayals of the assessment, such as a pie chart, a score on a test, or a photograph may help engage the family interest. The nurse can suggest possible goals but must carefully validate whether the family shares the same concerns and wants to work toward the goals suggested by the nurse. If the family is uninterested, then the nurse presents the assessment again to gain feedback about the client's perception of the situation. The feedback process continues until a concern and goal that are shared by the family are identified.

During the implementation phase, nursing roles include those of educator, facilitator of family decisions, liaison to community resources, provider of emotional support and direct care, and advocate for the client within the community systems, if necessary.

The goals of the nursing contacts are not to "fix" the family or to address all the problems of family members. Helping family members gain awareness of the distinctions between feelings and behaviors may curb some of the impulsivity and encourage members to think before they act. Unhealthy family behavior patterns are recognized by describing and tracking them with family members. They can then be reframed and sometimes modified to be more functional for the family.

Helping the family feel a sense of power to break through the hopelessness by working with them toward a small but achievable success empowers the family toward similar actions in the future (Dunst et al., 1988). However the possibility of additional problems is great, and continued support and recognition of the family's attempts and strengths are necessary. This must be balanced with the family's possible tendency to depend on the nurse when it needs to learn to develop itself (Table 10–4). The nurse becomes a compassionate and informed companion as the family struggles with its daily tasks of living.

Triangling is a fact of life with all families, but especially families that are anxious (see Chapter 9). Nurses cannot avoid triangles, but they can learn to manage themselves within them. When tension rises in the family, the tendency will be for a family member to try to escape uncomfortable feelings by pulling in a third or fourth or fifth person. This additional person serves to distract the family from its original tension. The distraction does not always help the family move toward a problem solution. When a community health nurse or anyone else is pulled into a triangle through the family's wish for that person to be closer and to take over, a calm and thoughtful presence can help diffuse the emotion. Instead of participating in the emotionality, the nurse should resist jumping in to help and instead be a thoughtful observer in the situation. Asking questions, maintaining neutrality, and demonstrating thoughtfulness will be what helps.

TABLE 10–4

Strategies for Working with Multiproblem Families

1. Foster continuity of care.
2. Be patient—don't expect instant solutions.
3. Help the family identify its strengths.
4. Work on small pieces of problems.
5. Help the family recognize opportunities for moving forward or doing it differently.
6. When all choices are undesirable, help the family cope more positively with the one they choose.
7. Ensure that all contacts are characterized by caring and respect.
8. Organize possible sources of tangible support.
9. Encourage the use of possible sources of intangible support.
10. Remember that the ultimate goal is empowerment of the family and development of individual self-esteem.

During the contact, nurses should be aware of their tendencies to feel hopeless, to discount the value of the time and effort spent with the family, or to feel angry and want to withdraw when family problems continue. Many nurses build in regular support by talking with colleagues or making a plan to take care of themselves in the midst of a heavy workload. Carefully defining a nursing role that includes realistic expectations of self is one way to help the nurse manage these feelings.

REALISTIC GOALS

The successful community health nurse will *not* be able to move all families toward health, but remembering the ways that successful families manage their lives and helping multiproblem families recognize that there may be other ways of managing family life is a useful strategy. It is unrealistic to believe that a family who may have had troubles for generations will be without concerns after limited nursing contact. Some examples of goals that can be achieved with multiproblem families are given in the sections that follow.

Selected Stressors Are Prevented or Reduced. The family may have many members with health or social problems. Not all these problems can be corrected. However, solid action aimed at one or two specific needs may improve the quality of the family's life. For example, one elderly man who had been cut off from his family in the community had multiple health problems, including emphysema, severe hypertension, fatigue, decubiti, depression, and nutritional deficits. His disorganized family had difficulty maintaining contact with him because of their own legal and parenting concerns and anger about past conflicts. The community health nurse worked on getting him a continued supply of food that he would eat (he rejected Meals on Wheels). His nutritional status improved, providing the basis for decreased fatigue, lower blood pressure, and healing of the decubiti. He was extremely worried about the physical safety of one of the preschool children of his daughter, who was abusing substances and neglecting her child. His sister agreed to care for the granddaughter in her home with the permission of the daughter who was not able to function as a parent. The family continued to have multiple problems, but two specific stressors were reduced, helping the family members to maintain health and safety that year.

The Support System Is Strengthened. Some families do not know the resources available to them or lack skills to access them. The nurse works at providing information or guiding the family through actions to access these resources, but some sources of support may be overlooked. Family members who appear dysfunctional may be able to do more than expected. Once support is started, feedback loops are set up that serve to continue the supportive behaviors. It feels good to be supported and it feels good to be acknowledged for the support. In one family an elderly grandmother had cancer and was being cared for in the home. The middle-aged mother was coping with caring for several preschool children, maintaining a job, and monitoring her 20-year-old retarded daughter. The daughter's help was enlisted to bathe and keep her grandmother company. She had not been counted on as a support in this family before, but once her potential was tapped, she was delighted to be asked. The mother got some respite for a time before the grandmother entered a hospice.

Family Organization Is Improved. The chaotic family may have little experience with a more ordered existence and may not recognize the benefits of simple structuring and rules. The very rigid family may never have experimented with a different way of doing things. Helping the family make minor changes in organization may help them move in the needed direction. For example, Marylee was 12 years old and was not attending school. She stayed home to take care of her mother who was often "ill." Her mother, who had dropped out of school herself at age 16, turned off the alarm in the mornings and slept late, and as a result Marylee missed the school bus. Repeated attempts by the school system to address the problem failed. With the community health nurse's help, Marylee's mother asked an older neighbor who rose early to call her every morning at 7:30 A.M. With the older neighbor's help, the mother began to see herself as able to parent Marylee, and as a result Marylee's school attendance improved.

Coping Processes Are More Adaptive. Many multiproblem families have learned dysfunctional coping behaviors as part of their lifestyle. For a family who tends to blame others or depend on others to help them out of any situation, the concept of planning and acting may be quite foreign. Drinking alcohol, "acting out," and procrastinating are examples of unhealthy coping behaviors. One family had a son, Andy, with spina bifida and was extremely dependent on various health care systems and social service agencies. They became angry any time there was a problem with Andy at school, with his catheter, with his wheelchair, or with his braces, blaming the agencies or others for not managing his care correctly. When a new set of braces caused a pressure sore on his skin, the community health nurse coached the mother to become active with the supply company who made adjustments. This success spurred the mother to change from anger and dependence to a more self-confident stance in dealing with her son's care.

Summary

Community health nurses interface with families in serious trouble within our communities. It is increasingly impossible to avoid multiproblem clients; in fact, the clients who need us the most have multiple problems. To gain access to these families, nurses need to examine their own values and approach families with respect and a willingness to allow them to define their care. Nurses who learn to expect less than perfection from themselves and the families they care for can be extremely influential as mutual progress is made in little steps. Restoring a family's sense of power and hope greatly enriches a nurse's satisfaction.

KEY IDEAS

1. Multiproblem families include families in crisis and families with chronic problems.
2. Some families can be supported through crisis and will regain their previous level of health.
3. Strategies for working with families in crisis include identifying stressors, reframing appraisals, locating resources, and considering alternative ways to cope.
4. Families at risk for multiple chronic problems include vulnerable families, families with negative choices, families in poverty, and families with disturbances in internal dynamics.
5. All families have some strengths that must be tapped for intervention to be successful.

6. Nurse–family interventions may be influenced by the family's previous negative contacts with the health care system. Strategies to counteract this include locating the family, creating trust, and building strength (Zerwekh, 1992).
7. A community health nurse makes choices about the level of intervention (individual, family subsystems, family as a unit, or family within the environment) based on the family assessment and on practical limitations to practice.
8. A community health nurse considers the level of family functioning when making choices about realistic goals and specific interventions.
9. The goals of nursing contact do not include trying to "fix" the family.
10. Realistic goals in families with multiple, chronic problems include reducing stressors, strengthening the support system, improving family organization, introducing more adaptive coping behaviors, and altering the environment.

GUIDELINES FOR LEARNING

1. In what ways do family environment, family dynamics, and family stress influence how an individual will cope and behave? What has been the greatest influence for you?
2. Pick a major social problem in which you already have some interest (e.g., pollution, global warming, poverty, teen pregnancy, drug abuse, violence). In what ways could a community health nurse intervene in these environmental issues to advocate a change for family health?
3. Read your local newspaper, paying particular attention to the events and crimes occurring that day. How many of these news items are related to symptoms in families—that is, families in which the family unit is unable to support its members? Do you agree that dysfunction or inadequacy in the family should be considered when someone is being judged for a crime? Why or why not?
4. In a small group, discuss the ways in which your family has coped with problems in the past. How much pileup of stress was there at that time? What resources did you use? What were your coping strategies? Would you do it this way again? What would have helped your family at that time? Could you envision help from a community health nurse? Why or why not?
5. Role play a visit with a community health nurse in which the family has multiple problems. Have someone set up the situation so that no matter what the nurse does, the situation seems unsolvable. Break and discuss your feelings and reactions to this.
6. Role play the same visit with the same family, but this time have the director set up the situation so that the family members are confidentially instructed to feel some hope and will attempt to work on a little piece of the issues. Break and discuss your feelings and reactions to this situation. What was different?
7. Identify which family you would be more comfortable working with—a family in crisis or a family who has chronic problems. Why?
8. Spend some time with magazines, scissors, and paste. Compose a collage that depicts the life of the family you are interacting with in the community. What does the collage evoke in you and in others in your group?

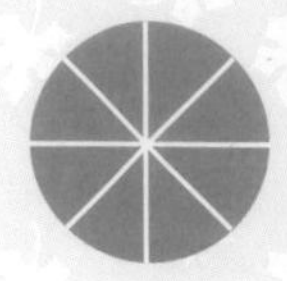

APPLYING THE NURSING PROCESS: *Working with a Multiproblem Family*

The Walker family consists of Edna, age 29; William, age 31; and their children, Mary, 13; Sean, 9; and Mark, 3½. The Walkers are a struggling urban family living in their third apartment within 2 years. William has a high school education but no formal job training. He has supported the family off and on in his job as a house painter. He has a back injury and works sporadically because of his physical problems and the limited availability of work. Their average annual income is $18,000. The Walkers' financial situation adds to the constant stress within the family. Although the Walkers' care for each other, their interactions are usually chaotic and tense.

Mr. and Mrs. Walker married when he was 18 and she was 16. Edna has an eighth grade education, having dropped out of school after experiencing learning problems. She is a very concrete learner, has never worked, and has no job skills. Edna is currently 70 pounds overweight and smokes about 1 pack of cigarettes a day. She spends most of her day caring for the children or talking on the telephone to her mother, who lives about 15 miles away. Edna's mother tries to be very supportive of the family but is getting older. She used to baby-sit and help the family out financially, but has not been able to do this recently because of her own health problems and her lack of transportation.

Mary, in the seventh grade, is a help to her mother. She has few outside interests other than watching television and occasionally cooking. Her younger brother, Sean, has been diagnosed with a learning disability (LD) and is failing in school. Mark, a preschooler, has asthma along with elevated blood lead levels.

The family's health problems require frequent clinic appointments, but the Walkers' automobile is often nonfunctional. Relations with the health care clinic are strained because of the clinic's perception that the Walkers are noncompliant. The stress of making it to these appointments leads to frequent cancellations and sporadic contact with the clinic.

Assessment

After receiving the referral, the community health nurse makes an appointment to meet the Walkers, but when she arrives no one is home. She later learns that the Walkers had gone earlier to the clinic for Mark's asthma appointment, but their automobile wouldn't start on the way home. At a second scheduled appointment, the Walkers again are not there. Later, by telephone, she finds out that Edna's mother fell and had to be taken to the hospital. The appointment is rescheduled. Edna is careful to be there and has obviously attempted to clean up the house and make herself presentable. She has on lipstick and has carefully combed her hair and set out cookies and coffee for the nurse.

Mary, who is home from school that day with a cold, pops in and out of the room during the visit. The nurse meets with Edna, William, and Mark; Sean is at school. William has just returned from trying to get temporary work, but he has been unsuccessful.

During the initial visit, the community health nurse asks questions, completes a Family Assessment Guide (Table 10–5), and has the family begin to help her construct a genogram (Fig. 10–1). She is also observing the family's interactions and the environment. She inquires about connections with community resources through use of an eco-map (Fig. 10–2*A*).

When the community health nurse first entered the house, William was in the bedroom. Edna yelled for him to come out several times and finally went back to the bedroom to get him, complaining about his behavior to the nurse. They sit on opposite sides of the room, with Edna doing most of the talking. Mark runs back and forth between them, carrying a piece of paper torn from the telephone book on which he is coloring.

The apartment, which is in a poorer section of the city, is on the third floor of an older building with trash in the yard. The stairs up to the apartment are dirty and unlit, and the paint is peeling. The Walkers' apartment is cheery, with some curtains and knickknacks. Space appears to be a problem, because some of the pots and pans are stored in a corner in the front room, the kitchen table is covered with bills and school books, and the family shares two bedrooms.

TABLE 10–5

Family Assessment Guide

I. IDENTIFYING DATA

Name Walker

Address

Phone

Household members (relationship, sex, age, occupation, education)

William	Father	M	31	parttime house painter	h.s.
Edna	Mother	F	29	homemaker	8th grade
Mary	Daughter	F	13	student 7th grade	
Sean	Son	M	9	student	
Mark	Son	M	3½		

Financial data (sources of income, financial assistance, medical care plans, expenditures) $18,000/year income; no health insurance; applied for medical funds for Children with Special Needs for Mark's medicines

Ethnicity English/Irish descent

Religion None practiced

Identified patient(s) Mark

Source of referral and reason Asthma clinic for repeated unkept appointments

II. GENOGRAM (see Fig. 10–2)
Include household members, extended family, and significant others
Ages or date of birth (DOB), occupation, geographic location, illnesses, health problems, major events
Triangles and characteristics of relationships

III. INDIVIDUAL HEALTH NEEDS

Identified health problems or concerns Wm.—back injury with pain; Edna—concrete learner, obese, smokes; Mary—little socialization; Sean—school failure

Medical diagnoses Sean—LD; Mark—asthma, elevated blood Pb

Recent surgery or hospitalizations Mark to E.R. ×3 in past 6 months for asthma

Medications and immunizations Mark up to date on immunizations; no asthma meds. in house and Rx not refillable

Physical assessment data Mark—T, 98.4°; P, 86; R, 18; breath sounds clear; no wheezing; good hydration

Emotional and cognitive functioning Mark—age-appropriate play

Coping Strained relations with asthma clinic due to unkept appts.; Edna frightened by Mark's asthma

Sources of medical care and dental care None, except well-child clinic and asthma clinic for Mark

Health screening practices

IV. INTERPERSONAL NEEDS

Identified subsystems and dyads Spousal, parent–child, sibling

Prenatal care needed NA

Parent–child interaction Little concern re: Sean's school failure

Spousal relationships Married 13 years; traditional spousal roles clear

Sibling relationships "Get along ok"

Concerns about elders Maternal grandmother (mgm) recently ill and hospitalized p̄ a fall

Continued

TABLE 10–5

Family Assessment Guide (Continued)

Caring for other dependent members NA

Significant others NA

V. FAMILY NEEDS

A. Developmental

Children and ages 13, 9, 3½

Responsibilities for other members Mary helps mother; has few outside interests

Recent additions or loss of members None

Other major normative transitions occurring now None

Transitions that are out of sequence or delayed Development of personal interests and peer relationships for Mary

Family proceeding at expected sequence Could use anticipatory guidance

Tasks that need to be accomplished Learning successes for Sean; socialization for Mary; school readiness for Mark

Daily practices for nutrition, sleep, leisure, child care, hygiene, socialization, transmission of norms and values

Adequate hygiene

Maternal gm was only baby-sitter

Nutrition not explored

Family planning used Tubal ligation

B. Loss or Illness

Non-normative events or illnesses Maternal gm in hospital

Reactions and perceptions of ability to cope Edna worried about care of her mother following hospital discharge

Coping behaviors used by individuals and family unit Cannot visit due to lack of transportation

Meaning to the family Threat

Adjustments family has made

Roles and tasks being assumed by members

Any one individual bearing most of responsibility

Family idea of alternative behaviors available

Level of anxiety now and usually

C. Resources and Support (see Fig. 10–3, eco-map)

General level of resources and economic exchange with community Low

External sources of instrumental support (money, home aides, transportation, medicines, etc.) Unreliable care; chronic financial stress; able to buy only necessities

Internal sources of instrumental support (available from family members) Maternal gm babysat before her illness

External sources of affective support (emotional and social support, help with problem solving) None

TABLE 10–5

Family Assessment Guide (Continued)

Internal sources of affective support (who in family is most helpful to whom?) mgm

Family more open or closed to outside? Does not actively seek resources

Family willing to use external sources of support? Yes

D. Environment

Type of dwelling 3rd floor apt., walk-up, dirty yard and stairs

Number of rooms, bathrooms, stairs, refrigeration, cooking 2 BR, 1 bath; working stove, refrigeration, heating; decorated; cluttered, due to inadequate storage

Water and sewage Public

Sleeping arrangements Parents together; boys together; Mary on folding bed in LR

Types of jobs held by members Painter

Exposure to hazardous conditions at job Yes—paint & height

Level of safety in the neighborhood Moderate crime & air pollution

Level of safety in household Peeling paint in hallway of 40-yr-old bldg; unlit stairs; working smoke detector; no pets; dust could be allergen for Mark

Attitudes toward involvement in community Only recently moved to apt.; "keep to themselves"

Compliance with rules and laws of society

How are values similar and different from immediate social environment?

E. Internal Dynamics

Roles of family members clearly defined? Yes

Authority and decision-making rest where? Health care with Edna

Subsystems and members (See "Interpersonal Needs" section)

Hierarchies, coalitions, and boundaries Mary helpful to Edna; spouses' activities are goal-directed and roles complement each other

Typical patterns of interaction ?Expression of feelings by children

Communication including verbal and nonverbal Spouses—some intense verbal interactions; Edna more vocal, complains

Expression of affection, anger, anxiety, support, etc. Anxiety, hope

Problem-solving style Deal with immediate needs

Degree of cohesiveness and loyalty to family members Cohesive, caring, loyal, "stick together"

Conflict management Edna complains, worries; Wm. seeks work and verbally withdraws; deny alcohol abuse or drug use

VI. ANALYSIS

Identification of family style Chaotic (see Chapter 9)

Identification of family functioning Tapia level II

What are needs identified by family? Edna—care for her mother, Mark's asthma, better housing; Wm.—work and car repair

What are needs identified by family health nurse? (See problem list in case study analysis)

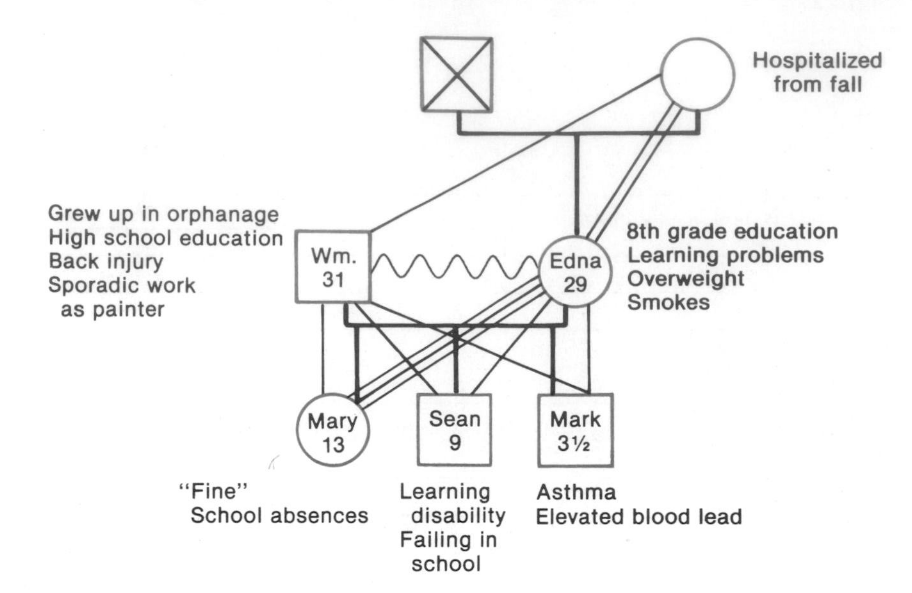

Figure 10–1 ● The Walker family genogram. (Adapted from Cain, A. (1981). Assessment of family structure. In J. Miller and E. Janosik (Eds.). *Family-focused care* (p. 117). New York: McGraw-Hill.)

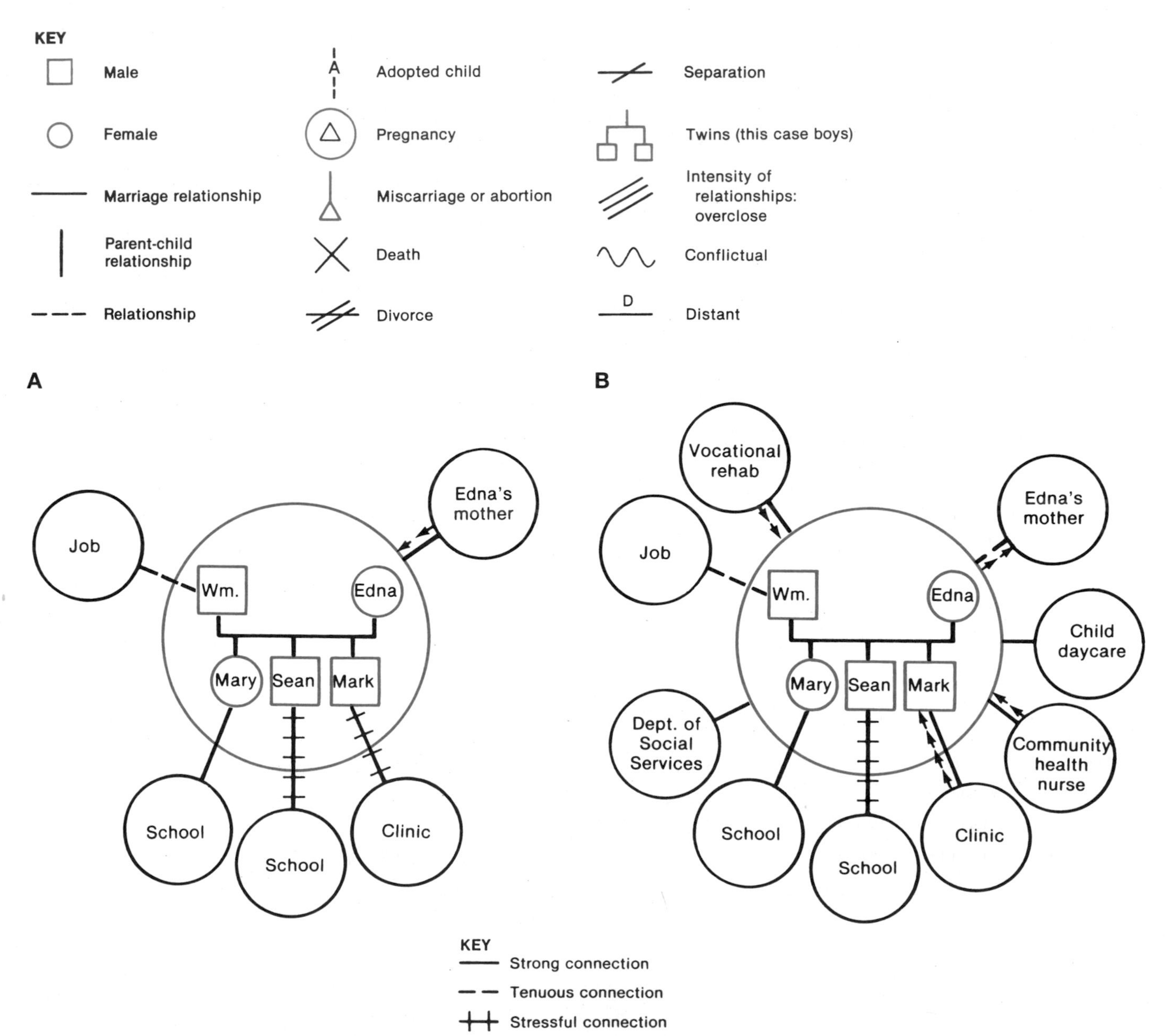

Figure 10–2 ● *A,* Eco-map of Walker family on first home visit. *B,* Eco-map of Walker family after 6 months of nursing care. (Adapted from Hartman, S. (1978). Diagrammatic assessment of family relationships. *Social Casework, 59,* 470.)

Analysis

On discussing the situation with the family, the community health nurse identifies the following family health needs: this family is experiencing demands from normal growth and development, is coping with illness and the external stress of the job market and the family's environment, and has inadequate resources. She does not believe there are disturbances in family dynamics. The nurse identifies the family style as chaotic but somewhat receptive and the family level of functioning as Tapia level II (see Chapter 9).

She specifies the following list of problems specific to individuals, subsystems, the family, and the environment:

William
- Impaired mobility related to previous back injury
- Chronic pain related to previous back injury

Edna
- Altered nutrition and obesity
- Impaired gas exchange and potential for illness related to smoking
- Altered learning

Mary
- Impaired socialization
- Disruption in completion of developmental tasks

Sean
- Altered learning
- Potential for impaired socialization and impaired self-concept

Mark
- Altered gas exchange related to asthma
- Lead poisoning
- Potential developmental delay

Subsystems
- Concern about mother's health and well-being
- Expenditure of resources for mother

Family Unit
- Compromised family coping
- Limited social contact

Environment
- Residence: presence of environmental hazards (lead)
- Income: difficulty buying necessities and no health insurance
- Neighborhood: moderate crime and pollution

Edna and William are asked their perception of what is happening and what they would like to work on. William is most concerned with finding work and keeping the automobile running. Edna is worried about her mother and how she will cope by herself when she is released from the hospital, and about Mark's asthma, which frightens her. She is less concerned with Sean's school problems or Mark's lead poisoning and thinks of Mary as doing fine. Her wish for the family is to get their own house with a yard for the kids to play in. When asked how she and William get along, she just shrugs her shoulders.

Planning

Before formulating a plan of care, the nurse analyzes the data and tries to determine priorities. She is concerned about what the family identifies as its needs and what she and the health care system can realistically do something about, and about setting some realistic goals. Together, she and the family come up with the following short-term goals:

- To contact the health care system of Edna's mother within the next 3 days and determine what plans are being made for care after discharge
- To arrange for alternative transportation for Mark and Edna to get to the clinic for next week's appointment
- To call the state vocational rehabilitation department to get information for William about job retraining

Long-term goals include safe care for Edna's mother, stabilization of the family income, appropriate treatment and family response for Mark's asthma, and a move to a dwelling without chipping paint. Goals that the community health nurse would like to achieve but are not yet seen as needs by the family include further assessment and family response to Sean's learning disability, support of Mark's developmental functioning, and increased socialization for Mary. Concerns about Edna's smoking and weight are also targets, as is the family's repertoire of coping strategies.

Implementation

Because the family is functioning at Tapia level II and the family style is considered chaotic, the community health nurse alters her approach to the family. She takes special care to set realistic short-term goals that can be achieved within a week. She is aware that the family style may necessitate frequent changes in goals and plans and is careful to keep her contract with the family clear and reasonable on both sides. Her goal is to take small steps so that the family can begin to see some successes and to pay special attention to pointing out these successes and what the family did to achieve them. She will shape and role model behaviors toward more successful coping. However, crises must be dealt with first. With this family, the unpredictable should be expected and must be considered as the family moves toward maintaining itself.

Result

After 6 months, the nurse and the family are able to see some successes. William has been evaluated by the vocational rehabilitation department and is waiting to hear about retraining as a security guard. Edna has heard about a program as a daycare mother and is considering a job herself. Her mother fell again and has been placed in a rehabilitation nursing home that is on the opposite side of the city. The family cannot get there very often but did visit her near Christmas.

Mark has been reevaluated in the asthma clinic, and medications have been prescribed. Edna gives the medicine more regularly now that the nurse has taught her how it helps prevent asthma attacks. Edna says she is more comfortable now because she can recognize these attacks earlier; she usually goes outside to smoke but has not cut down on her use of cigarettes. Overall, the family is now connected with more community resources (Fig. 10–2*B*).

Not much has changed with Mary or Sean, but the state department of social services is finding funds to help move the family into new housing because of Mark's lead poisoning. This housing does not have a yard, so this will remain Edna's dream for a while longer.

REFERENCES

Berne, A. S., Dato, C., Mason, D. J., & Rafferty, M. (1990). A nursing model for addressing the health needs of homeless families. *Image: Journal of Nursing Scholarship, 22*(1), 8–13.

Burr, W. (1973). *Theory construction and the sociology of the family.* New York: John Wiley & Sons.

Cain, A. (1981). Assessment of family structure. In J. Miller & E. Janosik (Eds.). *Family-focused care*, p. 117. New York: McGraw-Hill.

Carey, R. (1989). How values affect the mutual goal setting process with multiproblem families. *Journal of Community Health Nursing, 6*(1), 7–14.

Danielson, C., Hamel-Bissell, B., & Winstead-Fry, P. (1993). *Families, health, & illness: Perspectives on coping and intervention.* St. Louis: Mosby-Year Book.

Dunst, C., Trivette, C., & Deal, A. (1988). *Enabling and empowering families: Principles and guidelines for practice.* Cambridge, MA: Brookline Books.

Fox, M. (1989). The community health nurse and multiproblem families. *Journal of Community Health Nursing, 6*(1), 3–5.

Gillis, C. L. (1991). Family nursing research: Theory and practice. *Image: Journal of Nursing Scholarship, 23*(1), 19–22.

Haan, J., Kaplan, G., & Camacho, T. (1987). Poverty and health: Prospective evidence from the Alameda County Study. *American Journal of Epidemiology, 125*(6), 989–998.

Hartman, S. (1978). Diagrammatic assessment of family relationships. *Social Casework, 59,* 470.

Holmes, T. H., & Rahe, R. H. (1967). The social readjustment rating scale. *Journal of Psychosomatic Research, 11*(2), 213–218.

Karpel, M. (1986). Testing and promoting family resources. In M. Karpel (Ed.). *Family resources: The hidden partner in family therapy.* New York: Guilford Press.

Kerr, M., & Bowen, M. (1989). *Family evaluation.* New York: W.W. Norton & Co.

Lowe, M., & Freeman, R. (1981). Family coping index. In R. Freeman & J. Heinrich (Eds.). *Community health nursing practice.* Philadelphia: W.B. Saunders.

McCubbin, H., Cauble, A. E., & Patterson, J. M. (1982). *Family stress, coping, and social support.* Springfield, IL: Charles C Thomas.

Otto, H. (1973). A framework for assessing family strengths. In A. Reinhardt & M. Quinn (Eds.). *Family-centered community nursing* (pp. 87–93). St. Louis: C.V. Mosby.

Riess, D., & Oliveri, M. E. (1980). Family paradigm and family coping: A proposal for linking the family's intrinsic adaptive capacities to its responses to stress. *Family Relations, 29,* 431–444.

Tapia, J. (1972). The nursing process in family health. *Nursing Outlook, 20*(3), 267–270.

Wilson, H. S. (1989). Family caregiving for a relative with Alzheimer's dementia: Coping with negative choices. *Nursing Research, 38*(2), 94–98.

Zerwekh, J. V. (1992). Laying the groundwork for family self-help: Locating families, building trust, and building strength. *Public Health Nursing, 9*(1), 15–21.

BIBLIOGRAPHY

Brooker, C. (1990). The health education needs of families caring for a schizophrenic relative and the potential role for community psychiatric nurses. *Journal of Advanced Nursing, 15,* 1092–1098.

Campbell, J., & Humphreys, J. (1993). *Nursing care of survivors of family violence.* St Louis: C. V. Mosby

Eells, M. A. (1989). *Case studies in home health: Problem families, problem agencies.* Baltimore: Williams & Wilkins.

Flynn, C. P. (1990). Relationship violence by women: Issues and implications. *Family Relations. 39*(2), 194–198.

Garfinkel, I., & McLanahan, S. (1986). *Single mothers and their children: A new American dilemma.* Washington, DC: Urban Institute Press.

Heiney, S. (1988). Assessing and intervening with dysfunctional families. *Oncology Nursing Forum, 15*(5), 585–590.

Kupferschmid, B. J., Briones, T. L., Dawson, C., & Drongowski, C. (1991). Families: A link or liability? *Critical Care Nurse, 2*(2), 252–257.

Lewis, R. A. (1989). The family and addictions: An introduction. *Family Relations, 38*(3), 254–258.

Liepman, M. R., Silviaq, L. Y., & Nirenberg, T. D. (1989). The use of family behavior loop mapping for substance abuse. *Family Relations, 38*(3), 282–287.

Margolin, L., & Craft, J. L. (1989). Child sexual abuse by caretakers. *Family Relations, 38*(4), 450–455.

Satariano, H. H., & Briggs, N. J. (1989). The good family syndrome. *Pediatric Nursing, 15*(3), 285–286.

Quinn, P., & Allen, K. R. (1989). Facing challenges and making compromises: How single mothers endure. *Family Relations, 38*(4), 390–395.

Volk, R. J., Edwards, D. W., Lewis, R. S., & Sprenklc, D. H. (1989). Family systems of adolescent drug abusers. *Family Relations, 38*(3), 266–273.

SUGGESTED READINGS

Carney, P. (1992). The concept of poverty. *Public Health Nursing, 9*(2), 74–80.

Donabedian, D. (1980). What students should know about the health and welfare systems. *Nursing Outlook, 28*(2), 122–125.

Edelman, M. W. (1987). *Families in peril: An agenda for social change.* Cambridge, MA: Harvard University Press.

Haan, M., Kaplan, G., & Camacho, T. (1987). Poverty and health. *American Journal of Epidemiology, 125*(6), 989–997.

Jackson, A. (1993). Black, single, working mothers in poverty: Preferences for employment, well-being, and perceptions of preschool-age children. *Social Work, 38*(1), 26–34.

Lynch, I., & Tiedje, L. (1991). Working with multiproblem families: An intervention model for community health nurses. *Public Health Nursing, 8*(3), 147–153.

McElmurry, B., Swider, S., Grimes, M., Dan, A., Irvin, Y., & Lourenco, S. (1987). Health advocacy for young, low-income, inner city women. *Advances in Nursing Science, 9*(4), 62–75.

Moccia, P., & Mason, D. (1986). Poverty trends: Implications for nursing. *Nursing Outlook, 34*(1), 20–24.

National Commission on Children. (1991). *Beyond rhetoric: A new American agenda for children and families.* Washington, DC: U.S. Government Printing Office.

Presnecker, B. (1984). The poor: A population at risk. *Public Health Nursing, 1*(4), 237–249.

Schorr, L. (1989). *Within our reach: Breaking the cycle of disadvantage.* New York: Doubleday.

Zerwekh, J. (1992). Laying the groundwork for family self-help: Locating families, building trust and building strength. *Public Health Nursing, 9*(1), 15–21.

Zerwekh, J. (1992). The practice of empowerment and coercion by expert public health nurses. *Image: Journal of Nursing Scholarship, 24*(2), 101–105.

Unit III

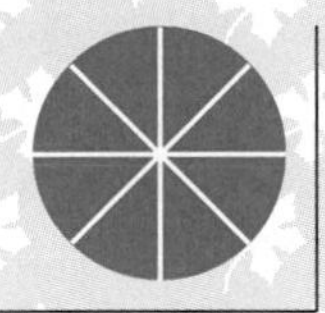

Community as Client

Chapter 11

Epidemiology: Unraveling the Mysteries of Disease and Health

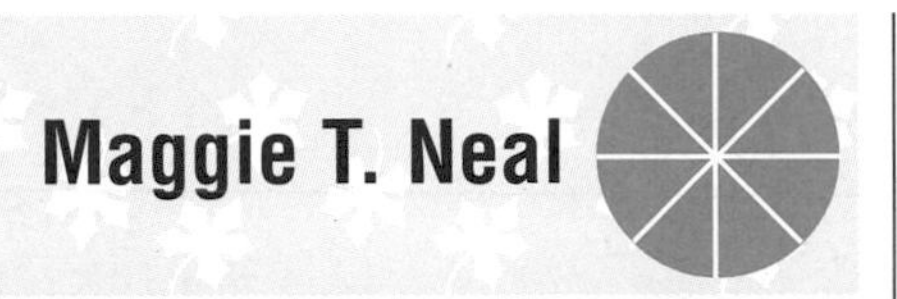
Maggie T. Neal

Continued

Focus Questions

How does the diagnosis of the health status of a population differ from an assessment of a family or an individual?

What is epidemiology?

How are data used in determining the health status of a community?

What statistical measures are used in epidemiology?

How are epidemiological concepts and/or methods such as incidence and prevalence or knowledge of the natural history of a disease used in assessing health, planning programs, and evaluating health care delivery?

What is known from epidemiological data about the overall health of the American population and aggregates?

"Too Much Heart Surgery?" "Where Do We Stand in the Fight against Cancer?" "What Doctors Don't Know about Women: NIH Tries to Close the Gender Gap in Research" "The Second 100,000 Cases of AIDS: United States, June 1981–December 1991" "Are We Becoming a Geriatric Society?" "Decline of Birth Rate in United States" "Immigration at an All-Time High" "Evaluation of Health: Haves and Have Nots"

Where does the information come from that informs the headlines above? Who collects it? How is it used in nursing and health care? The desire to understand health problems, conditions related to health, and the improvement of the well-being of a population requires a systematic approach to gathering factual information. Much of our knowledge about health phenomena and disease conditions comes from the basic and applied sciences such as microbiology, physiology, immunology, pathology, and sociology. However, *epidemiology* is the discipline that provides the structure for systematically studying health, disease, and conditions related to health status. Nursing and medical science may also be used to guide clinical practice and influence health outcomes. For example the Healthy Babies Program, which includes home visiting by a nurse during an infant's first year, was established to decrease infant mortality and promote health. Epidemiological concepts are used to understand and explain how and why health and illness occur as they do in human populations.

Interests of Population-Based Data

In community health nursing, the *community* or the *total population* under study replaces the individual as the focus of concern and study. Practicing nursing at the community level extends the boundaries of practice beyond those that are traditionally associated with caregiving activities. Caring effectively for the community as a client requires different skills and tools. The thinking and decision-making that a community health nurse uses to define the health status of a community are markedly different from those used in assessing individual patients or families. Furthermore, application of the nursing process to the entire community is complex and generally requires educational preparation at the graduate level.

The concepts and methods employed in assessing health status that affect program planning in health care, as well as analysis and applications of epidemiology data, form the basis of this chapter. An in-depth understanding of statistics is not required to understand epidemiology. Computation of the simple formulas used in this chapter requires only basic mathematical skills: addition, subtraction, multiplication, and division.

A FEW STATISTICS

The use of a formula to determine *rate* is essential to describe the population characteristic that is being studied (e.g., disease frequency, event, or condition). This description always includes a time specification (such as a calendar year), a specification of the person or the population at risk, and a place specification (such as a census tract, city, or county).

Rates and Ratios

A *rate* is a statistic used for describing an event, characteristic, or happening. In epidemiology a rate is used to make comparisons among populations or to compare a subgroup of the population (specific rate) with the total population. The numerator of a rate is the actual number of events and the denominator is the total population at risk. In epidemiology the rate is usually converted to a standard base denominator—such as 1000, 10,000, or 100,000—to permit comparisons between various population groups (Table 11–1).

The use of standard base rates makes it easier to compare the magnitude of an event (e.g., illness, death) in different population groups. For example, if city A had 125 teenage pregnancies in an at-risk population group of 120,602 female teenagers (14 to 19 years old), the rate of teenage pregnancies in city A would be expressed as 125 per 120,602. If city B had 492 teenage pregnancies in an at-risk population of 194,301 female teenagers, the rate of teenage pregnancies in city B would be 492 per 194,301 (see Table 11–1). Comparison of these two rates is very difficult as no common reference point exists. However, if these two rates were converted to a common at-risk population of 100,000, city A's rate would be 103 per 100,000, and city B's rate would be 253 per 100,000. Common base rates permit accurate comparisons and are much easier to understand.

Health statistics are sometimes reported as a *ratio,* which is simply the comparison of one number with another. In health statistics a ratio is often used to compare one at-risk population with another. Ratios are usually simplified by

TABLE 11–1

Rates and Ratios

Rates

A rate is:

$$\frac{\text{No. of events}}{\text{Population at risk}} \times 100{,}000 \text{ (or another standard base number)}$$

Example:

City A's teen pregnancy specific rate is arrived at by:

$$\frac{125 \text{ (No. of pregnancies)}}{120{,}602 \text{ (Population at risk)}} \text{ or } \frac{125}{120{,}602}$$

In epidemiology this rate is converted to a common base such as 100,000. This is accomplished by multiplying the specific rate by the common base:

$$\frac{125}{120{,}602} \times 100{,}000 = 103 \text{ or } 103 \text{ teenage pregnancies per } 100{,}000 \text{ teenage females 14–19 years old}$$

Converting City B's specific rate of 492/194,301 to a common base of 100,000:

$$\frac{492}{194{,}301} \times 100{,}000 = 253 \text{ or } 253 \text{ teenage pregnancies per } 100{,}000 \text{ teenage females 14–19 years old}$$

Ratios

Ratios are expressed on a common base, so the ratio of city A to city B is 103 to 253 (which is expressed as 103:253). Dividing 253 by 103 we get 2.4563, or a ratio of 1:2.4563, which we would express as approximately 1:2.5

reducing the numbers so that the smallest number becomes 1. To use the example of cities A and B, the ratio of teen pregnancies in city A to city B would be 103 (city A) to 253 (city B), or 103:253, which can be reduced to approximately 1:2.5; in other words, city B has approximately 2.5 times as many teenage pregnancies per 100,000 female teenagers aged 14 to 19 years as does city A.

Suppose you were told that there were more homicides in Los Angeles than in Washington, DC. How would you compare the rates, rather than just the numbers? Would you need to know the total population at risk for each city? In reality the 1992 murder rate for Los Angeles was 30.77 per 100,000 population as compared with 74.41 per 100,000 population in Washington, DC. The murder rate for Washington, DC, was higher than that for Los Angeles.

Using rates also has some disadvantages. Although using rates makes comparisons possible and easy, health planning also depends on the real numbers of population at risk represented by those rates. Even though city A has a lower teenage pregnancy rate than that of city B, the residents of city A may decide that a rate of 125 pregnancies is higher than desired. It would take considerable effort to target more than 120,000 female teenagers and their partners.

Measures of Morbidity and Mortality

Mortality (death rates) and *morbidity* (illness rates) statistics are collected routinely and used as indicators of the frequency of death or disease as they occur in time, place, and persons. The concept of morbidity also includes measures related to specific symptoms of a disease, days lost from work, and number of clinic visits. In the United States death records are required by law; they are tabulated by the National Center for Health Statistics and help determine trends in the United States.

Incidence and Prevalence Rates

Incidence refers to the rate at which a specific disease develops in a population. An incidence rate is the number of new cases of an illness or injury that occurs within a specified time. In contrast *prevalence* measures all of the existing cases at a given point of time. Prevalence includes the incidence plus all of the existing cases. The prevalence rate is influenced by how many people become ill and the number of people who die or do not recover (Figure 11–1).

Prevalence is important in determining measures of chronic illness in a population and is affected by factors that influence the duration of the disease. Thus, prevalence rates have relevance for planning for health care services, resources, and facilities; for determining health care personnel needs; and for evaluating treatments that prolong life.

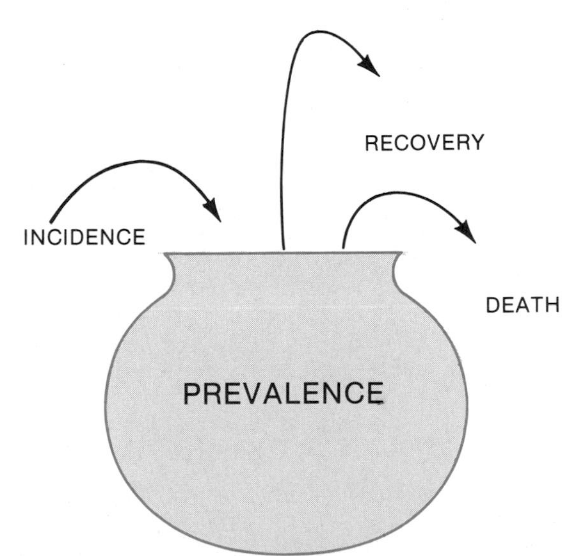

Figure 11–1 ● Prevalence pot: the relationship between incidence and prevalence. (Redrawn from Morton, R. F., Hebel, J. R., McCarter, R. J. (1990). *A study guide to epidemiology and biostatistics* (p 30.) (3rd ed.). Gaithersburg, MD: Aspen Publishers.)

Conversely incidence rates are used as tools for studying patterns of both acute and chronic illness. Incidence rates are important because they reflect a direct measure of the magnitude of new illness in a population and provide assessments about the risk associated with particular illnesses. Because they reflect only the development of a disease, incidence rates remain unchanged by new medical treatment patterns.

CRUDE, ADJUSTED, AND SPECIFIC RATES

A rate can be expressed for the total population (*crude* or *adjusted* rate) or for a subgroup of the population (*specific* rate). Table 11–2 presents the formulas for frequently used rates.

Age-specific and age-adjusted rates are often quite helpful in making comparisons among populations. For example, Boca Raton, FL, is a retirement community populated by a high proportion of persons older than 65 years. Orlando, FL, also has a significant population of retirees, but the personnel of many corporate headquarters and young people who work at Disney World also live there. Making a comparison of mortality between the two cities would not be justified unless one compared the death rates of 65-year-olds or 25-year-olds in each city. This comparison would be age-specific. If each age-specific rate in Boca Raton were compared with the age-specific rates in the standard population, the number of deaths of people in that age group in Boca Raton would then have been adjusted to reflect the age distribution of the standard population. The same adjustment would need to be completed using data from Orlando to ensure that any differences were not due only to a difference in the age distribution of the two cities. The same adjustments could be made for gender, race, and socioeconomic class if one wanted to exclude those effects in making comparisons among populations.

TABLE 11–2

Frequently Used Mortality Rates

$$\text{Crude death rate} = \frac{\text{Total No. of deaths during a year}}{\text{Total population at mid-year}} \times 1000$$

$$\text{Cause-specific death rate} = \frac{\text{Total No. of deaths from specific cause during a year}}{\text{Total population at mid-year}} \times 1000$$

$$\text{Age-specific death rate} = \frac{\text{Total No. of deaths from a specific cause}}{\text{Total mid-year population of the given age group}} \times 1000$$

$$\text{Maternal death rate} = \frac{\text{Total No. of maternal deaths}}{\text{Total No. of live births}} \times 1000$$

$$\text{Infant mortality rate} = \frac{\text{Total No. of deaths of children} <1 \text{ year}}{\text{Total No. of live births during the same year}} \times 1000$$

$$\text{Neonatal death rate} = \frac{\text{Total No. of deaths, birth to 28 days of age}}{\text{Total No. of live births plus fetal deaths during year}} \times 1000$$

$$\text{Fetal death rate} = \frac{\text{Total No. of deaths during 20–28 weeks' gestation}}{\text{Total No. of live births plus fetal deaths during year}} \times 1000$$

Types of Epidemiological Investigations

The study of epidemiology, because it involves the health of human beings, tends to use observational rather than experimental approaches to research design. Thus those engaged in epidemiological research frequently observe rather than manipulate variables believed to influence the health of the human population. This means that the researcher has far less control of the factors under study and that extraneous factors may also be included in the study design. Epidemiological studies, however, do identify nonrandom patterns of health and disease and serve as the basis for determining the circumstances in which experimental studies would be beneficial. They also are of value in planning and evaluating health care services. There are three major types of epidemiological studies.

Descriptive Studies. These studies customarily describe the amount and distribution of disease within a population. This approach relies primarily on the use of existing data and answers the following questions:

- Who is affected (person)?
- Where is the disease distributed in the human population (place)?
- When is the disease present (time)?
- What is the overall effect of the disease (population)?

Analytic Studies. In contrast analytic studies begin to answer questions about cause-and-effect relationships between potential risk factors and a specific health phenomenon or disease condition. Hypotheses, which are statements of possible relationships, are used to predict the causal association among the variables. Being able to predict risk thus points to factors that, if changed, may prevent the disease from occurring or reduce its risk. The hypotheses are tested through retrospective studies, cross-sectional studies, or prospective studies. If the evidence suggests that some relationships are appropriate for further study to confirm cause and effect, an experimental study, usually known as a clinical or experimental trial, may be conducted.

Experimental Trials. Experimental trials always begin with carefully designed questions, hypotheses, and research protocols that specify the criteria for selection of the people (subjects) to be studied, the procedures for random assignment of the experimental and control groups, the treatment procedure, the follow-up of subjects, and the details of the data analyses. In experimental studies the researcher always manipulates variables, such as a nursing intervention or a health teaching approach, with the experimental and control groups. Because of ethical concerns about not causing suffering or exacerbation of illness, experimental studies usually involve the testing of hypotheses related to disease prevention, health promotion, or, in some situations, the treatment of a specific disease.

Because community health nurses are asked to plan, implement, and evaluate health care services for specific populations, understanding epidemiological concepts and principles is important. For example, epidemiological investigations can evaluate the extent to which a program that is provided by nurse practitioners and designed to increase access to early prenatal care is successful in reducing prematurity and low birth weight. Epidemiological methods also may be used to evaluate the effectiveness of primary intervention strategies and thus improve nursing practices.

Understanding Aggregate Level Data

A primary focus of community health nursing is the definition of health-related problems (assessment) and the posing of solutions (interventions) for populations or aggregates of people. Population-level decision-making requires a different understanding than that used in direct caregiving to individuals. The questions for analysis are different. At the population level pertinent questions might be:

- What are the prevalence rates of cancer among various age, gender, and racial groups?
- Which subgroups have the highest incidences of cancer?
- Who is at high risk for development of cancer?
- What programs are available for cancer prevention and/or early detection?
- What would be required to further reduce the risk of cancer mortality or morbidity for the entire population?

Given the focus of community health on the well-being of the community, emphasis is necessarily placed on what makes a healthy community. These factors include the interrelationship between the health status of the population and the potential for healthy actions within the population, factors that influence health status, and the ability of the health care system to allocate appropriate resources and respond effectively to the needs of the population. The projected trend for health care reform calls for nurses to assume more responsibility for patients in the community. Therefore there is a more urgent need for nurses to understand and practice nursing at the population level.

In an attempt to respond effectively to the health care challenges of the 1990s, the U.S. Department of Health and Human Services (DHHS) published a report entitled *Healthy People 2000,* in which national objectives for health promotion and disease prevention were established (see discussion in Chapter 2). This report identifies the goals and priorities that health care planners and providers should work toward to improve the health of the U.S. population. Although the goals are directed toward healthier lives for all Americans, particular emphasis is given to special cohorts. A *cohort* is a group of people who share similar characteristics. For example, people born in the same decade represent an *age* cohort. *Healthy People 2000* has targeted certain cohort groups: "newborn babies, boys and girls, teenagers and young people, women and children, and people in their later years" (p. 9).

Concepts Related to Prevention, Health Promotion, and Disease

Three major concepts are crucial to understanding epidemiology: the natural history of disease, the levels of prevention, and the multiple causation of disease. To plan nursing interventions community health nurses need to know how epidemiologists and other health care planners conceptualize the natural history of disease and prevention.

THE NATURAL HISTORY OF DISEASE

Diseases evolve over time. Leavell and Clark (1965), in their classic description of the disease process, delineate two distinct periods: *prepathogenesis* and *pathogenesis* (Fig. 11–2). In the prepathogenesis period of a disease or condition, interactions occur between the person, the environment, and the causative agent that increase the potential for disease. In this stage no disease exists; however factors that increase risk are present. For example obesity in combination with a sedentary lifestyle and smoking increases a person's chances for development of coronary heart disease. Because some risk factors can be altered, understanding the natural history of a disease is important. Awareness of the presence of risk allows the nurse to initiate preventive measures against the disease or limit its development.

As pathological changes develop, the disease moves to the pathogenesis stage. Many diseases, such as acute or infectious diseases, run their course and a person experiences complete recovery. However changes resulting from chronic diseases or conditions may have long-term effects. Symptoms generally become more fixed and are less reversible as the disease continues. With advancing disease, functional changes may produce marked disability and lead to death.

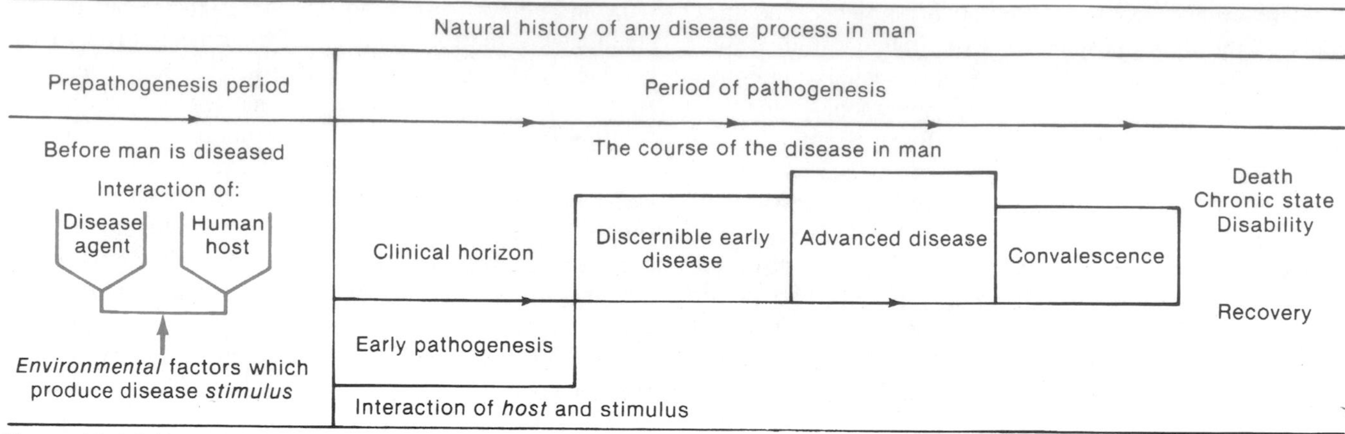

Figure 11–2 ● Natural history of disease. (Redrawn from Leavell, H. R., and Clark, E. G. (1965). *Preventive medicine for the doctor in his community: An epidemiologic approach* (p 18). New York: McGraw-Hill.)

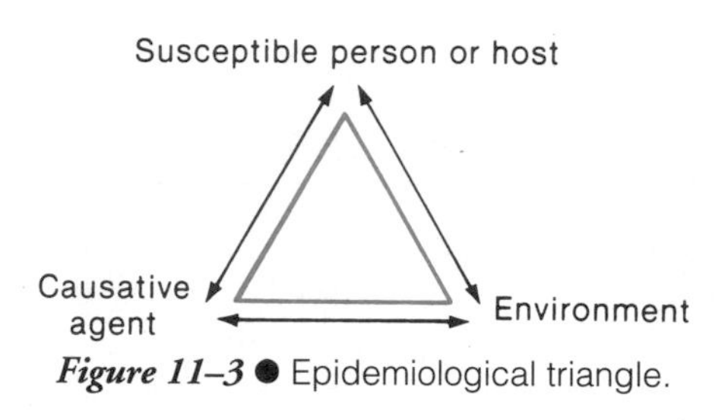

Figure 11–3 ● Epidemiological triangle.

Analyzing the natural history of a disease involves the use of the epidemiological triangle (Fig. 11–3). A change in any of these factors (the person, the causative agent, or the environment) has the potential to change the balance of health. When considering the person or host, demographic characteristics, the level of health and history of prior disease, genetic predisposition, states of immunity, body defenses, and human behavior should be examined (Table 11–3). Causative agents may include the presence or absence of biological, physical, chemical, nutritional, genetic, or psychological factors that have the ability to affect health and disease in the person. The environment includes anything external to the person or agent, including the presence of other persons or animals that potentially affect health and disease.

TABLE 11–3

Some Host, Agent, and Environmental Factors that Affect Health

Host Factors

Demographic Data: Age, gender, ethnic background, race, marital status, religion, education, and economic status
Level of Health: Genetic risk factors, physiological states, anatomical factors, response to stress, previous disease, nutrition, fitness
Body Defenses: Autoimmune system, lymphatic system
State of Immunity: Susceptibility versus active or passive immunity
Human Behavior: Diet, exercise, hygiene, substance abuse, occupation, personal and sexual contact, use of health resources, food handling

Agent Factors (Presence or Absence)

Biological: Viruses, bacteria, fungi, and their mode of transmission, life cycle, virulence
Physical: Radiation, temperature, noise
Chemical: Gas, liquids, poisons, allergens

Environmental Factors

Physical Properties: Water, air, climate, season, weather, geology, geography, pollution
Biological Entities: Animals, plants, insects, food, drugs, food source
Social and Economic Considerations: Family, community, political organization, public policy, regulations, institutions, workplace, occupation, economic status, technology, mobility, housing, population density, attitudes, customs, culture, health practices, and health services

LEVELS OF PREVENTION

Because disease occurs over time there are many potential points at which intervention may prevent, halt, or reverse the pathological change. A three-level model developed by Leavell and Clark (1965) based on the idea that disease evolves over time continues to be used in the conceptualization and structure of health programs (Fig. 11–4).

Primary Prevention. Primary prevention is aimed at altering the susceptibility or reducing the exposure of persons who are at risk for developing a specific disease. Primary prevention includes general health promotion and specific protective measures in the prepathogenesis stage that are designed to improve the health and well-being of the population. Nursing activities include health teaching and counseling to promote healthy living and lifestyles. Specific protective measures aimed at preventing certain risk conditions or diseases (such as immunizations, the removal of harmful environmental substances, or the use of car safety seats for infants and children) are also primary prevention activities.

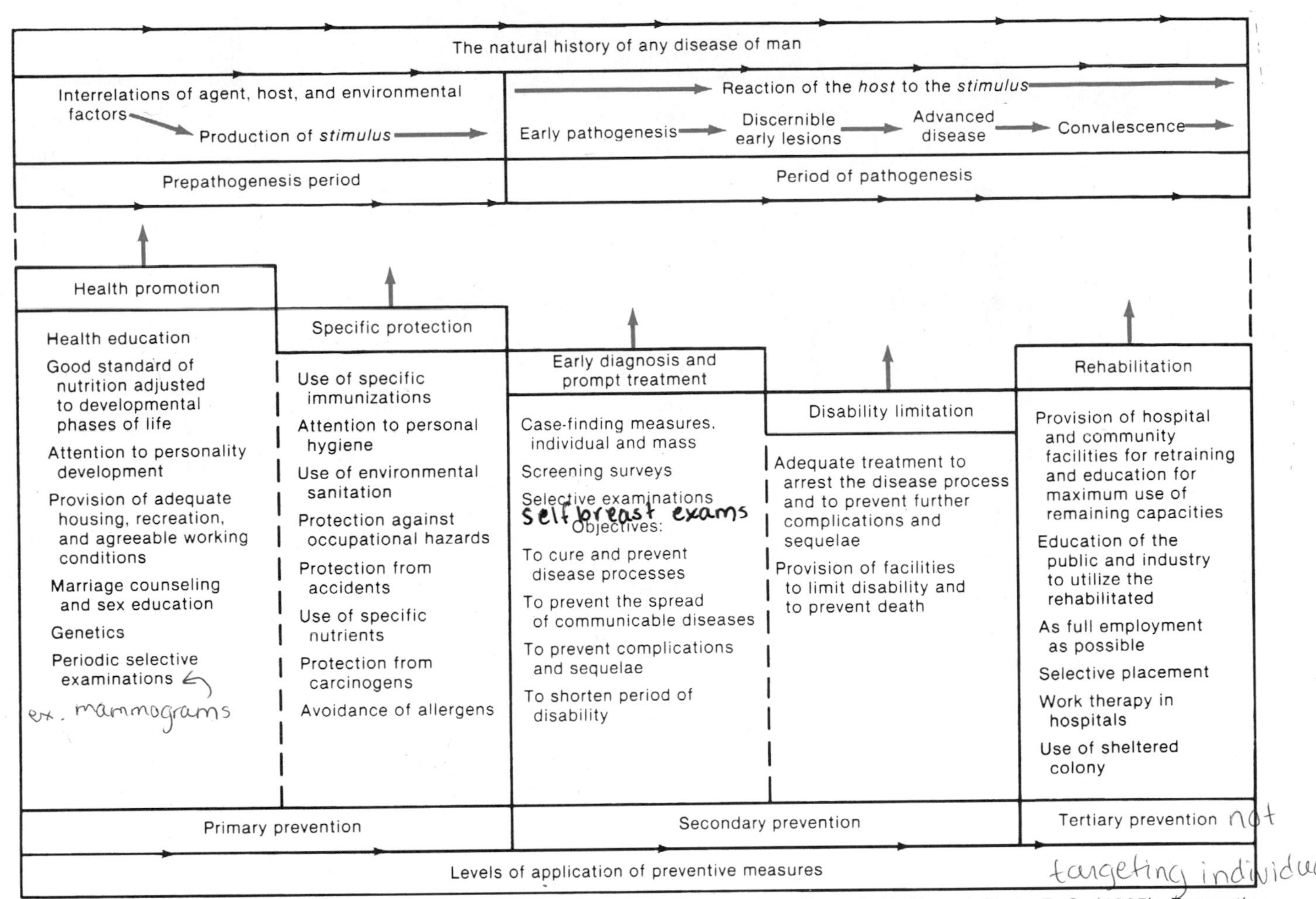

Figure 11–4 ● Levels of prevention in the natural history of disease. (Redrawn from Leavell, H. F., and Clark, E. G. (1965). *Preventive medicine for the doctor in his community: An epidemiologic approach* (p. 21). New York: McGraw-Hill.)

Secondary Prevention. Secondary prevention is aimed at early detection and prompt treatment either to cure a disease as early as possible or to slow its progression and prevent disability or complications. Screening programs in which asymptomatic persons are tested to detect early stages of a disease are the most frequent form of secondary prevention. Early case finding and prompt treatment activities are directed toward preventing the spread of communicable diseases, such as impetigo in a school. Preventing or slowing the development of a particular disease or condition and preventing complications from a disease, such as scoliosis in teenage girls, are also examples of secondary prevention.

Tertiary Prevention. Tertiary prevention is aimed at limiting disability in persons in the early stages of disease and at performing rehabilitation for persons who have experienced a loss of function due to a disease process or injury. Nursing activities include education to prevent deterioration of a person's condition, direct nursing care, and referrals to resources that can help patients minimize the loss of function.

MULTIPLE CAUSATION OF DISEASE

The theory of multiple causation of disease is critical to understanding epidemiological problems. Causality generally is thought of in terms of a stimulus or catalyst that produces an effect, result, or outcome. In epidemiology the interactions of the agent, person (host), and environment are analyzed by statistical measures to determine whether there is a causal relationship between various stimuli and health status. Understanding these interactions and relationships is even more important and complex as one considers the natural history of noninfectious diseases, chronic conditions, and the health and well-being of a population.

Vital and Health Statistics

A major source of information about a population comes from the vital statistics that are recorded about the population. *Vital statistics* is the term used for the data collected about the significant events that occur over a

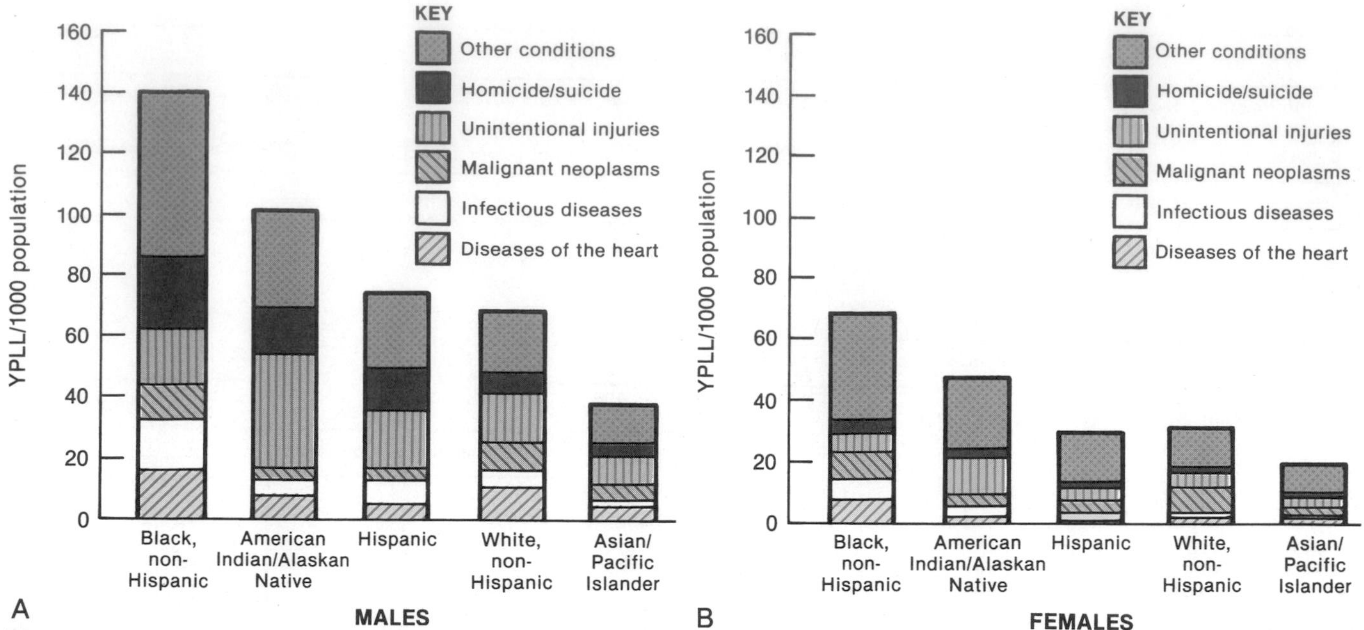

Figure 11–5 ● Rate of years of potential life lost (YPLL) before age 65 years, by race, Hispanic origin, and gender. (Redrawn from Desenclos, J-C. A., and Hahn, R. A. (1992, November 20). Years of potential life lost before age 65, by race, Hispanic origin and sex—United States, 1986–1988. *Morbidity and Mortality Weekly Report* (CDC/DHHS-PHS, *Vol. 41,* No. SS–6). Washington, DC: Government Printing Office.)

period of time within a population. The data used in epidemiology come from the ongoing registration of *vital* events, such as death certificates, birth certificates, and marriage certificates. These data are systematically collected by agencies such as the U.S. National Center for Health Statistics (NCHS), and the World Health Organization (WHO). Many other governmental agencies, such as the Centers for Disease Control and Prevention (CDC), the National Health Survey (NHS), and private groups, such as the Children's Defense Fund, also issue reports related to particular health concerns. One example of such a publication is the *Morbidity and Mortality Weekly Report* (*MMWR*) published by the CDC.

Another example of a report of this nature is a surveillance study by Desenclos and Hahn (1992), who examine years of potential life lost (YPLL) of persons younger than 65 years (Fig. 11–5). Premature mortality for the leading causes of death is identified for men and women by race and Hispanic origin. The rates of premature deaths differ greatly among racial and ethnic groups. Health care priorities and prevention strategies therefore need to consider the varying conditions among different aggregates. For example the authors suggest that mortality among young persons can be substantially reduced, if not prevented, through programs targeted to youth.

Use Figure 11–5, "Rate of Years of Potential Life Lost (YPLL) before Age 65 Years, by Race, Hispanic Origin, and Sex:—United States, 1986–1988" to compare rates among five racial and ethnic groups. Which group shows the highest premature mortality rate for men? For women? Which group shows the lowest premature mortality rate for men? For women? (You are correct if you answered that black non-Hispanic men and women have the greatest premature mortality and Asian/Pacific Islanders have the lowest premature mortality in the United States.)

The researchers note that homicide or suicide was responsible for 14% and 6% of the total YPLL in those younger than 65 years for non-Hispanic black males and females, respectively. For Native Americans, five conditions accounted for 48% and 34% of the total YPLL in those younger than 65 years for males and females, respectively. The conditions were (1) motor vehicle injuries, (2) other unintentional injuries, (3) suicide, (4) cirrhosis, and (5) diabetes. The rates for YPLL due to chronic disease for Hispanic males and females were lower than or similar to those for non-Hispanic whites, except for cirrhosis. The lower rate for Hispanic females was due to fewer suicides and unintentional injuries.

Health statistics such as morbidity data, unlike the death rate, are not systematically recorded in the United States. Therefore, morbidity statistics are less accurate than mortality statistics. The major sources of morbidity data come from hospital records, the notification system for reporting infectious diseases, and special surveys.

Table 11–4 represents the number of days per year that a person decreases normal activities for more than half a day because of illness or injury. This includes bed-disability, work-loss, and school-loss days. Using the total days of restricted activity between 1970 and 1989 as a measure, which year had the highest number of days of disability? Did children spend more days away from school in 1970 or 1989? What other interpretations are possible from the data in the table? (You are correct if you identified 1980 as the year with the most disability

TABLE 11–4

Days of Disability, by Type and Selected Characteristics: 1970 to 1989*

Item	Total Days of Disability (millions)						Days per Person					
	1970	1980	1985	1987	1988	1989	1970	1980	1985	1987	1988	1989
Restricted activity days[1]	2913	4165	3453	3448	3536	3693	14.6	19.1	14.8	14.5	14.7	15.2
Male	1273	1802	1442	1464	1487	1558	13.2	17.1	12.8	12.7	12.7	13.2
Female	1640	2363	2011	1984	2049	2135	15.8	21.0	16.6	16.1	16.5	17.0
White[2]	2526	3518	2899	2896	2969	3087	14.4	18.7	14.5	14.3	14.6	15.0
Black[2]	365	580	489	475	487	511	16.2	22.7	17.4	16.4	16.6	17.1
Hispanic[3]	(NA)	(NA)	228	226	253	278	(NA)	(NA)	13.2	12.0	13.0	13.2
Under 65 years	2331	3228	2557	2594	2657	2774	12.9	16.6	12.4	12.3	12.5	12.9
65 years and over	582	937	895	854	879	919	30.7	39.2	33.1	30.3	30.6	31.5
Northeast	709	862	689	684	667	669	14.5	17.9	13.8	13.6	13.5	13.7
Midwest	691	989	744	746	762	812	12.4	17.2	12.7	13.0	12.8	13.6
South	996	1415	1308	1220	1328	1392	15.9	19.8	16.3	15.0	16.1	16.7
West	518	899	712	797	779	820	15.6	22.0	15.7	16.0	15.6	15.8
Family Income:												
Under $10,000	(NA)	(NA)	893	756	754	694	(NA)	(NA)	25.8	24.2	26.6	26.5
$10,000 to $19,999	(NA)	(NA)	781	750	751	768	(NA)	(NA)	16.7	16.9	17.8	18.7
$20,000 to $34,999	(NA)	(NA)	791	761	734	752	(NA)	(NA)	12.1	12.3	12.3	13.3
$35,000 or more	(NA)	(NA)	568	685	726	798	(NA)	(NA)	9.9	9.9	9.7	9.9
Bed-disability days[4]	1222	1520	1436	1474	1519	1579	6.1	7.0	6.1	6.2	6.3	6.5
Male	503	616	583	595	607	652	5.2	5.9	5.2	5.2	5.2	5.5
Female	720	904	852	879	912	927	6.9	8.0	7.1	7.1	7.3	7.4
Under 65 years	959	1190	1064	1081	1107	1164	5.3	6.1	5.1	5.1	5.2	5.4
65 years and over	263	330	371	394	412	415	13.8	13.8	13.7	14.0	14.4	14.2
Work-loss days[5]	417	485	575	603	609	659	5.4	5.0	5.3	5.4	5.3	5.6
Male	243	271	287	299	307	322	5.0	4.9	4.8	4.8	4.8	5.0
Female	175	215	288	304	302	337	5.9	5.1	6.0	6.1	5.8	6.4
School-loss days[6]	222	204	217	198	222	260	4.9	5.3	4.8	4.4	4.9	5.7
Male	108	95	100	96	107	129	4.7	4.8	4.4	4.2	4.6	5.6
Female	114	109	117	102	115	131	5.1	5.7	5.3	4.6	5.2	5.7

From DHHS. (1992, December). *Vital and health statistics, current estimates from the National Health Interview Survey: 1991* (PHS Publication No. 93–1512, CDC Series 10, No. 184). Hyattsville, MD: U.S. Government Printing Office.

*Covers civilian noninstitutional population. Beginning 1985, the levels of estimates may not be comparable to estimates for 1970 and 1980 because the later data are based on a revised questionnaire and field procedures. Based on National Health Interview Survey.

NA = Not available. [1]A day when a person cuts down on his usual activities for more than half a day because of illness or injury. Includes bed-disability, work-loss, and school-loss days. Total includes other races and unknown income, not shown separately. [2]Beginning 1980 race was determined by asking the household respondent to report his race. In earlier years racial classification of respondents was determined by interviewer observation. [3]Persons of Hispanic origin may be of any race. [4]A day when a person stayed in bed more than half a day because of illness or injury. Includes those work-loss, school-loss days actually spent in bed. [5]A day when a person lost more than half a workday because of illness or injury. Computed for persons 17 years of age and over (beginning 1985, 18 years of age and over) in the currently employed population defined as those who were working or had a job or business from which they were not on layoff during the 2-week period preceding the week of interview. [6]Child's loss of more than half a school day because of illness or injury. Computed for children 6–16 years of age (beginning 1985, children 5–17 years old).

days and 1989 as the year in which children lost more days from school.)

Figure 11–6 presents 1991 data related to days of disability for persons of all groups by family income. Do lower-income families have fewer or greater numbers of days of disability? This pattern holds for bed disability and work or school loss. What might account for the difference? There is also regional variation in the days of disability in 1991 data. The Northeast has the lowest rate, at 13.1 per 1000; the Midwest, 15.2 per 1000; the West, 16.5 per 1000; and the South, 18.2 per 1000 (DHHS, 1992b, p. 111).

When seeking out sources of population or community data it might also be worthwhile to look to other organizations that routinely use health statistics, such as local health departments, hospitals, regional planning agencies, and other local and state governmental agencies.

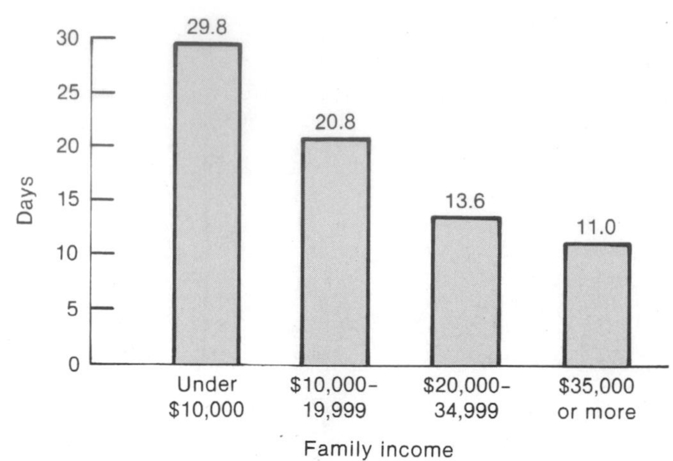

Figure 11–6 ● Days of disability per person, all ages, by family income, 1991. (Redrawn from U.S. Department of Health and Human Services (DHHS). (December 1992). *Vital and health statistics, current estimates from the National Health Interview Survey, 1991.* (No. 184, Dec 1992.) Hyattsville, MD: U.S. Government Printing Office.)

Demographic Data

Age, sex, race, social class, occupation, marital status, and religion are demographic characteristics that are frequently used when describing human populations. These factors contribute to variations in health status, health-related behaviors, and utilization of health care.

Major demographic findings, reported by the U.S. Bureau of the Census, provide specific information that describes the population. This information is collected every 10 years from the national census. In addition to the overall profiles of the population, e.g., age, gender, marital status, and educational level, many specific reports are issued each year. For example a report of national population trends and projections might include information about the overall population as well as information about the number of women of childbearing age, the baby boom generation (born between 1946 and 1964), and growth due to net immigration. This report may also

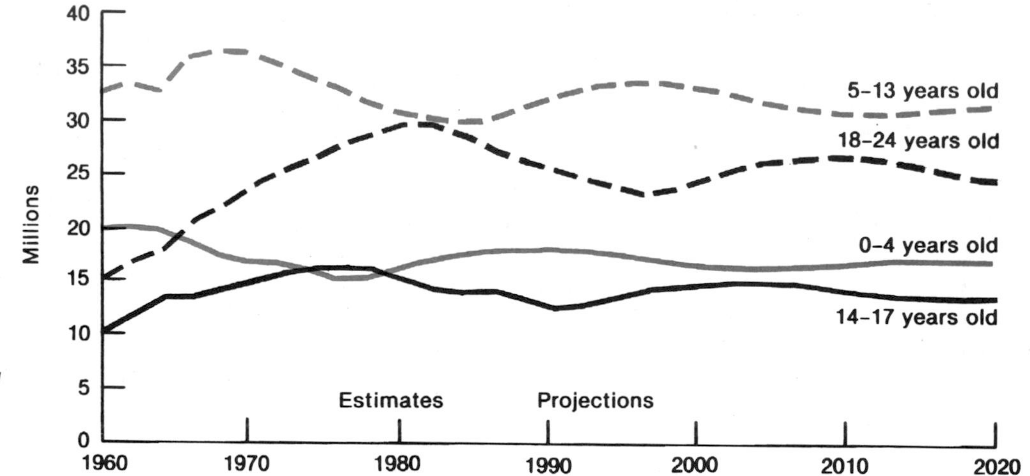

Figure 11–7 ● Trends in the population younger than 25 years: 1960–2020. (Redrawn from U.S. Bureau of the Census. (1989). *Population profile of the United States: 1989* (CPR, series p-23, No. 159, p. 7). Washington, DC: U.S. Government Printing Office.)

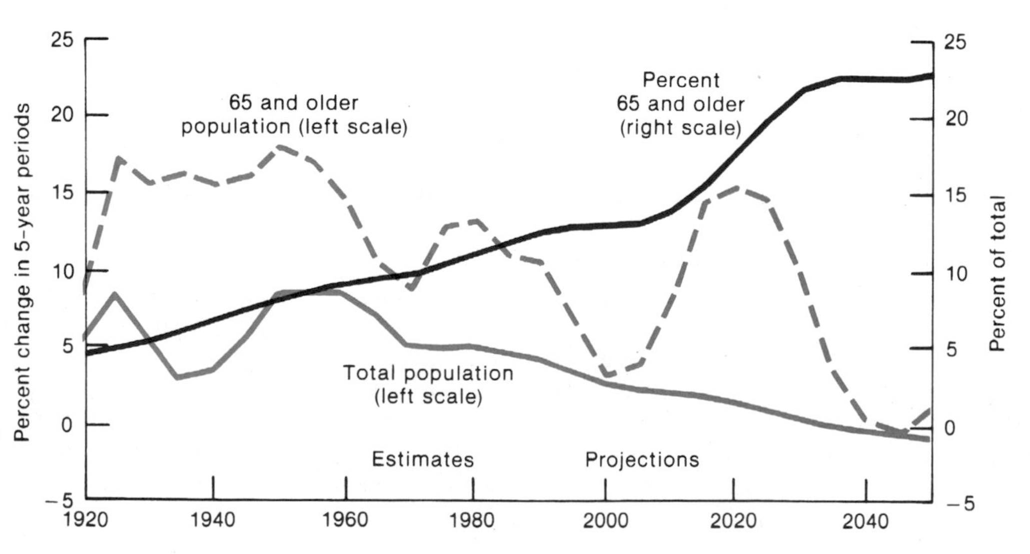

Figure 11–8 ● Trends in the total and 65-years-and-older populations: 1920–2050. (Redrawn from U.S. Bureau of the Census. (1989). *Population profile of the United States: 1989.* (CPR, series p-23, No. 159, p. 7). Washington, DC: U.S. Government Printing Office.)

include data related to the trends of the population younger than 25 years, such as preschool children (Fig. 11–7), the older-than-65-years group (Fig. 11–8), or life expectancy for a given birth year (Fig. 11–9). Community health nurses will find this information useful in planning health care services and anticipating the needs of target groups in the population.

THE AGING POPULATION

It is expected that the numbers of elderly persons will increase at a moderate rate until 2010 (Figs. 11–8 and 11–10). At that point the baby boom generation will enter the 65+ age group and the numbers will accelerate. When population pyramids between 1960 and 1990 are compared, the shift in age is apparent (Fig. 11–11). Because of the increased need for health services in this age group and the increasing proportion of persons older than 65 years, this information is important for community health nurses.

Although the overall growth of the population is expected to slow and possibly stop around 2045, the average life span continues to rise. The real and projected gains are presented in Fig. 11–9.

GENDER, RACE, AND LIFE EXPECTANCY

The information presented in Figure 11–9 has been converted to a table that allows comparisons of projected gains in average life expectancy (Table 11–5). Closely analyze the table and make hypotheses as to the difference in net gain.

- What might be some possible reasons for women living longer than men?

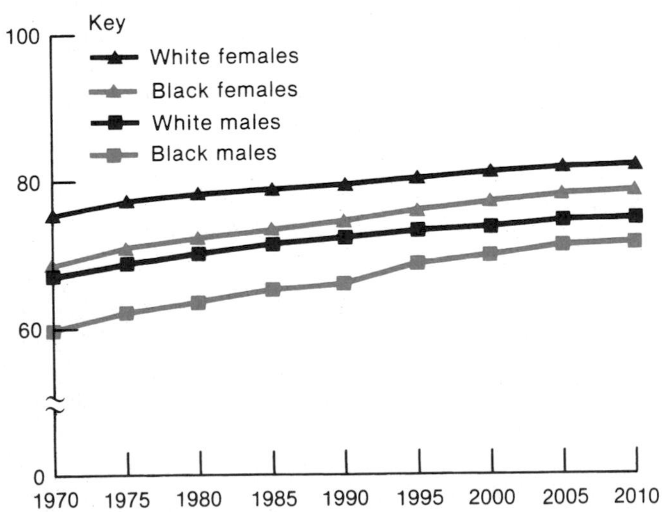

Figure 11–9 ● Life expectancy at birth for black and white males and females: 1970–2010. (From U.S. Bureau of the Census. (1992). *Statistical abstracts of the United States, 1992: The national data book* (112th ed.) (No. 103, p 76). Washington, DC: U.S. Department of Commerce, Economics, and Statistics Administration.)

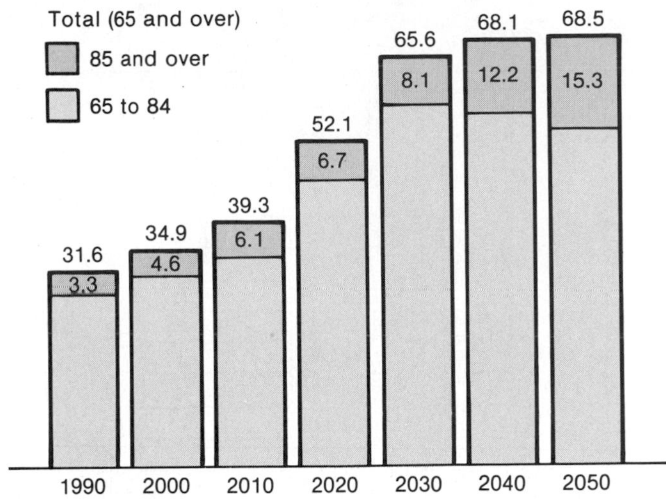

Figure 11–10 ● Projections of the elderly population by age. (Redrawn from U.S. Bureau of the Census. (1989). *Population profile of the United States: 1989.* (CPR, series p-23, No. 159, p. 40). Washington, DC: U.S. Government Printing Office.)

TABLE 11–5

Real and Projected Gains in Years of Life for Men and Women from 1970

	1990	2010 (Projected)	1990	2010 (Projected)
	All Men		All Women	
	72.0	74.4	79.2	81.3
1970	−67.1	−67.1	−74.7	−74.7
Gain in years	4.9	7.3	4.5	6.6
	White Men		White Women	
	73.4	74.9 (Projected)	79.3	81.7 (Projected)
1970	−68.0	−68.0	−75.6	−75.6
Gain in years	5.4	6.9	3.7	6.1
	Black Men		Black Women	
	66.0	71.4 (Projected)	74.5	78.5 (Projected)
1970	−60.0	−60.0	−68.3	−68.3
Gain in years	6.0	11.4	6.2	10.2

Data from U.S. Bureau of the Census. (1992). *Statistical abstracts of the U.S. 1992—The national data book* (112th ed.). Washington, DC: U.S. Government Printing Office, Publication No. 103, p. 67.

Give thought to what is presented in Table 11–5. Which groups are expected to experience the highest net gain between 1990 and 2010? Notice that black men and black women are expected to make the most gain.

Now make some guesses as to possible reasons for the higher gains for both black men and women.

- What might be a social reason for the difference? What is known about the relationship of socioeconomic status and health status?
- What reason related to health risk behavior might account for the difference? What is known about health screening patterns among the black population?

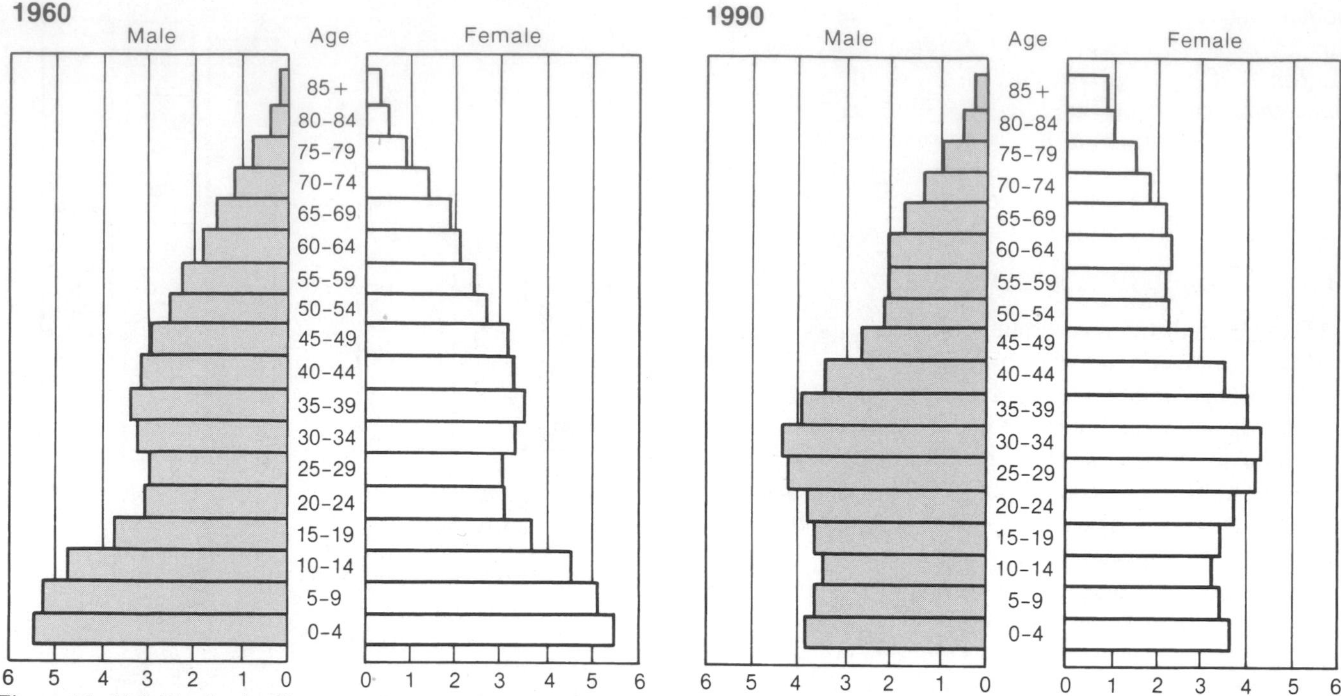

Figure 11–11 ● Distribution (in percent) of the U.S. population by age and sex: 1960 and 1990. (Redrawn from U.S. Bureau of the Census. (1992). *Households, families, and children: A 30-year perspective* (CPR, series p-23, No. 159, pp. 4–5). Washington, DC: U.S. Government Printing Office.)

- What health service barrier might contribute to the difference? Who have been the primary subjects of health care research?

Health-Related Studies Published by the Department of Commerce

To find out which area of the country is growing the fastest or which state is projected to have the highest median age in the year 2000 it would be wise to consult data from the U.S. Department of Commerce, which commissions such studies. The U.S. Department of Commerce publishes other records, including such information as city and urban growth and/or decline, household and family data, marital status and living arrangements, fertility among women, percentage of women in the labor force, labor force and occupation, poverty rates and figures, unemployment rates, and race and ethnicity.

For example the Hispanic population is growing rapidly in the United States; in fact this population is growing more rapidly than the non-Hispanic population. This population tends to be young and is highly concentrated in the southwestern states (63%). Fifty-five percent live in California and Texas alone.

A comparison of family structure between 1970 and 1990 shows that the proportion of families that are headed by married couples has declined for whites, blacks, and persons of Hispanic origin. Families headed by a single parent and with a female head of household have increased for all groups (Fig. 11–12).

The poverty level is another area for which data have been analyzed by the U.S. Department of Commerce. Figure 11–13 presents data based on the government-established poverty level. It is apparent that the rate of poverty declined dramatically during the 1960s (from 22.4% in 1959 to 12.1% in 1969). In the 1970s the rate fluctuated. From 1978 to 1983 the actual number of poor people increased again (from 24.5 to 35.3 million, or by 44%). The poverty rate in the 1990s is higher than at any time during the 1970s. Currently 36.9 million Americans (14%) are living in impoverished conditions.

Major Causes of Death*

Use of epidemiological data and biostatistics provides an important knowledge base for population-focused nursing practice. In addition the emphasis on more holistic care and health promotion requires an understanding of known risk behaviors and the raising of new questions about how to reduce the barriers associated with positive behavior change (Redland and Stuifbergen, 1993). The leading

* The survey of literature for articles relating to major causes of death was completed in September 1993.

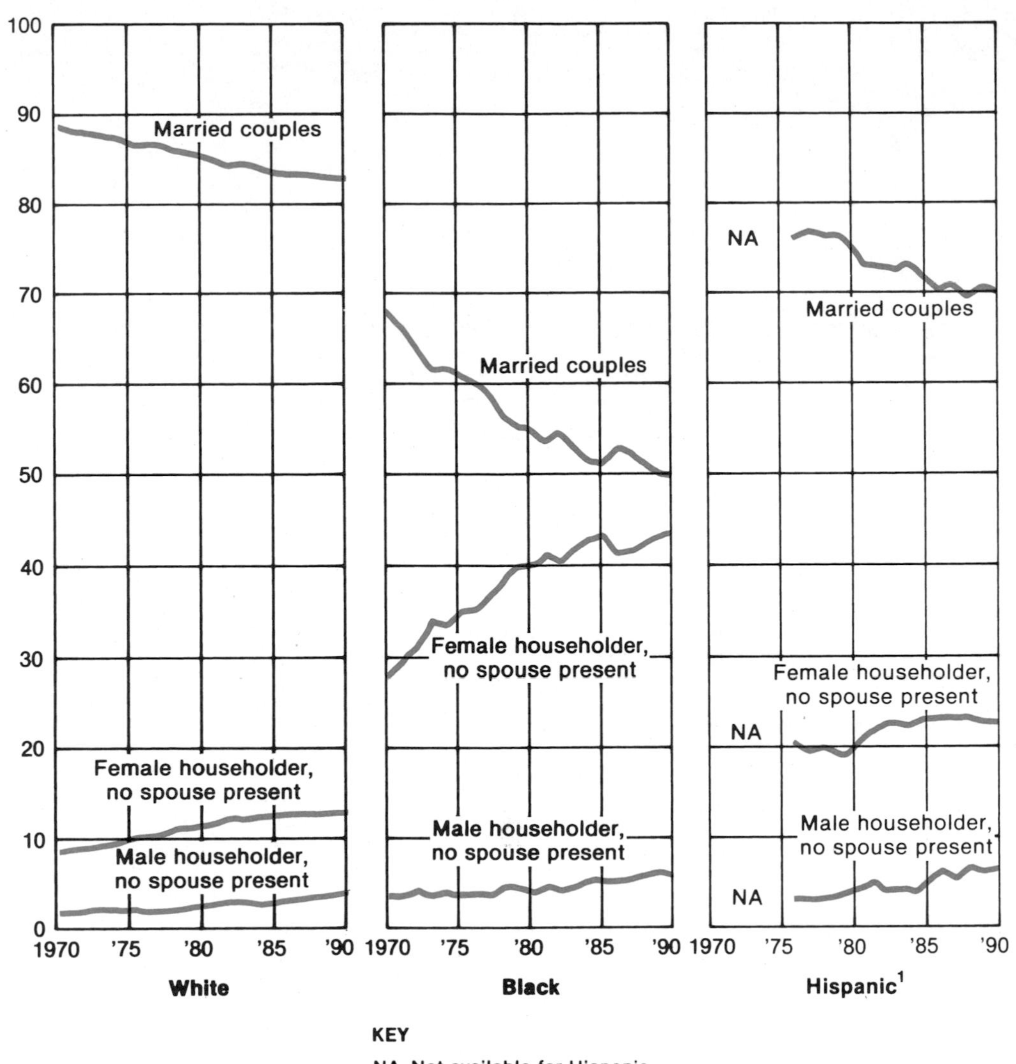

Figure 11–12 ● Type of family as a percentage of all family householders, by race and Hispanic origin: 1970–1990. (Redrawn from U.S. Bureau of the Census. (1992). *Households, families, and children: a 30-year perspective* (CPR, series p-23, No. 159, p. 16). Washington, DC: U.S. Government Printing Office.)

causes of death are frequently the focus of epidemiological study; however the bigger challenge is in understanding the factors that contribute to the development of the disease and/or death. McGinnis and Foege (1993) argue that major external (nongenetic) factors, which they have identified, are responsible for approximately half of the deaths in the United States. Table 11–6 lists these causes of mortality. McGinnis and Foege advocate a change in how causes of death are reported. For example when a person who smoked for 45 years officially dies of lung cancer, they would list the cause of death as cigarettes, not cancer. Their new list, based on the synthesis of research conducted between 1977 and 1993, reflects a growing trend of giving attention to prevention of the illness rather than to the treatment of the disease. Clearly the public health burden imposed by these causes will guide and shape future health policy priorities, including public health nursing priorities. These causes offer a different dimension to consideration of quality of life and causes of disease. The work of McGinnis and Foege validates nursing's strong commitment to disease prevention and the well-being of the overall population.

LEADING CAUSES OF DEATH IN THE UNITED STATES: 1992

In 1992, an estimated 2,177,000 deaths occurred in the United States. Although the estimated number of deaths is 1% higher than the number of deaths in 1991, the estimated rate for 1992 (853 deaths per 100,000) is the lowest death rate since 1982. The decrease in the death rate reflects a lower mortality for a number of causes of death, including heart disease, cerebrovascular accidents, accidents, and atherosclerosis. In contrast, provisional data for human

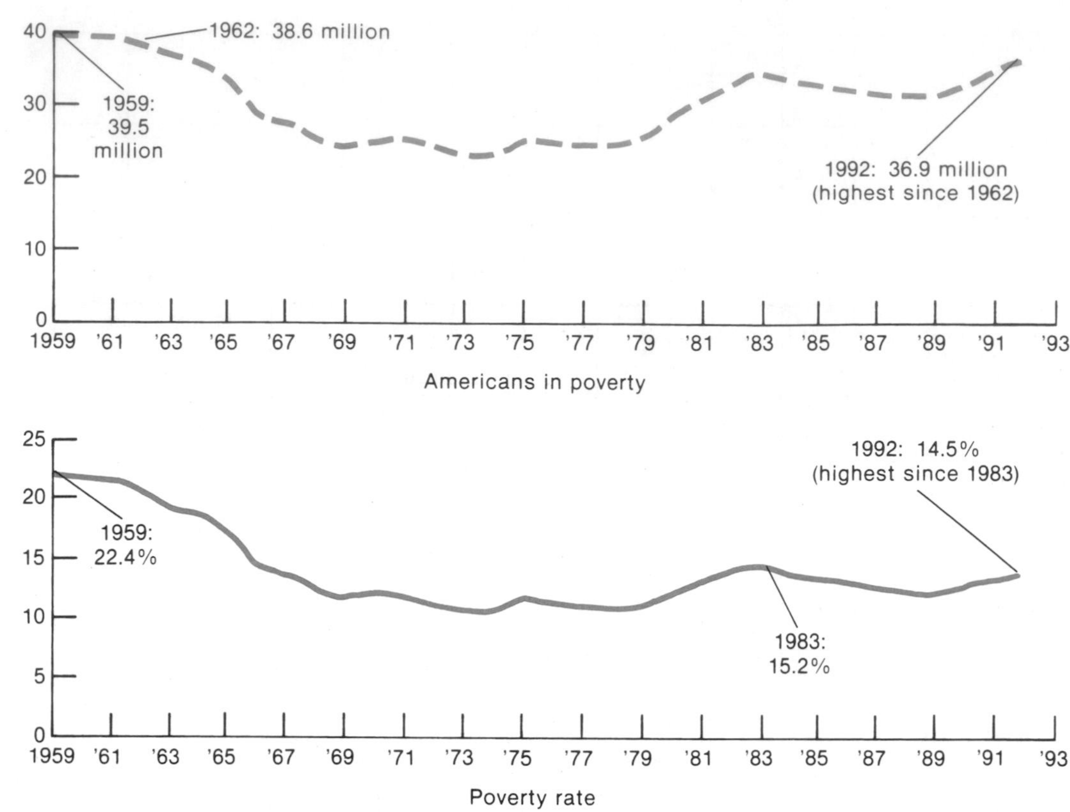

Figure 11–13 ● Americans in poverty. (Redrawn from Gugliotta, G. (1993, October 5). Number of poor Americans rises for third year. *Washington Post,* p. A6.)

TABLE 11–6

Actual Causes of Death in the United States in 1990

Cause	Deaths: Estimated No.*	Deaths: Percentage of Total Deaths
Tobacco	400,000	19
Diet/activity patterns	300,000	14
Alcohol	100,000	5
Microbial agents	90,000	4
Toxic agents	60,000	3
Firearms	35,000	2
Sexual behavior	30,000	1
Motor vehicles	25,000	1
Illicit use of drugs	20,000	<1
Total	**1,060,000**	**50**

From McGinnis, M. J., and Foege, W. (1993). Actual causes of death in the United States. *Journal of the American Medical Association, 270,* p. 2208.

*Composite approximation drawn from studies that use different approaches to derive estimates, ranging from actual counts (e.g., firearms) to population attributable risk calculations (e.g., tobacco). Numbers over 100,000 rounded to the nearest 100,000; over 50,000, rounded to the nearest 10,000; below 50,000, rounded to the nearest 5000.

immunodeficiency virus (HIV) infection reflects a 13% increase between 1991 and 1992 (CDC, 1993).

The 15 leading causes of death in 1992 reflect 86% of the total deaths in the United States (Table 11–7). The 1992 ranking of the three leading causes of death (heart disease, cancer, and cerebrovascular disease) and the 10th through 15th leading causes of death remain the same as in 1991. Chronic obstructive pulmonary disease (fifth in 1991; fourth in 1992) and accidents (fourth in 1991; fifth in 1992) changed rankings between 1991 and 1992. The same was true for HIV infection (ninth in 1991; eighth in 1992) and suicide (eighth in 1991; ninth in 1992). Pneumonia and diabetes mellitus remained in the sixth and seventh positions, respectively, for both years.

Heart Disease

In 1992 approximately 720,000 persons died of coronary heart disease (CHD). Risk factors or susceptibility to CHD are not random. Risk factors identified in the Framingham Study, begun in 1948, and other epidemiological investigations include (1) being male, (2) advanced age, (3) high serum lipid concentrations (especially the ratio of total cholesterol to high-density lipoprotein cholesterol), (4) high blood pressure, (5) smoking, (6) diabetes mellitus, (7) obesity, (8) specific

TABLE 11–7

Estimated Deaths, Death Rates, and Percent of Total Deaths for the 15 Leading Causes of Death: United States, 1992*

Rank	Cause of Death (ICD-9)	No.	Death Rate	Percent of Total Deaths
	All causes	2,177,000	853.3	100.0
1	Diseases of heart	720,480	282.5	33.1
2	Malignant neoplasms, including neoplasms of lymphatic and hematopoietic tissues	520,090	204.3	23.9
3	Cerebrovascular diseases	143,640	56.3	6.6
4	Chronic obstructive pulmonary diseases and allied conditions	91,440	35.8	4.2
5	Accidents and adverse effects	86,310	33.8	4.0
	Motor vehicle accidents	41,710	16.4	1.9
	All other accidents and adverse effects	44,600	17.5	2.0
6	Pneumonia and influenza	76,120	29.8	3.5
7	Diabetes mellitus	50,180	19.7	2.3
8	Human immunodeficiency virus infection	33,590	13.2	1.5
9	Suicide	29,760	11.7	1.4
10	Homicide and legal intervention	26,570	10.4	1.2
11	Chronic liver disease and cirrhosis	24,830	9.7	1.1
12	Nephritis, nephrotic syndrome, and nephrosis	22,400	8.8	1.0
13	Septicemia	19,910	7.8	0.9
14	Atherosclerosis	16,100	6.3	0.7
15	Certain conditions originating in the perinatal period	15,790	6.2	0.7
	All other causes	298,430	117.0	13.7

From CDC. (1993, September 28). Annual summary of births, marriages, divorces, and deaths: United States, 1992. *Monthly Vital Statistics Report.* (CDC/NCHS-PHS. *Vol. 40,* No. 13). Washington, DC: U.S. Government Printing Office.

*Data are provisional, estimated from a 10% sample of deaths. Rates per 100,000 population. Figures may differ from those previously published. Due to rounding, figures may not add to totals.

ICD-9 = Ninth revision, International Classification of Diseases, 1975.

electrocardiographic abnormalities, and (9) low vital capacity (Friedman, 1987; Castelli et al., 1992). Other studies include psychological factors, family history of CHD, and physical inactivity as characteristics that contribute to the development of CHD.

Cancer

More than 8 million Americans have a history of cancer. Cancer in 4 million of them was diagnosed 5 or more years ago, and they are considered to be *cured* (generally defined as being symptom-free for 5 years following treatment). With some forms of cancer a person is considered cured in a shorter period, and with other forms follow-up may be required for a longer period.

In 1992 cancer was diagnosed in approximately 1,130,000 people. This number does not include carcinoma in situ and basal and squamous cell skin cancers, which account for another 600,000 cases (American Cancer Society, 1992).

In 1992 approximately 521,000 people (or about 1400 per day) died of cancer; this is approximately 6000 more cancer-related deaths than occurred in 1991. According to the American Cancer Society (ACS) the cancer mortality rate in the United States has risen steadily since the mid-1940s. The major increase occurred in lung cancer while rates for other sites have declined or leveled off (Fig. 11–14).

About 4 of 10 persons (40%) will survive the "relative" 5-year time frame after treatment. This represents a gain from 1 in 5 (20%) in the 1930s and 1 in 3 (30%) in the 1960s when normal life expectancy is taken into consideration. The improved survival rate is used to document progress in early detection and treatment.

The importance of prevention should not be underestimated. It is known that "regular screening and self-exams can detect cancers of the breast, tongue, mouth, colon, rectum, cervix, prostate, testes, and melanoma at an early stage when treatment is more likely to be successful" (ACS, 1992, p. 1). These cancers represent about 50% of patients with recent diagnosis, of whom two thirds are expected to survive 5 years. It is believed that with early detection the survival rate could be 89%. In addition approximately 90% of the skin cancers could have been prevented by protection from ultraviolet radiation in sunlight. Furthermore cancer from cigarette smoking and heavy alcohol use could be totally prevented. The ACS estimated that in 1992 about 158,000 persons would die of cancer related to tobacco smoking and that about another 16,500 deaths would be related to excessive alcohol use, frequently in combination with cigarette smoking.

Human Immunodeficiency Virus Infection

Acquired immunodeficiency syndrome (AIDS) was first reported by health care providers in California and the Centers for Disease Control and Prevention (CDC) in June 1981 (CDC, 1981). In 1987, 50,000 cases of AIDS were reported. That number reached 100,000 by August 1989 and the cumulative total was 206,392 by December 31, 1991 (Fig. 11–15) (CDC, 1992a).

It is estimated that 8 to 10 million adults and 1 million children worldwide are infected with HIV. The World Health Organization (WHO) estimates that 40 million persons may be infected by HIV by the year 2000 (WHO, 1991). It is expected that AIDS will remain a major public health challenge in the next century.

By the end of 1991, 10 years after the first report, HIV infection had emerged as a leading cause of death among men and women younger than 45 years and in children 1 to 5 years in the United States (CDC, 1991c). Although homosexual and bisexual men account for the majority of persons who die of AIDS, persons who have received a

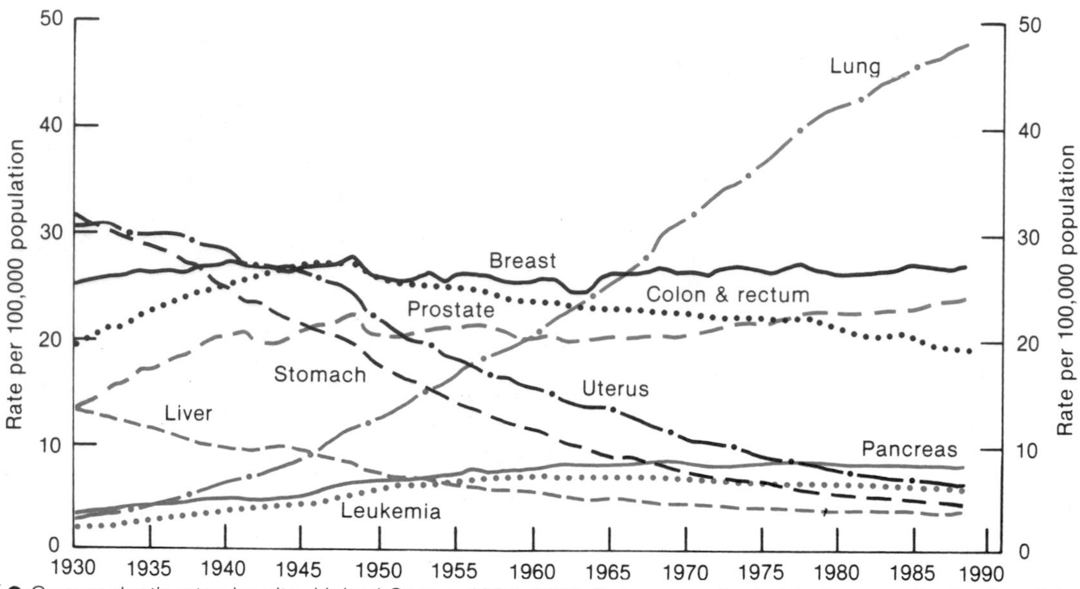

Figure 11–14 ● Cancer death rates by site, United States, 1930–1988. Rates are adjusted to the age distribution of the 1970 census population and are combined for both sexes, with the exception of breast and uterus (female population only) and prostate (male population only). (Redrawn from American Cancer Society. (1992). *Cancer facts and figures, 1992* (p. 3). Atlanta, GA: American Cancer Society.)

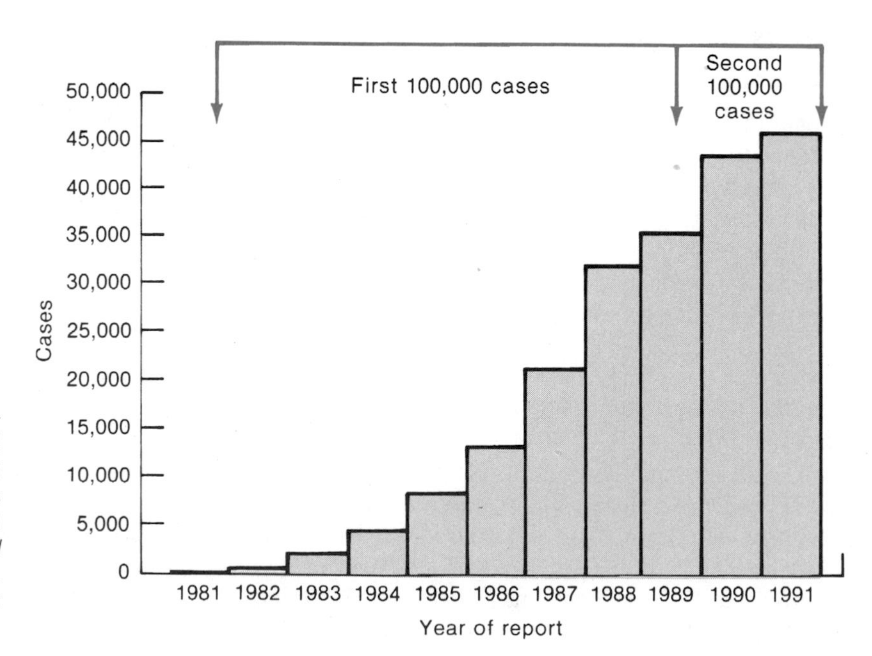

Figure 11–15 ● Cases of acquired immunodeficiency syndrome (AIDS), by year of report—United States, June 1981–December 1991. (Redrawn from CDC. (1992, January 7). The second 100,000 cases of acquired immunodeficiency syndrome—United States, June 1981 to December 1991. *Morbidity and Mortality Weekly Report* (CDC/PHS-DHHS, *Vol. 41,* No. 2, p. 28). Washington, DC: U.S. Government Printing Office.)

blood transfusion or blood product and children born to mothers with HIV also are represented in the death rates. People of all ages die of AIDS (Fig. 11–16) (*The National Data Book,* 1992, p. 63).

Sixty-one percent of the first 100,000 cases occurred among homosexual and bisexual men with no history of intravenous drug use (IDU) and 20% were females or heterosexual males with a history of IDU. Of the second 100,000 cases of AIDS, 55% occurred in homosexual and bisexual males with no history of IDU and 24% occurred in females or heterosexual males with a history of IDU. The second 100,000 persons with HIV reflect an increasing proportion of individuals who report heterosexual exposure. The change, although small (5% to 7%) between the first and the second 100,000 cases represents a 44% increase in heterosexual transmission (CDC, 1992).

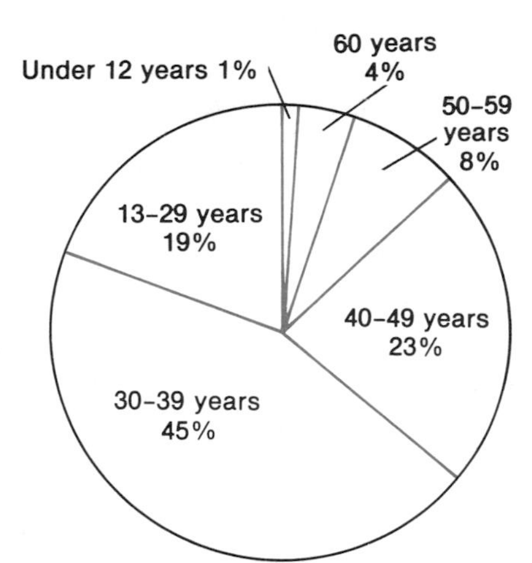

Figure 11–16 ● Distribution of AIDS deaths, by age: 1982–1991. (Redrawn from U.S. Bureau of the Census. (1992). *Statistical abstracts of the United States, (1992): The national data book* (112th ed.) (p. 63). Washington, DC: U.S. Department of Commerce, Economics and Statistics Administration.)

In 1993 the CDC reported that more women developed AIDS from heterosexual intercourse than from IDU (Fig. 11–17). Approximately 60% of the women had sex partners who had a history of IDU and the majority of the remaining women had sex partners who were bisexual men.

Education for prevention of HIV is critical for reducing the incidence of AIDS. It is known that men and women who have unprotected sexual contact with "multiple sexual partners and in the presence of other sexually transmitted diseases . . . particularly with partners known to have risks for HIV infection, are at increased risk for HIV infection" (CDC, 1992a, p. 29). A close analysis of expected trends suggests that heterosexual transmission in the non–drug-using population will account for an increasing number of cases in the next few years (Brookmeyer, 1991). This suggests that men and women need to know the drug and sex histories of their partners prior to sexual intercourse.

Table 11–8 includes characteristics of persons reported and diagnosed with AIDS in 1989 and 1990. This table will be used to answer the following questions.

- Which region of the country reported the largest percentage increase in this time period?
- In which groups of people did the largest proportionate increases occur from 1989 to 1990?
- In which two groups were the largest number of cases reported?
- What was the percentage increase of reported cases from 1989 to 1990?

Answers to the preceding questions, respectively, are as follows:

- The U.S. Territories and the South
- Women, persons between 5 and 19 years of age, blacks, Hispanics, persons living in the South, and persons exposed to HIV through heterosexual contact

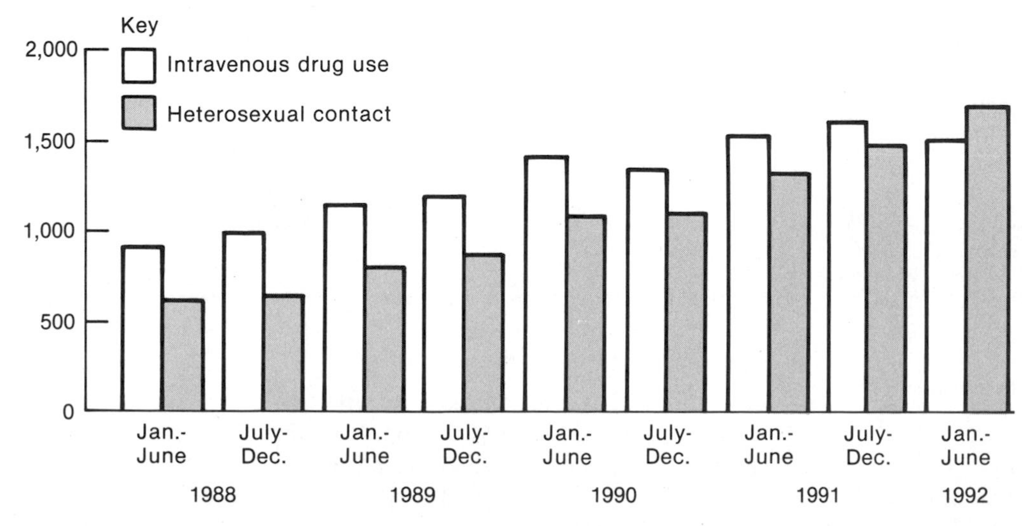

Figure 11–17 ● New cases of AIDS in women, attributed to intravenous drug use or heterosexual contact. (Redrawn from CDC. The second 100,000 cases of acquired immunodeficiency syndrome—United States, June 1981–December 1991. *Morbidity and Mortality Weekly Report* (CDC/PHS-DHHS, *Vol. 41,* No. 2, pp. 28–29). Washington, DC: U.S. Government Printing Office.)

TABLE 11–8

Characteristics of Reported Persons with AIDS and Percent Changes in Cases, by Year of Report and Year of Diagnosis: United States, 1989 and 1990

Category	1990 Reported Cases			*1989* Reported Cases	% Change 1989–1990	
	No.	*(%)*	*Rate**		*Reported*	*Diagnosed†*
Sex						
Male	38,082	(87.9)	30.9	31,282	21.7	5.9
Female	5,257	(12.1)	4.1	3,948	33.2	17.4
Age (years)						
0–4	622	(1.4)	3.3	533	16.7	2.3
5–9	120	(0.3)	0.6	89	34.8	33.0
10–19	208	(0.5)	0.6	149	39.6	17.0
20–29	8,338	(19.2)	19.7	6,992	19.3	5.9
30–39	19,722	(45.5)	46.8	16,260	21.3	4.7
40–49	10,026	(23.1)	33.5	7,640	31.2	13.6
50–59	3,013	(7.0)	13.4	2,518	19.7	4.1
≥60	1,290	(3.0)	3.1	1,049	23.0	13.5
Race/Ethnicity‡						
White	22,342	(51.6)	11.8	18,661	19.7	2.5
Black	13,186	(30.4)	42.5	10,336	27.6	12.0
Hispanic	7,322	(16.9)	31.9	5,829	25.6	13.3
Asian/Pacific Islander	260	(0.6)	3.8	239	8.8	–8.8
American Indian/Alaskan Native	71	(0.2)	4.0	63	12.7	23.1
Region						
Northeast	13,572	(31.3)	26.7	10,710	26.7	–2.2
Midwest	4,068	(9.4)	6.8	3,491	16.5	12.7
South	14,331	(33.1)	16.8	11,010	30.2	14.9
West	9,624	(22.2)	18.2	8,511	13.1	3.3
U.S. territories	1,744	(4.0)	46.2	1,508	15.6	31.0
HIV exposure category						
Male homosexual/bisexual contact	23,738	(54.8)	—	19,891	19.3	5.2
History of intravenous-drug use						
Women and heterosexual men	10,018	(23.1)	—	8,089	23.8	7.9
Male homosexual/bisexual contact	2,295	(5.3)	—	2,214	3.7	–2.7
Persons with hemophilia						
Adult/adolescent	340	(0.8)	—	289	17.6	–2.9
Child	31	(0.1)	—	25	24.0	16.7
Transfusion recipients						
Adult/adolescent	866	(2.0)	—	777	11.5	–1.0
Child	39	(0.1)	—	40	–2.5	–2.6
Heterosexual contacts	2,289	(5.3)	—	1,631	40.3	40.9
Born pattern II country§	422	(1.0)	—	379	11.3	–10.1
Perinatal	681	(1.6)	—	565	20.5	7.8
No identified risk	2,620	(6.0)	—	1,330	—	—
Total	43,339	(100.0)	17.2	35,230	23.0	7.2

From CDC. (1991, June 7). The HIV/AIDS epidemic: The first 10 years. *Morbidity and Mortality Weekly Report* (CDC/DHHS-PHS, *Vol. 40,* No. 22). Washington DC: U.S. Government Printing Office, p. 362.

*Per 100,000 population.

†Diagnosed cases adjusted for estimated delays in reporting.

‡Excludes persons with unspecified race/ethnicity.

§Persons born in countries where heterosexual transmission predominates.

- Whites and homosexual and bisexual men.
- 23% (35,230 to 43,339 cases)

Given the number of patients cared for by health care providers, few cases of occupational exposure have been reported (Table 11–9). The CDC monitors occupational transmission of HIV and circumstances surrounding the transmission. It is suspected that the number is greater than reported because some health care providers are not evaluated for HIV infection following exposure.

TABLE 11–9

Health Care Workers with Documented and Possible Occupationally Acquired HIV Infection, by Occupation: United States, through September 1992

Occupation	Documented	Possible
Dental worker, including dentist	0	6
Embalmer/morgue technician	0	3
Emergency medical technician/paramedic	0	7
Health aide/attendant	1	5
Housekeeper/maintenance worker	1	5
Laboratory technician, clinical	11	12
Laboratory technician, nonclinical	1	1
Nurse	12	14
Physician, nonsurgical	4	7
Physician, surgical	0	2
Respiratory therapist	1	1
Surgical technician	1	1
Technician/therapist, other than those listed above	0	3
Other health care occupations	0	2
Total	**32**	**69**

From CDC. (1992, October 30). *Morbidity and Mortality Weekly Report* (CDC/DHHS-PHS, *Vol. 41*, No. 43). Washington, DC: U.S. Government Printing Office, p. 824.

Health Profiles/Status and the Life Cycle

PATTERNS OF MORTALITY AND MORBIDITY DURING PREGNANCY AND INFANCY

The health status of the infant cannot be separated from that of the mother. Therefore factors related to the prenatal period are frequently addressed along with those that are present in the period immediately following birth.

The infant mortality rate, because of its sensitivity, is one of the most widely used statistics in determining the overall improvement in health in the United States; it is also used in making comparisons with international rates. Traditionally the high rate of infant mortality has been viewed as an indicator of unmet health needs and unfavorable environmental conditions. It is important to note that there has been a steady decline in the infant mortality rate; a drop from 29.2 per 1000 live births in 1950 to 9.2 per 1000 live births in 1990, and 8.5 per 1000 live births (provisional) in 1992 (CDC, 1991b; DHHS, 1992; CDC, 1993). In 1992, 34,400 actual infant deaths occurred. This improvement, however, still leaves the rate for the United States higher than that of other industrial countries.

The 1988 infant mortality rate was the lowest rate ever recorded in the United States. However, the disparities between minority and majority populations continues to be quite large. For white infants the mortality rate was 8.5 per 1000 live births (851 per 100,000) compared with 17.6 per 1000 live births for black infants (CDC, 1991b, p. 644). Table 11–10 lists in rank order the 10 leading causes of infant death by race. Four causes account for more than 50% of all infant deaths: conditions related to low birth weight, congenital anomalies, sudden infant death syndrome (SIDS), and respiratory distress syndrome. The four leading causes of infant death differ by race (see Table 11–10). Congenital anomalies account for 24.8% of the deaths of white infants. For black infants SIDS is the leading cause of death at 12.8%. Although the rank order of the four leading causes of death is different for black and white infants, the top four conditions account for 54.3% of all deaths among white infants and 45.3% of all deaths among black infants.

Low birth weight is associated with several preventable risks, including the lack of prenatal care, maternal smoking, use of alcohol and drugs, poor nutrition, and pregnancy before the age of 18 years. Lower socioeconomic and educational levels are also often linked with low birth weight. An expectant mother who received no prenatal care is three times more likely to give birth to a low-birth-weight infant. This is particularly true in the high-risk groups of adolescents and women living in poverty.

PATTERNS OF MORTALITY AND MORBIDITY OF CHILDHOOD

The rate of childhood deaths in the United States has dramatically declined since the mid-1950s, although the United States still has a higher rate of infant mortality than most other industrialized nations.

Infectious diseases such as polio, diphtheria, scarlet fever, measles, pneumonia, and whooping cough have been virtually eliminated through immunizations. According to WHO 7.5 million children die each year of diseases for which vaccines or effective treatments exist. However in the United States the infectious diseases category has been replaced by that of unintentional injuries, which are also largely preventable. From 1977 to 1989 there was a significant drop in the childhood death rate (23%), due mostly to the mandatory use of motor vehicle safety restraints for young children in all 50 states and the increased use of seat belts (Fig. 11–18). Still nearly half of unintentional injuries result from motor vehicle accidents. Drowning and fires are the other most frequent causes of injury-related deaths (National Center for Health Statistics [NCHS], 1992). The leading causes of death in children are presented in Table 11–11 (CDC, 1993, pp. 20–22).

Infectious diseases such as repeated tonsillitis, repeated ear infections, mononucleosis, hepatitis, meningitis, bladder or urinary tract infection, diarrhea or colitis, rheumatic fever, and pneumonia remain an important morbidity problem of childhood. Forty percent of all nonroutine visits

TABLE 11–10

Number of Infant Deaths, Mortality Rate per 100,000, and Percentage of Deaths Attributed to Each Cause, by Race: United States, 1988

Race/Rank Order	Cause of Death (ICD-9 Codes)	No.	Rate	% Distribution
Black				
1	Sudden infant death syndrome (798.0)	1520	226.2	12.8
2	Disorders relating to short gestation and unspecified low birth weight (765)	1478	219.9	12.5
3	Congenital anomalies (740–759)	1410	209.8	11.9
4	Respiratory distress syndrome (769)	957	142.4	8.1
5	Newborn affected by maternal complications of pregnancy (761)	509	75.7	4.3
6	Accidents and adverse effects* (E800–E949)	281	41.8	2.4
7	Infections specific to the perinatal period (771)	279	41.5	2.4
8	Newborn affected by complications of placenta, cord, and membranes (762)	268	39.9	2.3
9	Intrauterine hypoxia and birth asphyxia (768)	232	34.5	2.0
10	Pneumonia and influenza (480–487)	224	33.3	1.9
	All other causes (residual)	4,682	697.0	39.5
	All causes	**11,840**	**1762.0**	**100.0**
White				
1	Congenital anomalies (740–759)	6442	211.5	24.8
2	Sudden infant death syndrome (798.0)	3771	123.8	14.5
3	Respiratory distress syndrome (769)	2148	70.5	8.3
4	Disorders relating to short gestation and unspecified low birth weight (765)	1726	56.7	6.7
5	Newborn affected by maternal complications of pregnancy (761)	875	28.7	3.4
6	Accidents and adverse effects* (E800–E949)	638	20.9	2.5
7	Newborn affected by complications of placenta, cord, and membranes (762)	615	20.2	2.4
8	Infections specific to the perinatal period (771)	574	18.8	2.2
9	Intrauterine hypoxia and birth asphyxia (768)	527	17.3	2.0
10	Pneumonia and influenza (480–487)	387	12.7	1.5
	All other causes (residual)	8222	270.0	31.7
	All causes	**25,925**	**851.1**	**100.0**
Total†				
1	Congenital anomalies (740–759)	8141	208.2	20.9
2	Sudden infant death syndrome (798.0)	5476	140.1	14.1
3	Disorders relating to short gestation and unspecified low birth weight (765)	3268	83.6	8.4
4	Respiratory distress syndrome (769)	3181	81.4	8.2
5	Newborn affected by maternal complications of pregnancy (761)	1411	36.1	3.6
6	Accidents and adverse effects* (E800–E949)	936	23.9	2.4
7	Newborn affected by complications of placenta, cord, and membranes (762)	907	23.2	2.3
8	Infections specific to the perinatal period (771)	878	22.5	2.3
9	Intrauterine hypoxia and birth asphyxia (768)	777	19.9	2.0
10	Pneumonia and influenza (480–487)	641	16.4	1.6
	All other causes (residual)	13,294	340.0	34.2
	All causes	**38,910**	**995.3**	**100.0**

From CDC. (1991, September 20). Infant mortality—United States, 1988. *Morbidity and Mortality Weekly Report* (CDC/DHHS-PHS, *Vol. 40,* No. 37). Washington, DC: U.S. Government Printing Office.

*When a death occurs under "accidental" circumstances, the preferred term within the public health community is "unintentional injury."

†Includes races other than black and white.

to pediatricians are related to infectious diseases; 38% of children are reported to have had at least one of these diseases. Repeated ear infections are the most commonly reported condition. It is also of importance that girls are more than five times as likely to have bladder or urinary tract infections (CDC, 1991a).

Healthy development in childhood is a primary concern. Developmental problems and chronic physical conditions are on the rise among this age group. Children living in poverty are at high risk for these conditions. Hearing and speech impairment and lead poisoning present major threats to the well-being of children. Emotional and learning disorders are two other significant issues. In all of these areas, prevention through the establishment of healthy parenting, improvement of environmental conditions, and the establishment of healthy habits are paramount in improving the health profile of children.

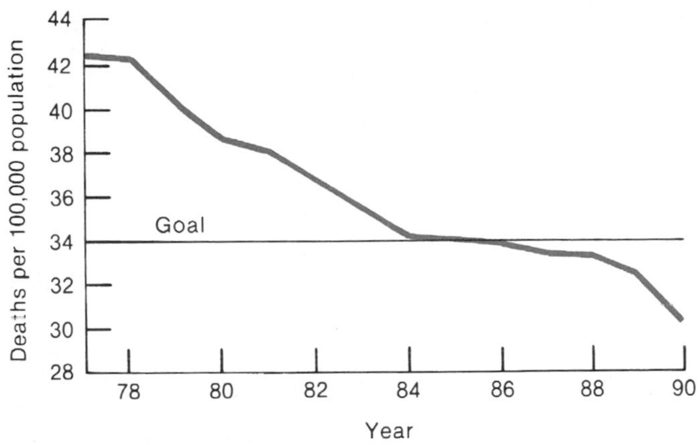

Figure 11–18 ● Death rates for children aged 1 to 14 years, 1977–1990 and 1990 goal (1990 data are provisional). (Redrawn from National Center for Health Statistics (NCHS). (Sept-Oct 1992). NCHS data line. *Public Health Reports* (*Vol. 107*, No. 5). Hyattsville, MD: U.S. Government Printing Office.)

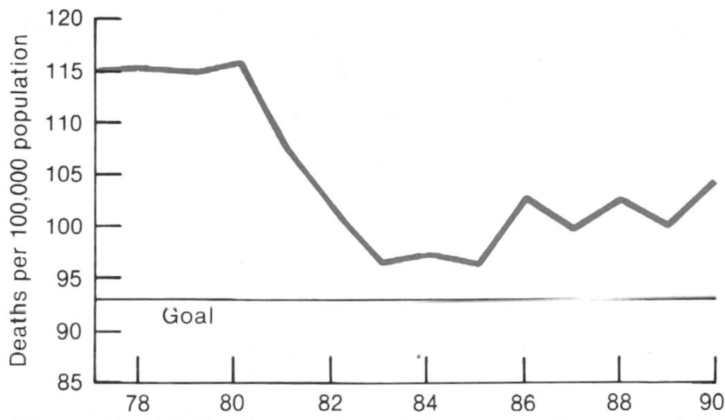

Figure 11–19 ● Death rates for adolescents and young adults aged 15 to 24 years, 1977–1990 and 1990 goal (1990 data are provisional). (Redrawn from NCHS. (Sept-Oct 1992). NCHS data line. (*Public Health Reports, Vol. 107*, No. 5). Hyattsville, MD: U.S. Government Printing Office.)

TABLE 11–11

Leading Causes of Death in Children*

Rank	Cause	Total	<1 Year	1–14 Years
1	Accidents	32.6	21.3	11.3
2	Pneumonia and influenza	18.8	18.1	10.7
3	Heart disease	15.9	14.8	1.1
4	Homicide	10.6	8.8	1.8
5	Malignant neoplasms	2.9	0	2.9
6	HIV†	0.6	—	—

Data from CDC. (1993, September 28). Annual summary of births, marriages, divorces, and deaths: United States, 1992. *Monthly Vital Statistics Report.* (CDC/NCHS-PHS, *Vol. 40,* No. 13). Washington, DC: U.S. Government Printing Office.

*Children defined as infants <1 year to 14 years. Rates per 100,000 of age-adjusted population.

†HIV tabulation is not broken down by age category.

PATTERNS OF MORTALITY AND MORBIDITY IN ADOLESCENTS AND YOUNG ADULTS

In those between 15 and 24 years of age, unintentional injuries are responsible for approximately 40% of deaths; 75% of these deaths involve motor vehicles. Alcohol is involved in more than half of fatal accidents. The mortality rates of adolescents and young adults are rising again after declining in the early 1980s (Fig. 11–19). Raising the minimum drinking age resulted in fewer motor vehicle accident deaths in the early 1980s. The upward trend that began in the mid-1980s is believed to be related in part to raising the speed limit on rural interstate highways and inconsistent use of seat belts.

Of great concern is the increasing rate of homicide deaths of young black men. A 74% increase in homicide deaths of black men occurred between 1985 and 1989. Homicide is the second leading cause of death in this age group, with the rate for black men being seven times the rate for white men (Fig.11–20). Race, however, is not an important risk factor when socioeconomic considerations are taken into account. Suicide, the second leading cause of death of white men in this age group, also rose during this time frame. Women of both races have relatively low suicide rates.

Other major health problems of this age group, such as cancer and heart disease, are overshadowed by unintentional injuries, homicide, and suicide (Figs. 11–21 and 11–22). However it is during this period that young people develop habits that have importance for health in later years. Lifestyle patterns related to nutrition, physical fitness and exercise, cigarette smoking and drug use, safety, and sexual conduct emerge during this period. These behaviors help to determine the rate of future chronic illness in this cohort of the population as it ages.

For example substance use and abuse, often initiated in young adulthood, persists until other health concerns arise. Young women are beginning to smoke at an earlier age and at almost the same rate as men (Fig. 11–23). Even though the overall percentage of those who smoke has declined from 48% in 1965 to 28% in 1988, significant numbers in this group continue to smoke. Educational level is a predictive factor for smoking (Fig. 11–24). Alcohol consumption, a major contributor to accidents and violence, also is linked to chronic disability. Experimentation with illicit drugs, though declining, continues to be a significant problem (DHHS, 1992, p. 17).

Unintended pregnancies and sexually transmitted diseases present health risks in this population. It is estimated that 78% of women and 86% of men have engaged in sexual intercourse before age 20 years. Eighty-four percent of all teenage mothers did not intend to become pregnant. These young women often do not finish school, have higher unemployment rates, deliver low-birth-weight infants, and lack adequate parenting skills (DHHS, 1992, p. 18).

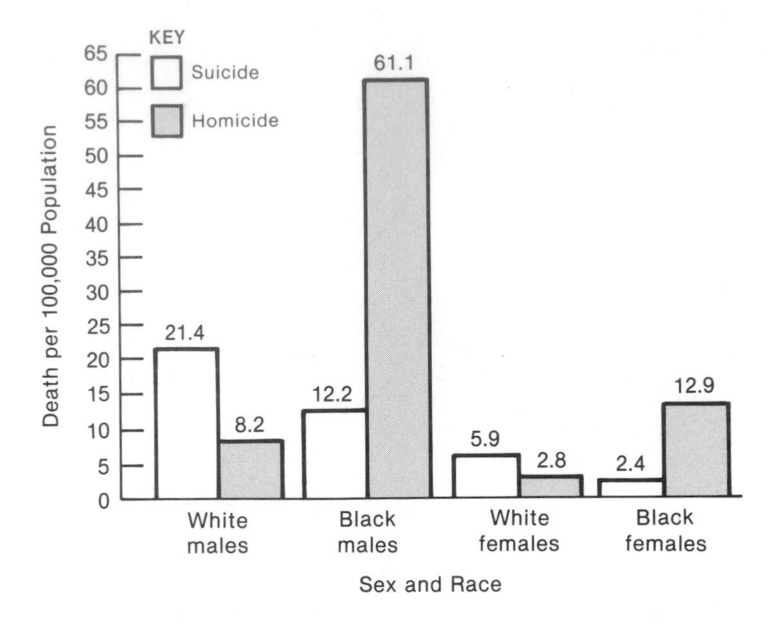

Figure 11–20 ● Death rates from suicide and homicide per 100,000 population, 1989. (Data from U.S. Bureau of the Census. (1992). *Statistical abstracts of the United States, 1992: The national data book* (112th ed.). Washington, DC: U.S. Department of Commerce, Economics and Statistics Administration.)

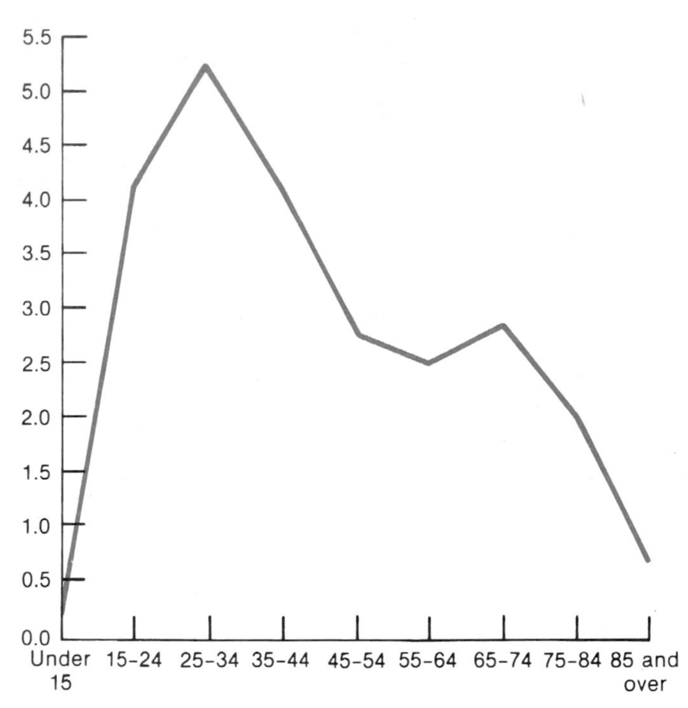

Figure 11–21 ● Death by suicide of males, all races by age, in thousands, 1989. (Data from US Bureau of the Census. (1992). *Statistical abstracts of the United States, 1992: The national data book* (112th ed.). Washington, DC: U.S. Department of Commerce, Economics and Statistics Administration.)

Prevention through health education and role-modeling is important for this age group. However education is not enough to bring about the desired changes in behavior. Aggressive counseling and support, especially for high-risk groups, is believed necessary to further reduce the problems of alcohol and drug abuse, school failure, delinquency, violence, unwanted pregnancies, and the development of future chronic disease.

PATTERNS OF MORTALITY AND MORBIDITY IN ADULTS

In the adult age group personal responsibility for maintaining health is paramount. All of the major health problems faced by those between 25 and 65 years old are preventable, totally or in part, through lifestyle or environmental changes. For example the dramatic decline in heart disease (40% decline), strokes (50% decline), and, to a lesser extent, accidents (30% decline) in this age group since 1970 is associated with reduced cigarette smoking, lower blood cholesterol levels, increased control of high blood pressure, decreased alcohol consumption, increased (mandatory) seat belt use, lower speed limits, and availability of air bags in automobiles (DHHS, 1992, pp. 20–22). Accompanying these lifestyle changes are several social norms that also increase the public's awareness of the relationship of risk to health. Reduced public acceptance of risks related to smoking have been the

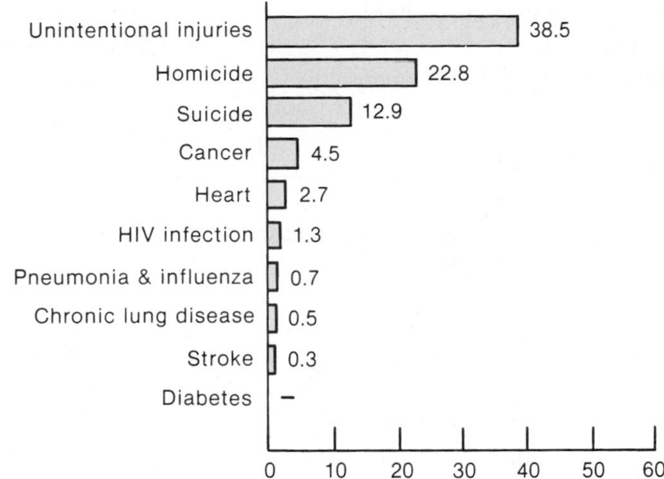

Figure 11–22 ● Leading causes of death for persons aged 15 to 24 years, 1992. Provisional, age-specific, and age-adjusted death rates for the ten leading causes of death per 100,000 population, estimated from a 10% sample of deaths. HIV = Human immunodeficiency virus. (Data from CDC. (1993, September 28). Annual summary of births, marriages, divorces, and deaths: United States, 1992. *Monthly Vital Statistics Report, 41,* 23–24.)

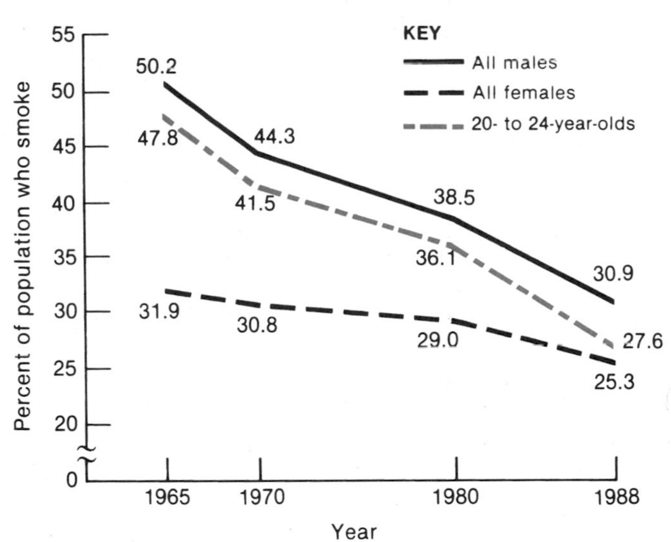

Figure 11–23 ● Cigarette smoking by gender, 1965–1988. (Data from US Bureau of the Census. (1992). *Statistical abstracts of the United States, 1992: The national data book* (112th ed.). Washington, DC: U.S. Department of Commerce, Economics and Statistics Administration.)

impetus for the establishment of anti-smoking laws and the creation of smoke-free work environments. Increased concern about drinking while driving has launched such movements as Mothers Against Drunk Drivers (MADD), and resulted in tougher regulations related to blood alcohol levels, stiffer penalties for driving while intoxicated, and raising of the drinking age.

Cancer has become the leading cause of death for those 35 to 64 years old as deaths from heart disease have decreased (Table 11–12). Although overall mortality rates for cancer have changed little since the mid-1950s, significant changes in some age groups and with selected cancers have occurred. Further changes are believed possible. For example it is estimated that smoking is responsible for 30% of cancer deaths, and another 35% (such as colon cancer) are thought to be associated with diet. Both of these cancers can be reduced through reduction of risky behaviors and aggressive screening. Screening and early diagnosis of breast and cervical cancer also have improved the survival rates of women (DHHS, 1992, pp. 20–22). Other lifestyle changes affecting this age group—for example cigarette smoking—are discussed earlier in the chapter.

Preventing much of the chronic disease affecting this age group is dependent primarily on individual beliefs and actions and to a lesser extent on societal norms and behavior. Increased awareness of risks and choices related to health promotion, preventive screening, and early diagnosis and treatment is essential. Many of these services are expected to be provided by nurses. It will be a major challenge to all health care providers to empower individuals to develop or modify lifestyle patterns that maintain health and prevent disease. The emphasis on individual responsibility, however, cannot ignore other significant factors beyond individual control. The environment, workplace standards, socioeconomic status, media images, educational level, and access to information and health care are all powerful influences that affect adult behavior and choices that support health.

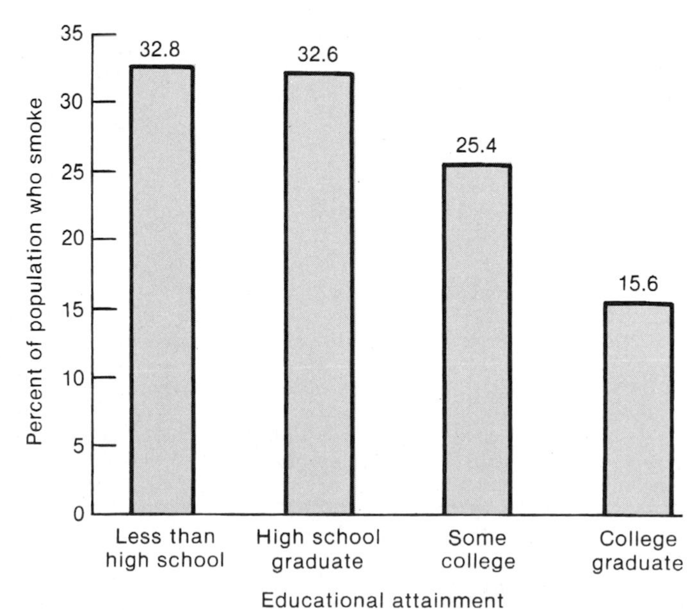

Figure 11–24 ● Cigarette smoking by educational attainment, 1988. (Data from U.S. Bureau of the Census. (1992). *Statistical abstracts of the United States 1992: The national data book* (112th ed.). Washington, DC: U.S. Department of Commerce, Economics and Statistics Administration.)

TABLE 11–12

Leading Causes of Death in Adults 25 to 64 Years Old, 1992*

Cause	Rate
25–34 Years	
Unintentional Injuries	31.8
HIV infection	23.4
Homicide	22.8
Suicide	14.2
Cancer	12.4
Heart disease	7.3
Stroke	1.8
Diabetes mellitus	1.4
Pneumonia and influenza	1.1
Chronic lung disease	0.6
35–44 Years	
Cancer	44.0
HIV infection	36.3
Heart disease	31.8
Unintentional injuries	28.0
Homicide	17.9
Suicide	14.4
Stroke	7.2
Diabetes mellitus	3.9
Pneumonia and influenza	3.1
Chronic lung disease	2.0
45–54 Years	
Cancer	148.6
Heart disease	112.7
Unintentional injuries	26.1
HIV infection	21.3
Stroke	16.9
Suicide	14.5
Homicide	12.6
Diabetes mellitus	12.1
Chronic lung disease	8.9
Pneumonia and influenza	5.4
55–64 Years	
Cancer	441.6
Heart disease	344.9
Chronic lung disease	48.2
Stroke	46.5
Diabetes mellitus	35.6
Unintentional injuries	31.7
Chronic liver disease and cirrhosis	28.0
Pneumonia and influenza	17.3
Suicide	14.5
Nephritis and nephrosis	8.7

From CDC. (1993, September 28). Annual summary of births, marriages, divorces, and deaths: United States, 1992. *Monthly Vital Statistics Report* (CDC/NCHS-PHS, *Vol. 41,* No. 13). Washington, DC: U.S. Government Printing Office, pp. 23–24.

*Provisional age-specific and age-adjusted death rates for the ten leading causes of death per 100,000 population. Estimated from a 10% sample of deaths.

PATTERNS OF MORTALITY AND MORBIDITY IN OLDER ADULTS

The proportion of persons older than 65 years will continue to increase, with the over-85 cohort having the most rapid growth. Individuals reaching 65 years now can expect to live into their early 80s. However, the substantive question facing these individuals is not as much a question of living as it is a question of the quality of one's remaining years of life. Even in this age group, increasing evidence suggests that some lifestyle changes can result in major health and quality-of-life benefits. The outcomes of the top three causes of death—heart disease, cancer, and stroke—can still be altered (Table 11–13). For example older smokers who quit smoking increase their life expectancy, reduce the risks associated with heart disease, and improve circulation and respiratory functioning (Office of Smoking and Health, 1989). Likewise it is believed that eating a nutritionally balanced diet, reducing weight, and decreasing sodium intake can reduce the risk of heart disease and

TABLE 11–13

Leading Causes of Death of Adults 65 Years and Older, 1992*

Cause	Rate
65–74 Years	
Cancer	870.3
Heart disease	852.2
Chronic lung disease	156.1
Stroke	134.5
Diabetes mellitus	76.6
Pneumonia and influenza	55.7
Unintenional injury	44.6
Chronic liver disease and cirrhosis	31.6
Nephritis/nephrosis	23.7
Septicemia	20.9
75–84 Years	
Heart disease	2175.3
Cancer	1359.1
Stroke	465.7
Chronic lung disease	323.6
Pneumonia and influenza	227.1
Diabetes mellitus	144.4
Unintentional injuries	95.8
Nephritis/nephrosis	71.8
Septicemia	60.9
Atherosclerosis	43.4
≥85 Years	
Heart disease	6513.2
Cancer	1768.3
Stroke	1575.2
Pneumonia and influenza	1034.1
Chronic lung disease	443.5
Unintentional injuries	267.3
Atherosclerosis	266.1
Diabetes mellitus	239.1
Nephritis/nephrosis	211.5
Septicemia	181.7

From CDC. (1993, September 28). Annual summary of births, marriages, divorces, and deaths: United States, 1992. *Monthly Vital Statistics Report* (CDC/NCHS-PHS, *Vol. 41,* No. 13). Washington, DC: U.S. Government Printing Office, pp. 23–24.

*Provisional age-specific and age-adjusted death rates for the ten leading causes of death per 100,000 population. Estimated from a 10% sample of deaths.

promote the maintenance of health. Chronic neuromuscular problems such as arthritis and osteoporosis, visual and hearing impairments, incontinence, digestive conditions, and dementia are all concerns of this age group. Because of the impact of illness on day-to-day living, prevention and preservation of function are desirable (DHHS/PHS, 1992, pp. 23–24).

A key to physiological decline is lack of physical activity. A large portion of this age group, 40%, report no participation in leisure-time physical activity, and only about 30% report participation in routine activities such as walking or gardening. Regular physical activity and exercise are associated with reducing the incidence of coronary heart disease, hypertension, non–insulin-dependent diabetes, colon cancer, depression, and anxiety (Caspersen, 1989). All of these chronic diseases are concerns of the age group of persons older than 65 years.

Primary health services for this age group include counseling for promotion and maintenance of healthy behaviors and prevention of life-limiting and life-threatening conditions. Control of hypertension, management of chronic conditions, and aggressive screening for skin, breast, cervical, and prostate cancer are important health services issues. Because the death rate for pneumonia and influenza increases in this age group, pneumococcal and influenza vaccines are encouraged.

Life changes in this age group frequently threaten a person's functional independence. Retirement, changes in family and social roles, illness, disability, loss of spouses and close friends, and changing support networks place one at risk for bereavement, loneliness, and low self-esteem—all associated with social isolation and depression.

Health Profiles/Status of Populations at High Risk

Improvement in the overall health of Americans requires special attention to the improvement of those persons at especially high risk. Understanding the differences between the total population and the low-income population, certain racial and ethnic minorities, and individuals with disabilities is one way to begin to address the gap in the health status and health care services of those groups. In discussing the groups included in this section, two caveats are important: First, data systems for collecting information at the national and state levels are, in many cases, quite limited (see Chapter 6). Thus, definitions, descriptions, and preventive interventions may be difficult at best. Second, the population subgroups are extremely heterogeneous, making generalizations about an entire cohort inappropriate unless reassessed at the local level. The data presented are intended to help identify broad risk groups and not to stereotype behavior of the particular group.

PATTERNS OF MORTALITY AND MORBIDITY OF PERSONS WITH LOW INCOMES

Approximately half of poor persons in the United States were younger than 18 years (40%) or older than 65 years (10.7%) in 1987 (U.S. Bureau of Census, 1989). Low socioeconomic status encompasses family groups or individuals who are unemployed, underemployed, or in low-wage jobs, as well as many single-parent families who live in substandard housing and have an educational achievement rate below that of the general population.

Poverty increases health risks in many ways. The death rates of poor persons are approximately twice the rates of persons above the poverty level. The incidences of disease and of some types of cancer are significantly higher. Poor individuals are more vulnerable to traumatic injury and death by violent crimes. Injuries in children are associated with fires, drowning, and suffocation. Infant mortality, discussed earlier, presents a unique health care problem in this group.

The patterns of vulnerability continue throughout adulthood and are evidenced by increased incidences of disease, injury, and death. Because many individuals in this group are not covered by health insurance plans, illnesses often are untreated and preventive services are underused, both of which are believed to be more costly to the public over the long term. Changing the health effects of income-related disparities is a challenging task. Although a difficult and time-consuming endeavor, it is an undertaking well worth the effort. The rewards will include lower health costs and improved health status of the U.S. population.

PATTERNS OF MORTALITY AND MORBIDITY AMONG MINORITIES

Predominant minority populations in the United States are blacks, Hispanics, Asians and Pacific Islanders, American Indians, and Alaska Natives (see Chapter 6). These categories, however, are oversimplifications of the diversity within each racial or ethnic group. There is great diversity between and among racial/ethnic groups, including characteristics associated with health status, such as lifestyle patterns, genetic influences, and health risks.

Black Americans

Many health risks of black Americans are associated with poverty. One third of blacks are below the poverty level, a rate three times higher than that of the white population. Blacks have a greater number of chronic conditions and activity limitations than whites of all ages (NCHS, 1991). Although increasing, life expectancy for blacks lags behind that of the total population. The leading causes of death due to chronic conditions are the same as for the majority of the overall population (Fig. 11–25). Heart disease, cancer, and stroke are the three leading causes of death for both blacks and whites; however, blacks do not live as long with these conditions. Only 38% of blacks reach the 5-year postdiagnosis mark compared with 50% of whites (DHHS, 1992, p. 33). For blacks, homicides were the fourth leading cause of death in 1992. Blacks also have higher rates for unintentional injuries and diabetes. Diabetes is almost 30% more frequent among blacks; females, especially those who are overweight, are at highest risk.

Both blacks and Hispanics are at greater risk of contracting AIDS and sexually transmitted diseases (see Chapter 19). Rates for other conditions, such as low birth weight, infant mortality and morbidity, and adolescent pregnancy, also show striking disparities among blacks when compared with rates of other groups in the total population (see Chapter 22). *Differences decrease dramatically for most diseases when death rates are adjusted for income level. This indicates that socioeconomic class, rather than race, is the primary contributing factor for the disparities in health status* (DHHS, 1992).

Health care–seeking behaviors of the black population are apparently different from those of the white population. Some of the difference is related to problems of access. Blacks do not receive adequate routine and preventive health care services. Blacks make less frequent visits to physicians; black mothers are twice as likely not to receive prenatal care until the last trimester of pregnancy, and more blacks receive medical care from clinics and emergency rooms. Changing patterns of access and delivery of health services is a major challenge if the frequency and severity of complications from illness is to be reduced. Universal access, one of the principal features of health care reform, is intended to address the disparity in services.

Hispanic Americans

Hispanics constitute the largest and fastest growing minority subgroup. This group is young (median age younger than 26 years compared with 33 years for the total population) and has a high birth rate. This group also has a small but significant migrant farmworker population, which requires special attention.

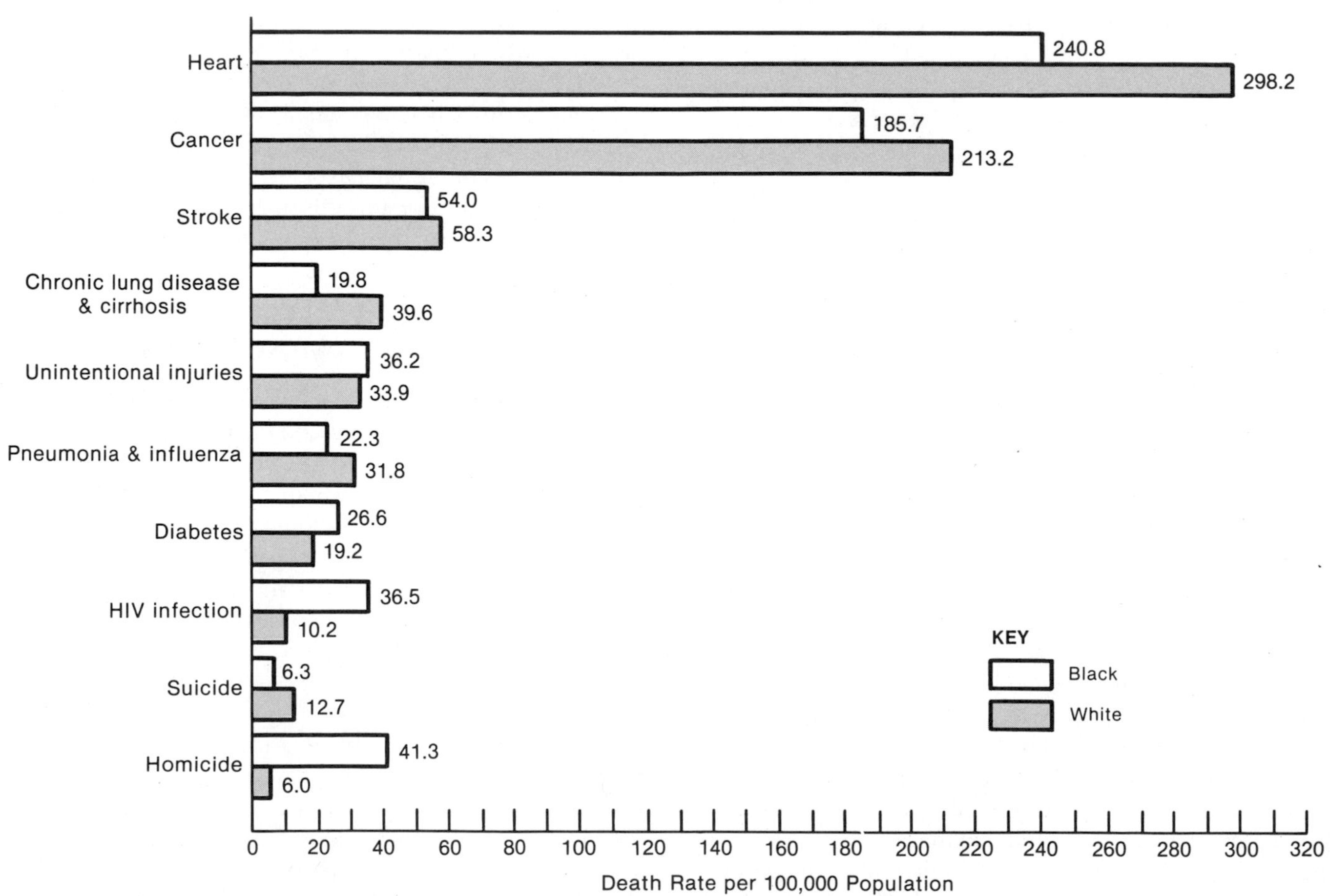

Figure 11–25 ● Leading causes of death for blacks compared with whites, 1992. Provisional, age-specific, and age-adjusted death rates for the ten leading causes of death per 100,000 population. Estimated from a 10% sample of deaths. (Data from Centers for Disease Control and Prevention. (1993, September 28). Annual summary of births, marriages, divorces, and deaths: United States, 1992. *Monthly Vital Statistics Report, 41,* 20–22.)

Hispanics are the second poorest minority group, and their health status is reflective of the influences of poverty. Hispanics actually have less access to health care and preventive health care services than other groups because more of them do not have health insurance. Language is another barrier to getting care.

As in the total population, the two leading causes of death in Hispanics are heart disease and cancer; however, the death rates associated with these diseases are higher than for non-Hispanics. Death rates for unintentional injuries, homicides, chronic liver disease and cirrhosis, and AIDS are higher than for whites, and deaths from suicide, stroke, and chronic obstructive pulmonary disease are lower than for whites. Smoking and alcohol consumption are major health risks, especially among Hispanic teenagers (DHHS, 1992a). The cultural, and therefore the health, profile of this group is very diverse. For example, Mexican Americans have a low rate of cerebrovascular disease, whereas the opposite is true for Puerto Ricans living in New York City. Cuban Americans are high users of prenatal services, but Mexican Americans and Puerto Ricans are not.

Asians and Pacific Islanders

Because health data are often collected using black/white racial categories and because of the small size of this minority group, consistent health status reports on Asians and Pacific Islanders is difficult. Local studies, in areas with a significant concentration, are used to identify health status and health risks.

As with other minority groups, health status within this cohort tends to be influenced by socioeconomic status and degree of acculturation. The risk of cancer is approximately the same as for the general population, but is higher in selected subgroups for certain types of cancer. For example, Native Hawaiian women have a higher rate of breast cancer, Southeast Asian men have a higher rate of lung cancer, and Southeast Asians in general have a liver cancer rate 12 times higher than that of the white population (DHHS, 1992a). For those who do get cancer, there is greater risk of death. The 5-year survival rates for Asian and Pacific Islanders are poorer than for whites (Horton and Smith, 1990).

The risk of having low-birth-weight infants exceeds that of whites for most of the subgroups for which data have been collected, although variation exists among the subgroups (Table 11–14). Likewise, infant mortality rates are variable across subgroups, with Japanese and Chinese having the lowest rates. Laotians have the highest rate, with more than 8 deaths per 1000 births (DHHS, 1992a).

Asian and Pacific Islander immigrants are at serious risk for two infectious diseases, tuberculosis (TB) and hepatitis B. Among Southeast Asian immigrants, the incidence of TB is 40 times higher than in the general population. Higher rates of hepatitis B place Asian immigrants at greater risk of serious side effects, such as chronic liver disease, cirrhosis, and liver cancer (DHHS, 1992a).

American Indians, Aleuts, and Eskimos

Native Americans suffer from a variety of illnesses that are preventable or ameliorated by early diagnosis and treatment. Many of the health problems are exacerbated by poverty and substance abuse. Detailed data have been collected on American Indians, who have much higher rates of alcoholism and related problems such as accidents, homicides, and suicides (Table 11–15). An estimated 75% of unintentional injuries and 54% of motor vehicle accidents among this group are alcohol related (DHHS, 1992a). As a result American Indians are at greater risk of early death than are members of the general population.

Heart disease and cancer rates are lower among American Indians, perhaps because they are generally diseases of older age. Cirrhosis and diabetes are the two

TABLE 11–14

Percentage of Low-Birth-Weight (LBW) Infants in Selected Subgroups of the American Population (as a Percentage of Live Births)

Race/Ethnic Group	% LBW Infants
White	5.7
Black	12.7
Asian/Pacific Islander	6.2
Chinese	5.0
Japanese	6.3
Hawaiian	6.6
Filipino	7.3
Hispanic	6.2
Mexican	5.7
Puerto Rican	9.3
Cuban	5.9
Central and South American	5.7

From Reedy, M.A. (Ed.). (1993). *Statistical record of Hispanic Americans.* Detroit: Gale Research Inc.

TABLE 11–15

Health Risks of American Indians Compared with U.S. Population

Health Risk	Comparison with Overall U.S. Population
1. Alcoholism	438% greater
2. Tuberculosis	400% greater
3. Diabetes mellitus	155% greater
4. Accidents	131% greater
5. Homicide	57% greater
6. Pneumonia and influenza	32% greater
7. Suicide	27% greater

From Indian Health Service. (1991). *Trends in Indian health.* Washington, DC: U.S. Government Printing Office.

chronic conditions that afflict American Indians at a higher rate than that of the general population. Diabetes is so common that in many tribes, 20% of members have the disease. In some Arizona tribes the incidence rate is as high as 40% of all adults (DHHS, 1992a).

American Indian children are at risk for many of the health problems associated with higher levels of poverty. Despite a poorer overall health status than that of the U.S. population, the infant mortality rate is lower. The Indian Health Service (IHS) reported an infant mortality rate of 9.7% when the rate for all U.S. infants was 10.1% (IHS, 1991).

Many of the health problems in Native Americans can be reduced or eliminated by early diagnosis and treatment, particularly TB, diabetes, and pneumonia. Some can be reduced or eliminated by changing patterns of behavior. Public health officials and Native American leaders are engaged in health projects aimed at reducing risky behaviors, improving lifestyle habits, and facilitating access and services for Native American populations.

Summary

This chapter has three objectives: (1) to provide a brief background relevant to the use of epidemiology in understanding health, disease, and conditions related to risk factors and health status; (2) to present an overview of the basic formulas and methods of epidemiological investigation; and (3) most importantly, to provide demographic data, vital statistics, and mortality and morbidity data about the health profiles of all age groups. Similar data are discussed for low-income and minority populations. Data on leading causes of death are current through 1992. Examples in the form of tables and figures have been provided, along with questions and answers, to assist the reader in interpreting the data.

Understanding the multiple factors that contribute to illness, injury, and premature death is necessary but not adequate for improving the health status of the U.S. population. Community health nurses use the knowledge of risk factors to shape health policy priorities and to positively influence the health profiles of those they serve.

Knowledge of major external factors (tobacco, diet, activity, alcohol and drug use, and sexual behavior) that contribute to the leading causes of death—heart disease, cancer, and stroke (HIV infection for adults under 45 years)—is insufficient for improving health. Changes in behavior by individuals and populations are often influenced by a supportive social environment, accessible services, and heightened attention to specific priorities through public policy debates.

Community health nurses develop population-focused nursing services based on knowledge of the epidemiological and demographic data. Aggregates or population groups are targeted for specific nursing care, which assists participation in health promotion and prevention activities; reduces premature death, disability, and illness; reduces disparities in health among population groups; and fosters healthy lives.

Resources for Epidemiological Information

Epi Info is a software package for handling and organizing epidemiological data and study designs. It includes features used by epidemiologists and may be freely copied and given to colleagues. Epi Info version 5.01, disks, and manual may be ordered for $35.00 from USD, Inc., 2475 A West Park Place, Stone Mountain, GA 30087.

Data on health care providers with occupationally acquired HIV infection are published in the CDC's *HIV/AIDS Surveillance Report.* Free copies are available from the CDC National AIDS Clearinghouse, P.O. Box 6003, Rockville, MD 20849–6003 (telephone: 1–800–458–5231).

KEY IDEAS

1. Epidemiology is the study of the health status of human populations.
2. Epidemiologists and nurse researchers use descriptive, analytic, and experimental research methods to study causative factors of illness, disability, and premature death; to describe the natural history of disease; to identify populations at risk for poor health; and to determine the effectiveness of screening, health education, and treatment measures.
3. Epidemiology is helpful to community health nurses for describing the health status of a population and the factors that contribute to its well-being, for targeting aggregates at risk of specific health conditions, and for evaluating the effectiveness of nursing interventions with populations.
4. Rates and ratios are statistics used to describe births, deaths, and the incidence and prevalence of disease and disability in populations.
5. The natural history of a disease is influenced by characteristics of the people (host), agents (biological, chemical, and physical), and environment that make up the epidemiological triangle.
6. Age, sex, race, social class, occupation, marital status, and religion are demographic characteristics frequently used when describing human populations. These factors contribute to variations in health status, health-related behaviors, and utilization of health care.

7. Much of the disparity in the health status of minority populations is linked with poverty.
8. Community health nursing involves attending to the health status of multiple subpopulations as well as to the total population.
9. Health care services and programs are aimed at three levels of prevention: primary, secondary, and tertiary.
10. Understanding the multiple factors that contribute to illness, injury, and premature death are necessary but not adequate for improving the health status of the U.S. population. A key challenge for community health nursing is to use knowledge of risk factors to shape health policy priorities and to positively influence the health profile of those they serve.

GUIDELINES FOR LEARNING

1. Obtain a copy of your local health department's annual report. See whether you can identify prevalent health needs/problems of your local community.
2. What are the five leading causes of death in your community? Are they similar to or different from the national mortality data?
3. Are there special cohort groups that have higher rates for morbidity or mortality? If so, what types of health problems contribute to the higher rates?
4. Are there higher or lower rates of infectious disease in your community compared with those in your state and those in the United States?
5. As a community health nurse, how would you prepare a plan to reduce health problems identified in activity 3 or 4 above? Whose support would you need to enroll to implement such a plan? How would you go about acquiring community support for your plan?

REFERENCES

American Cancer Society. (1992). *Cancer Facts and Figures—1992.* Atlanta, GA: Author.

Brookmeyer, R. (1991). Reconstruction and future trends of the AIDS epidemic in the United States. *Science, 253,* 37–42.

Caspersen, C. J. (1989). Physical activity epidemiology: Concepts, methods, and application to exercise science. *Exercise and Sport Sciences Review, 17,* 423–473.

Castelli, W. P., Anderson, K., Wilson, W. F., & Levy, D. (1992). Lipids and risk of coronary heart disease: The Framingham Study. *Annals of Epidemiology, 2*(1/2), 23–28.

Centers for Disease Control and Prevention (CDC). (1993, September 28). Annual summary of births, marriages, divorces, and deaths: United States, 1992. *Monthly Vital Statistics Report* (CDC/NCHS-PHS, *Vol. 40,* No. 13, 1–6). Washington, DC: U.S. Government Printing Office.

CDC. (1992a, January 17). The second 100,000 cases of acquired immunodeficiency syndrome—United States, June 1981–December 1991. *Morbidity and Mortality Weekly Report* (CDC/DHHS-PHS, *Vol. 41,* No. 2, 28–29). Washington, DC: U.S. Government Printing Office.

CDC. (1992b, October 2). Graphs and maps for selected notifiable diseases in the United States, 1991. *Morbidity and Mortality Weekly Report* (CDC/DHHS-PHS, *Vol. 41,* No. 39, 721–736). Washington, DC: U.S. Government Printing Office.

CDC. (1991a, October). *Incidence and impact of selected infectious diseases in childhood* (DHHS, series 10, No. 180). Hyattsville, MD: National Center for Health Statistics.

CDC. (1991b, September 20). Infant mortality—United States, 1988. *Morbidity and Mortality Weekly Report* (CDC/DHHS-PHS, *Vol. 40,* No. 37, 644–646). Washington, DC: U.S. Government Printing Office.

CDC. (1991c, June 7). The HIV/AIDS epidemic: The first 10 years. *Morbidity and Mortality Weekly Report* (CDC/DHHS-PHS, *Vol. 40,* No. 22, 357–363, 369). Washington, DC: U.S. Government Printing Office.

CDC. (1990, March 30). Mortality patterns—United States, 1987. *Morbidity and Mortality Weekly Report* (CDC/DHHS-PHS, *Vol. 39,* No. 12, 193–201). Washington, DC: U.S. Government Printing Office.

CDC. (1981). *Pneumocystis* pneumonia—Los Angeles. *Morbidity and Mortality Weekly Report* (DHHS-PHS, *Vol. 30,* 250–252). Washington, DC: U.S. Government Printing Office.

Department of Health and Human Services (DHHS), Public Health Service. (1992a). *Healthy people 2000: National health promotion and disease.* Washington, DC: U.S. Government Printing Office.

Prevention Objectives (DHHS Publication No. 91–50213). Washington, DC: U.S. Government Printing Office.

DHHS. (1992b, December). *Vital and Health Statistics: Current Estimates from the National Health Interview Survey, 1991* (DHHS publication No. 93–1512, CDC Series 10, No. 184). Hyattsville, MD: U.S. Government Printing Office.

Desenclos, J.-C. A. & Hahn, R. A. (1992, November 20). Years of potential life lost before age 65, by race, Hispanic origin and sex—United States, 1986–1988. *Morbidity and Mortality Weekly Report* (CDC/DHHS-PHS, *Vol. 41,* No. SS–6, 1–23). Washington, DC: U.S. Government Printing Office.

Friedman, G. D. (1987). *Primer of epidemiology.* New York: McGraw-Hill.

Horton, C. P., & Smith, J. C. (Eds.). (1990). *Statistical record of black America.* Detroit: Gale Research Inc.

Indian Health Service. (1991). *Trends in Indian health.* Washington, DC: U.S. Government Printing Office.

Leavell, H. R., & Clark, E. G. (1965). *Preventive medicine for the doctor in his community: An epidemiological approach.* New York: McGraw-Hill.

McGinnis, J. M., & Foege, W. H. (1993). Actual causes of death in the United States. *Journal of the American Medical Association, 270,* 2207–2212.

National Center for Health Statistics. (1991). *Health United States 1990.* Washington DC: U.S. Government Printing Office.

National Center for Health Statistics. (1992). National center for health statistics data line. *Public Health Reports* (September-October, *Vol. 107,* No. 5, 599–601). Hyattsville, MD: National Center for Health Statistics.

Office of Smoking and Health. (1989). *Reducing the health consequences of smoking: 25 years of progress. A report of the Surgeon General* (DHHS Publication No. CDC89–8411). Washington, DC: U.S. Government Printing Office.

Redland, A. R., & Stuifbergen, A. K. (1993). Strategies for maintenance of health-promoting behaviors. *Nursing Clinics of North America, 28,* 427–442.

Reedy, M. A. (Ed.). (1993). *Statistical record of Hispanic Americans.* Detroit: Gale Research Inc.

Statistical Abstracts of the United States. (1992). *The National data book* (112th ed.). Washington, DC: U.S. Government Printing Office.

U.S. Bureau of the Census. (1992). *Households, families, and children: A 30-year perspective* (CPR series p-23, No. 181). Washington, DC: U.S. Government Printing Office.

U.S. Bureau of the Census. (1989). *Population profile of the United States: 1989* (CPR series p-23, No. 159). Washington, DC: U.S. Government Printing Office.

World Health Organization. (1991, May). *In point of fact* (No. 74). Geneva, Switzerland: World Health Organization.

SUGGESTED READINGS

Austin, D., & Werner, S. (1982). *Epidemiology for the health sciences: A primer on epidemiologic concepts and their uses* (7th ed.). Springfield, IL: Charles C Thomas.

DHHS. (1990). *Healthy people 2000: National health promotion and disease prevention objectives.* Washington, DC: Government Printing Office.

Friedman, G. D. (1987). *Primer of epidemiology* (3rd ed.). New York: McGraw-Hill.

McGinnis, J., & Foege, W. (1993). Actual causes of death in the United States. *Journal of the American Medical Association, 270,* 2207–2212.

Valanis, B. (1986). *Epidemiology in nursing and health care.* Norwalk, CT: Appleton-Century-Crofts.

Chapter 12

Community Assessment

Jean O. Trotter, Claudia M. Smith, and Frances A. Maurer

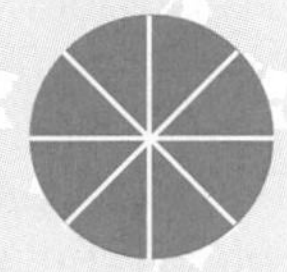

Focus Questions

What is community-focused nursing?

How are communities defined?

What are the critical attributes of a community?

How are groups and aggregates different types of populations?

How are spatial and relational boundaries different types of places?

What are goals of communities?

What are frameworks for assessing communities?

What is a general systems framework for assessing communities?

What are factors to consider in assessing the health of communities?

What are sources of data regarding communities?

What are approaches to community assessment?

How do community health nurses analyze community data?

The community health nurse is concerned with the health of the individual, the family, and the community. This unit focuses on applying the nursing process with the community as client. What is the role of the nurse in population-based nursing? What does it mean to be a nurse responsible for the health of a community? Where does one start?

Assessment, the first step of the nursing process, forms the foundation for determining the client's health, regardless of whether the client is an individual, a family, or a community. When nurses learn how to assess an individual client, they learn to use their senses of sight, touch, and sound to perform skills such as inspection, palpation, auscultation, and percussion. This chapter will discuss how the community health nurse uses senses such as touch, sight, sound, and smell, as well as cognition, past experiences, and other tools to make observations about the community. From these, data are analyzed to make diagnoses about the community's health status.

Through the process of community assessment, nurses will experience what it is like to be with people, to get to know them and their strengths and problems, and to work with them in planning and implementing programs to meet their unique needs. Just as all individuals and families are different, communities, too, are different. What makes one community different from another? To understand, nurses must get to know the community, its people, its purpose, and how it functions.

How does one go about getting to know a community? More specifically, how might you become familiar with a community? One way is to read about a community through newspapers, community histories, and objective statistical reports. Another way is to visit the community, talk to the people, attend meetings—that is, *be with* the people. A visit to or a walk or a drive through the community provides a "feel" for the community that cannot be obtained from just reading about it. Being in the community allows you to subjectively experience it and learn how community members experience their community.

Take a moment to reflect on this scene:

> You are driving down a city street on a warm, sunny day. The row houses you see are in various physical states; some are painted and appear to be cared for, while others are in disrepair and dilapidated; there is no grass, and the street is littered with trash. People are sitting on the steps and front porches, talking and watching the traffic pass by. A number of young adolescent females are sitting on the steps holding infants. Children of different ages are playing on the sidewalk and in the streets. The neighborhood is "alive" with noise and activity. As you continue your drive, you enter an area in which the houses are detached. There are small yards with green grass that is carefully maintained, and the streets are lined with lovely flowering trees. A few adults are working in their yards; a few children are playing in a nearby park. It is very quiet.

Two neighborhoods, geographically close but characteristically distant. Who lives in the two neighborhoods? What would it be like to live there? What would it be like to be a community health nurse responsible for the health of these communities?

Think about the community in which you live. How do other people see it? How would you describe it? What type of nursing care do you think your community needs?

Before we go any further, let's look at the meaning of a community. Is it only the neighborhood in which you live, or does it have other meanings?

Community Defined

If you were to ask five people to define the word *community,* you would probably get five different answers: "a place where people dwell;" "a group of people with common interests;" "a place with specific boundaries." Some may speak about an academic community, a religious community, a nursing community, while others may define community as the neighborhood or city in which they live. Who or which definition is correct?

It is difficult to formulate a definition of community that is precise and accurate, yet comprehensive. In this text, *community* is defined as *an open social system that is characterized by people in a place over time who have common goals* (Table 12–1). The term is applicable to a variety of situations. A community includes a place and groups and/or aggregates. An *aggregate* is defined as any number of individuals with at least one common characteristic (Williams, 1977). How a person defines community depends on the situation and that person's purpose. To community health nurses working for a county health department, community might mean a geographic area and its residents, such as the county or health district to which they are assigned. Nurses working with the homeless, the elderly, or a special interest group may define community as people with common characteristics (aggregate) within a specific place.

TABLE 12–1

Definitions

Community: An open social system characterized by people in a place over time who have common goals.

Group: Two or more persons engaged in an interdependent, purposeful relationship in which repeated face-to-face communication occurs. (Health-related purposes of groups include support, task accomplishment, learning, socialization and psychotherapy [Spradley, 1985].)

Population: A collection of individuals who share one or more personal or environmental characteristics, the most common of which is geographical location (Schultz, 1987). The terms *population groups* and *aggregates* are synonyms for population (Williams, 1977).

Population "at risk": An aggregate or population of humans who share a characteristic that places them in danger of health problems or illness (Schultz, 1987).

LITERATURE REVIEW

Community health literature offers a variety of definitions. Hillery (1955) reviewed 94 definitions of community and found that the most significant area of agreement was about the "possession of common end, norms, and means." Warren (1987) defines community as "a complex, interrelated structure of interaction patterns on the basis of which certain relevant functions are performed." Shamansky and Pesznecker (1981) provide an operational definition of community considering the following three factors: (1) *who* (people factors), (2) *where* and *when* (space and time factors), and (3) *why* and *how* (for what purpose?).

Anderson and McFarlane (1988) define community in terms of a core dimension (people) and eight subsystems: physical environment, education, safety and transportation, politics and government, health and social services, communication, economics, and recreation.

Other authors define community by describing types or categories. Communities may be geographically or socially bound (Burgess, 1983); categorized as emotional, structural, or functional (Archer, 1985); or defined in terms of relational and territorial bonds (Turner and Chavigny, 1988).

One of the most comprehensive definitions of community found in the recent community health literature is formulated by Higgs and Gustafson (1985): "A community is a group of people with a common identity or perspective, occupying space during a given period of time, and functioning through a social system to meet its needs within a larger social environment." This definition is most closely related to the concept of community discussed in this text.

CRITICAL ATTRIBUTES OF A COMMUNITY

For the purpose of this text, a community may be defined as a community if it includes three critical attributes or defining characteristics: people, place, and social interaction and/or common characteristics, interests, goals. All communities contain all three of these attributes.

People. Population is the most obvious of the necessary community attributes. The number of people included in the community depends on the other two critical attributes. It can be a relatively small number (a group of 20 pregnant adolescents enrolled in a clinic) or a large population (a city of 1,000,000). The ages, sex, ethnicity, religion, occupations, and socioeconomic status may be similar or diverse.

Place. Traditionally, communities were described in relation to geographic area. However, population aggregates such as the elderly, the poor, people with acquired immunodeficiency syndrome (AIDS) or any group whose members share one or more common characteristics, goals, or interests are sometimes used to identify a community for assessment purposes. Therefore, communities may be defined by one of two designations: geopolitical (spatial) or phenomenological (relational). Figures 12–1 and 12–2 illustrate some geopolitical and phenomenological communities.

Geopolitical. The *geopolitical* community is a spatial designation—a geographic or geopolitical area. This is the most traditional approach to the study of community.

Geopolitical communities are formed by either natural or man-made boundaries. A river, a mountain range, or a valley may create a natural boundary; for example, the Chesapeake Bay separates Maryland into the eastern and western shores. Man-made boundaries may be structural, political, or legal. Streets, bridges, or railroad tracks may create structural boundaries. City, county, or state lines create legal boundaries. Political boundaries may be exemplified by congressional districts or school districts.

Another type of man-made boundary is a census tract. The U.S. Census Bureau divides the United States into census tracts for the purpose of gathering demographic data about the U.S. population every 10 years. Census tract data are valuable in health planning. Census tract maps are available in libraries and health departments (Fig. 12–3).

Why does a community health nurse need to be concerned about geopolitical boundaries? A geopolitical view of community focuses the nurse's attention on the environment, housing, transportation, education, and political process subsystems. All of these are related to geographic locations as well as the population composition and distribution, health services, and resources and facilities. Statistical and epidemiological studies are frequently based on data from specific geopolitical areas.

Phenomenological. A *phenomenological* community is a relational designation. This "area" or "place" is less concrete than the geopolitical area, but is just as real to its members. It can be identified in terms of its "feeling of belonging." People in a phenomenological community have a group perspective that differentiates them from other groups. This identity may be based on culture, beliefs, values, common interests, characteristics, or goals. Examples of phenomenological communities include a group of people with common interests, such as a common religious conviction or professional or academic interest; with common beliefs, such as beliefs about human rights including women's rights or racial equality; or with a common goal, such as Students Against Drunk Drivers (SADD), whose common goal is to decrease alcohol-related accidents among student drivers.

Another example of a phenomenological community is a *community of solution.* This type of phenomenological community has special significance for health planning. The National Commission on Community Health Services (1966) suggested that where health services are concerned, the boundaries of each community are established by the

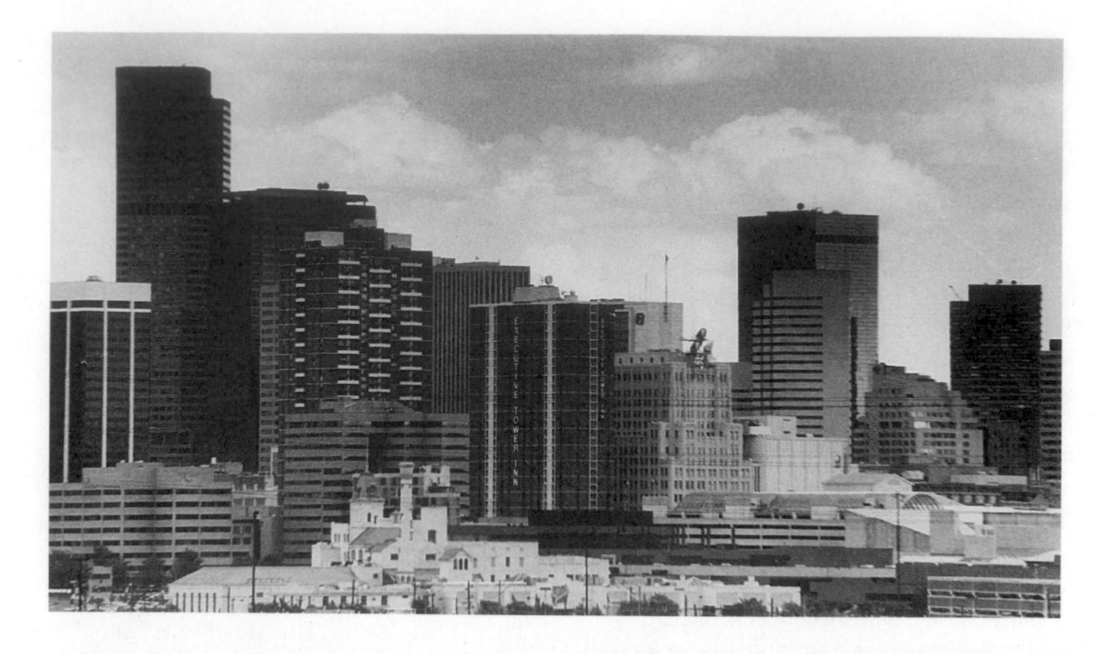

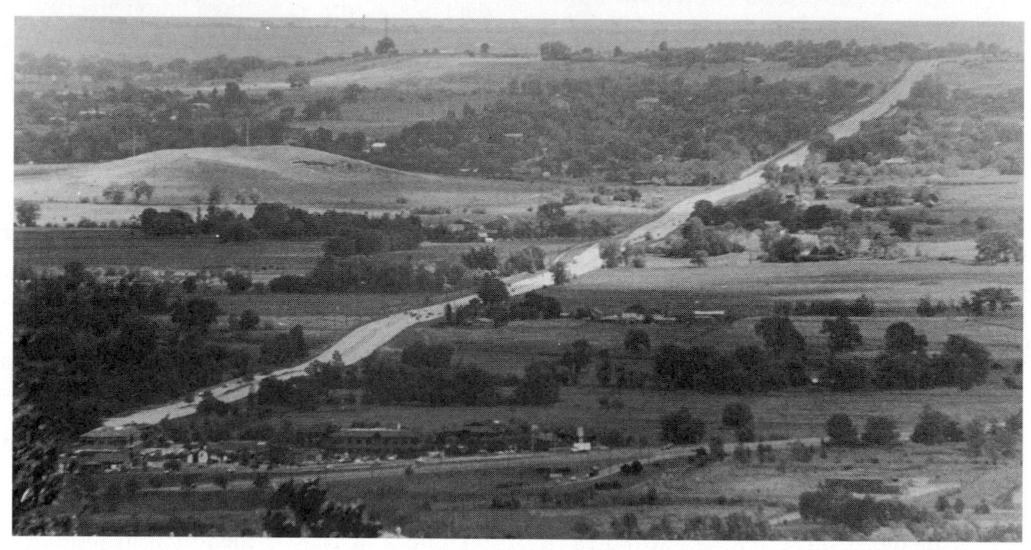

Figure 12–1 ● Geopolitical communities. In geopolitical communities, place is designated by a geographical or political boundary. The people who live, work, learn, and/or play there constitute the population. In most suburban and urban geopolitical communities, the individuals know only some of the residents on a face-to-face, personal basis. In less densely populated rural areas, most people may know each other on a personal basis.

boundaries within which a problem can be identified, dealt with, and solved. A community of solution includes (1) a *health problem shed* (i.e., an area that has similar health problems) and (2) a *health marketing area* (i.e., an area that has similar solutions to the problem or an adequate supply of health resources to meet the problem).

For example, an oil spill in the Chesapeake Bay would affect more than one county. It might affect parts of several counties in Maryland and Virginia. All the communities affected become the health problem shed. All the communities that join together and pool their resources to meet the need create a health marketing area. Figure 12–4 illustrates one city's communities of solution. The concept of a community of solution is especially important in coordinating health care and decreasing duplication and fragmentation of services.

Social Interaction and/or Common Interests, Goals, and Characteristics. Communities, like families, have their own patterned interaction among individuals, families, groups, and organizations; this interaction varies from community to community depending on needs and values. In a geopolitical community this may go beyond talking to one's neighbor and include interaction with agencies and institutions within the community. In a phenomenological

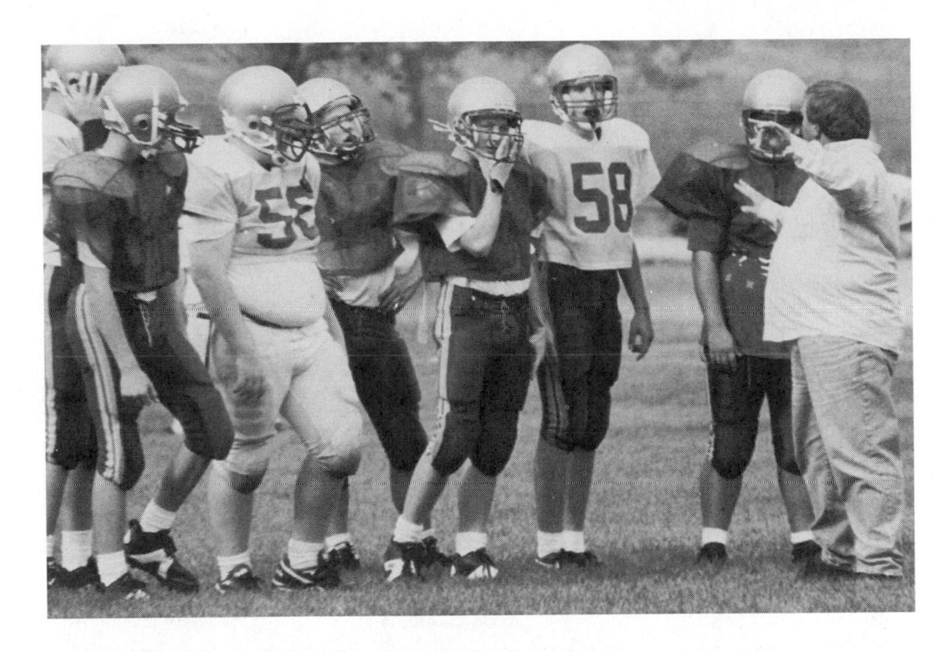

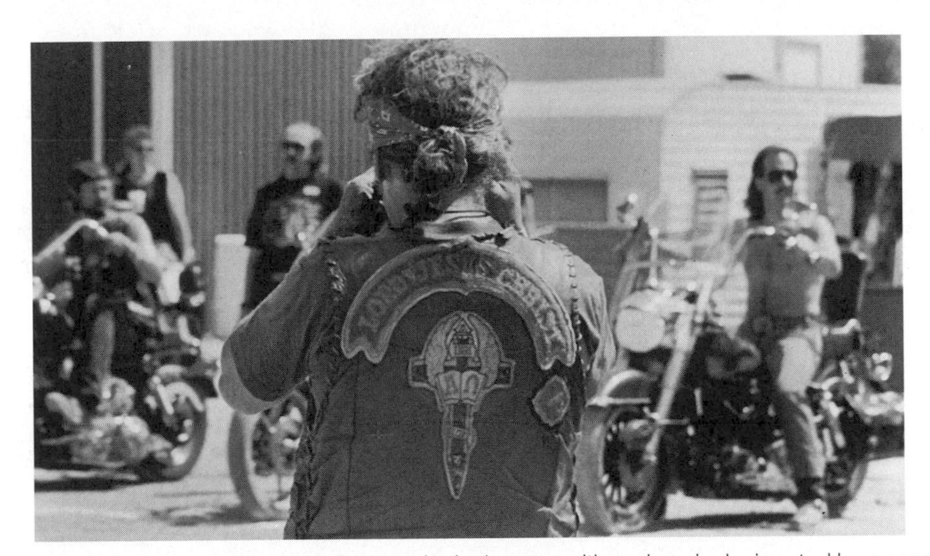

Figure 12–2 ● Phenomenological communities. In phenomenological communities, place is designated by a sense of belonging among its members. Although all human communities exist in a physical place, the members of a phenomenological community are bound together by their interpersonal connectedness rather than by geography. For example, individuals may belong to the U.S. military community, even though they live throughout the entire world. A sense of belonging occurs in phenomenological communities such as clubs, schools, gangs, senior centers, businesses, and churches and other religious organizations.

community, this attribute is inherent. A phenomenological community exists because there is a common interest or goal.

Each of us lives in a geopolitical community, but we may be members of several phenomenological communities. Figure 12–5 illustrates one individual's community membership.

Now that we have defined the concept of community, how do you approach the community as a client? How do you study it? There are many theoretical approaches to studying communities and community health nursing.

Community Frameworks

Perspectives on community come from many fields of study, including anthropology, sociology, epidemiology, social psychology, social planning, and nursing. Community health nurses have adapted and used theories from other disciplines. Several frameworks especially helpful in community health nursing include developmental, epidemiological, structural/functional, and systems.

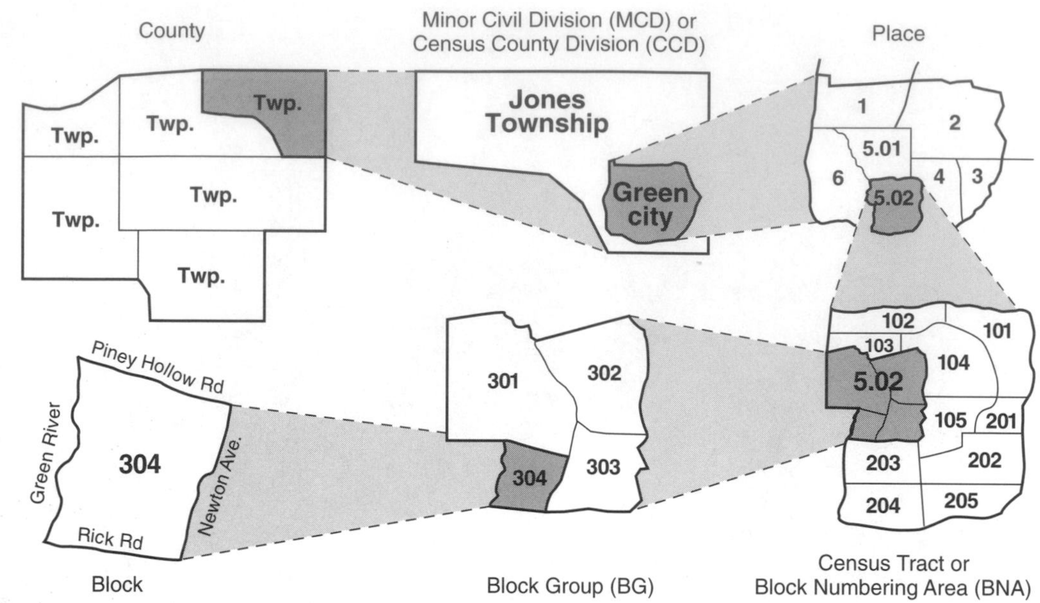

Figure 12–3 ● Census small-area geography map. (Redrawn from Bureau of the Census, U.S. Department of Commerce. (1993). *A guide to state and local census geography.* Washington, DC: Author, p. 21.)

DEVELOPMENTAL FRAMEWORK

With a developmental perspective to assessment, information about the community is collected from several points in time because communities change (McCool and Susman, 1990). Exploring the life history of the community allows the community health nurse to view the community in the context of its own past. For example, even if a community has inadequate resources for treatment of substance abuse, it may currently have many more resources than it did 5 years ago.

Changes in a community are related to the needs of the population, changes in the societal context, changes in the physical environment, and the history of the community

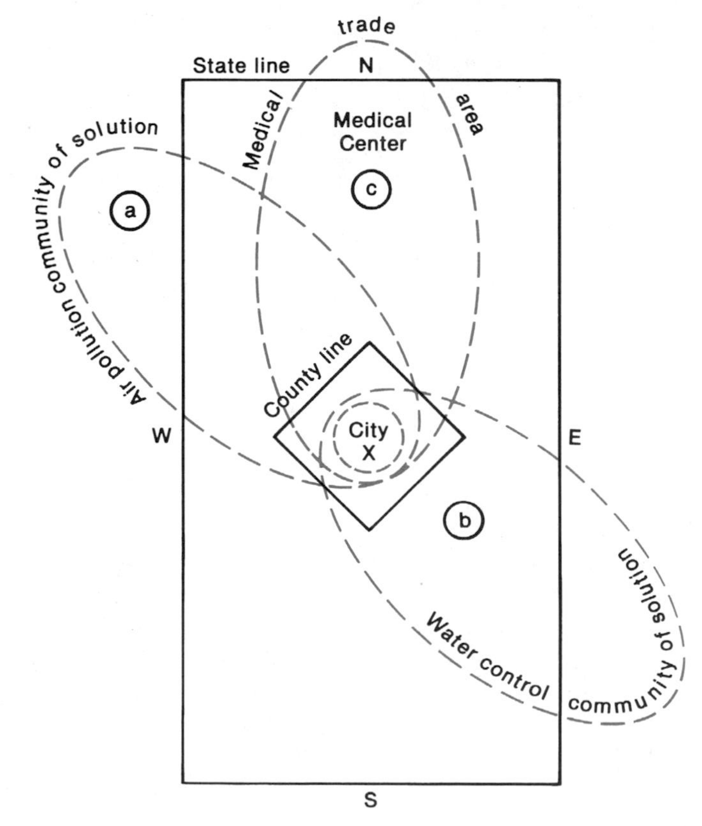

Figure 12–4 ● Communities of solution for City X. Note that health solution boundaries extend beyond city, county, and state lines. **a,** Because of air currents, air pollution may be displaced to the northwest. **b,** Because of the topography of the land, the water and sewage drains toward the southeastern portion of the state, which constitutes another "health problem shed." If the state and neighboring states joined together to solve the problem, this would constitute a health marketing area. **c,** A similar principle holds true for the medical trade area: the state emergency medical services system territory includes part of the adjoining state to the north. (Adapted from National Commission on Community Health Services: *Health is a community affair.* Cambridge, MA: Harvard Press, 1966.)

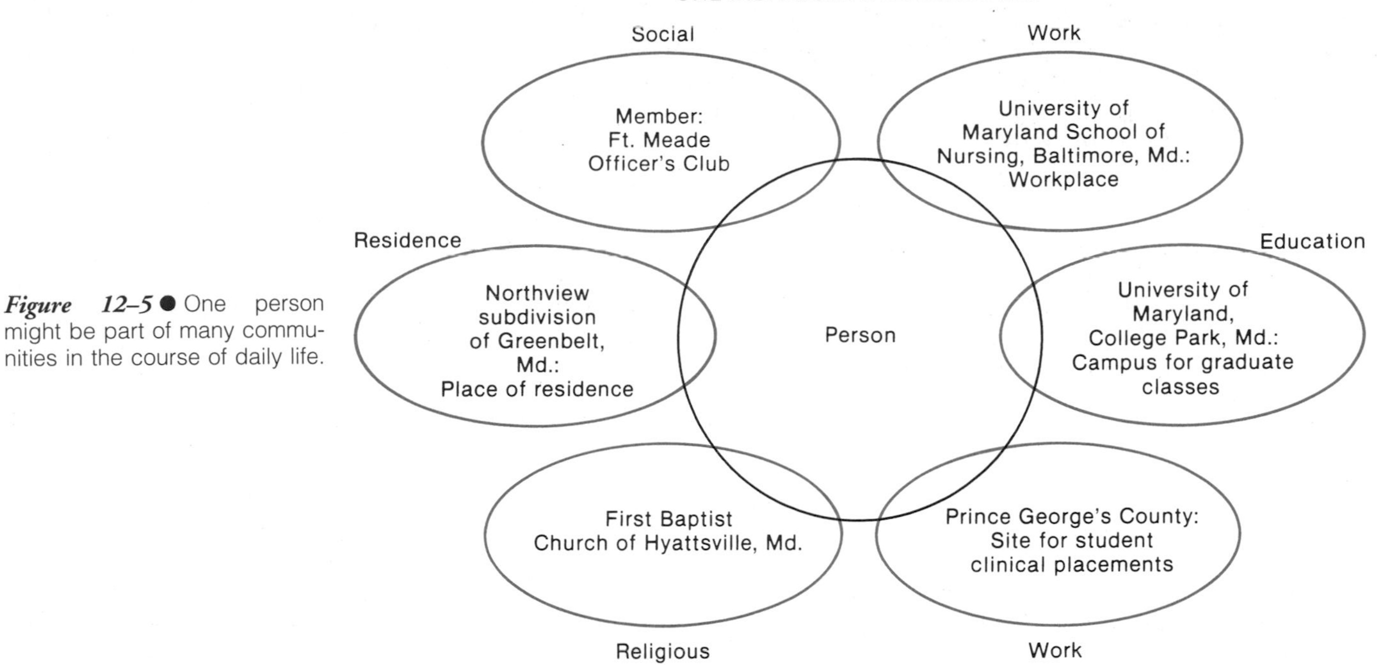

Figure 12–5 ● One person might be part of many communities in the course of daily life.

itself. For example, the U.S. population is currently aging; as the population ages, more health services are needed for the elderly. Loss of population within a community may result in decay of existing buildings. An incorporated area may change its form of governance from a city manager and council to a city mayor and council.

The development of a community is influenced by single events as well as trends. Events may be linked with the age of the community (e.g., the opening of the first local health department office), with changes in the environment (e.g., the closing of a business owing to shifts in the national economy), and with unexpected situations, such as a flood (McCool and Susman, 1990). Patterns of change may form trends. For example, trends in health status of the community members are identified by analyzing epidemiological data from several points in time.

EPIDEMIOLOGICAL FRAMEWORK

An epidemiological perspective focuses on the health of the population. In this approach to community assessment, the community health nurse identifies those at greater risk of illness, injury, disability, and premature death so that interventions can be targeted to help reduce their risk (Finnegan and Ervin, 1989). Interventions focus on prevention of problems.

A "recipe" does not exist for identifying which epidemiological data should be collected about a community. As discussed in Chapter 11, more data exist regarding mortality and the use of hospital services in the United States than exist about morbidity and the use of primary care services. However, we do know that health problems are not distributed evenly among all persons but instead vary with human characteristics such as age, gender, race, and socioeconomic status. Because this is so, it is important for nurses working with communities to consider the different health needs among various aggregates (e.g., elderly persons, pregnant women, workers in a specific occupation, and poor individuals). The concept of aggregate is essential when using an epidemiological approach to community assessment.

STRUCTURAL/FUNCTIONAL FRAMEWORK

Structural/functional approaches to community emerged from anthropology and sociology. As social systems, communities have structures, processes, and functions. Structures are the parts of the community, and their organization and processes are the interactional patterns that change with time. Functions are the purposes and actual outcomes that result from community structures and processes. This approach asks: What structures and patterns of human interaction foster community goal achievement?

The following functions of the community can be identified:

- Creation and distribution of goods and services
- Provision for socialization
- Control of social behavior
- Provision of a sense of identity and mutual support
- Coordination, control, and direction of activities to attain other community goals (Katz and Kahn, 1967; Warren, 1987)

These social functions that the community must perform may be arrived at through alternative social structures and processes. In other words, the same or similar results can be achieved in different ways. In systems language this is called *equifinality.* Communities differ by degree of autonomy, presence of service areas, psychological identification, and pattern of relationships (Warren, 1987).

Communities have differing degrees of autonomy in their ability to provide the basic functions for their members. A very large urban area might provide employment, a varied production of basic goods and services, its own police authority, and a network of formal groups that socialize and support the people. A suburban community might supply a strong social network and support of its members, but have few opportunities for employment within the community and essentially no formal production of goods. Such a community is dependent on a larger urban area for the function of production and distribution. A community may have multiple service areas. For example, the suburban community may consist of two school districts, one election district, and the market area of two hospitals. The degree to which members identify with the locale may be strong or weak.

A community's relationship with other communities and the larger society affect the community. For example, many of the structures within a community, such as a hospital, nursing home, or home health agency, may be owned by corporations outside the community. Currently, most communities must be concerned not only with their internal functioning, but also with their relationships to their social environments.

NURSING THEORIES

Most nursing theories were developed for individual clients, not communities (Hanchett, 1988; Marriner-Tomey, 1989). Many nursing theories view the community as the environmental system influencing individuals and families.

Only a few nursing theories view the community as client (Hamilton and Bush, 1988). Goeppinger and colleagues (1982) proposed the development of a community assessment tool using Cottrell's characteristics of a competent community as a framework. *Community competence* is based on eight variables: commitment, self–other awareness and clarity of situation definitions, articulateness, communication, conflict containment and accommodation, participation, management of relations with the larger society, and machinery for facilitating participant interaction and decision making (Cottrell, 1976). Most of these characteristics of a competent community are community processes that can contribute to the inclusion and participation of community members.

The theories of Johnson (1980), Roy (1984), King (1971), and Neuman (1982) may be used to view the community as client because they are based, in part, on general systems theory. As discussed in Chapter 1, general systems theory can be applied to any social system, including a community. Table 12–2 presents views of the health of a community from the perspective of these nursing theories.

TABLE 12–2

Perspective on the Health of Communities in Selected Nursing Theories

Theorist	Health of a Community
Dorothy Johnson	Successful community functioning and adjustment to environmental factors.
Sister Callista Roy	Effectiveness of the community in accomplishing its functions and adapting to external stimuli.
Imogene King	Quality interactions between individuals, groups, and the entire community that contribute to community functioning and development.
Betty Neuman	Competence of the community to function and maintain balance and harmony in the presence of stressors.

Data from Anderson, E., McFarlane, J., & Helton, A. (1986). Community-as-client: A model for practice. *Nursing Outlook, 34*(5); Hanchett, E. (1988). *Nursing frameworks and community as client—bridging the gap.* Norwalk, CT: Appleton & Lange; and Marriner-Tomey, A. (1989). *Nursing theorists and their work* (2nd ed). St. Louis: Mosby-Year Book.

The assessment tool used in this text is based on systems theory (Table 12–3). In addition, it incorporates aspects of a structural/functional framework by considering the goals of the community and analyzing internal community functioning. The tool also incorporates aspects of an epidemiological framework in the analysis of the health status of the people within the community.

Systems Framework for Community Assessment

The health of a given community is dependent on many factors. To determine how healthy a community is and what its health needs might be, the community health nurse must use a systematic approach to assessment. When nurses assess an individual client, they use a "head-to-toe," or body system, approach to assessment. To facilitate an organized, systematic approach to collecting data about the community as a client, this text presents a conceptual framework based on general systems theory. A systems analysis framework can help the nurse to decide what data to collect and how to organize them.

OVERVIEW OF SYSTEMS THEORY

Components of any system include boundaries, goals, set factors—physical and psychosocial characteristics, inputs, throughputs, outputs, and feedback. The external environment is referred to as the *suprasystem* (von Bertalanffy, 1968). An open system is constantly in the process of responding to internal and external stimuli and attempting to adapt and maintain a sense of balance.

TABLE 12–3

Community Assessment Tool

1. Identify the boundaries of this community.
   a. People
   b. Place
   c. Social interaction and/or common goals, interests, or characteristics
2. Identify the suprasystem and explain the importance of looking at the suprasystem during a community assessment.
3. Identify the goals of this community.
4. Describe the community's physical and psychosocial characteristics.
   a. Physical characteristics
      (1) How long has the community existed?
      (2) Obtain demographic data about the community's members (age, race, sex, ethnicity, housing, density of population).
      (3) Identify physical features of the community that influence behavior.
   b. Psychosocial characteristics
      (1) Religion
      (2) Socioeconomic class
      (3) Education
      (4) Occupation
      (5) Marital status
5. Which external influences (inputs) from the environment (suprasystem) are resources? Which are demands?

	Resources	Demands
Money:		
Facilities:		
Human services:		
Formal		
Informal		
Health information:		
Legislation:		
Values of suprasystem (i.e., what external values affect this community?):		

6. Internal functions (throughputs): Identify resources and demands within the community that influence its level of health.
   a. Economy
      (1) Formal and informal human services: What formal and informal human services are available within the community (resources)?
      (2) Money: What is the budget? How is revenue generated from within the community?
      (3) Facilities, equipment, goods: What health care facilities are available within the community? What does the community produce? What equipment/supplies does it have to produce its goods?
      (4) Education: How are members educated/socialized to function productively?
      (5) Analysis of economy subsystem functioning: What is the ratio of resources to demands?
      (6) How accessible, adequate, and appropriate are the services, facilities, finances, and education in this community?
   b. Polity: Describe the political system within the community used to attain community goals.
      (1) What is the basic organizational structure?
      (2) Who are the formal and informal leaders?
      (3) What is the pattern of decision making? How have decisions been made in the past?
      (4) What methods of social control are used?
      (5) Analysis of the polity subsystem: What is the ratio of demands to resources?
   c. Communication: Describe the communication within the community that fosters a sense of belonging and provides identity and support to its members.
      (1) Nonverbal communication: What is the "personality"/emotional tone of the community? How do people talk about their community? What clubs and organizations are present?
      (2) Verbal communication: What is the pattern of communication? Who communicates with whom? Is it vertical or horizontal? How is communication achieved? What is the form of communication? When does the communication occur?
      (3) Analysis of communication subsystem: How well does the community communicate a sense of identity or belonging to its members? How adequate is the communication?
   d. Values: Identify the ideas, attitudes, and beliefs of community members that serve as general guides to behavior.
      (1) Traditions: What traditions are upheld?
      (2) Subgroups: What subgroups or cliques are obvious in this community?
      (3) Environment: Describe the environment, and explain how it reflects values.
      (4) Health:
         (a) What types of health facilities are used? How often?
         (b) What are people's attitudes about health and health care professionals?
         (c) What priority do community members place on health?
      (5) Homogeneity vs. heterogeneity: Is the community homogeneous or heterogeneous in its beliefs and values?
      (6) Analysis of values subsystem: How well does the community provide guidelines for the behavior of its members?

Continued

TABLE 12–3

Community Assessment Tool *Continued*

7. Health behavior and health status (outputs):
   (Be sure to refer to the community assessment tool in Table 12–4 for this portion of the assessment, because there are some differences between the geopolitical community and the phenomenological community.)
   a. People factors:
      (1) Describe the general trends regarding size of community.
      (2) What are the trends in mortality and morbidity?
         (a) What is the mortality rate?
         (b) What are the major causes of death?
         (c) What major diseases/illnesses are present?
         (d) Who are the vulnerable groups? What are the risky behaviors?
         (e) What presymptomatic illness or problems might be expected?
         (f) What is the level of social functioning in this community?
         (g) What types of disabilities and/or impairments are present or might be found in this community?
   b. Environmental factors:
      (1) Physical environmental factors: What is the quality of the physical environment (air, water, housing, work or home environment)?
      (2) Social environmental factors: What is the emotional tone and stability of the population?
8. Describe feedback from the environment about the community's functioning.
9. Make inferences about the level of health of this community.
   a. What are some actual health problems or needs?
   b. What are some potential health problems or needs?
   c. How well is the community working to meet its health needs? What is its proposed action to meet its health needs?
   d. How has the community solved similar problems in the past?
   e. What are the strengths of the community?
10. Identify one actual or potential health need for which you, as a nurse, could plan an intervention.

Adapted from Community health faculty, Undergraduate Program, University of Maryland School of Nursing (1975). *Community assessment tool.* Baltimore: University of Maryland School of Nursing.

The model of community assessment presented here and illustrated in Figure 12–6 can be used to assess any type of community. The components of the systems model of assessing a community are defined as follows:

Boundaries: Factors that separate a community from its environment and maintain the integrity of the community.

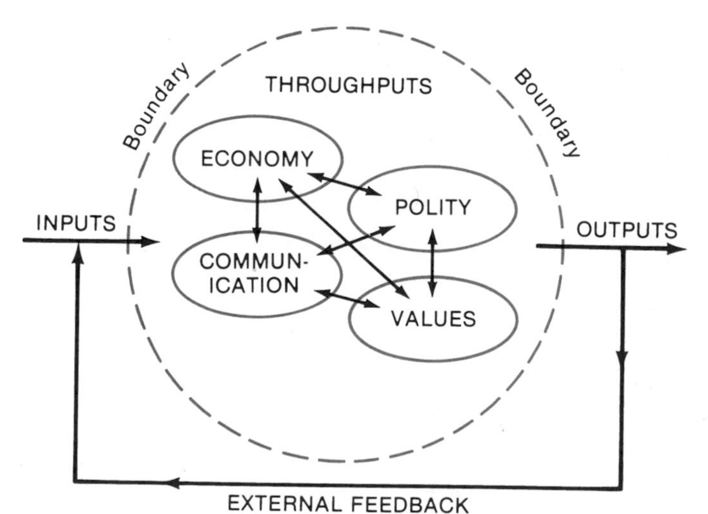

Figure 12–6 ● Community as system.

Goals: The purpose or reason for which the community exists.

Set factors: The physical and psychosocial characteristics of the community that affect behavior.

Inputs: External influences.

Throughputs: The internal functioning of the community, divided into four functional subsystems (University of Maryland, 1975): economy, polity, communication, and values.

Outputs: The health behavior and health status of the community.

Feedback: The information that is returned to the system regarding its functioning.

COMPONENTS TO ASSESS

Table 12–4 summarizes the assessment process, comparing and contrasting the geopolitical and phenomenological types of community. At the bottom of each section of the assessment, possible data sources are listed. Each component of the assessment will be discussed in more detail.

Boundaries

The first step in community assessment is to define the boundaries or parameters. Remember that a community is defined in terms of the three critical attributes or defining characteristics. The definition of a community determines

TABLE 12–4

A Systems Approach to Community Assessment

Geopolitical Community

I. Boundaries: The focus of a boundary in a geopolitical community is on place.
- A. Type of boundary
  - 1. What are the natural (e.g., river, mountain) or man-made parameters (e.g., railroads, streets, legal, census tracts)
- B. Permeability
  - 1. How open or closed is the system?
- C. Suprasystem
  - 1. What is the external environment that is most closely involved with the community? Examples:

Community	*Suprasystem*
Census Tract 2102	City of Baltimore
Adams Morgan neighborhood	Washington, DC

Sources of data: Maps, census tract maps, libraries, city clerks, health departments, printed material describing the community.

II. Goals
- A. Purpose
  - 1. What is the reason or purpose for which the community exists?

Sources of data: Charter of Incorporation, printed material about the community, interviews of key informants such as community leaders.

III. Set factors
- A. Physical/biological characteristics
  - 1. Length of time community has been in existence
  - 2. Pertinent demographic data
    - a. Age
    - b. Race
    - c. Sex
    - d. Ethnicity
    - e. Housing
      - (1) Type (single family)
      - (2) Ownership (rent or own)
      - (3) Condition
    - f. Density of population
      - (1) Rural, urban, suburban
      - (2) No. of people per housing unit
  - 3. Physical features of the community
- B. Psychosocial characteristics
  - 1. Religion
    - a. Religious preference of members
    - b. No. and type of churches
  - 2. Socioeconomic class
  - 3. Education
    - a. Educational level of members
    - b. No. and type of educational institutions
  - 4. Occupation
  - 5. Marital status

Sources of data: Census tract data, health planning agencies, libraries, city/county clerks, Chamber of Commerce, printed matter about the community, telephone books listing churches and schools, a visit to the neighborhood (for information on set factors of the community), written surveys, local realtors (for information on housing).

Phenomenological Community

I. Boundaries. The focus of a boundary in a phenomenological community is on criteria for membership.
- A. Criteria for membership
  - 1. Who can belong?
  - 2. What are the requirements or prerequisites for belonging to or attending this community?
  - 3. What are the common characteristics used by the health provider to place people in this aggregate?
- B. Permeability
  - 1. How open or closed is the system?
- C. Suprasystem
  - 1. What is the external environment that is most closely involved/associated with this community? Examples:

Community	*Suprasystem*
A Catholic School	Archdiocese or a particular parish
A senior center in Howard County	The Howard County Office on Aging

Sources of data: Interviews, printed material describing the community (e.g., pamphlets), philosophical and membership criteria statements.

II. Goals
- A. Purpose
  - 1. What is the reason or purpose for which the community exists?

Sources of data: Printed materials about the community, statement of philosophy and goals, interviews of key informants such as community leaders and community members.

III. Set factors
- A. Physical characteristics
  - 1. Length of time community has been in existence
  - 2. Pertinent demographic data
    - a. Age
    - b. Race
    - c. Sex
    - d. Ethnicity
    - e. Environment in which group meets
    - f. Density of population
      - (1) Relationship of no. of people to area
  - 3. Physical features of the community
- B. Psychosocial characteristics
  - 1. Religion
  - 2. Socioeconomic class
  - 3. Educational level
  - 4. Occupation
  - 5. Marital status

Sources of data: A visit to the community, health and membership records, surveys, interviews with key informants.

Continued

TABLE 12–4

A Systems Approach to Community Assessment *Continued*

Geopolitical Community	Phenomenological Community
IV. Inputs: Matter, energy, information from outside the community (suprasystem) that influence the community system; may be resources (R) or demands (D). A. Money B. Facilities available to the community but located outside the community 1. Health care 2. Transportation 3. Safety measures/emergency services (fire, police, ambulance) C. Human services 1. Formal (professional resources) 2. Informal (volunteers) D. Health information via printed material and mass media E. Legislation F. Values of the suprasystem *Sources of data:* Budget, local telephone book and newspapers list many facilities; health or social service directories; information and referral services; systematic tour of sites of service and organizations.	IV. Inputs: Matter, energy, information from outside the community (suprasystem) that influence the community system; may be resources (R) or demands (D). A. Money B. Facilities available to the community but located outside the community 1. Health care 2. Transportation 3. Safety/emergency measures C. Human services 1. Formal (professional resources) 2. Informal (volunteers) D. Health information via printed material and mass media E. Legislation F. Values of the suprasystem *Sources of data:* Interview, observation, local telephone book, newspapers, social service directories, budgets, interviews of key informants of suprasystem.
V. Throughputs: The internal processes within the community A. Economy: Production/goal attainment 1. Human services a. Formal b. Informal 2. Money a. What is the community's budget? b. How is revenue generated within the community? 3. Facilities and equipment 4. Education: How are members educated? *Note:* Lack of any of the above indicates a demand. *Analysis questions:* Are facilities, services, money and goods adequate, accessible, and coordinated? *Sources of data:* Budget, interviews, drive or walk through the community, telephone book and service directories.	V. Throughputs: The internal processes within the community A. Economy: Production/goal attainment 1. Human services a. Formal b. Informal 2. Money a. What is the community's budget? b. How is revenue generated within the community? 3. Facilities and equipment 4. Education: Is there continuing education within the group? How are members educated? *Note:* Lack of any of the above indicates a demand. *Analysis questions:* Are facilities, services, and equipment adequate, accessible, and coordinated? *Sources of data:* Budget, interviews, surveys.
B. Polity: Coordination, control, and direction of activities to attain system goals 1. Organizational structure: What is the organizational structure? 2. Leadership a. Who are the formal leaders? b. Who are the informal leaders? 3. Decision making/problem solving a. What is the decision-making process? b. Who have been the key decision makers for health issues? c. How have problems been approached and solved in the past? d. What problem-solving approaches have not worked in the past? 4. Social control: The rules and norms of a community that influence behavior. a. Rules: Local laws/control measures often enforced through police, law agencies, courts, and the government. b. Norms: Social sanctions enforced by neighborhood, school, or church. *Sources of data:* Organizational chart and charter, interviews and meetings with the community, laws	B. Polity: Coordination, control, and direction of activities to attain system goals 1. Organizational structure: What is the organizational structure? 2. Leadership a. Who are the formal leaders? b. Who are the informal leaders? 3. Decision making/problem solving a. What is the decision-making process? b. Who have been the key decision makers for health issues? c. How have problems been approached and solved in the past? d. What problem-solving approaches have not worked in the past? 4. Social control: The rules and norms of a community that influence behavior a. Rules: Legal control enforced by by-laws, policies, and procedures. b. Norms: Social sanctions enforced by the group. *Sources of data:* By-laws, procedure and policy books, attending meetings, being with the group
C. Communication: Provision of identity and support to members 1. Nonverbal a. What is the "personality" or emotional tone of the neighborhood? (1) Is it different at different times of the day?	C. Communication: Provision of identity and support to members 1. Nonverbal a. What is the "personality" or emotional tone of the group?

TABLE 12–4

A Systems Approach to Community Assessment *Continued*

Geopolitical Community	Phenomenological Community
2. Verbal a. Who communicates with whom? (1) Horizontal (2) Vertical b. How is communication achieved (e.g., newspaper, television, radio, newsletter, posters, fliers, person to person, informal gatherings, formal meetings)? c. What is the focus of the communication? d. When does the communication occur (e.g., meeting dates, frequency of newsletters, and meetings)?	2. Verbal a. Who communicates with whom? (1) Horizontal (2) Vertical b. How is communication achieved (e.g., newsletters, person-to-person, classes, committees, bulletin boards, kiosks, telephone)? c. What is the focus of the communication? d. When does the communication occur (e.g., meeting dates, frequency of communication)?
Sources of data: Interviews, newspapers, kiosks, meetings, visit to community	*Sources of data:* Interviews, newsletters, meetings, classes, committees, being with the community
D. Values: Socialization 1. Traditions a. What traditions are upheld? b. Are kinship bonds strong, or is each person expected to deal with his or her own problems?	D. Values: Socialization 1. Traditions a. What traditions are upheld? b. How are birthdays, holidays, or transitional events celebrated?
2. Subgroups a. Are there identifiable subgroups with their own special values, life customs, and problems (e.g., Little Italy, Chinatown, drug culture)?	2. Subgroups a. Are there subgroups or cliques?
3. Environment: Is the environment neat and well kept, or is little attention paid to aesthetics?	3. Environment: Is the environment neat, well kept, and aesthetically pleasing, or is little attention paid to aesthetics?
4. Health a. What type of health facilities are used? b. How often are they used? c. What are the attitudes about health, health care, and health professionals? d. What priority does health have?	4. Health a. How do members define health? b. What type of health facilities are used? c. How often are they used (preventive care vs. crisis only)? d. What are their attitudes about health, health care, and health professionals?
5. Is the community homogeneous or heterogeneous in relation to its values?	5. Is the community homogeneous or heterogeneous in relation to its values?
Sources of data: Surveys of agencies to determine utilization, surveys of community members, newspapers, and community announcements	*Sources of data:* Observation and interaction with members, charts, or records, surveys of members
VI. Outputs: Measurable, health-related behaviors that are released from the community to the environment.	VI. Outputs: Measurable health-related behaviors that are released from the community to the environment.
People Factors	*People Factors*
A. General trends 1. What is the relationship between birth and death rates? 2. What is the relationship between immigration and emigration rates? 3. What are the changes in demographic characteristics (set factors) such as age, sex, race, occupation, marital status, educational levels? 4. Mobility: How often and how easily do people move in and out of the community?	A. General trends 1. What was the original size of the community? Has the community remained stable, grown, or decreased in size? 2. What are the changes in demographic characteristics (set factors) such as age, sex, race, occupation, marital status, educational achievement?
B. Trends in mortality and morbidity 1. What is the mortality rate? 2. What are the major causes of death? 3. What are the major diseases/illnesses present in the community?	B. Trends in mortality and morbidity 1. What is the mortality rate? 2. What are the major causes of death, or what would you expect to be the leading cause of death? (Consider age and other set factors.) 3. What diseases/illnesses are present or expected to be present in this type of community? (Consider age and other set factors.)
4. What are the number and location of vulnerable or at-risk aggregates (e.g., poor, homeless, elderly, or malnourished individuals; migrants; selected occupational groups; or risky behavior such as intravenous drug abuse for HIV)?	4. What risky health behaviors are present?

Continued

TABLE 12–4

A Systems Approach to Community Assessment *Continued*

Geopolitical Community	Phenomenological Community
5. What is the prevalence of presymptomatic illness (e.g., no. of people with increasing blood pressure, blood cholesterol, or blood sugar levels)?	5. What is the prevalence of presymptomatic illness (e.g., no. of people with increasing blood pressure, blood cholesterol, or blood sugar levels)? Estimations may be made on the basis of special surveys or part of a screening program.
6. What is the level of social functioning? a. Dependency ratio: $\frac{\text{Population less than 18 years + population over 65 years}}{\text{Population between 18 and 65}}$	6. What is the level of social functioning? Look at dependency needs or no. of people who are dependent on others for assistance (financial or other). Example: If you have 15 senior citizens in a center who need help with ambulation and three who are independent, the community has high dependency needs.
7. Disabilities and impairments	7. Are disabilities or impairments present (e.g., children with learning disabilities in a school; visual or auditory impairment in a school or elderly group; or elderly individuals who might use aids such as wheelchairs)?
Sources of data: Local and state vital statistics (available through local and state health departments); *MMWR (Morbidity and Mortality Weekly Report),* published by the Centers for Disease Control and Prevention (available at libraries or by supscription); the U.S. census report (available at libraries and health departments); reports of screening programs; interviews with key informants.	*Sources of data:* Agency or community records, interviews with key informants, review of the literature pertaining to aggregates (e.g., literature about elderly individuals will provide information about most morbidity and mortality).
Environmental Factors	*Environmental Factors*
A. Physical factors B. Social factors *Sources of data:* Visit to community; reports such as Air Quality Index (AQI).	A. Physical factors B. Social factors *Sources of data:* Visit to community

its boundaries. This is an essential first step, because the boundary, as the "skin" or outside limit of the client, determines what data the nurse will collect as part of the community and what data are inputs into the community from the outside environment (the suprasystem).

Boundaries, like skin in the individual, maintain the integrity of the system and regulate the exchange between a community and its external environment, the suprasystem. Exchanges between the client and its environment are in the form of matter, energy, or information.

Boundaries of a geopolitical community are spatial and concrete. They can be natural or man-made, as discussed earlier. Because the boundaries of geopolitical communities are real and concrete, they are often visible on maps. For example, the Potomac River and the Maryland state line can be visualized on a map as indicators of the boundaries of Washington, D.C.

The boundaries of phenomenological communities are more relational or conceptual than are geopolitical boundaries and usually relate to the reason the community exists or the criteria for membership. To determine the boundary of a phenomenological community, one would ask the following questions: Why does the community exist? Who can belong? What criteria are necessary for membership? What brings the members together? For example, the boundary of the nursing community would be its criterion for membership—that is, one must be a nurse to belong.

The Morgan Center, a nutrition center for frail elderly persons, is a phenomenological community consisting of 25 senior participants, a site manager, and three staff members. To attend Morgan Center, the participants must be 65 years of age or older, live in Allen County, be classified as frail (having difficulty with at least one activity of daily living [ADL]), and be continent. What are the boundaries of this phenomenological community? Remember that a community's purpose and situation define the community. In this situation we could define the community as an aggregate of elderly (the frail elderly) attending Morgan Center. The criteria for membership (65+ years, residents of Allen county, frail, continency) determine the boundaries. We could also define the community as Morgan Center, including the frail elderly, the site manager, and the staff. Either definition is correct, depending on the reason or purpose for the assessment. However, it is imperative that the parameters of the community be defined because they determine what data will be collected. In the first situation, the nurse will collect data about frail elderly persons only, and the site manager and the staff will be external influences (inputs) to the community; in the second example, the nurse will collect data about frail elderly persons, the site manager, and the staff as part of the community. Boundary definition is especially important when examining the external influences (inputs) and the internal processes (throughputs) of a community.

Permeability of Boundaries. Community boundaries have varying degrees of permeability. The boundaries of any system may be relatively permeable (open) or impermeable (closed). For example, entrance or membership into a religious community may be contingent on certain beliefs and rituals, making the boundary impermeable to someone who does not hold these beliefs. In a phenomenological community, the criteria for membership often define the boundary's permeability or openness. A geographical community may have housing available only at the $250,000 level and higher. If so, the boundaries are impermeable to someone of a low socioeconomic status. Communities that have a greater variety of housing would be open to more people.

The openness or closedness of a community has implications for health planning. A very closed, rigid system is resistant to change, whereas an open, flexible system is more receptive to change and to help from the health care delivery system. If boundaries are too open, the identity of the system may become blurred or the community identity obliterated entirely.

Suprasystem. Once you have determined the boundary of the community, anything outside the boundary becomes the suprasystem. No system (individual, family, or community) can exist in isolation. Therefore, every client system operates within a larger system, known as the suprasystem, which is defined as the environment outside the client system that affects the system. The suprasystem of the geopolitical community is more concrete to identify. For example, the immediate suprasystem of Ridgely's Delight, a neighborhood in Baltimore, is Baltimore itself. The suprasystem of Baltimore is the state of Maryland. It is usually easier to identify a specific suprasystem for a geopolitical community than it is for a phenomenological community.

In a phenomenological community the suprasystem becomes anything outside of the community that affects or is affected by the community. It is sometimes difficult to identify a single suprasystem for a phenomenological community. For example, what is the suprasystem for an aggregate such as the elderly individuals in Orange County? It might be the Orange County Office on Aging, or it could be more than that. One would look at sources of inputs (external influences) from the larger society, such as legislation, services, and money, that influence (positively or negatively) the elderly community. For some phenomenological communities, however, it may be possible to identify a specific suprasystem. For example, Girl Scout Troop No. 201 is a phenomenological community; its suprasystem is the Girl Scouts of Central Maryland.

Goals

Goals of communities vary with the type of community, but in general they are focused on maximizing the well-being of members, promoting survival, and meeting the needs of the community members. What are the goals of the community in which you live? Are they to provide safe housing for residents? A goal of the Morgan Senior Center might be to provide socialization for its members. The community health nurse can assess the goals of the community by asking questions such as, "What is the purpose of the community?" and by asking to see a written statement of the community's philosophy and goals, if available.

Set Factors

Set factors are the physical/biological and psychosocial characteristics of the community. These are often referred to as demographics.

Physical Characteristics. Physical characteristics include (1) the length of time the community has been in existence; (2) pertinent demographic data about the community's members (e.g., age, race, sex, ethnicity, housing, density of population); and (3) physical features of the community that influence behavior.

The length of time the community has been in existence (the age of the community) has implications regarding stability, health services, and needs. A very new community may have few services simply because the supply has not caught up with the demand. On the other hand, communities that have been in existence for a long time may have many resources, or they may have resources that reflect past population needs but not the current needs (if population shifts have occurred).

Pertinent demographic data such as age, race, sex, ethnicity, and density of the population have significant meaning in the planning of health care and services. By looking at the age, race, and sex of members of the community, the community health nurse can make some inferences about possible health needs. A community with a large population of elderly individuals will have very different needs from those of a community with a predominantly young population. Generally, elderly individuals need more services than younger persons. Race is a factor in certain diseases (e.g., sickle cell anemia in the black population). A population with an unusually high number of females will need women's health care services, and a community with a high number of adults may need blood pressure screening programs to detect early hypertension.

Ethnicity is reflected in customs, beliefs, and values and may affect how the community addresses certain health practices. It is important for the community health nurse to understand these customs and beliefs when assessing needs and planning interventions. In some areas, the cultural and ethnic backgrounds of the population have become the basis for the community. Some cities have sections that reflect the ethnic and cultural heritage of certain groups (e.g., Little Italy and Chinatown in San Francisco). Groups such as the Sons of Norway, the Sons of Italy, and the Polish Home Club have formed phenomenological communities on the basis of their ethnic and cultural heritage.

The type, condition, and amount of housing and density of the population are environmental factors that have implications for health. Crowded living conditions have long been associated with the increased transmission of some communicable diseases (e.g., tuberculosis, pediculosis). It is also important to note the condition of the housing and whether the housing is available and financially accessible to people in the community. The type and condition of housing may say a lot about the resources and values of the people living in the community.

In a phenomenological community, one might look at the environment or the place in which the group meets. This takes into consideration the environmental factors and the aesthetics that contribute to or interfere with members' ability to feel comfortable in the physical environment.

Physical features of the community can influence the community's behaviors. A community with fences around all houses demonstrates a value of privacy and may imply little social interaction or the presence of dogs or pools. A school with open classrooms influences the interaction among students. Other physical features such as living or working in a community with toxic substances may influence the level of health of the residents or workers.

Psychosocial Characteristics. Psychosocial characteristics that affect the emotional tones of the community include religion, socioeconomic class, education, occupation, and marital status.

Religious affiliation has an important effect on health beliefs and practices. For example, a predominantly Catholic community would most likely not be very receptive to information on birth control, whereas a Protestant community might.

Socioeconomic level has significant implications for both the level of health and members' ability to pay for services. For example, people living below the poverty level are prone to many illnesses related to insufficient nutrition and have need for more health services. A community with a high proportion of people in a low socioeconomic class will have less financial access to health care than communities with higher income levels.

Another factor to consider is the educational level of the community, because it has a significant effect on health resources and the types of programs planned. The health learning needs of a community with a mean educational level of eighth grade will be quite different from those of a community with primarily college graduates. Higher educational levels are associated with more preventive health care behaviors.

Knowing the occupations of members of the community provides information about diseases for which they may be at risk. For example, a coal mining community may be more at risk for lung diseases, whereas a "white collar," high-technology community might be more at risk for stress-related conditions such as coronary artery disease.

Thus, looking at some demographic information can provide the nurse with some idea of the possible health needs of the community. This is the basis for aggregate health planning—that is, looking at a number of people with common characteristics and planning programs to meet their unique needs.

At this point you may be asking, "Where do I get information about the community's set factors?" A visit to the neighborhood often provides information about the set factors of the community. Formal data may be obtained by using already collected data such as census tract information or county, city, and state planning statistics found at the local libraries or planning boards or city or county clerk offices. The Chamber of Commerce often provides printed materials about the community that may reflect some set factors. Telephone books often list denominations of churches and numbers and types of schools. In a phenomenological community, sources of data are health and membership records, surveys, interviews, and observations made on visiting the community.

Inputs (External Influences)

All communities, like individuals and families, have external influences that affect their functioning. In systems terminology the external influences are called *inputs*. Inputs are matter, energy, and information, any of which may be physical and/or psychosocial in origin, that come from outside the community—that is, from the suprasystem. Inputs may be either resources (assets or strengths) or demands (liabilities or weaknesses) on the community and may be imperative or voluntary. For the purpose of organization, inputs are grouped into the following categories: money, facilities, human services, health information, legislation, and values of the suprasystem.

Money. Communities may receive money from outside the community. For example, money may come from taxes, state or federal funds, contributions, grants, or endowments provided to the community from outside. When assessing a given community, the nurse will want to find out what sources of outside funding, if any, are available to the community. Community health nurses are especially interested in money that may be used to fund health services.

Facilities. It is important to look at the institutional facilities located outside the community that may be available to the community. This includes health care facilities such as hospitals, health maintenance organizations, nursing homes, home care agencies, and clinics, as well as facilities promoting safety and transportation.

In addition to finding out what facilities are present in the external environment, it is important to find out how accessible the facilities are to members of the community with which the nurse is working (Urrutia-Rojas and Aday, 1991). For example, if a nurse is working with a group of low-income pregnant women in a rural area and finds that a prenatal clinic is available, he or she will also need to know whether the clinic is geographically and financially accessible. Is public transportation available at a reasonable cost, or do patients need an automobile to get to the clinic? Does insurance exist to pay for the care? Do the women perceive that they are treated with respect and receive quality care from the health care providers? Even a beautifully furnished clinic will not meet the people's needs if they cannot get there to use the facility or perceive that they are not wanted there.

Human Services. Human services and resources may be formal or informal. Formal human services refer to professional resources such as nurses, physicians, and the local health department. Informal human resources reside in the general population and usually volunteer their services. For example, many rural communities formerly had women who served as midwives. These women were lay people who volunteered to help with childbirth in their community. Often church groups take on informal human service functions. There are also many volunteer support groups for a variety of health conditions (e.g., Alcoholics Anonymous). Folkhealers may exist as well.

When assessing a community, the nurse should identify the formal and informal human resources in the suprasystem affecting the community. For example, there may be physicians and nurses outside of the community who will see the members of the community (resource), or there may be no physicians in the larger suprasystem who will accept members of the community who are on medical assistance (demand).

Health Information. Health information may be communicated to the community in a variety of ways, such as through printed matter, radio, television, or person to person. If the suprasystem has certain information that would help the community, yet does not have an effective way to get this information to community members, this absence of a method of communication would be a demand. Find out what health information is available and how it is disseminated.

Legislation. The suprasystem has many laws, policies, and procedures that may affect a community in either a positive (resource) or a negative (demand) manner. A geopolitical community has laws governing environmental pollution and zoning issues, all of which affect the health of a community. A phenomenological community will also be affected by external legislation and policies and procedures. For example, some legislation affects the health and health care of the elderly (e.g., the Older American Act and Medicare legislation). When working with a community, the nurse should ask, "What are the external laws that affect this community? How do they affect this community positively and negatively?"

Values of the Suprasystem. Every system has its own values. The suprasystem's values may be consistent or inconsistent with the values of the community. It is important for nurses to know the values of the suprasystem and to be able to identify whether they are congruent or incongruent with the values of the community with which they are working. If the two sets of values are consistent, they will not conflict, and the suprasystem will be more supportive of any changes needing to be made; however, if the community's values are inconsistent with those of the suprasystem, there will be conflict.

Because the external influences come from the suprasystem, it is important to obtain data about the suprasystem. Where can these data be found? A review of the suprasystem budget, local telephone book and newspapers, health or human service directories, information and referral services, systematic tours of services and agencies, interviews with key informants, and legal and policy and procedure books provide a wealth of information about inputs into the community.

Throughputs (Internal Functions)

Throughputs are defined as the internal structures and processes of the community itself. For the purpose of data collection and analysis, the throughputs, or internal processes, are divided into four functional subsystems: economy, polity, communication, and values (University of Maryland, 1975). There may be resources and demands within each of these subsystems.

Economy. *The goal of the economy subsystem is production and distribution of goods and services.* This takes into consideration such categories as human services; money; facilities, equipment, and goods; and education. These are the same factors discussed in the assessment of inputs. However, the factors are now assessed within the community itself.

Human Services. Human services available within the community may be either formal (nurses and physicians) or informal (volunteers). What human services are available within the community to meet the community's health needs? Are services adequate and sufficiently accessible to meet the community's needs, or are services available only to a certain segment of the population, such as those who can afford to pay or who have transportation? Are the human services responsive to the needs of the community?

Money. What is the budget? How does the community get its money? How is revenue generated from within the community? What are the fund raising activities?

Facilities, Equipment, and Goods. What health care facilities (e.g., hospitals, clinics, home health agencies, nursing homes, daycare centers) are available within the community? How are they used? Are they accessible, appropriate, and adequate for the population in the community?

Does the facility have the equipment and supplies it needs to produce its goods? What does it produce? What is its contribution to the larger society? For example, is this a high-technology geopolitical community that supplies research and development, or is it a phenomenological community, such as Mothers Against Drunk Driving (MADD), that provides support to its members and information to the larger suprasystem? These are examples of positive production (resources). It is possible for a community to produce a negative effect on the larger society. For example, a community of drug abusers may produce a negative effect (demand) on the system and the suprasystem.

Education. Education assists people to learn how to function productively in society, and therefore, it is included in this subsystem. How are the members educated? In a geopolitical community we can look at the number and types of schools as well as the level of education. In a phenomenological community, we look at needs for education of the group and what type of education is taking place. For example, what education is being provided to pregnant teenagers about their pregnancy?

In addition to assessing these factors, we need to begin to analyze the findings. Are the resources outweighing the demands? Are the finances, services, facilities, and education appropriate, accessible, and adequate to members of the community? What is the ratio of demands to resources?

Polity. *The goal of polity is coordination, control, and direction of activities to maintain the community and attain the system goals.* In our society, the formal government, as well as the informal leadership, serves this function. The polity subsystem of a community provides organizational structure, leadership, decision making, and social control to its members in return for members' compliance and support.

Organizational Structure. The organizational structure represents the way in which a population group has organized to facilitate collective action and to exert some control over its collective behavior. An organizational chart of a community will provide information about how the community is organized, its formal leadership positions, and its decision-making process. How is the community organized? Is it an incorporated city with a mayor and city council? Is it a charter government? Is it a volunteer group with no elected leaders?

Leadership. Both formal and informal leadership are present in any group; it is important to identify both types. Who are the formal leaders? Formal leaders may be elected or appointed. They have the authority in decision making, but informal leaders often have the power. To effect any kind of change, one must have a good understanding of both the formal and informal leadership dynamics. For example, if a strong leader pattern prevails, attention should be placed on reaching and convincing the leaders before any attempt is made to contact the target population (i.e., the population in which change is desired).

Decision Making or Problem Solving. It is important to find out how the community approaches its problems and its pattern of decision making. To effect any type of change, one must know not only whom to approach, but also how the community has acted in the past to solve its problems.

What is the decision-making process? Who have been the key decision makers for health issues? How have problems been approached and solved in the past? What problem-solving approaches have not worked in the past? Answers to these questions will provide a basis for determining the action pattern of the community and how capable it will be at solving its problems (Freeman and Heinrich, 1981). They will also give the nurse a clue as to what role is necessary in planning health programs. A community that is quite independent and can function with a minimal amount of assistance will need a partnership role. A dependent community may need the nurse to take a more active and direct role in developing leadership skills of community members.

Social Control. *Social control* refers to the rules and norms of a community that affect behavior. The rules in a geopolitical community usually refer to local laws or control measures, often enforced through police, law agencies, courts, and the government; examples include curfews, speed limits, and "blue laws." In a phenomenological community, the rules are the control enforced by bylaws, policies, and procedures.

The norms in a geopolitical community are social sanctions enforced by the members of the neighborhood and by institutions such as the schools and churches, whereas in a phenomenological community, the norms are enforced by the group (e.g., peer pressure among adolescents).

Communication. *The goal of the communication subsystem is to provide identity and support to its members—that is, to provide a sense of belonging.* People in the community offer group participation in exchange for support and identity from the community.

The communication subsystem refers to the many affective relationships that exist among community members. These relationships provide the emotional tone of the community. Emotional tone is communicated through nonverbal and verbal communication.

Nonverbal Communication. What "personality" or "emotional tone" is communicated to you when you visit the community? Does it feel warm and inviting? Does it feel cold and hostile? How do members describe their community? What are the nonverbal messages being communicated by the community to the external environment and between community members? How are strangers and newcomers treated?

Verbal Communication. Who communicates with whom? Is communication horizontal (egalitarian) or vertical (hierarchical)? How is communication achieved (e.g., by newspaper, television, radio, newsletters, posters, fliers, person-to-person communication, informal gatherings, formal meetings)? What is the focus of the communication? Is it business or goal directed, social, or a combination? When does the communication occur?

Values. *The goal of the values subsystem is to provide guidelines for behavior.* This component addresses the general orienting principles that guide the socialization and behavior of members of the community. Community members accept and conform to the standards of the community in return for approval. It is important to examine patterns of behavior that reflect values, beliefs, standards, culture, and ethnic background (see Chapter 6), as these help to determine the health action pattern of the community. The patterns of behavior that are examined include traditions, presence of identifiable subgroups, aesthetics/environment, health, and homogeneity of the group.

Traditions. Some communities are steeped in tradition, while others have few traditions. Traditions often reflect the ethnic background of a community's members and can also vary with the age of the community. A new, young community may have no or only a few traditions, whereas an older community may have many long-standing traditions. The celebration of traditions often provides a sense of identity to a community's members and stability to the community.

Therefore, when assessing a community a nurse may need to address the following questions: Are traditional ways followed, or is individuality stressed? Are kinship bonds strong, or is each individual expected to cope with his/her own problems? What traditions are upheld? How are they celebrated?

Subgroups. Subgroups may be present within a community. For example, subgroups may exist based on ethnic/racial identity, social class, and age of community members. These identifiable subgroups have their own values, customs, problems, and strengths.

Aesthetics/Environment. Observation of the environment can tell you a lot about what the people value. That is, do they value clean, tidy environments that are pleasing to the eye, or is the environment in decay or disrepair, with little or no attention given to the aesthetics (because the focus is on survival and basic life support instead)?

Health. People vary in relation to the value and priority they place on health. To assess needs and plan health care, nurses must know what the community values in the way of health. Even though health care professionals value preventive health, a given community may not. The people in the community may have some very different ideas about what they want in a health program. If health care professionals do not consider the community's needs and values, then health care programs will not be effective. Therefore, it is important to address such questions as: What types of health facilities are used? How often are they used? What are the attitudes about health, health care, and health care professionals? What priority do members place on health? How is health defined by community members?

Homogeneity. Is the community homogeneous or heterogeneous in its beliefs and values? Communities may be very similar in their values or very diverse. The level of homo- or heterogeneity affects the community health nurse when planning care. In more heterogeneous communities interventions need to be tailored to the various subgroups and aggregates.

Outputs (Health Behavior/Health Status)

Outputs include measurable, health-related behaviors that are exchanged from the community to the environment. This is often referred to as *health status.* The health status of the community includes two interrelated factors: people and environment.

It is important to look at these health behaviors not only at one point in time, but to examine trends in behavior. We will look first at people factors and then at environmental factors.

People Factors. The people factors that the community health nurse needs to investigate include general trends, trends in mortality (death) and morbidity (illness), the presence of vulnerable groups or aggregates with at-risk behaviors, the prevalence of presymptomatic illness, and the level of social functioning.

Growth Trends. The stability and growth of the community have implications for health and health planning. Therefore, it is important to look at the current size of the community and compare it with its original size or size at a particular point in time. Is it growing or decreasing in size? What is the relationship between the birth and death rates (geopolitical community)? What is the relationship between immigration and emigration? What are the changes in demographic characteristics? Is the community becoming a younger or an older population or staying the same? How mobile is the population?

Trends in Mortality and Morbidity. Trends in mortality and morbidity are indicators of a community's health status. The medical cause of death is a valuable indicator. For example, a high infant mortality rate may reflect evidence of inattention to or lack of value for preventive health care and identifies a need to provide preventive prenatal health services. However, medical cause of death alone may be inadequate, because the cause of disease may be related to personal or social phenomena. For example, extreme poverty is a social condition that contributes to the cause of death. In the example just given, the high infant mortality rate may be due to a combination of inadequate preventive health services and malnutrition related to poverty.

Epidemiological questions the community health nurse will want to address are: What are the trends related to death and illness? What is the mortality rate? What are the major causes of death? What major diseases are present in the population? What is the prevalence/incidence of diseases?

Mortality. Consider the number of deaths, age-specific rates of death, and the major causes of death in the community. If working with a geopolitical community, this information can be obtained from local and state vital statistics and health departments. Also, *Morbidity and Mortality Weekly Report (MMWR),* published by the Centers for Disease Control and Prevention (CDC), is available at libraries or by subscription.

Morbidity. It is important to know what diseases and conditions are present in a community and their incidence/prevalence. For a geopolitical community this could be done by reviewing statistics collected officially. In a phenomenological community, one would need to collect data by surveying records, preparing questionnaires, or arranging interviews. In the United States, morbidity data are not systematically collected and so are sketchy and inadequate in scope.

Vulnerable Aggregates/Risky Behavior. What risky or vulnerable types of behavior are present in this community? There may be groups within a geopolitical community who do not have a disease or condition requiring medical care, but do have a personal or social condition that makes them unusually susceptible or lowers their ability to deal with disease or disability. Examples include the homeless, people living below the poverty level, multiproblem families, the malnourished, and pregnant adolescents.

Risky behaviors include behaviors that place people at risk for disease. For example, intravenous (IV) drug use is a risky behavior associated with the human immunodeficiency virus (HIV); cigarette smoking increases the risk of lung cancer; driving without a seat belt is associated with vehicular trauma.

Prevalence of Presymptomatic Illness. What is the prevalence of presymptomatic illness in a community? It is difficult to get precise data on the prevalence of presymptomatic illness, but one can make estimates based on special surveys or screening programs. Some examples of presymptomatic illness are increased blood pressures, increased blood cholesterol levels, and numbers of seropositive HIV individuals.

Level of Social Functioning. What is the level of social functioning in a community? The level of social functioning refers to the quality of life and the relationship of dependency to independency in a community. If a large number of people are dependent on a small number for support or help, the demand on the community for resources is much greater than if the proportion is balanced. People may be dependent for a variety of reasons, such as age, lack of finances, illness, or disability. For example, a community that has a high preponderance of elderly individuals will need more health facilities and services because of the increased medical needs of that age group.

As you learned in the previous chapter, ratios are used to show relationships. A dependency ratio shows the proportion of dependents to independents. An example of a dependency ratio is shown below.

$$\text{Dependency ratio} = \frac{\text{Population under 18 years} + \text{Population over 65 years}}{\text{Population between 18 and 65 years}}$$

To calculate the dependency ratio, add the total number of people younger than 18 years plus the total number of people older than 65 years and divide by the total number of people between the ages of 18 and 65.

For example, Elmhurst has a population of 6784 people. According to the census information, there are 1604 people under the age of 18 and 2422 people over the age of 65. The dependency ratio, therefore, is

$$\frac{1604 + 2422}{2758} = 1.45$$

That means that there are almost 1½ dependent people for each person considered to be able to care for others.

Disabilities and Impairments. Are disabilities or impairments present? These can be physical or emotional. People with impairments or disabilities require special care from the community. Therefore, it is important to identify numbers of people and types of impairments or disabilities to be able to identify whether their needs are being met by the community or further services are necessary.

Environmental Factors. Environmental factors include the physical and the social environment. Indicators of the health status of the physical environment include the air, food, and water quality; the adequacy of housing; and the quality of the home and work site (see Chapter 24). Solid waste disposal and hazardous waste disposal are also relevant.

Indicators of the health status of the social environment include the emotional tone of the community, the stability of the population (i.e., an extremely mobile population or rapid turnover of members in either a geopolitical or phenomenological community can be a measure of dissatisfaction and instability within the community), and the reported quality of life in the community. The quality of life may include personal satisfaction with the community, as well as measures of community competence previously discussed in this chapter.

Feedback

Feedback may be internal or external. Internal feedback is information from within the community itself that helps the community monitor its functioning. For example, if the city council receives information that tax revenues are lower than projected, the city may need to modify its budget and reduce spending.

External feedback is information from the suprasystem and larger environment about a community's functioning. Such information provides an opportunity for the community to modify itself, adapt to changing environmental conditions, and negotiate interchanges with its environment. For example, community health nurses within a local health department may receive information about new state regulations that require directly observed medication therapy for persons with newly diagnosed tuberculosis. Such information would necessitate that the nurses institute these services. Dialogue between nurses in the local and state health departments and with community members would help determine realistic ways to initiate such services. In this case, feedback from the suprasystem mandates that the community institute new services in response to changing regulations.

Tools for Data Collection

Community health nurses can use a systems analysis framework to guide data collection for a community assessment. Where does one go to collect all these data? What tools are needed? A very important tool is the use of self, particularly your senses. Of course, an automobile or other means of travel, a map, and a few resource materials are also very helpful.

SELF

Use your eyes, ears, nose, hands, and body to inspect, "auscultate," "palpate," and "percuss" the community. You can tell a lot about a community just by using your own senses.

- Use your eyes to inspect the community. What do you see? What do the people look like? What are they doing? What does the environment look like?
- Use your nose to smell the environment. Is it pleasant? Polluted? Fresh? Stale?
- Use your ears to "auscultate" the community. What are the people saying? Is the community loud or quiet?
- Use your body to "palpate" and "percuss" the community. What is the "feeling" of the community? Is it warm, open, and friendly or cold, hostile, and suspicious?

During your visit to the community, talk to the people—the community members and leaders, health care professionals, clergy, real estate agents, and business people. They can tell you a lot about the community. Read about the community in newspapers, literature, or printed materials put out by the community or by other organizations. Look for bulletin boards, kiosks, or information centers where community activities and information are posted.

EXISTING DATA SOURCES

National Sources

There are many sources of demographic and epidemiological data already collected. The National Center for Health Statistics, a federal agency established to collect and disseminate data about the health of U.S. residents, conducts the National Health Interview Survey. Many other agencies and organizations collect data on specific diseases, conditions, or aggregates. Table 12–5 provides a listing of some of these data sources. *The United States Government Manual,* available from the U.S. Government Printing Office in Washington, D.C., is a good reference for information about federal programs and agencies that have health data.

The U.S. Census Bureau collects information on the demographic characteristics (age, sex, race, socioeconomic level, marital status, educational level, housing, and morbidity and mortality of certain diseases) of the U.S. population every 10 years. These are very valuable data, but if you are using 1990 data in the year 1998, the data may need to be supplemented with other, more current data. State and local planning offices use a variety of statistical methods to estimate the size of populations between censuses. The census data are helpful for viewing patterns over time to identify trends. Census tract information is available at the reference section in some libraries and local and state health departments.

Many special interest groups collect and publish data about their particular group. For example, the American Heart Association, the American Lung Association, and Mothers Against Drunk Drivers all have publications that provide useful information about the topic and the aggregate characteristics.

Longitudinal research is being done with large populations in several areas of the United States. Although these populations are not national samples, they are large community samples that allow conclusions to be made about demographic risk factors and the long-term effects of various health-related behaviors on morbidity and mortality. Schools of public health are conducting longitudinal epidemiological studies in several communities, including Alameda, CA; Evans County, GA; Framingham, MA; and Ypsilanti, MI. Findings appear in health research and professional journals.

TABLE 12–5

Sources of Health and Population Data*

National Center for Health Statistics, Hyattsville, MD

Vital Statistics of the United States

Compiles detailed statistics at the city, county, state, and national levels on births, marriages, divorces, and deaths. Published in book form approximately 2 years after the reporting year ends.

Monthly Vital Statistics Report

Provides provisional up-to-date tallies on births, marriages, divorces, and deaths on a monthly basis. Data are usually published 3 to 5 months after data are gathered.

Vital and Health Statistics Series

For community health nursing practice:

Series 5, *Comparative International Vital and Health Statistics.* Compares U.S. vital and health statistics with other countries.

Series 10, *Data From the National Health Interview Survey.* A continuing national household interview survey that reports on illness; accidental injuries; disability; the use of hospital, medical, dental, and other services; as well as other health-related topics. Examples:

No. 184, *Current Estimates from the National Interview Survey.* Includes incidence of acute conditions and episodes of persons injured, disability days, physician contacts, prevalence of chronic conditions, limitation of activity, and self-assessed health status. Data estimates are reported by subgroups of population, including by age, sex, race, income, and geographic region. This publication is updated yearly.

No. 180, *Incidence and Impact of Selected Infectious Diseases in Childhood.*

No. 177, *Impairments Due to Injuries: United States 1985–1987.*

Series 11, *Data from the National Health Examination Survey and the National Health and Nutrition Examination Survey.* Data collected by direct examination, testing, and measurement of national samples of population are the basis for estimates of prevalence of specific diseases and their distribution in the U.S. population with respect to physical, physiological, and psychological characteristics. This series has infrequent publications. Example:

No. 241, *Clinical Chemistry Profile Data for Hispanics, 1982–1984.* Published in December 1992.

Series 13, *Data on Health Resources Utilization.* Provides data on the utilization of health manpower and facilities providing long-term care, hospital care, and family planning services.

For advanced practice and nursing researchers:

Series 1 reports describe general programs of the National Center for Health Statistics, its offices and divisions, and the data collection methods used. Reports include questionnaires, surveys, sampling, and other data collection techniques used.

Series 2 reports on data evaluation and methods research.

Series 4 Documents and committee reports. Present the final reports of major committees such as the *Report on Recommended Model Vital Registration Law.*

Advance Data from Vital and Health Statistics

Special Reports concentrating on a specific health issue or topic. Examples:

No. 221, *Recent Trends in Adolescent Smoking, Smoking-Uptake Correlates, and Expectations About the Future.*

No. 218, *Serious Mental Illness and Disability in the Adult Household Population: United States, 1989.*

No. 216, *AIDS Knowledge and Attitudes for January–March 1991.*

No. 201, *Characteristics of Persons with and without Health Care Coverage: United States, 1989*

Health, United States

Annual report presented to the President and Congress. In 1992, the report entitled, *Health, United States, 1992 and Healthy People 2000 Profile* highlighted the status of the 2000 Health Objectives.

Bureau of the Census, Washington, DC

Current Population Reports, Series P-25. Reports on population estimates and projections with local, state, and national summaries.

Current Population Reports, Series P-23, Special Studies. Detailed report on specific issues or characteristics of populations or aggregate groups. Examples:

P23-178 Sixty-Five Plus in America (August, 1992). Provides health, mortality, economic, geographic, and social characteristics of elderly individuals in the United States.

P23-179 Studies in Household and Family Function (September, 1992). Descriptive analyses of the shifts in family composition and living arrangements over the past 25 years.

P23-180 Marriage, Divorce, and Remarriage in the 1990s (October, 1992). Retrospective review and look at current trends related to marriage and fertility of adults in the United States.

Current Population Reports, Series P20. Population characteristics reports for subgroups of the population. Example:

P20-471 The Black Population in the United States (March, 1992). Reports on black Americans, including demographics such as family composition, occupation, income, poverty rates, education levels, percentage of population, geographic distribution, and marital status.

P20-472 Residents of Farms and Rural Areas: 1991. Reports on farm populations and demographic characteristics with respect to geographic distribution, age, sex, marital status, income, and educational level.

P20-463 Geographical Mobility: March 1990 to March 1991. Reports on mobility characteristics of subgroups of population by age, race, education, and geographic location.

Statistical Abstract of the United States. Annual publication of summary statistics on the social, political, and economic organization of the United States. Includes population; vital statistics; health and nutrition; education; health insurance coverage; human services; and federal, state, and local government finances

Public Health Service, Centers for Disease Control and Prevention

Morbidity and Mortality Weekly Report (MMWR). Publishes provisional and summary data on reportable infectious diseases and other health concerns by state. Reports include special topics of health concern related to trends, control or treatment recommendations, and other health-related discussions. *MMWR* is available by subscription. It can also be found at local or state health departments and in some libraries.

*Most states have at least one library designated as a depository for government publications. Your local librarian can refer you to the nearest depository.

State and Local Sources

Chapter 11 defines vital and demographic data. Local and state health departments collect and disseminate information about the vital statistics in their localities. County and city planning and zoning boards often have current demographic data and a list of many resources. Health departments, agency records, libraries, business people, clergy, telephone books, and service directories are all additional sources of information.

Many local areas publish a community resource guide that includes resources within a given geographic area. These books are often written in an annotated bibliography format and are very valuable resources to a community health nurse. Check with the health department or the health and welfare council in your area to see if one is available.

SURVEYS

If you cannot locate sources of data for the community under study, you may need to develop a survey to obtain needed information. This is especially true when working with segments of a geopolitical community where the only data available may be for a larger area than the community segment under study. Surveys are also needed in a geopolitical community when different, more specific information is desired. In a phenomenological community, it may be necessary to develop data collection tools because data may not be available.

Surveys include a series of questions asked by the investigator to obtain information from individuals within a population. Questions help describe the prevalence, distribution, and interrelationships of health and illness conditions, beliefs, attitudes, knowledge, or health-related behaviors within a population (Polit and Hungler, 1993).

The purpose of a survey might be to collect demographic data, obtain information on strengths and problems, conduct a needs assessment, identify utilization patterns of services and facilities, or determine health interests of community members. The survey may be written or verbal. Written surveys can be mailed or conducted on a person-to-person basis. Low return rates and the cost of mailing are the major disadvantages of mailed surveys. Interviews or questionnaires often yield additional valuable information, as there is direct contact with community members. However, surveys, whether done by mail, face-to-face, or on the telephone, are time consuming.

If communities have small populations, it is best to attempt to survey the entire population. When surveying the entire population is impractical because of time, cost, or difficulty reaching the community members, random sampling of the community is recommended (Polit and Hungler, 1993). Random sampling allows the results from the sample to be generalized to the entire population.

Whenever you develop a tool or survey, be sure to first perform a pilot study with a small sample of a "like population." That is, if you are planning to survey elementary school children, have five or six children of the same age complete the survey. The pilot study helps determine whether the survey was tailored to the characteristics of the study population with respect to reading level and the time needed to complete it. In addition, the pilot study can help illuminate any ambiguous or confusing directions or whether there are any questions that allow different interpretations.

Either the survey format or specific questions might need to be altered based on the results of the pilot study. Directions may need to be clarified, the time allowed may need to be lengthened, or the survey itself may need to be shortened. Questions may need to be modified to reduce confusion or to obtain more detailed information.

When conducting a knowledge survey, it would be helpful to know if the pilot group could answer all or most of the questions without a health intervention. For example, if you were planning a health education program on safety and found that the pilot group could correctly answer most of the questions, the value of proceeding with your intervention as initially designed would be in question. You might conclude that no knowledge deficit really exists or that you need to increase the sophistication of the material to be taught.

INTERVIEWS

Interviews with key informants—people in the community and leaders of the community—are very valuable sources of data. These interviews can provide focus as well as a great deal of information. The community health nurse should use every opportunity to interact with the people in the community. They are the richest sources of information about their health status, interests, community problems and strengths, and possible solutions.

COMMUNITY FORUMS

Community forums provide an opportunity to obtain input from members of the community regarding their opinions about needs, services, or specific topics. Forums can be open to the entire community or focused on a small segment or subgroup of the community. The advantage of the forum approach is that it is a relatively cost efficient and effective way of obtaining opinion data from the community.

Focus groups are conversations held in a group with a small number of people (usually seven to ten) to identify different perceptions and viewpoints about a subject (Krueger, 1988). Focus groups are usually held with more than one group to identify patterns in perception. For example, focus groups might be held in a community early in the assessment process to identify patterns or themes

TABLE 12–6

Pros and Cons of Data Collection Methods

Data Collection Method	Pros	Cons
Surveys		
Written	Reliable and valid	Low return rate; costly (i.e., mailing and printing costs)
Verbal (person to person or by telephone)	Good return rate; participants may provide additional information which is valuable.	Time consuming
Interview of key informants	Inexpensive; valuable subjective data that may be difficult to obtain on written survey.	Biased view
Community forums	Provide opportunity for wide variety of community members to supply input on wide range of topics regarding community; may find an otherwise unidentified need.	May be difficult to keep the forum from becoming a grievance or gripe session
Census tract data	Readily available; show trends over time	Collected only every 10 years
Preexisting reports and publications	Readily available; show trends over time	May not include data for specific community being assessed by nurse.

regarding perceived community strengths and health problems.

As you can see, there are many types of data collection. Only a few examples have been used here. Table 12–6 summarizes the pros and cons of the various methods of data collection.

Approaches to Community Assessment

Just as assessment of the individual or family can be approached in a variety of ways, so also can assessment of the community be approached in several ways. The approach taken depends on the type of community and the reason for the assessment.

COMPREHENSIVE NEEDS ASSESSMENT APPROACH

As its name implies, the comprehensive needs assessment is the most thorough assessment of the community; it is also the most traditional and the most time consuming. In the comprehensive approach, the nurse begins with the total community (geopolitical or phenomenological) and uses a systematic process to assess all aspects of the community to identify or validate actual and potential health problems.

PROBLEM-ORIENTED APPROACH

In the problem-oriented approach, the community health nurse assesses a community in relation to a specific topic or health problem. The nurse begins the process with the problem or topic area and then assesses a specific community in relation to that subject. For example, a group of nursing students were very interested in AIDS. They chose the topic and reviewed the literature to identify potential communities with which to work. Although IV drug abusers and the homosexual population might be obvious aggregates or groups to work with, the literature also stressed the need for health teaching prevention programs among adolescents and female sexual partners of IV drug users. The students chose an adolescent population of 11th graders and assessed the population in relation to the topic. As a result of a survey, they determined that a knowledge deficit regarding HIV transmission existed, and a primary prevention program was developed.

FAMILIARIZATION APPROACH

Familiarization involves studying data already available on a community (e.g., census tract data, surveys, or other official data from the health departments). This approach helps the community health nurse focus on special populations (aggregates or groups) that have similar characteristics and may have health needs. Table 12–7 in the geopolitical case study illustrates existing census tract data. From these data one sees that there are many children and adolescents living in this census tract. Having identified the youth as a target population, the community health nurse would focus the assessment on this aggregate.

Analysis

The areas of consideration for data analysis include community strengths, major problems, major health-related problems, current and proposed community action for problem resolution, and the community's pattern of action involving past problems.

In applying a systems analysis to the data, three parameters are used to make inferences about the level of health:

1. There must be congruency between the physical, psychological, and social data and imperatives.
2. The community requires a minimum of energy to function (efficiency).

TABLE 12–7

1990 Census Tract Data for Census Tract 1 in City X (to Use with Geopolitical Community Case Study)

	Census Tract 1	
	Number	*Percentage**
I. Population statistics	7924	
A. Total population		
B. General characteristics		
1. Race		
White	8	0.1
Black	7899	99.7
2. Age (years) by sex		
Males		
Total	3408	43.0
Under 5	548	6.9
5–9	743	9.4
10–19	1280	16.2
20–34	401	5.1
35–54	293	3.7
55–64	89	1.1
65–74	33	0.4
75 and above	21	0.3
Females		
Total	4516	57.0
Under 5	522	6.6
5–9	782	9.9
10–19	1323	16.7
20–34	930	11.7
35–54	701	8.8
55–64	140	1.8
65–74	80	1.0
75 and above	41	0.5
3. Persons per household	mean = 4.48	
4. Type of family		
Total no. families	1586	
Families with children under 18	1363	85.9
Husband–wife families	471	29.7
Families with other male head	42	2.6
Families with female head	1002	63.2
5. Marital status		
Male		
Total (over 14)	1502	
Single	878	58.4
Married	543	36.2
Separated	39	2.6
Widowed	31	2.1
Divorced	11	0.7
Female		
Total (over 14)	2577	
Single	1036	40.2
Married	572	22.2
Separated	582	22.6
Widowed	246	9.6
Divorced	141	5.5
C. Social characteristics		
1. Nativity, parentage, and country of origin		
All persons	7924	
Native of United States	7838	98.9
Native of foreign country or mixed	82	1.0
Foreign born	4	0.1
2. School enrollment	3785	
Elementary	2544	67.2
High school	834	22.0
College	108	2.9

*Numbers may not add to 100% due to rounding or missing data.

	Census Tract 1	
	Number	*Percentage**
3. Years of School Completed		
Persons 25 and over	2217	
No school completed	50	2.3
Elementary, 1–4	194	8.8
Elementary, 5–7	531	24.0
Elementary, 8	333	15.0
High school, 1–3	615	27.7
High school, 4	427	19.3
College, 1–3	47	2.1
Colege, 4 or more	20	0.9
Median school years completed	9	
4. Mobility of residents, 1985–1990		
Same house	3791	50.1
Different house		
Central city	1744	22.0
Other part of SMSA†	72	0.9
Outside SMSA	20	0.3
Abroad	11	0.1
Unknown	2116	26.7
5. Means of transportation and place of work		
Total no. of workers	1620	
a. Transportation		
Private auto (driver)	234	20.6
Private auto (passenger)	245	15.1
Bus	931	57.5
Subway, train	0	0
Walk	102	6.3
Work at home	0	0
Other	8	0.5
b. Place of work		
Inside SMSA	1149	70.9
City X central business district	118	7.3
Remainder of City X	874	54.0
Surrounding counties	156	9.6
Outside SMSA	14	0.9
Not reported	457	28.2
D. Labor force characteristics		
1. Employment status		
Male		
Age 16 and over	1285	
In labor force	832	64.7
Female		
Age 16 and over	2334	
In labor force	938	40.2
2. Occupation		
Total employed (age 16 and over)	1596	
Professional, technical, and kindred workers	90	5.6
Managers and administrators	37	2.3
Sales workers	75	4.7
Clerical and kindred workers	260	16.3
Craftsmen, foremen, and kindred workers	136	8.5
Operatives	365	22.9
Laborers	125	7.8
Service workers	403	25.3
Private household workers	105	6.6

*Numbers may not add to 100% due to rounding or missing data.
†SMSA, Standard Metropolitan Statistical Area.

Continued

TABLE 12–7

1990 Census Tract Data for Census Tract 1 in City X (to Use with Geopolitical Community Case Study) *Continued*

	Census Tract 1	
	Number	*Percentage**
E. Income characteristics		
1. Mean income	$14,220	
2. Source of income		
No. of families	1525	
a. Wage or salary	806	52.8
b. Self-employed	18	1.2
c. Farm self-employed	0	0
d. Social Security	200	13.1
e. Welfare	501	32.9
3. Income below the poverty level		
No. of families	742	48.7
II. Housing characteristics		
Total units	1770	
Vacancy status	6	0.3
Owner occupied	138	7.8
Renter occupied	1626	91.9
Lacking plumbing	9	0.5
Number of rooms		
1–2	21	1.2
3–4	1013	57.2
5–8	734	41.5
9 or more	2	0.1
Median	4.3	
Persons per room		
1.00 or less	1035	58.7
1.01–1.50	534	30.3
1.51 or more	195	11.1
Contract rent (per month)		
Less than $150	21	1.5
$150–199	41	3.0
$200–249	471	34.6
$250–299	489	36.0
$300–349	239	17.6
$350–399	96	7.1
$400–449	0	0
$450 or more	1	0.7
No cash rent	2	1.5
	Number	*Rate per 1000*
III. Vital statistics		
A. Births		
Total live births	140	18
Neonatal deaths (before 28 days of age)	3	21.4
Infant deaths (before 1 year of age)	2	14.2
Premature single live births	20	3
Single live births	140	18
Live births to mothers		
Below 17 years of age	32	4
Below 20 years of age	67	17
Live births to mothers		
With inadequate prenatal care	11	78.6
With less than tenth grade education	33	235.7
Live births to mothers with five or more children	23	164

	Census Tract 1	
	Number	*Rate per 100,000*
B. Mortality†		
Total deaths	36	454
Maternal deaths	1	13
Coronary heart disease	7	88
Cancer	7	88
Stroke	0	0
Diabetic deaths	2	25
Liver cirrhosis	2	25
Influenza and pneumonia	1	13
Drug dependence	1	13
All accident deaths	3	38
Motor vehicle deaths	0	0
Homicide deaths	7	88
Suicides	1	13
Congenital anomalies	4	50
IV. Morbidity: reportable diseases		
Total incidence	498	6285
Tuberculosis (all forms)	2	25
Syphilis	19	240
Gonorrhea	462	5830
Hepatitis B	3	38
Hepatitis A	1	13
Chickenpox	11	139
Mumps	2	25
Rubella	1	13
Salmonellosis	7	88
Shigellosis	2	25
Streptococcal infection	1	13
Lead poisoning	1	13
Bacterial meningitis	1	13
HIV	7	88

*Numbers may not add to 100% due to rounding or missing data.
†Rates not adjusted for age.

3. The health status behaviors must be satisfying to the aggregate or group and to people in the community (University of Maryland School of Nursing, 1975).

Physical imperatives include safe air and water. Nonabusive interpersonal relationships are an example of a psychosocial imperative. For an example of efficiency, communities X and Y have similar health behavior trends regarding the incidence of heart disease in their communities. However, the average length of hospital stay in community X and the cost of treatment are 20% higher than in community Y. From this one can infer that community X is not operating as efficiently as community Y. Similarly, a community may appear to have an acceptable level of health, but community members may express dissatisfaction about the way they are treated at health care facilities. From this one can infer that the community is not functioning up to its capacity because it is not meeting one of the parameters.

It is through analysis of the relationships between the component parts of a system and the system's external environment (suprasystem) that the health status of the community may be determined, its health needs identified, priorities established, and programs planned and implemented. The next chapter focuses on analysis of the data and planning and implementing appropriate interventions.

Summary

This chapter has discussed the study of community as a client system. Before beginning to assess a community, it is essential that the nurse define the community. There are three defining characteristics: people, place, and social interaction and/or common interest, goals, or characteristics. Place is further defined as being of two types, geopolitical or phenomenological.

After defining the community, systems theory was utilized as a basis to formulate a conceptual framework to study community. The model includes boundaries (the defining characteristics of the community); goals; set factors (physical and psychosocial characteristics); inputs, or external influences on the community; throughputs, which are conceptualized as four internal functioning subsystems of the community (economy, polity, communication, and values); outputs, or level of health or health behaviors; and feedback.

Approaches to community assessment, sources of data, and tools were presented. Two applications of the nursing process (one geopolitical and one phenomenological) are presented at the end of the chapter.

KEY IDEAS

1. Community health nurses assess communities to determine the critical health needs as a basis for planning and implementing effective nursing care.
2. A community contains three essential elements: people, place, and social interaction and/or common characteristics.
3. An organized framework for gathering data will help the community health nurse comprehensively assess a community and identify missing information.
4. Developmental, epidemiological, structural-functional, and systems frameworks may be used to assess communities. This text uses a systems framework for community assessment.
5. The first step in community assessment is determining the community's boundaries. The boundaries help the nurse identify which processes and resources are *internal* to the community and which affect the community from the *external* environment, or suprasystem.
6. Influences from the suprasystem and the internal processes of the community may be positive (resources) or negative (demands).
7. For the community health nurse, the process of data collection in community assessment may include observation, interviews, review of community records, reading local newspapers and periodicals, examining government documents, review of the professional literature, and surveys of community members.
8. A community health nurse may approach community assessment comprehensively or focus on a preselected health problem or aggregate.

The following two applications describe a geopolitical community and a phenomenological community. Use the community assessment tool in Table 12–3 to organize the data available for each community. Then compare your assessments with the completed assessment tools included for each of the applications.

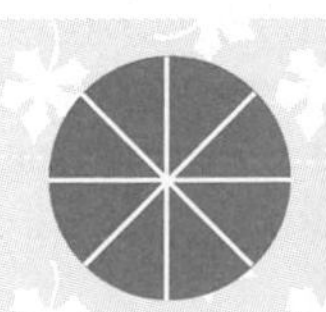

APPLYING THE NURSING PROCESS: *A Geopolitical Community**

Census Tract 1 (CT 1), located in City X, is bounded on the north by First Avenue, on the south by Tenth Avenue, on the west by A Street, and on the east by J Street. Although this CT is zoned for residential use, previously existing stores are allowed to remain but cannot expand. Most people within this CT do not know that CT boundaries exist. Therefore, they do not form any real bonds based on location alone. Neighborhood school yards and recreation centers, a library, a multipurpose center, and

*Adapted from Kidd, C. (1985). *Case study: Geopolitical community.* Baltimore, MD: University of Maryland School of Nursing, Undergraduate Program.

churches help to contribute a sense of community. Several clubs and organizations within the CT also contribute to a sense of community, including various church groups, Boy/Girl Scouts, the urban 4H Club, the senior citizens center, the Young Men's Christian Association (YMCA), Big Brothers/Sisters, and a soup kitchen. Primarily churches within the CT are Baptist, Methodist, or storefront churches. Several church leaders are recognized by this community as community leaders.

CT 1 is located in an inner city. The streets look relatively clean, but some alleys and backyards have litter and broken glass. Stray dogs abound, and there are places for rats to breed. The crime rate is almost twice that of City X. Property crime rates are higher than violent crime rates. A police station is located within the CT, and a fire station is nearby. Emergency medical services are coordinated by the city. A Neighborhood Watch Program has recently been implemented to attempt to reduce crime. This program resulted from combined efforts of the local police, church leaders, school officials, and the city council. City X has a mayor and a city council, with one city council member basically representing CT 1.

CT 1 suffers from moderate air and noise pollution. The major source of pollutants is traffic, which contributes sulfur dioxide, carbon monoxide, and hydrocarbons. Several industries, an airport, and a train station are located within a 10-mile radius of this CT and also contribute pollutants. Residents benefit from both city water and a city sewage system. Drinking water is chlorinated and fluoridated.

In times of need, community members tend to turn to certain people within the community for advice and assistance. These include church leaders, the director of the YMCA, a worker at the soup kitchen, the manager of Paul's Corner Store, and the owner of Gibby's Pawn Shop.

Within the CT are numerous small businesses such as restaurants, barber shops, cleaners, fast-food carry-outs, corner markets, pawn shops, and taverns. Numerous appliance, bakery, clothing, discount department, drug, florist, food, furniture, hardware, hobby, industrial supplies, jewelry, liquor, shoe, and wig stores are located within the CT. Most local stores extend credit but are also more expensive than larger stores outside of the CT. Local food stores accept food stamps. Several large shopping centers/malls are located outside the CT; some are accessible by bus, while others are accessible only by automobile. The CT is part of one school district composed of six elementary schools (grades K–5), two junior high schools (grades 6–8) and one senior high school (grades 9–12).

Two public health nurses (PHN) from the nearby district office of the city health department are assigned to provide nursing services to these schools. One nurse is assigned to the elementary schools, while the other is assigned to the junior and senior high schools. Each nurse spends 1 day (8 hours) per week divided among her assigned schools. According to state law the nurses must follow up on designated communicable diseases and required immunizations as their top priorities. Health problems commonly referred to the nurses include communicable diseases and rashes, minor first aid problems, pregnancy, chronic illnesses (e.g., diabetes, seizure disorders, and asthma), head lice, personal hygiene, and dental problems; requests for birth control information and vision screening are also made.

Occasionally the public health nurse teaches a class or large group on a health-related topic. Within four blocks of the CT is a Head Start Program offering daycare for children aged 2½ to 5 years from 7:00 A.M. to 5:30 P.M. Monday through Friday. There is a waiting list, and families must be eligible on the basis of income.

There are one physician (general practice), one dentist, and one podiatrist within the CT. A Planned Parenthood office is located outside the CT but is accessible via the bus line. The district office of the city health department is located a few blocks from the CT and provides maternity, well-baby, well-child (through age 6), sexually transmitted disease (STD), immunization, and chest radiography services. Home visiting services are provided to home health care clients and to some clients as follow-up to clinic services.

Located next to the district health department is the Inner City Community Mental Health Center, which provides five basic services: therapy, partial hospitalization, crisis intervention, referral to inpatient psychiatric settings, and consultation. The Inner City Nursing Home is a 314-bed long-term care facility that offers skilled nursing care for convalescent, chronically ill, and aged patients. Although it is located near the CT, the occupants of the facility are drawn from a much larger geographical area.

The majority of CT residents utilize one or more of three public and/or nonprofit hospitals. Hospital emergency department (ED) services are used extensively for acute care; hospital outpatient department (OPD) services are used less frequently. These three hospitals accept all third-party reimbursements and "charity cases." Outside the CT but within a 20-mile radius are various other health care facilities including two private home health agencies, six hospitals (some private and some public), and numerous physician and dentist offices (most requiring payment at the time of service). Health- and social-related associations and organizations outside the CT, but providing services to those who need it, include the Agricultural Extension Service, American Cancer Society, American Diabetic Association, American Heart Association, American Red Cross, Association for Retarded Citizens, Birthright, Child Development Center, Childbirth Education Association, Crisis Intervention, Services for Children with Special Needs, Drug Abuse Center, Family and Children's Society, Family Crisis Center, Goodwill Industry, Health and Welfare Council, La Leche League, League for the Handicapped, Legal Aid Bureau, American Lung Association, Meals on Wheels, National Association for the Advancement of Colored People (NAACP), National Foundation, March of Dimes, Poison Control Center, Public Housing Authority, Rape and Family Abuse Center, Right to Life, Salvation Army, United Way, and Vocational Rehabilitation Center.

Table 12–7 presents 1990 census tract data for Census Tract 1. Use these numerical data and the CT description to complete an assessment of this geopolitical community.

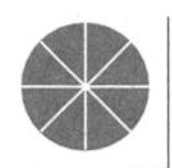

Geopolitical Community Assessment of CT 1

BOUNDARIES

- People: Residents of census tract 1, 7924 people.
- Place: This is a geopolitical community with defined borders:

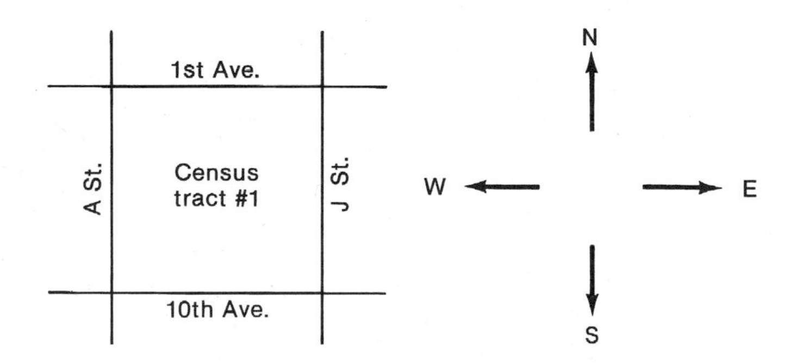

- Common interests or goals: The residents live in the same area.
- Suprasystem: City X. Look at the suprasystem to identify the resources and demands from outside the community (inputs) that affect the community.

GOALS

The goals of any geopolitical community are to promote the survival and maximize the well-being of the community. No specific goals are listed in the description.

SET FACTORS

Physical Characteristics.

1. Length of existence is not identified but could be determined by a review of city history.
2. Demographic data (refer to Table 12-7 for the source of the answers provided in this section):
   - Age: The largest age group is 10 to 19 years old (1280 males + 1323 females = 2603 of 7924 total population, or 33%).
   - Race: Almost exclusively black (99%).
   - Sex: There are more females (57%) than males (43%) in the community.
   - Ethnicity: The community consists of mostly native-born citizens of the United States (98.9% native-born children of native-born parents).
   - Characteristics of housing: Most rent (1626 of 1770 households, or 92%) and live in small housing units. The median number of rooms is 4.3. Most pay between $199 and $299 per month (471 + 489 = 960 of 1626 renters, or 59%).
   - Density of population: The population is rather dense, with an average of 4.48 persons in each household.
3. Physical features of the community: CT is urban, relatively clean, residential and business area.

Psychosocial Characteristics.

1. *Religion:* The two denominations with the most number of churches are Baptist and Methodist.
2. *Socioeconomic class:* This community is poor, with a mean income of $14,220. Forty-nine percent of families live below the poverty level (742 of 1525), and 33% are on welfare (501 of 1525).
3. *Education:* The median level of education is ninth grade; only 3% of those 25 and over have some college education (67 of 2217).
4. *Occupation:* The three largest job categories for workers in this community are service jobs, operative jobs, and clerical positions.
5. *Marital status:* Most of the eligible residents (those 14 years or older) are either married or single. Twenty-seven percent of persons report that they are married (1115 [543 males + 572 females] of the eligible population of 4079 [1502 males + 2577 females]). Forty-seven percent report their marital status as single (1914 [878 males + 1036 females] of 4079). Note that there is a discrepancy between the number of males and females who list their marital status as either married or single. The community health nurse would want to explore the reasons for such a discrepancy to reach a clearer understanding of the marital status of community residents.
6. *Family composition:* This community consists primarily of young families, the majority of which are headed by single females. Thirty percent of households are headed by a husband and wife; 63% are headed by single females. Eighty-six percent of all households have children under the age of 18 years.

INPUTS

	Resources	Demands
Money	No information is given about budget inputs or financial demands on the community from the suprasystem. The community health nurse should attempt to gather additional data on the question.	
Facilities	Inner City Community Mental Health Center	
	Inner City Living Home	Living Home not exclusive to community.
	Shopping centers and malls	Shopping access limited.
	District office of city health dept.	
	Planned Parenthood Office	
	Six hospitals	
	Two private home health care agencies	
	Industry, airport, and train station may provide employment.	Contribute pollutants to the community.
Human services		
Formal	Numerous physicians and dentists	
	All social and health agencies listed at the end of the community description (e.g., Poison Control Center and American Cancer Society)	
	City water and sewer	
	Emergency medical services	
	Head Start Program	
	Bus transportation	
Health information	May be provided by the same social and health agencies listed at the end of the community description. The nurse would need to find out which of these do and do not provide health information and education to the community.	
Legislation	No information is available at this time. However, the community health nurse should be aware of or attempt to discover which city legislation affects the community (e.g., City X Board of Education would determine school policies and plans and direct the activities of all schools in the city, including those in this community).	
Values		Crime rate of City X is less than that of the CT. City X's environmental pollutants affect the community.

THROUGHPUTS (INTERNAL FUNCTIONS)

Economy.

	Resources	Demands
Formal human services	Public health nurses in schools Scouts Urban 4H Club Big Brothers/Sisters Police	Services of school nurses are limited.
	One physician, one dentist, one podiatrist	Not adequate to meet the needs of the community. No daycare facilities, community colleges, or technical schools in the community.
Informal human services	Church groups Number of small businesses that extend credit and accept food stamps	Higher prices in local stores
Facilities, equipment, goods	Schools Churches Recreational centers Library Senior Citizen Center YMCA	No parks or shopping malls Lack of cars for transportation High property crime rate Environmental hazards such as stray dogs and rats
Money	Little is known about this topic. One area to explore would include an appraisal of the money acquired and spent within the community. Because this community is part of a larger city, the budget for infrastructure support would come from the city. Information could be obtained about the taxes collected from residents of this community and that amount compared with the money spent by the city on providing services to the community. Is more money collected by the city than is spent on community needs, or is more money spent on community needs than is collected from residents?	
Education	Little is known about how members are socialized and educated to function productively. It is known that the education level of this community is low, and that many members are below the poverty level. Many of those who are employed are employed in occupations that require little advanced education.	

Analysis of Economy: This community has relatively few resources to meet the health-related needs of its members. It has a relatively weak economy in terms of goods and services, with a number of demands that are not being met. In planning health services for this community, funding would need to be considered. The nurse should explore getting funding sponsors or city funding or should pursue grants from philanthropic and government sources.

Polity.

- Organizational structure: the community is part of City X; it does not have its own organizational structure.
- Leaders: The formal leaders include the local representative to the city council, church leaders, and local business owners. The informal leaders include the manager of the corner store, the pawn shop owner, the worker at the soup kitchen, and the director of the YMCA.
- Patterns of decision making: Because this community is only a portion of the larger city, probably many of the decisions that affect it are made from outside the community. For example, the City Board of Education makes the decisions related to the local schools. Some of the questions a nurse might want to ask to get additional information in this category would include: Does the councilman meet with other leaders and community members to address concerns and problem solve, or does he or she make decisions without community input? How have past decisions been made? The Neighborhood Watch program started with the combined efforts of local police, church leaders, school officials, and the city councilman.
- Methods of social control: In any geopolitical community, the rules are enforced by the police. Norms are established by schools, churches, neighborhood expectations, family standards of conduct, and peer group influences. The nurse would need to interview community members to get a sense of the norms set by the community; no information is available at this point.

Analysis of Polity: This community has a mix of formal and informal leaders, but little is known about the norms representative of the community. The nurse would need more data to complete an assessment of polity. In planning health care for the community, the nurse would be especially interested in discovering which community norms might be compatible with health care or health-seeking behavior.

Communication.

- Nonverbal: Residents feel a sense of community or belonging. There are numerous clubs and organizations.
- Verbal: Informal communication wherever people gather and talk (e.g., the corner store, in churches, and in other group activities). A bulletin board is used to post notices, but it is not known if there are any community newspapers or periodicals.

Analysis of Communication: There appears to be a variety of opportunities for social gathering and exchange of information. There is little evidence to suggest that the community has the capacity to communicate easily with all its members (e.g., a newspaper). In planning health care, the nurse should be aware of the usual avenues of communication within the community so that she or he can use them to gather and disburse information to members.

In reference to communication on health-related matters, the nurse would want to know if community residents express their needs and concerns to health care providers and whether health care providers seek out or listen to community concerns. Do health care providers communicate among themselves? Are they involved in coordinating services? Or do providers determine the care and service needs by themselves? More information is needed.

Values.

- Traditions: There is no information in the description on community traditions.
- Subgroups: There are a number of subgroups and aggregates that can be identified by church attendance, age, and education. With the number of churches within the community, there appears to be a subgroup of individuals who are actively involved in religous practices. The age of the population would indicate that there is also a substantial number of young individuals (< 18 years old) as a subgroup. Single mothers as heads of household are another aggregate, and the median educational level reflects a large subgroup with minimal high school experience.
- Environment: The streets are clean. Back alleys and backyards are littered with debris and glass, providing a haven for rats. There are stray dogs. The crime rate is higher than that in the city, and residents are subject to both property and violent crime. The environment is relatively stark, and adherence to certain laws (e.g., littering or leash laws) is lax. The higher crime rate indicates a community that may contain a higher proportion of residents who are less concerned with adhering to laws related to private property and personal safety than is contained in the city as a whole.
- Health: Community residents tend to rely on community hospitals for their health care needs. The emergency department is used more frequently than the outpatient department, indicating that members place a greater priority on acquiring health care services when ill than on seeking preventive health care. Nothing is known from the data about the residents' attitudes toward health professionals.
- Homogeneity vs. heterogeneity: This community appears to be very homogeneous with respect to race, socioeconomic status, education, and residential maintenance. With the existing high crime rate and the organization of a Neighborhood Watch program, it appears that the community is divided in its attitudes toward crime; however, many residents appear to be concerned about personal safety.

Analysis of Values: Because of the degree of homogeneity, it appears that community members share similar values. Church groups and church attendance are valued, as is parenthood. Community members are moderately concerned about the physical appearance of their property. Education and preventive health care are not especially valued, based on the level of education and the type of health care services used. The nurse would need to consider community values in planning health programs or services to ensure community participation.

OUTPUTS (HEALTH BEHAVIORS AND HEALTH STATUS)

People Factors.

- Size: There is inadequate information to identify trends related to the size of the community. The nurse would need population statistics over several time periods to determine whether this community is growing, losing members, or remaining relatively stable. It is known that the total births during this time are greater than the total deaths. It is also known that a majority of those residents who were surveyed reported that they live in the same home or in a different home in the same general area. The two factors seem to indicate a growing population that is not very mobile but remains within the community limits.
- Mortality and morbidity: The mortality rate is 454 per 100,000 population. The three most common causes of death are heart disease, cancer, and congenital anomalies. The most common communicable diseases are gonorrhea, syphilis, and chickenpox. Several vulnerable or high-risk groups can be identified: pregnant teenagers and their infants, sexually active teens, and poor individuals.
- This community has many young mothers. The nurse can use pregnant teenagers to illustrate some of the presymptomatic illnesses or problems that might be expected in this community: poor nutrition and anemia, inadequate prenatal care, poor self-efficacy, and inadequate family support systems. Why would these problems be expected? The nurse can use research to identify potential problems associated with specific situations. Chapter 22 documents research findings that identify the social and health-related impacts of pregnancy.
- Social functioning: The level of social functioning can be measured by calculating the dependency ratio:

$$\frac{\text{No. of persons under 20} + \text{No. of persons over 65}}{\text{No. of persons age 20 through 64}} \times 100$$

For this community the dependency ratio is

$$\frac{5373}{2554}\left(\frac{548 + 743 + 1280 + 522 + 782 + 1323 + 33 + 21 + 80 + 4}{401 + 293 + 89 + 930 + 701 + 140}\right) = 2.1 \times 100 = 210$$

This community is very dependent on its adult members.

- Types of disabilities or impairments present or expected: Congenital anomalies are known to be the third leading cause of death for this community. The nurse can expect that there would also be a number of infants who survive with congenital health problems. In addition, from the literature it is known that teenage mothers have a greater number of infants with learning disabilities, so this community might be expected to experience this problem. To validate this expectation the nurse could survey families, Head Start, and school officials.

Environmental Factors.

- Physical environment: Housing is crowded and not well kept. The air contains a number of pollutants (i.e., sulfur dioxide, carbon monoxide, and hydrocarbons). The city provides sewer and chlorinated and fluoridated water. We do not have additional information about the quality of the water supply.
- Social environment: The community is relatively stable; many residents have remained in the area for some time, but they are subjected to a high rate of crime and the stress that accompanies concern for personal and family safety.

Level of Health.

- Actual needs: A number of health needs can be identified from the existing data, including congenital anomalies; maternal, infant, and neonatal deaths; sexually transmitted diseases, particularly syphilis, gonorrhea, and HIV; poverty; heart disease; deaths from drugs and cirrhosis; cancer; chickenpox; and air pollution.

- Potential needs: A knowledge deficit about community resources and the unacceptability or inaccessibility of community resources may exist. The ratio of deaths from drugs and cirrhosis suggests that drug and alcohol use is higher than national rates. Congenital anomalies might be related to fetal alcohol syndrome, but more information is needed about the types of such anomalies before this can be determined.
- Community action: Some community action has been taken related to crime reduction, but community action related to health needs is not available. One way to ascertain the community's response to health needs would be to determine how the community has acted to solve other health-related problems, or if it has not acted to solve past health problems. Either way the nurse will have information that will help determine whether the community can effectively address health issues.

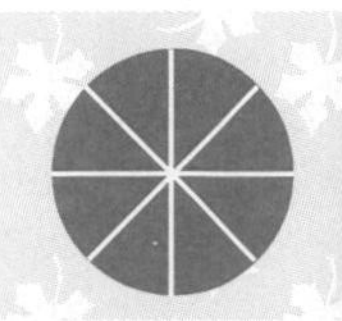

APPLYING THE NURSING PROCESS: *Phenomenological Community**

Northview, a public high school (grades 9–12), is located in Census Tract 1 in City X; it is one of 10 public high schools in that city. Northview school district encompasses all of Census Tract 1. Most of the students who attend Northview walk to school or take the city bus.

The school is a two-story red brick building built in 1953. The building and its grounds, which consist of a parking lot, an athletic field, and a small area of grass, cover one city block. The school is situated between B and C Streets and between Second and Third Avenues. The main entrance to the school is on B Street. When approaching the school, one is struck by the rather stark appearance of the complex—no trees, little grass, mostly concrete—and a moderate amount of litter (paper, broken glass, and beverage cans) around the schoolyard.

The interior of the building is very traditional in appearance. The long halls, lined with lockers on either side, are painted a pale yellow; the floors are tiled, and the windows have grates over them for security. The entrance area next to the administrative offices has a display of trophies won in various sports events, and a kiosk or bulletin board that lists the football schedule and various notices for students, faculty, and visitors. The first floor consists of the administrative offices, health room, counselors' offices, auditorium, music room, gymnasium, cafeteria, kitchen, faculty lounge area, a few small classrooms, and a "common area." Students describe the common area as "their" place. It is located just outside of the gymnasium, so it is also convenient to use when there are ballgames. The area resembles a small teen center and is the only area of the school in which students are permitted to smoke. The second floor consists of classrooms and a large media center. Lockers and bathrooms are on both floors. The bathrooms have a lot of graffiti on the walls but are fairly clean. The classrooms have a traditional appearance, with green chalkboards, individual chairs with arm desks, a teacher's desk, and some visual materials such as posters and signs. In several rooms hanging maps and screens appear to be in disrepair. The classrooms were designed to hold 30 to 35 students. The basement consists of the physical maintenance plant, the science laboratories, and the industrial arts classrooms. The stairways are at the ends of the halls.

The staff at Northview includes the principal, Mr. Johnson; 32 teachers; three full-time and two part-time counselors; a psychologist who visits weekly or when called; a community health nurse from the local health department who spends one-half day per week at the school; a truancy officer who covers three schools; secretaries; cooks; janitors; and volunteers who staff the health room. The teachers are members of the teachers' union and are active in its activities.

The mean age of the teachers is 28 years of age. Most of the teachers are women and have been teaching fewer than 10 years. The student:teacher ratio is 1:26, but this includes special

*From Trotter, J. (1985). *Description of a phenomenological community: A case study.* Baltimore, MD: University of Maryland School of Nursing, Undergraduate Program.

education and resource teachers. The average class size is 35. Each teacher is involved as a home room advisor along with having a regular teaching assignment. The home room is a 20-minute period at the beginning of each day. Each teacher is assigned approximately 25 students as advisees. The home room period serves as an attendance and announcement time, as well as a time for some small group activities.

The enrollment at Northview is 834: 275 ninth graders (140 female and 135 male), 240 tenth graders (122 female and 118 male), 200 eleventh graders (102 female and 98 male), and 119 twelfth graders (61 female and 58 male). The enrollment was 852 last year. The students range in age from 13 to 19; 817 of the students are black, and 17 are of Asian descent. The religion is predominantly Protestant.

Northview is an active school with many organizations, clubs, and activities. Joanne Riley, president of the Parent–Teacher Association (PTA), states, "It is very difficult getting a lot of the parents involved." The PTA meets once a month, and the average attendance is 30. The Student Government Association (SGA) is composed of representatives elected from each of the four classes. They meet weekly to determine student policies and to plan and coordinate student activities. The president of the SGA, Pat Smith, says the biggest problem he sees is that a lot of kids drop out of school as soon as they can. "It's hard to get some of these students involved in school activities. Take Harry over there [he points to a boy standing in hall with about five other students around him]—whatever he says goes with many of the problem kids. Yeah, we definitely have two kinds of kids here—ones who want to better themselves and ones who are here because they have to be." He also says that students are very proud of their football team, which has won the regional championship for the last 3 years. The school publishes a monthly newspaper, *The Viewer,* and an annual yearbook. The school is very active in sports (football, basketball, track, and baseball) and has other activities such as drama club, dance club, chorus, band, and cheerleading. Many of the clubs and organizations have fund-raisers to help support their activities. School dances are held at intervals during the school year, usually associated with special events such as the Homecoming game or Valentine's Day. School-wide assemblies are held during the school day about three times per year.

Because Northview is part of the public school system, it must adhere to certain guidelines set forth by state and local authorities. These include the following policies:

1. All children must attend school until age 16.
2. Students must have at least 20 credits to graduate (one physical education, three social studies, two mathematics, two science, four English, and eight elective credits).
3. All students must pass mastery tests in reading and mathematics to graduate from high school.
4. Each school year must consist of a minimum of 180 instructional days.
5. All high schools in City X are in session from 8 A.M. to 3 P.M., with 30 minutes for lunch.

The budget is determined by the City X school board. Funds for the public schools are tax supported (city and state) and are allocated to schools based on a formula that considers full-time-equivalent students (FTEs). This year the budget was cut in capital equipment areas and in the areas of sports.

The school is organized by departments. Each department has a chairperson who is a faculty member as well as a "team leader." Each team or department makes decisions about how to present the material, but the material must be within the overall curriculum guidelines. All faculty report to the principal. At Northview there are 11 departments: Art, Business, English, Foreign Languages, Home Economics, Industrial Arts, Mathematics, Music, Physical Education, Science, and Social Studies. The physical education teachers are responsible for teaching the health component of the curriculum. Occasionally, the community health nurse will teach a class on a health-related topic.

The community health nurse spends one-half day per week at the school. Because it is not always the same day each week, the school principal announces over the public address system when the nurse is in the building. The nurse then sees students in the health room based on self-referrals or referrals from teachers or other school personnel. The health problems most commonly referred to the nurse include communicable diseases and rashes, first aid problems, pregnancy, chronic illnesses, personal hygiene, dental problems, and eating disorders (obesity and anorexia); requests for birth control information and vision screening are also made.

During a recent visit to the school, some of the following comments/concerns were overheard:

Students:

- "I can't wait until I get out of here. I'm quitting school as soon as I can."
- "I sure hope we win the trophy again this year."

- "My period is 3 weeks late; I think I might be pregnant. Do you know where I can get an abortion? My dad would kill me if he knew about it!"
- "I heard that if you take the pill too long, it does something to your blood."
- "Did you hear what happened to Angie? She got some kind of terrible infection from wearing a tampon. I sure hope that doesn't happen to me."

Teachers:

- "If we don't get our raise this year, I'm quitting teaching."
- "We just can't handle all of these kids unless we get more help in the classroom."
- "I'm really concerned about the increasing number of pregnancies among our girls. Last year there were 38, and there are already 45 this year. It's such a shame—they don't have any way to continue their schooling. They drop out of school before the baby is born, and even though they say they're planning to come back, there's no one to take care of the baby."
- "I really think we need to do something about the increasing number of substance abuse and sexually transmitted disease cases."
- "You know these students don't go for regular health and dental checkups; they only go when they're sick or have problems."

Principal:

- "I'm really pleased about how well our program is working to reduce absenteeism." (Last year the principal and the PTA worked together to identify components of the problem and then petitioned the school board for additional funds for a truancy officer, who works with volunteers to check on absent students.)

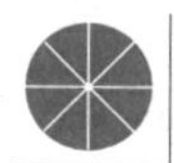

Phenomenological Community Assessment of CT 1

BOUNDARIES

- People: Students (834) and staff, consisting of one principal, 32 teachers, five counselors, janitors, and cooks.
- Place: One city block in City X, Census Tract 1, between B and C Streets and 2nd and 3rd Avenues.
- Common interests or goals: Students' education; for staff, education and employment.
- Criteria for membership: Students must have completed eighth grade; teachers, counselors, and staff must meet the employment criteria set by the school system for their occupation, unknown to us.
- Suprasystem: City X school system and the Board of Education.

GOALS

Education of students, grades 9 through 12. The nurse may find other goals described in the school's written philosophy.

SET FACTORS

Physical Characteristics.

1. In existence since 1953.
2. Demographic data:
    - Ages: Students, 13 to 19 years; faculty mean age, 28 years.
    - Race: Students: 817 black (98%); 17 Asian descent (2%). Staff and faculty: unknown.
    - Sex: Students, 425 (51%) females; 409 (49%) males.
    - Ethnicity: Unknown; predominantly black student body.
    - Housing: Very little information is available about the housing situation of community members; it is known only that this is a city environment. (However, the nurse could observe the housing and review census tract data.)
    - Density of population: Teacher-to-student ratio is 1:35; classrooms are slightly crowded, as they were built to hold 30 to 35 students.
3. Physical features of the community: Fairly young, fairly large student group; traditional school building.

Psychosocial Characteristics.

1. *Religion:* Mostly Protestant
2. *Socioeconomic class:* No data. (The nurse could ask the principal and review census tract data.)
3. *Education:* Students, grades 9 through 12; faculty, presumably college education (the nurse should check this); staff, no information available.
4. *Occupation:* Faculty, teachers and counselors; staff includes secretaries, cooks, and janitors.
5. *Marital status:* No information, but the nurse could expect that most of the students are single.

INPUTS

	Resources	Demands
Money	Taxes fund budget Fund-raisers from PTA	A smaller budget than previous year's budget.
Facilities	There are facilities in the surrounding census tract, but no information is available in this description.	No information.
Human services		
Formal	Community health nurse, ½ day/wk Psychologist Truancy officer	Not full time.
Informal	Volunteers PTA	Probably a lack of resources to assist pregnant teenagers to stay in school.
Health information		City school district does not require sex education courses in the curriculum. Lack of information related to abstinence and birth control.
Legislation	Laws related to attendance, mastery examinations, no. of credits for graduation, curriculum, and no. of instructional days. Immunization requirements for students not described. Union laws for teachers.	
Values of suprasystem	Information related to budget.	Budget adjustments indicate that school board values sports less than the community, and with only ½ day/wk of funding for the nurse, it appears health is not a high priority.

THROUGHPUTS (INTERNAL FUNCTIONS)

Economy.

	Resources	Demands
Formal human services	Principal Teachers Counselors Staff	Fewer teachers than needed based on teacher dissatisfaction and student: teacher ratio.
Informal human services	Volunteers in health room. (Some people would place this resource here, others in "Inputs".)	No resources for unwed mothers. No formal health education program.
Money	No information about amount of money generated within the community. Fundraising within certain clubs. No information on how money is spent.	
Facilities	Description indicates adequate space, classrooms, common area for students, faculty lounge, health room.	Lack of audiovisual equipment. Some equipment in classroom in disrepair.
Education	Mastery examinations are a criterion for productivity. The curriculum appears to provide educational opportunities for students who wish to go on to college, as well as for students who are interested in jobs immediately out of high school (business, industrial arts); further assessment is necessary.	

Analysis of Economy: There is a mix of resources and demands. The community is struggling with budget and personnel problems that affect the provision of services. There are volunteers, and for the most part there are adequate facilities. Any new health programs would have to be inexpensive or require additional fund-raising.

Polity.

- Organizational structure:

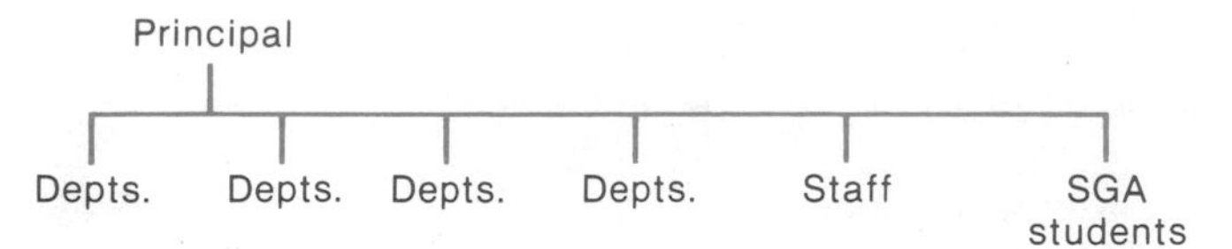

- Leaders: The formal leaders are the principal, the department chairpersons, and the SGA president. Informal leaders include Harry, the leader of the "problem" students.
- Patterns of decision making: Decisions regarding the curriculum are made within the departments following school system guidelines. An example of a past decision is that made regarding absenteeism. In this decision some efforts at democratic decision making were probable, as the principal enlisted the PTA and school board. No other data are available.
- Methods of social control: Rules regarding attendance come from the suprasystem, with the SGA and PTA particularly mentioned in relation to absenteeism. Students are allowed to smoke only in the common area.

Analysis of Polity: The data are sparse, but it seems that there are a variety of formal leaders and only one informal leader. The formal leaders are resources, but the informal leader is not considered a positive leader by the formal leaders. There are norms of conduct and no real information to suggest whether they are being largely ignored or violated, with the exception of absenteeism and dropping out. When planning for health care services, there are a variety of leaders and groups who need to be involved.

Communication.

- Nonverbal: Teachers appear frustrated, while students cannot wait to leave. SGA activity indicates that some students are engaged in school. The school seems to support sports activities, and there are many clubs and student organizations (i.e., Drama Club, Dance Club, Chorus, Band, and cheerleading). There are several special events, such as homecoming, throughout the year.
- Verbal: No mention of school-wide announcements, but there is a bulletin board. The principal has established a task force with other personnel to study the drop-out rate. There is some evidence of democratic or horizontal communication, but most communication appears to be vertical; this needs further exploration. Announcements are made during the home room period, a school newspaper is published monthly, and a school yearbook is published annually. School assemblies are held three times a year.

Analysis of Communication: There is a mix of resources and demands, but many more resources are identified. There are a variety of verbal and nonverbal communication patterns and a variety of planned activities. Low morale would need to be considered when suggesting new health activities. Time would need to be spent empowering faculty and students.

Values.

- Traditions: School dances associated with special events (Homecoming, Valentine's Day) and sports events.
- Subgroups: Student activities groups, sports groups, Harry's group, and the SGA.
- Environment: Window grates for security; trophies displayed; moderate litter on the school campus; common area for student use/relaxation; the description does not indicate that the complex is poorly maintained.
- Health: Facilities consist of a health room, but there is no description of supplies or environment. With regard to attitudes about health care, health priority, and health care professionals, generally students seek crisis-oriented care. Students appear to consider the nurse a valuable resource for health care and information. Some students do not appear to value

preventive care (i.e., there is a need for birth control information, and the pregnancy rate is high). Interviews or surveys are necessary to get additional information.

- *Homogeneity vs. heterogeneity:* The description indicates that the students are racially homogeneous. Socioeconomic status is not known; the nurse would need additional information. Attitudes toward school and education appear to be polarized (i.e., some students are active in school organizations and pursue education, others drop out). No information is available to make an assessment about the staff.

Analysis of Values: The school values traditions, safety, and sports. Students are very homogeneous and therefore are more likely to have similar values than those in another community with more widely variant characteristics. The school appears to be moderately concerned with cleanliness. The health care provider is valued, but preventive health care behavior is not a priority. If preventive health issues are linked with sports, some students may be interested.

OUTPUTS (HEALTH BEHAVIORS AND HEALTH STATUS)

People Factors.

- *Size:* Slightly fewer students than 2 years ago. No additional information is available.
- *Mortality and morbidity:* The number of students enrolled decreases with grade level. There is no information on how many students have died in recent years. There is also no information about the reason for leaving the school or causes of death, if any have occurred. Major diseases and conditions are communicable diseases (specific diseases unknown) and rashes, accidents requiring first aid, pregnancy, chronic illnesses (none specified), dental problems, and eating disorders. There is no information about the incidence and prevalence of these problems.

  Presymptomatic illness or problems that might be expected in students as per the literature include substance abuse; sex education needs; access to birth control; depression and suicide; pregnancy; sexually transmitted diseases; trauma and violence; and communicable diseases such as mononucleosis, upper respiratory illnesses (URIs), and, if population underimmunized, measles.

  Vulnerable or high-risk groups include pregnant teenagers (45 of 425 girls, or 11% [national rate in 1985 was 7% {USDHHS, 1990}]), teenage parents, dropouts, substance abusers (including smokers), and sexually active teenagers.
- *Social functioning:* School attendance is problematic but may be improving, according to the principal.
- *Types of disabilities or impairments present or expected:* Learning disabilities are likely to be present because the school has special education classes. No additional information is available, but a likely source would be health room records and children with individualized education plans related to disabilities.

Environmental Factors.

- *Physical environment:* Appears adequate from the description, except some classes may be crowded.
- *Social environment:* Teachers appear dissatisfied, indicating a stressful environment.

Level of Health.

- *Actual needs:* Substance abuse; sexually transmitted diseases; pregnancy; health information needs related to hygiene, birth control, sexual abstinence; teenage parenting.
- *Potential needs:* Depression, accident rate.
- *Community action:* No information is supplied, but remarks about health-related needs seem to indicate there is little action addressing health issues.

GUIDELINES FOR LEARNING

① Write a definition of community. Does it include the three critical attributes? Does your definition relate more to a geopolitical or a phenomenological community?

② Draw a diagram depicting the communities to which you belong. Do you work or attend school in the same geopolitical community in which you live? How many phenomenological communities are you a member of? In which communities do you receive health care?

③ Interview at least two members from the same community regarding their perceptions of the health of their community members and the community's competence. Compare and contrast their responses. What questions emerge for further assessment?

④ Use the responses in guideline 3 above to begin to develop a survey you might use with more community members.

⑤ Use the community assessment tool presented in this chapter to assess a community. Start by identifying whether it is a geopolitical or phenomenological community.

⑥ Using the demographic characteristics of a community and epidemiological and nursing literature, predict what health problems are likely to exist in that community.

⑦ Suppose that a state survey of public schools indicates increasing rates of alcohol and tobacco use among middle school students. The parents and school administrators deny there is a problem in the school in Community A. As a school nurse, how might you begin to explore whether there is a problem in this community school?

REFERENCES

Anderson, E., & McFarlane, J. (1988). *Community as client: Application of the nursing process.* Philadelphia: J.B. Lippincott.

Archer, S. (1985). *Community health nursing* (3rd ed.). Monterey, CA: Wadsworth Health Services.

Burgess, W. (1983). *Community health nursing practice.* Norwalk, CT: Appleton-Century-Crofts.

Community health faculty, Undergraduate Program, University of Maryland School of Nursing. (1975). *Community assessment tool.* Baltimore: University of Maryland School of Nursing.

Cottrell, L. (1976). The competent community. In B. Kaplan, R. Wilson, & A. Leighton (Eds.). *Further explorations in social psychiatry* (p. 195–209). New York: Basic Books.

Finnegan, L., & Ervin, N. (1989). An epidemiological approach to community assessment. *Public Health Nursing, 6*(3), 147–151.

Freeman, R., & Heinrich, J. (1981). *Community health nursing practice.* Philadelphia: W.B. Saunders.

Goeppinger, J., Lassister, P., & Wilcox, B. (1982). Community health is community competence. *Nursing Outlook, 30,* 464–467.

Hamilton, P., & Bush, H. (1988). Theory development in community health nursing: Issues and recommendations. *Scholarly Inquiry for Nursing Practice: An International Journal, 2*(2), 145–160.

Hanchett, E. (1988). *Nursing frameworks and community as client: Bridging the gap.* Norwalk, CT: Appleton & Lange.

Higgs, Z., & Gustafson, D. (1985). *Community as a client: Assessment and diagnosis.* Philadelphia: F.A. Davis.

Hillery, G. (1955). Definitions of community: Areas of agreement. *Rural Sociology, 20,* 118–120.

Johnson, D. (1980). The behavioral system model for nursing. In J. Riehl & C. Roy (Eds.). *Conceptual models for nursing practice* (2nd ed.). New York: Appleton-Century-Crofts.

Katz, D., & Kahn, R. (1966). *The social psychology of organizations.* New York: John Wiley & Sons.

Kidd, C. (1985). *Description of a geopolitical community: A case study.* Baltimore: University of Maryland School of Nursing.

King, I. (1971). *Toward a theory for nursing: General concepts of human behavior.* New York: John Wiley & Sons.

Krueger, R. (1988). *Focus groups: A practical guide for applied research.* Newbury Park, CA: Sage Publications.

Marriner-Tomey, A. (1989). *Nursing theorists and their work* (2nd ed.). St. Louis: Mosby–Year Book.

McCool, W., & Susman, E. (1990). The life span perspective: A developmental approach to community health nursing, *Public Health Nursing, 7*(1), 13–21.

National Commission on Community Health Services. (1966). *Health is a community affair.* Cambridge, MA: Harvard University Press.

Neuman, B. (1982). *The Neuman systems model: Application to nursing education and practice.* Norwalk, CT: Appleton-Century-Crofts.

Polit, D., & Hungler, B. (1993). *Essentials of nursing research: Methods, appraisal, and utilization* (3rd ed.). Philadelphia: J.B. Lippincott.

Roy, C. (1984). *Introduction to nursing: An adaptation model* (2nd ed.). Englewood Cliffs, NJ: Prentice-Hall.

Schultz, P. (1987). When the client means more than one. *Advances in Nursing Science, 10*(1), 71–86.

Shamansky, S., & Pesznecker, B. (1981). A community is . . . *Nursing Outlook, 29*(3), 182–185.

Spradley, B. (1985). *Community health nursing: Concepts and practice.* Boston: Little, Brown.

Trotter, J. (1985). *Description of a phenomenological community: A case study.* Baltimore: University of Maryland School of Nursing.

Turner, J., & Chavigny, K. (1988). *Community health nursing: An epidemiological perspective through the nursing process.* Philadelphia: J.B. Lippincott.

University of Maryland School of Nursing. (1975). *Conceptual framework,* Baltimore: University of Maryland School of Nursing.

Urrutia-Rojas, X., & Aday, L. (1991). A framework for community assessment: Designing and conducting a survey in a Hispanic immigrant and refugee community. *Public Health Nursing, 8*(1), 20–16.

U.S. Department of Health and Human Services. (1990). *Healthy people 2000: National health promotion and disease prevention objectives.* Washington, DC: US Government Printing Office.

von Bertalanffy, L. (1968). *General systems theory.* New York: George Braziller.

Warren, R. (1973). *Perspectives on the American community.* Chicago: Rand-McNally.

Williams, C. (1977). Community health nursing—what is it? *Nursing Outlook, 25*(4), 250–254.

BIBLIOGRAPHY

American Nurses' Association (1980). *A conceptual model of community health nursing.* ANA Publication No. CH-10, 2M. Washington, DC: Author.

American Public Health Association (1980). *The definition and role of public nursing in the delivery of health care.* Washington, DC: Author.

Braden, C. (1984). *The focus and limits of community health nursing.* Norwalk, CT: Appleton-Century-Crofts.

Bureau of Census (1990). *1990 Census of population and housing.* Washington, DC: U.S. Department of Commerce.

Lyon, L. (1987). *The community in urban society.* Chicago: The Dorsey Press.

Milio, N. (1971). *9226 Kercheval: The storefront that did not burn.* Ann Arbor, MI: The University of Michigan Press.

Rauckhorst, L., Stokes, S., & Mezey, M. (1980). Community and home assessment. *Journal of Gerontological Nursing, 6*(6), 319–327.

U.S. Department of Health and Human Services. (1985). *Report of the Consensus Conference on the Essentials of Public Health Nursing Practice and Education.* Rockville, MD: Author.

White, M. (1982). Construct for public health nursing. *Nursing Outlook, 30*(9), 527–530.

World Health Organization. (1974). *Community health nursing, report of a WHO expert committee.* Geneva, Switzerland: Author.

SUGGESTED READINGS

Anderson, E., McFarlane, J., & Helton, A. (1986). Community-as-client: A model for practice. *Nursing Outlook, 34*(5), 220–224.

Andrews, A., & Engelke, M. K. (1985). Rural home environment assessment: Implications for community health nurses. *Home Healthcare Nurse, 3*(5), 39–44.

Balacki, M. (1988). Assessing mental health needs in the rural community: A critique of assessment approaches. *Issues in Mental Health Nursing, 9*(3), 299–315.

Bausell, B. (1985). A national survey assessing pediatric preventive behaviors, *Pediatric Nursing, 11,* 483–444.

Davis, J. (1986). Using participant observation in community based practice. *Journal of Community Health Nursing, 3*(1), 43–49.

Dever, A. (1980). *Community health analysis: A holistic approach.* Rockville, MD: Aspen.

Finnegan, L., & Ervin, N. (1989). An epidemiological approach to community assessment. *Public Health Nursing, 6*(3), 147–151.

Goeppinger, J., Lassiter, P., & Wilcox, B. (1982). Community health is community competence. *Nursing Outlook, 30,* 464–467.

McCool, W., & Susman, E. (1990). The life span perspective: A developmental approach to community health nursing. *Public Health Nursing, 7*(1), 13–21.

Stein, K., & Eigsti, D. (1982). Utilizing a community data bank system with community health nursing students. *Journal of Nursing Education, 21*(3), 26–32.

Chapter 13

Community Planning and Intervention

Jean O. Trotter, Claudia M. Smith, and Frances A. Maurer

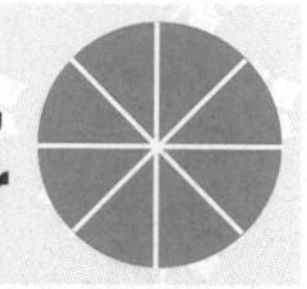

Focus Questions

What is the history of contemporary health planning in the United States?

What are the responsibilities of community health nurses in planning health-related changes with communities?

How do models of community organization relate to health planning?

What principles and steps can assist the nurse and community to develop an effective plan?

What are examples of community diagnoses?

How are priorities determined in health planning with communities?

What is a target population?

What are major types of interventions typically planned by community health nurses?

What are strategies for implementing plans?

Population-Based Health Planning

Health planning is a continuous social process by which data about clients are collected and analyzed for the purpose of developing a plan to generate new ideas, meet identified client needs, solve health problems, and guide changes in health care delivery (Ruybal, 1978). To date you have primarily been responsible for developing a plan of care for the individual client. How do you go about developing a plan of action to meet the health needs of a community? How is it different from planning for the health of an individual or a family? What types of nursing actions and interventions are appropriate for the community?

This chapter introduces the process of planning and implementing *population-based* health care. It describes the components of and steps used in program planning, types of interventions appropriate for the community level, and the responsibilities of the community health nurse in planning and implementing care with populations.

CONCEPTS AND DEFINITIONS

Population-based health planning is the application of a problem-solving process to a particular population. In population-based health planning, communities are assessed, needs and problems are prioritized, desired outcomes are determined, and strategies to achieve the outcomes are delineated.

The persons for whom you desire change to occur are referred to as the *target population.* Planning care for groups or aggregates results in programs, and hence the term *program planning* is often used when planning care at the community level.

Programs may be aimed at primary, secondary, or tertiary levels of prevention. For example, a health education program about safer sex is aimed at preventing sexually transmitted diseases through health promotion measures (primary prevention); a program to screen preadolescent girls for scoliosis is geared toward early detection and treatment (secondary prevention); and an exercise program for stroke victims to limit or minimize their disability is an example of a tertiary level of prevention.

Population-based health planning can range from planning health care for a small group of people to planning care for a large aggregate or an entire city, state, or nation. The planning process described in this chapter is applicable to all types of communities (phenomenological and geopolitical) and to all levels of planning (local, state, national, and international). Health planning can be proactive or reactive. The goal is to use a more proactive approach and for nurses to be an integral part of the planning process.

HISTORY OF U.S. HEALTH PLANNING

The history of health planning in the United States has come full circle in the past few decades. Before the 1960s, health planning occurred primarily at the state level, but beginning in the 1960s health planning was emphasized at the federal level. In 1966 the Comprehensive Health Planning and Public Health Service Amendment (PL 89-749) was passed to enable states and local communities to plan for better health resources. However, problems inherent in the law and inadequate funding allocation for its implementation stimulated further legislation.

The National Health Planning and Resources Development Act of 1974 (PL 93–641) was designed to provide funding for nationwide health planning that would improve health status and care in local communities and attempt to reduce costs. It created a national network of health system agencies and statewide coordinating councils responsible for health planning. The goals of this act were to prevent unneeded or duplicate services, encourage new services based on a regional needs assessment, decrease fragmentation of services, coordinate resources, and reduce costs.

With the 1980 presidential election, the political climate shifted. There was a desire to reduce the size of the federal government as well as the influence the federal government had on states. The Reagan administration proposed eliminating federal planning requirements by 1982 and encouraged states to make their own planning decisions. Currently there is no federal mandate for community health planning; however, the federal health objectives for the year 2000 suggest targets for local communities and states to consider (U.S. Department of Health and Human Services, 1990).

Improved technology and increased life span have resulted in increasingly heavy demands on the health care delivery system. Costs of health care continue to escalate, and the need for long-term comprehensive care is increasing. With these escalating costs, health planning has become economically focused.

Since the 1980s federal legislation has been enacted to decrease the costs of inpatient care. The Omnibus Budget Reconciliation Act of 1980 was enacted to encourage the use of noninstitutional services, such as home health care, to fight escalating costs. The Prospective Payment system (PL 98-12) initiated in 1983 drastically changed hospital billing and altered patterns of inpatient hospital stays. No longer are patients kept in the hospital until they are well; instead, they are kept only until they are "stable." It has become a "treat-them-and-street-them" philosophy of care (Trotter, 1987).

The second half of the 1980s brought federally mandated budget control and cutbacks of domestic spending through the Gramm-Rudman Balanced Budget and Deficit Control Act of 1985. It is a challenge to all health care professionals to plan and implement cost-effective health care programs, programs that truly meet the needs of the people they serve. There is no room for waste or fragmentation. Health care professionals must find ways to meet the challenge, and nurses must become more cognizant of the health care planning process and their role within it.

The 1992 presidential election offered new opportunities for nurses to be involved in efforts to reform the nation's health care system (American Nurses' Association, 1991). Debate continues about the degree to which government should be involved in health planning and whether federal or state planning is preferred (see Chapter 3). Some states have passed their own health care legislation ensuring access to health care and identifying standard health benefit packages. The focus of these planning efforts has been on access to health care and financing mechanisms.

Health care planning for specific geopolitical communities continues at the state and local levels. Community health nurses are involved with specific communities to assess community needs, explore how the *Healthy People 2000* objectives apply to specific geopolitical or phenomenological communities, and develop plans to meet the health care needs of the people.

RATIONALE FOR NURSING INVOLVEMENT IN THE HEALTH PLANNING PROCESS

Florence Nightingale and Lillian Wald pioneered health planning based on an assessment of the health needs of the communities they served (see Chapter 2). Also, nurses have long been involved in implementing programs planned by other disciplines. Both the American Nurses' Association (1980) and the American Public Health Association (1980) state that the primary responsibility of community health nurses is to the community or population as a whole and that nurses must acknowledge the need for comprehensive health planning to implement this responsibility. Both professional organizations identify program planning as a primary function of the community health nurse.

In addition to mandates from professional organizations, there are several reasons nurses should be involved in program planning. Nurses make up more than one third of all health care workers in the United States and implement the majority of health care programs. Our involvement in numerous and diverse health programs has given us experience in seeing what works and what does not. This experience helps to identify difficulties that can be avoided in the future.

Nurses spend a greater amount of time in direct contact with their clients than any other health care professionals. We are with the clients in the community, gaining first-hand information about their health, their lifestyles, their needs, and what it is like to be a member of that community. This exposure to the community places us in the unique position of possessing valuable information useful to the planning and implementation of successful health programs.

Not only do nurses make up a large portion of health care providers, they are also a large portion of health care consumers in the United States. With the emphasis on consumer participation in health planning, nurses are in a unique position to make an impact in the planning of population-focused health programs.

NURSING ROLE IN PROGRAM PLANNING

Planning for change at the community level is more complex than that at the individual level. There are more components to the client system and more people and more complex organizations involved. Therefore, community health planning often takes a multidisciplinary approach, which requires excellent teamwork and thorough communication. The roles of collaborator, coordinator, and facilitator are very important when working with the community as client.

It is necessary to *collaborate* with people from the community to validate nursing diagnoses made from the assessment; to plan *with,* not *for* the community; and to enlist community members' support and assistance in implementing change. If the community is not involved from the very beginning, the program may not be effective. Just as you will have better compliance and outcome from planning care with an individual client, so, too, you will have a more successful program if you involve the community in the assessment and planning phases.

The *coordinator* role emerges when working with a variety of community members and organizations within and outside of the community. The nurse is in a key position to coordinate the activities and *facilitate* the community's ability to achieve a higher level of health. However, to affect change at the community level, one must understand community organization.

Planning for Community Change

To effectively plan and implement programs at a community level, it is important for the community health nurse to understand how the community works, how it is organized, who are its key leaders, how the community has approached similar problems, and how other programs have been introduced in the past. The role of the health care professional who is facilitating the community organization process with regard to a specific health need or problem is one of working with the community members. To be an effective change agent in applying the nursing process, the nurse must be aware not only of the community and how it works, but also of methods of community organization that facilitate change.

COMMUNITY ORGANIZATION MODELS

According to Rothman (1978), there are three models of community organization practice designed to facilitate change in a community: community development, social planning, and social action. The three models can be used separately or in combination. Although they are presented here in pure form, in reality they are generally combined. Social planning is the model most used by community health nurses and other public health care practitioners since the 1970s. However, community development approaches used by Lillian Wald and others during the 19th century, as well as during the 1960s, are reemerging as models for community empowerment.

Each model contains four components: goals, strategy, practitioner role, and medium of change. Table 13–1 summarizes the salient points from each of the three models. A thorough understanding of the components is necessary in planning for change in a community. Each model involves community change.

Community Development Model

The community development model is an approach designed to create conditions of economic and social progress for the whole community and involves the community in active participation. The community development approach is also referred to as the *locality development approach* because of its work within the community. The community/locality development model is a "grass roots" approach that uses a democratic decision-making process, encourages self-help, seeks voluntary cooperation from the members, and develops leadership within the group (Milio, 1971). In this approach, community members believe they have some control over their destiny and therefore become actively involved. The change strategy is characterized by "We know we have a problem, let's get together and discuss it." The theory underlying this model is that if people are involved in determining their own needs and desires, they will become more active in solving their problems than if someone else comes in and solves the problems for them. If they are more active in working out solutions to their own problems, they will be more satisfied with the solution and will continue to expend energy to make it work. That is, if they are "vested" in the solution, they will have more of a commitment to it.

This approach, then, has the potential of having the longest lasting effect of the three models to be discussed. However, it is also the most time consuming to initiate, because it takes time to discuss the problems, to make decisions democratically, and to develop leadership within the group that will be able to sustain the program. Therefore, even though the community/locality development approach to community organization is successful, it may not always be used in pure form because of the amount of time it takes to accomplish the action.

Social Planning Model

The social planning approach emphasizes a process of rational, deliberate problem solving to bring about controlled change for social problems. This is an "expert" approach in which knowledgeable people (experts) take responsibility for solving problems. The degree of community involvement may be very small or very great. (The greater the involvement, the more successful the outcome will be.) The social planning approach is characterized by "Let's get the facts and proceed logically in a systematic

TABLE 13–1

Three Models of Community Organization Practice According to Selected Practice Variables

Variables	Community Development	Social Planning	Social Action
Goal categories of community action	Self-help; community capacity and integration (process goals)	Problem solving with regard to substantative community problems (task goals)	Shifting of power relationships and resources; basic institutional change (task or process goals)
Basic change strategy	Broad cross section of people involved in determining and solving their own problems	Fact gathering about problems and decisions on the most rational course of action	Crystallization of issues and organization of people to take action against "enemy" targets
Salient practitioner role	Enabler-catalyst; coordinator; teacher of problem-solving skills and ethical values	Fact gatherer and analyst; program implementer; facilitator	Activist-advocate; agitator; broker; negotiator; partisan
Medium of change	Manipulation of small task-oriented groups	Manipulation of formal organizations and of data	Manipulation of mass organizations and political processes

From Rothman, J. (1978). Three models of community organization practice. In Cox, F., Erlich, J., Rothman, J., & Tropman, J. (Eds.). *Strategies of community organization: A book of readings* (pp. 25–45). Itasca, IL: Peacock Publications.

manner to solve the problem." Pertinent data are considered before decisions are made about a feasible course of action to meet the need.

Agencies and organizations frequently use this approach as they attempt to bring about desired change. The legislative and regulatory process is one example of a social planning approach. Problems are identified; data are collected; and bills are introduced into local, state, or national legislative bodies to effect change.

The social planning approach can be very effective, but it has one major pitfall: the potential for lack of community involvement. Much money has been spent and many health programs have failed because experts have planned programs *for* rather than *with* the community. It is important for the health planners, the nurse experts, to develop a partnership with the community for effective health care planning.

Social Action Model

The social action approach is a process in which a direct, often confrontive action mode seeks redistribution of power, resources, or decision making in the community and/or a change in the basic policies of formal organizations. In this approach one group of people or segment of an organization or community is feeling "oppressed," and the organization or community is viewed as needing basic changes in its institutions or practices. Aggressive actions may be taken to facilitate these changes. This approach, which is direct and often confrontive and radical, may be characterized as "Let's organize to rectify an imbalance of power." In the 1960s the social action approach was used a great deal. The civil rights movements and protests against the Viet Nam War were examples of the social action approach. Current examples include welfare rights organizations and advocacy groups for the homeless, as well as some antiabortion groups.

Change Theory

Each of the community organization models involves change. Change can be threatening and stressful or exciting and rewarding. Understanding some theory about planned change will provide a guide to use in the planning process.

Lewin describes change as being a three-stage process: unfreezing, moving, and refreezing (cited in Dever, 1980). In the first stage, unfreezing, a need for change is felt. The stimulus for the perceived need may be within the client or come from an outside force. A disequilibrium exists or is created, making a disruption in the status quo (unfreezing), and change is initiated. Moving, the second stage of the change process, occurs when the proposed change is tried out by the people involved, old actions are questioned, and attitude changes occur, creating movement toward acceptance of the proposed change. This is a vulnerable time for the people involved, because change is threatening and anxiety producing. They will need help and support while trying out the proposed change. Refreezing, the third stage of the change process, occurs when the change is established and accepted as a permanent part of the system. Stabilization of the situation occurs. Lewin also describes forces that facilitate (driving forces) or impede (restraining forces) change. Driving forces must exceed restraining forces for change to occur.

Structures for Health Planning

Several structures or schemes have been developed by national organizations to help communities plan for improving their health. These structures encourage collaborative partnerships and comprehensive assessments as building blocks for community health planning.

Planned Approach to Community Health (PATCH) is a program initiated by the Centers for Disease Control and Prevention (Association for the Advancement of Health Education [AAHE], 1992). PATCH attempts to engage entire geopolitical communities in a comprehensive assessment of their health needs rather than focusing solely on high-risk groups or those served by a specific health institution. PATCH depends on the participation of citizens; the cooperation of several organizations within the community; and vertical integration of local, state, and federal government resources.

The Institute of Action Research for Community Health (IARCH) at the University of Indiana School of Nursing is helping cities in the United States adopt The World Health Organization's Healthy Cities project (Flynn et al., 1992; World Health Organization, 1991). The Healthy Cities project seeks to promote the health of urban communities through developing local leadership, innovative health programs, and effective coordination of resources (World Health Organization, 1991). IARCH (1993) publishes a quarterly newsletter, *CITYNET*, that helps cities exchange information about their strategies and successful projects.

Assessment Protocol for Excellence in Public Health (APEX-PH) (1991) is a planning workbook published by the National Association of County Health Officials especially for use by local health departments in planning with geopolitical communities. APEX-PH is discussed in more detail in Chapter 30.

Healthy Communities 2000: Model Standards (American Public Health Association, 1991) is a publication designed to help individuals, local health departments, and community planning groups tailor the *Healthy People 2000* objectives to the needs and resources of a specific community. These objectives were introduced in Chapter 2, and examples are provided throughout the text relative to specific community health problems. *Healthy Communities 2000* was developed under the direction of representatives from several public health associations and the U.S. Public Health Service. Two nurses were a part of the work group, and drafts of the document were circulated for review by community health nurses and other public health professionals. The document reprints the *Healthy People 2000* objectives, including national criteria and target populations. It also includes additional objectives that assist the community to decide how to attain the desired health outcomes, as well as indicators that can be used to measure achievement of the objectives. Figure 13–1 illustrates the format of the document.

Steps of Program Planning

The planning process consists of a series of specific steps. Although each of these steps is necessary, the steps do not have to occur in the exact sequence given. Occasionally several steps may be undertaken simultaneously, or they may occur in a slightly different order. Identification of the planning group may occur much earlier in the sequence. The steps are as follows:

1. Assessment
2. Analysis of data
3. Diagnosis

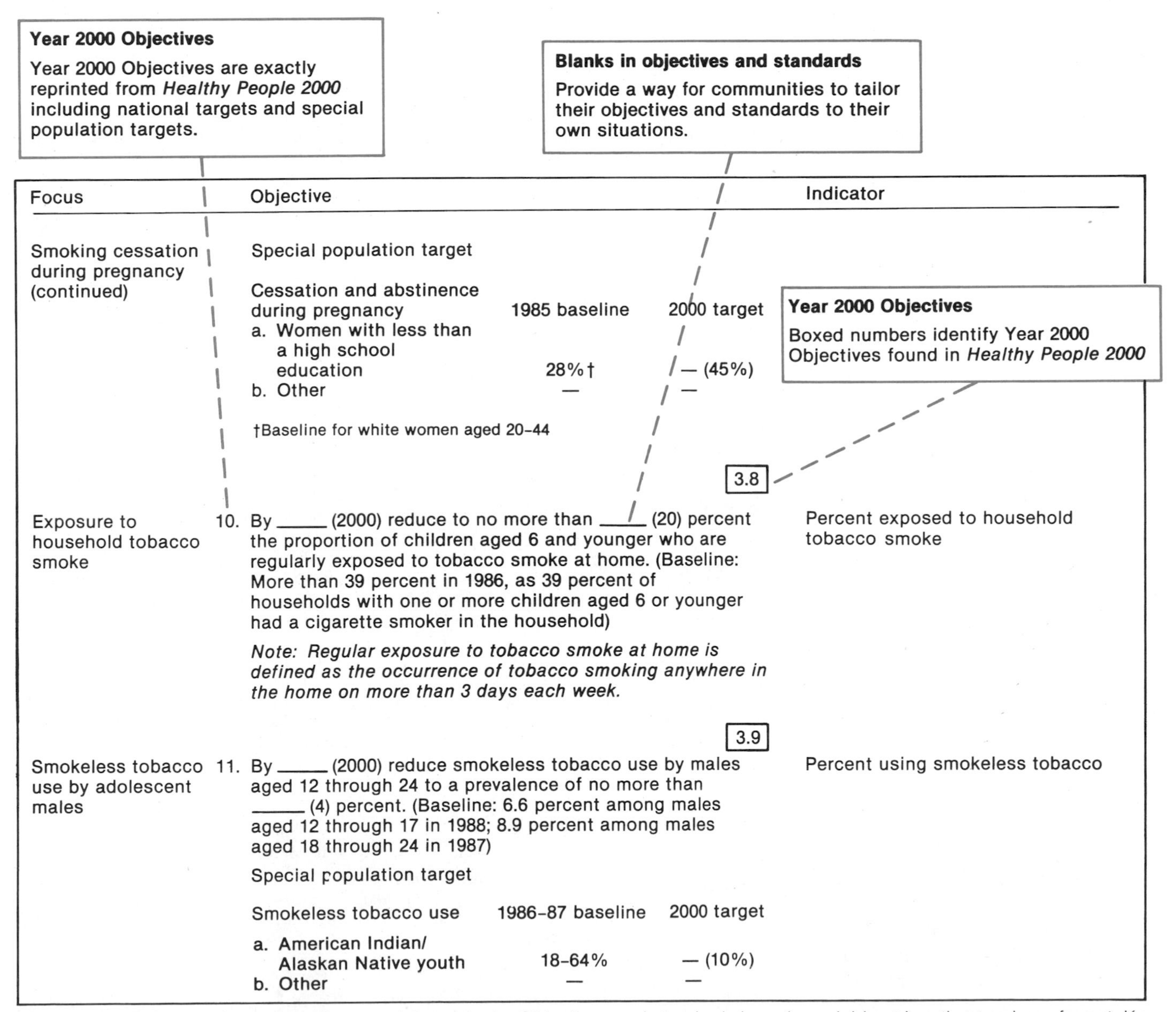

Figure 13–1 ● Quick reference guide to model standards. Objectives and standards have been laid out in a three-column format. Key features are explained in insets. (Redrawn from American Public Health Association. (1991). *Health communities 2000—Model standards: Guidelines for community attainment of the year 2000 objectives* (pp. xxx–xxxi). Washington, DC: Author.)

Continued

Categories for objectives and standards

Objectives and standards have been organized in each Priority Area using the following categories:
- Health status
- Risk reduction
- Services and protection
- Community surveillance

Model standards

Community-oriented objectives to give guidance for how to achieve objectives suggested in *Healthy People 2000.*

Services and protection objectives

3.14

Community planning	13. By ____ (2000) the community will develop a plan (increase to 50 the number of states with plans) to reduce tobacco use, especially among youth. (Baseline: 12 states in 1989)	Existence of plan Documented implementation of plan
Citizen involvement	14. By ____ the community will have a broad-based coalition that meets on a regular basis to plan and implement programs to reduce tobacco-related deaths and morbidity.	a. Existence of a coalition with a defined structure and membership b. Presence of a plan for coalition activities c. Records of coalition activities and programs implemented d. Defined process for evaluation of coalition activities and programs
Tobacco use prevention and cessation programs	15. By ____ the community will be served by tobacco use prevention and cessation programs, including: a. Public information campaigns	Presence in community of: a. Public information campaigns b. Health provider education programs
Tobacco use prevention and cessation programs (continued)	b. Health provider education, referral, and cessation programs c. School health education programs d. Other community intervention strategies	c. Patient education programs d. Telephone "hotline" and referral services e. School tobacco and health education programs f. Inventory of appropriate community resources g. Programs targeted for community-specific special populations

Focus information

Provides a way for readers to quickly identify topics of interest.

Indicators

Suggest measures for achievement of objectives and standards.

Figure 13-1 Continued ● See legend on previous page.

4. Validation
5. Prioritization of needs
6. Identification of the target population
7. Identification of the planning group
8. Establishment of the program goal
9. Identification of possible solutions
10. Identification of alternative solutions
11. Identification of resources
12. Selection of the best intervention strategy
13. Delineation of specific objectives
14. Delineation of the intervention work plan
15. Planning for program evaluation

Steps 8 through 15 are called *operations planning* by some (Hale et al., 1994).

ASSESSMENT

A thorough, accurate assessment of the community is the first essential step in program planning. Adequate assessment of the community will provide clues to determine the importance of the need and the appropriateness of the intervention to the community. The information presented in Chapter 12 provides a framework for community assessment and assessments of a geopolitical and a phenomenological community.

ANALYSIS OF DATA

A systematic analysis of the data collected is necessary to identify the problems, needs, strengths, and trends in the community. It is always helpful to categorize the data first to identify the inferences that are descriptive of actual and/or potential health problems. The community assessment described in Chapter 12 provides a framework in which to categorize the data about community functioning. Within each subsystem nurses identify resources (strengths) and demands (weaknesses), looking not only at whether something is present, but also to what extent, how it is working, and how it relates to the past and future to provide an idea of trends over time. Nurses also consider the health status of the population.

In addition to illustrating the community's strengths and weaknesses, an analysis will provide information about demographic and personal characteristics, which are important to consider when planning and implementing health programs. For example, if you are working with a group of senior citizens enrolled in a senior center and your assessment indicates that there is a potential risk for injury by fire, what other factors would you look for in the assessment data before you plan a fire prevention program? One factor that comes to mind is the educational level. Knowing the educational level provides you with information about the appropriate level at which to plan the teaching interventions. The level of disability and social functioning indicates whether there are visual or hearing impairments that might affect the type of teaching strategy you use. Also, if many seniors are in wheelchairs or need assistive devices, you would focus the program on fire safety involving limited mobility and would need to modify practice sessions to the participants' level of ability. In other words, analysis of community data provides information not only about what is needed, but also about what will be appropriate in the intervention.

Ways to Display Data for Analysis. As shown in Chapter 11, there are a variety of ways to display data, which aids in the analysis process. Graphs, charts, histograms, and mapping techniques are some of the most common visual displays.

It is important to obtain as much data as possible specific to the target population. Table 13–2 includes the age and sex of people living in Census Tract 1 and City X. Census Tract 1 data are included in City X totals, but as can be seen, Census Tract 1 is quite different from City X. The population of the census tract is younger than the total city population, and data from the city cannot be used to describe the residents of the census tract. If you looked at City X data only and thought the data would apply specifically to Census Tract 1 this would not be accurate.

TABLE 13–2

Comparison of Age by Sex of Populations in Census Tract 1 and City X, 1990

	Census Tract 1		City X	
Statistic	*Number*	*Percentage*	*Number*	*Percentage*
Total population	7924	100	905,759	100
Age by sex (years)				
Males				
Total	3408	43.0	427,467	47.2
Under 5	548	6.9	38,512	4.3
5–9	743	9.4	44,204	4.9
10–19	1280	16.2	84,037	9.3
20–34	401	5.1	85,373	9.4
35–54	293	3.7	95,793	10.6
55–64	89	1.1	41,788	4.6
65–74	33	0.4	25,938	2.9
75 and above	21	0.3	11,822	1.3
Females				
Total	4516	57.0	478,292	52.8
Under 5	522	6.6	37,567	4.1
5–9	782	9.9	43,502	4.8
10–19	1323	16.7	86,668	9.6
20–34	930	11.7	95,611	10.6
35–54	701	8.8	108,122	11.9
55–64	140	1.8	48,920	5.4
65–74	80	1.0	36,165	4.0
75 and above	41	0.5	21,737	2.4

DIAGNOSIS

After analyzing the data, it is time to make a definitive statement (diagnosis) stating what the problem is or the needs are. Nursing diagnoses for communities may be formulated regarding

- Inaccessible and unavailable services
- Mortality and morbidity rates
- Communicable disease rates
- Specific populations at risk for physical or emotional problems
- Health promotion needs for specific populations
- Community dysfunction
- Environmental hazards (American Nurses' Association, 1986).

The format of the problem statement varies depending on the philosophy of the agency conducting the assessment. For example, problems or needs may be stated very simply in epidemiological terms, such as "a high rate of adolescent pregnancies," whereas other times you may be asked to state the problem or need as a nursing diagnostic statement.

Nursing diagnosis is a relatively new aspect of nursing practice that has evolved since 1973 as a result of the efforts of the North American Nursing Diagnosis Association (NANDA, 1991). The initial NANDA classification system of nursing diagnoses focused on the physical needs of individual clients and was severely criticized because it was not applicable to the family and community situations faced by community health nurses (Hamilton, 1983; Muecke, 1984). Over the years the NANDA classification system has expanded to include biological-psychological-social needs of individuals and families but is still criticized by many for not adequately addressing the community as client. The most recent effort of the National Group for the Classification of Nursing Diagnosis has been the emergence of a taxonomy of nursing diagnoses into 11 functional health patterns (Gordon, 1982). Tools have been developed to assess the community using the functional health pattern typology (Gikow and Kucharski, 1987; Wright, 1985).

Other classification systems have been developed in an attempt to address the community. One example is the Omaha Classification System, written by community health nurses for community health nursing practice. It was designed by the Omaha Visiting Nurse Association and is especially applicable to the home setting because it focuses on physiological and psychosocial problems, but also considers more environmental and community factors than are considered in the NANDA system (Martin and Scheet, 1993).

Because community health nursing is concerned with health promotion, others have developed ways to add wellness diagnoses to the problem-focused diagnoses of NANDA. Neufield and Harrison (1990) recommend that wellness nursing diagnoses for aggregates and groups include three components: the name of the specific target population, the healthful response desired, and related host and environmental factors. For example:

> high school students with children have the potential for responsible parenting; this potential is related to a desire to learn about child development (host factor) and the presence of a family life education curriculum and an availability of teachers (environmental factor).

Currently, there is a move to develop nursing diagnoses pertinent to the community as client; these may eventually be incorporated into the NANDA classification scheme and accepted by the National Group for the Classification of Nursing Diagnosis. It is hoped that this can be achieved and that separate schemes, which would further divide nursing specialties, can be avoided.

How does one formulate a community-focused nursing diagnosis? A diagnosis is a statement that synthesizes assessment data. It is a label that describes a situation (state) and implies an etiology (reason). A nursing diagnosis limits the diagnostic process to those diagnoses that represent human responses to actual or potential health problems that are within the legal scope of nursing practice (Anderson and McFarlane, 1988).

There are three components to a nursing diagnosis: a descriptive statement of the problem, response, or state; identification of factors etiologically related to the problem; and signs and symptoms that are characteristic of the problem (Carpenito, 1993).

Using this information, let us take a moment to try to state nursing diagnoses for some problems on the community level.

Situation 1

Howard County is a suburban county with a rapidly increasing number of elderly people. The assessment data indicate the presence of only one taxicab company serving that area. There is no public bus system.

Obviously, the problem is lack of transportation, but how might this be worded in nursing diagnosis format?

Suggestion

Inadequate transportation services for senior citizens of Howard County related to:

- lack of funds for public transportation

or

- recent increase in the population age 60 years and more.

The same diagnosis can be rewritten to be more consistent with the NANDA classification:

> Altered health-seeking behaviors related to inadequate transportation services for senior citizens.

However, inadequate transportation probably also affects other areas of seniors' lives such as socialization and community participation. If this were validated through further assessment, an additional diagnosis might be:

Impaired social interactions related to inadequate transportation for senior citizens.

Situation 2

Students in Johnson High test very low on an acquired immunodeficiency syndrome (AIDS) awareness survey. Further investigation reveals that no information is provided to the students, and the parents do not want information taught in the school. Ninety-eight percent of the students stated that they do not believe they are in any danger of getting human immunodeficiency virus (HIV).

Suggestion

Lack of knowledge about AIDS in high school students related to:

- inadequate information provided in school curriculum
  or
- parental attitudes about the disease
  or
- perceived perception that they are not at risk for the disease.

Situation 3

Assessment data indicate that a high number of children at Little Joy Daycare Center have low hematocrit levels and median household incomes less than $12,000. Both parents and children scored very low on a nutrition game.

Suggestion

High prevalence of low hematocrit levels among children at Little Joy Daycare Center related to:

- lack of information about foods high in iron
  or
- low median household income of families whose children attend Little Joy Daycare Center.

This diagnosis can also be rewritten to be more consistent with NANDA:

Altered health maintenance among children at Little Joy Daycare Center related to lack of knowledge about foods high in iron and low median household income.

VALIDATION

It is important to validate data and nursing diagnoses with the community. Do community members really see this as a problem? If so, do they desire a solution? Or have they adjusted to the problem and therefore may be resistant to change? For example, people living in a run-down housing area in a large city are offered better housing in a new project. However, many people choose to remain where they are rather than leave their friends and move to a strange environment. They have adapted to the problem and are, for a variety of reasons, resistant to possible solutions. The restraining forces (friendships and fear of the unknown) are greater than the driving forces (desire for newer housing). Many programs have failed because the professionals planned care based on their own values and perceptions of the problem and did not validate clients' perceptions of the problem and their desire for change. Perhaps if the residents had been involved in the decisions to move together, there would be less resistance.

How is validation with the community carried out? Validation may be done in a variety of ways. You might choose to use a questionnaire, conduct a personal interview, and/or make appointments with key community leaders or informants. Also, community members need to be included in planning groups.

PRIORITIZATION OF NEEDS

The community assessment identifies needs and problems. However, not all needs can be met simultaneously; priorities must be determined. Prioritization can be based on many factors, such as the seriousness of the problem, the desires/concerns of the community, time, cost, and availability of resources. Obviously a life-threatening situation, such as a nuclear spill, will have priority over other less life-threatening situations. The American Public Health Association has identified the first five of the following six factors to consider when determining priority of health needs at the community level (American Public Health Association, 1961).

1. Degree of community concern.
2. Extent of existing resources for dealing with the problem (e.g., time, money, equipment, supplies, facilities, human resources).
3. Solubility of the problem.
4. Need for special education/training measures.
5. Extent of additional resources and policies needed.
6. Degree to which community health nursing can contribute to the planning process.

When attempting to prioritize the community's needs, it is important to use your assessment data and the nursing literature to answer questions such as: How concerned is the community? Are there enough resources to deal with the problem? Is it possible to solve the problem? What additional education and training measures, if any, will be needed to solve the problem? What additional resources will be needed? Are there any existing policies that need to be changed or modified for the problem to be solved? Are community health nurses likely to be effective? It is possible that after answering these questions, priorities will change from those identified initially.

IDENTIFICATION OF THE TARGET POPULATION

The term *target population* is used to describe the identified group or aggregrate in which change is desired as the result of a program or intervention. Sometimes an assessment is conducted on an entire community—as was done with "City X" and "Northwood High" in Chapter 12. However, intervention can also target one segment of the population. For example, City X has a high rate of gonorrhea. If a community health nurse planned a program to decrease gonorrhea among high school students in Census Tract 1, the males and females enrolled in high school in Census Tract 1 would be the target population—that is, the group in which the nurse wishes to effect change. Can you identify the target population in the following examples? What is the community?

- *Example 1:* A program to decrease alcohol-related automobile accidents among students at Jackson High.
- *Example 2:* An exercise program for the frail elderly at Hebron House Senior Center.
- *Example 3:* A health education program about first aid for 10- and 11-year-old girls enrolled in Girl Scout Troop No. 26.

Students, the frail elderly, and 10- and 11-year-old girl scouts can be identified as the target population in the three respective examples. Did you list Jackson High, Hebron House Senior Center, and Girl Scout Troop No. 26 as the phenomenological communities? If so, you are correct.

Can the target population and the community ever be one and the same? Even though they are listed separately in the above examples, it is possible for the community and the target population to be one and the same. Remember that Chapter 12 stressed how important it is to define the community, because the parameters delineated in the definition determine what data to collect. Therefore, the community could be defined as the students enrolled at Jackson High. If this is the case, the community and the target population would be one and the same. Likewise, the frail elderly at Hebron House and the 10- and 11-year-old girls of Troop No. 26 could be designated as the community; again, the community and target population would be the same.

IDENTIFICATION OF THE PLANNING GROUP

The nature and extent of the community's needs will determine who should be involved in developing the plan. Consideration should be given to (1) those for whom the plan is designed—that is, the consumers; (2) those who are concerned with the health problems; (3) those who appear best able to contribute resources to the plan; and (4) those who are most likely to follow through in carrying out the plan of action. The size of the planning group must also be considered. For logistical reasons, it is obvious that everyone concerned with the problem cannot personally be involved as a member of the planning group. However, the interests of those who are concerned must be considered and handled in a representative manner throughout the planning process.

TABLE 13–3

Guidelines for Who Should Be Involved in the Planning Group

- Broad segments of the community, whenever possible, to provide widespread base of support for the program
- Leaders and others who control financial resources and have the legal authority to deal with the problem
- People in a position to promote acceptance of the program (e.g., media representatives, key community leaders, and influential community members)
- Those who will implement the program
- Those who will be affected by the program
- Those who are most likely to offer resistance
- Specialists in the area who can contribute to the group's understanding of the problem and knowledge of possible alternative solutions

It is also important to identify the "opposition" early in the planning process and attempt to get them involved. It is much better to involve them in the planning process than to wait until the program is implemented and then face opposition and program failure.

General Guidelines. Community members need to be included early in the assessment phase. However, an expanded or a different group may be created to help plan a specific program; this group may be formed before or after the target population is identified. Considerations about who should be involved in the planning group are summarized in Table 13–3.

ESTABLISHMENT OF THE PROGRAM GOAL

The program goal is a comprehensive statement of intent or purpose. There is a difference between the program goal and the objectives. The goal is stated very generally and gives no indication of possible means of achieving the desirable outcome (McKenzie and Jurs, 1993). Objectives, however, are stated in terms of a specific outcome that contributes in some way to the achievement of the goal. The following are two examples of program goals:

1. To improve health knowledge regarding AIDS
2. To decrease infant mortality rate

These are broad statements of purpose, not specific and measurable objectives.

After the program goal is established, health planners will have to meet to discuss possible ways to achieve the goal and a feasible time frame within which to accomplish the goal.

IDENTIFICATION OF POSSIBLE SOLUTIONS

It is at this point in the process that the planning group has a "brainstorming" session to examine various strategies and to identify the pros and cons of each strategy for this particular community. What might work for one community may be inappropriate for another. There are several factors that influence the appropriateness of strategies. Physical, psychological, social, cultural, economic, and political considerations all affect the appropriateness of strategies to solve a problem in any given community.

Physical factors include demographic characteristics (set factors) such as the age, race, and sex of the population. For example, a health education program that uses a series of speakers might be appropriate for an adult population, whereas a group of children might need a more action-oriented, active participation program such as a puppet show or a game.

The major area of concern in relation to psychological factors is motivation. How will the strategies being proposed affect the community's motivation? Will members perceive this as helping or hindering the solution of the problem? Persons' perceptions of a problem and individual motivational factors are very important indicators of their health behavior. People will accept strategies or programs that are consistent with their value system and that they perceive as helping the problem. For example, many prevention-oriented programs have been aimed at people living in impoverished conditions. Many of these programs have failed because the people responsible for the programs did not consider motivational factors. Studies show that poverty contributes to an orientation to the present rather than to the future. Therefore, people living in impoverished conditions tend to be more crisis or treatment oriented rather than prevention oriented.

What motivates people to accept or oppose a strategy? A variety of factors can influence acceptance or opposition. Opposition can be based on a rational decision-making process or an irrational emotional process. It is important to ask, "Does the solution to the problem conflict with any basic religious or cultural beliefs held by this segment of the population?" For example, a program on birth control for adolescents may meet with much opposition from parents and/or some churches. As another example, opposition to AIDS education may exist within a school because many parents do not want sex education taught in the school.

Perceived vulnerability is another source of emotional opposition to programs. If people feel threatened, they may oppose the planned change. Although there is always a small portion of the population that will oppose any change, it is important to identify who might feel threatened by or vulnerable to the proposed action. Once these people are identified, the nurse can plan to work with them to explain the plan and solicit their help and cooperation rather than their opposition.

Social practices influence the acceptability of certain programs in a community. Understanding the community's social values and beliefs enables the nurse to plan a program that will be more consistent with these beliefs. For example, a rural community with a long history of self-sufficiency may prefer to raise money internally to fund a new program, rather than apply for a grant from the state health department.

Cultural, ethnic, and religious values influence how people accept health care plans. People will not accept programs that are incongruent with their cultural, ethnic, and religious practices.

The level of education is crucial in knowing what type of interventions to plan. The level of education influences whether the nurse will plan a program that has a lot of reading or a visual, nonreading program. When printed materials of any kind are used in the intervention or to promote the program, it is very important that the reading level be considered (see Chapter 18).

Economic factors are also a consideration. We live in a very cost-conscious era in which people ask, "Is the strategy cost effective?" If it is not, the nurse will probably have to plan a more cost-efficient alternative. Remember that cost effectiveness refers to time and resources as well as money. Generally, the least costly alternative will be the most popular, but there are times when an alternative that is more costly in money but saves time or resources will be favored.

What about political factors? You have heard people say, "It will probably go through this year because this is an election year," or "This would not be a very good proposal in this administration." These statements refer to the political climate and the importance of knowing when to propose certain programs. In election years, programs and strategies that appeal to the greatest number of voters for a politician in a given area would be more powerful strategies than ones that appeal to a small minority of the voting population. It is also extremely important to know what community leaders and elected officials favor and to approach them for their support early on. Knowing how to write letters to elected officials to elicit their support or to influence their vote is very important.

Power is closely associated with politics. Milio (1981) describes organizational effectiveness as the capacity of an organization to bargain for scarce resources. Whoever has the most power gets the resources.

IDENTIFICATION OF ALTERNATIVE SOLUTIONS

While looking at possible solutions, it is also important to look at alternative ways to meet the identified need. Discussing the options in relation to the need and the identified resources is an important part of planning.

IDENTIFICATION OF RESOURCES

The nurse should identify the resources within the community as well as outside the community that can be utilized to help solve the problem. This includes both human and nonhuman resources. Human resources can provide expertise and people. Nonhuman resources include funding, facilities, supplies, and equipment. It is much better to know ahead of time that personnel, funding, or needed supplies are insufficient than to abort the mission for lack of resources after the intervention is begun.

SELECTION OF THE BEST INTERVENTION STRATEGY

The nurse should select the best strategy for this population within the context of resources and time available. There is almost always more than one way to solve a problem. The key in this step of the planning process is to be able to select the best strategy for this population within the context of available resources.

Having decided on a course of action, it is time to plan the details of the intervention. The first step is to delineate specific, measurable objectives.

DELINEATION OF SPECIFIC OBJECTIVES

Objectives for health programs include outcome objectives, process objectives, and management objectives (Hale et al., 1994). *Outcome objectives* address the health status or health behaviors desired in the target population or community. *Process objectives* specify the implementation activities and health care delivery that are necessary to achieve the desired changes in health status and/or health behavior. *Management objectives* define the structures needed to carry out the process objectives.

For outcome objectives to be useful, they must meet a variety of criteria. Outcome objectives should

- identify the program participants (WHO),
- describe specific behavior program participants will exhibit to demonstrate accomplishment of the objectives (WHAT),
- describe the condition in which participants will demonstrate accomplishment (WHERE AND TO WHAT EXTENT),
- describe the standard performance expected to indicate accomplishment (HOW MUCH), and
- describe the time frame (WHEN) (Mager, 1962; Gronlund, 1970).

How does writing objectives for the community differ from writing objectives for an individual client? The same criteria must be met, but community-focused objectives are written for the group or aggregate. When working with an individual client, the nurse may state the following objective:

> After watching a film on diabetes, the client will state at least three signs of hyperglycemia.

How would a similar objective be stated if the nurse was working with a group of diabetic patients? One example might be:

> After watching a film on diabetes, 90% of the participants enrolled in the diabetic education program will state at least three signs of hyperglycemia.

What is the difference? When working with the community, the nurse must consider the group and indicate whether all of the group or a certain portion of the group need to demonstrate the action. Examples of specific behavioral objectives written for the community can be seen in Table 13–4. This table further illustrates the

TABLE 13–4

Behavioral Objectives

SAMPLE OUTCOME GOAL:

At least 40% of the smokers among mothers enrolled in the Central City Mom and Tots Center will have modified their smoking habits by June 1997.

Determine specific behavioral objectives: include who, behavior, condition, criteria, and when.

SAMPLE OBJECTIVE (criterion-referenced)

Given a smoking modification program, at least 80% of the interested mothers will devise and implement a contract to modify their smoking habits by the fifth week of the program.

1. Who—Description of group participants	Interested mothers
2. Behavior—Description of the behavior the participants will exhibit to demonstrate accomplishment of the objectives	Devise and implement a contract to modify smoking habit
3. Condition—Description of condition in which participants will demonstate accomplishment	Given a smoking modification program
4. Criteria—Standard of performance expected to indicate accomplishment	At least 80% will actively participate
5. When—Description of time frame	By the fifth week of the program

SAMPLE OBJECTIVES (norm-referenced)

After the presentation by the nursing students, the target population will demonstrate a statistically significant increase in knowledge as measured by a paper-and-pencil pretest and posttest.

1. Who—Description of group participants	The target population
2. Behavior—Description of the behavior the participants will exhibit to demonstrate accomplishment of the objectives	As measured by a paper-and-pencil pretest and posttest
3. Condition—Description of condition in which participants will demonstrate accomplishment	After the presentation by the nursing students
4. Criteria—Standard of performance expected to indicate accomplishment	Will demonstrate a statistically significant increase in knowledge

difference between criterion- and norm-referenced objectives.

In criterion-referenced outcome objectives, the objectives specify the behaviors desired in the target population or community. For example, the pregnancy rate of Census Tract 1 will be reduced to 40 pregnancies per 1000 female teenagers in 3 years. In norm-referenced objectives, the desired outcome is compared with another population or an ideal. For example, the pregnancy rate of female teenagers in Census Tract 1 will be no higher than the national rate of pregnancies per 1000 female teenagers in 3 years. The population could also be compared with itself: The teen pregnancy rate of Census Tract 1 will be reduced 50% in 3 years.

Process objectives specify incremental activities or service delivery that will lead to attainment of outcome objectives (Hale et al., 1994). These objectives are monitored in short time intervals to ensure that the program is on course to meet outcome objectives and program goals. The following is an example of a process objective:

> Seventy-five percent of Northview High students will participate during the spring semester in an education session on reducing risky sexual behavior.

Such an objective would contribute to attainment of the program goal: to reduce risky sexual behavior among high school students.

Management objectives are concerned with funding; personnel; program support, such as equipment and record keeping; and publicity (Hale et al., 1994). The following is a management objective:

> The health department will hire three community health nurses for school health within 4 months.

DELINEATION OF THE INTERVENTION WORK PLAN

In this step the nurse will need to plan the basics of the intervention and take into consideration the specific what, how, who, when, and where (Table 13–5). A good plan will have the following questions answered *before* any intervention:

- WHAT actions are to be done?
- HOW are the actions to be accomplished?
- WHAT resources (equipment, space, money) are needed?
- WHO is responsible for the accomplishment of each action?
- WHEN will each action occur?
- HOW MUCH TIME will it take to accomplish the action?
- WHERE will the actions take place? This includes obtaining the place and determining how much space is needed.

TABLE 13–5

Steps in Establishing a Work Plan

1. Identify the specific target population to be served by the program.
2. Specify the number of people to be served during various time periods. (This is called *utilization.*)
3. Sequence the interventions logically, and specify when they are to be phased in and who is responsible to do so (perhaps using a Gantt Chart).
4. Determine the personnel needed. Anticipate their learning needs regarding implementing the program. (For example, if a program is to screen pregnant women for risk of abuse, nurses would need to know the factors indicating increased risk.)
5. Identify space, equipment, educational materials, and disposable supplies needed.
6. Develop a budget, including revenue sources and costs of personnel, equipment and supplies, publicity, use of buildings, and administrative services.
7. Develop mechanisms for managing the entire program, including supervising personnel, administering the budget, monitoring the planned sequence of activities (work plan), and conducting formative evaluation.
8. Develop mechanisms to communicate with interested parties and include them in program monitoring and decision making.

This work plan includes specific process and management objectives discussed earlier in the chapter.

Taking the time to make a detailed work plan in the beginning will save time and will make for a much smoother working phase. There is nothing more frustrating, or embarrassing, than coming to the intervention phase and realizing that a very basic detail is missing.

PLANNING FOR PROGRAM EVALUATION

Evaluation is the last step of the nursing process. All too often it is not even thought about until the end. However, plans must also be made for evaluation. Evaluation is needed *throughout* the program to measure progress, as well as at the end to measure the overall value, adequacy, efficiency, outcomes of the program, and effectiveness. Evaluation is a continuous feedback process that provides the stimulus for changes in the system.

Program evaluation is the process of determining whether the program is achieving its purpose, whether it should be continued or terminated, and how it can be improved or better managed (Hale et al., 1994). Process and management objectives are evaluated throughout the program to ensure that planned activities are being accomplished. Outcome objectives are measured primarily at the end of the program to determine whether the program goal was attained.

There are many approaches to program evaluation. Chapter 14 is devoted to exploring different methods of program evaluation in detail. It is sufficient to mention in this chapter that a plan for program evaluation must be seen as an essential step in the planning process so that

TABLE 13–6

Pitfalls and Keys to Success in Implementing Health Programs

Pitfalls to Success
Inaccurate assessment
Nonvalidation of data with community
No community involvement
Insufficient resources
Lack of coordinated planning
Lack of leadership
Poor communication
Keys to Success
Thorough, accurate assessment
Validation of assessment data with the community
Involvement of the community
Sufficient resources
Well-thought-out plan with coordination among team members
Good leadership
Open communication

systematic program evaluation becomes a reality, not merely an afterthought. Table 13–6 summarizes some keys to success and pitfalls in planning and implementing health care for communities.

TOOLS USED TO PRESENT AND MONITOR PROGRAM PROGRESS

During implementation of the plan, it is important to evaluate progress. A visual guide to present and measure program progress is often helpful. Several tools are used to chart activity and anticipate management problems in the implementation phase. The three that will be discussed here are the Gantt Chart, the Program Evaluation and Review Technique, and the Program Planning Budget System (Rowland and Rowland, 1992).

Gantt Chart

Henry Gantt developed the Gantt Chart during World War I to identify the process needed to accomplish a result. Starting with a final work result, major steps necessary to obtain the result are projected backward from results to actions; their timing and sequence are then considered (Drucker, 1974). The Gantt Chart considers the concepts of events and time (Fig. 13–2). The events are listed down the left side of the chart. Time is represented across the chart for each event by lines showing when the event is to start and when it is to be completed.

Program Evaluation and Review Technique

The Program Evaluation and Review Technique (PERT) is a network programming method developed during the 1950s through a joint effort between the U.S. Navy and private industry (Lockheed Aircraft Corporation and BoozAllen & Hamilton, Inc.) for the Polaris Missile project. PERT also looks at the concepts of events and time and is particularly useful for very large scale projects.

The intent of PERT is to:

- focus attention on key developmental parts of the program;
- identify potential program problems;
- evaluate program progress toward goal attainment;
- provide a prompt, efficient reporting method; and
- facilitate decision making.

There are three steps to PERT:

1. Identification of specific program activities.
2. Identification of resources to accomplish these activities.
3. Determination of the sequence of activities for accomplishment (Roman, 1969).

PERT uses a flowchart designed to estimate the time it should take to complete specific events necessary to complete the entire project. Events are shown on a chart by shapes (circles, ovals, squares, or triangles) with numbers. The number is not necessarily a sequential number. That is, number 3 does not have to occur after number 2. The numbers designate a task, not a sequential order. The activities to complete the events are the time-consuming element. Time is represented on the chart by lines and arrows. Unlike the Gantt Chart, each line has three different numbers representing three time estimates: optimistic, most likely, and pessimistic. "Optimistic" is the shortest amount of time possible to complete the activity if everything goes perfectly; "most likely" is the most likely amount of time needed to complete the activity; and "pessimistic" is the longest amount of time the activity might take (Rakich et al., 1992).

Planning, Programming, and Budgeting System

The Planning, Programming, and Budgeting System (PPBS) is an economical method of expressing a program plan. It is an outcome-oriented accounting system designed to determine the most efficient method of resource allocation to attain measurable objectives (LaPatra, 1975).

The three components of the PPBS are as follows:

1. *Planning:* Formulation of objectives and identification of alternatives and methods for accomplishing the objectives.
2. *Programming:* Delineation of resources for each identified alternative.
3. *Budgeting:* Assignment of dollar values to the resources required for the program implementation.

Although it was designed by the U.S. Department of Defense to plan broad-scale programs, the PPBS can be used as a framework to plan programs for smaller organizations and population groups.

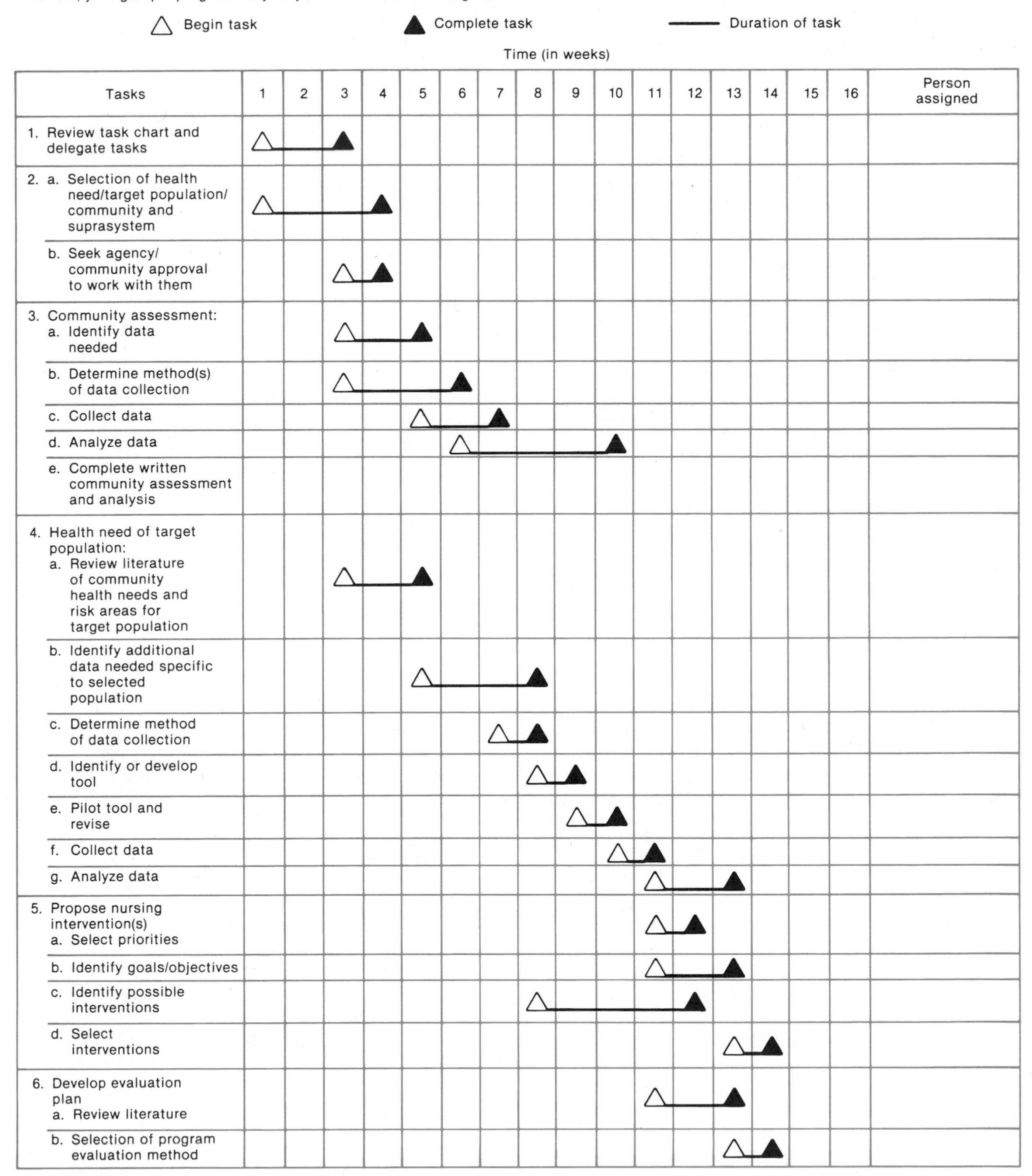

Figure 13–2 ● Example of a Gantt chart, which specifies time frame, tasks, and persons assigned to work on each task. Time frames listed are suggested task allotment intervals; actual intervals may vary. (Adapted from Community Health Nursing Faculty, Undergraduate Program. (1985). *Syllabus for nursing 325.* Baltimore: University of Maryland School of Nursing.)

Implementation

Implementation is the action portion of the plan; in other words, the plan states what will occur in the implementation. Mobilizing people and resources to activate the plan of action is a challenging task for the community health nurse.

The role of the nurse during implementation varies based on the type of program, the community, and the community organization methods used. Throughout the implementation phase, the nurse continues to collaborate and coordinate. The role of facilitator increases because the nurse must facilitate the community's sense of ownership of the program. Active participation of the community is essential to the success of the program; the health program will be successful *only* if the community "owns" it. The nurse facilitates ownership by getting key people involved from the beginning and by facilitating increased involvement in the program. Therefore, the nurse's role may change during implementation as the community begins to take on more responsibility.

Implementation results in change, which can be stressful and threatening. Resistance to change is natural and inevitable, because every system attempts to maintain dynamic equilibrium. Change brings an initial state of disequilibrium. However, if the people in the community have been involved from the beginning in a plan that affects them, informed about the benefits of the plan for them, and convinced of the value of the plan, they are less apt to offer resistance.

In many health programs, it is community health nurses who perform the interventions and manage the program. Community health nurses often conduct health education and screening programs and provide primary health care. Community health nurses manage programs by supervising personnel, administering the budget, ordering equipment, maintaining program records, and ensuring that planned interventions are accomplished.

TYPES OF INTERVENTIONS

Just as there are many different types of interventions for the individual, so, too, there are a variety of interventions for the community as client. There are several major types of community health intervention programs, including the following:

- Health education programs
- Screening programs
- Establishment of services
- Policy setting and implementation
- Increasing community self-help
- Increasing power among disenfranchised individuals

Health Education Programs

Much intervention at the community level is aimed at educating people about their health (see Chapter 18). Health education programs can be geared toward one or more of the three levels of prevention. Programs provide information on how to prevent illness, promote health, care for those illnesses, and minimize the effects of illness or injury.

The teaching methodology must be appropriate to the community. It is important to use different methods of presentation that appeal to many senses (not just the lecture method, which is the least effective method). U.S. society has been described as a media society. Use media that are well received by a given age group (e.g., for young children, use a puppet show or coloring books to teach content). Be creative! One example of a creative health promotion program is a population control music video designed for adolescents in which the lyrics suggest birth control behaviors. This creative effort was designed by The Johns Hopkins Population Center for reaching populations in other countries. It has been very popular in the Philippines and was released in Mexico.

Screening Programs

Screening programs are designed to provide early detection and diagnosis of health problems (see Chapter 17). It is important to remember that screening does not prevent the disease, but merely identifies risk factors or early signs so that appropriate treatment intervention may be obtained.

It is very important to note here that when planning a screening program, referral and treatment resources must be included as part of the intervention. It is not enough to say, "You have a problem." The nurse must also provide information about how and where to go for help.

Establishment of Services

Many community health programs focus on establishing the services needed to meet the health needs of a given population. Some examples of services are school health clinics, home health care nursing services, grocery shopping services for home-bound elderly individuals, and establishment of adult daycare centers for elderly persons. Bremer (1987) has described the establishment of a community health nursing service to promote the health of elderly individuals in their homes and to prevent disability.

With the advent of nurse practitioners in the 1970s, contemporary community nursing centers began to emerge. In a study by the National League for Nursing, 170 community nursing centers were identified in 31 states (Barger and Rosenfeld, 1993). More than half were affiliated with another organization, often a school of nursing, while the rest were free standing. The study found that community nursing centers provide direct access to nursing services such as primary care, assessment and screening, education, case management, and counseling. The centers tend to provide care for traditionally underserved populations such as children and poor, elderly, and homeless individuals. Approximately 30% of the care is paid for directly by clients, almost 50% is paid for by insurance or gifts, and 20% is uncompensated.

Policy Setting and Implementation

A community may have needs that must be met by policy changes (Williams, 1983). These changes might include legislation at the local or state level. Interventions that focus on policy setting may include lobbying, building coalitions, and participating in the political process. For example, a group of nurses initiated mandatory seat belt legislation as a result of the deaths and injuries they witnessed in emergency departments. In St. Louis, public health nurses were successful in getting the jurisdiction for a lead poisoning control program returned to the health department (Kuehnert, 1991). Previously, the responsibilities for lead screening and control had been transferred from the health department to the private sector, resulting in lower screening rates and a higher prevalence of lead poisoning.

Increasing Community Self-Help

Locality development strategies focus on strengthening the processes that involve community members in solving their own problems (Rothman, 1978). These strategies do not result immediately in new educational programs on a specific health topic or in new services or policies. Instead, the short-term results among community members include increased self-confidence, increased levels of problem-solving skills, and new or strengthened communication and problem-solving networks and coalitions. Milio's (1971) work with the Mom and Tots Center in Detroit is a classic example of this form of community development. Another example is the Rural Elderly Enhancement Program in Alabama, in which nurses initiated a project to develop community volunteer coalitions; provide accessible and safe water, housing, and transportation; and conduct needs assessments of elderly persons and school-age children (Farley, 1993). Table 13–7 illustrates some of the results of the volunteer coalitions.

TABLE 13–7

Community Participation in the Alabama Rural Elderly Enhancement Program

Volunteer Coalition	Services
Housing	Builds steps, ramps, porches for elderly individuals; replaces roofs, windows.
Fund raising	Helps elderly individuals buy medications and obtain transportation and public water.
Education	Volunteers who are trained by nurses provide health education.
Helping hand	Volunteers who are trained by nurses provide friendly visits and homemaking, personal, and respite care.
Tutoring and enrichment	Conducts after-school and summer programs for children in the arts, sciences, and reading.

Data from Farley, S. (1993). The community as partner in primary health care. *Nursing and Health Care, 14*(5), 244–249.

Increasing Power among Disenfranchised Individuals

Strategies that shift the power balance within or among communities can empower disenfranchised individuals. The power balance can be shifted if the ability of community members to help themselves is increased. However, often the institutionalized structures of the community must also be changed if the population is to have more equal access to community power. One example is the attempt to restructure employment opportunities so that a working adult is guaranteed a wage above the poverty level (National Commission on Children, 1991).

STRATEGIES FOR IMPLEMENTING PROGRAMS

There are several strategies for implementing programs on the community level.

Single Action. In the single action approach, programs are implemented one time for a very specific purpose. Sometimes this is all that is necessary or all that resources will allow.

Phasing. It is sometimes necessary or advantageous to phase programs in over a period of time. This is often used in very large programs and in programs in which a multitude of resources are needed. Sometimes the problem is so multifaceted that it takes several different stages of interventions to solve it.

Collaboration and Networks. Collaborative efforts between disciplines and agencies can be very effective and efficient when planning care at the community level. A partnership between agencies and personnel results in better use of resources and often a much stronger program. A great deal more can be accomplished when resources are pooled.

A group of nine senior nursing students enrolled in a community health nursing course at the University of Maryland used the strategy of collaboration when they conducted their community project. The initial assessment revealed a need to plan an exercise program for frail elderly individuals attending Hebron House Nutrition Center in Howard County, Maryland. The nursing students collaborated with the county Office on Aging, the university, and the county cable television station to produce a videotape of exercises for frail elderly persons. All three groups profited from the collaborative effort. The students gained valuable experience working with multiple disciplines and multiple agencies. The Hebron House community gained a video exercise program that is used three times weekly, and the cable television station gained a show that aired on television three times weekly for home-bound frail elderly individuals (Trotter et al., 1987).

Coalitions. A coalition is a temporary union for a common purpose. Coalitions are effective strategies at the local, state, and national political levels and often are aggregate oriented. For example, there are coalitions for women's health issues.

KEY IDEAS

1. Health planning is a social process used by multiple disciplines to promote the health of populations and the competency of communities.
2. Health interventions planned for groups and aggregates are often called *programs.* Programs may be single actions, but more often are ongoing interventions involving several different activities and phases.
3. Steps in health program planning are consistent with the nursing process and include assessment, analysis, planning, implementation, and evaluation.
4. Community health planning based on community assessment is a basic element of community health nursing.
5. Community health nurses work in partnership with other professionals, community leaders, and community members to plan and implement health care based on a community assessment.
6. Community nursing diagnoses address the community members' responses to actual and potential health problems. There is no single classification system for nursing diagnoses for communities.
7. Program goals are broad statements of desired health outcomes. Outcome, process, and management objectives contribute to goal attainment.
8. Community health nurses use *Healthy People 2000* objectives and *Healthy Communities 2000* standards as guides to develop goals and objectives for health programs in specific communities.
9. Community health nurses often implement and manage community health programs.
10. Common health care interventions performed by community health nurses include provision of primary care, health education, screening, policy formation, establishment of new nursing services, and community empowerment.
11. Planning health programs for communities includes planning for evaluation.

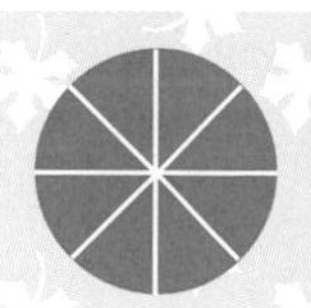

APPLYING THE NURSING PROCESS: *Health Planning for a Phenomenological Community*

In this case study we use the community assessment of Northview High School in Chapter 12 to plan and begin to implement health programs. Many of the steps of program planning discussed earlier in this chapter are evident.

A community health nurse, Marian Fields, is assigned full time to two high schools, Northview and South Central high schools. This is a new assignment for her. She is expected to spend 5 days each 2-week period at each school. Previous to her appointment, the health department provided a nurse for ½ day per week at each school. Her job description includes staffing a health room to address the complaints of ill students, maintaining the health and immunization records on all students, administering medication and providing treatments as ordered for chronically ill students (e.g., nebulizer treatments for asthmatic students), assisting with classroom instruction on health-related issues, and developing programs to address the major health-related concerns of the high school students.

Through the assessment of Northview High School in Chapter 12, the following health issues emerged:

- Substance abuse, including smoking
- Communicable diseases and rashes

- Injuries necessitating first aid
- Insufficient birth control information
- Unprotected sexual activity
- Teenage pregnancy
- Lack of daycare for infants of teenage parents
- High dropout rates for pregnant teens
- Sexually transmitted diseases
- Vision screening
- Chronic illnesses
- Personal hygiene
- Dental problems
- Obesity and anorexia

Ms. Fields decides to concentrate her initial program efforts on a single health issue rather than attempt to address all the health problems of the high school at one time.

Prioritization

In selecting a health need for intervention, the community health nurse should consider how many students are affected by the problem, as well as the degree of risk associated with the problem. Risky sexual behavior is selected as the priority problem because it is of concern to both parents and faculty, community health nurses can contribute to the solution, and risky sexual behavior can be changed. Addressing risky sexual behavior also has the potential to contribute to other health status outcomes as well. The nurse's ultimate goal is to change the health status of her community by lowering the rates of teen pregnancy and sexually transmitted disease through reducing the number of students engaging in unprotected sexually activity.

Target Population

The target population is the students attending Northview High School.

Planning Group

Ideally the planning group at Northview should include the following:

- The consumers (students in the high school)
- Those who are concerned with the problem (faculty, administrators, members of the Parent-Teacher Association [PTA])
- Those with resources (health department, board of education)
- Those who will implement the plan (community health nurse, physical education teacher)

In this situation, Ms. Fields is charged by the principal to develop a plan and then bring it to him and the school board for consideration. She is able to arrange several meetings with a group consisting of some faculty (including the physical education teacher), health department personnel, and student representatives.

Possible Solutions

During the meetings, participants brainstorm the following possible solutions to the problem:

- Teen clinic on site
- Teen clinic near the school
- Educational program regarding sexually transmitted diseases and containing contraceptive information
- Educational program without contraceptive information
- Simulation experience: caring for a child (to increase motivation to avoid pregnancy)
- Peer counseling/partnership program
- Interviews with teenage parents to see why they got pregnant
- Inviting teenagers with sexually transmitted diseases or the human immunodeficiency virus to speak (to increase perceived vulnerability to disease)
- Participatory programs to strengthen identity and self-efficacy and identify own goals/values

Program Goals

After much discussion, the group incorporates a number of solutions into a two-phase program design. The first phase is to develop a comprehensive sex education program aimed at changing risky health behaviors. The second phase is to improve access to health services for sexually active students.

Phase 1: A Sex Education Program

Ms. Fields is responsible for designing the educational program. She reviews the literature on teenage pregnancy, use of birth control, sexual activity, attitudes, and knowledge level. Because there are various opinions about the inclusion of sexually transmitted disease and contraceptive information in a sexual education program for adolescents, Ms. Fields needs to identify the community's position on these topics. From conversations with parents she knows that many would support inclusion of this information in the educational program. She meets with the principal to determine his position. He informs Ms. Fields that he will support inclusion of the topics and that the school superintendent has informed him that five of seven school board members will support that position.

To validate that Northview High School students' needs are similar to the needs identified in the literature, the nurse designs a questionnaire to distribute to a sample of students. The aim of the questionnaire is to assess the level of student knowledge about the selected topics to tailor the educational program for the students at Northview High School. Her survey reveals that students are knowledgeable about the mechanics of sexual intercourse, and most acknowledge the importance of protection during sexual intercourse; nevertheless, they continue to engage in risky behavior and show knowledge deficits on a number of topic areas included in the following nursing diagnoses.

Nursing Diagnoses/Problems

1. Population at risk for health problems owing to a high rate of sexual activity (more than 50% of students sampled report engaging in sexual intercourse).
2. Knowledge deficit related to the risks of pregnancy during sexual activity.
3. Inconsistent use of birth control.
4. Knowledge deficit related to functioning of various birth control mechanisms.
5. Knowledge deficit related to signs, symptoms, and potential consequences of untreated sexually transmitted diseases.

Nursing Goals and Actions

The *program goals* are as follows:

- Provide students with the skills needed to explore the benefits and risks of engaging in sexual activity during adolescence.
- Increase the knowledge level of students about sexually related information so that students can make informed choices about behavior.

Problem 1 Outcome Objective. Consistent with the *Healthy People 2000* objectives, reduce the number of students who begin sexual activity and increase the number of students who postpone beginning sexual activity until they are older.

The *nursing actions* are as follows:

1. Develop a seminar discussion program with student participation that explores the reasons students begin or continue to engage in sexual activity.
2. Identify the benefits and risks of beginning sexual activity.
3. Provide skills development exercises that help students practice declining sexual advances.
4. Develop a peer network that will support students who choose not to engage in sexual activity.

Problem 2 Outcome Objective. Increase student knowledge about the process of conception.
The *nursing actions* are as follows:

1. Explore the physiological process of conception.
2. Examine the "myths" associated with preventing pregnancy during sexual intercourse and physical intimacy.

Problems 3 and 4 Outcome Objective. Increase student knowledge about birth control methods. The *nursing actions* are as follows:

1. Review various birth control methods.
2. Discuss the benefits and risks of each method.
3. Identify the risk of pregnancy for each method.
4. Hold a discussion seminar that explores with students common reasons why some opt not to use birth control.
5. Link the myths associated with reduced risk of pregnancy, inconsistent contraceptive use, and actual pregnancy risks.

Problem 5 Outcome Objective. Increase student knowledge of sexually transmitted disease. The *nursing actions* are as follows:

1. Review common sexually transmitted disease signs and symptoms.
2. Review treatment and potential complications of common sexually transmitted diseases.
3. Provide seminar discussion to explore with students issues and concerns related to these health issues; correct misconceptions.
4. Relate the best ways to reduce the risk of sexually transmitted disease.

Implementation

Ms. Fields identifies a number of resources to assist with the program she has designed. The physical education teacher is willing to assist with the lecture portion of the program but does not want to conduct seminar discussions. The health department is willing to provide a social worker and a clinical psychologist to implement the first discussion groups and assist high school staff to become more comfortable with the discussion process. In addition, the health department is willing to provide posters, brochures, and other visual aids for classroom instruction.

Ms. Fields presents her plan to the principal, who agrees that the plan is appropriate and sends it to the school superintendent for review. The superintendent, with the principal and Ms. Fields in attendance, presents the plan to the school board, and it is approved by one vote. The principal assigns a volunteer biology teacher to help with classroom instruction. Ms. Fields intends to implement the program at the start of the second term, after the students return from winter vacation.

Process Objective. Seventy-five percent of students will participate in the instructional program during the spring semester.

Phase 2: Improve Student Access to Health Services, Including Services to Address Risky Sexual Behavior

To validate the need for additional adolescent health services, Ms. Fields surveys the resources for teen health services in the surrounding geopolitical communities. She finds that there is a community health center nearby. This site provides services to well children under the age of 6, prenatal care to pregnant women, and family planning services. There are no services aimed specifically at adolescent health problems. Teens can be served at the site for pregnancy and family planning, but the clinic has not had the resources to actively target teens. From the assessment of the high school community (see Chapter 12), Ms. Fields knows that support services for teen parents are inadequate; many do not continue with school, many drop out. The surrounding census tract consists of families with moderately low income. Many are "gray area" families —that is, they have no health insurance but do not qualify for state medical assistance because their income exceeds the eligibility criteria. There are two general practitioners in the community, both with heavy patient loads. These practitioners do treat adolescent members of families in their practice, but restrict the number of families who are unable to pay for services. Care is acutely focused rather than preventive in nature. Both practitioners report that they do not have the time or resources to target teens or emphasize preventive health practices. There are no other medical professionals practicing within the community boundaries.

Nursing Diagnoses

1. Inadequate services to provide adolescent health care.
2. Inadequate services to address primary prevention with respect to pregnancy and sexually transmitted diseases.
3. Inadequate support services for teenage mothers with respect to daycare, parenting skills, and continuation of their educational program.

Nursing Goals and Actions

The *program goals* are as follows:

- Improve health services for adolescents.
- Improve support services for teenage parents, especially teenage mothers.

Problems 1 and 2 Outcome Objective. Provide adequate health care services to students within 24 months.

The *nursing actions* are as follows:

1. Convene a committee of community and suprasystem representatives and health care providers to identify the types of health services needed.
2. Have the committee brainstorm ways to provide these services, including addressing the issues of cost and access.
3. Develop a proposal for providing health care services to the teenage population.
4. Present the proposal to the school board for approval.

Implementation

The proposal to improve health care services for adolescents resulted in a recommendation for a school-based clinic. This proposal was taken to the school board, which held hearings. A vocal minority of census tract residents opposed a school-based clinic because they were not in favor of providing contraceptives in a school-based setting. The committee then altered its plan to improve services to adolescents through the community health center. Funding for a pilot project was approved as a joint effort of the local school district and the health department, with each contributing $25,000. In addition, the health department will provide the space and the services of one community health nurse to staff the program. The program can use any existing equipment at the health center, but new equipment and other support personnel will have to come out of the program budget. The adolescent program is projected to start in approximately 3 months. Ms. Fields is in the process of developing a referral mechanism for students seen through the school health suite who require further medical attention or seek services not currently offered through student health services. Evaluation will be needed as the project unfolds.

Problem 3 Outcome Objective. Develop support services for teenage parents that will facilitate their educational progress and the well-being of their children within 18 months.

The *nursing actions* are as follows:

1. Meet with representatives of the teachers and administrative staff to identify problem areas for continued education.
2. Meet with a sampling of young mothers and fathers to help identify problem areas and the types of services they feel would be most beneficial to their educational advancement.
3. Convene a committee of professionals, students, and community representatives and leaders. Report your results with problems 1 and 2 above, assist the committee to develop a proposal for support services, and have committee members present the proposal to the school board.

Implementation

Ms. Fields met with both professionals and students in an effort to identify the problems associated with continued schooling during and after pregnancy. Some of the problems identified included the following:

- No in-school child daycare;
- Limited daycare options in the community and the cost of those options;
- Student families who are unable to provide daycare because of their employment responsibilities;
- Poor preparation for parenting, including information related to managing infant illness, hygiene, infant growth and development, and discipline techniques; and
- Lack of emotional support for continued schooling, especially among peers.

Ms. Fields is in the process of meeting with the committee to explore the information she has collected. Several parents of adolescent mothers, two teachers from the high school, a nurse practitioner from the community health center, and a minister active in adolescent counseling have agreed to serve on the committee, as well as two high school students who are mothers of infants. Ms. Fields would like to get representatives from the local school board and/or academic administrators to complete the committee. Her efforts to date have taken half of the academic year. She hopes to have the committee intact and the work completed before the end of the school year.

Process Objectives. Several process objectives were developed for Phase 2 consistent with the community standards suggested by the American Public Health Association (1991).

1. Two years from inception of the adolescent health program, 75% of Northview High School students referred to the program will receive services at the health center or be referred to other community-based services to meet their needs.
2. Within two years, all adolescent parents will have access to affordable, certified child care.
3. Within two years, all adolescent parents who remain in school will be encouraged to attend a school-based parenting skills program.

GUIDELINES FOR LEARNING

① Based on the assessment of Census Tract 1 in Chapter 12, apply the steps for program planning. Be sure to identify who needs to be involved in the planning process to ensure its success. Rewrite the health problems as nursing diagnoses. Develop at least one program goal and related outcome and process objectives. Discuss your rationale for selecting the priority problem that you did.

② Attend a community meeting at which health concerns or health programs are discussed. Identify the key persons involved, and discuss with several why they are interested in health care. Identify differing points of view. Think about alternative solutions that might provide common ground—in other words, that would include as many points of view as possible.

③ Interview a community health nurse who has been involved in establishing a new health program. Discuss who was involved; how long the process took; and what the sources of money, equipment, and space were. Ask the community health nurse why the program was successful. Ask what aspects were unsuccessful and what might have been done differently.

④ Consider which model of community organization you are more inclined to use: locality development, social planning, or social action. What values and experiences contribute to your preference?

⑤ Read a major newspaper, watch the national news on television, or use other resources to identify examples of locality development, social planning, and social action. What are the advantages and disadvantages of each model for community change? How long range were the outcomes? What aspects of planning and implementing were especially difficult?

REFERENCES

American Nurses' Association (ANA). (1986). *Standards of community health nursing practice.* Washington, DC: Author.

American Public Health Association (APHA). (1991). *Healthy communities 2000—Model standards: Guidelines for community attainment of the year 2000 national health objectives.* Washington, DC: Author.

ANA. (1991). *Nursing's agenda for health care reform.* Washington, DC: Author.

ANA, Division on Community Health Nursing. (1980). *A conceptual model of community health nursing.* Washington, DC: Author.

Anderson, E., & McFarlane, J. (1988). *Community as client: Application of the nursing process.* Philadelphia: J.B. Lippincott.

APHA, Committee on Public Health Administration. (1961). *Guide to a community health study* (2nd ed.). Washington, DC: Author.

APHA, Public Health Nursing Section. (1980). *The definition and role of public health nursing in the delivery of care.* Washington, DC: Author.

Association for the Advancement of Health Education. (1992). PATCH: Planned Approach to Community Health. *Journal of Health Education, 23*(3), 1–192.

Barger, S., & Rosenfeld, P. (1993). Models in community health care:Journal of Health Education, 23(3), 1–192. Findings from a national study of community nursing centers. *Nursing and Health Care, 14*(8), 426–431.

Bremer, A. (1987). Revitalizing the district model for the delivery of prevention-focused community health nursing services. *Family and Community Health, 10*(2), 1–10.

Carpenito, L. (1993). *Nursing diagnosis: Application to clinical practice,* (5th ed). Philadelphia: J.B. Lippincott.

Dever, G. E. (1980). *Community health analysis. A holistic approach.* Germantown, MD: Aspen.

Drucker, P. (1974). *Management: Tasks, responsibilities, practices.* New York: Harper & Row.

Farley, S. (1993). The community as partner in primary health care. *Nursing and Health Care, 14*(5), 244–249.

Flynn, B., Rider, M., & Bailey, W. (1992). Developing community leadership in healthy cities: The Indiana model. *Nursing Outlook, 40*(3), 121–126.

Gikow, F., & Kucharski, P. (1987). A new look at the community: Functional health pattern assessment. *Journal of Community Health Nursing, 4*(1), 21–27.

Gordon, M. (1982). *Nursing diagnosis: Process and application.* New York: McGraw-Hill.

Gronlund, N. E. (1970). *Stating behavioral objectives for classroom instruction.* New York: Macmillan.

Hale, C., Arnold, F., & Travis, M. (1994). *Planning and evaluating health programs: A primer.* Albany, NY: Delmar Publishers.

Hamilton, P. (1983). Community nursing diagnosis. *Advances in Nursing Science, 5*(3), 21–35.

Institute of Action Research for Community Health. (1993). *CITYNET.* Indianapolis, IN: Author.

Kuehnert, P. (1991). The public health policy advocate: Fostering the health of communities. *Clinical Nurse Specialist, 5*(1), 5–10.

LaPatra, J. W. (1975). *Health care delivery systems: Evaluation criteria.* Springfield, IL: Charles C Thomas.

Mager, R. F. (1962). *Preparing objectives for programmed instruction.* San Francisco: Fearon Publishers.

Martin, K., & Scheet, N. (1993). *The Omaha System: Applications for community health nursing.* Philadelphia: W.B. Saunders.

McKenzie, J., & Jurs, J. (1993). *Planning, implementing, and evaluating health promotion programs: A primer.* New York: Macmillan.

Milio, N. (1971). *9226 Kercheval: The storefront that did not burn.* Ann Arbor, MI: The University of Michigan Press.

Milio, N. (1981). *Promoting health through public policy.* Philadelphia: F.A. Davis.

Muecke, M. (1984). Community health diagnosis in nursing. *Public Health Nursing, 1*(1), 23–35.

National Commission on Children (1991). *Beyond rhetoric: A new American agenda for children and families.* Washington, DC: U.S. Government Printing Office.

Neufield, A., & Harrison, M. (1990). The development of nursing diagnoses for aggregates and groups. *Public Health Nursing, 7*(4), 251–255.

North American Nursing Diagnosis Association. (1991). *Taxonomy I revised with official diagnostic categories.* St. Louis: Author.

Rakich, J., Longest, B., & Darr, K. (1992). *Managing health services organizations* (3rd ed.). Baltimore: Health Professions Press.

Roman, D. (1969). The PERT System: An appraisal of program evaluation review technique. In H. Schulberg, A. Sheldon, & F. Baker (Eds.), *Program evaluation in the health fields.* New York: Behavioral Publications.

Rothman, J. (1978). Three models of community organization practice. In Cox, F., Erlich, J., Rothman, J., & Tropman, J. (Eds.). *Strategies in community organization: A book of readings.* Itasca, IL: F.E. Peacock Publishers.

Rowland, H., & Rowland, B. (1992). *Nursing administration handbook* (3rd ed.). Gaithersburg, MD: Aspen Publishers.

Ruybal, S. (1978). Community health planning. *Journal of Family and Community Health, 1,* 9–13.

Trotter, J. (1987, October). Home care: For people or for profit? Presented at the annual meeting of the American Public Health Association, New Orleans, LA.

Trotter, J., Walp, J., Hunt, S., & Madachy, P. (1987, October). A moving collaborative effort. Paper presented at the annual meeting of the American Public Health Association, New Orleans, LA.

U.S. Department of Health and Human Services. (1990). *Healthy people 2000: National health promotion and disease prevention objectives.* Washington, DC: U.S. Government Printing Office.

Williams, C. (1983). Making things happen: Community health nursing and the policy arena. *Nursing Outlook, 31,* 225–228.

World Health Organization. (1991). *City networks for health.* Geneva, Switzerland: Author.

Wright, C. (1985). Computer-aided nursing diagnosis for community health nurses. *Nursing Clinics of North America, 20*(3), 487–495.

BIBLIOGRAPHY

Alinsky, S. (1971). *Rules for radicals: A pragmatic primer for realistic radicals.* New York: Random House.

Aydelotte, M., Barger, S., Branstetter, E., Fehring, R. Lingren, K., Lundeen, S., McDaniel, W., & Riesch, S. (1987). *The nursing center: Concept and design.* Washington, DC: American Nurses' Association.

Batra, C. (1992). Empowering for professional, political, and health policy involvement. *Nursing Outlook, 40*(4), 170–176.

Clark, H. M. (1986). A health planning simulation game. *Nurse Educator, 11*(4), 16–20.

Courtney, R. (1987). Community practice: Nursing influence on policy formation. *Nursing Outlook, 35*(4), 170–173.

Eigsti, D. G., Stein, K. Z., & Fortune, M. (1982). The community as client in planning for continuity of care. *Nursing and Health Care, 3*(5), 251–253.

Maglacas, A. (1988). Health for all: Nursing's role. *Nursing Outlook, 36*(2), 66–71.

Martinson, I., Jamieson, M., O'Grady, B, & Sime, M. (1985). The block nurse program. *Journal of Community Health Nursing, 2*(1), 21–29.

Moccia, P. (1988). At the faultline: Social activism and caring. *Nursing Outlook, 36*(1), 30–33.

Lundeen, S. (1993). Comprehensive, collaborative, coordinated, community-based care: A community nursing center model. *Family and Community Health, 16*(2), 57–65.

Stolte, K. (1986). A complementary view of nursing diagnosis. *Public Health Nursing, 3*(1), 23–28.

SUGGESTED READINGS

American Nurses' Association. (1986) *Standards of community health nursing practice.* Washington, DC: Author.

American Nurses' Association, Council of Community Health Nurses. (1986). *Community-based nursing services: Innovative models.* Washington, DC: Author.

American Pubilc Health Association. (1991). *Healthy communities 2000—model standards: Guidelines for community attainment of the year 2000 national health objectives.* Washington, DC: Author.

Association for the Advancement of Health Education. (1992). PATCH: Planned Approach To Community Health. *Journal of Health Education, 23*(3), 1–192.

Farley, S. (1993). The community as partner in primary health care. *Nursing and Health Care, 14*(5), 244–249.

Flynn, B., Rider, M., & Ray, D. (1991). Healthy cities: The Indiana model of community development in public health. *Health Education Quarterly, 18,* 331–347.

Schorr, L. (1989). *Within our reach: Breaking the cycle of disadvantage.* New York: Anchor Books, Doubleday.

U.S. Department of Health and Human Services. (1990). *Healthy people 2000: National health promotion and disease prevention objectives.* Washington, DC: U.S. Government Printing Office.

Chapter 14

Evaluation of Nursing Care with Communities

Claudia M. Smith

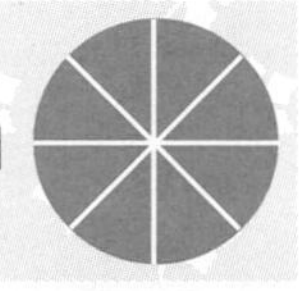

Focus Questions

What are the responsibilities of a community health nurse generalist in evaluation of nursing care with communities?

What are steps in evaluation?

What questions can be answered by evaluation?

What outcomes are indicators of the effectiveness of nursing interventions with communities?

How does evaluation of nursing care with communities compare with evaluation of care with families and individuals?

How can evaluation of process be used to improve the operation of nursing programs?

How is evaluation used to modify nursing care with communities?

What methods and tools are used in evaluation?

Responsibilities in Evaluation of Nursing Care with Communities

Evaluation is the process by which a nurse judges the value of nursing care that has been provided. As with any type of nursing care the community health nurse seeks to determine the degree to which planned goals were achieved and to describe any unplanned results.

The purpose of the evaluation is to facilitate additional decision-making. After an evaluation it might be possible to conclude that what had been done could not have been done better, that the goals were reached, and that the goals were mutually desirable to the nurse and the community members. This would be cause for celebration. As a result of another evaluation it might be possible to conclude that alterations are needed in the plan of care to more effectively reach the desired outcomes. Or it might be possible to conclude that, although goals were reached, the cost in money, time, or other resources was too expensive for the nurse or the community members.

Evaluation is based on several assumptions: first that nursing actions have results, both intended and unintended; second that nurses are accountable for their own actions and care provided; and third that different sets of actions result in resources being used differently (i.e., some nursing interventions use more resources than others).

Evaluation involves two parts: measurement and interpretation. Many different schemes or models exist for organizing ideas about evaluation, which may result in confusion among people who use different terminology for similar concepts.

Basic to the nursing process, however, is the notion of measuring whether planned goals were achieved. Synonyms for this activity and its result are *outcome attainment* (Donabedian, 1980), *performance evaluation* (Suchman, 1967), *results of effort,* and *evaluation of effectiveness* (Deniston and Rosenstock, 1970). The question that the nurse attempts to answer is, *Were the planned goals achieved?*

Another basic notion addresses the quality of the results and the process that contributed to the results. Some terms used to express this idea are *appropriateness, adequacy,* and *efficiency* (Table 14–1). These terms each describe different aspects of measuring quality. The following are some questions that may be asked about quality. *How and why did the interventions work? Were the nurses' actions ethical? Did the nurses address the most important goals? Did the nurses involve community members and recipients as participants (American Nurses' Association [ANA], 1986)? Were resources used wisely? How many needs and goals did the plan actually address?*

TABLE 14–1

Definitions

Appropriate—Suitable for a particular occasion or use; fitting
Adequate—Able to fill a requirement; sufficient or satisfactory
Effective—Producing an expected result; productive
Efficient—Acting effectively with minimum waste or effort; exhibiting a high ratio of output to input
Side effect—A secondary and usually unfavorable effect
Result—A consequence; outcome; a particular ending
Satisfaction—Fulfillment; gratification of a need or desire

RESPONSIBILITIES OF BACCALAUREATE-PREPARED COMMUNITY HEALTH NURSES

According to the ANA (1986), community health nurses with bachelor's degrees in nursing (community health nursing generalists) are expected to work with community health nurse specialists and community members in evaluating "responses of the community" to nursing interventions.

The responsibilities of community health nurses for evaluation of nursing care with communities vary depending on the size and complexity of the community and whether the community is geopolitical or phenomenological (see Chapter 12). Baccalaureate-prepared community health nurses are expected to work with community members, community health nurse specialists, and multidisciplinary teams to evaluate nursing care with geopolitical communities. Community health nurse generalists may also work with multidisciplinary teams and nurses who engage in quality assurance and accreditation reviews. Baccalaureate-prepared community health nurses will be more capable members of evaluating teams if they have been introduced in their education to ideas and skills in evaluating nursing care with communities (ANA, 1980).

There will be times when a baccalaureate-prepared community health nurse is working with a small phenomenological community, such as a senior center or school; it is likely that in this case the community health nurse can evaluate his or her own performance with minimal assistance from a supervisor and peers. Either independently or with help from supervisors community health nurses are expected to evaluate the effectiveness of intervention programs that involve teaching, direct physical care, and screening and referral.

Regardless of the type or size of community the members themselves are involved in planning and conducting the evaluation, as they are in all steps of the nursing process (ANA, 1986). It is impossible to measure many health outcomes without the judgment of the community members themselves.

FORMATIVE AND SUMMATIVE EVALUATION

When is nursing care with communities evaluated? Evaluation of the effectiveness of care that takes place after the interventions have been performed is known as *summative* evaluation because the nurse is evaluating the *sum,* the "bottom line," the end results. Summative evaluation involves measurement of community responses to nursing care and interpretation of the degree to which planned goals were met. Summative evaluation usually consists of measurement of outcomes and goal attainment.

Summative evaluation may also take place several months or years after nursing care has been provided. This evaluation seeks to determine whether there has been a long-term impact on the health status and the health responses of the community.

Formative evaluation is evaluation that occurs throughout the nursing process but before evaluation of the outcomes of care. This evaluation occurs during the *formation* of the nursing care and during its actual delivery. In other words formative evaluation considers the day-to-day provision of programs of nursing care. It is formative evaluation that allows ongoing modification of nursing practices.

COMMUNITY INVOLVEMENT

Because the community members are involved in evaluation, at least part of the evaluation must occur in the clients' community. Mutuality is an important aspect of evaluation. Because much of the impact of the community health nurse is indicated by self-care and lifestyle changes of community members, a nurse must document and validate outcomes directly with community members. Also, it is possible that, although goals have been achieved, some negative or unexpected results have also occurred. It is essential that the nurse explore the perceptions of community members to discover and validate the meaning of the experience. It is important to determine how satisfied community members are with both the outcomes and the nursing interventions.

Stakeholders are those who have expectations about nursing care, but who are not directly involved in its delivery. For example, there are those whose approval was necessary, those who contributed money or supplies, those who volunteered to assist, and those (such as "competitors") on whom the presence of nursing services had an impact. Stakeholders in a community immunization campaign might be the county health officer, a retail pharmacist who donates syringes, a local pediatrician who is concerned about financial competition, and parents of those immunized. Community health nurses need to identify the stakeholders and invite them to participate in evaluation.

STANDARDS FOR A GOOD EVALUATION

Standards for evaluation of nursing care with communities have been formulated by the ANA (1986):

1. The employing agency is to provide supervision, consultation, and general evaluation plans for the generalist community health nurse.
2. The community members are to participate in the evaluation.
3. The nursing care is to be revised based on the evaluation.
4. Evaluation is to be documented so that the record can strengthen nursing practice and knowledge.

Steps in Evaluation

Evaluation is a process that includes several steps: planning, collecting the data, analyzing and interpreting the

TABLE 14–2

Steps in Evaluation

Plan the Evaluation

1. Review goals and objectives.
2. Meet with stakeholders to identify which evaluation questions should be answered.
3. Develop a budget for evaluation.
4. Determine who will conduct the evaluation.
5. Develop the evaluation design: What will be done?
6. Decide which evaluation instruments will be used to collect information.
7. Analyze how the evaluation questions relate to the goals and objectives.
8. Analyze whether the questions of stakeholders are addressed.
9. Determine when the evaluation will be conducted; develop a time line.

Collect Evaluation Data

10. Develop specific processes for collecting data through questionnaires, review of records or documents, personal interviews, telephone interviews, and observation.
11. Determine who will collect the data.
12. Pilot the data collection instruments.
13. Refine the instruments based on data from the pilot.
14. Identify the sample of persons from whom evaluation data will be collected.
15. Collect the data.

Analyze the Data

16. Determine how the data will be analyzed.
17. Determine who will analyze data.
18. Analyze the data, generate several interpretations, and make recommendations.

Report the Evaluation

19. Determine who will receive results.
20. Determine who will report the findings.
21. Determine format for the report.
22. Discuss how the findings will affect the program.
23. Determine which findings will be included in the report.
24. Distribute the report.

Implement the Results

25. Plan how the results will be implemented.
26. Identify who will implement the results.
27. Determine when the results will be implemented; develop a time line.

Adapted from McKenzie, J., & Jurs, J. (1993). *Planning, implementing, and evaluating health promotion programs: A primer* (pp. 195–196). New York: Macmillan.

data, providing recommendations, reporting the results, and implementing the recommendations (McKenzie and Jurs, 1993). Table 14–2 identifies evaluation activities in greater detail related to each of the major steps.

Questions Answered by Evaluation

Evaluation of nursing care with communities involves evaluation of programs of care for populations. Program evaluation includes evaluation of outcomes (program goals and outcome objectives) as well as evaluation of the structures and processes used to achieve the outcomes (Hale et al., 1994). The ANA considers *outcomes, structures,* and *processes* as the primary categories of criteria to be used to measure the quality of nursing care. *Outcomes* are the end results; *structures* are the social and physical resources; and *processes* are the "sequence of events and activities" (ANA, 1986, p. 18) used by the nurse during the delivery of care.

Table 14–3 describes the following five categories of questions that can be answered by evaluation: (1) outcome attainment, also called effectiveness; (2) appropriateness of care; (3) adequacy of care in relation to the scope of the problem; (4) relationship of resources to results, also called efficiency; and (5) process. This set of questions includes the criteria of outcome, structure, and process evaluation and adds appropriateness and adequacy. Questions of appropriateness and adequacy evaluate the nursing care program in relationship to the community health needs. Efficiency addresses the relationship of outcomes to structures and processes. Each of these sets of evaluation questions are discussed in more detail.

EVALUATION OF OUTCOME ATTAINMENT

Evaluation of outcome attainment, also called effectiveness, addresses the results of nursing care. Change toward predetermined goals, as well as unplanned effects, may have occurred, including changes in the population, the health care system within the community, or the environment (see Table 14–3). Table 14–4 identifies several variables that can be used as outcome measures of community health. Changes can occur in the population's

TABLE 14–3

Questions Answered by Evaluation

Variable	Questions	Examples of Measurement
1. Outcome attainment	Did change occur? To what degree was progress made toward the goal? What are actual effects on clients? What unintended outcomes occurred?	Numbers and rates of children immunized Numbers of cases of cancer found on Papanicolaou smears Changes in attitudes regarding people with acquired immunodeficiency syndrome (AIDS) Reduction in teenage pregnancy rate
2. Appropriateness	Did the goals fit the need? Are the goals and plans acceptable to the community? Are the plans likely to achieve the goals? Does the plan duplicate existing efforts?	Plan of care compared wth clinical nursing knowledge Community preferences
3. Adequacy	To what degree does the intervention meet the total amount of need? Were some people not served?	Rate of effectiveness multiplied by number of people exposed to service Outcomes relative to total needs in population Degree to which need was a priority
4. Efficiency		
Cost-effectiveness	What resources were used? Is there a better way to attain the same results? What resources were necessary to attain results?	Relation of effort to outcome Output/input Money Time Personnel Client convenience
Benefit-cost analysis	Do the benefits justify the use of resources?	
5. Process	What did nurses do? When? Where? How many people were reached? Why were there successes and/or failures? What contributed to the results? What methods were used?	Numbers of clinics/week or month Numbers of home visits Amount of money spent Education content taught and strategies used Numbers of people attending screening sessions

Data from Deniston, O., & Rosenstock, I. (1970). Evaluating health programs. *Public Health Reports, 85,* 835–840; Donabedian, A. (1980). *The definition of quality and approaches to its assessment, Vol. 1.* Ann Arbor, MI: Health Administration Press; Freeman, R. (1963). *Public health nursing practice* (3rd ed.). Philadelphia: W.B. Saunders; and Suchman, E. (1967). *Evaluative research: Principles and practice in public service and social action programs.* New York: Russell Sage Foundation.

TABLE 14–4

Possible Outcome Measures

Possible Outcome Measures
1. Knowledge
2. Behaviors, skills
3. Attitudes, commitment to action
4. Emotional well-being
5. Health status (epidemiological measures)
6. Presence of health care system services and components
7. Satisfaction/acceptance regarding the program interventions
8. Presence of policy allowing, mandating, funding
9. Altered relationship with physical environment

knowledge, behavior and skills, attitudes, emotional well-being, and health status.

When evaluating the health of a community it is necessary to consider more than the outcomes of the population. Because the interaction of people in their environment facilitates or hinders health, such variables as the presence of health services, the satisfaction and acceptance of such programs, the presence of policies, and a harmonious balance with the environment must also be considered. Each of these variables, which is used as an outcome measure of the health of communities, is discussed in more detail.

Knowledge

A great deal of patient teaching and health education is evaluated by measuring the health-related information that the individual, group, or population has obtained. Although information alone does not result in behavior changes, having information will often increase the possibility of behavior changes. For example, just because a father knows how to prepare infant formula in the proper concentration and with adequate asepsis does not ensure that he will actually do so. However, if he does not have that information, the only way he could prepare the formula would be by trial and error or by chance. Having the information increases the probability that it will be prepared properly.

When evaluating populations, surveys may be used to determine knowledge about specific health-related topics. Such surveys may be conducted as interviews or through written questionnaires (Polit and Hungler, 1993). When working with populations the community health nurse is interested in the proportion of the population that was reached by the teaching and the proportion that retained the information presented. Having information is not sufficient for healthy living; the information must be put to use.

Behaviors and Skills

Integrating health-related behaviors and skills into daily living affects health status. Raising children; caring for an elderly bed-bound family member; seeking a prostate examination; and preparing nutritious foods require action. Such actions are labeled *competent* or *skilled* if they are consistent with existing knowledge and if they are performed in an effective and efficient manner.

Health behaviors may change as a result of interventions performed by community health nurses (see Chapters 16 and 18 for more details regarding health promotion and health teaching).

When evaluating health behaviors of populations the nurse's interest is in the proportion of the population who engage in such behaviors. The usual way to collect information about health behaviors is to ask people what they do. However, people do not always provide accurate reports, as they may have forgotten information or want to "look good" to the surveyor.

Time and money often limit the degree to which behavior change can be measured. Observing the behavior of populations helps confirm the accuracy of what is reported; however, this takes much more time and money. Asking people to make a contract with themselves to make a commitment to specific actions has been shown to increase the likelihood that the actions will be performed (Sloan and Schommer, 1991). Therefore, when it is not possible to measure actual behavioral changes of populations, community health nurses can measure the degree to which people commit to specific actions.

Attitudes

Attitudes include opinions and preferences about ideas, people, and things. Persons have attitudes about the concept of health and the ways in which health may be attained and maintained. Because attitudes predispose the selection of some actions over others, attitudes are a health-related measure. For example, if a population generally views health as the ability to perform work, people may take cold medication to allow them to feel well enough to go to work. However, they may not alter their high-cholesterol diets because their current diets do not interfere with their immediate ability to work.

Community attitudes also predispose the population to support or work against various policies and services. For example, if the dominant community attitude toward criminals is that they should be punished and live stark lives, there may be little support for prison health services. If the predominant community attitude is that health prevention can reduce human suffering and dollars spent for sickness care, there may be more support for prison health services.

Attitudes toward health and health behavior can be changed through planned or spontaneous experiences. Attitudinal change is also called *emotional* or *affective learning*. Attitudes of populations can be measured before and after an intervention to determine whether affective learning has occurred. Changes in attitude may predispose people to change their behaviors. For example, as more members of a population adopt the attitude that smoking is undesirable, smoking rates decrease.

Emotional Well-Being

Emotional well-being in a population can be measured by the proportion of members who experience self-esteem and satisfaction with their lives. Emotional well-being of a community can be measured also by assessing the structures and processes that exist to strengthen human development and connectedness. For example, a group of nursing students initiated a "reminiscence group," during which residents of a nursing home could reflect on and share their life experiences. The students' initial assessment indicated that the residents rarely communicated with each other, even when in the same room; had few visitors; and reported that they did not "feel at home." After several weekly meetings the nursing students observed that the participants initiated conversation more with each other, and several of the residents reported "feeling at home."

Criteria for emotional well-being of a community also include the degree of acceptance and cohesion among members and patterns of support, socialization, and decision-making. When community members participate in the decision-making that leads to goal achievement, perceptions of self-efficacy are enhanced. *Self-efficacy* is the belief that one can influence one's environment and circumstances. Self-efficacy contributes to self-concept and is necessary if community members are to have an impact on their health.

Health Status

The ultimate measure of the effectiveness of health services and programs is the health status of the population. Community health programs seek to reduce premature deaths, disabilities, and injuries. Health status is measured using epidemiological statistics about morbidity and mortality (see Chapter 11). More recently there have been attempts to measure increases in positive health that occur after nursing interventions. To measure positive health, the community health nurse focuses on what is desirable, rather than on the reduction of health problems. Two examples of such measurements are the percentage of the population with normal blood pressure and the percentage of the population engaging in safer sex.

Presence of Health-Related Services

Community health nursing interventions may be directed toward establishing new services and programs or strengthening the continuity of care among existing services. Such interventions may be measured by the presence of new health services and by the increased numbers of people receiving care. For example, in one senior center, the community health nursing students noted that the population was not engaging in physical exercise. Knowing that nursing students could not be assigned permanently at that site, the students developed a videotape of exercises for the elderly. Copies were made for all of the senior centers in the suburban county. This resulted in multiple senior centers having access to professionally led, appropriate exercises. As a result of the nursing interventions, a new service was available for senior citizens.

Satisfaction/Acceptance

Health-related services may exist in a community but not be effective because the people within the community do not accept the service. The perceived quality of interpersonal relationships is an important factor in strengthening client satisfaction. For example, if the members of the community do not feel that they are treated with dignity when they attend a clinic, they are likely to stop attending. They will transfer to another service, if one exists, or they may even go without care to avoid the negative experiences. Even when the care provided through a nursing program is effective, more people may be reached if the program is also tailored to be satisfying to the participants.

Geographic accessibility, waiting time, and cost are other factors that contribute to a population's satisfaction with nursing programs. When nurses are aware of the culture of the population, clients are likely to be more satisfied.

Satisfaction with services can be measured through interviews and questionnaires. Questionnaires have the advantage of being anonymous. Questions may be as simple as asking, *What do you like about coming to this clinic? What would you change?*

Policies

Policies are expressions of goals and rules that exist within a community; they are expressions of values (Diers, 1985). Policies may be decided by persons within governments, formal organizations (such as the ANA, the American Heart Association, and nonprofit volunteer clinics), businesses, and informal groups. Interpersonal and political power influence the creation and maintenance of policies.

Community health nurses, often in collaboration with others, can use the existence of health and social policy as one measure of the effectiveness of interpersonal and political power. New policy may be created or an existing policy may be defended or changed. Policy may mandate, allow, or initiate actions that affect a community's health. For example, during recent state budget cuts, one state nurses' association passed a resolution advocating that budget cuts not be made in health programs for the poor and disabled. Such organizational policy served as a guide for nurses who were lobbying their state legislators to disallow cuts in medical assistance, provide basic health care for all, and fund positions for school nurses who care for children with disabilities.

Altered Relationships with the Environment

Elimination or reduction of environmental hazards is one measure of the effectiveness of programs directed toward providing a safer environment. For example, the removal of trash in a vacant lot reduces breeding grounds for rats and other wild animals while also removing physical and chemical hazards. Additionally the effectiveness of a community educational program about environmental hazards may result in reduced dumping. Reductions in environmental hazards result in fewer accidents and injuries.

Reductions in consumption and waste are other measures of environmental health. More efficient use of resources is the goal. For example, increasing the numbers of people who weatherize their homes or participate in recycling demonstrates the effectiveness of conservation programs. Community health nurses may be instrumental in collaborating to establish such programs or in referring people to existing programs.

Because the basic standard of living is associated with health behaviors and health status, the level of poverty in a community can be used as one measure of the community's health. The level of poverty directly relates to both the physical and the social environments (Haan et al., 1987). Therefore, changes in the level of poverty can be used as a measure of the effectiveness of public health activities to improve the basic standard of living within the community.

EVALUATION OF APPROPRIATENESS

Appropriateness may be defined as how well the nursing planning and interventions fit the assessed health need. The community health nurse considers the appropriateness of both the goals and the interventions. Table 14–3 includes some questions used in the evaluation of the appropriateness of nursing care.

Goals are usually more appropriate when the community health nurse has accurately assessed health needs of the population, readiness to change, and resources available. The *Healthy People 2000* objectives (U.S. Department of Health and Human Services [DHHS], 1990) are targets that guide local communities in selecting specific goals and objectives for health programs. When the assessment and planning have been conducted in partnership with the community members, the nursing care is more likely to be appropriate. At times the community health nurse must wait until after the intervention has been accomplished to evaluate whether the specific goals and objectives were realistic for a given community. Just as each individual is unique, so is each community.

The interventions are usually more appropriate when the community health nurse is familiar with the literature that describes what has worked well with similar populations. Nursing case studies and experimental research are helpful in suggesting ideas for interventions within a specific community. For example, it is known that strengthening the decision-making skills of adolescents is helpful in preventing drug use and unprotected sex. Exercise has been shown to slow the progression of osteoporosis in postmenopausal women. Consequently each of these interventions would be evaluated as appropriate with their respective populations.

EVALUATION OF ADEQUACY

The community health nurse also evaluates the adequacy of both the goals and the interventions. Adequacy addresses the degree to which goals and interventions are sufficient to achieve the desired change. Table 14–3 includes some questions related to adequacy.

Even when care is appropriate, it may be inadequate. Nursing care is inadequate when there is not enough of that care as compared with the total population need. For example, community health nurses who provide outreach to identify pregnant women, refer them for prenatal care and nutrition programs, and teach them about the importance of nutrition are engaged in appropriate nursing care. Prenatal care and improved nutrition are ways to increase the birth weight of infants. However, such care may be inadequate if there are far more pregnant women than can be reached by the number of community health nurses. Such care may also be inadequate if the women are "found" but the prenatal and nutrition services have long waiting lists. When nursing services are appropriate but inadequate to meet the need, nurses should consider other interventions, such as creating community awareness that additional services are needed.

EVALUATION OF EFFICIENCY

Efficiency is related to evaluation of structure because it is a measure of the relationship of resources to outcomes. Resources may include the nurses themselves, equipment, facilities, policies or legal authority, organizational features, and environmental features (ANA, 1986). Money, time, and emotional energy are other resources.

Table 14–3 also includes some questions to ask when considering efficiency. For example, when evaluating the efficiency of a well-child clinic, the community health nurse might ask whether equipment exists that is not used, how many doses of immunizations were wasted, whether the layout of the clinic prevents unnecessary walking yet provides privacy, or whether heat escapes out the door each time it is opened.

The money, time, and other resources of the population must also be considered. Interventions may be efficient for nurses but inefficient for individuals and their families. Are

TABLE 14–5

Questions to Ask in Process Evaluation of Health Programs

Is the target population being reached? If not, what outreach or publicity may be needed? What evidence exists that the program is acceptable to the target population?
How many people have been served? How does this compare with projections of desired utilization? What should be done if the demand for services exceeds the current capacity?
Are the program activities being phased in on time? If not, what modifications in the time line are needed?
What are the staff development needs of the nurses and other personnel? What aspects of the intervention are difficult to implement and require further education?
Are the planned resources being received? Have the budget revenues continued as planned? Are the program expenditures within the proposed budget? Have equipment and materials been received? Have interested persons volunteered as they said they would?
Have the planned interventions been carried out? If so, to what degree do they meet professional standards?
Have any of the planned interventions not been implemented? If so, what are the barriers? Can these interventions be omitted because the objectives are being achieved without the interventions? Or should the interventions still be initiated?
What concerns have emerged regarding communication, decision-making, and participation? Are all interested parties still involved and informed about the program's progress? How do they perceive the program?

parents tired when they reach the clinic because they could not afford a sitter for the other children? Are parents dissatisfied with the information they receive because the language of the nurses and pamphlets is "over their heads"?

PROCESS EVALUATION

Process evaluation focuses on how well the health-related program is operating and is linked to the original plan (Patton, 1982). The questions included in Table 14–5 help analyze how well the planned program is actually being implemented. Answering the questions helps the community health nurse refine and manage the program. Process evaluation is concerned with clinical nursing care, but it also focuses on administrative and fiscal issues (Meany-Handy, 1985). Evaluation of the process of implementing the program is formative, because it occurs throughout the life of the program.

Uniqueness in Evaluation of Nursing Care with Communities

CRITERIA FOR EFFECTIVENESS

In goal-based evaluation of populations, criteria for success are written in terms of *percent of population,* not an individual or a family. Because more than one individual is being evaluated, the population must often be sampled. In large populations a random sample of at least 10% to 20% of persons will be useful. With small populations it is most helpful if the nurse can obtain information from all members, or as many as possible. One hundred percent participation is rare, however.

More time and personnel may be needed to evaluate the care provided to populations or communities. Because of the numbers of people in the population, there may be a need for more than one person to collect the information for evaluation. More time may also be required to ensure that the evaluators are following the same procedures, which increases interobserver reliability (Polit and Hungler, 1993).

For care provided to individuals and families, the evaluation is documented on the legal record of the respective client. When evaluating care provided to populations, the results are usually reported as statistics for the aggregate or as a case study (without identifying the specific participants).

Because populations include multiple individuals or families, the criteria for measuring goal achievement may compare the population with another population; measurements must be available for both populations to make the comparison. This is often called *normative referencing.* The population may be compared with itself before and after the implementation. If change occurred, the nurse would expect to see an increase or decrease in one or more outcome measures. The population also may be compared with an entirely different population, such as the average for the United States. For example, if a population had an incidence of prostate cancer higher than the average rate in the United States, the goal might be to reduce the incidence of prostate cancer to the national rate.

Criterion-referenced evaluation measures the extent to which specific objectives are reached at the level desired by the planner. Most of the *Healthy People 2000* objectives are criterion-referenced objectives. The following is a criterion-referenced objective targeted toward mothers of infants and preschool children: In a smoking modification program, at least 30% of the mothers will devise and implement a contract to modify their smoking habits by the fifth week of the program. If 30% of the mothers do so, the objective will have been achieved. The mothers are not compared with other populations. (Chapter 13 provides more examples of normative-referenced and criterion-referenced objectives.)

There is no easy way to determine what the criteria should be. Sometimes, for example, if the desired behavior is essential for safety, the criteria are high. For example, 100% of participants will hold the infant with the head higher than the stomach and burp the infant during feeding, so that the infant does not choke. When a nurse believes that all of the participants should know how to demonstrate the skill, then the behaviors should be as clear as possible.

TABLE 14–6

Tool to Assess Clients' Interests

Put a check mark (✓) by the three things that you want to learn about most.

_____ What is the difference between medicine and street drugs?

_____ What can street drugs do to my body?

_____ How can I say no to drugs?

_____ What can I do to feel good without using drugs?

_____ Why do people use drugs?

_____ Other ____________________

____

The criteria for proper holding need to be explicit in this objective.

However, it is usually not realistic for 100% of the participants to reach the objectives. In group education sessions there are usually a few people who are not interested that day, not feeling well, or are distracted so that they do not participate fully. Even when the participants are interested in learning, the teaching may not be sufficient for them to learn. They may need different learning strategies or more time. If the desired learning is complex or requires a change in lifestyle, nurses should expect a lower percentage of the population to achieve the objective. For example, 14% to 45% of smokers who quit are able to abstain for 12 months (Pirie and others, 1992).

Criteria for desirable outcomes can be selected because they reflect the clients' interests. For example, elementary school children were given an interest inventory to determine what they most wanted to learn related to drugs (Table 14–6). Their answers helped nursing students establish both the objectives of and the content for the teaching sessions.

Criteria for desirable outcomes also can be selected because they constitute the next logical step. For example, after parents have learned to take the temperature of their infant, they should know which temperatures to report to the pediatrician, clinic, or nurse practitioner.

SOURCES OF EVALUATION DATA

The nursing process is to be mutual with the entire population or their representatives. Consequently evaluation of community health nursing practice involves participants from the community (ANA, 1986). As part of the planning for evaluation, decisions must be made regarding who will be involved in the evaluation.

Some evaluation questions can be answered by the nurse alone and others can be answered best when others' perspectives are solicited. When measuring effectiveness the community health nurse ensures that the relevant outcome measures are collected from the target population. At times it will also be helpful to collect information from others close to the target population. For example, in a smoking cessation program, the community health nurse may also collect information about smoking habits from other members of the participants' households (this would be done with the participants' permission).

Epidemiological mortality and morbidity data often are obtained from other health care team members who collected the information. If the goal is a health system change, such as the establishment of a clinic, a visit to the new clinic and interviews with both the health providers and the population receiving care will be useful.

The community health nurse can evaluate efficiency with information from both the nurses implementing the health care program and the population who received care. Nurses can best describe the effort that they contributed: Who did what? How many times? With how many people? The participants themselves can best describe their efforts in terms of time, money, and physical and emotional energy. To evaluate efficiency, both effort and outcomes must be measured and considered together.

Dissatisfaction occurs most frequently when expectations are not met. Nurses should expect dissatisfaction to be expressed by those who perceive that care is inappropriate, inadequate, inefficient, or ineffective. At times the care provided by community health nurses may be both effective and relatively efficient, yet contribute to the dissatisfaction of some. There are many stakeholders who have expectations about nursing care, yet who are not directly involved in its delivery. The more the community health nurse is aware of stakeholders' expectations during the planning phase, the fewer surprises there will be. Intermittent contact with all interested parties throughout

TABLE 14–7

Data in a Written Evaluation Report

1. Indicate baseline health status/behaviors of client population.
2. Indicate baseline resources and methods currently being used to address the health problem.
3. List the health-related goals and objectives.
4. Describe the nursing interventions (effort). Enumerate what actions were completed. If an educational strategy is being evaluated, include both the actions completed and the content taught.
5. Indicate things that were planned but *not* done.
6. Specify other changes in the environment that could have affected the health outcomes (such as changes in funding, a television health education campaign, or the closing of a clinic).
7. Describe what behaviors indicate goal achievement and the degree to which the need is resolved.
8. Describe the level of satisfaction of those involved and identify actual and potential resistance.
9. Indicate any modifications that were made in the goals.
10. Discuss the relationship of effort to outcomes—efficiency.
11. Include interpretations and judgments.
12. Make recommendations.

the process will allow early identification of misunderstandings, negotiation, and revision of the process to balance the interests of many. At times it is impossible to satisfy everyone.

RECORDING EVALUATIONS

Table 14–7 identifies data that are to be included in a written record of the evaluation of nursing care with communities. This documentation describes what actually occurred, provides a historical record from which to study trends, and provides a basis for deciding whether programs should be continued and how they might be modified.

Analyzing Evaluation Data

Distinctions should be made among facts, interpretations, judgments, and recommendations when discussing and presenting the results of an evaluation (Patton, 1982). Factual findings include data (e.g., the program has served 50 clients during the first 2 months). Interpretations are statements about interrelationships, reasons, and meanings (e.g., the clients have shown up because of the public service announcements on the radio). Judgments are evaluations made in the context of values and include statements about the desirability or undesirability or goodness or badness of the data and interpretations (e.g., I'm really disappointed that we haven't reached 100 clients already). Recommendations are suggested actions based on the facts, interpretations, and judgments. A recommendation in this situation might be to increase the publicity to double the numbers of clients served in the next 3 months.

Modification of Nursing Care with Communities

Communities are dynamic and complex. Each human being exists within a community and is an agent of his or her own needs, desires, and self-expression. Social interaction among *multiple* human beings is even more complex. Consequently because nursing care is created through the processes of human interaction, it must be continuously evaluated and revised. As the membership of the population changes, so do health status, health risks, health needs, and interests.

Community health nursing practice occurs within physical, political, economic, cultural, and social contexts. A change in any one of those contexts results in changes in all other aspects of the community system. While nurses implement the planned care, there are a multitude of changes that occur simultaneously in their environments. Therefore, formative evaluation helps community health nurses to modify all steps of the nursing process.

Evaluation Methods and Tools

DESIGNS FOR EVALUATION OF EFFECTIVENESS

Case descriptions and quasi-experimental designs may be used to evaluate the effectiveness of community health nursing interventions with communities (Kosecoff and Fink, 1982). A case description examines the community, health goals, community health nursing interventions, and outcomes. The evaluation described in this chapter can be used to develop a case description. The case evaluation design allows a thorough description of the situation and is especially helpful in creating a history of the process, communicating information about a new or a demonstration program to others, and documenting both formative and summative evaluations. With a case description, the community health nurses cannot prove that it was the nursing intervention that led to the specific health outcomes. However, there are ways to evaluate the likelihood that the outcomes were the result of the nursing interventions: (1) the implementation can occur shortly after assessment so that developmental maturation does not account for the change; (2) the population members can be asked whether they participated in other activities from the time of assessment until the time of evaluation; and (3) the nurse can be alert to other community changes that might have contributed simultaneously to the health outcomes (Kosecoff and Fink, 1982).

The time-series design is a quasi-experimental method in which information is collected about the same population more than once (Kosecoff and Fink, 1982). The steps of the nursing process include assessment, pre-test, implementation, evaluation (post-test), and later evaluation. Such a design allows pre-test and post-test results to be compared to demonstrate that change did occur. Additionally the later evaluation indicates whether or not the change was lasting; this evaluation considers permanency of results, also called *impact.*

Evaluation research attempts to discover links between implementations and health results, including the meaning of the experience to the participants. The goal of empirical evaluation research is to establish that interventions are causally linked to desired outcomes. Such knowledge is generalizable to similar situations and can assist community health nurses in selecting which intervention strategies are likely to work best. Such information helps persuade funding sources that their money will be well spent.

Because human beings are diverse, evaluation research also seeks to find what works best with different populations. How are the results different with women and men, or young and old? For example, empirical research indicates that young children learn best through participation. Interpretive evaluation research seeks to describe the meaning of the experience to the participants. When nurses understand the perceptual and cultural meanings that the

TABLE 14–8

Checklist Tool for Evaluating Behaviors Related to Infant Feeding

This tool can be used to observe parent or caregiver behavior related to infant formula feeding. An item is checked when the behavior is observed during a feeding session.

_____	Responds to hunger cues almost always
_____	Uses clean bottle/nipple/formula
_____	Changes or washes nipple if contaminated
_____	Holds infant
_____	Holds bottle so that air is not allowed in nipple *or* uses collapsible bag bottles
_____	Burps infant
_____	Stops at _____ oz. or sooner if infant is full

nursing care has for the participants, nurses are better able to modify care. The care can become more beneficial and satisfying for the recipients.

TOOLS FOR EVALUATION OF EFFECTIVENESS

The category of health outcome that is being measured will help determine the tools that will be used. Often the tools are the same ones that are used to measure change with individuals; however, the community health nurse is now collecting the information from large numbers of people.

Behavior change is best measured through observation. Some parenting programs, for example, have used videotapes of parent-child interactions to collect information about aspects of parenting; the tapes are then given to the parents as a reward for participation. Criteria used to interpret parenting skills can take several forms. Table 14–8 includes a checklist that can be used to record the presence or absence of specific parenting actions. Table 14–9 addresses similar actions but rates the quality of the parenting based on constellations of behaviors.

Oral or written questions are usually used to collect information on factual knowledge and attitudinal learning. The same questions can be used to measure both, but the scoring is different. Table 14–10 provides examples of questions that are modified to measure factual knowledge or attitudes.

TABLE 14–9

Rating Tool for Evaluating Behaviors Related to Infant Feeding

Client demonstrates proper infant feeding by responding to infant hunger cues, preparing clean bottle/nipple/formula, holding infant, preventing sucking of air, and feeding no more than _____oz.

Score 1	Score 3	Score 5
Sometimes responds to cry	Usually responds to hunger cues	Always responds to hunger cues
Often uses contaminated nipples and dirty bottles	Occasionally uses contaminated nipples and dirty bottles	Uses clean equipment; changes nipple if contaminated
Usually props infant	Usually holds infant	Never props bottle
Allows sucking of air	Usually does not allow air in nipple	Prevents air in nipple
Feeds continuously	Stops at _____oz. to burp infant	Stops at _____oz. to burp infant

EFFICIENCY ANALYSIS

The efficiency of programs can be evaluated using cost-effectiveness and benefit-cost analyses. Both consider the resources used in relation to outcomes.

In cost-effectiveness the cost per unit of outcome is determined. For example in a home health agency the average cost per home visit can be determined if costs and number of home visits are recorded. Similarly, the average cost per maternity clinic visit or the average cost of providing prenatal nursing care can also be computed. The costs must be computed and the value of the outcomes must be estimated (Schalock and Thornton, 1988). To accurately compare the cost-effectiveness of programs, the acuity of patient problems must be similar for the two programs. Cost-effectiveness analysis is often used to address the

TABLE 14–10

Questions Modified to Measure Knowledge and Attitude

Knowledge:

For each item, circle either True or False.

1. True or False: Use of condoms during sexual intercourse can help prevent HIV infection.
2. True or False: Environmental tobacco smoke can reach a fetus during the mother's pregnancy.

Key: 1. True; 2. True.

Attitude:

For each item, circle Yes if you agree with the statement and circle No if you disagree with the statement.

1. Yes or No: Condoms should be used by sexually active individuals to prevent HIV infections.
2. Yes or No: Pregnant women should be encouraged to avoid environmental tobacco smoke.

Alternative Attitude Format:

Circle the response that indicates the intensity with which you agree or disagree with each item.

1. Condoms should be used by sexually active individuals to prevent HIV infections.

   Strongly Agree   Agree   Uncertain   Disagree   Strongly Disagree

2. Pregnant women should be encouraged to avoid environmental tobacco smoke.

   Strongly Agree   Agree   Uncertain   Disagree   Strongly Disagree question, *Can similar outcomes be achieved with less cost?*

Benefit-cost analysis also considers the resources used in relation to the resulting outcomes. However, benefit-cost analysis asks, *Are the outcomes achieved worth the cost incurred?* A number of difficulties are encountered in completing a benefit-cost analysis (Schalock and Thornton, 1988). First such an analysis is difficult to do because it requires that a dollar value be placed on the benefits (outcomes) and health programs often produce some intangible effects. Not all outcomes can be quantified in terms of dollars. For example what is the dollar value of improved self-esteem? Second to provide justice (i.e., to correct an inequity in access to health care), the provision of care may be more important than whether it is efficient. Third the value of benefits must be considered from several perspectives. For example, the provision of home visits to families with infants can benefit the infant, the parent, and society. If only the cost of care versus the immediate health outcomes is considered (e.g., having up-to-date childhood immunizations) the benefits may not seem worth the cost. However, if the long-term benefit of preventing hospitalization and disability from measles and the benefit of high immunization levels within the community are considered, the benefits are greater.

Costs of programs include the direct costs of services, administrative costs, and the costs of increased demand on related services (Schalock and Thornton, 1988). For example, costs of an immunization program include direct cost of nursing services, equipment, educational material, and biological agents; indirect costs include record-keeping, utilities and building maintenance, salaries of administrative personnel, and publicity. There may also be increased health care costs related to identification, referral, and treatment of health problems among the children who come for immunizations.

The costs that clients incur in terms of time, energy, and money should be considered in benefit-cost analyses. However, current methods of benefit-cost analysis often ignore this human impact, especially for families with ill members. For example, care of ill persons in the home costs the health care system less than care in a hospital or nursing home. However, for some families the cost of caring for their family member at home is expensive in terms of lost wages and/or emotional stress.

Evaluation of efficiency helps community health nurses refine programs so that more services are provided with the same dollars, or the same services are provided at a lower cost. Dollars saved can be channeled to serve more people or to fund other health programs. Because community health nurses directly provide the care in many health programs, they are likely to have evidence of the less tangible benefits of the services. It is important that they contribute this information to any benefit-cost analysis. Because there is no precise estimation of the benefits, community health nurses can help expand the discussion to include quality-of-life issues.

Summary

Evaluation of nursing care with communities seeks to determine whether health has improved. Were the desired health goals reached? How much progress was made toward the goals? What themes, patterns, and results emerged? What side effects were evident? Evaluation of care is primarily descriptive and interpretive.

Community health nurses want to know that they are making a positive contribution to the lives of those they serve. It is motivational for nurses to learn that their practice has contributed to improvements in the health of populations, the structures of care, or the environment. Such personal knowledge affirms the value of the nurses' care. Evaluation more importantly provides information to help community health nurses improve their nursing practice.

KEY IDEAS

1. The responsibilities of community health nurses include the evaluation of nursing care provided to communities.
2. Evaluation involves several steps including planning the evaluation, collecting the data, analyzing and interpreting the data, reporting the evaluation, and implementing the suggestions.
3. Evaluations are conducted to demonstrate that goals and objectives are being achieved; to make decisions about continuing, expanding, or ending specific programs of nursing interventions; to improve nursing care so that goals and objectives are achieved efficiently; and to improve nursing care so that it is acceptable to the community.
4. Health-related programs have goals, outcome objectives, process objectives, and administrative objectives.
5. Formative evaluation is conducted during the process of nursing care delivery to modify and improve the program. Summative evaluation occurs at the end of the program to determine whether goals and outcome objectives were achieved.
6. Community members are to be involved in evaluation. Stakeholders are those who may be affected by the nursing interventions, including those who contribute resources and those who receive the care.
7. An essential part of evaluation is determining effectiveness: whether the goals and outcome objectives have been achieved. Indicators of the effectiveness of nursing care include knowledge, behavior and skills, attitudes, emotional well-being, morbidity and mortality rates, the presence of

services or health policies, client satisfaction, and human/environment relationships.

8. Programs of nursing care should be appropriate to the assessed community needs.
9. Community health nurses seek to develop programs of nursing care that are adequate to the scope of community needs.
10. Programs of nursing care need to be efficient: the resources need to be used wisely to achieve the desired outcomes.
11. Evaluation of process objectives helps monitor and improve programs of nursing care. Process evaluation addresses the degree to which the program of interventions is being carried out as planned.
12. Evaluation enables the improvement of nursing care with communities.

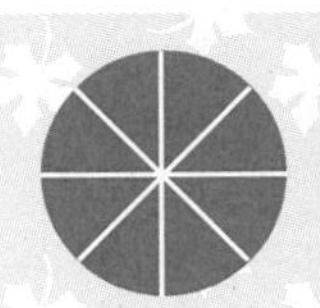

APPLYING THE NURSING PROCESS: *Evaluation at Northview High School*

The following evaluation is based on the program of nursing care for Northview High School described in the application of the nursing process in Chapter 13.

Phase I: A Sex Education Program

Nursing Diagnoses/Problems

1. Population at risk for health problems owing to high rate of sexual activity
2. Knowledge deficit related to the risks of pregnancy during sexual activity
3. Inconsistent use of birth control
4. Knowledge deficit related to functioning of various birth control mechanisms
5. Knowledge deficit related to signs, symptoms, and potential consequences of untreated sexually transmitted diseases

Program Goals

Provide students with the skills needed to explore the pros and cons of engaging in sexual activity during adolescence

Increase the knowledge level of students about sexually related information so that students can make informed choices about behavior

Problem 1 Outcome Objective. Consistent with the *Healthy People 2000* objectives, reduce the number of students who begin sexual activity or increase the number of students who postpone beginning sexual activity until they are older

Problem 2 Outcome Objective. Increase student knowledge about the process of conception

Problems 3 and 4 Outcome Objective. Increase student knowledge about birth control methods

Problem 5 Outcome Objective. Increase student knowledge of sexually transmitted disease

Process Objective

Seventy-five percent of students will participate in the instructional program during spring semester

Evaluation Plan

Ms. Fields is responsible for formulating an evaluation plan. In consultation with the others involved in implementing the program (teachers, psychologist, social worker) an evaluation plan is developed. A series of four evaluation methods are decided on to measure the outcomes (effectiveness) of the program:

1. Observations and interviews with participants in the seminar discussion and peer network programs to evaluate Problem 1
2. A post-test to measure knowledge levels to evaluate Problems 2, 3, 4, and 5
3. A survey to measure sexual activity and practices to evaluate Problem 1
4. A summary evaluation of the effectiveness of the entire sex education program

Collection of Evaluation Data

1. Ms. Fields attended two of the seminar discussions led by the social worker to observe student/leader interactions and student responses. Additionally, the students were asked to evaluate the seminars using a five-question evaluation survey to measure satisfaction with room provided for additional comments. Ms. Fields and the psychologist devised an interview tool to guide the evaluation process of the peer support program.
2. A 20-question post-test was developed by Ms. Fields and the other two teachers in the sex education program. The post-test measured knowledge in the area of pregnancy risks; appropriate use of birth control; and the signs, symptoms, and potential consequences of untreated sexually transmitted disease.
3. A random sampling survey was conducted of the student population who received the intervention program. It measured sexual behavior 3 months after the program.
4. Summary evaluation of the program included evaluation steps 1, 2, and 3 above as well as interviews with the principal, teaching staff, and counselors; an assessment of the number of students affected; and the time and materials necessary to accomplish the program.

Analysis of the Data

1. Evaluation of the seminar discussion group indicated that approximately 70% of the students in attendance were actively engaged in the guided discussion. They asked and answered questions and raised issues during the discussion. The student evaluation of the seminars indicated that 80% felt the seminars were informative and 65% said the discussions were helpful in aiding their decision-making process related to initiating or continuing sexual activity, in analyzing the role of peer pressure in the decision-making process, and in clarifying their position on the issues. About 10% of students thought the discussions were useless, and 12% reported they did not feel comfortable engaging in the discussion process.

   The peer support program was intended to support students in their decision to remain celibate or postpone sexual activity. Students were happy with the peer program. They reported a variety of responses from other students including inquiry and ridicule. The members felt that the program helped them to be comfortable with their decisions. The peer group continues to meet, and the number of new members increased by 5%.
2. The post-test results indicated that students were able to differentiate between pregnancy risk situations and those that had less risk of pregnancy, and were able to identify birth control methods, pros and cons of various methods, and failure rates. They improved in the area of knowledge about sexually transmitted disease, but were not able to link specific health complications with selected diseases.
3. The survey of a random sample of students administered 3 months after the program revealed that students were using condoms with greater frequency during sexual activity and that the use of a concurrent birth control method had increased about 10%. There was essentially no change in the numbers of students reporting sexual activity.
4. Summary evaluation indicated that the peer program was working well for those who had joined. The seminar discussion and teaching intervention reached all intended students (sophomores, juniors, and seniors), or 75% of the high school enrollment. Teachers reported they were pleased with the instructional portion of the program, but thought that adding audiovisual materials, including a film, would be useful to the learning process. They were still uncomfortable leading the seminar discussions. Overall the planned interventions had worked well. Recommendations: (1) Continue the program for all grades, with an emphasis on the incoming freshman class and the new sophomores who had missed the intervention during this school year. (2) Add to audiovisual budget to upgrade available instructional media. (3) Continue peer support program and encourage expanded enrollment in the program. (4) Provide a summer in-service program to increase teacher expertise with seminar discussion of sexual issues.

Report Evaluation Results

Ms. Fields prepared a written report of the evaluation results, which she presented to the principal in a personal meeting. The principal reviewed the report and concurred with the results. He presented the report and recommendations to meetings of the PTA and the school board. Ms. Fields was asked to attend both meetings and participated in the discussion.

Implement Recommendations

The PTA was satisfied with progress in the sex education program and voted to provide funding support to improve audiovisual materials and contribute to a teacher in-service program. The school board has taken the report under advisement and is expected to decide on a course of action by the end of the summer. This will be too late to provide a summer in-service for interested teachers.

Phase II: Improve Student Access to Health Services Including Services to Address Risky Sexual Behavior

Nursing Diagnoses/Problems

1. Inadequate services to provide adolescent health care
2. Inadequate services to address primary prevention with respect to pregnancy and sexually transmitted diseases
3. Inadequate support services for teenage mothers with respect to daycare, parenting skills, and continuation of their educational program

Program Goal

Improve health services for adolescents and improve support services for teenage parents, especially teen mothers

Problems 1 and 2 Outcome Objective. Provide adequate health care services to students within 24 months

Problem 3 Outcome Objective. Develop support services for teenage parents that will facilitate their educational progress and the well-being of their children within 18 months

Process Objectives

Several process objectives were developed for Phase II consistent with the community standards suggested by APHA (1991)

1. By 2 years from inception of the adolescent health program, 75% of Northview High School students who are referred to the program will receive services at the health center or be referred to other community-based services to meet their needs
2. Within 2 years all adolescent parents will have access to affordable certified child care
3. Within 2 years all adolescent parents who remain in school will be encouraged to attend a school-based parenting skills program

Evaluation Plan

To address Problems 1 and 2, Ms. Fields and the committee proposed and received funding to improve adolescent health services situated within the local health center and to develop a community referral mechanism for students seen in the school health suite who need further medical care. To address Problem 3, Ms. Fields received input from interested parties (teachers, school staff, teenage parents) and intends to convene a committee to develop a proposal for support services.

The formative evaluation plan consists of reviewing the progress on these two efforts with individuals involved in the process.

Collection of Evaluation Data

Ms. Fields met with the staff of adolescent services to review progress. She, health department personnel, and the principal reviewed her written plan for implementing referrals from the health suite. Ms. Fields and the vice-principal reviewed her progress on convening the committee to address support services for teenage parents.

Analysis of the Data

Adolescent health services will be operational in 2 weeks. The staff is in place, and all the requested supplies have been ordered. The existing equipment provided by the health department is in place and is operational. The service center originally planned to begin providing care in March, but implementation was delayed because of late-arriving equipment and the health department's delay in designating a nurse to staff the service. Ms. Fields does have an adequate plan for community referrals, which includes all agencies and professional personnel who are willing to provide care for free or at a reduced rate. Unfortunately, the two general practitioners in the community are unwilling to assume care for any more patients at reduced fees at this time. Ms. Fields has enlisted the help of other professionals in an effort to identify other physicians who might be willing to assist with the project.

Ms. Fields has been only partially successful in gathering her committee to look at teenage parent support services. She has consulted with local community leaders (an alderman, three church pastors, and two local business owners) and enlisted their help in recruiting volunteers. She is hoping to have a complete committee in place in 1 month.

Report Evaluation Results

At this point, the individuals who need to know the results of the efforts are involved in the review of progress and are informed about the status of the efforts.

GUIDELINES FOR LEARNING

1. Based on the plan of nursing care that you developed for C.T. 01 using the first Guidelines for Learning in Chapter 13, design an evaluation plan. Who are the stakeholders who need to be involved in the evaluation process? How will you evaluate program effectiveness? What will you include in your formative process evaluation?
2. Reflect on your own experience with a health program (e.g., health education, screening, clinical care). Why did you seek care from that program? What were your goals? What was helpful to achievement of your goals? What contributed to your satisfaction and/or dissatisfaction? How would you modify the program if you were the nurse involved?
3. Based on the incidence of teenage pregnancy and sexually transmitted diseases, including human immunodeficiency virus (HIV) infection, a school system has decided to permit the distribution of condoms to high school students who request them. The school board has voted for the policy and its meetings were open to the public. A vocal minority of parents are upset by the policy because they believe sexual abstinence should be the school's policy. They also believe that the family is the place for sex education. What point of view do you hold in this ethical question? What alternative courses of action would be possible if you were the school health nurse? What would you choose to do, and why?
4. Interview a community health nurse to determine how child health or other clinic programs are evaluated. What data are routinely collected and what questions are answered? To what degree does the nurse participate in the collection and interpretation of the evaluation data? How are the data used to modify the program?

REFERENCES

American Nurses' Association (ANA). (1980). *ANA social policy statement.* Washington, DC: Author.

ANA. (1986). *Standards of community health nursing practice.* Washington, DC: Author.

Deniston, O., & Rosenstock, I. (1970). Evaluating health programs. *Public Health Reports, 85,* 835–840.

Diers, D. (1985). Policy and politics. In D. Mason & S. Talbott (Eds.). *Political action handbook for nurses* (pp. 53–59). Menlo Park, CA: Addison-Wesley.

Donabedian, A. (1980). *The definition of quality and approaches to its assessment* (Vol. 1). Ann Arbor, MI: Health Administration Press.

Freeman, R. (1963). *Public health nursing practice* (3rd ed.). Philadelphia: W.B. Saunders.

Haan, M., Kaplan, G., & Comacho, T. (1987). Poverty and health: Prospective evidence from the Alameda County study. *American Journal of Epidemiology, 125,* 989–998.

Hale, C., Arnold, F., & Travis, M. (1994). *Planning and evaluating health programs.* Albany, NY: Delmar Publishers.

Kosecoff, J., & Fink, A. (1982). *Evaluation basics: A practitioner's manual.* Beverly Hills, CA: Sage Publication.

McKenzie, J., & Jurs, J. (1993). *Planning, implementing, and evaluating health promotion programs: A primer.* New York: Macmillan Publishing Company.

Meany-Handy, J. (1985). Quality assurance in community health nursing. In S. Archer & R. Fleshman (Eds.). *Community health nursing* (3rd ed.) (pp. 214–230). Monterey, CA: Wadsworth Health Sciences.

Pirie, P., McBride, C., Hellerstedt, W., Jeffery, R., Hatsukami, D., Allen, S., & Lando, H. (1992). Smoking cessation in women concerned about weight. *American Journal of Public Health, 82*(9), 1238–1243.

Polit, D., & Hungler, B. (1993). *Essentials of nursing research: Methods, appraisal, and utilization* (3rd ed.). Philadelphia: J.B. Lippincott.

Schalock, R., & Thornton, C. (1988). *Program evaluation: A field guide for administrators.* New York: Plenum Press.

Sloan, M., & Schommer, B. (1991). The process of contracting in community health nursing. In B. Spradley (Ed.). *Readings in community health nursing* (4th ed.) (pp. 304–312). Philadelphia: J.B. Lippincott.

Suchman, E. (1967). *Evaluative research: Principles and practice in public service and social action programs.* New York: Russell Sage Foundation.

U.S. Department of Health and Human Services. (1990). *Healthy people 2000: National health promotion and disease prevention objectives.* Washington, DC: U.S. Government Printing Office.

BIBLIOGRAPHY

Anderson, E., & McFarlane, J. (1988). *Community as client: Application of the nursing process.* Philadelphia: J.B. Lippincott.

Archer, S. E. (1974, September-October). PERT: A tool for nurse-administrators. *Journal of Nursing Administration, 4,* 26–32.

Donabedian, A. (1985). *The methods and findings of quality assessment and monitoring: An illustrated analysis.* Ann Arbor, MI: Health Administration Press.

Goeppinger, J., Lassiter, P., & Wilcox, B. (1982). Community health nursing is community competence. *Nursing Outlook, 30,* 464–467.

Mason, E. (1984). *How to write meaningful nursing standards* (2nd ed.). New York: John Wiley.

Patton, M. (1982). *Practical evaluation.* Newbury Park, CA: Sage Publications.

Patton, M. (1990). *Qualitative evaluation and research methods* (2nd ed.). Newbury Park, CA: Sage Publications.

Pickett, G., & Hanlon, J. (1990). *Public health administration and practice.* St. Louis: Mosby-Year Book.

Rossi, P., & Freeman, H. (1982). *Evaluation: A systemic approach* (2nd ed.). Beverly Hills, CA: Sage Publications.

Stufflebeam, D., & Shinkfield, A. (1985). *Systematic evaluation: A self-instructional guide to theory and practice.* Boston: Kluwer-Nijhoff Publishing.

RECOMMENDED READINGS

American Nurses' Association. (1986). *Standards of community health nursing practice.* Washington, D.C.: Author.

Price, J., & Vincent, P. (1976). Program evaluation: What to ask before you start. *Nursing Outlook, 24,* 84–87.

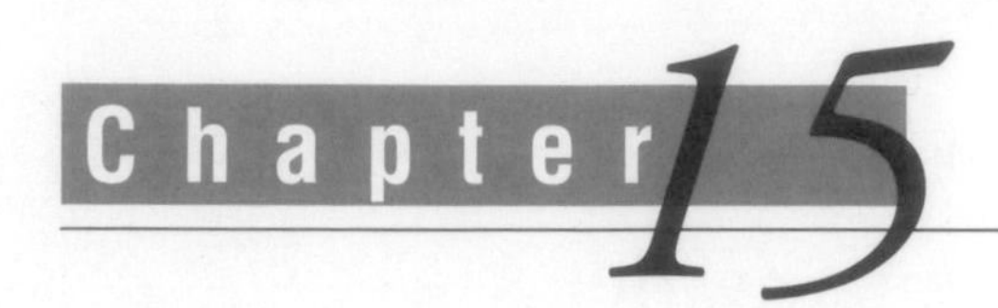

Chapter 15

Nursing in a Disaster

Barbara Santamaria

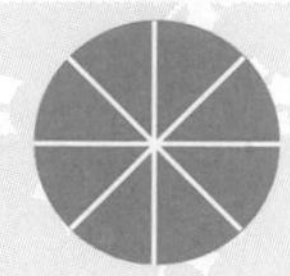

Focus Questions

What happens when a disaster occurs? Who is in charge?

What are the common physical and psychosocial effects on disaster victims and workers?

What are the responsibilities of community health nurses in disaster nursing?

What are the agencies that may be involved in pre-disaster planning?

What is your emergency preparedness plan? Your family's plan?

Overview of Disaster

The many disasters that have occurred during the 1980s and 1990s have brought the need for emergency preparedness to the attention of the American public. Historically, Americans have prepared for emergencies only in times of national threat, such as during World War II and in the early 1960s when Russia showed its technical superiority with Sputnik. However, the occurrence of Hurricanes Hugo in South Carolina and Andrew in Florida and of multiple earthquakes in California has created a concern across the country for preparedness to meet disasters, both natural and man-made.

Disaster has many forms: a school bus crash in Kentucky killing 24 children; Hurricane Elena hitting the Gulf Coast and driving 81,000 people to shelters; Hurricane Andrew leaving 180,000 people homeless in Florida; and a wrecked tanker truck or railroad car spilling dangerous chemicals into the air and onto the ground, requiring the evacuation of nearby residents. The Iraqi invasion of Kuwait with the kidnapping of foreign nationals and deliberate environmental damage was yet another disaster. Successful efforts to address these and other disaster situations demand sophisticated preplanning measures and a well-coordinated implementation effort during the actual diaster situation. Comprehensive planning requires that personnel have contingency plans to meet any and all stituations that may arise during and after the actual disaster occurs.

Definition of Disaster

The American Red Cross (ARC) defines a disaster as "an occurrence, either natural or man-made, that causes human suffering and creates human needs that victims cannot alleviate without assistance" (American Red Cross, 1975). The Disaster Relief Act of 1974 (PL 93–228) defines a major disaster as "any hurricane, tornado, storm, flood, wind driven water, tidal wave, earthquake, volcanic eruption, landslide, mudslide, snowstorm, drought, fire, explosion, or other catastrophe in any part of the United States which in the determination of the President causes damage of sufficient severity and magnitude to warrant major disaster assistance above and beyond emergency services by the Federal Government to supplement the efforts and available resources of the State and Local Governments, and private relief organizations in alleviating the damages, loss, hardship and suffering caused by the disaster" (Federal Emergency Management Agency, 1983). Table 15–1 provides examples of some major disasters experienced by communities in the United States during the 6-year period from 1985 to 1991. A major disaster is more likely to create a mass casualty incident rather than a multiple casualty incident. A *multiple casualty incident* is one in which fewer than 100 persons are injured. Multiple casualties generally strain but do not overwhelm

TABLE 15–1

Major Disasters, 1985–1991

Date	Type of Accident and Location	No. of Deaths
May 31, 1985	Storm and tornadoes in Pennsylvania and Ohio	74
Aug. 2, 1985	Plane crash at Ft. Worth/Dallas airport	135
Nov. 4–5, 1985	Floods in West Virginia, Pennsylvania, and East Coast	65
Aug. 31, 1986	Two-plane collision over Los Angeles	82
April 24, 1987	Collapse of apartment building construction in Bridgeport, CT	28
Aug. 16, 1987	Plane crash in Detroit, MI	156
Oct. 17, 1989	Earthquake in San Francisco area	61
Jan. 25, 1990	Plane crash in Cove Neck, NY	73
Feb. 1, 1991	Two-plane collision on the ground, Los Angeles	34
March 4, 1991	Plane crash in Colorado Springs, CO	25
Sept. 3, 1991	Fire at food processing plant in Hamlet, NC	25
Oct. 21, 1991	Brush fires in Oakland, CA	25

Data from National Safety Council (1992). *Accident facts.* Washington, DC: U.S. Government Printing Office.

the resources available to care for them. A *mass casualty incident* is a situation that significantly overwhelms the available facilities and resources.

When there are mass casualties, a community or region usually will require the assistance of emergency personnel and resources from other communities or states. Hurricane Hugo is an example of a disaster in which entire communities required outside assistance to address the needs of their citizens.

Epidemiology of Disaster

TYPES OF DISASTERS

Epidemiology is the study of the patterns of disease occurrence in human populations and the factors that influence these patterns (Lilienfeld and Lilienfeld, 1980). Disaster may be studied and analyzed using the epidemiological framework of agent, host, and environment in an attempt to predict, prevent, or control the outcome of a disaster. Essentially there are two types of disasters: natural and man-made. Both types will vary in intensity, severity, and impact.

Natural disasters include hurricanes, tornadoes, flash floods, blizzards, slow-rising floods, typhoons, earthquakes, avalanches, epidemics, and volcanic eruptions. Man-made disasters include war, transportation accidents, food or water contamination, and building collapse. Fire may be either man-made or naturally occurring. The Los Angeles fires of 1993 that destroyed many homes and businesses resulted from a combination of both man-made and natural causes: they were started by an arsonist and then were exacerbated by weather conditions (i.e., a dry summer season and high winds).

DISASTER AGENTS

To apply the epidemiological framework in a disaster situation, the *agent* is the physical item that actually causes the injury or destruction. Primary agents include falling buildings, heat, wind, rising water, and smoke. Secondary agents include bacteria and viruses that produce contamination or infection after the primary agent has caused injury or destruction.

Primary and secondary agents will vary according to the type of disaster. For example, a hurricane with rising water can cause flooding and high winds; these are primary agents. The secondary agents would include damaged buildings and bacteria or viruses that thrive as a result of the disaster. In an epidemic, the bacteria or virus causing a disease is the primary agent rather than the secondary agent.

HOST FACTORS

In the epidemiological framework as applied to disaster, the host is humankind. Host factors are those characteristics of humans that influence the severity of the disaster's effect. Host factors include age, immunization status, preexisting health status, degree of mobility, and emotional stability. Individuals most severely affected by a disaster are elderly persons, who may have trouble leaving the area quickly; young children whose immune systems are not fully developed; and persons with respiratory or cardiac problems. For example, a fire in a nursing home is potentially more lethal than a fire in a college dormitory. In a fire situation, elderly individuals in the nursing home are at greater risk because they are less physically fit and more susceptible to smoke and other consequences than are young college students.

ENVIRONMENTAL FACTORS

Environmental factors that affect the outcome of a disaster include physical, chemical, biological, and social factors. Physical factors include the time when the disaster occurs, weather conditions, the availability of food and water, and the functioning of utilities such as electricity and telephone service. Chemical factors influencing disaster outcome include leakage of stored chemicals into the air, soil, ground water, or food supplies. Biological factors are those that occur or increase as a result of contaminated water, improper waste disposal, insect or rodent proliferation, improper food storage, or lack of refrigeration owing to interrupted electrical services. Social factors are those that contribute to the individual's social support systems. Loss of family members, changes in roles, and the questioning of religious beliefs are social factors to be examined after a disaster.

PSYCHOLOGICAL FACTORS

Psychological factors contribute to the effect of the disaster on individuals. Psychological factors are closely related to agent, host, and environmental conditions. The nature and severity of the disaster affect the psychological distress experienced by the victims. The existence and length of a warning period and physical proximity to the actual site of the disaster influence the amount of psychological distress experienced by victims. The closer an individual is to the actual site of the disaster and the longer the individual is exposed to the immediate site of the disaster, the greater the psychological distress that individual will experience.

The victim's perception of the disaster is the strongest influence on the type of psychological response to a disaster that individual will experience. Individuals experience disasters in relation to how significantly they are directly affected. An individual who perceives a disaster to be less severe than it is will probably have a less severe psychological reaction than a person who perceives the situation as catastrophic (Richtsmeir and Miller, 1985). An individual's perception of a disaster may change over time as the person begins to acknowledge the full impact of the disaster. The human mind is capable of allowing perceptions to be only as disastrous as the mind can cope with at a given time.

Demi and Miles (1983) have identified both situational and personal factors that influence an individual's response to a disaster. Situational variables include the amount of warning time before disaster occurs, the nature and the severity of the disaster, physical proximity to the disaster, and the availability of emergency response systems. An individual's reaction to a disaster will be greater if there is little or no warning, the disaster is man-made, the extent of damage and death is great, the victim is in close physical proximity to the disaster site, and support systems are limited. Personal variables include psychological proximity, coping ability, losses, role overload, and previous disaster experience. An individual's risk of developing severe psychological consequences is greater if that person is emotionally close to the individuals affected, has compromised coping abilities, has experienced many losses, feels overloaded in his or her role, or has never before experienced a disaster.

According to Demi and Miles (1983), psychological reactions fall into three categories: mild to severe, normal to pathological, and immediate to delayed. A reaction may be severe, normal, or mild and yet abnormal. A few people will be so overwhelmed by the trauma that they will experience extreme psychological distress immediately. Others, despite their intense involvement in the disaster, may appear unaffected psychologically during both the impact and postimpact phases. These people may be using denial and repression as defenses to handle their thoughts and feelings. All disaster victims and workers may need referral and follow-up with a mental health care professional to restore them to their pre-disaster mental health level.

Some of the more common psychological reactions to a disaster include depression, sadness, fear, anger, phobias, guilt, and irritability. Feelings of guilt may arise in survivors when many victims have died. Fear of death or of another disaster occurring is a frequently seen reaction. Anger may be exhibited as general irritability or full-fledged rage and may be directed toward the cause of the disaster, displaced onto the support system, or directed inward. Anxiety may be demonstrated by hyperalertness, trembling, palpitations, and tenseness. Depression is often demonstrated by frequent crying, insomnia, decreased interest in relationships, loneliness, and feelings of worthlessness.

Individuals may suffer impaired intellectual functioning, have difficulty concentrating, or making decisions, and experience impaired memory. Psychosomatic complaints and mental illness are also responses to disaster situations and are evidenced by loss of appetite, fatigue, intestinal upset, sleep disorders, and muscular weakness. Preexisting medical conditions are frequently exacerbated by disaster.

If survivors do not recognize and deal effectively with these feelings, they may suffer numbness and exhaustion. Individual responses to disaster are unique, and survivors should be counseled accordingly. The psychological stress experienced as a result of a disaster may have long-term effects, such as interpersonal or social problems. Some individuals may turn to alcohol or drugs in an attempt to relieve the stress they feel. Others may have difficulty resuming their usual routines and relationship patterns.

POSTTRAUMATIC STRESS DISORDER SYNDROME

Posttraumatic stress disorder (PTSD) syndrome is identified in the third edition of the *Diagnostic and Statistical Manual of Mental Health Disorders* (American Psychiatric Association, 1980). This syndrome was first recognized in veterans of the Vietnam War; it is now known that it may occur after a number of traumatic events, including war, terrorism, kidnapping, and disasters. Three criteria define the syndrome. First, the trauma must be universally recognized. Second, the individual must reexperience the trauma through flashbacks, dreams, or triggering events. Third, the individual must demonstrate psychic impairment (i.e., either numbing or decreased interest in normal events). In addition, victims of PTSD experience two or more of the following symptoms: hyperalertness or exaggerated startle response, sleep disturbance, survival guilt, decreased concentration, impaired memory, and avoidance behavior. Reminders of the trauma increase the symptoms in victims of this syndrome. Community nurses and others involved in treating clients after disasters should be aware that the symptoms of PTSD may not be evident for some time after the actual event has occurred. Health personnel need to be sensitized to the possibility of PTSD in survivors of disasters.

Phases of a Disaster

There are three phases to any disaster. The actions of emergency personnel and other health professionals depend on which phase of the disaster is at hand.

PREIMPACT PHASE

The preimpact phase is the initial phase of the disaster, prior to the actual occurrence. A warning is given at the sign of the first possible danger to a community. Many times there is no warning, but with the aid of weather networks and satellites, many meteorological disasters can be predicted.

The earliest possible warning is crucial in preventing loss of life and minimizing damage. This is the period when the emergency preparedness plan is put into effect. Emergency centers are opened by the local Civil Defense Authority. Communication is a very important factor during this phase; disaster personnel will call on amateur radio operators, radio and television stations, and any available method to alert the community and keep it informed. The community must be educated to recognize the threat as serious. When communities experience false alarms several times, members may not take future warnings very seriously.

The role of the nurse during this warning phase is to assist in preparing shelters and emergency aid stations and establishing contact with other emergency service groups.

IMPACT PHASE

The impact phase occurs when the disaster actually happens. It is a time of enduring hardship or injury and of trying to survive. This is a time when individuals help neighbors and families at the scene, a time of "holding on" until outside help arrives. The impact phase may last for several minutes (e.g., after an earthquake, plane crash, or explosion) or for days or weeks (e.g., in a flood, famine, or epidemic).

This phase must provide for preliminary assessment of the nature, extent, and geographical area of the disaster. The number of persons requiring shelter, the type and number of needed disaster health services anticipated, and the general health status and needs of the community must be evaluated.

The impact phase continues until the threat of further destruction has passed and the emergency plan is in effect.

If there has been no warning, this is the time when the Emergency Operation Center (EOC) is established and put in operation. The EOC is the operating center for the local chapter of the American Red Cross. It serves as the center for communication with other government agencies, the center for recruitment of health care providers to staff shelters, and the liaison center for working with other volunteer agencies. Shelters are opened, and every shelter has a nurse as a member of the disaster action team (DAT). The nurse is responsible for assessing health needs and providing physical and psychological support to victims in the shelters. During the impact phase injured persons are triaged, morgue facilities are established and coordinated, and search and reunion activities are organized.

POSTIMPACT PHASE

Recovery begins during the emergency phase and ends with the return of normal community order and functioning. For persons in the impact area this phase may last a lifetime (e.g., victims of the atomic bombing of Hiroshima). The victims of a disaster go through four stages of emotional response:

1. *Denial:* During the first stage, the victim may deny the magnitude of the problem or, more likely, will understand the problem but may seem unaffected emotionally. The problems created by the disaster are being denied or have not fully "registered." The victim may appear unusually unconcerned.
2. *Strong emotional response:* In the second stage, the person is aware of the problem but regards it as overwhelming and unbearable. Common reactions during this stage are trembling, tightening of the muscles, sweating, speaking with difficulty, weeping, heightened sensitivity, restlessness, sadness, anger, and passivity. The victim may want to retell or relive the disaster experience over and over.
3. *Acceptance:* During the third stage, the victim begins to accept the problems caused by the disaster and makes a concentrated effort to solve them. He or she feels more hopeful and confident. It is especially important for victims to take specific actions to help themselves and their families.
4. *Recovery:* The fourth stage represents a recovery from the crisis reaction. Victims feel that they are back to normal. Routines become important again. A sense of well-being is restored. The ability to make decisions and carry out plans returns. Victims develop a realistic memory of the experience (Richtsmeir and Miller, 1985).

EFFECTS OF DISASTER ON THE COMMUNITY

Not only are individuals affected physically and emotionally by a disaster, but also the entire community is affected. According to the American Red Cross (1989), the most important disruptions are the following:

- Public service personnel are overworked.
- Lifelines are interrupted, including telephone systems, television and radio broadcasting, transportation, and water and sanitation services.
- Resources such as food and medical supplies are depleted.
- Rumors run rampant and are hard to check.
- Public and private buildings may be damaged.

In a disaster, the social and psychological reactions of individuals are closely interwoven with those of the community. According to the American Red Cross (1987), the four phases of a community's reaction to a disaster are as follows:

- *Heroic phase:* strong, direct emotions focusing on helping people to survive and recover
- *Honeymoon phase:* a drawing together of people who simultaneously experienced the same catastrophic event.
- *Disillusionment phase:* feelings of disappointment because of delays or failures when promises of aid are not fulfilled. People seek help to solve their own personal problems rather than community problems.
- *Reconstruction phase:* a reaffirmation of belief in the community when new buildings are constructed. However, delays in this process may cause intense emotional responses.

Dimensions of a Disaster

Disasters have a number of dimensions in which they may differ: predictability, frequency, controllability, time, and scope or intensity. These dimensions influence the nature and possibility of preparation planning, as well as response to the actual event.

PREDICTABILITY

Some events are more easily predicted than others. Advances in meteorology, for example, have made it more feasible to accurately predict the probability of certain types of natural, weather-related disasters (e.g., tornadoes, floods, and hurricanes), while others, such as earthquakes, are not as easily predicted. Man-made disasters, such as explosions or wrecks, are also less predictable. Whenever an event is predictable, authorities and emergency personnel have more time to prepare for the situation than when an event is not foreseeable (i.e., spontaneous).

FREQUENCY

Although natural disasters are relatively rare, they appear more often in certain geographical locations. Residents of the gulf coast of the United States live in what is commonly referred to as "hurricane alley." These people are at greater risk for experiencing a hurricane than someone who lives in Alaska. California residents are at greater risk for earthquakes, and people who live near large river systems are at greater risk for flooding than people who live elsewhere. The National Weather Service has calculated that Texas and Oklahoma experience more tornadoes than other states. However, the greater frequency of natural disasters may or may not prepare citizens for their occurrence. Some citizens become immune to repeated warnings and are less likely to seek shelter to protect themselves and their property when warned. Other citizens take each warning seriously and regularly take appropriate safety precautions.

CONTROLLABILITY

Some situations allow for prewarning and control measures that can reduce the impact of the disaster; others do not. The Midwest floods of 1993, for example, allowed for some control and mitigating actions. Emergency planners were able to control some of the effects of the flooding by sandbagging levees and river banks to reduce the effects of water damage, and by deliberately blasting dikes and dams to divert flood waters to less populated areas. The immediate impact on people was reduced by the ability of emergency personnel to organize evacuations and reduce the risk of injury and death.

The Los Angeles earthquake of 1994 did not allow for prewarning and immediate precautionary actions, but other types of control measures are available. Mitigating measures can be implemented well in advance of potential disasters. The enactment of building standards and codes intended to reduce the harmful effects of a disaster are one example. More stringent fire safety measures (e.g., smoke detectors, sprinkler systems, and improved fire doors) have made more newly constructed buildings safer in the event of an actual fire. Newer buildings with more stringent construction codes survived the most recent San Francisco earthquake with less structural damage than older buildings built before these codes were implemented. Los Angeles was in the process of retrofitting its freeway system to strengthen highway resistance to earthquake damage when the 1994 earthquake hit the area.

TIME

There are several characteristics of time as it relates to the impact of a disaster: the speed of onset of the disaster, the time available for warning the population, and the actual length of time of the impact phase. It is more difficult to prepare for very sudden events. A flash flood, for instance, may catch many unaware, while the gradual flooding in the Midwest in 1993 allowed more time for preparation. When there is a lengthy period of warning, more protective measures can be introduced. For example, several days' warning allows authorities in low coastal areas to evacuate vulnerable communities before a hurricane hits. Tornadoes do not offer such lengthy warning periods. The impact phase of the disaster may last for minutes, hours, or even days. The most damage is generally caused by the worst possible combination of time factors: a rapid onset, no opportunity for warning the populace, and a lengthy duration of the impact phase.

SCOPE AND INTENSITY

A disaster may be concentrated in a very small area or involve a very large geographical region, usually affecting many more people. A disaster can be very intense and highly destructive, causing many injuries, deaths, and property damage, or less intense, with relatively little damage done to property or individuals. Sometimes a relatively small disaster may be extremely disruptive to a large segment of the community. For example, an explosion at a water purifying plant may cause minimal injury to property and personnel at the plant, but may reduce or eliminate the water supply for an entire community for days or even weeks.

Disaster Management: Responsibilities of Agencies and Organizations

The key to effective disaster management is predisaster planning and preparation.

PLANNING

Planning for a disaster involves five major areas: the use of technology to forecast events, the use of engineering to reduce risks, public education on potential hazards, a coordinated emergency response, and a systematic assessment of the effects of a disaster to better prepare for the future (Merchant, 1986). Responsibility for addressing these five areas of disaster planning are shared by local, state, federal, and voluntary agencies.

The principles of disaster planning have been outlined in a publication from the Civil Defense Preparedness Agency, Department of Defense (Dynes et al., 1972). Planning includes the following:

- A continuous process
- A knowledge base
- A focus on principles
- Anticipatory guidance
- Reducing unknown situations
- Evoking appropriate actions
- Overcoming resistance

Governmental, environmental, technical, and economic resources are involved in predisaster preparation. Community education and "mock disaster" exercises are part of any well-designed preparation plan. As potential team members, nurses should play an active role in preparing for disasters by participating in community planning and mock disaster exercises. Nurses can volunteer or may be required by their job to take part in disaster preparation. The local chapter of the American Red Cross offers disaster nursing training sessions for nurses who are required to participate or are interested in disaster care. Nurses can also function as primary teachers in affecting community understanding of the necessity of preparation for disasters. Disaster plans must be practiced, evaluated, and updated at regular intervals by all participants in disaster preparation.

Established organizations provide many of the community services needed in a disaster. Organizations providing health care include hospitals, nursing homes, and government agencies such as health departments. Table 15–2 lists some of the organizations that are involved in disaster planning and relief. Disaster preparation must include a plan for coordinating efforts between response groups within a community or between communities. Clear lines of authority, specified tasks and duties, definite channels of communication, and explicit decision-making roles are needed.

TABLE 15–2

Disaster Agencies

Federal Agencies

1. Federal Emergency Management Agency
   Federal Central Plaza
   500 C St. S.W.
   Washington, DC 20472
   (202) 646–2500
2. U.S. Army Corps of Engineers
   20 Massachusetts Ave. N.W.
   Washington, DC 20314–1000
   (202) 272–0660
3. Department of Health and Human Services
   200 Independent Ave. S.W.
   Washington, DC
   (202) 475–0257

International Disaster Relief Agencies

1. American Red Cross
   430 17th St. N.W.
   Washington, DC 20006
   (202) 737–8300
2. Disaster Relief International
   27 La Patera Lane
   Santa Barbara, CA 93117
3. International Reserve Committee
   600 Executive Blvd. Suite 608
   Rockville, MD 20852
   (800) 638–8079

All national agencies have state and local offices that respond to disasters; the local group is the source of immediate response. If the disaster exceeds both local and state resources, including the private sector and volunteer organizations, the state may request aid from other states or the federal government.

Local Volunteer Organizations

1. Boy Scouts of America
2. Goodwill Industries
3. Mennonite Disaster Service
4. Volunteers of America
5. Seventh Day Adventist
6. Church of the Brethren

Local Governments and Communities

Local governments are responsible for the safety and welfare of their citizens. They act to protect the lives and property of the citizens, protect public health, carry out evacuating rescues, and maintain public works. Local disaster response organizations should include local area government agencies such as fire departments, police departments, public health departments, public works departments, emergency or civil defense services, and the local branch of the American Red Cross.

Communities should have an emergency operations plan. This is accomplished by assessing the community's potential for disaster. Geological hazard surveys and risk assessments for floods, transportation accidents, and fires are conducted. Local planning efforts include contingency action plans for various types of disaster situations, designation of an overall field commander, and identification of community resources that can be used in a disaster. The plan is developed and tested in mock disaster exercises and then revised and refined. Disaster response organizations should meet regularly under the direction of local civil defense authorities.

Area hospitals develop their own action plan for handling small community disasters such as a school bus accident or a large apartment fire. They are also involved in community planning preparation for larger scale disasters that require a coordinated community effort. Local volunteer organizations such as the Boy Scouts, Girl Scouts, Jaycees, Veterans' Associations, and church groups can be considered as additional resources to be used as the need arises. Local health care professionals who do not participate in community organizations that are officially involved in disaster planning may be called on to volunteer their services during an emergency.

State Governments

State governments provide financial support to local governments. For disaster planning purposes, if the disaster involves more than one local jurisdiction, the state may also coordinate services. Usually there is one state agency designated as the command center for state-coordinated efforts. When a disaster happens, the state governor may have some state agencies (e.g., state police; National Guard; state emergency or civil defense services; and state health, welfare, and social service agencies) work directly on disaster relief. Most states also have a state coordinator to manage fire department resources and personnel.

Federal Government

The federal government generally enacts laws and provides funds to support state and local governments. The Public Disaster Act of 1974 (PL 93–288) provided for consolidation of federal disaster relief activities and funding under a single agency. Thus, the Federal Emergency Management Agency (FEMA) was established in 1979 as the coordinating agency for all available federal disaster assistance. FEMA is the focal point in the federal government for emergency planning, preparedness, mitigation, response, and recovery. The agency works closely with state and local governments by funding emergency programs and providing technical guidance and training.

The National Disaster Medical System (NDMS) is composed of the Department of Health and Human Services, the Department of Defense, FEMA, and state and local governments. NDMS, which is designed to deal with medical care needs in disasters of great intensity and scope, has three main objectives: to provide medical assistance to a disaster area in the form of medical assistance teams, medical supplies, and equipment; to evacuate patients that cannot be cared for in the affected area to other predetermined locations, and to provide a national network of hospitals that are designated to accept patients in the event of a national emergency.

For disaster relief, the federal government has many other agencies and programs; only a few are listed here. The National Guard provides transportation, assistance with evacuations, and police services when local or area police resources are strained or overwhelmed by disaster needs. The U.S. Department of Housing and Urban Development's temporary housing program helps families either relocate or repair their homes. The Small Business Administration has a disaster program that helps both businesses and families by providing government-guaranteed loans to assist in their recovery. The Individual Family Grant Program provides grants of up to $5000 to families to assist in their recovery.

American Red Cross

The American Red Cross (ARC) was founded in 1881 by Clara Barton. It is a voluntary agency that was granted a charter on January 5, 1905, by the U.S. Congress. This charter was reaffirmed by Congress in the Disaster Relief Acts of 1970 and 1974 and in the administrative regulations established for carrying out those Acts. The charter gives the ARC the authority to act as the primary voluntary national disaster relief agency for the American people and to be ready for immediate action in every part of the United States.

The legal grant of power and imposition of duties on the ARC are clear. Its jurisdictional lines with respect to coordinated efforts with other federal agencies has been ensured by federal statute and a variety of memoranda of understanding with federal agencies. This federal legislation applies only to those emergencies and major disasters that have been declared as such by the President. On a national level and in many communities, the ARC acts to coordinate the disaster relief efforts of a variety of voluntary agencies. The federal grant of authority to the ARC makes unnecessary the issuance of special permission or a license by state or local governments for the ARC to activate and carry out its relief program. The ARC has created the following five programs to meet the human needs of a disaster:

1. *Damage Assessment:* The first task after a disaster strikes is to survey the damage or undertake a damage assessment. This is defined as "the gathering of immediate and accurate information about the physical damage resulting from a disaster" (American Red Cross, 1985).
2. *Mass Care:* Providing shelter and food is called *mass care* by the ARC. Such care includes the following:
   - *Food provision:* Food is provided at shelters or feeding stations or may be taken by mobile units to disaster areas.
   - *Shelter provision:* Mass shelters may be established in schools, public buildings, hotels, motels, or churches.
   - *Supply provision:* Personal hygiene articles, toilet articles, and/or cleaning supplies may be provided.
3. *Health Services:* Disaster health services will try to meet the emotional and medical needs of victims and disaster workers by providing medical, nursing, and health care in shelters and emergency aid stations; blood and blood products; emergency medical and hospital supplies; assistance to public health officials; and assistance to families in finding available health services.
4. *Family Services:* Family Services is an emergency assistance program to help families resume living by providing food (paying for groceries or arranging for meals in a restaurant), clothing (paying for clothing, shoes, or winter coats), shelter (paying temporary hotel or motel costs or assisting with payment of rent, security deposits, utility deposits, and temporary home repairs), medical needs (assisting in procurement of prescriptions, eyeglasses, dentures, foods for special diets, and prostheses), household furnishings (providing items necessary to permit the family to return home, such as emergency furniture, cooking and eating utensils, linens, and necessary appliances), and occupational supplies and equipment (tools, uniforms, and other items needed to help the wage earner to return to work). All ARC assistance is free and is provided through funds donated by the American people.
5. *Disaster Welfare Inquiry Service:* Disasters frequently disrupt communication, to the dismay of friends and families outside the disaster area. The ARC Disaster Inquiry Service gathers information about the disaster area, what and who were affected, and individuals killed or injured and makes this information available to concerned relatives through their local ARC chapter.

PREVENTION AND MITIGATION

Certain types of disasters, particularly man-made ones, may be preventable. Other disasters are not preventable, but their impact may be mitigated. Some disasters have been prevented by the enforcement of good building codes or by proper land and water management. Many man-made disasters could be prevented by observing proper safety precautions, including regular equipment maintenance. Local, state, and federal laws do address some of the safety aspects of building codes; proper maintenance of equipment and supplies; and the correct storage, use, and transportation of chemicals.

Public education is another strategy that can be used to reduce the impact of dangerous situations. In areas that are prone to certain types of disaster situations, public education can alert the community how best to prepare for such situations in advance of an actual event. Community health nurses may be involved in such efforts, which may include instruction regarding proper safety precautions, proper storage of emergency supplies, and first aid courses to prepare the public to care for injuries in the event of an actual emergency. Public communication systems such as radio and television routinely broadcast information about how people can obtain information in the event of an actual disaster situation.

Early warning systems alert the public to the probability of immediate danger and help to reduce the impact of predictable disasters such as hurricanes or tornadoes. They may also provide information on an evacuation plan or other immediate actions that improve the chance of survival and reduce the probability of injuries.

EMERGENCY RESPONSE

The primary goals of disaster management are to prevent or minimize death, disability, suffering, and loss on the part of disaster victims. How these goals are achieved will vary with the type of disaster and the type of rescue worker. Police officers and firefighters will have an entirely different focus than health care workers.

Emergency Operation Center and Emergency Medical System

Preplanning mandates the designation of a command center and coordinated interactions among various response personnel. In the event of a disaster situation, the emergency operations center (EOC) becomes operational. Each community determines the locale and personnel involved in their EOC; a typical organizational chart is provided in Figure 15–1. The EOC includes health personnel from the local emergency medical system (EMS). These personnel will be involved in treating people at the scene of the disaster as well as at other designated locations, including local hospitals.

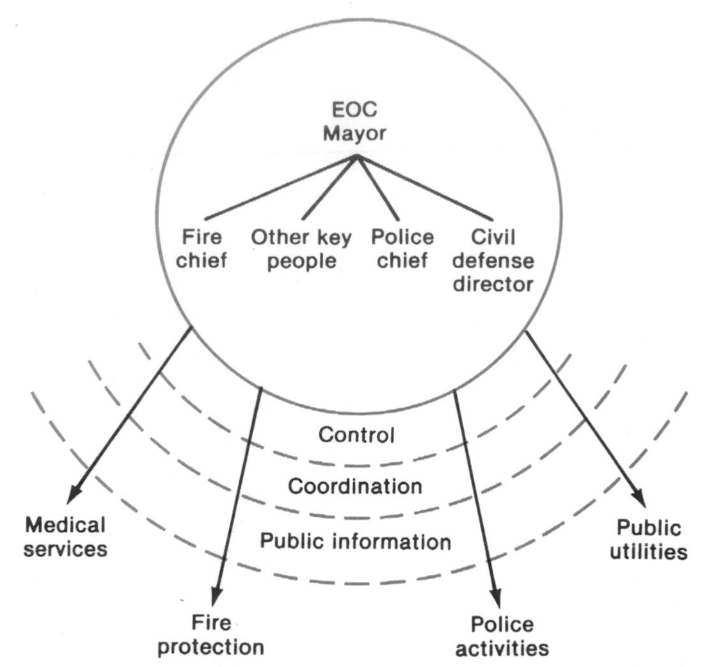

Figure 15–1 ● Organizational chart of emergency operation center (EOC). (Redrawn from Federal Emergency Management Agency. (July 1972). *Disaster operations: A handbook for local governments.* CPG–1–6. Washington, DC: Author.)

Principles of Disaster Management

According to Garb and Eng (1969), there are eight fundamental principles that should be followed by all who have a responsibility for helping the victims of a disaster. It is critical that rescue workers use these principles in proper sequence, or they will be ineffective and possibly detrimental to disaster victims. The eight basic principles are as follows:

1. Prevent the occurrence of the disaster whenever possible.
2. Minimize the number of casualties if the disaster cannot be prevented.
3. Prevent further casualties from occurring after the initial impact of the disaster.
4. Rescue the victims.
5. Provide first aid to the injured.
6. Evacuate the injured to medical facilities.
7. Provide definitive medical care.
8. Promote reconstruction of lives.

The first two actions are designed to control or mitigate the results of the disaster and have already been addressed. Preventing further casualties after initial impact depends on evaluating and lessening any unsafe conditions present after the disaster. For example, access to unstable buildings and washed-out bridges must be prevented, and contamination of water and food supplies must be averted or corrected. Conditions such as these need to be assessed rapidly and the dangers removed or isolated immediately to prevent further injury and death. Periodic physical assessments of the disaster scene are essential to make certain the area is safe. These activities are generally carried out by local utility personnel, firemen, and other individuals trained in structural assessment.

Rescue involves locating and freeing trapped victims and then evacuating them to a safe place. An effective rescue and evaluation team with good leadership skills is essential for saving lives after a disaster. First aid must be provided to victims with life-threatening injuries to prevent death. Complications and death may be avoided if adequate first aid is given.

Evacuation of victims must be done in an orderly but timely fashion. Many factors will affect evacuation and must be considered by the nurse. These include availability of transport vehicles, condition of the roads leading to advanced care facilities, time between disaster impact and arrival at the hospital (many hospitals need at least 1 hour to be prepared to meet disaster needs), and availability of adequate staff to handle the most seriously injured. Usually the destination of disaster victims is determined by the EOC after it has communicated with the receiving hospitals.

Provision of definitive medical care depends on an existing disaster plan and adequately trained disaster personnel. Hospitals must have well-honed disaster plans to meet the needs of large groups of victims in a short time. These plans should be practiced at least twice each year. The plans should include activities for disasters that occur internally as well as externally. An internal disaster is a catastrophic event occurring on the medical center grounds and resulting in multiple injuries. An external disaster is a catastrophic event occurring off the medical center grounds and resulting in multiple injuries for which the hospital would need to provide emergency care. To meet the accreditation requirements of the Joint Commission on Accreditation of Healthcare Organizations, all hospitals must have disaster plans, hold disaster drills, and regularly evaluate these plans and activities.

Finally, the reconstruction of the victim's life begins with initial care and continues until the victim has recovered. This may take days, months, or years. Victims and disaster workers must receive adequate psychological counseling and emotional support to be able to effectively return to normal living.

Triage

There are several times during the emergency response in which triage may be necessary to best determine the needs of injured victims. *Triage* is a French word meaning "sorting" or "categorizing." The term first came into use during World War I when casualties were sorted during battle. During a disaster, the goal is to maximize the number of survivors by sorting the treatable from the untreatable victims. In a disaster, the potential for survival and the availability of resources are the primary criteria used to determine which patients receive immediate treatment. In a disaster situation, saving the greatest number of lives is the most important goal. Triage may take place during the rescue operation at the scene of the disaster, and again at each stage of transport for the disaster victims.

Prioritizing of victims for treatment can be done in many ways; some communities use color coding (American Red Cross, 1982). Probably the best and most easily understood four-category system is the first-priority, second-priority, third-priority, and dying-or-dead system:

1. Red — most urgent, first priority
2. Yellow — urgent, second priority
3. Green — third priority
4. Black — dying or dead

First-priority patients have life-threatening injuries and are experiencing hypoxia or nearing hypoxia. Examples of injuries in this category include shock, chest wounds, internal hemorrhage, head injuries producing increased loss of consciousness, partial- or full-thickness burns over 20% to 60% of the body surface, and chest pain. Patients with catastrophic head or chest injuries do not fall into this category because they have a poor chance of survival.

Second-priority patients have injuries with systemic effects and complications but are not yet in shock or hypoxic. The patients appear stable enough to withstand a 30- to 60-minute wait without immediate risk. Examples of injuries in this category include multiple fractures, open fractures, spinal injuries, large lacerations, partial- or full-thickness burns over 10% to 20% of the body surface, and medical emergencies such as diabetic coma, insulin shock, and epileptic seizure. Patients with second-priority status may need to be observed closely for signs of shock, at which time they would be recategorized to first priority.

Third-priority patients have minimal injuries unaccompanied by systemic complications. Usually these patients can wait several hours for treatment without danger. Examples of injuries in this category include closed fractures, minor burns, minor lacerations, sprains, contusions, and abrasions.

Dying or dead patients are hopelessly injured patients or dead victims. These patients have catastrophic injuries (e.g., crushing injuries to the head or chest) and would not survive under the best of circumstances. These patients create the greatest difficulty, because failure to treat patients conflicts with nursing philosophy. In a disaster, triage must give the chance of survival to the greatest number of victims rather than to one individual. Death is a common occurrence during a disaster. A person who has died is placed in the lowest priority category. Personnel and equipment must be reserved for the greatest number of viable patients.

Ideally, triage leads to appropriate and definitive care for all victims. However, this can occur only if the cause of the multiple casualties is quickly controlled so that rescue teams may care for the injured in an organized manner. If the disaster conditions continue or if secondary events such as fires or building collapses occur, the rescue effort will be disrupted and the treatment of victims will be inhibited. It is an ongoing process of evaluating the victims, with transportation out of the area a primary goal.

Many different personnel are involved in the triage operation. Each person must know his or her exact role. Nurses and other emergency personnel are often used as triage officers instead of physicians, because physicians are administering emergency care to the more critical victims.

Community Nursing's Responsibilities in a Disaster

PLANNING

Nursing Care Goals for Disaster Nursing

Disaster nursing can be defined as the adaptation of professional nursing skills in recognizing and meeting the nursing, physical, and emotional needs resulting from a disaster. The overall goal of disaster nursing is to achieve the best possible level of health for the people and the community involved in the disaster.

Disaster nursing is as multifaceted as the demands of the disaster that must be met. Much depends on the location of the nurse at the time the disaster occurs. If the nurse is in the center of the disaster area, she or he may need to help with evacuation, rescue, and/or first aid until the immediate needs are met.

Hospital nurses will be needed to care for disaster victims as they are brought in for acute care problems. Most frequently, community health nurses are the first called by the ARC to report to shelters providing care for disaster victims.

The community health nurse brings the principles of both public health and community health nursing to bear during the stress of a crisis. The nurse must counsel, teach, assess, and be able to delegate to others tasks that the nurse would normally perform. In the shelters, the nurse in charge evaluates health care needs, establishes nursing care priorities and plans for health care supervision, prepares for isolation of persons with suspected communicable diseases and in general oversees the health and well-being of all shelter personnel.

Developing a Response Plan: Primary Prevention

A response plan should be concerned with delivering emergency health care as efficiently and as quickly as possible. To that end, community nurses should know in advance all community medical and social agency resources that will be available during a disaster. They should know where equipment and supplies have been stored and their prearranged role and rendezvous site.

Most agencies have a disaster notification network to alert personnel. Staff must follow a protocol of notification so that all available personnel are alerted or called to duty when the need arises. A good notification network should include a contingency plan for cases in which some personnel may not be reachable. In that way, the communication network is not disabled. Nonresponders are simply bypassed, and the notification process continues.

If possible, when disasters are predictable or probable, health care personnel should be prewarned or placed on alert. Having personnel on alert status, reduces the response time during the actual disaster.

Another important element of a response plan is the designation of an alternative reporting site for health care workers. In the event of a major disaster, some designated sites may be destroyed or damaged. A good plan will include alternative response sites to which workers can report.

Emergency personnel should be *very familiar* with the equipment and supplies they will use in the event of an actual disaster. In addition to mock disaster drills that allow personnel to practice procedures and set up equipment, a periodic check of equipment and supplies should be part of the response plan. Some of the supplies are perishable and need to be restocked at regular intervals. If supplies are not actually unpacked at regular intervals, health care personnel may be disconcerted during a disaster to find that damaged, destroyed, or outdated supplies represent a significant portion of what they have to work with.

Education

Health promotion programs to encourage community preparation for disaster events should be part of the planning preparation for nurses in the community. Public education efforts should be geared toward safety, self-help, and first aid measures. A good education program should include information about proper storage of food and water, rotation of canned goods to ensure use before expiration dates, and safety precautions for water use (e.g., boiling water if equipment is available or using bottled water when plumbing is not working or tap water is not safe to drink).

A good first aid program should include information about the types of supplies needed in a home first aid kit (Table 15–3). First aid teaching programs should be geared toward helping the public become prepared to address trauma injuries such as fractures, bleeding, and burns. While the general public cannot be prepared to deal with sophisticated injuries, a sound knowledge of first aid will help most families cope with the most likely injuries in a disaster situation.

TABLE 15–3

Items for First Aid Kit

Acetaminophen (Tylenol), adult and child formula or aspirin
Alcohol preps or antiseptic spray
Antacid (low sodium) tablets
Aromatic spirits of ammonia
Eye wash
Hydrogen peroxide
Isopropyl alcohol
Antidiarrheal agent (e.g., Kaopectate)
Laxative
Emetic agent (e.g., Ipecac)
Activated charcoal (for use if advised by Poison Control Center)
Bar of soap
Moistened towelettes
Gauze pads, assorted sizes
Gauze rolls
Adhesive tape
Adhesive bandages
Latex gloves
Petroleum jelly
Triangular bandages
Scissors
Tweezers
Sewing needle and thread
Safety razor blades
Safety pins assorted sizes
Thermometer

Adapted from American Red Cross. (June 1991). *Your Family Disaster Supplies Kit*. Washington, DC: Author.

Every family in the community should be encouraged to have a personal preparedness plan (Table 15–4). This plan should consist of the following items:

- Emergency telephone numbers
- Battery-operated radio
- Working flashlight
- First aid kit
- Medical information (allergies, blood types, prescription medications)
- Physician names, addresses, and telephone numbers
- Persons to be notified in an emergency

Family members should have a prearranged site at which to reassemble in case they are forced to evacuate a dwelling from different exits. This simple plan can save confusion and the unnecessary injuries that often occur when family members attempt to reenter a dwelling to look for others who have already evacuated.

A public awareness campaign to alert residents about the types of supplies to bring with them to designated shelters will help supplement emergency supplies and make shelter living a little more palatable. Brown et al. (1988) surveyed Hurricane Elena evacuees in one Florida county. Residents indicated that food, blankets, pillows, prescription medication, personal grooming items, portable chairs, and a radio would be useful supplies to improve comfort in shelter living. For people who have ample warning before evacuation, Hayes et al. (1990) recommend bringing diversionary recreational equipment such as crossword puzzles, card games, drawing materials, and toys.

TABLE 15–4

What Family Members Should Know in an Emergency

How and where to turn off utilities
How to escape and where to go
Where to meet with family members in case of separation (e.g., at a neighbor's house or across the street from the front door)
Plans for care of pets (pets are not allowed in shelters)
Safety precautions for various kinds of disasters (e.g., fire, hurricane, etc.)
A list of necessary items in the event of a disaster. The items on this list may include medications, dentures, or eyeglasses; special food or infant formula; sturdy shoes and clothing for cold or inclement weather; identification; checkbook, credit cards, driver's license, and other important papers; blankets; favorite toys and extra clothing for children.

Adapted from American Red Cross. (November 1991). *Emergency Preparedness*. Washington, DC: Author.

EMERGENCY CARE

During the impact phase of a disaster, nurses and other emergency personnel are usually advised to remain in place and not attempt to provide care until the situation has stabilized. In weather-related or predictable disasters such as hurricanes or tornadoes, emergency personnel may be asked to evacuate the site of the pending disaster as a safeguard so that they can render assistance after the disaster has struck. This is often a very difficult request for health care personnel to follow. Many are torn between their duty and the real need to remain with family members. Nurses and other health care personnel need to determine in advance which course of action they intend to pursue and, when necessary, clarify their intent with supervisory personnel.

Survey Assessments

After a severe disaster, survey teams are assigned to make a rapid assessment of the casualties and damage to infrastructure. Health personnel are assigned to survey teams, and often nurses function as health assessment personnel. Nurses who function on assessment teams are expected to perform casualty damage assessments, *not* render immediate first aid. This may also be problematic for some community health nurses, whose first instinct will be to render immediate care. Nurses who function on survey teams should expect to remain with their primary assignment. The information obtained from survey assessments is crucial to help the EOC determine the emergency needs and plan for the equipment and personnel necessary to address those needs.

Emergency Assessment

During the assessment process, data are collected and analyzed so that a nursing diagnosis can be made. In a shelter, emergency aid station, or morgue, the following areas should be part of the nursing assessment:

1. The individual's health problems, both current and past. Priority for care is always given to the seriously ill or injured. Crisis intervention techniques are used for those persons in dire distress.
2. Past and present health problems of the general population and trends in health care needs. Trends in health care needs must be identified in all settings to identify problem-solving strategies. Information about the population that must be assessed includes age and population proportion of elderly individuals and very young children, ethnicity, and the primary language spoken.
3. The surrounding physical environment. Are there safety hazards? What is the existing level of sanitary conditions? Are roads open and passable? Is weather a factor? The physical environment must be assessed not only for disaster victims, but also for disaster workers.

Determining Immediacy of Care

Based on the assessment, goals should be established for health care, and plans for meeting those goals should be made. In an emergency aid station, planning for the individual focuses on whether care can be provided at the station or only at an acute care hospital; this is done via triage, which was addressed earlier in the chapter. Discharge planning is necessary and begins when a victim enters the shelter. Plans must be made for health care supervision and for transfer to regular community health care facilities as needed. Plans must also be made to deal with dead victims, notify and provide grief counseling for families, and arrange for burial.

Major Health Concerns After a Disaster

After a major disaster producing severe disruption of community services and dislocation of citizens, a number of health-related concerns are present. Some of these can be anticipated and addressed in pre-disaster planning. Table 15–5 lists a number of the health and social issues related to specific types of disasters. In addition, any major disruption can expect to have repercussions that have health-related consequences, including potential overcrowding in shelters and other types of community living arrangements, decreased personal hygiene and sanitation because of reduced services and privacy, increased personal injuries and malnutrition, potential contamination of food and water supplies, and disruption of public health services. Nurses working with a community disrupted by disaster can anticipate these types of problems and plan to reduce the health hazards associated with them via activating community resources, ensuring adequate sanitation facilities and on-the-spot health education to reduce health and sanitation hazards, initiating immunization programs to reduce the spread of communicable diseases, and overseeing nutritional and hydration programs to ensure adequate minimum standards for the population under care. During disaster situations nurses must help individuals make the most of their health care, help maximize the populations' health, and find ways to improve the environment.

Role at Emergency Aid Stations

Nurses are involved in providing care at emergency aid stations. According to the ARC Disaster Services regulations and procedures that govern the activities of the ARC, "at least one registered nurse must be present at all times while the emergency aid station is open" (American Red Cross, 1988). ARC defines the functions of the Disaster Health Service nurse in charge as follows (American Red Cross, 1989):

- Arranging with the volunteer medical consultant for initial and daily health checks based on the health needs of shelter residents
- Establishing nursing care priorities and planning for health care supervision
- Planning for appropriate transfer of patients to community health care facilities as necessary
- Evaluating health care needs
- Arranging for secure storage of supplies, equipment, records, and medications and periodically checking to see whether material goods must be ordered
- Requesting and assigning volunteer staff to appropriate duties and providing on-the-job training and supervision
- Consulting with the shelter manager on the health status of residents and workers and identifying potential problems and trends
- Consulting with the food supervisor regarding the preparation and distribution of special diets, including infant formulas
- Planning and recommending adequate staff and facilities when local health departments initiate an immunization program for shelter residents
- Establishing lines of communication with the health service officer
- Arranging with the mass care supervisor for the purchase and replacement of essential prescriptions for persons in the shelter

Psychological Needs of Victims

Disasters produce physical, social, and psychological consequences that are exhibited to various degrees in different persons, families, communities, and cultures

TABLE 15–5

The Effects of Disaster on Individuals and Communities

Phase	Most Common Health Effects: *Physical Effect*	Most Common Health Effects: *Psychosocial Effects*	Effects on Community	Effects on Health Care Delivery System	Red Cross Health Services Supplementation
TORNADO					
Preimpact	Usually a warning period *Victims:* Aggravation of chronic illness or condition; stress-related symptoms	Usually a warning period *Victims:* Stress	Public services overtaxed Telephone system overloaded Transportation problems Communications problems	Little need for health care	
Impact	*Victims:* Wounds (all types); bone, muscle, and joint injuries; fractures; aggravation of chronic illness or condition; obstetrical complications; stress-related symptoms; death	*Victims:* Stress; crisis reaction; grief *Workers:* Stress; burnout syndrome	Utilities disrupted Communications disrupted Transportation disrupted Public buildings damaged Families separated and homeless Sanitation disrupted	Ambulances and rescue squads overburdened or unable to get through Sources of care overburdened and access impeded due to debris on roads Need for blood and blood products Damage to hospitals and nursing homes	Disaster action teams Emergency aid stations Shelters Temporary infirmaries Morgues Hospial contacts
Postimpact	*Victims and Workers:* Complications secondary to above; respiratory problems, including upper respiratory infections and those associated with fiberglass; clean-up wounds; gastrointestinal problems; aggravation of chronic illness or condition; stress-related symptoms	*Victims:* Stress; crisis reaction; grief *Workers:* Stress; burnout syndrome	Utilities disrupted Goods depleted Services overburdened Communications problems Temporary services implemented Overabundance of unusable donated clothes, toys, and other articles	Possible overburdening of sources of health care Possible overburdening of environmental health workers Interruption of home health services Scarcity of medical supplies and personnel	Red Cross service center FEMA Disaster Assistance Center Shelters Temporary infirmaries Emergency aid stations Hospital contacts Home visits
HURRICANE					
Preimpact	Aggravation of chronic illness or condition; obstetrical complications; wounds (evacuation); muscle injuries from moving heavy objects; stress-related symptoms	*Victims and workers:* Stress	Public services disrupted due to evacuation Transportation and communications problems Resources depleted	Planning and preparedness activities	Shelters Emergency aid stations Hospital contacts Temporary infirmaries
Impact	*Victims and Workers:* Asphyxia due to drowning; wounds; bone, joint, and muscle injuries; aggravation of chronic illness or condition; stress-related symptoms	*Victims:* Stress; crisis reaction *Workers:* Stress; burnout syndrome	Utilities disrupted Communications and transportation problems Public buildings damaged Public services disrupted Families separated and homeless Sanitation disrupted	Sources of care overburdened or inoperable Ambulances and rescue squads overburdened and unable to get through Possible increased need for blood and blood products Damage to hospitals and nursing homes	Disaster action teams Emergency aid stations Hospital contacts Temporary infirmaries Morgues Home visits

continued

TABLE 15–5

The Effects of Disaster on Individuals and Communities *Continued*

Phase	Most Common Health Effects: Physical Effect	Most Common Health Effects: Psychosocial Effects	Effects on Community	Effects on Health Care Delivery System	Red Cross Health Services Supplementation
Postimpact	*Victims and workers:* Complications secondary to above; respiratory problems; upper respiratory infections; gastrointestinal problems; clean-up injuries; animal, snake, and insect bites; skin irritations and infections; aggravation of chronic illness or condition; obstetrical complications; stress-related symptoms	*Victims:* Stress, crisis reaction; grief *Workers:* Stress; burnout syndrome	Restored services interrupted Goods depleted Services overburdened Temporary services implemented	Continued overburdening of health care facilities and health care providers Possible overburdening of environmental health workers Mass immunization clinics Interruption of home health services Scarcity of medical supplies	Shelters Temporary infirmaries Emergency aid stations Home visits Red Cross service center FEMA Disaster Assistance Center
EARTHQUAKE					
Preimpact	Threat may be present to those who live on a fault; usually no warning	Possibility of stress	Preparedness planning	Preparedness planning	Preparedness planning
Impact	High incidence of mortality and morbidity *Victims:* Stress-related symptoms; wounds; bone, joint, and muscle injuries; death; burns from explosions	*Victims:* Stress; crisis reaction; grief *Workers:* Stress; burnout syndrome	Public services overtaxed Utilities disrupted Communications disrupted Transportation disrupted Public buildings damaged Families separated and homeless Sanitation disrupted	Ambulances and rescue squads overburdened Facilities overburdened or damaged Increased need for blood and blood products Power loss	Shelters Temporary aid stations Morgues Hospital contacts
Postimpact	After secondary disaster such as aftershock: *Victims:* Wounds; clean-up injuries; gastrointestinal and respiratory problems; aggravation of chronic illness or condition; obstetrical complications; stress-related symptoms	*Victims:* Stress; crisis reaction; grief *Workers:* Stress; burnout syndrome	Utility services interrupted Goods depleted Services overburdened Communications problems Temporary services implemented	Possible overburdening of health facilities, health care providers, and environmental health workers Mental health facilities overtaxed Scarcity of medical supplies Overabundance of donated and outdated medical supplies Mass immunizations Loss of facilities	Shelters Emergency aid stations Temporary infirmaries Hospital contacts Home visits Red Cross service center FEMA Disaster Assistance Center

From American Red Cross. (1982). *Participant Workbook.* 3076–A. Washington, DC: Author.

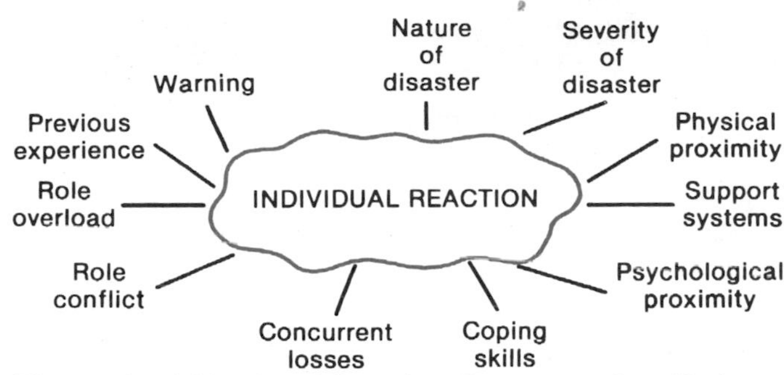

Figure 15–2 ● Variables influencing disaster reaction. (Redrawn from Demi, A. S., Miles, M. S. (1983). Understanding psychologic reactions to disasters. *Journal of Emergency Nursing, 9*(1), 12.)

depending on their past experiences, coping skills, and the scope and nature of the disaster (Fig. 15–2). Because most people affected by a disaster pass through predictable stages of psychological response, nurses and other health care professionals can anticipate and prepare for the needs of the victims (Demi and Miles, 1983). The following victims of a disaster are more likely to need crisis intervention than others:

- Those who have lost one or more family members
- Those who have suffered serious injury
- Those who have a history of a psychiatric disorder
- Those who have lost their home or possessions
- Those who have been previously institutionalized for a mental illness
- Those who have suffered a pre-disaster stress
- Those who are poor or on a fixed income
- Elderly individuals
- Members of minority groups
- Those who have not handled previous crises in a healthy way, especially those who have been hostile or self-destructive during a previous crisis
- Those without adequate support systems

The reactions of individuals to disasters vary greatly. The speed of onset, severity, and duration of symptoms are determined by many personal variables. Despite psychological distress, many people can function effectively during the impact phase of disaster but will later experience severe emotional distress. Some people will be so overwhelmed by the disaster that they will experience immediate extreme distress. Others, despite their involvement, may appear unaffected through the impact and emergency phases. These persons may utilize defenses of repression and denial to handle this distress. To function effectively, nurses and other disaster workers use some of these defenses during a disaster (Richtsmeir and Miller, 1985). Demi and Miles (1983) emphasize that there is no single correct way to react to a disaster. Both immediate and delayed reactions can be pathological without appropriate support and intervention. However, early post-disaster reactions are more easily recognized, and adequate treatment is usually provided, whereas delayed reactions, such as PTSD, are less frequently recognized and can go untreated.

Most victims will have some psychological reaction to the disaster situation. These reactions are usually transient, and many victims recover on their own with support from volunteer workers and family members. The most important thing emergency personnel can do for victims is to recognize that they have a legitimate reason for their reactions and emotions and to work toward providing them with emotional support. A psychological assessment by the nurse will aid in identifying those individuals more prone to severe psychological distress.

It is critical that survivors of a disaster each be assessed for the level of psychological stress they are suffering and the degree of impairment they are experiencing in their physical and emotional health and productive functioning. Individuals suffering minimal distress usually need support only from family and friends. Those who suffer a moderate amount of distress usually need the help of a support group or short-term counseling. Persons with severe distress may need extensive therapy.

At the disaster site or primary triage point, simple support measures can alleviate the psychological trauma experienced by survivors (Richtsmeir and Miller, 1985). These measures include the following:

- Keeping families together, especially children and parents
- Assigning a companion to frightened or injured victims, or placing victims in groups where they can help each other
- Giving survivors tasks to do to keep them busy and reduce trauma to their self-esteem
- Providing adequate shelter, food, and rest
- Establishing and maintaining a communication network to reduce rumors
- Encouraging individuals to share their feelings and support each other
- Isolating victims who demonstrate hysterical or panic behavior

Some persons will need more intensive support. Whenever possible, community mental health nurses will be an important asset to the health care team to assist in meeting the psychosocial needs of victims. A quick psychological assessment guide is a useful tool to help emergency personnel determine the psychological state of victims (Table 15–6). Individuals at risk of suffering psychological crisis after disaster may not seek help even if they need it. Therefore, it is essential that the nurse assess the stress level of victims, make other rescue team members aware of this, and refer those victims that need help to appropriate professional counselors. The nurse, as a member of the disaster team, participates in rescue operations and acts as a case-finder for persons suffering psychological stress,

TABLE 15–6

Disaster Stress Reaction Assessment*

1. Has client experienced a disastrous event? ______ Yes ______ No
2. Was this event generally outside the range of human experience? ______ Yes ______ No
3. Would this event evoke symptoms in almost everyone exposed to it, even those who have been emotionally healthy previously? ______ Yes ______ No

If answer to first three questions is yes, client may be experiencing a disaster stress reaction. Continue assessment.

4. Does client have any of the following symptoms? (Place a check next to each symptom experienced.)
   ______ a. Reexperiencing disaster through recurrent intrusive recollections or dreams
   ______ b. Reexperiencing disaster in response to environmental triggers
   ______ c. Feeling of unreality, numbness, or lack of responsiveness to events
   ______ d. Decreased interest in previously significant people
   ______ e. Decreased interest in previously meaningful activities
   ______ f. Hyperalertness
   ______ g. Increased startle response
   ______ h. Guilt about surviving disaster or about behavior during disaster
   ______ i. Difficulty concentrating and/or remembering
   ______ j. Avoiding activities or places that stimulate recollection of disaster
   ______ k. Worsening of symptoms with exposure to events that symbolize or resemble disaster experience

Three or more of these symptoms indicate high likelihood of client's having a disaster stress reaction.

Other symptoms not diagnostic of disaster stress reaction, but that may accompany the reaction, are the following:

______ Increased irritability
______ Unpredictable explosions of aggressive behavior
______ Impulsive behavior (if a change from previous pattern)
______ Overwhelming sadness

From Demi, A. S., & Miles, M. S. (1983). Understanding psychologic reactions to disaster. *Journal of Emergency Nursing 9,* 13–16.

*Items derived from the text of the *Diagnostic and statistical manual of mental disorders* (3rd ed.). Washington, DC: American Psychiatric Association, 1980, pp. 236–239.

intervening to help the victim deal effectively with the stress.

RECOVERY

During the recovery phase of a disaster, nurses are involved in efforts to restore the community to normal. Referral of injured victims for rehabilitation and convalescence is important to reduce the chances of long-term disability. Psychosocial needs must be addressed. In addition to identifying those in need of longer term counseling, nurses must link victims with support agencies to help with food, clothing, and shelter needs. Depending on the extent of damage to the community and the injuries of victims, the recovery phase can be relatively quick or can extend over a long period of time. Community recovery from the Los Angeles earthquake of 1994 is expected to take years. The San Francisco area has still not completely recovered from the earthquake of 1989.

It is very important for all emergency response personnel to learn from each disaster in order to improve response to the next emergency situation. For this reason, evaluation is an essential element of any disaster plan. Evaluation should include assessment of the effectiveness of the immediate response, determination of the impact of the disaster on the community, follow-up of victims to determine how well victim needs were met by the services provided, and assessment of the impact of the disaster on response personnel. The evaluation may result in new priorities, goals, and care plans.

PERSONAL RESPONSE OF CARE PROVIDERS TO DISASTER

Disaster workers are often overlooked when those affected by a disaster are considered. Many disaster workers report being overwhelmed by the devastation and the extent of personal injuries. They may feel unqualified to cope with some of the medical emergencies presented. In major disasters, many work without relief for 24 to 36 hours. If they are residents of the affected community, they must deal with personal losses and concerns for friends and relatives in addition to working with the people under their care.

Health care workers are subject to the same concerns and emotional traumas as other community residents, yet are expected to function in a health care capacity (Laube, 1985). Chubon (1992) examined the responses of community health nurses during the aftermath of Hurricane Hugo in 1989. She reports that the nurses experienced conflict between family and work-related responsibilities. Many expressed feelings of anger, grief, and frustration about their personal losses. Supportive colleagues eased the stress for health care workers. The ARC encourages disaster workers to go through a debriefing process after their disaster work is complete. This process may consist of one or several sessions and is designed to help health care workers recognize and deal with the personal impact of the disaster.

ETHICAL AND LEGAL IMPLICATIONS

There are no laws specifically defining the scope of practice for nurses during a disaster. However, there are guideline sources, including the state's Nurse Practice Act, professional organization standards, a state attorney's opinions, and current and common practice laws. All nurses should be familiar with the Nurse Practice Act in the state where they live and work, not only for disaster purposes but also for the general practice of nursing.

Although it does not have standards for disaster nursing, the American Nurses' Association, has standards for emergency nursing practice. Although these are professional, not legal, standards, common thinking will protect the nurse working within these standards of practice.

For nurses working with the ARC, protection is provided under the federal mandate. The authority vested in the ARC makes unnecessary the issuance of special permission or a license by state or local governments for the ARC to activate or carry out its relief program. No state, territory, or local government can deny the right of the ARC to render its services in accordance with the congressional mandate and its own administrative policies.

As a volunteer during a disaster, a nurse in most situations would be covered by the "Good Samaritan" Acts of the state. The purpose of the Good Samaritan Acts are to encourage medically trained persons to respond to medical emergencies by protecting them from liability through grants of immunity.

Conclusion

Community health nurses provide encouragement, care, and support to community members during a disaster and are uniquely qualified to meet the challenges of disaster nursing. They are able to deal with unexpected events, rapid changes, and intense demands for nursing service. They must be prepared to apply innovative problem-solving techniques to emotionally charged situations under poor environmental conditions and with frequent interruptions.

KEY IDEAS

1. Disasters can be naturally occurring or man-made.
2. Individuals respond in many different ways to the disaster experience, and emergency care providers are not immune to personal responses to the experience.
3. A significant amount of disaster preparedness is taken up with preplanning and mock exercises to prepare response personnel for an actual event.
4. During the preimpact phase of a disaster, nurses and other designated disaster relief personnel can initiate shelter preparation in the event of a significant warning interval; if not, they remain on alert and wait for the event to occur.
5. Local, state, federal, and voluntary agencies should be involved in community disaster planning efforts.
6. The American Red Cross is responsible for resident relief during disasters, including shelter operations, health care, and relief supplies for workers in the field.
7. Community health nurses are an integral part of the disaster planning and implementation effort. They are involved as planners, educators, direct caregivers, and assessment supervisors. They may serve as community survey assessors or triage officers after the disaster has occurred.
8. Evaluation and reassessment of the actual disaster relief effort is a crucial part of disaster management efforts. The information gathered by a thorough evaluation should be used to strengthen the community's response plan to better meet the next emergency situation.

GUIDELINES FOR LEARNING

1. Call your local branch of the American Red Cross and ask what kind of activities related to disaster relief the agency has undertaken in the past 5 years.
2. Identify your local command emergency operation center. If you are unsure about how to find this information, call your local police or fire department and ask for the information.
3. Ask other health personnel if they have had personal experiences taking care of victims in disaster or emergency situations.
4. Consider what your response might be in an emergency situation. What if you witnessed a car or bus wreck? If you were driving by, would you stop? If no, why not? If yes, what would you do first? If you were home and heard about the wreck on a radio news bulletin, would you report to work? Would you report to work if your supervisor called and asked you to come in? If you were not employed, would you call the Red Cross and volunteer your professional services? Would you go to the scene?

5. Research a major disaster that has occurred in the United States during the past 5 years. Identify the health needs of the population. According to your research accounts, was the disaster handled efficiently by the disaster health personnel? Were any areas singled out as needing improved performance? Can you identify any areas for improvement based on your readings?

REFERENCES

American Psychiatric Association. (1980). *Diagnostic and statistical manual of mental health disorders* (3rd ed.). Washington, DC: Author.

American Red Cross. (July 1972). *Disaster operations: A handbook for local governments.* CPG–1–6. Washington, DC: Author.

American Red Cross. (1975). *Disaster relief program.* 2235. Washington, DC: Author.

American Red Cross. (1982). *Participant workbook.* 3076-A. Washington, DC: Author.

American Red Cross. (1985). *Disaster services, regulations and procedures.* 3066. Washington, DC: Author.

American Red Cross. (1987). *Disaster services, regulations, and procedures.* Washington, DC: Author.

American Red Cross. (1988). *Disaster services, regulations and procedures.* Washington, DC: Author.

American Red Cross. (1989). *Disaster services, regulations and procedures.* 3076-1A. Washington, DC: Author.

American Red Cross (June 1991) *Your Family Disaster Supplies Kit.* Washington DC: Author.

American Red Cross (November 1991) *Emergency Preparedness.* Washington DC: Author.

Brown, S. T., Kurtz, A. W., Turley, J. P., & Gulitz, E. 1988. Sheltering and response to evaluation during Hurricane Elena. *Journal of Emergency Nursing, 14*(1), 23–26.

Chubon, S. J. (1992). Home care during the aftermath of Hurricane Hugo. *Public Health Nursing, 9*(2), 97–102.

Demi, A. S., & Miles, M. S. (1983). Understanding psychological reactions to disaster. *Journal of Emergency Nursing. 9*(1), 13–16.

Dynes, R. R., Quarantelli, E. L., & Kreps, G. A. (1972). *A perspective on disaster planning.* Washington, DC: Defense Civil Preparedness Agency, U.S. Department of Defense.

Federal Emergency Management Agency. (1981). *Disaster operations: A handbook for local governments.* Washington, DC: U.S. Government Printing Office.

Federal Emergency Management Agency. (1983). *Disaster assistance program.* D R and R–18 program guide. Washington, DC: U.S. Government Printing Office.

Garb, S., and Eng, E. (1969). *Disaster handbook* (2nd ed.). New York: Springer.

Hayes, G., Goodwin, T., & Miars, B. (1990). After disaster: A crisis support team at work. *American Journal of Nursing Feb.*(2) 90, 61–64.

Laube, J. (1985). Health care providers as disaster victims. In J. Laube and S.A. Murphy (Eds.), *Perspectives on disaster recovery.* Norwalk, CT: Appleton-Century-Crofts.

Lilienfeld, A. M., & Lilienfeld, D. A. (1980). *Foundations of epidemiology.* New York: Oxford University Press.

Merchant, J. A. (1986). Preparing for disaster. *American Journal of Public Health. 76*(3), 233–235.

National Safety Council. (1992). *Accident facts.* Washington, DC: U.S. Government Printing Office.

Richtsmeir, J. L., & Miller, J. R. (1985). Psychological aspects of disaster situations. In L. M. Garcia (Ed.), *Disaster nursing.* Rockville, MD: Aspen.

BIBLIOGRAPHY

Applebaum, S. (1981). *Stress management for health care professionals.* Rockville, MD: Aspen.

Ciuca, R., Downie, C. S., & Morris, M. (1977). When disaster happens. *Journal of Nursing, 77,* 454–456.

Demi, A. S., & Miles, M. S. (1984). An examination of nursing leadership following a disaster. *Topics in Clinical Nursing, 6*(1), 63–78.

Garcia, L. (1985). *Disaster nursing, planning, assessment and intervention.* Rockville, MD: Aspen.

Komnenick, P., & Feller, C. (1991). Disaster nursing—College of Nursing, Arizona State University. *Annual Review Nursing Research, 9,* 123–134.

Ward, P. M., Eck, C. A., & Sanguino, T. F. (1990). Emergency nursing at the epicenter: The Loma Prieta earthquake. *Journal of Emergency Nursing, 16*(4), 49A–55A.

SUGGESTED READINGS

Brown, S. T., Kurtz, A. W., Turley, J. P., & Gulitz, E. (1988). Sheltering and response to evacuation during Hurricane Elena. *Journal of Emergency Nursing, 14*(1), 23–26.

Chubon, S. H., (1992). Home care during the aftermath of Hurricane Hugo. *Public Health Nursing, 9*(2), 97–102.

Clayton, G. M., Martin, P., Poon, L. W., Lawhorn, L. A., & Avery, K. L. (1993). Survivors. *Nursing and Health Care, 14*(5), 256–260.

Demi, A. S., & Miles, M. S. (1983). Understanding psychologic reactions to disaster. *Journal of Emergency Nursing, 9*(1), 13–16.

Farrell, M. (1990). A nurses' experience on a disaster-preparedness team. Department of Nursing, University of New Hampshire. *International Nursing Review, 37*(6), 358–362, 270.

Hanson, C. (1990). Going on a Red Cross disaster assignment: The Huntsville tornado. *Journal of Emergency Nursing, 16*(4), 66A–69A.

Hayes, G., Goodwin, T., & Miars, B. (1990). After disaster: A crisis support team at work. *American Journal of Nursing, Feb.*(2) 90, 61–64.

Miles, M. S., Demi, A. S., & Mostyn-Aber, P. (1984). Rescue workers' reactions following the Hyatt Hotel disaster. *Death Education, 8,* 315–331.

Murphy, S. A. (1984). After Mount St. Helens: Disaster stress research. *Journal of Psychosocial Nursing, 22*(7), 9–18.

Parker, S. (1990). Public health nurses bring special disaster relief skills. *California Nurse, 86*(1), 6.

Unit IV

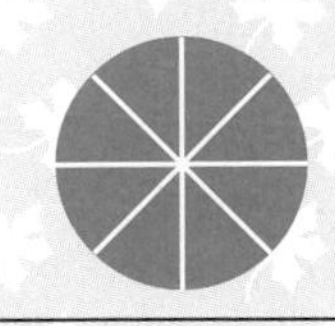

Tools for Practice

Chapter 16

Health Promotion and Risk Reduction in the Community

Mary Ellen Lashley

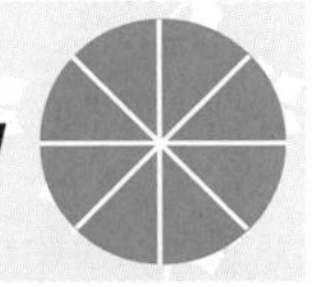

Focus Questions

What does it mean to be healthy?

What is the difference between promoting health and preventing illness?

What models help explain health-related behaviors?

What influences the health of a society?

What are the major national policies for health promotion?

What are the responsibilities of the community health nurse in promoting health and preventing illness in the community?

Over the years Americans have improved their efforts to prevent illness and promote health and longevity. Currently there is a trend toward improved health and self-care in American society. This trend is evident on both an individual and a community level. In 1989, for example, improvements were noted in the efforts of Americans to limit consumption of high cholesterol food, avoid driving while drinking, use seat belts, and reduce cigarette smoking (The Prevention Index, 1989). Even so, 50% to 75% of the mortality in the U.S. population results from lifestyles damaging to health (Gallagher and Kriedler, 1987). Controlling fewer than 10 risk factors (such as poor diet and exercise, smoking, and drug and alcohol abuse) can prevent between 40% and 70% of premature deaths, one third of all cases of acute disability, and two thirds of all cases of chronic disability (United States Department of Health and Human Services) [USDHHS], 1990b).

As consumers take a more active role in wellness, government funding and services are also shifting toward illness prevention and health promotion. *Healthy People,* a 1979 publication, represented the first United States Surgeon General's report on health promotion and disease prevention in the nation. This report proposed a national strategy for improving the health of Americans by identifying major health problems and setting national goals to reduce death and disability. However, there was no national strategy for implementation of this plan, and the percentage of federal health care dollars devoted to prevention efforts has not increased.

Health promotion is a major goal of community health nursing practice. Community health nurses facilitate health in the population through direct nursing interventions aimed at health promotion and disease prevention and through advocacy and political action for greater public and private support of prevention programs. In this chapter, the concept of health is explored in greater depth, and major influences on health are examined. Theoretical models are presented that attempt to explain health-related behaviors. National policies related to health promotion and risk reduction are reviewed, and types of health promotion and risk reduction programs are examined. Finally, the responsibilities of the community health nurse in facilitating health promotion are explored using the nursing process.

The Meaning of Health

The concept of health has been defined in a variety of ways. Historically, health and illness were viewed as extremes on a continuum, with the absence of clinically recognizable disease being equated with the presence of health. In 1974 the World Health Organization defined health in terms of total well-being and discouraged the conceptualization of health as simply the absence of disease.

More contemporary definitions of health have emphasized the relationship between health and wellness. Although health may be viewed as a static state of being at any given point in time, *wellness* is the process of moving toward integration of human functioning; maximization of human potential; self-responsibility for health; greater self-awareness and self-satisfaction; and wholeness in body, mind, and spirit (Clark, 1986; Dunn, 1961; Murray and Zentner, 1985).

Four perspectives on health clarify alternative conceptualizations of health and provide direction for developing goals for health promotion (Smith, 1981):

1. The *eudaemonistic perspective* defines health as the realization of one's potential for complete development. *Eudaemonistic* is a term derived from the Greek word *eudemon,* meaning "fortunate" or "happy." In this model, illness is seen as an impediment to happiness or good fortune.
2. The *adaptive model* of health defines health as the ability to interact effectively within the physical and social environment. The disease state thus represents a failure in adaptation and ineffective coping with environmental changes.
3. The *role performance model* of health views health as the ability to perform social roles. Illness is determined by the capacity to function and perform one's daily activities.
4. The *clinical model* views health as the absence of physiological disease or the absence of disequilibrium. Persons with clinical symptoms of disease are not considered healthy from this perspective.

These models represent progressive development of the concept of health from the narrowly defined clinical focus to the broader, eudaemonistic perspective, which is currently more widely accepted in nursing. Even this perspective, however, views illness as an impediment to self-actualization rather than as a potential growth-promoting experience. Therefore, persons having each of these perspectives on health will be motivated differently to pursue health promotion (Table 16–1).

Another term commonly found in health promotion literature is the notion of *holistic health.* Persons who view health from a holistic perspective focus on the biopsychosocial dimensions of health, seeing persons as interrelated with others and with their environment. The focus of holistic health is on acceptance and harmony of body, mind, and spirit (Murray and Zentner, 1985). Unlike the eudaemonistic perspective, an illness experience is not necessarily viewed as an impediment to self-actualization but can actually become a growth-promoting and potentially beneficial experience.

Health promotion is the process of assisting persons to enhance their well-being and maximize their human potential. The focus of health promotion is on changing patterns of behavior to promote health rather than to simply avoid illness. The goal of health promotion is to enable

TABLE 16–1

Examples of Differing Conceptions of Health

Health Focus	Motivation	Client Statement	Nursing Response
Eudaemonistic	Motivated by joy and self-fulfillment.	"To be healthy is to realize my full potential."	Explore with client health-promoting behaviors such as diet, exercise, or recreational activities that foster self-esteem and a sense of personal accomplishment.
Adaptive	Motivated by altering oneself or the risks in the environment as situations change (i.e., engaging in stress reduction, dietary or exercise programs, or community recycling; reducing exposure to environmental hazards).	"I get sick when I am no longer able to cope with the stresses in my environment."	Explore with client lifestyle or environmental changes that can be made to protect health and reduce the risk of illness.
Role performance	Motivated by being able to fulfill responsibilities at work, play, home, community.	"As long as I can work and fulfill obligations to my family and my job, I consider myself healthy."	Reinforce influence of health promotion and risk reduction behaviors on ability to fulfill role expectations.
Clinical	Motivated by the absence of diagnosable disease.	"If I eat better I can avoid getting a heart attack."	Conduct routine health screening to foster early detection of disease. Stress health-promoting behaviors that may prevent the onset of disease.

persons to exercise control over their well-being and to ultimately improve their health. Health promotion involves focusing on persons and populations as a whole and not solely on people at risk for specific diseases (Kickbusch, 1986). Health promotion is appropriate for everyone.

Influences on Health

Many factors influence health. These factors are integrated into an individual's lifestyle. *Lifestyle* refers to the way people live their lives and involves patterns of work, play, eating, sleeping, and communicating (Gallagher and Kriedler, 1987). A healthy lifestyle is easier to maintain when healthful patterns of behavior are learned early in life. Therefore, the family plays a critical role in the development of health beliefs and behaviors. Healthy lifestyle behaviors that are shaped by familial and sociocultural influences include routine exercise patterns, sound nutritional practices, regular seat belt use, avoidance of harmful substances (e.g., tobacco, alcohol, drugs), stress management, protection from harmful environmental agents, and routine medical and dental evaluations. When assisting persons to move to a higher level of wellness through health promotion activities, the community health nurse must examine the biological, environmental, and sociocultural influences affecting their health and well-being (Murray and Zentner, 1985).

Biological Influences. *Biological* or *genetic* endowment influences susceptibility to illness. Genetic inheritance involves such physical characteristics as sex; skin, eye, and hair color; facial structure; and height and weight. Certain diseases are more common in one sex or race than another, but illness related to age, sex, or race may also be influenced by cultural, ethnic, and environmental factors. Similarly, physical features such as height and build may also be environmentally influenced. Thus, because many of these factors exist or operate simultaneously, it is often difficult to determine the relative influence of genetics and the environment on the risk of developing disease.

Environmental Influences. *Environmental* influences contribute to or detract from the ability of persons to develop to their optimum potential. It is estimated, for example, that adverse conditions in the physical environment (e.g., air, food, and water pollution) directly or indirectly cause approximately one half of all cancers (Murray and Zentner, 1985).

When examining environmental influences on health, the physical, psychological, and sociocultural environments must be considered. Factors in the *physical* environment that influence health include weather and climatic conditions, noise, light, air, food, water, and exposure to toxic substances. (See Chapter 24 for an in-depth discussion of environmental health issues.) The *psychological* environment includes the person's perception of his or her environment and is influenced by the behavior of others, which contributes to self-esteem, conveys intimacy or distance, and promotes or hinders communication.

Factors in the *sociocultural* environment that influence health include the historical era in which one lives, values of family and significant others, social institutions (e.g., governments, schools, and churches), socioeconomic class, occupation, and social roles that encourage or diminish the importance of preventive health practices. For example, an industrial worker may be exposed to toxic or carcinogenic substances that render him or her susceptible to different types of illness. In addition, health resources may be available only in more affluent communities, which diminishes access to services by persons of lower socioeconomic status. In the United States, higher education and higher socioeconomic class are associated with greater participation in health promotion activities. (See Chapter 6 for a discussion of cultural influences.)

The *health care system* is another important aspect of the environment that must be considered when determining the health potential of a society. Health care systems focus in varying degrees on prevention, cure, and rehabilitation in an effort to improve the health of society. Approximately 18% of all Americans and 31% of Americans without private or public health insurance have no access to primary health care (USDHHS, 1990a). Lack of funding or availability of such services may mean that pregnant women receive little or no prenatal care, children do not receive immunizations, and diseases go undetected. This lack of care has a tremendous impact on the health of a society. For this reason, one of the nation's health care goals for the year 2000 is to achieve access to preventive services for all Americans.

Health services may be directed toward primary, secondary, or tertiary levels of prevention. *Primary prevention* is aimed at preventing the onset of disease or disability by reducing risks to health, decreasing vulnerability to illness, and promoting health and well-being. *Secondary prevention* is aimed at diagnosis and treatment of illness at an early stage, thereby halting further progression of disease and assisting persons to return to normal functioning. Secondary prevention includes case finding and screening of high-risk groups for the presence of disease. *Tertiary prevention* focuses on the restoration of optimal functioning once a condition becomes irreversible by limiting the extent of disability that may occur and by assisting clients to function at an optimal level within the constraints of their existing disabilities. The focus of this chapter is on primary prevention to promote health and prevent illness in an individual, family, or community. (See Chapter 11 for an in-depth discussion on levels of prevention.)

National Policy

Health promotion is a social project, not solely a medical enterprise. Societies have a political responsibility to strengthen the link between health and social well-being. An integration of government, major interest groups (environmental, industrial, medical, labor, educational), and community forces is needed to establish and maintain public policy and community action that promotes the health of individuals, families, and communities in society.

The ability of the health care system to engage in health promotion is often determined by national legislation and policies that provide economic and political support for health promotion services in the community. Pender (1987) notes that less than 5% of the federal health care budget is spent on illness prevention and health promotion.

FOCUS ON HEALTH PROMOTION

Healthy People, the first U.S. Surgeon General's Report on Health Promotion and Disease Prevention, was instrumental in identifying major health problems of the nation and in setting national goals for reducing death and disability. The central message of this report was that the health of the nation could be improved by individual and collective action in public and private sectors and by promoting a safe, healthy environment for all Americans (*Healthy People,* 1979).

In 1980 the United States Department of Health and Human Services published a second document entitled *Promoting Health/Preventing Disease: Objectives for the Nation.* This document set forth specific objectives for meeting the national health care priorities established in the Surgeon General's report. These priorities included reduction in hypertension, family planning, pregnancy and infant health, immunizations, reduction in sexually transmitted diseases, preventive health services, toxic agent control, occupational safety and health, accident prevention, dental health, infectious disease control, reduction in smoking and alcohol and drug abuse, improved nutrition, increased exercise and fitness, improved stress management, and control of violent behavior. The objectives set out in this report were targeted for completion in 1990. *Prevention 89/90: Federal Programs and Progress,* published by the Office of Disease Prevention and Health Promotion of the United States Department of Health and Human Services, reported on the progress made toward meeting the 1990 objectives. The report concluded that, based on an analysis of trends in infant, childhood, adolescent, and adult mortality, the nation met most of its overall 1990 goals (USDHHS, 1990b).

Another significant federal publication related to health promotion was the Office of Disease Prevention and Health Promotion's 1988 publication entitled *Disease Prevention/Health Promotion: The Facts.* This publication examined demographic trends and recommendations related to nutrition, fitness, stress, toxic agent control, major causes of disease, and risks to health in the United States. In addition, the *Surgeon General's Report on Nutrition and Health* (1988) examined the state of the nation's nutritional health. This report concluded that there is a disproportionate consumption of foods high in fat among Americans and made the following recommendations:

- Limit consumption of foods high in calories, fat, cholesterol, and sugar.
- Maintain desirable body weight.
- Minimize alcohol consumption.
- Increase consumption of complex carbohydrates and fiber.
- Decrease sodium intake.
- Increase consumption of foods high in calcium for adolescents and adult women.
- Increase iron-rich food consumption for children, adolescents, and women of childbearing age.
- Provide for fluoridation of community water systems to prevent tooth decay.

Healthy People 2000 updated the major health problems of the nation and included specific health objectives for the year 2000. The general goals advocated in this report include: (1) increasing the span of healthy life for all Americans, (2) reducing health disparities among Americans, and (3) achieving access to preventive health care services for all Americans. The national health objectives for the year 2000 developed from these goals address the areas of health promotion, health protection, clinical preventive services, and priorities for system-wide improvements in surveillance and data systems. Age-related objectives target children, adolescents and young adults, adults, and older adults. Priority objectives include improving health status through a reduction in morbidity and mortality; promoting risk reduction interventions; increasing public awareness of health risks and preventive measures; educating professionals regarding the importance of prevention and of providing preventive services; and increasing comprehensiveness, accessibility, and quality of services for health promotion and protection (USDHHS, 1990a, 1990b). (See Table 16–2 for selected objectives targeting health promotion priorities.)

NATIONAL SURVEYS OF HEALTH PROMOTION

The federal government and private organizations have conducted a number of surveys to determine health promotion behavior patterns in the nation. For example, in 1981 the National Survey of Personal Health Practices and Health Consequences was conducted by the Office of Health Information, Health Promotion, Physical Fitness and Sports Medicine and by the Division of Environmental Epidemiology of the National Center for Health Statistics. The survey revealed that the majority of Americans agree that improving nutrition, maintaining ideal body weight, engaging in regular exercise, and decreasing smoking would improve the health of Americans (Pender, 1987).

More recently, *The Prevention Index '89* noted improvements in major health-promoting behaviors of Americans. This report summarized the sixth annual nationwide study commissioned by *Prevention* magazine and based on a Harris Survey. The prevention index is a measure of the effort of Americans to prevent accidents and disease and promote health and longevity. Adults reported decreases in smoking, excessive consumption of dietary salt and sugar, and recreational drug use; an increase in seat belt use; improved efforts to limit cholesterol intake; and an increase in regular breast self-examination practice and Papanicolaou smears.

The U.S. Public Health Service Office of Disease Prevention and Health Promotion coordinates the efforts of public and private sectors to reduce the risks of disease and promote the nation's health. This office publishes general public information, health policy papers, and conference proceedings.

These government and private efforts represent a national trend toward making prevention of disease and promotion of health a higher health care priority. Federal government initiatives have stressed health care cost containment, improved quality of care, and improved access to care. Emphasis has also been placed on individual choice and responsibility for one's health.

Health Models

Health status is influenced by biological, environmental, and sociocultural factors. These multiple influences on health ultimately determine the type and extent of personal health behaviors. A *model* is a related set of statements or concepts that describe, explain, or predict phenomena (Flynn and Heffron, 1984). A variety of theoretical models have been proposed in an attempt to describe, explain, or predict preventive health behaviors.

HEALTH BELIEF MODEL

The Health Belief Model, which has been widely used to explain wellness and illness behaviors, was created in the 1950s and has since been revised and tested extensively (Becker, 1974; Hochbaum, 1956; Rosenstock, 1974). Proponents of the Health Belief Model contend that individuals will take action to avoid disease states. Actions are motivated by (1) the sense of personal *susceptibility* to a disease, (2) the perceived *severity* of a disease, (3) the perceived *benefits* of preventive health behaviors, and (4) the perceived *barriers* to taking actions to prevent a disease. Potential barriers may include fear, pain, cost, inconvenience, or embarrassment (Rosenstock, 1974).

The client's perception of health status and the value placed on taking preventive action may also be affected by *demographic* variables (age, sex, race, ethnicity), *sociopsychological* variables (social class, peer pressure, attitude toward medical authorities), and *structural* variables (personal experience with disease, knowledge of disease).

TABLE 16–2

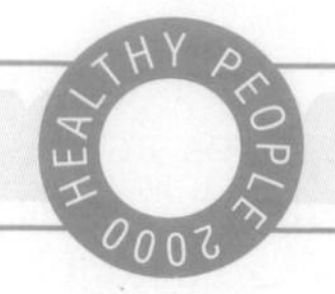

*National Objectives for Selected Health Promotion Priorities**

PHYSICAL ACTIVITY AND FITNESS

1. Reduce overweight to a prevalence of no more than 20% among people age 20 and older and no more than 15% among adolescents age 12 through 19. (Baseline: 26% aged 20 and older, 15% aged 12 through 19 in 1976–1980)
2. Increase to at least 30% the proportion of people age 6 years and older who regularly (preferably daily) engage in light to moderate physical activity for at least 30 minutes per day.
3. Reduce to no more than 15% the proportion of people age 6 years and older who engage in no leisure time physical activity. (Baseline: 24% aged 18 and older in 1985)
4. Increase the proportion of worksites offering employer-sponsored physical activity and fitness programs as follows:

50–99 employees	20%	(1985 Baseline: 14%
100–249 employees	35%	23%
250–749 employees	50%	32%
≥ 750 employees	80%	54%)

5. Increase to at least 50% the proportion of primary care providers who routinely assess and counsel their patients regarding the frequency, duration, type, and intensity of each patient's physical activity practices. (Baseline: 30% of sedentary patients counseled in 1988)

NUTRITION

1. Reduce growth retardation among low-income children age 5 years and younger to less than 10%. (Baseline: Up to 16% in 1988)
2. Reduce dietary fat intake to an average of 30% of calories or less and saturated fat intake to an average of less than 10% of calories among people age 2 years and older.
3. Decrease salt and sodium intake so that at least 65% of home meal preparers cook without adding salt, at least 80% of people avoid using salt at the table, and at least 40% of adults regularly purchase foods modified or lower in sodium. (Baseline: 54%, 68%, and 20% respectively)
4. Reduce iron deficiency to less than 3% among children age 1 through 4 and among women of childbearing age.
5. Increase to at least 75% the proportion of mothers who breast-feed their infants in the early postpartum period and to at least 50% the proportion who continue breast-feeding until their infants are 5 to 6 months old. (Baseline: 54% and 21% respectively)
6. Increase to at least 90% the proportion of restaurants and institutional food service operations that offer identifiable low-fat, low-calorie food choices, consistent with the Dietary Guidelines for Americans.
7. Increase to at least 90% the proportion of school lunch and breakfast services and child care food services with menus that are consistent with the nutrition principles in the Dietary Guidelines for Americans.
8. Increase to at least 75% the proportion of primary care providers who provide nutrition assessment and counseling or referral to qualified nutritionists or dietitians. (Baseline: Physicians provide diet counseling to 40 to 50% of patients in 1988)

TOBACCO

1. Reduce cigarette smoking to a prevalence of no more than 15% among people age 20 years and older. (Baseline: 29% in 1987)
2. Reduce the initiation of cigarette smoking by children and youths so that no more than 15% become regular cigarette smokers by age 20 years. (Baseline: 30% in 1987)
3. Reduce to no more than 20% the proportion of children age 6 years and younger who are regularly exposed to tobacco smoke at home. (Baseline: 39% in 1986)
4. Establish tobacco-free environments and include tobacco use prevention in the curricula of all elementary, middle, and secondary schools, preferably as part of quality school health education. (Baseline: 17% of schools banned smoking in 1988; 75% had curricula)
5. Increase to at least 75% the proportion of worksites with a formal smoking policy that prohibits or severely restricts smoking at the workplace. (Baseline: 54% of medium and large companies in 1987)
6. Enact in all 50 states comprehensive laws on clean indoor air that prohibit or strictly limit smoking in the workplace and in enclosed public places. (Baseline: 12 states in 1990)
7. Increase to at least 75% the proportion of primary care and oral health care providers who routinely advise cessation and provide assistance and follow-up for all of their tobacco-using patients. (Baseline: 52% of internists counseled 75% of their smoking patients in 1986)

PRIMARY CARE

1. Provide quality K–12 school health education in at least 75% of schools.
2. Provide employee health promotion activities in at least 85% of workplaces with 50 or more employees.

(Also see last objective under each section above.)

*From United States Department of Health and Human Services. (1990). *Healthy people 2000: National health promotion and disease prevention objectives. Summary report.* Washington, DC: U.S. Government Printing Office.

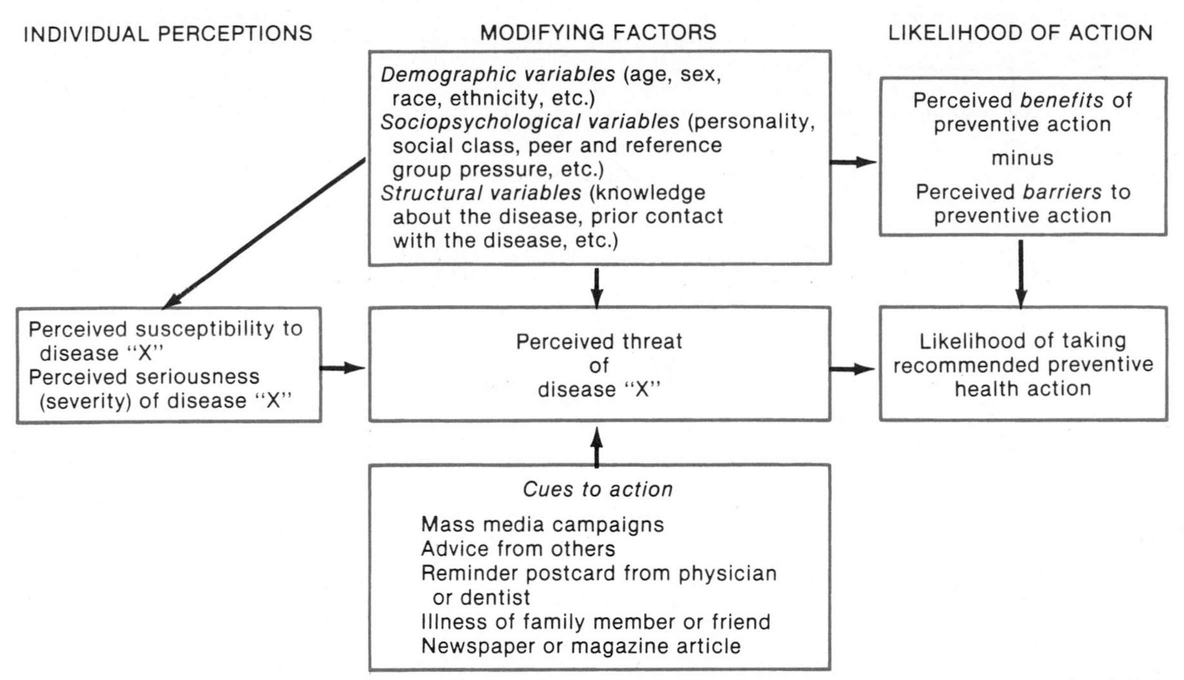

Figure 16–1 ● Health Belief Model. (From Becker, M. (1974). *The health belief model and personal health behavior* (p. 7). Thorofare, NJ: Charles B. Slack.)

Internal cues (detecting a breast lump) or *external cues* (advice from significant others, exposure to a media campaign) may also serve to motivate healthful behaviors (Fig. 16–1).

Empirical research demonstrates that the attitude and belief dimensions of the Health Belief Model do predict individuals' health-related behavior. When an illness or injury is perceived to be serious and barriers are low, individuals are more likely to seek medical care and follow the suggested treatment. In addition, individuals are most likely to engage in preventive health behavior when barriers to care are low and they perceive that they are susceptible to an illness or injury (Janz and Becker, 1984).

It is important for community health nurses to assess what clients perceive to be barriers to engaging in preventive behaviors or obtaining medical care. In addition to helping clients decrease those barriers, nurses can provide information that gives the client an accurate understanding of his or her susceptibility.

The Health Belief Model is directed more toward health-protecting behaviors than health-promoting behaviors. *Health-protecting* behaviors are behaviors that protect persons from problems that jeopardize their health and well-being, rather than behaviors that improve health by fostering personal development or self-actualization. Immunizing the population against infectious disease and reducing exposure to environmental health hazards are examples of health-protecting behaviors. Many health behaviors, such as management of dietary intake, exercise, and stress management, serve a dual function by both promoting and protecting health.

HEALTH PROMOTION MODELS

Whereas the Health Belief Model may account for those actions taken to prevent disease, Pender (1987) proposes a health promotion model that attempts to account for those behaviors that improve well-being and develop human potential. Pender contends that health promotion behaviors are determined by *cognitive–perceptual factors* (which include individual perceptions of the importance of health, control over health, definition of health, and perceived benefits and barriers to health-promoting behaviors), *modifying factors* (which include demographic, biological, interpersonal, and environmental–situational factors, as well as learned health-promoting behavior patterns), and *internal and external cues to action* (Szafran, 1989; Pender, 1987). Pender's model represents a diversity of biological, sociocultural, cognitive, and environmental factors affecting health promotion behavior (Figure 16–2).

HUMAN ECOLOGICAL MODELS

Ecological views of health examine determinants of health based on interrelated biological and social systems. Kulbok (1985) has proposed a Resource Model of Preventive Health Behavior, which represents a socioecological perspective of preventive health behavior. Kulbok contends that there is no single determinant of positive health actions. Instead, the likelihood of practicing preventive health behaviors increases with greater social and health resources available to individuals. Social resources include social status, education, and income. Health resources include perceived health status, energy level,

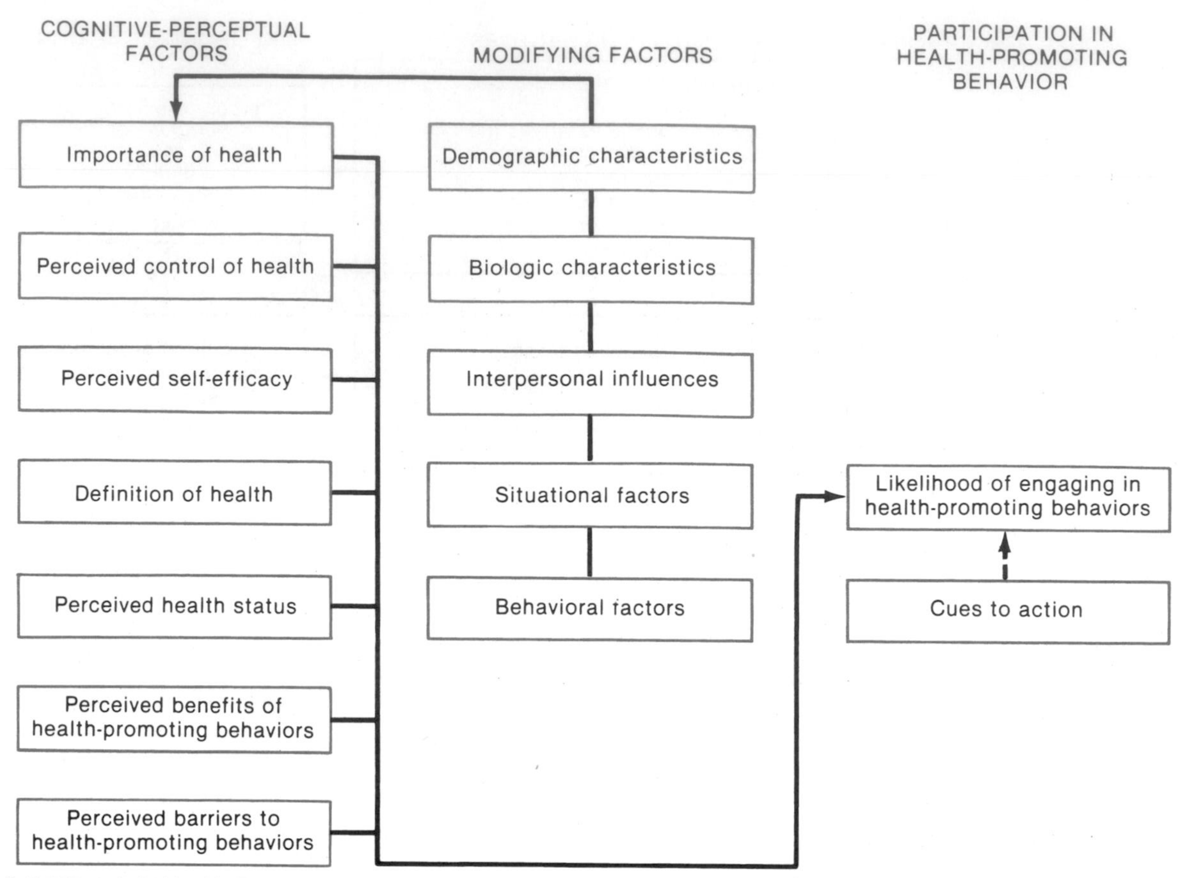

Figure 16–2 ● Pender's Health Promotion Model. (From Pender, N. (1987). *Health promotion in nursing practice* (p. 58). Norwalk, CT: Appleton & Lange.)

concern over health, participation in social groups and religious services, extent of positive friendships and family relationships, and a sense of general psychological well-being. Preventive health behaviors are defined in this model as actions taken voluntarily to promote and maintain health (Kulbok, 1985).

Shaver (1985) proposes an integrated and holistic human ecological model of health and wellness. In this model, host factors (i.e., personality, gender, age, cognitive ability, and physiological processes) are integrated with environmental factors (i.e., social support, cultural norms, energy exchange, life events, space, and time) to assess vulnerability, risk, and personal response to actual or potential health needs. These biopsychosocial approaches allow for a more comprehensive and individualized assessment on which to plan care to maximize health and promote the development of human potential (Shaver, 1985). This model is very similar to the epidemiological triad (see Chapter 11), except that it does not separate the "agent" from related host and environmental factors to identify a specific causative factor that promotes or prevents an individual from engaging in preventive health behaviors.

The models used to explain preventive health behaviors tend to be action oriented. Persons evaluate and respond to their perceived needs and subsequently act by taking preventive action or adopting health-promoting behaviors. Even so, because the models have as their end point a change in behavior, actual health outcomes or documented improvements in health are not directly addressed (Woods, 1989). For example, in applying the Health Belief Model to breast cancer, a woman may feel personally susceptible to developing breast cancer owing to risk factors such as age and family history. She may realize the disease is serious and appreciate the benefit of routine mammography and breast self-examination. In response to a media campaign in her community (external cue) or to palpating a breast lump (internal cue), she may act by seeking mammography screening. As a result of this behavior, the disease may be detected early and treated, and hopefully the woman will go on to live an active and healthy life. Here the theoretical model would need to take into account the possible health outcomes as a result of adopting preventive health behaviors. Continuing work on theoretical models and their application to research is needed to better understand the relationship between changes in behavior and the actual effects of behavior modification on health status.

Health Promotion and Risk Reduction Programs

A variety of programs have been implemented in communities to reduce the risk of disease for individuals and groups in society. *Health promotion programs* seek to increase the level of well-being and promote self-actualization of individuals and aggregates by advocating behaviors that seek to expand the potential for health and personal development. The goal of health promotion programs is to enable persons to positively act in their environment by creating conditions that nurture and promote health. *Risk reduction programs,* however, are directed toward facilitating health protective behaviors, which enable persons to react to threats in the environment through early identification and avoidance of risks (Pender, 1987). Thus, risk reduction programs are more reactive in their intent and are directed toward preventing illness by identifying, avoiding, and reducing risks to health or by detecting illness early, before the onset of symptoms. (See Chapters 17 and 24 for in-depth discussions on risk reduction and environmental influences.) The benefits of community approaches to prevention are summarized in Table 16–3.

The community health nurse develops, implements, and evaluates health promotion and risk reduction programs in schools, worksites, hospitals, churches, and community settings. When planning programs for wellness in the community, it is important to develop partnerships with those persons who are most likely to be affected by the program and to promote a sense of cooperation, collaboration, and teamwork between groups (Office of Disease Prevention and Health Promotion, 1988; Clark, 1986). Those incentives that are most likely to motivate persons to participate in programs should be chosen; these may include tangible gifts, socialization, or certification for participation.

Programs should emphasize self-responsibility for wellness behaviors. The location and duration of the program should be realistic and convenient, and the goals of the individuals and the organizations involved should be considered. Programs may address personal, occupational, family, social, and environmental well-being. Adequate provision must be made for following up persons enrolled in the program to evaluate the effectiveness of interventions (Clark, 1986).

TABLE 16–3

Benefits of Community Prevention Programs

1. Opportunity to reach the masses and effect widespread changes in social norms.
2. Increased public awareness of the importance of health promotion.
3. Increased cost efficiency of group intervention compared with one-to-one contacts.
4. Ability of the program to serve as an environmental cue, triggering healthful behaviors.
5. Ability of the program to promote the development of an environment of social support for health promotion.
6. Opportunity to evaluate the effectiveness of health promotion programs and to generalize findings to a wide range of demographic characteristics.

Data from Pender, N. (1987). *Health promotion in nursing practice* (2nd ed.). Norwalk, CT: Appleton & Lange.

PROGRAMS FOR INDIVIDUALS

There are a number of settings in which health promotion programs may be successfully implemented; these are determined by client focus. The client focus may be individual, family, or population centered. Individual health promotion programs are dependent on an accurate assessment of individual needs and risks to health based on biological, psychological, social, cultural, environmental, developmental, and situational variables.

Research has demonstrated that certain groups of individuals are more likely to engage in health-promoting behaviors. For example, older adults have more health-promoting lifestyles, a greater sense of responsibility for their health, better nutritional practices, and manage stress more effectively than do young or middle-aged adults (Walker et al., 1988). Women, regardless of their ethnic affiliation, tend to define health in terms of ability to achieve life goals, reach one's optimal potential, experience greater self-awareness and sense of purpose, and move toward harmony of mind and body (Fugate-Woods et al., 1988). These views correspond to a more eudaemonistic perspective of health, suggesting that women may be more responsive to the philosophy and goals undergirding health promotion programs.

Socioeconomic status also exerts a great impact on individual health. Persons with low incomes, for example, have been found to have death rates that are twice those of persons with income levels above the poverty line. The incidence of heart disease is 25% greater for low-income persons compared with the general population. The incidence of cancer also increases as family income decreases (USDHHS, 1990a).

Individualized health promotion strategies are based on assumptions that personal lifestyle is the cause of many diseases and disabilities and that persons are responsible for making informed decisions about their health (*Healthy People,* 1979). These decisions, however, can be made only in the context of available, affordable health care. Table 16–4 lists the major health concerns for persons at different stages of growth and development

TABLE 16–4

Threats to Individual Health and Individual Health Promotion Strategies Across the Life Span

Age Level (yr)	Major Threats to Health	Health Promotion Strategies
Infant (Birth to 1)	Low birth weight Congenital disorders Birth injuries Accidents Sudden infant death syndrome	Provide comprehensive prenatal care. Foster early detection of developmental delays. Promote effective parent–child relationships. Educate parents on health risks in infancy.
Children (1 to 14)	Accidental injury Motor vehicle accidents Learning, sensory–perceptual (hearing, vision, speech), or behavioral disorders Poor nutrition Child abuse Lead poisoning Communicable diseases Dental health	Promote early childhood development programs (Head Start). Promote effective parent–child relationships. Provide nutrition, accident, home and environmental safety, and growth and development education. Advocate for programs that provide nutritious meals at school, food stamps, and income supplements. Maintain parental awareness of need for immunizations and support community immunization programs. Teach importance of brushing, flossing, limiting sweets, and adequate community water fluoridation to prevent tooth decay. Begin educating children on lifelong habits of health promotion and health protection.
Adolescent and young adult (15 to 24)	Violent death or injury (accidents, homicide, suicide) Substance abuse Sexually transmitted diseases (STDs) HIV infection Unwanted pregnancy	Encourage use of safety belts, use of helmets when riding motorcycles, and abiding by speed limits. Educate regarding maladaptive effects of alcohol and drugs. Advocate for comprehensive mental health services in community. Advocate for greater control of firearms in community. Expand STD services (screening, case-finding, health education, counseling). Provide maternal, infant, prenatal, and family planning services. Educate on prevention of HIV infection.
Adults (25 to 64)	Chronic disease Cancer Cardiovascular disease Hypertension Smoking Stress Mental illness Periodontal disease Accidents Alcohol abuse HIV infection	Encourage regular exercise and fitness, sound nutritional practices, and routine health screening for chronic illness. Teach effective stress reduction, management, and coping skills. Promote dental health and mental health services. Educate on accident prevention, alcohol abuse, and HIV prevention.
Older adults (65 and older)	Chronic disease Cancer Cardiovascular disease Sensory impairments Loss and depression Accidents	Educate on home safety to prevent accidents and reduce risk of falls. Promote integrated system of gerontological services in community.

Data from *Healthy people: The Surgeon General's report on health promotion and disease prevention* (1979). Washington, DC: United States Department of Health and Human Services; and United States Department of Health and Human Services. (1990). *Healthy people 2000: National health promotion and disease prevention objectives. Summary report.* Washington, DC: U.S. Government Printing Office.

and appropriate strategies for promoting health at each level. (The reader is also referred to Chapter 6 for a more in-depth discussion of cultural influences on health.)

PROGRAMS FOR FAMILIES

The community health nurse works with families to promote health and prevent disease. Families are often the basis for the development of positive health habits throughout life, as parents can encourage healthy personal habits by their children. For example, nearly half of all childhood deaths are due to unintentional injuries such as motor vehicle accidents, drownings, and fires (USDHHS, 1990a). Educating parents on home safety hazards, use of child safety seats, and injury prevention may ensure a safer environment for children through parental intervention in hazard reduction, parental modeling, and reinforcement of lifelong health practices. Table 16–5

TABLE 16–5

Nurse's Role in Health Promotion and Disease Prevention Through Stages of Family Development

Stage	Nursing Role
Couple	Counselor on sexual and marital role adjustment Teacher and counselor in family planning Teacher of parenting skills Coordinator for genetic counseling Facilitator in interpersonal relationships
Childbearing family	Monitor of prenatal care and referrer for problems of pregnancy Counselor on prenatal nutrition Counselor on prenatal maternal habits Supporter of amniocentesis Counselor on breast-feeding Coordinator with pediatric services
Family with preschool and school-age children	Monitor of early childhood development; referrer when indicated Teacher in first aid and emergency measures Coordinator with pediatric services Supervisor of immunizations Counselor on nutrition and exercise Teacher in problem-solving issues regarding health habits Participant in community organizations for environmental control Teacher of dental care hygiene Counselor on environmental safety in home Facilitator in interpersonal relationships
Family with adolescents	Teacher of risk factors to health Teacher in problem-solving issues regarding alcohol, smoking, diet, and exercise Facilitator of interpersonal skills with teenagers and parents Direct supporter, counselor, or referrer to mental health resources Counselor on family planning Referrer for sexually transmitted disease Participant in community organizations on disease control
Family with young or middle-age adults	Teacher in problem-solving issues regarding lifestyle and habits Participant in community organizations for environmental control Case-finder in the home and community Screener for hypertension, gynecological disease (e.g., Pap smear, breast examination), cancer signs, mental health, and dental care Counselor on menopausal transition for husband and wife Facilitator in interpersonal relationships among family members
Family with older adults	Referrer for work and social activity, nutritional programs, homemakers' services, etc. Monitor of exercise, nutrition, preventive services, and medications Supervisor of immunization Counselor on safety in the home

From McCarthy, N. (1990). Health promotion and the family. In C. Edelman & C. Mandle (Eds.). *Health promotion throughout the life span* (2nd ed.) (p. 113). St. Louis: Mosby–Year Book.

describes responsibilities of the community health nurse to promote health and prevent disease in families experiencing developmental changes across the life span.

PROGRAMS FOR POPULATIONS IN COMMUNITIES

The community health nurse may also develop and implement programs that reach larger aggregates in the community. Major types of community health promotion programs include school, workplace, church, hospital, and community-wide programs.

School-Based Health Promotion. School-based health promotion programs can facilitate health promotion behaviors by encouraging the development of health-promoting habits early in life that, in turn, foster long-term health-promoting behaviors. Successful school health promotion programs are based on an understanding of human behavior and developing partnerships with persons who will be most affected by the program (e.g., students, families, peers, faculty and staff, affiliating agencies). Such programs contribute to overall community health promotion efforts by developing a sense of individual and social responsibility for health, promoting an understanding of health and disease, reinforcing positive attitudes toward wellness, encouraging informed decision-making in matters of health, and structuring the environment and social influences to support health promotion behaviors (Pender, 1987; *Healthy People,* 1979).

Williams and colleagues (1980) describe a school-based health promotion–risk reduction program that integrates health education, screening, and special interventions for high-risk students with a behavior-oriented health curriculum. The program assumes that for a healthier lifestyle to be adopted, health-related behaviors must be taught in childhood. The curriculum is based on the developmental capabilities of the children. Classroom activities extend to the home, family, and community and stress forming a positive self-image, developing decision-making skills for health matters, and increasing awareness of self-responsibility for health. Topics for study focus on nutrition, dental health, exercise and fitness, and substance abuse. Evaluation is based on changes in knowledge, attitude, and behavior relative to health-promoting activities. (The reader is also referred to Chapter 28 for an in-depth discussion of school health nursing.)

Workplace Health Promotion. The workplace has become a major channel for health promotion activities and as such has received national attention. One of the nation's goals for the year 2000 is to provide employee health promotion activities in at least 85% of workplaces with 50 or more employees (USDHHS, 1990b). In 1987 the United States Department of Health and Human Services conducted a national survey of worksite health promotion to determine the extent and scope of health promotion and risk reduction activities in worksites across the United States. The study found that approximately 66% of worksites with more than 50 employees had at least one health promotion activity in place. The most frequently reported activities are summarized in Table 16–6.

Numerous positive outcomes act as incentives for employer and employee participation in health promotion activities. Incentives for employers include reduced rates of employee absenteeism because of improved health status, increases in employee productivity, decreases in use of medical insurance benefits and workers' compensation for illness and accidents, decreases in employee turnover, decreases in accidents, and decreases in premature morbidity and mortality. Incentives for employee participation include the promotion of a safe work environment, improved access to services, convenient service location, company payment for services, and availability of services on company time. Prizes, awards, or rewards may also be offered as incentives for participation. Barriers to participation may include the cost of service, time away from work, and lack of motivation or interest (*National Survey of Worksite Health Promotion Activities,* 1987; Verderber et al., 1987).

TABLE 16–6

Worksite Health Promotion Activities

Most Frequently Reported
Smoking cessation (36% of worksites)
Health risk assessment (30% of worksites)
Back care (29% of worksites)
Stress management (27% of worksites)
Exercise and fitness (20% of worksites)
Nonworksite accident prevention (20% of worksites)
Other Important Worksite Health Promotion Activities
Hypertension control
Weight control
Nutrition education
Alcohol, drug abuse, and mental health counseling
Toxic substance management*
Management of HIV and biological hazards*

*Added to list by chapter author.

From *National survey of worksite health promotion activities.* (1987). Washington, DC: Office of Disease Prevention and Health Promotion.

Church-Based Health Promotion Programs. Churches are ideal locations for reaching groups in the community with health promotion programs. Churches emphasize the spiritual dimension of health. When combined with programs that promote physical and mental health, churches truly serve to promote the total spectrum of health and well-being. Stuchlak (1992) describes a church-based health fair experience known as *Toning the Temple.* Based on a review of morbidity statistics in the local health department, a church planning group decided to conduct a health fair that focused on prevention of heart disease, stroke, cancer, and accidents. Some of the activities at the church-based health fair included instruction in relaxation techniques and low-fat diets, blood pressure screening, glucose checks, cardiopulmonary resuscitation instruction, aerobics demonstrations, and cancer and pulmonary function screenings. The health fair was announced at the morning services for two Sundays preceding the event, and fliers were posted throughout the church. The fair was held immediately following the church service. After the health fair, changes were noted in the behaviors and activities of church members and groups. For example, low-fat refreshments were more routinely served during church socials, and the church began to sponsor more exercise-related events. In addition, rules prohibiting smoking were enforced for groups using the church building.

Increasingly, nurses are assuming formal positions within churches to more effectively minister to the physical, emotional, and spiritual needs of their congregations. The "parish nursing" concept, originated by Dr. Granger Westberg (1990), a Lutheran minister, recognizes the value of nursing as an essential ministry of the church. Parish nurses can be found organizing health fairs, making home visits, conducting blood pressure screening clinics, and providing counseling and referral services to clients within the local church body. Parish nurses may hold office hours before or after church services, thus making themselves accessible to persons within the congregation.

Hospital-Based Health Promotion Programs. Hospital-based health promotion programs may be employee, client, or community focused. Health promotion activities may be targeted to clients who are recovering from illness and wish to maintain their health and prevent rehospitalization. The hospital may also be responsive to the health promotion needs of the larger community by offering programs to the general public.

The increased visibility of the hospital in the community may serve as an incentive for hospital involvement in health promotion activities. Hospital administrators may find these community outreach programs to be financially lucrative, as health promotion programs draw potential new clients and attract media attention.

Health Promotion in Geopolitical Communities. Community-wide health promotion and disease prevention programs utilize health care, educational, recreational, social, and governmental resources to develop and implement programs that enhance the well-being of large population groups. Community-centered programs have been credited with enhancing opportunities for social support and information exchange in the community and for exerting a significant impact on social policy. Goals for health promotion in geopolitical communities include decreasing morbidity and mortality in the community, achieving widespread community risk reduction, promoting cost-effective community-wide health promotion, and promoting and sustaining health promotion efforts in the organizational network of the community. Community programs influence social policy by (1) providing a basis for evaluating the effectiveness and generalizability of programs to larger groups in society; (2) promoting collaboration and communication among resources in the community; (3) changing societal norms and values through positive, mass influence; and (4) promoting a holistic approach to health care (Pender, 1987).

In the 1970s, the World Health Organization began to coordinate and promote the establishment of comprehensive community-based prevention programs as pilot projects for possible nationwide application. The North Karelia Project of Finland, the Multiple Risk Factor Intervention Trial (MRFIT), and the Stanford Heart Disease Prevention Program in California are examples of such programs. In these epidemiological studies, comprehensive prevention efforts are directed toward selected communities. Studies are then conducted to determine the impact of large-scale health promotion and disease prevention programs on the prevention of morbidity and mortality from selected diseases in a community (Puska et al., 1983).

Interventions in these large-scale studies may include the use of mass media and community health education programs to increase public awareness of health risks and prevention practices, counseling, lifestyle assessments, church and social group involvement, training of health professionals, and reorganization of public services to target high-risk populations. (See Tables 16–7 and 16–8 for an example of a community-centered prevention effort targeted at smoking cessation and smoking cessation suggestions.)

TABLE 16–7

Community-Wide Smoking Cessation

In developing a preventive health program targeted at community-wide smoking cessation, it is important to take into account the magnitude of the problem in the population. Tobacco use is the single most preventable cause of death in the United States, accounting for one of every six deaths in the nation. Cigarette smoking accounts for 21% of all coronary heart disease deaths, 30% of all cancer deaths, and 87% of lung cancer deaths. Smoking is associated with low birth weight in infants, an increased risk of spontaneous abortion, and increased fetal and neonatal mortality. Despite this, however, 25% of pregnant women smoke during their pregnancy.

Although cigarette smoking has declined markedly in the United States since the 1960s, smoking rates remain high in blacks, blue-collar workers, and persons with less formal education (USDHHS, 1990a). The health and productivity costs of smoking are estimated to be $38 to $45 billion a year (Office of Disease Prevention and Health Promotion, 1988).

Involuntary, passive, or second-hand smoking refers to a nonsmoker's exposure to environmental tobacco smoke. Passive smoke has been found to increase the risk of lung cancer and other diseases in nonsmokers and of severe respiratory illness, such as asthma and upper respiratory infections, in children. A national objective for the year 2000 is to reduce cigarette smoking prevalence to no more than 15% of adults (USDHHS, 1990a).

In developing a community-wide smoking cessation program, the community health nurse enlists the participation of schools, worksites, churches, and hospitals. Nurses can work with businesses and community organizations to set standards for institution-wide smoke-free environments. The community health nurse may lead public education campaigns to (1) address the hazards of smoking to smokers, nonsmokers, pregnant women, and children and (2) to teach methods of smoking cessation. Because nurses are often viewed as role models of healthful behaviors in the community, it is also important that nurses who smoke have access to resources in the workplace, such as smoking cessation programs, to assist them in their smoking cessation efforts. The public should also be informed of the hazards of smokeless tobacco.

In the schools, the community health nurse may offer smoking cessation programs to encourage a tobacco-free school environment. Table 16–8 presents concrete suggestions for assisting clients in smoking cessation. Finally, the community health nurse should support legislation and policies that advocate for smoke-free public places, smoking restriction laws (such as advertising and sales restrictions on youth), and excise taxes that support health promotion and smoking prevention programs.

Health Promotion and the Nursing Process

The community health nurse assists persons and groups to become more self-directed and motivated in taking

TABLE 16–8

Smoking Cessation Suggestions

- Keep a notebook of current and past successes. Use the list as a reminder of your ability to succeed in new ventures.
- Identify a personal reason for quitting smoking other than "because it's bad for me."
- Make a list of things that are personally pleasurable; choose one as a reward (instead of a cigarette) when feeling uncomfortable or bored.
- Keep a log of each cigarette lit, including the purpose; focus on smoking the cigarette and the sensations occurring during and after smoking.
- Put cigarettes in an unfamiliar place.
- Every time a cigarette is reached for, ask, Do I really want this cigarette? Do I really need this cigarette? What can I do instead of smoking this cigarette?
- Develop and pre-practice responses to peer pressure to smoke, including, Come on, one won't hurt; Smoking makes you independent, like an adult; Here, have one; and Are you a sissy? Take an assertiveness course if necessary to develop the skill of saying no.
- Smoke with the hand opposite from the one usually used.
- Buy cigarettes only by the pack, not by the carton.
- Buy different brands of cigarettes and avoid smoking two packs of the same brand in a row.
- Stay away from friends who smoke and from places where people smoke.
- End all meals with foods not associated with smoking (e.g., a glass of milk or half a grapefruit rather than a cup of coffee or a drink).
- Switch to decaffeinated coffee or tea or bouillon.
- When using cigarettes as an energizer, substitute six small high-protein meals, sufficient sleep, a glass of milk, a piece of fresh fruit, fruit or vegetable juice, exercise or movement, or a relaxation exercise.
- Have carrot sticks, celery, or sunflower seeds ready to chew instead of smoking a cigarette.
- Eat more foods (e.g., vegetables, seeds, fruits) that leave the body alkaline and reduce the urge to smoke.
- Write a list of stress enhancers; learn structured relaxation and stress reduction approaches to deal with each stressor.
- Use affirmations such as, I no longer smoke; I can quit; and It's getting easier and easier to think about quitting smoking. Tell six people.
- Use deep breathing exercises or breathe for centering when the urge for a cigarette appears.
- Work with a peer who can be called for positive feedback when the urge for a cigarette occurs. Be sure the peer is positive about your ability to quit and does not nag or induce guilt.
- Ask friends and co-workers not to leave cigarettes around or offer them.
- When the urge for a cigarette occurs, picture the word *STOP* in large red letters.
- Ask for a hug instead of having a cigarette.
- Choose a time to stop smoking when a peak mental or physical performance is not expected.
- Write a contract and sign it with a trusted person so that continuing to smoke will prove embarrassing or will result in great loss.
- Read articles and books by people who have successfully quit smoking or helped others to do so.
- When feeling depressed, talk with people who have successfully quit smoking, and ask them why they are glad they quit.

From Murray, R., & Zentner, J. (1985). *Nursing assessment and health promotion strategies throughout the life span* (4th ed.) (p. 611). Norwalk, CT: Appleton & Lange.

actions that promote and maintain health and well-being. The community health nurse also utilizes the nursing process to promote health and prevent disease in the community. In general, the responsibilities of the community health nurse in health promotion include the following:

- Acting as a role model for wellness behaviors (see Chapter 1 for a more in-depth discussion on self-care)
- Mobilizing the client to meet personal wellness goals
- Fostering client self-responsibility and commitment to self-care
- Teaching self-care practices that enhance nutrition, fitness, stress management, development of satisfying relationships, and environmental health and safety
- Facilitating client problem solving, creativity, assertiveness, and communication skills
- Facilitating the development of social supports to meet client health promotion goals (Clark, 1986)

APPRAISAL AND ASSESSMENT

The first step of the nursing process is assessment. The community health nurse must assess the client's health care needs and health promotion behaviors to best determine the major health risks that could potentially affect the client's overall health and well-being. In assessing needs, the community health nurse must also examine social, environmental, and cultural influences on health behaviors of families and communities.

A variety of methods may be used to assess health promotion behaviors and health risks in a community. A comprehensive health promotion and risk reduction assessment should include a complete health history and periodic routine health maintenance examinations. Physical fitness evaluations and nutrition assessments provide valuable data to assess overall health status. Health risk appraisals may be used to collect data on individual health risks and health behaviors and to determine an individual's risk of developing certain illnesses over his or her lifetime.

Health Risk Appraisal

The *health risk appraisal* (HRA) (also termed the *health hazard appraisal* [HHA]) is a method for estimating an individual's risk for disease or death based on demographic, behavioral, and personal characteristics (Pender, 1987; Clark, 1986). The HRA identifies individual characteristics affecting life expectancy (Acquista et al., 1988). HRA tools estimate the odds that a person with a given risk factor will become ill or die from a selected disease over a given time span.

HRAs have both assessment and motivational purposes. One goal of the HRA is to collect and organize personal health data to provide an accurate, individualized assessment of risk factors that may lead to health promotion. A second major goal of the HRA is to stimulate the necessary behavioral changes that may reduce health risks (Acquista et al., 1988; Doerr and Hutchins, 1981).

The HRA was first developed in the early 1970s. Based on the medical model, the HRA focused on assessment of risk for specific disease entities and was primarily intended for physician use. However, since that time, a number of HRA tools have been published that reflect broader interests such as health attitudes, social supports, stressful life events, and coping strategies. In addition, special versions of HRAs have been developed for different age groups (Williams et al., 1980).

The Holmes and Rahe (1967) Social Readjustment Rating Scale is a well-known tool used to assess the stressful effects of significant life events on persons (Table 16–9). It is based on the assumption that stressful events may precipitate illness or have an additive effect in contributing to illness. The scale has been used to identify links between stressful life events and the development of illness; high scores on the tool have been found to predict the occurrence of illness. However, the scale has been criticized for reflecting a historical or cultural bias. The scale requires periodic updating to reflect societal changes that influence stressful life experiences. The scale has also been criticized for failing to distinguish between desirable and undesirable life events (Muir-Ryan, 1988). Events that have a negative meaning to an individual tend to produce greater distress. In addition, the scale does not seem to take into consideration that because individuals are unique, events may be perceived as stressful in different ways by the persons who experience them. Moreover, the scale does not account for factors that mediate the degree of distress a person experiences in a stressful situation. Factors such as receiving support or counseling to deal with a painful divorce or the death of a spouse may help persons cope more effectively with a potentially devastating life experience.

Finally, the life stress scales do not differentiate between discrete life events, such as divorce, and the strain produced from occupying major roles in life (i.e., spouse, employee, parent). Strains are "hardships, challenges, and conflicts or other problems that people come to experience as they engage over time in normal social roles" (Pearlin, 1983, p. 8). The strains experienced from occupying major social roles are ongoing and are not solely associated with a major crisis event.

Research on the identification of stressful life events has also been conducted on individuals across the life span, including children and adolescents (Muir-Ryan, 1988; Swinford and Webster, 1989; Yamamoto, 1979; Coddington, 1972). Stress and coping behaviors are specific to the child's age and developmental level. For example, among preadolescents, the most frequently reported stressful life events include conflicts with parents, concerns over self-image, difficulties in peer group relationships, and geographic mobility (Lewis et al., 1984).

TABLE 16–9

Social Readjustment Rating Scale

Rank	Life Event	Mean Value
1	Death of spouse	100
2	Divorce	73
3	Marital separation	65
4	Jail term	63
5	Death of close family member	63
6	Personal injury or illness	53
7	Marriage	50
8	Fired at work	47
9	Marital reconciliation	45
10	Retirement	45
11	Change in health of family member	44
12	Pregnancy	40
13	Sex difficulties	39
14	Gain of new family member	39
15	Business readjustment	39
16	Change in financial state	38
17	Death of close friend	37
18	Change to different line of work	36
19	Change in number of arguments with spouse	35
20	Mortgage over $10,000	31
21	Foreclosure of mortgage or loan	30
22	Change in responsibilities at work	29
23	Son or daughter leaving home	29
24	Trouble with in-laws	29
25	Outstanding personal achievement	28
26	Wife begins or stops work	26
27	Begin or end school	26
28	Change in living conditions	25
29	Revision of personal habits	24
30	Trouble with boss	23
31	Change in work hours or conditions	20
32	Change in residence	20
33	Change in schools	20
34	Change in recreation	19
35	Change in church activities	19
36	Change in social activities	18
37	Mortgage or loan less than $10,000	17
38	Change in sleeping habits	16
39	Change in number of family get-togethers	15
40	Change in eating habits	15
41	Vacation	13
42	Christmas	12
43	Minor violations of the law	11

From Holmes, T., & Rahe, R. (1967). The Social Readjustment Rating Scale. *Journal of Psychosomatic Research, 11*(10), 216.

Health risk appraisals enable the community health nurse to individualize assessment of risks and to recommend behavior changes compatible with a healthier lifestyle. In addition, HRAs can be administered to large groups and can be generated and processed by computers.

Appraisals usually begin with a questionnaire that identifies factors contributing most directly to individual risk. HRA instruments include questions regarding age, sex, ethnic background, personal and family history of disease, and lifestyle factors (smoking, drinking, exercise, driving practices, seat belt use, and job stress). Physical measures such as blood pressure and weight may be assessed, and blood tests may be obtained. In addition, risk factors for diseases that are amenable to early detection efforts are noted. For example, a 65-year-old woman who is found to have a family history of breast cancer may be counseled to have annual professional breast examinations and mammograms and to perform monthly breast self-examinations (see Chapter 17).

Personal data are compared with mortality data from cohort groups who share similar characteristics. Risk factors are weighted to determine the magnitude of the risks using (1) statistical formulas based on professional, medical, or actuarial judgment; (2) average risks for the population; and (3) established epidemiological and mathematical rules and assumptions.

Data are then analyzed through a computer program to produce an individual risk appraisal which includes the client's actual *chronological age,* the client's *risk age* (i.e., the estimated life expectancy, given the effects of present risks on health), and the client's *achievable age* (i.e., the lower risk age that may be achieved through a change in behavior) (Doerr and Hutchins, 1981; Goetz and McTyre, 1981). For example, a 55-year-old male client may have a risk age of 62 years owing to a 30-year smoking history, a sedentary lifestyle, and a strong family history of cardiovascular disease. However, the client may be informed that if he stops smoking and begins an exercise program, his achievable age is 53. In other words, by adopting a healthier lifestyle, his health status would be similar to that of a 53-year-old.

The community health nurse is responsible for evaluating the accuracy of HRA instruments in assessing individual risk factors and motivating lifestyle changes (Doerr and Hutchins, 1981). More research is needed to investigate the validity of tools in assessing risks, motivating changes in behavior, and determining whether risk reduction is maintained over time.

In addition, community health nurses have an ethical responsibility to provide feedback, education, and appropriate follow-up for identified risks. This follow-up must be planned into community health promotion programs that use HRA instruments. Individuals may be notified in writing or through follow-up counseling sessions on the findings of their health risk appraisals. Recommendations for lifestyle changes or for seeking follow-up medical evaluation should be explained to each participant.

Additional HRAs that take into account positive states of health need to be developed, refined, and tested (Doerr and Hutchins, 1981). Indeed, many HRAs have been criticized for focusing primarily on health protection or prevention behaviors that are based on a risk reduction model rather than on a health promotion or enhancement model (Walker et al., 1987). The community health nurse can research and develop tools that reflect these positive health states.

Lifetime Health Monitoring Program

Breslow and Somers (1977) developed the Lifetime Health Monitoring Program to focus on a lifetime schedule or series of packages for individual preventive procedures. The program identifies the major health goals and professional services needed throughout each level of development from pregnancy and the prenatal period to infancy, school age, adolescence, and young, middle, and older adulthood. Lifetime health monitoring programs' recommendations are influenced by the unique characteristics of the target group. Recommendations for screening procedures may be altered for groups with a higher risk for particular illnesses than the general population in that age category. For example, community health nurses working with lower socioeconomic groups may develop lifetime health monitoring recommendations reflective of the higher incidences of heart disease, cancer, and infectious diseases in their client populations. Occupational health nurses may develop recommendations consistent with the higher incidence of tobacco and alcohol abuse, stress-related illness, and other client problems more prevalent in their practice settings.

Unlike the HRA, the Lifetime Health Monitoring Program utilizes clinical and epidemiological criteria to identify health goals and services appropriate to different age groups. The program does not focus on assessing individual risks, but instead examines specific recommendations for different targeted age groups. Periodic updating of lifetime health monitoring programs is needed to reflect current epidemiological trends and screening recommendations.

Lifestyle Assessments and Wellness Inventories

Lifestyle assessments and *wellness inventories* are wellness-focused appraisals that place greater emphasis on promoting health rather than identifying risk factors for specific diseases. Lifestyle assessments focus on daily patterns of behavior that affect health and over which the individual has some control (Walker et al., 1987). The Healthstyle Self-Test is an example of a lifestyle assessment that focuses on smoking, alcohol and drug use, nutrition, exercise, fitness, stress management, and safety (Fig. 16–3).

The Health Promoting Lifestyle Profile (HPLP) is another instrument designed to measure health-promoting lifestyle behaviors. The HPLP focuses on lifestyle behaviors and perceptions related to nutrition, exercise, interpersonal support, stress management, health responsibility, and self-actualization (Walker et al., 1987).

Wellness inventories, which examine a comprehensive range of health-promoting lifestyles, are very similar to lifestyle assessments. They tend to be focused more on health promotion than are health risk appraisals, which deal primarily with health-protecting behaviors. Wellness in-

Healthstyle: *A Self-Test*

All of us want good health. But many of us do not know how to be as healthy as possible. Health experts now describe *lifestyle* as one of the most important factors affecting health. In fact, it is estimated that as many as seven of the ten leading causes of death could be reduced through common-sense changes in lifestyle. That's what this brief test, developed by the Public Health Service, is all about. Its purpose is simply to tell you how well you are doing to stay healthy. The behaviors covered in the test are recommended for most Americans. Some of them may not apply to persons with certain chronic diseases or handicaps, or to pregnant women. Such persons may require special instructions from their physicians.

Cigarette Smoking

If you never smoke, enter a score of 10 for this section and go to the next section on *Alcohol and Drugs.*

	Always	*Sometimes*	*Almost Never*
1. I avoid smoking cigarettes.	2	1	0
2. I smoke only low tar and nicotine cigarettes *or* I smoke a pipe or cigars.	2	1	0
Smoking Score:			

Alcohol and Drugs

	Always	*Sometimes*	*Almost Never*
1. I avoid drinking alcoholic beverages *or* I drink no more than 1 or 2 drinks a day.	4	1	0
2. I avoid using alcohol or other drugs (especially illegal drugs) as a way of handling stressful situations or the problems in my life.	2	1	0
3. I am careful not to drink alcohol when taking certain medicines (for example, medicine for sleeping, pain, colds, and allergies), or when pregnant.	2	1	0
4. I read and follow the label directions when using prescribed and over-the-counter drugs.	2	1	0
Alcohol and Drugs Score:			

Eating Habits

	Always	*Sometimes*	*Almost Never*
1. I eat a variety of foods each day, such as fruits and vegetables, whole grain breads and cereals, lean meats, dairy products, dry peas and beans, and nuts and seeds.	4	1	0
2. I limit the amount of fat, saturated fat, and cholesterol I eat (including fat on meats, eggs, butter, cream, shortenings, and organ meats such as liver).	2	1	0
3. I limit the amount of salt I eat by cooking with only small amounts, not adding salt at the table, and avoiding salty snacks.	2	1	0
4. I avoid eating too much sugar (especially frequent snacks of sticky candy or soft drinks).	2	1	0
Eating Habits Score:			

Exercise/Fitness

	Always	*Sometimes*	*Almost Never*
1. I maintain a desired weight, avoiding overweight and underweight.	3	1	0
2. I do vigorous exercises for 15-30 minutes at least 3 times a week (examples include running, swimming, brisk walking).	3	1	0
3. I do exercises that enhance my muscle tone for 15-30 minutes at least 3 times a week (examples include yoga and calisthenics).	2	1	0
4. I use part of my leisure time participating in individual, family, or team activities that increase my level of fitness (such as gardening, bowling, golf, and baseball).	2	1	0
Exercise/Fitness Score:			

Stress Control

	Always	*Sometimes*	*Almost Never*
1. I have a job or do other work that I enjoy.	2	1	0
2. I find it easy to relax and express my feelings freely.	2	1	0
3. I recognize early, and prepare for, events or situations likely to be stressful for me.	2	1	0
4. I have close friends, relatives, or others whom I can talk to about personal matters and call on for help when needed.	2	1	0
5. I participate in group activities (such as church and community organizations) or hobbies that I enjoy.	2	1	0
Stress Control Score:			

Safety

	Always	*Sometimes*	*Almost Never*
1. I wear a seat belt while riding in a car.	2	1	0
2. I avoid driving while under the influence of alcohol and other drugs.	2	1	0
3. I obey traffic rules and the speed limit when driving.	2	1	0
4. I am careful when using potentially harmful products or substances (such as household cleaners, poisons, and electrical devices).	2	1	0
5. I avoid smoking in bed.	2	1	0
Safety Score:			

A

Figure 16–3 ● Healthstyle: a self-test. *A*, Test. .

Continued

What Your Scores Mean to YOU

Scores of 9 and 10

Excellent! Your answers show that your are aware of the importance of this area to your health. More important, you are putting your knowledge to work for you by practicing good health habits. As long as you continue to do so, this area should not pose a serious health risk. It's likely that you are setting an example for your family and friends to follow. Since you got a very high test score on this part of the test, you may want to consider other areas where your scores indicate room for improvement.

Scores of 6 to 8

Your health practices in this area are good, but there is room for improvement. Look again at the items you answered with a "Sometimes" or "Almost Never." What changes can you make to improve your score? Even a small change can often help you achieve better health.

Scores of 3 to 5

Your health risks are showing! Would you like more information about the risks you are facing and about why it is important for you to change these behaviors. Perhaps you need help in deciding how to successfully make the changes you desire. In either case, help is available.

Scores of 0 to 2

Obviously, you were concerned enough about your health to take the test, but your answers show that you may be taking serious and unnecessary risks with your health. Perhaps you are not aware of the risks and what to do about them. You can easily get the information and help you need to improve, if you wish. The next step is up to you.

YOU Can Start Right Now!

In the test you just completed were numerous suggestions to help you reduce your risk of disease and premature death. Here are some of the most significant:

Avoid cigarettes. Cigarette smoking is the single most important preventable cause of illness and early death. It is especially risky for pregnant women and their unborn babies. Persons who stop smoking reduce their risk of getting heart disease and cancer. So if you're a cigarette smoker, think twice about lighting that next cigarette. If you choose to continue smoking, try decreasing the number of cigarettes you smoke and switching to a low tar and nicotine brand.

Follow sensible drinking habits. Alcohol produces changes in mood and behavior. Most people who drink are able to control their intake of alcohol and to avoid undesired, and often harmful, effects. Heavy, regular use of alcohol can lead to cirrhosis of the liver, a leading cause of death. Also, statistics clearly show that mixing drinking and driving is often the cause of fatal or crippling accidents. So if you drink, do it wisely and in moderation. *Use care in taking drugs.* Today's greater use of drugs—both legal and illegal—is one of our most serious health risks. Even some drugs prescribed by your doctor can be dangerous if taken when drinking alcohol or before driving. Excessive or continued use of tranquilizers (or "pep pills") can cause physical and mental problems. Using or experimenting with illicit drugs such as marijuana, heroin, cocaine, and PCP may lead to a number of damaging effects or even death.

Eat sensibly. Overweight individuals are at greater risk for diabetes, gall bladder disease, and high blood pressure. So it makes good sense to maintain proper weight. But good eating habits also mean holding down the amount of fat (especially saturated fat), cholesterol, sugar and salt in your diet. If you must snack, try nibbling on fresh fruits and vegetables. You'll feel better—and look better, too.

Exercise regularly. Almost everyone can benefit from exercise—and there's some form of exercise almost everyone can do. (If you have any doubt, check first with your doctor.) Usually, as little as 15–30 minutes of vigorous exercise three times a week will help you have a healthier heart, eliminate excess weight, tone up sagging muscles, and sleep better. Think how much difference all these improvements could make in the way you feel!

Learn to handle stress. Stress is a normal part of living; everyone faces it to some degree. The causes of stress can be good or bad, desirable or undesirable (such as a promotion on the job or the loss of a spouse). Properly handled, stress need not be a problem. But unhealthy responses to stress—such as driving too fast or erratically, drinking too much, or prolonged anger or grief—can cause a variety of physical and mental problems. Even on a very busy day, find a few minutes to slow down and relax. Talking over a problem with someone you trust can often help you find a satisfactory solution. Learn to distinguish between things that are "worth fighting about" and things that are less important.

Be safety conscious. Think "safety first" at home, at work, at school, at play, and on the highway. Buckle seat belts and obey traffic rules. Keep poisons and weapons out of the reach of children, and keep emergency numbers by your telephone. When the unexpected happens, you'll be prepared.

Where Do You Go From Here:

Start by asking yourself a few frank questions: *Am I really doing all I can to be as healthy as possible? What steps can I take to feel better? Am I willing to begin now?* If you scored low in one or more sections of the test, decide what changes you want to make for improvement. You might pick that aspect of your lifestyle where you feel you have the best chance for success and tackle that one first. Once you have improved your score there, go on to other areas.

If you already have tried to change your health habits (to stop smoking or exercise regularly, for example), don't be discouraged if you haven't yet succeeded. The difficulty you have encountered may be due to influences you've never really thought about—such as advertising—or to a lack of support and encouragement. Understanding these influences is an important step toward changing the way they affect you.

There's Help Available. In addition to personal actions you can take on your own, there are community programs and groups (such as the YMCA or the local chapter of the American Heart Association) that can assist you and your family to make the changes you want to make. If you want to know more about these groups or about health risks, contact your local health department or the National Health Information Clearinghouse. There's a lot you can do to stay healthy or to improve your health—and there are organizations that can help you. Start a new HEALTHSTYLE today!

For assistance in locating specific information on these and other health topics; write to the National Health Information Clearinghouse.

National Health Information Clearinghouse
P.O. Box 1133
Washington, D.C. 20013

B

Figure 16–3, continued ● *B,* Scoring and suggestions. (From Office of Disease Prevention and Health Promotion (1981). *Healthstyle: A self-test* (Publication No. H0012). Washington, DC: National Health Information Center.)

ventories encourage disease prevention by focusing on health enhancement and promotion activities. For example, the Clark Wellness Self-Assessment enables clients to assess their own nutritional and fitness practices, stress level, environmental influences, and impact of relationships on health (Clark, 1986) (Table 16–10). Lifestyle assessments and wellness inventories assist clients to identify ways to promote their own health and personal well-being.

DEVELOPING A HEALTH PROMOTION PLAN OF CARE

After a comprehensive assessment of lifestyle, health behaviors, and specific risks to health, the community health nurse develops a health promotion plan of care with clients in the community. The process of developing an individualized plan for health promotion includes the following:

TABLE 16–10

Wellness Self-Assessment

Directions: Read the statements for each dimension of wellness; circle the number that most appropriately resembles the importance of each statement to you and your well-being and your current interest in changing your lifestyle, as follows:

1. I am already doing this. (Congratulate yourself!)
2. This is very important to me and I want to change this behavior now.
3. This is important to me, but I'm not ready to change my behavior right now.
4. This is not important in my life right now.

Nutritional Wellness				
I maximize local fresh fruits and uncooked vegetables in my eating plan.	1	2	3	4
I minimize the use of candy, sweets, sugar, and simple carbohydrates.	1	2	3	4
I eat whole foods rather than processed ones.	1	2	3	4
I avoid foods that have color, artificial flavor, or preservatives added.	1	2	3	4
I avoid coffee, tea, cola drinks, or other substances that are high in caffeine or other stimulants.	1	2	3	4
I eat high-fiber foods daily.	1	2	3	4
I have a good appetite, but I eat sensible amounts of food.	1	2	3	4
I avoid crash diets.	1	2	3	4
I eat only when I am hungry and relaxed.	1	2	3	4
I drink sufficient water so my urine is light yellow.	1	2	3	4
I avoid foods high in saturated fat, such as beef, pork, lamb, soft cheese, gravies, bakery items, fried foods, etc.	1	2	3	4
I use bottled water or an activated carbon filtration system to ensure safe drinking water.	1	2	3	4
Fitness and Wellness				
I weigh within 10% of my desired weight.	1	2	3	4
I walk, jog, or exercise vigorously for more than 20 minutes at least three times per week.	1	2	3	4
I seem to digest my food well (no gas, bloating, etc.)	1	2	3	4
I do flexibility or stretching exercises daily and always before and after vigorous exercise.	1	2	3	4
I am satisfied with my sexual activities.	1	2	3	4
When I am ill, I'm resilient and recover easily.	1	2	3	4
When I look at myself nude, I feel good about what I see.	1	2	3	4
I use imagery to picture myself well and healthy every day.	1	2	3	4
I use affirmations and other self-healing measures when ill or injured or to enhance my fitness.	1	2	3	4
I avoid smoking and smoke-filled places.	1	2	3	4
Stress and Wellness				
I sleep well.	1	2	3	4
I have a peaceful expectation about my death.	1	2	3	4
I live relatively free from disabling stress or painful, repetitive thoughts.	1	2	3	4
I laugh at myself occasionally, and I have a good sense of humor.	1	2	3	4
I use constructive ways of releasing my frustration and anger.	1	2	3	4
I feel good about myself and my accomplishments.	1	2	3	4
I assert myself to get what I need instead of feeling resentful toward others for taking advantage of or intimidating me.	1	2	3	4
I can relax my body and mind at will.	1	2	3	4
I feel accepting and calm about people or things I have lost through separation.	1	2	3	4
I get and give sufficient touch (hugs, etc.) daily.	1	2	3	4
Wellness Relationships and Beliefs				
I have at least one other person with whom I can discuss my innermost thoughts and feelings.	1	2	3	4
I keep myself open to new experiences.	1	2	3	4
I listen to others' words and the feelings behind the words.	1	2	3	4
What I believe, feel, and do are consistent.	1	2	3	4
I allow others to be themselves and to take responsibility for their thoughts, actions, and feelings.	1	2	3	4
I allow myself to be me.	1	2	3	4
I live with a sense of purpose.	1	2	3	4

Continued

- identifying personal/family/community self-care strengths;
- identifying personal health goals and areas for improvement;
- prioritizing goals for behavior change based on perception of desirability or difficulty in reaching goals;
- identifying systems for reward or reinforcement of behavior;
- determining barriers to desired behavior changes;
- making a commitment to the proposed behavior change; and
- developing a plan for implementation (Pender, 1987; Borus et al., 1982)

TABLE 16–10

Wellness Self-Assessment *Continued*

Wellness and the Environment				
I have designed a wellness support network of friends, family, and peers.	1	2	3	4
I have designed my personal living, playing, and working environments to suit me.	1	2	3	4
I work in a place that provides adequate personal space, comfort, safety, direct sunlight, and fresh air and limited air, water, or material pollutants; or I use nutritional, exercise, or stress reduction measures to minimize negative effects.	1	2	3	4
I avoid cosmetics and hair dyes that contain harmful chemicals.	1	2	3	4
I avoid pesticides and the use of harmful household chemicals.	1	2	3	4
I avoid x-rays unless serious disease or injury is at stake, and I have dental x-rays for diagnostic purposes only every 3 to 5 years.	1	2	3	4
I wear a good sunscreen ointment when exposed to the sun.	1	2	3	4
I use the earth's resources wisely.	1	2	3	4
Commitment to Wellness				
I examine my values and actions to see that I am moving toward wellness.	1	2	3	4
I take responsibility for my thoughts, feelings, and actions.	1	2	3	4
I keep informed on the latest health/wellness knowledge rather than relying on experts to decide what is best for me.	1	2	3	4
I wear seat belts when driving and insist that others who drive with me do so also.	1	2	3	4
I ask pertinent questions and seek second opinions whenever someone advises me.	1	2	3	4
I know which chronic illnesses are prominent in my family, and I take steps to avoid incurring these illnesses.	1	2	3	4
I work toward achieving a balance in all wellness dimensions to enhance my sense of well-being and satisfaction.	1	2	3	4

From Clark, C. (1986). *Wellness nursing: Concepts, theory, research, and practice* (pp. 36–38). New York: Springer.

This process of care planning is appropriate for both individuals and aggregates. However, when planning care for aggregates, it is particularly important to develop partnerships with community members, achieve consensus on health goals appropriate to the community, and gain commitment from key community leaders in supporting health promotion efforts (see Unit III).

INTERVENTION STRATEGIES

When using the nursing process for health promotion, there are six key guidelines to consider during the implementation phase:

1. Increase knowledge by disseminating information related to health.
2. Consider everyday life situations and contexts for health promotion activities.
3. Develop environments conducive to health.
4. Strengthen social networks and supports.
5. Use diverse but complementary approaches in promoting health.
6. Involve the population as a whole, not just those at risk for a specific disease (Kickbusch, 1986).

Information Dissemination. There are a variety of strategies to consider when implementing health promotion programs. Information dissemination refers to mass communication of health promotion information to the community in the most effective and efficient manner. Information may be disseminated through the use of mass media, billboards, brochures, posters, or exhibits; often information is disseminated through a health fair. A *health fair* is a community event offering health screenings, information, resources, and counseling and referral services in a location that is convenient and accessible to community members.

The goal of information dissemination programs is to inform the community of ways to promote health and prevent disease. Information dissemination is a consciousness-raising activity that alerts the community to health-damaging behaviors and attempts to motivate the community to adopt healthier lifestyles. Examples of information dissemination programs include posters and commercial announcements on prevention of human immunodeficiency virus (HIV) infection, articles in local newspapers on diet and fitness recommendations to improve cardiovascular health, and billboards and bumper stickers encouraging seat belt use. Although information dissemination programs are a helpful approach to promoting health in the community, information alone is insufficient to effect large-scale, community-wide behavioral change. For example, despite widespread dissemination of literature on HIV prevention, the incidence of acquired immunodeficiency syndrome (AIDS) continues to grow in the United States, particularly among intravenous drug abusers and their heterosexual partners.

Lifestyle Modification. Lifestyle modification is a more comprehensive approach to effecting changes in health promotion behaviors. Lifestyle modification programs encourage self-responsibility for health and represent the action phase of health behavior. Assisting clients to implement lifestyle changes often necessitates frequent contacts between the health professional and the client. The community health nurse serves as a change agent, suggesting alternative behaviors and referring the client to resources in the community to facilitate positive lifestyle changes. Lifestyle modification programs may incorporate measures to improve self-confidence, assertiveness, and decision-making and promote flexibility to change (Fromm and Trustem, 1989).

Environmental Restructuring. Environmental restructuring is an approach that facilitates healthful lifestyles and creates environments conducive to information dissemination and health appraisal and assessment. Environments are restructured to optimize the healthful conditions existing in the environment. Restructuring may also mean increasing the availability of healthful options in the community by providing greater opportunities and resources to engage in health-promoting behaviors (Pender, 1987).

The community health nurse can educate communities on potentially harmful agents in the physical environment and on ways to eliminate, reduce, or minimize threats to health (Wiley, 1989). The community health nurse may be involved in restructuring the physical environment to *protect* health by (1) teaching families to avoid using toxic aerosol products without ventilation, (2) promoting smoking cessation programs, (3) establishing smoking guidelines in public buildings, (4) supporting legislation that promotes waste recycling and water and energy conservation, and (5) teaching families to monitor and limit routine x-ray exposure (Keller, 1989).

The environment may also be improved aesthetically, socially, and economically to *promote* or enhance health. For example, overcrowding may contribute to physical (infectious disease) and psychological (anxiety) disturbances. *Proxemics* is the study of the ways in which persons structure and use space. Color, light, temperature, and space must be considered when creating attractive and comfortable environments for persons to live and work (Moss, 1989). (See Chapter 24 for a more in-depth discussion of environmental health concerns.)

Strengthening Social Support. The sociocultural environment may also contribute to health promotion and community wellness. In examining the concept of social support, Roth (1989) differentiates between social networks and social supports. *Social networks* focus on the number of relationships or contacts a person has, whereas *social support* refers to the supportive value of the interactions within these relationships.

Social support may take the form of intimacy, caregiving, providing advice and information, or assisting with problem-solving. Social support may reinforce a positive self-concept and facilitate healthful coping behaviors and lifestyles. Social networks differ in the type and degree of social and cultural support they provide for health promotion (Roth, 1989). The community health nurse works with the client to create a growth-promoting environment that enhances self-esteem and well-being.

The community health nurse works to enhance the extent and quality of sociocultural supports by (1) assisting individuals, families, and communities to strengthen existing support systems; (2) providing new opportunities for meaningful social interactions (i.e., by developing school programs that teach children ways to keep and make friends, work cooperatively with others, and resolve differences peaceably); (3) improving the supportive quality of social networks; (4) mobilizing formal (health care, social organizations) and informal (family, friends, neighbors) support systems to enhance and maintain health; and (5) anticipating future needs for expanded supportive services in the community (Roth, 1989).

Public–Private Partnerships. Creating a community environment of support for health promotion also requires partnerships between the public and private sectors. The community health nurse should advocate and promote legislation that provides the funding and resources needed to conduct community health risk assessment and health education programs, promote environmental health and safety, enhance existing support systems in the community, and promote research on health promotion and risk reduction. The community health nurse may mobilize consumer interest groups, businesses, community agencies, and other organizations to influence lawmakers to develop and support policies that result in the adoption of laws and programs that foster health promotion.

EVALUATION

The evaluation of health promotion and risk reduction programs involves a process of systematic data collection, analysis, and interpretation to make informed decisions regarding program effectiveness, continuation, or revision. Evaluation of preventive programs for individuals, families, and communities is imperative to determine whether program goals have been met and whether the program has been effective in meeting the health needs of the targeted group (Borus et al., 1982). Evaluation may be ongoing and continuous with the assessment and intervention phases. Health promotion or risk reduction programs may be evaluated while they are in operation and after the program is completed.

Although individuals, families, and the community as a whole may benefit from preventive programs, the criteria for evaluating the success of programs differ depending on the client focus. Individuals and families, for example, may experience more direct and readily applicable benefits (e.g., better health and increased life satisfaction) from participating in preventive programs. (See Table 16–11 for criteria for evaluation of health promotion and risk reduction programs that focus on individuals and families.) Perceived life satisfaction, self-esteem, social support, and life stress may be measured using published instruments and scales available in social science and health literature

TABLE 16–11

Criteria for Evaluation of Health Promotion Programs for the Individual or Family

1. Improved health status
2. Improved communication among members
3. Increased income owing to increased employment
4. Higher levels of work productivity
5. Decreased personal expenditures for health
6. Reported increases in life, work, and family satisfaction
7. Satisfying use of leisure time
8. Reduced dependency on family members
9. Improvements in self-esteem
10. Decreased reported life stress
11. Increased awareness and use of supportive social networks

Data from Borus, M., Buntz, C., & Tash, W. (1982). *Evaluating the impact of health programs: A primer.* Cambridge, MA: MIT Press.

TABLE 16–12

Criteria for Evaluation of Health Promotion Programs in the Community

1. Reduced community-wide morbidity and mortality rates
2. Decreased number of days (on an aggregate level) missed from work owing to disability or illness
3. Decreased incidence of preventable communicable diseases
4. Decreased disability days, insurance usage, and unemployment owing to health reasons
5. Increased social satisfaction, quality of life, and self-esteem on an aggregate level
6. Decreased health care costs and reported hospitalizations
7. Decreased antisocial behaviors (arrests, driving while intoxicated)
8. Decreased monies spent on alcohol, drugs, and cigarettes in community
9. Decreased rates of divorce and domestic violence
10. Reported increases in exercise, fitness, nutrition, and other health promotion behaviors

Data from Borus, M., Buntz, C., & Tash, W. (1982). *Evaluating the impact of health programs: A primer.* Cambridge, MA: MIT Press.

(Robinson et al., 1991). Evaluation of health promotion programs on a community level is based on an epidemiological model. (See Table 16–12 for evaluation of health promotion programs in the community.)

Evaluation data may be collected from analysis of vital statistics, observations, questionnaires, and other records. Evaluation of health promotion and risk reduction programs allows the community health nurse to determine whether the benefits of the program outweigh the costs of time, money, and resources devoted to the project and to rate how the program compares with alternative programs and interventions that may be equally feasible and cost-effective.

The effectiveness of a health promotion or risk reduction intervention in a particular group may be measured by comparing that group with a control group that did not receive the intervention to determine whether the goals of the program would have been achieved in the absence of the intervention (Schulberg et al., 1969). Based on evaluation of the program's effectiveness, implications for changes in social and health policy may be made.

Summary

Statistics indicate that 50% to 75% of the mortality in the United States population results from lifestyles that are damaging to health (Gallagher and Kriedler, 1987). In 1979 the U.S. Surgeon General proposed a national strategy for improving the health of Americans by identifying major health problems and setting national goals to reduce death and disability. Currently the United States has set new goals for the year 2000 to maximize the health of the U.S. population. These goals center on increasing the span of healthy life, reducing health disparities, and achieving access to preventive services for all Americans.

Contemporary definitions of health emphasize the notion of integration of human functioning and the maximization of human potential. Assisting persons to move to a higher level of wellness through health promotion activities necessitates an examination of biological, sociocultural, and environmental influences affecting health. Models of health that take into account these socioecological influences allow for a comprehensive and holistic assessment of factors influencing human health. Moreover, the value placed on health by a society may be evidenced by political legislation and economic support that advance health in the community.

The community health nurse is responsible for assessing, planning, implementing, and evaluating health promotion and risk reduction programs in schools, workplaces, hospitals, churches, and the community at large to enhance social well-being, reduce risks to health, and promote personal development and self-actualization. Such programs should be based on a thorough assessment of health hazards, risks to health, and lifestyle patterns that promote health and well-being. Health risk appraisals, lifetime health monitoring programs, lifestyle assessments, and wellness inventories represent methods for comprehensively assessing health beliefs, risks, and practices.

Intervention strategies for community health promotion include information dissemination, lifestyle modification, environmental restructuring, sociocultural support, and political action. These strategies are evaluated on an ongoing basis to determine the effectiveness of health promotion and risk reduction interventions in enhancing and maintaining community health and well-being. The evaluation of program effectiveness provides a foundation for effecting needed change in social and health policies and practices that promote societal wellness.

KEY IDEAS

1. Controlling fewer than 10 risk factors (such as poor diet and exercise, smoking, drug and alcohol abuse) can prevent between 40% and 70% of premature deaths, one third of acute disability, and two thirds of chronic disability.
2. Health promotion involves focusing on persons and populations as a whole and not solely on people at risk for specific diseases.
3. Health promotion is a social project and not solely a medical enterprise.
4. The ability of the health care system to engage in health promotion is determined by national legislation and policies that provide economic and political support for health promotion services in the community.
5. Continuing work on health models and their application to research is needed to better understand the relationship between changes in behavior and the actual effects of behavior modification on health status.
6. The community health nurse applies the nursing process in developing and sustaining health promotion and risk reduction programs throughout the community to promote community health and well-being.

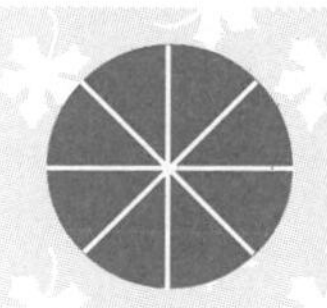

APPLYING THE NURSING PROCESS: *Initiating a Workplace Health Promotion Program*

Ms. W. is an occupational health nurse working in a steel plant. Over the years she noted a high incidence of hypertension; heart disease; cancer of the larynx, throat, and lung; and substance abuse in her client population. Ms. W. grew increasingly concerned about these statistics. Although a few screening programs were available in the facility (e.g., blood pressure screening, chest radiographs) to detect disease at an early stage, Ms. W. believed that a need existed for a comprehensive program that intervened before the onset of disease.

Assessment

After securing agreement and support from the management, Ms. W. worked in partnership with her employer to assess her clients' health risks, perceptions of need, and receptivity to a worksite health promotion program. She developed a questionnaire designed from a socioecological perspective of health to investigate employee health perceptions, determinants, and behaviors. She discovered that the majority of her clients defined health in terms of role performance. As one steel worker noted "I feel I'm healthy as long as I can work." She also found that 70% of respondents did not routinely engage in health promotion activities because of cost, poor access, lack of knowledge, or inconvenience of health promotion services. Ms. W. also administered an HRA tool to all employees who frequented the worksite clinic.

She analyzed the data using the epidemiological triad as a model. Identified host risk factors included an increased risk of morbidity and mortality based on age, family history, smoking, drug and alcohol use, stress, and poor nutrition and fitness patterns. In addition, individuals lacked knowledge of health promotion behaviors and risks to health. Identified environmental hazards included concerns over exposure to air pollutants and chemicals in the workplace, lack of access to affordable workplace health promotion services, and lack of supportive social networks to encourage healthful behaviors. Based on these findings two nursing diagnoses were developed:

1. Health maintenance, altered; related to multiple personal and environmental risks to health and lack of access to health promotion services.
2. Knowledge deficit related to health promotion and risk reduction behaviors.

Planning

Ms. W. presented the findings of her study to the administration. Company executives were hesitant to provide funding and resources necessary for the development of a worksite health promotion program until Ms. W. provided evidence from other studies that health promotion in the workplace has been found to reduce rates of employee absenteeism, improve worker productivity, decrease the use of medical insurance and workers' compensation claims, and improve employee morale and company image.

Ms. W. formed a committee consisting of steel worker employees and administrative and support personnel at different levels of the corporation. The committee agreed that priority should be placed on addressing smoking cessation, alcohol and drug abuse, stress management, exercise and fitness, nutrition, accident prevention, and reduction of environmental hazards. The committee also decided that services would be offered on site and on company time as an incentive for participation. The following goals were developed for the program:

1. Six months after initiation of the program, the number of days missed from work owing to disability or illness will decrease by 20%.
2. In 6 months, at least 70% of employees participating in the program will report improvements in job satisfaction, self-esteem, and feelings of well-being.
3. In 12 months, employee health care costs and hospitalizations will have decreased by at least 25%.

Implementation

Under Ms. W.'s direction and coordination, the committee developed a worksite health promotion program. Information about the program was disseminated throughout the corporation through brochures, posters, and mass mailings. The program included educational programs on fitness, nutrition, stress management, accident prevention, and reduction of environmental hazards (i.e., toxins, air pollutants, noise). Smoking cessation programs were offered at convenient times during the day and evening. Support groups were developed for employees to share concerns, discuss work-related issues, and promote supportive social relationships. Monthly activities (e.g., ballgames, picnics) were planned for employees and their families to provide opportunities for meaningful social interaction and promote a spirit of community. Mental health counseling services were offered on site to assist clients experiencing marital, family, or occupational stress. Supervisors and executive personnel met to discuss ways to restructure the environment to optimize health and enhance the aesthetics of the workplace.

Evaluation

After the program was in operation for 6 months, the committee began to analyze data to evaluate the program's effectiveness. Evaluation occurred at 6-month intervals while the program was in operation. Data revealed the following:

- a 25% decrease in number of days missed from work as a result of disability or illness;
- a 30% increase in reports of job satisfaction, self-esteem, and feelings of well-being;
- a 25% decrease in reported health care costs and hospitalizations; and
- a 30% decrease in reported antisocial behaviors (e.g., arrests, driving while intoxicated, incidents of domestic violence).

Employees also reported a 15% decrease in tobacco use (chewing and smoking) and a 10% reduction in alcohol and drug use. In addition, 30% of employees reported maintenance of a nutrition and fitness regimen 1 year after the program was in operation. Ms. W. also noted a 20% decrease in the number of clinic visits owing to on-the-job accidents and a decreased incidence of hypertensive episodes during blood pressure screening clinics.

Less progress was reported in the area of environmental restructuring. Although standards of safety were reportedly more closely adhered to, lack of fiscal resources was cited as a major deterrent to securing improvements in lighting, temperature, and work space to produce a more comfortable, attractive, and aesthetically pleasing environment. Still, measurable improvements in employee health, well-being, and productivity were substantial enough to justify continued employer support of the program.

GUIDELINES FOR LEARNING

1. Develop a health promotion plan for a client using one of the models of health presented in this chapter. Compare your plan with that of a fellow classmate who has chosen another model of health. What similarities or differences do you notice between the plans of care? To what extent are differences related to factors in the specific client? How does the model influence development of your care plan?
2. Talk with an individual client, family member, or colleague, exploring their ideas about health. Ask them to describe to you what it means to be healthy. Have them relate to you a personal experience in which they felt "better than ever" or "on top of the world." What was this experience like for them? Are their conceptions of health consistent with a eudaemonistic; role performance; adaptive; or clinical, disease-oriented perspective? What might have influenced their perceptions of health?
3. Explore conceptions of wellness and illness with persons from different socioeconomic, occupational, or cultural groups. What similarities or differences exist among these persons? What influences the meaning of wellness or illness to different individuals?
4. Reflect in writing on your perception of what it means to be healthy. Share your reflections with an individual experiencing acute or chronic illness.
5. Complete a wellness assessment or health risk appraisal tool. What risks to health are you able to identify in your own attitudes and behaviors? Identify one personal high-risk behavior that you routinely engage in, and attempt to modify your lifestyle in this area for 1 week. What was this experience like for you? What facilitated or hindered your ability to effect a healthful behavior change?
6. As an industrial health nurse working in a textile factory, you are responsible for planning and implementing health care programs in your facility. Major health needs of your client population include substance abuse, respiratory problems, hypertension, cancer, and back injuries. Although you would like to develop programs reflecting primary, secondary, and tertiary levels of prevention for all the major health needs, inadequate fiscal and human resources prevent you from doing so. Given the scarcity of resources, what health needs would you address first, and why? What level of prevention would your program target? What are the positive and negative implications of your decisions? What additional information do you need to gather to prioritize health needs effectively?

REFERENCES

Acquista, V., Wachtel, T., Gomes, C., Salzillo, M., & Stockman, M. (1988). Home based health risk appraisal and screening program. *Journal of Community Health, 6*(1), 43–52.

Becker, M. (Ed.). (1974). *The health belief model and personal health behavior.* Thorofare, NJ: Charles B. Slack.

Becker, M., Haefner, D., Kasl, S., Kirscht, J., Maiman, L., & Rosenstock, I. (1977). Selected psychosocial correlates of individual health related behaviors. *Medical Care, 15*(5), 24.

Borus, M., Buntz, C., & Tash, W. (1982). *Evaluating the impact of health programs: A primer.* Cambridge, MA: Massachusetts Institute of Technology.

Breslow, L., & Somers, A. (1977). The lifetime health monitoring program: A practical approach to preventive medicine. *The New England Journal of Medicine, 296*(11), 601–608.

Clark, C. (1986). *Wellness nursing: Concepts, theory, research, and practice.* New York: Springer.

Coddington, R. (1972). The significance of life events as etiologic factors in the diseases of children—II: A study of a normal population. *Journal of Psychosomatic Research, 16,* 205–213.

Doerr, B., & Hutchins, E. (1981). Health risk appraisal: Process, problems, and prospects for nursing practice and research. *Nursing Research, 30*(5), 299–306.

Dunn, H. (1961). *High level wellness.* Arlington, VA: R. W. Beatty.

Flynn, J., & Heffron, P. (1984). *Nursing: From concept to practice.* Bowie, MD: Brady Communications.

Fromm, C., & Trustem, A. (1989). Self responsibility. In P. Swinford & J. Webster (Eds.), *Promoting wellness: A nurse's handbook* (pp. 61–99). Rockville, MD: Aspen Publishers.

Fugate-Woods, N., Laffrey, S., Duffy, M., Lentz, M., Sullivan-Mitchell, E., Taylor, D., & Cowan, K. A. (1988). Being healthy: Women's images. *Advances in Nursing Science, 11*(1), 36–46.

Gallagher, L., & Kriedler, M. (1987). Nursing and health: Maximizing human potential throughout the life span. Norwalk, CT: Appleton & Lange.

Goetz, A., & McTyre, R. (1981). Health risk appraisal: Some methodologic considerations. *Nursing Research, 30*(5), 307–313.

Healthy people: The Surgeon General's report on health promotion and disease prevention. (1979). DHEW Publ. No. (PHS) 79-55071, Washington, DC: Department of Health, Education, and Welfare.

Hochbaum, G. (1956). Why people seek diagnostic x-rays. *Public Health Reports, 71,* 377–380.

Holmes, T., & Rahe, H. (1967). The Social Readjustment Rating Scale. *Journal of Psychosomatic Research, 11,* 213–218.

Janz, N., & Becker, M. (1984). The health belief model: A decade later. *Health Education Quarterly, 11*(1), 1–47.

Keller, D. (1989). Wellness in the global environment. In P. Swinford & J. Webster (Eds.). *Promoting wellness: A nurse's handbook.* Rockville, MD: Aspen Publishers.

Kickbusch, I. (1986). Health promotion: A global perspective. *Canadian Journal of Public Health, 77,* 321–326.

Kulbok, P. (1985). Social resources, health resources, and preventive health behavior: Patterns and predictions. *Public Health Nursing, 2*(2), 67–81.

Lewis, C., Siegel, J., & Lewis, M. A. (1984). Feeling bad: Exploring sources of distress among pre-adolescent children. *American Journal of Public Health, 74*(2), 117–122.

McCarthy, N. (1990). Health promotion and the family. In C. Edelman & C. Mandle (Eds.), *Health promotion throughout the life span* (pp. 110–132). St. Louis: C. V. Mosby.

Moss, V. (1989). Wellness in the immediate environment. In P. Swinford & J. Webster (Eds.), *Promoting wellness: A nurse's handbook* (pp. 185–211). Rockville, MD: Aspen Publishers.

Muir-Ryan, N. (1988). The stress coping response in school age children: Gaps in the knowledge needed for health promotion. *Advances in Nursing Science, 11*(1), 1–12.

Murray, R., & Zentner, J. (1985). *Nursing assessment and health promotion strategies throughout the life span* (4th ed.). Norwalk, CT: Appleton & Lange.

National survey of worksite health promotion activities. (1987). Washington, DC: Office of Disease Prevention and Health Promotion.

Office of Disease Prevention and Health Promotion. (1981). *Healthstyle: A self test.* (Publ No. H0012). Washington, DC: National Health Information Center.

Office of Disease Prevention and Health Promotion. *Disease prevention/health promotion: The facts.* (1988). Palo Alto, CA: Bull Publishing.

Olds, R. (1988). Promoting child health in a smoke-free school: Suggestions for school health personnel. *Journal of School Health, 58*(7), 26–29.

Pearlin, L. (1983). Role strains and personal stress. In H. B. Kaplan (Ed.). *Psychological stress: Trends in theory and research* (pp. 3–32). New York: Academic Press.

Pender, N. (1987). *Health promotion in nursing practice* (2nd ed.). Norwalk, CT: Appleton & Lange.

The Prevention Index '89: Summary report. (1989). Emmaus, PA: Rodale Press.

Promoting health/preventing disease: Objectives for the nation. (1980). DHHS Publ. No. (PHS) 0-349-256. Washington, DC: Department of Health and Human Services.

Puska, P., Salonen, J., Tuomilento, J., Nissinen, A., & Kottke, T. (1983). Evaluating community-based preventive cardiovascular programs: Problems and experiences from the North Karelia project. *Journal of Community Health, 9*(1), 49–64.

Robinson, J., Shaver, P., Wrightsman, L., & Andrews, F. (Eds.). (1991). *Measures of personality and social psychological attitudes.* New York: Academic Press.

Rosenstock, I. (1974). The health belief model and preventive health behavior. *Health Education Monographs, 2,* 354–385.

Roth, P. (1989). Family social support. In Bomar, P. (Ed.). *Nurses and family health promotion: Concepts, assessment, and interventions* (pp. 90–102). Baltimore: Williams & Wilkins.

Schulberg, H., Sheldon, A., & Baker, F. (Eds.). (1969). *Program evaluation in the health fields.* New York: Behavioral Publications.

Setting nationwide objectives in disease prevention and health promotion: The United States experience. (1986). Washington, DC: Office of Disease Prevention and Health Promotion.

Shaver, J. (1985). A biopsychosocial view of human health. *Nursing Outlook, 33*(4), 186–191.

Smith, J. (1981). The idea of health: A philosophical inquiry. *Advances in Nursing Science, 3*(3), 43–50.

Stuchlak, P. (1992). Toning the temple: A church-based health fair. *Journal of Christian Nursing, 9*(3), 22–23.

The Surgeon General's report on nutrition and health. (1988). DHHS Publ. No. (PHS) 88-50210. Washington, DC: Department of Health and Human Services.

Swinford, P., & Webster, J. (Eds.). (1989). *Promoting wellness: A nurse's handbook.* Rockville, MD: Aspen Publishers.

Szafran, K. Family health protective behaviors. In Bomar, P. (Ed.). (1989). *Nurses and family health promotion: Concepts, assessment, and interventions* (pp. 258–287). Baltimore: Williams & Wilkins.

United States Department of Health and Human Services. (1990a). *Healthy people 2000: National health promotion and disease prevention objectives. Summary report.* Washington, DC: U.S. Government Printing Office.

United States Department of Health and Human Services. (1990b). *Prevention 89/90: Federal programs and progress.* Washington, DC: U.S. Government Printing Office.

Verderber, S., Arch, M., Arch, D., Grice, S., & Gutentag, P. (1987). Wellness health care and the architectural environment. *Journal of Community Health, 12*(2,3), 163–175.

Walker, S. N., Sechrist, K. R., & Pender, N. J. (1987). The health promoting lifestyle profile: Development and psychometric characteristics. *Nursing Research, 36*(2), 76–81.

Walker, S., Volkan, K., Sechrist, K., & Pender, N. (1988). Health promoting lifestyles of older adults: Comparisons with young and middle-aged adults, correlates and patterns. *Advances in Nursing Science, 11*(1), 76–90.

Westberg, G. (1990). *The parish nurse.* Minneapolis: Augsburg Fortress.

Wiley, D. (1989). Family environmental health. In Bomar, P. (Ed.). *Nurses and family health promotion: Concepts, assessment, and interventions* (pp. 293–319). Baltimore: Williams & Wilkins.

Williams, C., Carter, B., & Eng, A. (1980). The "know your body" program: A developmental approach to health education and disease prevention. *Preventive Medicine, 9,* 371–383.

Woods, N. (1989). Conceptualizations of self care: Toward health oriented models. *Advances in Nursing Science, 12*(1), 1–13.

Yamamoto, K. (1979). Children's ratings of the stressfulness of experiences. *Developmental Psychology, 15*(5), 581–582.

BIBLIOGRAPHY

Bomar, P. (Ed.). (1989). *Nurses and family health promotion: Concepts, assessment, and intervention.* Baltimore: Williams & Wilkins.

Edelman, C., & Mandle, C. (1990). *Health promotion throughout the life span* (2nd ed.). St. Louis: C. V. Mosby.

Health promotion and disease prevention initiatives. (1990). *Primary Care Perspectives, Spring,* 1–2.

SUGGESTED READINGS

Butler, F. (1987). Minority wellness promotion: A behavioral self-management approach. *Journal of Gerontological Nursing, 13*(8), 23–28.

Olds, R. (1988). Promoting child health in a smoke-free school: Suggestions for school health personnel. *Journal of School Health, 58*(7), 26–29.

Stuchlak, P. (1992). Toning the temple: A church-based health fair. *Journal of Christian Nursing, 9*(3), 22–23.

Chapter 17

Screening and Referral

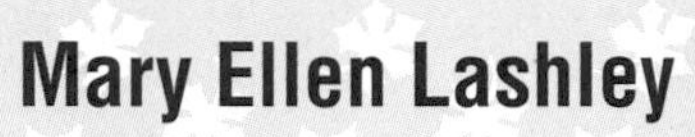

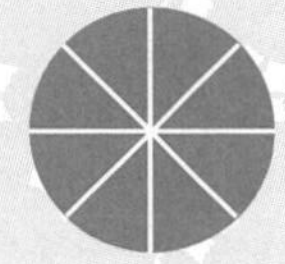

Focus Questions

What is the value of screening in maintaining the health of persons in the community?

How is screening linked to health promotion and maintenance?

What principles guide the selection, development, implementation, and evaluation of screening programs?

What are the responsibilities of the community health nurse in selecting, establishing, implementing, and evaluating screening programs?

What is the relationship between screening and referral?

What are the responsibilities of the community health nurse in the referral process?

Perhaps as at no other time Americans are experiencing a heightened awareness of the importance of maintaining healthy lifestyles and preventing illness. The plethora of fitness centers, health food stores, employee wellness programs, and health maintenance organizations attests to this fact. Moreover health has become not only socially acceptable and desirable but also "politically correct." Politicians and lawmakers who desire favor with their constituencies must deal with issues relating to the health of the American people.

Increasingly the nation is demanding a system of universal health care for all of its citizens. In addition the document *Healthy People 2000: National Health Promotion and Disease Prevention Objectives* represents a significant national initiative for improving the health of the nation. This document, produced under the auspices of the U.S. Public Health Service, lists the nation's objectives for promoting health and preventing disease by the year 2000. Major goals identified in the document include: increasing the healthy life span of Americans, reducing health disparities, and achieving access to preventive services (U.S. Department of Health and Human Services [DHHS], 1990a). Such a national focus on health challenges and stimulates those in the health care professions to take action to improve the health of the nation through health promotion and disease prevention, early diagnosis, and treatment of illness.

An essential component in maintaining the health of a community is early detection of disease. Although ideally one hopes to prevent disease, not all diseases are completely preventable. For example although some risk factors associated with the development of heart disease are known and can be avoided (high-fat diet, smoking, sedentary lifestyle), others are unmodifiable (age, sex, family history). For this reason it is essential that diseases that cannot be completely prevented are detected early in their natural history when they are more amenable to treatment. In this way complications from advanced disease can be prevented. The key to improvements in health care for the nation's citizens may lie not in the high cost of technology for treating advanced disease but in the early identification of illness and prevention of more serious morbidity (Doerr and Hutchins, 1981).

Secondary prevention is aimed at the early detection and treatment of illness. *Screening* is a major secondary prevention strategy. When previously unrecognized illnesses are identified through screening, it is essential that referrals are made for follow-up diagnosis and treatment. In this chapter the concept of screening is explored. The varied contexts in which persons are screened for illness are discussed. Finally the responsibilities of the community health nurse in the screening and referral process are articulated.

Definition of Screening

Screening is defined as the "presumptive identification of unrecognized disease or defect by the application of tests, examinations, or other procedures that can be applied rapidly and inexpensively to populations" (Valanis, 1986, p. 327). The goal of screening is to correctly differentiate between persons who have an illness, developmental delay, or other health alteration and those who do not.

Screening involves several key terms. Screening is aimed at the *presumptive* identification of disease. In other words if a screening test is positive (abnormal), one can only *presume* that the disease *may* be present. A screening test, in itself, is not sufficient to establish a positive diagnosis of disease. This is because a single screening test, taken in isolation, is not always 100% accurate. For example inaccuracies in test measurement can lead to false-positive or -negative test results. For this reason when a screening test is positive a referral is made for follow-up diagnostic testing to confirm whether, in fact, the disease is present.

Screening tests detect previously *unrecognized* disease. This means that screening tests are often conducted on seemingly healthy populations. Persons undergoing screening tests may be asymptomatic of disease and unaware that a problem potentially exists. Herein lies the value of screening. The goal of a screening test is to detect disease in an earlier stage than it would be if the client waited for clinical symptoms to develop before seeking help.

Screening is conducted through the application of *tests and procedures.* These tests can be applied *rapidly* and *inexpensively* to *populations.* In other words these tests should be appropriate for administration to a large group of people. To screen large groups in a timely manner, a test must be able to be administered rapidly and with ease. Tests should be relatively inexpensive, so that persons are more likely to take advantage of them.

Mass screening is used to denote the application of screening tests to large populations. These groups may be typical of the general population or may be selectively at a higher risk for certain diseases (Valanis, 1986). Since mass screening of the general population is often costly and does not necessarily detect enough new cases of disease to balance the cost of screening, some authorities feel that money may be better spent on targeting selected populations known to be at high risk for certain illnesses (Beck et al., 1988). For example, a community health nurse conducting a screening program at a senior citizen high-rise apartment building would be dealing with a group of people who are selectively at higher risk for developing certain diseases by virtue of their age.

Case-finding is screening that occurs on an individual or one-on-one basis. Case-finding attempts to use screening tests to identify previously unrecognized disease in *individuals* who may present to the health care provider for health maintenance checks or for an unrelated complaint (Valanis, 1986). A good example is when the community health nurse makes a home visit and checks the blood pressure of each member of the family. In this instance the nurse may detect previously unrecognized disease in family members who are unaware that a problem even exists.

Multiphasic screening is used to denote the application of multiple screening tests on the same occasion (Valanis, 1986). A health fair held at a shopping mall, for example, may include blood pressure, glaucoma, vision, diabetes, and anemia testing. Persons may rotate to different stations and receive a battery of tests during a single visit. An advantage of multiphasic screening is convenience to the participant. A disadvantage is the increased number of false-positive test results that occurs simply by the large number of screenings (Valanis, 1986).

Screening and the Natural History of Disease Model

The benefits of screening are evident when viewed in the context of the natural history of disease model (see Chapter 11). This model proposes that every disease has a natural history or life story. For example, a disease has a beginning or point of conception. Allowed to progress untreated, a disease runs its course. Finally the disease ends in some way (either through death, disability, or recovery of the person). A disease's natural history is divided into two periods: (1) the prepathogenesis period (before the disease begins) and (2) the pathogenesis period.

To have an impact on the natural history of disease, several strategies are proposed. *Primary prevention* strategies are aimed at preventing the disease from beginning by the avoidance or modification of risk factors. Primary prevention targets the *prepathogenesis* stage in the natural history of disease model. *Secondary prevention* strategies target the *pathogenesis* period (i.e., the period after the disease has begun). Secondary prevention strategies aim to detect the disease early in its course, when it is more amenable to treatment. Finally *tertiary prevention* strategies focus on rehabilitation and prevention of complications arising from advanced disease. Screening therefore targets the early pathogenesis period when a disease is present, detectable, and more amenable to treatment (Valanis, 1986).

Criteria for Selection of Screening Tests

Table 17–1 lists important principles to consider in deciding which screening tests should be used and to whom screening efforts should be directed (Gupta, 1990; Valanis, 1986).

VALIDITY OF SCREENING TESTS

Validity is defined as the ability of the screening test to correctly distinguish between persons with and without the disease. If a screening test were 100% valid, it would never have a false-positive or -negative reading. It would always be positive in those people who had the disease and negative in those people who did not. Statistically, the validity of a screening test can be measured. These measures are *sensitivity* and *specificity*.

Sensitivity is the ability of a screening test to identify persons who have the disease. Statistically it is measured using the following formula:

$$\frac{\text{No. of true-positive test results}}{\text{No. of people with disease (true-positive + false-negative)}}$$

Notice that the denominator in this equation (all people with the disease) includes two screening test results. Persons with the disease could have a screening result that is either true positive (i.e., they do in fact have the disease) or false negative (i.e., the screening test is normal but they do in fact have the disease). The greater the number of false-negative test results, the lower the sensitivity (Valanis, 1986).

Specificity is the ability of the screening test to identify persons who are normal or without disease. Statistically specificity is measured using the following formula:

$$\frac{\text{No. of true-negative results}}{\text{All persons without disease (No. of true-negative + false-positive results)}}$$

Notice that in this case persons who are healthy could have one of two test results: They could have either a true-negative finding (i.e., they do not have the disease and the test findings are normal) or a false-positive finding (i.e., they do not have the disease, but their screening test result is positive). The greater the number of false-positive test results, the lower the specificity (Gupta, 1990; Valanis, 1986).

It would be ideal if a screening test could be 100% sensitive and 100% specific. However, this combination of

TABLE 17–1

Criteria for Selection of Screening Tests

Principle	Explanation
The disease being screened for should be a significant health problem in the targeted population.	Significance is measured both through epidemiological data (e.g., the frequency of illness in the population, morbidity and mortality rates, rates of disability) and by the meaning and significance of the illness to the population being screened (e.g., recent media campaign heightening public awareness and concern, concern over discomfort from disease, financial cost of disease).
The screening test should be able to identify the disease at an earlier stage in its natural history than would be the case if one waited for clinical symptoms to develop.	Criteria for establishing an abnormal test result are well defined and highly sensitive and specific.
An effective treatment should exist for the disease being screened for.	Generally, it is believed that only diseases that can be treated effectively should be screened for. An exception to this was human immunodeficiency virus (HIV) infection, in which case early recognition of the disease prevented transmission to others and thereby protected public health, even before drug treatment was available for infected individuals.
The screening tests should be safe, simple to administer, cost effective, and acceptable to the client population.	For example, highly invasive tests, such as sigmoidoscopy, are generally not considered cost effective, simple to administer, acceptable to clients, or safe for use (owing to potential for bowel perforations) in *mass screening* programs.
Provisions should be made for follow-up diagnosis and treatment of persons with positive test results.	A screening program should not be conducted unless adequate community resources are available to deal with the outcome of positive test results. This is a potential ethical dilemma, since persons who are notified of an abnormality have a right to follow-up counseling and referral. If no resources exist in the community, the community health nurse has a responsibility to advocate for funding for such resources and to mobilize needed resources so that community health and well-being are protected.
The screening test should, be *reliable* and *valid* in detecting the disease.	See text discussion.

Data from Gupta, K. (1990). Screening and health maintenance. In C. Edelman & C. Mandle, (Eds.). *Health promotion throughout the life span* (2nd ed.) (p. 156). St. Louis: Mosby–Year Book; and Valanis, B. (1986) *Epidemiology in nursing and health care.* Norwalk, CT: Appleton-Century-Crofts.

accuracy and precision in measurement is not realistic. For this reason screening tests are not used to positively confirm a diagnosis and are not considered to be diagnostic. A margin for error inevitably exists in all screening tests (Gupta, 1990; Pickett and Hanlon, 1990; Valanis, 1986). The sensitivity and specificity of a test are often determined by the manufacturer of the test, who may select a higher cutoff value to improve specificity or a lower cutoff value to improve sensitivity (Bluestein and Archer, 1991).

Consider a diabetes screening clinic. If the normal blood glucose level ranges from 70 to 120 mg/dl and any level greater than 70 mg/dl were considered abnormal, what would happen to the sensitivity and specificity of the screening test? Since it is highly unlikely that anyone with diabetes would have a blood glucose level lower than 70 mg/dl, sensitivity would approach 100%. However, normal individuals with blood glucose levels between 70 and 120 mg/dl would be considered potentially diabetic; their positive test result would give a false picture of the presence of diabetes. Specificity would then go down. Therefore the relationship between sensitivity and specificity is inverse. The greater the sensitivity, the lower the specificity and vice versa. The more sensitive a test is made, the less specific it becomes.

Is it better to have a high sensitivity and a moderate or low specificity? Or should attempts be made to improve specificity even though sensitivity may be compromised? The answer to these questions depends on the disease being screened for and the physical, psychological, and financial impact of false-positive versus false-negative test results. In the case of diseases that are potentially fatal if not detected early, sensitivity may be more important. However the psychological trauma and financial cost of being labeled incorrectly as having a disease can be devastating. For example if a patient receives news that he is human immunodeficiency virus (HIV)–positive and later commits suicide, a false-positive reading has had significant and even fatal consequences. In this case high specificity is as important as high sensitivity.

RELIABILITY OF SCREENING TESTS

Reliability refers to the consistency or reproducibility of test results over time and between examiners. A test is reliable when it gives consistent results when administered at different times and by different persons (Gupta, 1990). For example a community health nurse monitors the blood pressure of a health fair participant. She or he obtains a reading of 190/110 mm Hg. She or he seeks another nurse to check the findings. The second nurse obtains a reading of 120/80 mm Hg. In this instance, the blood pressure results do not evidence good reliability. Here reliability may have been affected by the skill level of the examiners involved, degree of sensory impairment of the examiner, or condition of the equipment in use. Checking equipment, monitoring the correct procedure of examiners, or altering environmental noise level could improve the reliability of the screening test in this example. Reliability is an important consideration in selecting a screening test, and actions can be taken to improve the reliability of screening test results.

Contexts for Screening

Screening programs may be targeted to individuals (i.e., case-finding) or to populations (i.e., mass screening). By screening clients on an individual level, more time and attention may be given to the analysis of individual risk factors. The selection of screening tests may be individualized based on the provider's knowledge of the client's personal history and risk factors.

SCREENING OF INDIVIDUALS

A routine health maintenance examination is one example of a multiphasic, case-finding intervention. Periodic health checkups include a comprehensive health history, physical examination, and relevant laboratory and diagnostic studies. Additional tests may be considered based on an analysis of individual risk factors. Counseling and referral are vital components of the health examination.

Since most screening tests detect disease before the onset of clinical symptoms, the health history may have limited usefulness. However a health history can identify significant risk factors in personal or family history that may increase the risk of illness. Physical examinations have been found to detect as much as 60% of unrecognized disease (Gupta, 1990) such as hypertension and cancer. The frequency of periodic health examinations may vary depending on age, sex, or other risk factors. Table 17–2 presents a sample screening adult physical assessment tool.

TABLE 17–2

Screening Adult Physical Assessment Tool

General Survey: Apparent vs. actual age, sex, race, posture, gait, apparent health and nutritional status, general observations of behavior and affect
Vital Signs:
Height/Weight:
Mental Status: Orientation, recall, affect, attention, alertness
Integument: Color, lesions, dryness, moisture, vascularity
Head: Shape, size, symmetry, abnormalities
Eyes: Shape, size, pupillary constriction and accommodation, color, lesions, moisture (conjunctiva, sclera), visual acuity, peripheral vision, extraocular movements
Ears: Shape, size, position, lesions, auditory acuity
Mouth/Throat: Lesions, color, moisture, breath odor, exudate
Lymph: Lymphadenopathy (examine head/neck region, axilla, inguinal areas)
Cardiac: Point of maximum impulse, heart sounds (normal S_1, S_2; abnormal gallops, rubs, murmurs), apical heart rate, irregular rhythms, jugular venous distention
Respiratory: Lung sounds; chest size, shape, expansion; respiratory rate, depth, effort; use of accessory muscles; pursed-lip breathing
Peripheral vascular: Color of skin, mucous membranes, and nailbeds; central and peripheral pulses (strength, quality, symmetry); peripheral edema
Gastrointestinal: Abdomen: color of skin, shape, lesions, symmetry, umbilicus, tenderness, masses, bowel sounds
Genitourinary: Bladder percussion and palpation, examination of external structures
Reproductive: Testicular examination, pelvic examination, breast examination, Papanicolaou smear
Neurological: Coordination, gait, cranial nerve assessment, fine motor movements, sensation
Musculoskeletal: Range of motion of extremities, muscle strength and tone, palpation of joints, bilateral hand grasps, spinal curvatures

SCREENING OF POPULATIONS

On a population level, choice of screening tests is based on general sociodemographic rather than individual risk factors. A nurse planning a health fair in a local women's center, for example, may include screening for breast cancer. An individual attending the health fair may not be at an increased risk of developing breast cancer, based on age or personal and family history. Nevertheless, because the population group as a whole has been determined to be at risk, screening mammograms are made available.

Age, gender, and ethnicity factors have an impact on the risk status of a population. For example breast cancer is much more common in women than in men, and the risk of developing breast cancer increases with age. Black males are at a higher risk of developing malignant hypertension than are women or white males. Teenagers and young adults have a higher incidence of sexually transmitted diseases than that of the general population. Osteoporosis is more common in white postmenopausal women than in other population groups.

To determine what screening tests should be administered, the community health nurse must assess the risks inherent in the target population. What diseases are the target population most at risk of developing? Are these diseases easily screened for? Epidemiological literature provides information about the incidence of various illnesses, defects, and injuries in relation to sociodemographic factors.

MAJOR HEALTH THREATS IN THE GENERAL POPULATION

The two leading causes of death in the general adult population are heart disease and cancer. These diseases account for 58% of deaths in adults in the United States (DHHS, 1990b). Together, heart disease, malignant neoplasms, accidents, and stroke account for 80% of deaths of persons of all ages in the United States (DHHS, 1990b).

Cardiovascular Disease

The principal risk factors for heart disease and stroke include hypertension (blood pressure 140/90 mm Hg or higher), elevated serum cholesterol level (240 mg/dl or higher), cigarette smoking, obesity, family history of atherosclerotic disease, advancing age, and being male (DHHS, 1990b). Since half of these risk factors are modifiable, cardiovascular disease is highly amenable to prevention efforts. Selected national objectives for reducing the risk of cardiovascular disease through secondary prevention measures are presented in Table 17–3.

Hypertension. Hypertension has the highest prevalence of any cardiovascular disease in the United States. Hypertension affects approximately 30% of adults in the United States. Controlling hypertension therefore can significantly decrease mortality from heart disease and stroke (DHHS, 1990a, 1990b).

In 1972 the National Heart, Lung, and Blood Institute (NHLBI) initiated the National High Blood Pressure Education Program. This program has coordinated the efforts of federal government and national health organizations to identify and control hypertension. Since 1972 there has been a significant decline in the mortality rate from stroke. The National High Blood Pressure Education Program is credited with producing this trend. Still although the influence of hypertension on the development of cardiovascular disease is known by over 90% of the public, a much lower percentage of those with high blood pressure are aware that they have this condition (DHHS, 1990b). A national health objective for the year 2000 is to increase the control of high blood pressure in at least 50% of persons with hypertension (DHHS, 1990a). The Joint National Committee on Detection, Evaluation, and Treatment of High Blood Pressure has established criteria and guidelines for referring persons with high blood pressure to a source of medical care (National Institutes of Health [NIH], 1993) (Table 17–4). Screening programs aimed at the early identification of hypertension contribute greatly to the early diagnosis and treatment of this potentially fatal condition by making persons aware of their blood pressure status and by referring those with elevated readings for follow-up diagnosis and treatment.

Serum Cholesterol. Recently the media have greatly increased consumer awareness of the influence of serum cholesterol level on the development of coronary heart disease. However although nearly 75% of adults are aware that a high serum cholesterol level is a risk factor for the development of heart disease, only 17% know their own blood cholesterol level (DHHS, 1990b). Approximately 60 million adults in the United States are estimated to have

TABLE 17–3

Selected National Health Promotion Objectives for the Year 2000 to Reduce the Risk of Cardiovascular Disease

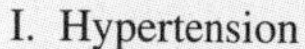

I. Hypertension
1. Increase to at least 50% the proportion of people with high blood pressure whose blood pressure is under control. (Baseline: 24% in 1982–1984)
2. Increase to at least 90% the proportion of people with high blood pressure who are taking action to help control their blood pressure. (Baseline: 79% in 1985)
3. Increase to at least 90% the proportion of adults who have had their blood pressure measured within the preceding 2 years and can state whether their blood pressure was normal or high. (Baseline: 61% in 1985)

II. Serum Cholesterol
1. Reduce the mean serum cholesterol level among adults to no more than 200 mg/dl.
2. Reduce the prevalence of blood cholesterol levels of 240 mg/dl or greater to no more than 20% among adults. (Baseline: 27% in 1976–1980)
3. Increase to at least 60% the proportion of adults with high blood cholesterol levels who are aware of their condition and are taking action to reduce their blood cholesterol to recommended levels. (Baseline: 30% in 1988)
4. Increase to at least 75% the proportion of adults who have had their blood cholesterol checked within the preceding 5 years.
5. Increase to at least 75% the proportion of primary care providers who initiate diet and, if necessary, drug therapy at levels of blood cholesterol consistent with current management guidelines for patients with high blood cholesterol levels.

Data from United States Department of Health and Human Services. (1990). *Healthy People 2000: National health promotion and disease prevention objectives* (summary report). Washington, DC: U.S. Government Printing Office.

TABLE 17–4

Recommendations for Selected Adult Health Screenings

Breast Self-Examination*

Indicated once a month for women older than 20 years

Clinical Breast Examination*

Women younger than 40 years: every 3 years
Women 40 years and older: every year

Mammography*

Baseline for women between 35 and 39 years
Every 1 to 2 years between ages 40 and 49 years
Annually after age 50 years

Digital Rectal Examination for Colon Cancer*

Every year after age 40 years

Stool for Occult Blood*

Every year after age 50 years

Sigmoidoscopy*

Every 3 to 5 years after age 50 years (following two initial negative tests 1 year apart)

Papanicolaou Test and Pelvic Examination*

Annually for women 18 years and older or for all women who are sexually active. After three or more consecutive normal examinations, Papanicolaou test may be performed less frequently at discretion of provider

Testicular Self-Examination*

Monthly for postpubertal males

Prostate Examination*

Digital rectal examination with examination of prostate every year after age 50 years (however, client should be receiving digital rectal examinations after age 40 years for colon cancer)
Prostate-specific antigen (PSA) blood screening test recommended annually for men older than 50 years; the blood level of PSA is elevated in men with prostate cancer
Transurethral ultrasound and biopsy considered if above tests are abnormal

Blood Pressure†

Classification of Hypertension

Normal: Systolic less than 130 mm Hg; diastolic less than 85 mm Hg
High Normal: Systolic 130 to 139 mm Hg; diastolic 85 to 89 mm Hg
Mild Hypertension (Stage 1): Systolic 140 to 159 mm Hg; diastolic 90 to 99 mm Hg
Moderate Hypertension (Stage 2): Systolic 160 to 179 mm Hg; diastolic 100 to 109 mm Hg
Severe Hypertension (Stage 3): Systolic 180 to 209 mm Hg; diastolic 110 to 119 mm Hg
Very Severe Hypertension (Stage 4): Systolic 210 mm Hg or above; diastolic 120 mm Hg above

Recommendations for Referral to a Source of Medical Care

Diastolic

Less than 85 mm Hg: recheck in 2 years
85 to 89 mm Hg: recheck in 1 year
90 to 99 mm Hg: refer for follow-up within 2 months
100 to 109 mm Hg: refer for follow-up within 1 month
110 to 119 mm Hg: refer for follow-up within 1 week
120 mm Hg or above: refer immediately for follow-up care

Systolic

Less than 130 mm Hg: recheck within 2 years
130 to 139 mm Hg: recheck in 1 year
140 to 159 mm Hg: recheck within 2 months
160 to 179 mm Hg: refer for follow-up within 1 month
180 to 209 mm Hg: refer for follow-up within 1 week
210 mm Hg or above: refer immediately for follow-up care

Cholesterol‡

Less than 200 mg/dl: desirable
200 to 239 mg/dl: borderline high
240 mg/dl or greater: high
Check once every 5 years or more frequently if indicated

Continued

TABLE 17–4

Recommendations for Selected Adult Health Screenings *Continued*

Blood Glucose Testing§

Annually for high-risk individuals (i.e., family history, personal history of glucose intolerance); otherwise during routine medical examinations

Eye Examinations and Glaucoma Testing||

Every 3 to 5 years for black persons age 20 to 39 years (other healthy adults require less frequent examinations; black persons are at higher risk of glaucoma); every 2 years for persons aged 40 to 64 years; every 1 to 2 years for persons 65 years and older

Purified-Protein Derivative Skin Test (PPD)¶

Annually for high-risk groups (i.e., HIV-positive persons, known contact with tuberculosis patient, immunosuppressed persons, persons who live or work in long-term care facilities or work in hospitals or schools, foreign-born persons from countries with high tuberculosis rates). Otherwise as indicated

*American Cancer Society recommendations (American Cancer Society, no date: a, no date: b, 1980, 1987, 1990a, 1990b, 1990c, 1991, 1993).
†Recommendations from National Institutes of Health (NIH). (1993). *The fifth report of the Joint National Committee on Detection, Evaluation, and Treatment of High Blood Pressure* (NIH Publication No. 93–1088). Washington, DC: U.S. Government Printing Office.
‡American Heart Association. (1989). *Cholesterol and your heart.* Dallas: Author.
§Cooper, G. (1980). Diagnosis: Diabetes. *Diabetes Forecast.* Alexandria, VA: American Diabetes Association.
||*Diagnostic testing guidelines for healthy individuals.* (1992). Clifton, NJ: Clinicians Publishing Group.
¶American Lung Association. (1991). *Facts about tuberculosis.* New York: Author.

serum cholesterol levels that place them at high risk of coronary heart disease. The mean cholesterol level for adults in the United States is 213 mg/dl (DHHS, 1990a).

In 1985 the NHLBI initiated the National Cholesterol Education Program to increase public awareness of the relationship between cholesterol and heart disease. The program also provided detailed guidelines for treatment of individuals with elevated serum cholesterol levels. Surveys indicate that approximately 56% of adults know that a diet high in saturated fat increases serum cholesterol. However, only 15% know that a desirable blood cholesterol level is lower than 200 mg/dl (DHHS, 1990b). A national health objective for the year 2000 is to reduce serum cholesterol to an average of no more than 200 mg/dl (DHHS, 1990a). Initiating cholesterol screening programs in the community may assist in the prevention of heart disease through early identification of at-risk persons and counseling and referral of high-risk individuals for further intervention aimed at modifying dietary fat consumption, instituting exercise programs, or initiating pharmacotherapy, if indicated, to reduce blood lipids levels.

Obesity. Another risk factor in the development of heart disease is obesity. Obesity is present in approximately 25% of the general population. An increased prevalence of obesity has been found in low-income and minority populations. Dietary fat is a major contributor to the development of obesity (DHHS, 1990b). By obtaining height, weight, and percent body fat measurements (i.e., triceps skinfold test, computerized analyses), persons who are overweight may be identified and referred for nutritional and fitness counseling.

Smoking. Persons who smoke cigarettes have been found to die of heart disease at a rate 70% higher than that of nonsmokers (DHHS, 1990b). Pulmonary function studies are conducted to measure damage to respiratory function that may be caused by smoking or by other lung diseases. A spirometer can be used to screen for compromised respiratory functioning. Screening for pulmonary dysfunction with prompt referral to smoking cessation programs and medical providers for follow-up may halt progression of heart and lung disease caused by the harmful effects of tobacco. Despite the benefits of pulmonary function studies, persons who smoke should be referred to smoking cessation programs regardless of their pulmonary status.

Cancer

Cancer is the second leading cause of death in the United States (DHHS, 1990a). It is a significant health problem in the U.S. population. Table 17–5 lists selected national health objectives for the early detection and treatment of breast, uterine, cervical, and colorectal cancer.

Lung Cancer. Lung cancer is the leading cause of cancer deaths and the most prevalent form of cancer. Approximately 85% of lung cancers are attributed to cigarette smoking (DHHS, 1990a). Although two thirds of lung cancer deaths in 1986 occurred in males, the number of lung cancer deaths now surpasses the number of breast cancer deaths in females (DHHS, 1990b). A national health objective for the year 2000 is to slow the rise in lung cancer deaths to achieve a rate of no higher than 42 per 100,000 population (DHHS, 1990a).

Breast Cancer. Breast cancer is the second most common cause of cancer in women. Risk factors in the development of breast cancer include advanced age, family history, early menarche, late menopause, and late or no childbearing (DHHS, 1990a, 1990b). Early diagnosis is essential to breast cancer survival. Ninety percent of persons with diagnosed localized breast cancer survive at least 5 years after diagnosis, whereas only 68% of those with lymph node involvement and 18% of those with distant metastases

HEALTHY PEOPLE 2000

TABLE 17–5

Selected National Health Objectives for the Year 2000 for Early Cancer Detection

1. Increase to at least 75% the proportion of primary care providers who routinely counsel patients about tobacco use cessation, diet modification, and cancer screening recommendations.
2. Increase to at least 80% the proportion of women aged 40 years and older who have ever received a clinical breast examination and a mammogram, and to at least 60% those aged 50 years and older who have received them within the preceding 1 to 2 years. (Baseline: 36% and 25% respectively in 1987)
3. Increase to at least 95% the proportion of women aged 18 years and older with uterine cervix who have ever received a Papanicolaou (Pap) test, and to at least 85% those who received a Pap test within the preceding 1 to 3 years. (Baseline: 88% and 75% respectively in 1987)
4. Increase to at least 50% the proportion of people aged 50 years and older who have received fecal occult blood testing within the preceding 1 to 2 years, and to at least 40% those who have ever received proctosigmoidoscopy. (Baseline: 27% and 25% respectively in 1987)
5. Increase to at least 40% the proportion of people aged 50 years and older visiting a primary care provider in the preceding year who have received oral, skin, and digital rectal examinations during one such visit.
6. Ensure that Pap tests meet quality standards by monitoring and certifying all cytology laboratories.
7. Ensure that mammograms meet quality standards by monitoring and certifying at least 80% of mammography facilities. (Baseline: 18–21% in 1990)

Data from United States Department of Health and Human Services. (1990). *Healthy people 2000: National health promotion and disease prevention objectives* (summary report). Washington, DC: U.S. Government Printing Office.

survive 5 years after diagnosis (DHHS, 1990a, 1990b). Screening efforts aimed at the early detection of breast cancer include breast self-examination, breast examination by a health professional, and mammography. Mammography is the most sensitive screening tool available for early detection (Gupta, 1990). Screening mammography and professional breast examination together are estimated to produce a 30% reduction in mortality from breast cancer in women older than 50 years (DHHS, 1990a). A national health objective for the year 2000 is to have at least 60% of women age 50 years and older receive clinical breast examinations and mammography every 2 years (DHHS, 1990a).

Colorectal Cancer. Following lung cancer, colorectal cancer is the second leading cause of cancer deaths in the nation (DHHS, 1990a). Annual digital rectal examinations are recommended for persons older than 40 years to detect colon cancer. Annual fecal occult blood testing is recommended after age 50 years. Sigmoidoscopic examinations for colorectal cancer are recommended every 3 to 5 years after the age of 50 years (after two consecutive negative examinations) (American Cancer Society [ACS], 1990a). A national health objective for the year 2000 is to have at least 50% of persons 50 years and older receive fecal occult blood testing every 1 to 2 years (DHHS, 1990a).

Cancer and Ethnicity in the United States. The incidence and mortality rates from cancer are disproportionately higher in blacks than in whites. Blacks have a higher than average risk of developing cancers of the lung, larynx, throat, respiratory tract, prostate, bladder, kidney, and pancreas. Black males have the highest incidence of prostate cancer in the world. Black populations have also been found to be less knowledgeable about cancer risks than the general population (DHHS, 1990b).

Cancer incidence is lower in Mexican-Americans and Native Americans than in white or black Americans (ACS, 1991). However, the rates of stomach, gallbladder, and cervical cancer are much higher in Mexican-Americans than in white Americans. Chinese, Japanese, and Filipinos have overall cancer incidence and mortality rates lower than those of American whites or blacks. The differences in cancer rates between ethnic populations have been attributed, in part, to the influence of lifestyle and genetic factors on the development of disease (ACS, 1991).

Early detection programs are particularly critical in economically disadvantaged and minority populations, where the incidence of cancer is high and knowledge, use, or availability of both primary and secondary preventive measures is low (DHHS, 1990b). For example fewer than 25% of low-income women, especially poor women of color, in the United States have ever had a mammogram.

In response to the increased incidence of cancer in the nation, the National Cancer Institute developed the Cancer Prevention Awareness Program. The goal of this program is to reduce cancer mortality rates by as much as 50% by the year 2000. Special emphasis is being targeted to black Americans as an identified high-risk group for the development of cancer.

National Objectives and Recommendations

Table 17–4 presents national recommendations for screening of common health problems in the general adult

TABLE 17–6

Screening Tests for Selected Populations*

General Adult Population	School-Age Children
Blood pressure Colorectal cancer (stool for occult blood) Breast cancer (breast self-examination, mammography [as indicated]) Glaucoma Visual acuity Hearing Diabetes (glucometry) Cervical cancer (Papanicolaou smear) Testicular cancer (testicular self-examination) Height/weight Dentition Podiatry assessment (elderly population) Mental status assessment (e.g., depression) Skin check Tuberculosis (purified protein–derivative [PPD] skin test)	Vision Hearing Blood pressure Scoliosis Height/weight Tuberculosis (PPD skin test) Dental health Urinalysis Hematocrit or hemoglobin
Adolescents and Young Adults	***Preschool Children***
Sexually transmitted diseases Papanicolaou smear Breast self-examination Testicular self-examination Blood pressure Vision Hearing Height/weight Dental health Mental health (depression, schizophrenia, eating disorders) Tuberculosis (PPD skin test) Urinalysis Hematocrit or hemoglobin	Vision Hearing Growth and development (e.g., Denver Developmental Screening Test [DDST], speech and language, head circumference up to age 2 years) Height/weight Tuberculosis (PPD skin test; initial PPD skin test at age 1 year) Blood pressure initially at age 3 years Initial dental referral at age 3 years Urinalysis Hematocrit or hemoglobin
	Infant/Neonate
	Height/weight Growth and development (e.g., DDST, head circumference) Urinalysis Hematocrit or hemoglobin Phenylketonuria (PKU) test, which is a test to detect an inborn metabolic defect caused by an enzyme deficiency; if untreated, PKU can cause mental retardation; a PKU screening test is usually indicated shortly after birth and at 2 to 4 weeks of age; testing guidelines are dictated by state law Blood lead level at 9 to 12 months, then annually unless at high risk

Data from American Academy of Pediatrics. (1991, July). Recommendation for preventive pediatric care. *American Academy of Pediatrics News.*
*In all population groups, periodic age-appropriate physical examinations are indicated.

population. Table 17–6 lists screening tests that may be appropriate to administer to selected target populations based on an analysis of age and other sociodemographic risk factors. Figure 17–1 presents guidelines for scoliosis screening, a common health problem in school-age children.

SETTINGS FOR SCREENING

The places vary in which screening programs are conducted. Individual case-finding may occur in the home, clinic, or office. To access groups, screening programs are frequently held in public places, such as in schools, churches, businesses, hospitals, shopping malls, community centers, and apartment complexes. Such accessibility helps to provide essential screening services to people where they live and work. A *health fair* is a type of screening program that usually includes a number of exhibits, resources, and services including screening tests specific to the targeted population, general health information, booths and exhibits from health-related community organizations, and counseling and referral services. Whether it is through individual case-finding or mass screening of populations, the community health nurse is in a key position to establish and implement screening programs in the community.

Community Health Nurse's Role in Screening

The community health nurse often assumes responsibility for establishing and implementing screening programs in the community that promote the early detection and recognition of illness. Using the nursing process the community health nurse is able to plan and implement screening programs that truly benefit the community being served.

ASSESSMENT

Initially the community health nurse must determine the need for a screening program by identifying the at-risk population. Determining risk status of an individual or community is based on an analysis of sociodemographic characteristics. What is the mean age of the population? What is the distribution of males to females? What is the ethnic composition of the community? Are there cultural practices or characteristics that place the population at a higher risk of developing certain diseases? What environmental or occupational hazards may predispose the community to illness? In asking these questions the community health nurse is in essence performing a community assessment to determine the needs and risks of the targeted population (see Chapter 12).

In addition to considering risks, the community health nurse should determine the *resources* available in the community. For example what screening programs are already in place in local hospitals, senior centers, worksites, schools, churches, or other locations in the community? The community health nurse should avoid replicating existing screening programs in the community, provided they are culturally acceptable and physically and financially accessible. If there are insufficient screening programs in the community, the community health nurse then investigates resources for establishing new programs. (See Table 17–7 for specific questions to ask to assess community needs and resources.)

The tests used in screening programs need to be selected with caution. Before deciding on the types of screening to be offered, the community health nurse needs to assess whether necessary screening equipment is available. Are there established procedures for administering selected screening tests? The community health nurse must gain knowledge and expertise of the specific screening proce-

What is Scoliosis?

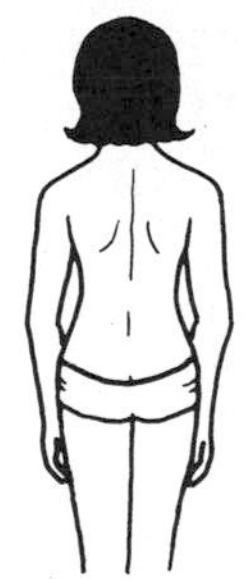

Normal
- head centered over mid-buttocks
- shoulders level
- shoulder blades level, with equal prominence
- hips level and symmetrical
- equal distance between arms and body

1a

Possible Scoliosis
- head alignment to one side of mid-buttocks
- one shoulder higher
- one shoulder blade higher with possible prominence
- one hip more prominent than the other
- unequal distance between arms and body

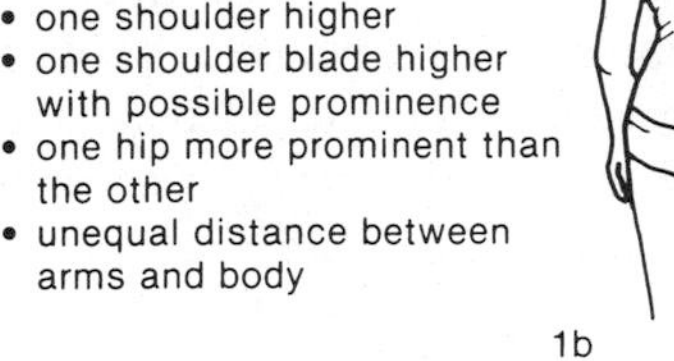

1b

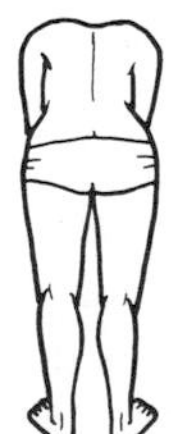

Normal
- both sides of upper and lower back symmetrical
- hips level and symmetrical

2a

Possible Scoliosis
- one side of rib cage and/or the lower back showing uneven symmetry.

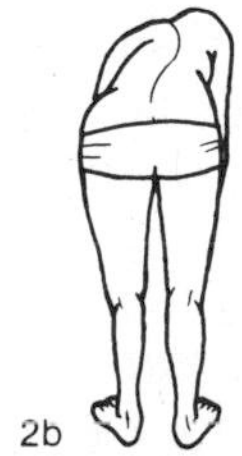

2b

- Scoliosis is a sideways (lateral) curving of the spine.
- One in 10 persons will have scoliosis. Two to three persons in every 1000 will need active treatment for a progressive condition. In one out of every 1000 cases surgery may be necessary.
- Frequent signs are a prominent shoulder blade, uneven hip and shoulder levels, unequal distance between arms and body, and clothes that do not "hang right."
- Eight percent of scoliosis cases are idiopathic (cause unknown). Scoliosis tends to run in families and affects more girls than boys.
- Spinal curvature is best dealt with when a young person's body is still growing and can respond to one or a combination of treatments (body brace, electro stimulation, etc.). You, your physician and/or your school screening program (now required in many schools) can perform a 30-second annual screen during these growing years. (See diagrams.) Mild cases may not need treatment, but must be monitored.
- Kyphosis (round back) may occur in developing adolescents. It should be screened for and may need to be treated.
- An annual 30-second screening for scoliosis and kyphosis during the bone-growing years can make the difference between a preventable condition and a disability in adult years.

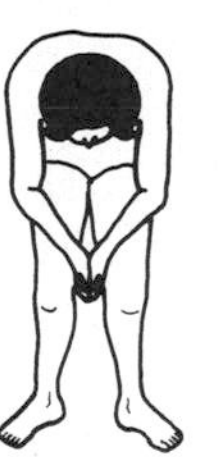

Normal
- even and symmetrical on both sides of the upper and lower back

3a

Possible Scoliosis
- unequal symmetry of the upper back, lower back, or both

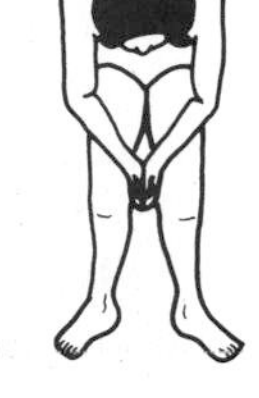

3b

Also Screen for Kyphosis:

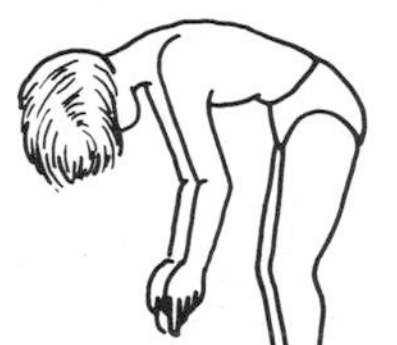

Normal
- smooth symmetrical even arc of the back

4a

Possible Kyphosis ("round back")
- lack of smooth arc with prominence of shoulders and round back.

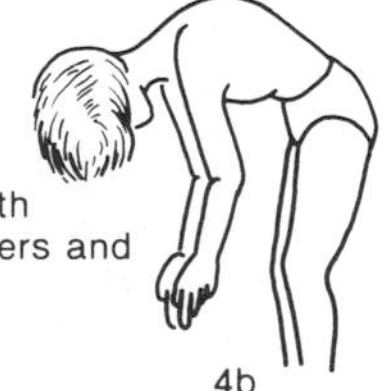

4b

Screen Out Scoliosis!
If one or more physical features suggest scoliosis or kyphosis, professional diagnosis must be sought.

Figure 17–1 ● Guidelines for scoliosis screening. (From National Scoliosis Foundation. (1990). *One in every 10 persons has scoliosis.* Watertown, MA: Author.)

TABLE 17–7

Assessing Resources to Support Screening Programs

Consider the following questions when assessing resources to support a screening program:

1. Is funding available to support a health fair or a wellness program in the local community?
2. What is the cost of implementing such a program?
3. What are the personnel and equipment needs to run screening booths or health education exhibits?
4. Is volunteer support available in the health care community to provide needed services or to loan screening equipment?
5. Are diagnostic and treatment services available to refer clients in whom presumed illness is detected?
6. What facilities are available for follow-up of persons who receive abnormal screening results?
7. Are key community leaders supportive of the program?

dures and appropriate use of equipment to ensure accurate measurement and test administration. In selecting screening tests the community health nurse should also follow the criteria outlined earlier in this chapter, which address issues of significance, cost-effectiveness, validity, treatment availability, safety, and client acceptance.

Finally it is important to assess the appropriate time and site for conducting a screening program. When and where will the community health nurse have the most access to the target population? When screening large populations it is important to estimate the number of people who will likely participate and to have the necessary space and personnel to accommodate the anticipated numbers. If the community health nurse wishes to target selected high-risk populations, he or she usually selects places where the aggregates are readily located. For example a retirement community or senior citizen high-rise is an excellent location for targeting elderly populations. Health fairs conducted in schools access school-age children and adolescents. Screening in the workplace accesses persons who may be selectively at high risk owing to certain occupational health hazards. Finally mobile vans may be used to bring important health screenings to a community.

NURSING DIAGNOSIS

The end point of assessment is the nursing diagnosis. Nursing diagnoses relevant to screening for unrecognized illness are numerous. Many of these are potential diagnoses, as a disease that goes unrecognized has potential adverse health consequences. A general nursing diagnosis for screening might be: *potential for injury related to undiagnosed, untreated illness in the community.*

PLANNING

After assessing the community's health needs and resources the community health nurse is ready to plan a screening program. First program priorities and goals need to be established. To identify problems accurately and set goals meaningful to the community, persons who are most likely to be influenced by the program should have a voice in program development. Key persons who will help in securing needed resources or who will be implementing the program need to have input in the planning process, including health care personnel, volunteers, and community leaders. Persons who can help to inspire acceptance of the program in the community are also valuable assets in promoting community involvement and participation.

The community health nurse must also design easy-to-use forms for documenting screening data. A written form documenting screening test results, normal parameters, and counseling and referral information should be developed and given to the participant for use in the screening program. (See Table 17–8 for sample form.) This form should also include biographical data on the participant. Additional information such as health history data and participant health goals may also be included. The form provides the written documentation of test results and health instructions for both the participant and the provider and is important for subsequent participant follow-up and for program evaluation.

Alternatives for screening programs are examined based on personnel, time, space, equipment, and cost considerations. Original plans may require modification due to insufficient funding or resources to implement an ideal program. For example during a period of scarce resources, voluntary contributions, in terms of money and personnel, often decrease.

Let us say that an occupational health nurse wants to develop a screening program for a large manufacturer. She or he establishes a task force that consists of representation from administration, employees at all levels of the industry, and health care providers in the employee health suite. The task force assesses the perceived health care needs of the target population, the extent of interest in conducting a worksite screening program, and the resources available to conduct the program. Health care personnel note a high incidence of hypertension in their employee health population. Workers express concern that they do not have the time to attend a screening program. The committee considers alternatives to holding a 1-day health fair during a designated time period. Management officials note that limited space and funding are available to conduct the program, but that the administration is willing to schedule all employees on a rotating basis through the employee health suite for hypertension screening. Open hours are held in conjunction with the rotating schedule provided by the managers to maximize convenience and accessibility of the screening program to all interested employees. Volunteer support is solicited from outside agencies to assist in implementing the program.

The next step is to establish program goals and objectives. Goals are broad statements of purposes or aims; objectives are more specific outcome criteria to measure

TABLE 17–8

Sample Screening Form

Biographical Information		
Date:		
Participant name:		
Address:		
Telephone number:		

Health History		
Have you or anyone in your family ever had (circle answer)		
Heart disease:	Yes	No
Cancer:	Yes	No
Anemia:	Yes	No
High blood pressure:	Yes	No
Lung disease:	Yes	No
Do you smoke?	Yes	No
(Amount):		
Do you drink alcohol?	Yes	No
(Amount):		

Screenings	Normal Range	Participant Result
Blood pressure	140/90 or less	(Ex:130/80
Weight	140 to 180 lb (varies with height, sex)	200 lb
Cholesterol	Less than 200 mg/dl	230 mg/dl)

Participant health goals: ______________________________

____

____

Recommendations and/or referrals: ______________________________

____

Signature of health screener: ______________________________

the effectiveness of the program. In this example the task force establishes the following goal: to improve the health status of employees through early detection and treatment of hypertension. The specific objectives include: (1) One month following the screening program, all participants who received abnormal test results will have received follow-up diagnostic testing and treatment, if indicated. (2) In 6 months the incidence and prevalence of hypertension will have increased by 5% in the target population. Note here that if a screening program is effective, the incidence and prevalence of the disease being screened for will increase. This is because screening results in the early detection of previously unrecognized illness and therefore increases the numbers of new and existing cases of a disease. However, mortality from the disease, and complications from the disease (i.e., stroke, heart attack) should decrease, as early detection and treatment improve survival rates and health outcomes. (3) In 1 year the number of days of absenteeism, number of disability days, and rate of hospitalization for illnesses resulting from complications of hypertension will decrease by 20%.

IMPLEMENTATION

After assessing the secondary prevention needs of the target population and planning a screening program to address these needs, the community health nurse is ready to implement the program plan. To implement a successful mass screening program, it is often helpful to use media resources to disseminate information about the program to the community. Flyers, mass mailings, and local advertisements in newspapers or on radio and television help to inform the target population of the program's existence. Media coverage of the program should be done at least several weeks in advance to ensure that information about the program is disseminated throughout the community. Coverage should include the location, dates, and times of the program; services offered through the program; fees, if any, that may be required from the participant for obtaining selected screening tests or services; and any additional preparatory instructions that the client may need. For example if blood tests are offered in the screening program, participants may need to be informed that they should fast at least 8 to 12 hours before receiving the blood test. (See Table 17–9 for an example of a public service announcement.)

Partnerships may be formed with volunteer and community organizations, health care providers, and other interested persons to assist with program implementation. Often local businesses or organizations may agree to co-sponsor a mass screening program. Those who will be working in the program need to be notified of their agreed-on responsibilities and participation in the screening program. Persons administering selected screening tests may need to be trained in test administration. A training session may need to be conducted with persons who will be administering selected screening tests to better ensure accuracy in test measurement and to improve reliability of test findings. Training may occur at a time separate from the actual program date, or persons may be asked to arrive an hour or two earlier on the date of the program to review procedures. The community health nurse should formally notify persons working in the screening program in writing to remind them of the intended date, time, and location of the program and to articulate their agreed-on role in the program.

Often the site where the program is to be held will need to be set up to accommodate the anticipated number of participants and to provide tables, chairs, or other equipment for service providers. Consideration must also be given to persons with disabilities to ensure access to all stations. Booths may be set up so that persons can move in a logical manner from station to station as they make their way toward the exit. A microphone may be used to direct the flow of traffic. Service providers should be asked to arrive early to allow time for orientation and set-up and to provide a time for questions and answers.

When the program begins, the community health nurse should be available to circulate among stations and to address any last-minute problems, such as individuals who fail to show up. In this instance the community health nurse may need to reorganize service providers to fill in gaps and to run selected stations during peak flow times.

Another potential problem is the discovery of a severely abnormal test result. It is also important to have established protocols for emergency intervention—such as finding a blood pressure of 240/130 mm Hg in a participant—so it is clear to all providers when immediate referral to another care source is indicated. Referral guidelines may be based on national criteria, such as those of the Joint National Committee on Detection, Evaluation, and Treatment of High Blood Pressure (NIH, 1993). Service providers who discover an abnormally high reading should contact the screening program coordinator for the appropriate course of action. Participants should not leave until they have secured the number of a health provider appropriate to deal with their identified problems.

Nutrition is an important consideration when conducting a mass screening program. If the program is scheduled for the entire day, persons working in the program will need meals and rest breaks. Free lunches may be provided by local businesses or restaurants as a community service or in exchange for advertising. If blood tests are part of the screening program, participants may be required to fast the night before, and afterward orange juice, cookies, crackers, or snacks should be provided.

The facility in which the program is conducted should be capable of accommodating large numbers of people, both in terms of space and rest room facilities. An exception to this rule is the use of mobile vans, which bring screening services directly to neighborhoods, schools, or worksites.

TABLE 17–9

Public Service Announcement

Public service announcements are messages on behalf of nonprofit groups presented like advertisements

Advantages

Aired free by radio or television
Reach mass audience
Identify sponsoring group(s)
On television, visual aids can be used

Disadvantages

Station determines if and when message is aired
Must be presented to station several weeks before airing
Each station may have specific requirements
Must be brief: 30-second spot = 75 words

Content

Discuss how listeners will benefit
Give next step
Name sponsoring groups
Tell listeners to call for more information

Example of 45-Second Announcement

Would you like to know what your blood pressure is? Has it been a while since you had your vision checked?

If so, come to the health fair on Saturday, April 18 at Valley View Mall from 1:00 to 8:30 P.M.

The health department and the Junior Chamber of Commerce are sponsoring this health fair for you, your friends, and your family. Representatives from many health groups will be on hand to conduct screening tests and teach you how to improve your health!

For more information call ______________ at *123–1234*

Although schools, churches, workplaces, malls, and community centers are usually equipped to deal with large aggregates, remember that the program may draw more people than some facilities can accommodate.

At the completion of the program the community health nurse may wish to tally the number of forms received (indicating the number of participants attending). Forms may be numbered ahead of time for ease in counting. Forms should be sorted so that persons with abnormal test results are placed in a separate file for subsequent follow-up. In a case in which screening test results are not known at the completion of the program (e.g., laboratory blood tests may take several days or weeks to process), a mechanism may need to be devised to ensure that persons responsible for follow-up are notified of additional abnormal test results.

EVALUATION

Evaluation, an essential component of screening programs, is conducted to justify continued program operation and funding from outside parties, to improve service delivery, or to determine the impact of the program on community health. Evaluation includes both *process* and *outcome* dimensions. *Outcome* evaluation refers to the actual end results of the program. Were program objectives achieved? Common outcome criteria for screening programs reflect such epidemiological trends as an increased incidence and prevalence of disease (note that a secondary prevention measure, when effective, actually increases the number of reported cases of disease), increased numbers of persons receiving medical care, decreased mortality from disease, reduced disability and decreased incidence of advanced disease complications, and decreased health care costs for treatment of advanced disease.

Process evaluation focuses on actual program performance regardless of whether the goals that have been set for the program are achieved, including the number of people served by the program, number of volunteer hours needed to conduct the program, reliability and validity of screening tests, efficiency in test administration and reporting of results to participants, and choice of appropriate location and timing of program in terms of community interest and convenience to community members.

Evaluation data may be obtained from analyzing epidemiological data, a follow-up survey of participants, feedback from service providers who worked the screening program, and feedback from community agencies to which referrals from the screening program were made. Program evaluation enables the community health nurse to determine whether the benefits of the program outweigh the cost of time, money, and resources devoted to the program and to rate how the program compares with alternative interventions that may also be effective in maintaining the health of the community (Borus et al., 1982).

Screening program participants may be compared with a control group that did not receive the screening intervention to determine the effectiveness of the screening program and its impact on changes in health status in the community. It is possible for example that, although the community receiving screening services evidences improved health outcomes, a community serving as a control group may also demonstrate improvements in health that are unrelated to the screening program. In other words, program goals may have been achieved regardless of the screening (or therapeutic) intervention (Shulberg et al., 1969). Such questions may be addressed through controlled studies that compare the impact of a therapeutic intervention (or the absence of an intervention) on similar at-risk populations.

Screening and the Referral Process

Referral, an essential component of any screening program, is the process of directing persons to resources to meet needs. It is essential that clients participating in a screening program obtain appropriate counseling and referral for follow-up of any abnormal test results. In fact it is considered unethical to obtain data that indicate an individual might be ill and to do nothing about it. Therefore, appropriate follow-up counseling and referral are essential to any screening program. Often a separate counseling and referral station is provided in a health fair setting, and participants are required to move through this station prior to leaving the health fair. At the counseling and referral station, trained volunteers review all the findings from the health fair with the participant, reinforcing appropriate health maintenance activities and ensuring that the participant understands the meaning of his or her test results, including the need for follow-up evaluation if indicated.

Participants must be advised that a screening program is not a substitute for receiving ongoing health supervision from a health care provider. In many screening programs participants are given written information that highlights this fact. It is not uncommon for persons participating in screening programs to feel that they have been checked over and found healthy.

ESTABLISHING CRITERIA FOR REFERRAL

The community health nurse establishes criteria or guidelines for initiating referrals. Screening test results that fall outside of normal parameters and require follow-up evaluation are an important criterion for referral. For example, any participant with a blood pressure reading above 140/90 mm Hg or a serum cholesterol level above

200 mg/dl should be referred for follow-up. Finally it is essential that the criteria for referral are clearly articulated to those in a mass screening program who are responsible for reviewing screening test results and findings with the participant.

ESTABLISHING A RESOURCE DIRECTORY

Participants who have identified needs that require further intervention are referred to organizations and programs in the community that are capable of providing the needed services. When possible, clients should be given a choice of providers if more than one exists. The community health nurse planning a mass screening program should maintain a list of community health organizations and programs to which persons may be referred. A comprehensive resource directory, listing all local community agencies and service organizations, is invaluable for any community health nurse to have. Information on community resources may be obtained through local and state health departments, local information and referral centers, police and fire departments, libraries, local government offices, or the local Chamber of Commerce. (See Table 17–10 for a guide for surveying health agencies that can be used to create a resource directory.)

The directory should be kept up to date and include: (1) the name, address, and telephone number of the agency; (2) hours of operation; (3) major services provided; (4) eligibility requirements for utilization of services; (5) procedure for activating services; (6) source of funding for the program and payment mechanisms; (7) the name of the director or head of the agency and those of other important contact persons; and (8) a statement reflecting the general impressions received when interacting with the agency.

TABLE 17–10

Guide for Surveying Health Agencies

Name of Agency:
Address:
Telephone number:
Hours and days open:
Major topic area of concern: (E.g., developmental delay, cancer)
Major purpose of service:
- Direct patient care
- Payment for client care
- Information and education
- Research
- Referral of clients and coordination
- Other (e.g., provide equipment)

Description of major services provided:
Procedure for initiating referral:
- Must client be referred by a doctor or health care professional?
- Does it help if a health worker calls first for client?
- What information or papers should client have for referral?
- Is the interview with the client over the telephone or in person?
- Are there waiting lists or limits on services received?

Cost of service and payment mechanisms:
- Government money
- Fees
- Donations, private funds, endowments
- Fund-raising campaigns
- Other

Types of service providers:
- Volunteer (trained, untrained)
- Secretaries, clerks
- Health or other professional workers
- Ancillary staff (e.g., aids)
- Other

Director of program or agency: (Include name, title, telephone number)
Other relevant contact persons:
General impressions of agency: (Consider atmosphere, degree of receptivity, promptness in responding to referral, courtesy, client satisfaction)

Modified from Smith, C. (1982a). *Guide for surveying health agencies.* Baltimore: University of Maryland School of Nursing.

INVESTIGATING PROCEDURE FOR INITIATING REFERRAL

Whether it is in the context of case-finding or a mass screening program, the community health nurse should be aware of the procedure for initiating referrals to a recipient agency or organization. For example, can a referral be made over the telephone by the client or the health care provider? Does the referral need to be in writing? Must specific forms be completed? Ideally it is helpful to give the client the name of a contact person in the agency who may be able to direct the client appropriately through the correct procedures for obtaining needed services.

DETERMINING CRITERIA FOR SERVICE ELIGIBILITY

The criteria for service eligibility should be assessed before initiating a referral, since some agencies have specific criteria for acceptance of their client populations. For example, local health departments will often serve only the residents of a particular locale or region. Local departments of aging provide services to elderly residents. Some government programs, such as medical assistance and Aid to Women, Infants, and Children (WIC), are provided only to those clients who meet specific eligibility criteria (such as income level, verification of need, age, gender, or other health criteria).

INVESTIGATING PAYMENT MECHANISMS

The community health nurse should also be aware of payment mechanisms required by referral agencies. For example, does the agency accept Medicare or medical assistance as payment in full? Do fees need to be paid immediately on delivery of the service? A working knowledge of the policies and procedures of the agency to which the client is being referred can assist the community health nurse to make more appropriate referrals based on the client's unique needs and resources. The client is also better informed of the agency's practices and is more likely to have realistic expectations of what services the agency is capable of providing.

In some instances it may also be appropriate to provide information about the client to the recipient agency. Information that the recipient agency may require may include basic biographical information (name, address, telephone number, age), purpose of the referral, specific needs identified by the nurse or client, and the role expected of the recipient agency. The community health nurse should identify what the client has been told regarding his or her role in the referral. The recipient agency should also have the signature and title of the referring person and the referring agency's address and telephone number where the recipient agency can obtain additional information (Smith, 1982b). If the client is not eligible for services owing to an inability to pay, the community health nurse may need to seek out other resources in the community (such as philanthropic or service organizations) to assist with payment. Civic groups such as the Lions Club, Rotary, or Knights of Columbus may provide donations or financial support to a client in need.

ASSESSING CLIENT RECEPTIVITY

The community health nurse also needs to assess the client's receptivity to the referral. Is the referral acceptable to the client and likely to be followed up on? Has the client had a previous negative experience with the agency to which he or she is being referred? What has the client been told about his or her role in the referral? Are there particular beliefs, values, or cultural biases that prevent the client from using the services of the agency? Additional barriers to acceptance of a referral may include differences in perception of needs between client and health care provider, lack of transportation to access the program or service, competing demands and responsibilities (e.g., child care, working hours) that make it difficult for the client to establish contact and keep appointments with the agency, or inadequate finances to pay for needed services.

EVALUATING EFFECTIVENESS OF REFERRAL

Persons referred for additional services should be contacted after the screening program to see whether they followed through with the referral (Table 17–11). Based on information obtained from the evaluation of the referral process, the type or extent of referrals or the information provided during the referral process may be modified. If this is the first time the nurse has referred a client to the agency or service, the community health nurse should also contact agency personnel to see whether they thought the referral was appropriate and to determine whether they have recommendations regarding future referrals.

TABLE 17–11

Evaluating the Effectiveness of a Referral

Dimension	Evaluation Question
Effectiveness	Was the recipient agency able to meet the client's need or provide the necessary services?
Appropriateness	Did the client encounter any obstacles to receiving care, such as ineligibility for services or inability to pay for services? If the client did not carry out the referral, what barriers prevented him or her from doing so?
Adequacy	What was the client's satisfaction with the services received? To what extent was the client's need met as a result of services provided by the agency? What additional measures can be taken to more effectively address these concerns and ultimately meet the client's needs?
Efficiency	Was it difficult for the client to establish contact with the agency and to obtain needed services in a timely manner?

Data from Smith, C. (1982b). *Letter of referral: Role of nurse in communication with the recipient agency (collaboration).* Baltimore: University of Maryland School of Nursing.

KEY IDEAS

1. Screening is an important secondary prevention strategy. The purpose of screening is to detect diseases in an early stage of development when they are more amenable to treatment.
2. The settings for administration of screening interventions are diverse and variable and depend on the client focus. Screening programs may be geared to individuals or populations.
3. Case-finding is the application of screening tests to individuals on a one-on-one basis.
4. Mass screening is the application of screening tests to large groups or populations.
5. Consider the following questions when selecting screening tests:
   - How significant is the disease being screened for?
   - What is the cost vs. benefit of screening?
   - How acceptable is the test to participants?
   - What is the test's reliability and validity?
   - How easy is it to administer the test?
   - Does the test detect disease at an early stage?
   - Is treatment available for the disease being screened for?
6. To determine what diseases should be screened for in a community the community health nurse as-

sesses the major health risks in the target population and the available constraints to and resources for implementing a screening program. Goals and objectives that specify desired outcome criteria for the screening program are developed.

7. The community health nurse implements the screening program in partnership with community members, volunteers, and health care providers.
8. Evaluation of the effectiveness of a screening program is based on analysis of epidemiological data and feedback from participants and collaborating agencies.
9. It is imperative that every screening program include counseling and referral services. The community health nurse coordinating a screening program must provide for participant follow-up to ensure that referrals were followed up on and that the client received the appropriate therapeutic intervention.
10. In making referrals the community health nurse must investigate the procedure for initiating referrals; determine criteria for service eligibility; assess client receptivity; investigate payment mechanisms; and evaluate the effectiveness of the referral.

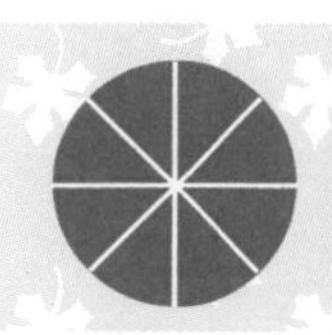

APPLYING THE NURSING PROCESS: *Organizing a Health Fair*

A community health nurse is assigned to a geographic district in which there is a large elderly population. Her experience with home visits to clients reveals that many of the elderly residents in the community regularly attend the local senior center and are very interested in maintaining personal health and fitness. However, because they live on a fixed income, they find it difficult to meet their basic living expenses. Owing to financial constraints, many clients hesitate to see their personal health care providers unless they become ill. They also cite difficulty with transportation as a major deterrent to seeking routine preventive health care.

Based on an analysis of sociodemographic risk factors, the community health nurse determines that this population is at risk of illness from such chronic diseases as hypertension, heart disease, stroke, and cancer. Since many of these diseases can be prevented or treated effectively if diagnosed early, the community health nurse decides to conduct a health fair. She selects the local senior center as the desirable location for the fair, because it is highly accessible and well utilized by the target population.

Planning

In planning the fair, she elicits the help of key community leaders, the director of the senior center, and senior residents in the community who will likely benefit from the program. These individuals meet as a planning committee and identify program goals, resources, and constraints. The general goal for the screening program is to promote and maintain the health of elderly residents in the community through early detection and treatment of disease.

The director of the senior center indicates that members of the center would be very willing to volunteer their services to assist with the implementation of the program. The community health nurse investigates the extent of support from others in the health care community and elicits the help of local nursing students. The community health nurse selects appropriate screening tests to administer based on cost factors, client acceptance, availability, and reliability. She decides to conduct screenings for hypertension, diabetes, glaucoma, vision, hearing, podiatry, colorectal cancer, height and weight, and cholesterol level. In addition volunteers from the local ACS and American Heart Association are asked to participate and run booths with information on heart disease, breast self-examination, mammography, and testicular self-examination. Other local community and health organizations are invited to participate and to distribute information. The local chapter of the American Association of Retired Persons and the local department of aging are asked to explain their programs, services, and resources. Equipment for vision examinations is provided through the Society for the Prevention of Blindness. A local audiologist agrees to conduct hearing screenings. A local medical laboratory agrees to administer blood tests for cholesterol and diabetes.

The community health nurse establishes a list of community resources and guidelines for counseling and referring participants in the screening program in whom abnormal screening test results are found. Guidelines for referral are based on nationally established criteria for normal test results. Nursing students at the local university are asked to conduct blood pressure screening and to run the counseling and referral station.

Implementation

The community health nurse asks that health fair workers arrive early on the day of the fair for a general orientation. At this time it is discovered that the representative from the local chapter of the department of aging is ill and will be unable to attend. The community health nurse modifies her original plan; she provides persons at the counseling and referral station with the address and telephone number for general information on the department of aging for distribution to interested residents.

Evaluation

During the health fair the community health nurse circulates between stations to assess progress and address any problems that may develop. At the completion of the health fair, participants are asked to complete an evaluation form, indicating their satisfaction with the health fair.

After the health fair the community health nurse compiles a list of participants with abnormal test results and conducts follow-up telephone calls 2 to 3 weeks later to determine whether individuals have followed through with counseling and referral recommendations.

Six months following the health fair the community health nurse surveys all participants to elicit data on the impact of the screening program on health status. She notes that participants report greater awareness of the need for early detection. Several participants indicate that because of the screenings, previously unrecognized diseases such as hypertension, diabetes, and glaucoma were detected and treated early. These participants report no complications from advanced disease, and believe that early detection greatly improved their current health status. In addition the community health nurse surveys the nurse practitioner in the senior center's medical clinic to obtain feedback on perceived helpfulness of the mass screening program. The nurse practitioner reports an increased incidence of hypertension and diabetes owing to early detection but a decrease in mortality and disability from complications of advanced disease states. Based on the positive evaluation findings, the community health nurse recommends that the local department of aging hold health fairs for the elderly population in the community at convenient and accessible locations on an annual basis.

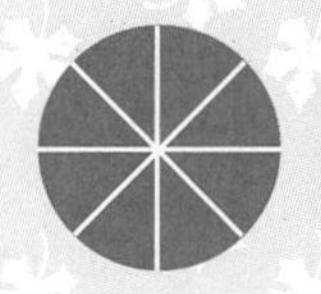

APPLYING THE NURSING PROCESS: *Case-Finding*

A nurse practitioner works in an employee health clinic at a steel plant. A 52-year-old black male client comes in for an employee health physical. The client states he is in good health and denies symptoms of illness, but his family has a history of stroke, heart disease, and diabetes. He acknowledges cigarette smoking of three packs a day for 20 years. Based on an analysis of individual risk factors, the nurse practitioner performs a comprehensive physical examination, with special emphasis on blood pressure status and cardiac, respiratory, and peripheral vascular assessments. In addition she monitors blood glucose and serum lipid levels and performs an electrocardiogram. Based on these screening tests the nurse practitioner finds that the client is overweight and has elevated blood pressure and serum cholesterol and serum glucose levels. The electrocardiogram is within normal limits. The client is counseled regarding his risk factors and is referred to his medical provider for follow-up diagnosis and treatment.

The nurse practitioner contacts the client 1 week later to assess whether the client has followed through in seeking medical evaluation. The client reports that he returned to his medical provider and was placed on a low-fat diabetic diet and an exercise program. In addition he reports being referred to a smoking cessation program.

Three months later the nurse practitioner sees the client for a follow-up employee health check. The client reports adhering to his prescribed regimen and feeling more energetic and less fatigued. The nurse practitioner contacts the client's provider, who reports that the client's blood glucose and serum cholesterol levels and blood pressure have all returned to normal limits and that the client has lost 10 lb. He continues to smoke but has reduced his consumption to two packs of cigarettes per day.

GUIDELINES FOR LEARNING

1. Select a family member, patient, or group in your community (e.g., church members, members of an organization to which you belong). Assess the risk factors in the chosen individual or group. Identify screening tests that would be appropriate to administer to this individual or group based on the criteria for selection of screening tests outlined in the chapter.
2. Interview a friend or family member on her or his perception of the meaning and value of screening and early diagnosis of disease in personal health. To what extent does this individual engage in secondary prevention? When was the last time she or he had a physical examination or other recommended screening tests, considering individual risk factors? What motivates the individual to take advantage of health screenings? What barriers prevent her or him from complying with general recommendations for health screening?
3. Compare perceptions of the value of screening between individuals from different socioeconomic or cultural backgrounds. Are there similarities or differences? What do you think accounts for the differences?
4. Analyze your own personal risk factors for developing illnesses that are amenable to early detection and treatment (e.g., heart disease, cancer, diabetes). Consider demographic variables and personal and family health history in your risk assessment. What screening recommendations are applicable to you? To what extent are you compliant with these screening recommendations? What factors have an impact on your decision to seek screening services?
5. Reflect on a time when you were referred for assistance in meeting an unmet need. What was the nature of the referral? What was it like for you to be referred? To what extent did you follow through on the referral? What affected your decision-making and behavior related to your acceptance of the referral? What was the outcome of the referral?
6. A community health nurse working in a hypertension screening clinic discovers a client with dramatically high blood pressure. In attempting to make a referral for follow-up care, the community health nurse discovers that the client has no financial access to treatment. In what way does this situation constitute an ethical dilemma for the nurse? What can the community health nurse do to resolve this dilemma?

REFERENCES

American Academy of Pediatrics. (1991, July). Recommendations for preventive pediatric care. *American Academy of Pediatric News.*

American Cancer Society (ACS). (no date: a). *Cancer facts for men: What you can do to protect yourself against cancer.* Atlanta: Author.

ACS. (no date: b). *Cancer facts for women.* Atlanta: Author.

ACS. (1980). *Cancer related checkups.* Atlanta: Author.

ACS. (1987). *Special touch: A personal plan of action for breast health.* Atlanta: Author.

ACS. (1990a). *Colorectal cancer: Go for early detection.* Atlanta: Author.

ACS. (1990b). *For men only: What you should know about prostate cancer.* Atlanta: Author.

ACS. (1990c). *For men only: Testicular cancer and how to do TSE (a self exam).* Atlanta: Author.

ACS. (1991). *Cancer facts and figures for minority Americans—1991.* Atlanta: Author.

ACS. 1993). *Cancer facts and figures—1993.* Atlanta: Author.

American Heart Association. (1989). *Cholesterol and your heart.* Dallas: Author.

American Lung Association. (1991). Facts about tuberculosis. New York: Author.

Beck, S., Breckenridge-Potterf, S., Wallace, S., Ware, J., Asay, E., & Giles, R. (1988). The family high-risk program: Targeted cancer prevention. *Oncology Nursing Forum, 15*(3), 301–306.

Bluestein, D., & Archer, L. (1991). The sensitivity, specificity, and predictive value of diagnostic information: A guide for clinicians. *Nurse Practitioner, 16*(7), 39–45.

Borus, M., Buntz, C., & Tash, W. (1982). *Evaluating the impact of health programs: A primer.* Cambridge, MA: MIT Press.

Cooper, G. (1980). Diagnosis: Diabetes. *Diabetes Forecast,* Alexandria, VA: American Diabetic Association.

Diagnostic testing guidelines for healthy individuals. (1992). Clifton, NJ: Clinicians Publishing Group.

Doerr, B., & Hutchins, E. (1981). Health risk appraisal: Process, problems, and prospects for nursing practice and research. *Nursing Research, 30*(5), 299–306.

Gupta, K. (1990). Screening and health maintenance. In C. Edelman, & C. Mandle (Eds.). *Health promotion throughout the life span* (2nd ed.) (pp. 156–172). St. Louis: Mosby–Year Book.

National Institutes of Health. (1993). *The fifth report of the Joint National Committee on Detection, Evaluation, and Treatment of Blood Pressure* (NIH Publication No. 93–1088). Washington, DC: Author.

National Scoliosis Foundation. (1990). One in every 10 persons have scoliosis. Watertown, MA: National Scoliosis Foundation.

Pickett, G., & Hanlon, J. (1990). *Public health: Administration and practice* (9th ed.). St. Louis: Mosby–Year Book.

Shulberg, H., Sheldon, A., & Baker, F. (Eds.). (1969). *Program evaluation in the health fields.* New York: Behavioral Publications.

Smith, C. (1982a). *Guide for surveying health agencies.* Baltimore: University of Maryland School of Nursing.

Smith, C. (1982b). *Letter of referral: Role of nurse in communication with the recipient agency (collaboration).* Baltimore: University of Maryland School of Nursing.

U.S. Department of Health and Human Services (USDHHS). (1990a). *Healthy people 2000: National health promotion and disease prevention objectives. Summary report.* Washington, DC: U.S. Government Printing Office.

USDHHS. (1990b). *Prevention 89/90: Federal programs and progress.* Washington, DC: U.S. Government Printing Office.

Valanis, B. (1986). *Epidemiology in nursing and health care.* Norwalk, CT: Appleton-Century-Crofts.

SUGGESTED READINGS

Ailinger, R. (1984). Hypertension screening for Hispanics. *Journal of Community Health Nursing, 1*(4), 265–270.

Andrews, A., Benedict, R., & Krupa, K. (1982). A pilot occupational health screening program provided by baccalaureate nursing students. *Occupational Health Nursing, 30*(1), 29–33.

Finney, C. (1991). Measurement issues in cholesterol screening: An overview for nurses. *Journal of Cardiovascular Nursing, 5*(2), 10–22.

Kineon, E., & Campbell, J. (1992). Rural health screening: A case study in coordination. *Nursing Connections 5*(1), 43–48.

Lashley, M. (1987). Predictors of breast self-examination practice among elderly women. *Advances in Nursing Science, 9*(4), 25–34.

Leatherman, J., & Davidhizar, R. (1992). Health screening on a college campus by nursing students. *Journal of Community Health Nursing, 9*(1), 43–51.

Oda, D., & Boyd, P. (1988). The outcome of public health nursing services in a preventive child health program: Phase I. Health assessment. *Public Health Nursing, 5*(12), 209–213.

Skipper, M., & Douglas, K. (1986). An opportunity for partnership: Door-to-door lead paint screening. *Caring, 5*(12), 38–42.

Stanton, A. (1987, March). Care of the elderly: Happy birthday . . . screening the well elderly and their careers. *Community Outlook 20–21,* 24.

Young, C., & Gottke, S. (1985). Multiphasic health screening for the rural elderly. *Home Healthcare Nurse, 3*(3), 41–42, 44–46.

Chapter 18

Health Teaching

Gail L. Heiss

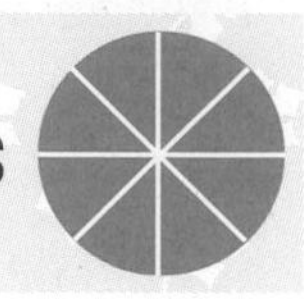

Focus Questions

What is the distinction between patient education and health education?

How do the *Healthy People 2000* objectives affect the role of the community health nurse?

How does the community health nurse identify health education needs? What impact does the community environment have on these learning needs?

What teaching strategies should the nurse use with the identified target group for education? Should the nurse use more than one strategy?

How does the nurse determine the appropriateness of educational aids such as print or audiovisual materials for the learners?

What community resources are available to enhance health education?

How will the nurse know whether the teaching strategies have been effective?

The process of health teaching in the community has been a distinct function of the community health nurse since the origins of community health nursing. Lillian Wald, in her accomplishments in family-centered nursing, promoted health teaching as a means of preventing illness by promoting healthy lifestyle behaviors (Kaufman et al., 1988). The concept and practice of teaching patients in the community has been evolving since the mid-1890s and continues to change with the profession of nursing.

New challenges in health promotion and disease prevention face the community health nurse. For example traditional health education for childbearing women and for children is now complicated by the increase in teenage pregnancies, child abuse, and family violence. The need also exists for communities to educate their members on the resurgence of tuberculosis and the increase of sexually transmitted diseases.

This chapter provides the community health nurse with the concepts and tools needed to develop and implement community health education programs. With the opportunity for health education, members of the community will have the resources and support to strive for personal, family, and community health.

The Health Teaching Process

DEFINITIONS

Patient Education

It is helpful to differentiate between patient education and health education. The term *patient education* is normally used to describe a series of planned teaching-learning activities designed for individuals, families, or groups who have an *identified alteration in health.* The nurse uses a systematic process to assess patient learning needs that relate to the health problem, and then implements the teaching plan to accomplish changes in attitude or behavior (Redman, 1988).

Health Education

Health education focuses on health promotion and disease prevention. The role of the community health nurse includes educating people to avoid disease, to make lifestyle changes, and to improve their health and that of their families, the environment, and the community. The difference between patient education and health education is that health education is directed toward individuals or groups who are *not* experiencing an alteration in health. Community assessment identifies individuals, families, and groups who would benefit from additional information on healthy behaviors. Health education empowers individuals and target groups for self-care, self-help, self-improvement, and improvement of the community (Spellbring, 1991).

POLICIES

American Nurses' Association

In the American Nurses' Association (ANA) Social Policy Statement (1980) and the ANA Standards of Practice (1991) the nursing profession expresses the belief that health can be promoted through education. Both of these documents mandate that nursing interventions promote health through the use of teaching-learning opportunities and the utilization of appropriate resources. Even more specific to the community health nurse are the ANA Standards of Community Health Nursing Practice (1986). These standards outline health education as a distinct intervention. The health education nursing interventions are implemented in partnership with community members, community leaders, and other health care providers.

Financial Reimbursement

Nurses quite possibly have the greatest opportunity to implement education programs because of the extensive amount of time they spend with individuals and families in the community. Currently the structure of the insurance companies in the United States is based on reimbursement for illness care rather than for wellness promotion. Reimbursement is available for physician-ordered education relating to existing illness. However there is no method for direct reimbursement of the nurse who provides education as a health promotion intervention. The failure of insurance companies to reimburse unless the education is ordered by the doctor degrades the role of the nurse as a health educator. It also negates the client's efforts to achieve self-care and wellness (Rankin and Duffy, 1983).

Community educational programs are sometimes offered for a fee. Individuals who value self-care and health will often pay out of pocket for educational programs such as weight management or childbirth education. In this case the nurse does receive payment for teaching and preparation time. Unfortunately persons who cannot afford to pay for educational services are excluded.

Some nurses provide health education as a part of their job, and are reimbursed with a salary. This may include occupational health nurses, school nurses, or nurses in the traditional public health setting. In addition to planning group education, these nurses often have a caseload of families and individuals who need direct care and home visits. Careful time management is required for planning and implementing health education.

EXPANDING OPPORTUNITIES

The current call for reform of the health care delivery system is providing the community health nurse unique opportunities to shape the future. Community-based programs that take a more positive approach to health and wellness are needed. Nurse entrepreneurs can use the

TABLE 18–1

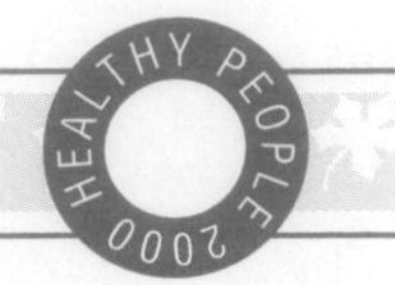

Objectives Relevant to Health Education

Physical Activity and Fitness

Increase the proportion of worksites offering employer-sponsored activity and fitness programs

Nutrition

Increase to at least 50% the proportion of worksites with 50 or more employees that offer nutrition education and/or weight management (baseline: 17% offered nutrition education and 15% offered weight control activities in 1985)

Tobacco

Increase to 50 the number of states with plans to reduce tobacco use, especially among youth (baseline: 12 states in 1990)

Family Planning

Increase to at least 85% the proportion of young persons aged 10 through 18 years who have discussed human sexuality, including values surrounding sexuality, with their parents and/or have received information through other parentally endorsed sources, such as school, religious, or youth programs (baseline: 66% of young persons aged 13 through 18 years discussed sexuality with their parents in 1986)

Violent and Abusive Behavior

Extend coordinated, comprehensive violence prevention programs to at least 80% of local jurisdictions with populations of more than 100,000

Educational and Community-Based Programs

1. Increase to at least 20% the proportion of hourly workers who participate regularly in employer-sponsored health-promotion activities
2. Increase to at least 90% the proportion of people aged 65 years and older who had the opportunity during the preceding year to participate in at least one organized health-promotion program through a senior center, life care facility, or other community-based setting serving older adults
3. Establish community health-promotion programs that separately or together address at least three of the *Healthy People 2000* priorities and reach at least 40% of each state's population
4. Increase to at least 50% the proportion of counties that have established culturally and linguistically appropriate community health promotion programs for racial and ethnic minority populations
5. Increase to at least 90% the proportion of hospitals, health maintenance organizations, and large group practices that provide patient education programs, and to at least 90% the proportion of community hospitals that offer community health programs addressing the priority health needs of their communities (baseline: 60% of community hospitals offered community health promotion programs in 1987)

From U.S. Department of Health and Human Services (1990). *Healthy people 2000: National health promotion and disease prevention objectives. Summary report.* Washington, DC: U.S. Government Printing Office.

public demand for health education to develop and market educational programs that meet population needs. Nurses working in community health agencies can use the health education trends to expand their job description and advance professionally. Nurses can also work politically to influence public policy regarding development and funding of health education programs.

Health promotion through health education and utilization of resources is also of interest to the nurse in the occupational setting. The occupational nurse can work with distinct groups to assess health needs and provide education about, for example, stress management, smoking cessation, or nutrition. The nurse is also an important link between employees and community resources.

Some of the best examples of identifiable health needs and education opportunities are evident in the document *Healthy People 2000: National Health Promotion and Disease Prevention Objectives* (U.S. Department of Health and Human Services, 1990). Behavioral change through education is a common theme. Of particular interest to the community health nurse are the objectives pertaining to educational and community-based programs (Table 18–1).

Research Results: What Works in Client Health Education?

Research on health education has been extensive. Some of the most prominent public health research regarding individuals' adherence to health promotion activities was initiated in the 1950s by Becker, Hochbaum, Kegeles, and Rosenstock (Rosenstock, 1974) (see also Chapter 16). According to their research, participation in prevention activities such as education programs will influence health behaviors. However research questions regarding how much and what type of education is most influential remain unanswered.

MULTIPLE TOOLS AND METHODS

There is no doubt that health education works, and that actual changes in behavior and attitude occur following health education interventions. The research efforts of Lindeman (1988) have established that preoperative education influences recovery from surgery. The research revealed that patient education worked using a variety of strategies such as lecturing, modeling, or providing printed material, and that all methods were equally effective in increasing skills or knowledge level. Unfortunately little research is available to determine how effective any of these strategies is in maintaining change over a long period, which is often the goal of health education.

Continued research is needed concerning the effectiveness of group vs. individual instruction. Cost-saving efforts in health care delivery are a priority. If research proves that cost-saving group education is equally effective, the role of the community health nurse in groups will expand accordingly.

INDIVIDUALIZATION AND REPETITION

Individual characteristics such as age, social status, and educational level influence teaching effectiveness and long-term health behaviors (Lindeman, 1988). Standard lecture methods that do not consider these or other individual differences are relatively ineffective in teaching self-care. Therefore the educational program should be individualized to meet the learner's needs. Some individualized approaches such as behavior modification, contracting, operant conditioning, fostering self-efficacy, and provision of regular feedback and reinforcement are possibly more effective for achieving long-term results, but need to be researched (Oberst, 1989).

Repetition increases learning. Adherence to health-promoting behaviors is best achieved when the education is repetitive and reinforced at different times (Lindeman, 1988). Although it is generally accepted that repetition and reinforcement enhance learning, the amount of repetition needed for various learners has not been quantified.

Technologies such as computer-assisted instruction, home video, audio recordings, and cable television can be used to individualize, repeat, and reinforce education. Technology may save nursing time, but its effectiveness should be studied (Smith, 1989).

SUPPORT SYSTEMS

The effectiveness of group instruction should be analyzed. The presence of a peer group can enhance learning by providing encouragement to the learners as they try new behaviors and by giving positive reinforcement when goals are met. Also teaching a supportive family instead of just one family member is more effective in achieving learning objectives (Bille, 1981).

Health education methods in groups are most useful when used in combination, such as a lecture followed by a demonstration and a discussion. During the educational program the teacher may use almost every teaching strategy. This combination of methods is likely to enhance group cohesiveness and group support. Research indicating the best combination of strategies for groups is not available.

Nursing Assessment of Health-Related Learning Needs

The development of content, strategies for teaching, and evaluation of the effectiveness of the health education program should be carried out in a systematic manner to achieve the most effective results. This systematic method is the teaching-learning process. The teaching-learning process parallels the nursing process (Fig. 18–1). The nurse will use both the nursing process and the teaching-learning process to intervene for community health promotion.

COMMUNITY LEARNING NEEDS

To create a health education program for a community, both the needs of the community and the learning needs of the individual participants should be assessed. Assessment of the community is based on epidemiological and demographic data, as well as the observations of health care personnel in the community (see Chapter 12). The need for community education can be assessed using the four classifications of educational needs as described by Atwood and Ellis (1971):

1. A real need is one that is based on a deficiency that actually exists.
2. An educational need is one that can be met by a learning experience.
3. A real educational need indicates that specific skills, knowledge, and attitudes are required to assist the client in attaining a more desirable condition.
4. A felt need is recognized as important by the learner.

The combined community assessment and educational needs assessment provide the impetus for planning a health education program.

TEACHING PROCESS
Identify learning needs and readiness to learn
Learning diagnosis
Behavioral objectives
Teaching
Evaluate achievement of behavioral objectives
ASSESSMENT
DIAGNOSIS
GOALS
INTERVENTION
EVALUATION
NURSING PROCESS
Health screening, identification of the health need. If the patient needs to learn, use the teaching process.
Nursing diagnosis. May include knowledge deficit.
All goals related to the health need. Some are learning goals.
All nursing actions.
Evaluate continuing health needs. Evaluate ability for self care. Evaluate continued need for teaching.

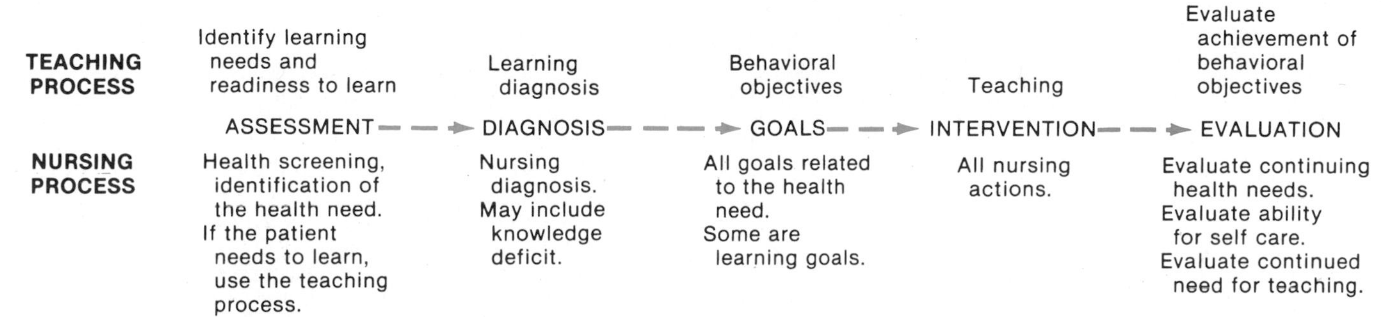

Figure 18–1 ● Relationship of the teaching and the nursing processes.

A model that combines community assessment and educational planning is the PRECEDE model. PRECEDE is an acronym for *p*redisposing, *r*einforcing, and *e*nabling *c*auses in *e*ducational *d*iagnosis and *e*valuation (Green et al., 1980). *Predisposing* factors are characteristics of the learner; these include knowledge, attitudes, and perceptions that motivate health-related behavior. *Enabling* factors are environmental resources and learner skills that facilitate or hinder attainment of health behaviors. *Reinforcing* factors are actual or expected rewards and feedback a learner receives following a health behavior. These three types of factors influence health-related behavior, which in turn contributes to the presence or absence of health problems that are linked with quality of life.

Most of the seven phases of the PRECEDE model begin with a diagnosis. In each phase the health educator looks to the preceding cause and factors that influence the diagnosis. The educator answers "why" a situation is occurring before planning the educational intervention. Analysis of the causes of the health problem helps eliminate the risk of planning ineffective interventions based on guesswork.

The phases of the PRECEDE model are similar to the nursing process. Phases 1 through 4 involve assessment, phase 5 is priority setting and planning, phase 6 is implementation, and phase 7 is evaluation (Table 18–2).

ASSESSMENT OF THE LEARNER

Assessment of the learner is essential to planning the educational program. Assessment of the learner also helps to facilitate the learner's acceptance and use of the teaching being offered. Within the community the learner may be an individual, family, or group. Initial assessment of the learner is often referred to as *assessment of the learner's readiness to learn*. Redman (1984) describes two aspects of readiness: emotional and experiential.

Emotional Readiness

Emotional readiness is the learner's motivation, or the willingness to put forth the effort needed to learn. Motivation to learn is based on attitudes and beliefs about health-related behaviors.

Motivation may be internally or externally reinforced. Internal motivation describes satisfaction in health-promoting activities based on the belief that the action is useful or enjoyable. External motivation must constantly be reinforced by rewards or praise. "Internal motivation is longer lasting and more self-directive than is external motivation" (Redman, 1988, p. 36). For example an individual who joins a weight loss group is more likely to achieve and maintain a weight loss if she or he joins the

TABLE 18–2

Phases of the PRECEDE Model Sample Community Educational Plan

Phase	Questions	Example
Phase I: Social diagnosis	What are the general concerns of the population?	Teenagers "hang out" at local stores
Phase II: Epidemiological diagnosis	What are the specific health problems?	Alcoholism and drug abuse Car accidents related to intoxication Asthma
Phase III: Behavioral diagnosis	What are health-related behaviors?	Underage drinking Illegal drug use Smoking
Phase IV: Educational diagnosis	What are predisposing, enabling, and reinforcing factors?	*Predisposing:* Teenagers desire to belong to peer groups *Enabling:* Cigarettes, alcohol, and drugs can be purchased *Reinforcing:* Teenagers who do not use substances are excluded by other teenagers
Phase V: Analysis of educational diagnosis	Which of the priority factors will be focused on during education?	Teenagers' desire to belong Belief that substance use is necessary to belong Community accessibility of substances
Phase VI: Administrative diagnosis	What specific objectives and resources are needed for health education?	**For Teenagers** *Objective:* Adolescents will explore alternative ways of being together *Resources:* Young adult small group facilitators needed **For Community** *Objective:* Community leaders will provide substance-free recreation sites and programs *Resources:* Community education at civic associations and local government meetings regarding adolescent needs
Phase VII: Evaluation	What are the results of education?	Civic club sponsors sports and games in substance-free site within 3 months Thirty percent of teenagers attend and report reduced smoking and drug use

Data from Green, L., Kreuter, M., Deeds, S., & Partridge, K. (1980). *Health education planning: A diagnostic approach.* Palo Alto, CA: Mayfield Publishing.

group to satisfy her or his own need for health, wellness, and self-esteem (internal motivation). If she or he joins the group to receive the rewards of buying new clothes or garnering the praise of others (external motivation), the person is less likely to maintain the weight loss.

Experiential Readiness

Experiential readiness includes the client's background, skill, and ability to learn (Redman, 1984). Assessment of the client's background includes cultural factors, the home environment, and socioeconomic status. This background information is useful in describing current health behaviors and the learner's ability to use education to change behavior.

Client skills and self-perception of skills are part of experiential readiness. A client who is learning to bathe a newborn needs both coordination and the belief that he or she can learn. It is also useful to assess how clients prefer to learn procedures or skills. Based on past experience, do clients prefer to try themselves, correcting their own mistakes, or do they prefer to be led through the process step by step several times until they feel confident?

Finally, in determining experiential readiness, the client's ability to learn should be assessed. Most pertinent is determination of the client's educational level. Direct

TABLE 18–3

Assessment of Readiness to Learn: Questions for the Nurse to Ask the Learner

Emotional Readiness
What sorts of things do you currently do or try to do to keep healthy?
Assesses attitudes about health promotion and disease prevention, sense of control over the ability to stay healthy, self-satisfaction in health-seeking behaviors
What things in your life make it hard to keep healthy?
Assesses perceptions of stressors or barriers to health-promotion activities, cost of healthy behaviors
Why did you join this health education group?
Assesses internal or external motivation to learn
What would you like to know more about?
Indicates priorities
What personal health goals do you hope to attain by the end of the experience?
Assesses expectations for the future, patient's interest in learning
Experiential Readiness
Background
Tell me about yourself, your family, and your lifestyle; include your ethnic or cultural origins, and your cultural beliefs about health and illness
Describes current health behaviors, cultural traditions that may influence adherence to health-promotion behaviors
Skills
Learning a Manual Skill
How would you describe your ability to learn this skill?
How would you describe your manual dexterity at the present?
How much practice do you usually need to master a new skill?
Assesses the learner's actual and perceived manual dexterity and coordination
Learning a Concept
How do you feel about learning these new ideas?
How often do you need something repeated before you feel comfortable with a new idea?
How do you think you learn best: by hearing? by seeing? by doing? by a combination of these?
Ability to Learn
What is your level of education? What did you study in school?
What subjects did you enjoy the most?
Assessment of formal level of education is not always sufficient; assessment of ability to read should be done utilizing a readability formula
How is your sense of sight? hearing? speech?
Do you trust your memory? What things, if any, do you find it difficult to remember? What do you do when you cannot remember?
Assesses ability to memorize information
To what degree is your ability to concentrate influenced by the surroundings, e.g., noise, people?
Assesses adequacy of the educational environment
How long can you concentrate before getting tired?
Assesses the need for short or long teaching sessions and the need of periodic breaks
Which of the following things have you said about yourself: I heard it, but it just didn't register. I heard it, but my mind went blank. I can tune everything else out.
Assesses the ability of the learner to listen carefully and attentively.

Adapted from Stromborg, M., & Cohen, R. (1991). Evaluating written patient education materials. *Seminars in Oncology Nursing, 7*(2), 125–134.

questioning related to years of formal education is useful but does not always provide complete and accurate information. For example although a client may have completed college, if she or he did not study medicine or nursing she or he may not understand complex medical terminology. In addition reading ability and learning disabilities should be considered (Table 18–3).

FACTORS IN A GROUP OF LEARNERS

The community health nurse frequently implements health education programs with groups of learners. The group may originate from the community at large to participate in an advertised education program; the group may also originate as a result of screening and identification of families with a health need. The nurse needs to utilize some principles of group process to plan and implement the health education program (Tables 18–4 and 18–5).

Background, skills, abilities, and motivations are different for each group member. An assessment of each learner's readiness to learn before the first group meeting is useful for determining group composition. If an individual assessment before the group meeting is not possible, some introductory time during the first meeting could be used to assess readiness to learn.

This gathering of emotional and experiential readiness data will assist in planning content for future group meetings. The nurse should document these data, and may want to ask a colleague to record the information while he or she is leading the group. Taking notes could distract from the important task of establishing rapport.

TABLE 18–4

Factors in a Group of Learners

Type of Membership
Homogeneous Membership
Members have similar learning needs, abilities, and learning style.
Some homogeneity is needed so members "feel" they belong, e.g., age, sex, background. No one member should "stand out" as different.
Planning of educational strategies may be easier for the nurse.
Heterogeneous Membership
Variation between members regarding learning needs, abilities, and learning style.
Differences between members may enhance learning by allowing members to listen and understand the experiences of others.
Very large groups can be divided into smaller learning "clusters" based on learning needs. "Clusters" can reconvene for large group sharing.
Small "clusters" can prevent members from being bored or overwhelmed (either of which can decrease motivation to attend the group).
Stability of Membership
Assessment of learning needs, and selection of members, provides less dissatisfaction and more stability of group.
Time-limited behavioral change groups have a more stable membership than continuing community groups such as Weight Watchers, La Leche League, or Parents Without Partners.
Assumption of Roles
Roles within the group influence communication and can support behavioral change.
Awareness of roles can assist the nurse in balancing participation of members and resolving conflict.

TABLE 18–5

Roles in Groups

Leader—Guides and directs group activities
Coordinator—Clarifies ideas, offers suggestions to demonstrate relationships between ideas; harmonizes activities of members
Follower—Passive member, frequently an audience in decision-making situations, accepts authority of others
Task Specialist—Helps group move toward achievement of group goals; focuses group movement
Evaluator—Measures group decisions and achievements against group standards and goals
Information and Opinion Giver—Requests data, opinions, and ideas related to the problem
Gatekeeper—Controls access to the group; limits entrance of outsiders
Energizer—Stimulates the group toward higher achievement
Peacemaker—Reconciles conflict between group members to eliminate dysfunction of the group

Adapted from Janosik, E. H., & Phipps, L. B. (1982). *Life cycle group work in nursing.* Monterey, CA: Wadsworth.

Constructing Health Education Lesson Plans

The next step in the teaching-learning process is the construction of the health education lesson plan. In the initial phase of the teaching-learning process, the nurse assesses "what" the learner wants or needs or is able to accomplish. The next step, the creation of the lesson plan, begins with the statement of results the nurse wants the learner to achieve. This statement is a *behavioral objective.* The result of the education may be a change in attitude, skill, behavior, or knowledge, but must be stated *before* the actual teaching begins.

BEHAVIORAL OBJECTIVES

Behavioral objectives reflect changes in the learner that are observable or measurable. If the behavioral objectives are properly written, they will be a useful tool in evaluation of educational outcomes. It is important to remember that behavioral objectives are statements of what the learner achieves, and not a statement of the teacher's activities.

Behavioral objectives accomplish the following (Grolund, 1970):

1. Provide direction for the teacher and indicate to others the "instructional intent"
2. Guide the selection of course content, teaching strategies, and teaching materials
3. Facilitate evaluation of the educational program, because evaluation measures the achievement of the objectives
4. Guide the student's learning by specifying what she or he is expected to do at the conclusion of the program

When writing behavioral objectives it is acceptable to state a main objective in behavioral terms that guide large segments of learning. This main objective is followed by more specific supporting objectives. The supporting objectives should represent all of the actions necessary to accomplish the main objective (Redman, 1988). Main objectives in the community may closely parallel the *Healthy People 2000* objectives, with supporting objectives specific to the community in which the program is implemented. Some guidelines and examples of behavioral objectives appear in Tables 18–6 and 18–7.

Behavioral objectives are classified in three "domains" of learning: cognitive (intellectual), psychomotor (motor skills), and affective (attitudes and emotions) (Bloom, 1956). All behavioral objectives fit in one of the domains of learning.

By assessing learning needs the nurse can evaluate the need for behavioral objectives in the cognitive, affective, or psychomotor domain. All three domains of learning are usually necessary to incorporate a new health behavior into the learner's life. Nurses generally desire learners to do the following:

1. Cognitively apply information
2. Perform skills with some guidance and, eventually, independently
3. Value the learning enough to use it

TABLE 18–6

Guidelines for Writing Behavioral Objectives

1. Begin each objective with an active verb (examples: discuss, name, compare, describe, predict)
2. State the objective as a learner outcome, not as a teacher outcome or intent
3. Include only *one* outcome per objective to facilitate evaluation of outcomes
4. Be sure the stated objectives are appropriate for the learners' needs and abilities

From Grolund, N. E. (1970). *Stating behavioral objectives for classroom instruction.* New York: Macmillan.

SELECTING CONTENT

Selection of the content of the health education program depends on the following:

1. The needs identified by the target group of learners
2. Determination by the nurse of what the group needs to know
3. Constraints placed on the nurse by the health care delivery system

Needs of the learners lead to the development of the behavioral objectives. Behavioral objectives lead to development of the content of the health teaching program. When developing the content of the program, the nurse consistently refers to the behavioral objectives for guidance. Behavioral objectives that were carefully developed from the needs assessment and that include learning in all

TABLE 18–7

Sample Behavioral Objectives

Following the health education program entitled "Low-Fat Meals for Your Family," the participant will:

Poorly Phrased Behavioral Objectives	Well-Phrased Behavioral Objectives
Cognitive Domain	
• Understand the importance of a healthy diet • Know what high-fat foods the family eats	• Describe the health benefits of a low-fat diet • Name at least three foods or recipes enjoyed by the family that are high in fat
Psychomotor Domain	
• Cook meals without as much fat • Buy low-fat foods	• Rewrite the "family favorite" recipe using low-fat ingredients • When shopping compare nutrition labels of popular snack foods (such as cookies and chips) • Increase the percentage of purchased foods that are low-fat
Affective Domain	
• Adjust successfully to the new family eating patterns • Appreciate the relationship between food and comfort	• Predict the family reactions to low-fat meals and snacks • Discuss possible solutions to family resistance to change

three domains will lead to the development of a teaching plan that is tailored to the needs of the target group.

It has been recommended when planning the educational program to start with the information that the group is seeking, even if that information is not the most important component of the health education. By meeting the immediate need to know, the nurse captures interest and motivates for further learning. In addition if the information the group is seeking is not addressed, the learners may not be able to concentrate on priority information being taught (Gessner, 1989).

The nurse independently determines some of the content of the health education program. Although the learner's or group's assessment of their own learning needs have been expressed, their list of learning needs may not be comprehensive. The nurse's expertise is useful for identifying information and attitudes needed for behavioral change that members of the group did not identify. For example the nurse may conduct a group for pregnant adolescents, with the overall goal of decreasing child abuse and neglect by adolescent parents. Group-identified learning needs may focus on the psychomotor aspects of new infant care and attitudinal changes necessary to becoming responsible parents. The group might not identify the relationship between infant crying, development of infant self-comforting behaviors, and abusive behaviors exhibited by some parents in reaction to infant crying. It is the nurse's responsibility to include these concepts and positive health behaviors in the educational plan.

The health care delivery system places constraints on health education programs. Time and money are limited resources and often influence the length of a program. The nurse needs to be selective in planning content so the most important concepts and knowledge about how to use the information are included at the outset of the educational program. Additional content is included if time and money permit.

The nurse also needs to plan use of educational materials within the constraints of a budget. Although the use of purchased print and audiovisual materials may enhance the program, content may still be effectively taught using less expensive teaching aids prepared by the nurse or the institution (the preparation of teaching aids is discussed later in the chapter).

The insurance industry also places restrictions on health education programs. The nurse must remember that some educational programs are reimbursed by third-party payers only if the content is approved by the insurer or is ordered by a physician. Alteration of content is sometimes required for compliance with these limitations.

SELECTING TEACHING STRATEGIES

Selection of the teaching strategy or technique to achieve the behavioral objectives is the next step in planning the health education program. Teaching techniques must be suitable to the size, composition, and learning abilities of the group. Consideration for cultural differences and community values is necessary. Differences in learning needs that were assessed previously influence the selection of the teaching strategy. Strategies should be suitable to the subject matter. Numerous teaching strategies that are useful in group education and factors that influence their selection are presented in Table 18–8.

EVALUATION STRATEGIES

To evaluate the health education process two components are assessed: learner outcomes and teacher effectiveness.

Learner Outcomes

Assessment of the learner outcomes is based on achievement of the behavioral objectives. If it is properly written, each objective is measurable. Actual performance of the desired behavior provides the evaluation data. The overall goal of community health education programs is typically to teach a health-promoting activity that is incorporated into the learner's lifestyle.

Direct observation by the nurse provides some indication of success, but actual measurement of the lifestyle change is often done by the participant. An example of this may be the outcome of health education to promote cardiovascular health. If the educational program was limited in length, the nurse may not be able to observe changes in the individual's pulse rate or blood pressure before the end of the program. Adherence to the actual behavioral objective of daily walking for 30 minutes is known only by the learner. The participant provides subjective reports of lifestyle changes. Long-term evaluation is possible, but cardiovascular changes over time may be influenced by other factors in addition to the health education program.

The use of a journal can provide data regarding adherence to health-promoting activities. However, keeping a journal requires a high level of commitment by the learner, and may not be a truthful representation of actual behaviors. In addition, although performance of health behaviors is the overall goal, journals do not measure increased cognitive knowledge.

Measurement of cognitive knowledge is best achieved through use of questionnaires or standardized testing. Although this method of evaluation yields usable data for comparison of groups, it is not always recommended. Questionnaires can be time-consuming and the learner must know how to read. Standardized tests have the same limitation for learners who cannot read, and may remind adult learners of their childhood school days. A negative experience using a questionnaire or test could prevent adult learners from seeking health education groups in the future.

TABLE 18–8

Teaching Techniques for Use in Groups of Learners

LECTURE: Traditional presentation
Advantage: Effective in large groups; good for lower-level cognitive learning
Disadvantage: Students are passive; students with increased intellectual ability may be bored
USE OF EXAMPLES: Begin with simple and progress; select examples based on common life experiences of the group
Advantage: Useful for clarification; students may be able to provide examples to verify learning
Disadvantage: Failure to relate the example to principles being taught results in learners remembering *only* the example
DISCUSSION: Often used to achieve objectives in the affective domain
Advantage: Active participation of the learner; assists learner to focus, analyze, generalize
Disadvantage: Not as effective in large groups; students in certain settings such as a lecture hall may not be able to hear the peer discussion
ROLE MODELING: Provides members with model for learning; also known as identification
Advantage: Learner is able to observe someone with desirable traits
Disadvantage: Need to carefully select nurse leader who possesses the desirable traits
POSITIVE REINFORCEMENT: Useful when teaching a group with high anxiety level
Advantage: Increases participation in discussion because members feel valued
Disadvantage: Reinforcement must be related to learner accomplishment, not the learner
DEMONSTRATION AND GUIDED PRACTICE: Effective for learning psychomotor skills
Advantage: Encourages involvement; safe place to make mistakes
Disadvantage: Difficult for left-handed learners
SIMULATION: Applies previously learned knowledge; use for psychomotor skills practice and affective learning
Advantage: Active participation; increases motivation and interest
Disadvantage: Limited use for cognitive learning
ROLE PLAYING: Provides exploration of attitudes and problem-solving skills
Advantage: Active participation; comparison of own beliefs to those of others
Disadvantage: Time consuming; need experienced leader to focus the discussion
SUPPORT GROUPS: Highly effective for attitude and behavioral change when used with cognitive teaching
Advantage: Decreases sense of "aloneness"; member differences provide model for new behaviors
Disadvantage: Group can become "stuck" in self-pity
CONTRACTING: Written or verbal; emphasizes outcomes
Advantage: Allows for differences in learner needs; can monitor change over time
Disadvantage: Learners with limited self-discipline will have difficulty adhering to contract
STRESS-REDUCTION EXERCISES: Reducing anxiety increases cognitive and affective learning
Advantage: Applicable to most learning situations; can become part of regular mental health
Disadvantage: Nurse needs to be comfortable with technique
COMPUTER-ASSISTED INSTRUCTION: Individualizes learning needs
Advantage: Useful for cognitive and affective learning; voice-generated instruction useful to overcome reading disabilities
Disadvantage: Equipment costly; initially may need highly individualized instructor time

Data from De Muth, J. (1989). Patient teaching in the ambulatory setting. *Nursing Clinics of North America, 24*(3), 645–655; de Tornay, R., & Thompson, M. (1982). *Strategies for teaching nursing* (2nd ed.). New York: John Wiley & Sons; Joyce, B., & Weil, M. (1980). *Models of teaching* (2nd ed.). Englewood Cliffs, NJ: Prentice-Hall; and Redman, B. (1988). *The process of patient education.* St. Louis: Mosby–Year Book.

A more positive method of evaluation is to put questions into a "game-show" format to use with groups.

In a small group environment it is appropriate to evaluate behavioral outcomes by interviewing each member of the group. A structured interview could be used to collect data about personal behavioral successes. These data would be uniform and provide for a simple analysis. However, if a structured interview were used, some of the personal successes and benefits of the instruction might not be included.

In contrast to a structured interview, if each member is interviewed informally he or she might share more personal behavioral successes. Personal successes shared informally during the group meetings provide motivation for other group members. Informal sharing about achievement of behavioral objectives also provides information about difficulties the learners are having and their satisfaction with the learning experience. The nurse is able to determine which objectives are difficult for the participants to achieve and can revise the educational strategies appropriately.

Evaluation and revision of health education programs is required of the community health nurse to adhere to the ANA Standards of Community Health Nursing Practice (ANA, 1986). Members of the community should be involved in the evaluation process. The evaluation should lead to the development of new databases for community planning. A prime example of continued evaluation and revision is the continued modification of the health goals for the nation.

Continued research is needed on evaluating the effectiveness of health education. This research is closely tied to program evaluation and is achieved with studies of population groups over time (see Chapter 14 for more information on evaluation methods).

TABLE 18–9

Teacher Effectiveness Sample Evaluation Tool

	Strongly Agree	Agree	Can't Decide	Disagree	Strongly Disagree
Circle the appropriate number					
1. The nurse listened to my concerns.	5	4	3	2	1
2. The nurse understood what I needed to learn.	5	4	3	2	1
3. I was able to ask questions.	5	4	3	2	1
4. The nurse used language I could understand.	5	4	3	2	1
5. There was enough variety during the sessions to make them interesting.	5	4	3	2	1
6. The nurse used examples that were familiar to me.	5	4	3	2	1
7. I had enough opportunity to participate.	5	4	3	2	1
8. The nurse valued my contributions to the group.	5	4	3	2	1
9. The nurse knew the subject matter.	5	4	3	2	1

Teacher Effectiveness

Teacher effectiveness influences the achievement of behavioral outcomes. Teacher performance can be evaluated through observation by a peer, review of videotapes of the teaching session, or by assessment by the learners.

When working with groups, teacher effectiveness can be enhanced using co-leaders. Co-leaders who have mutual trust and respect can learn from one another as they use various teaching strategies. It is particularly useful to pair a novice teacher with one who is more experienced. If the novice teacher is using a new technique, effectiveness will be enhanced through feedback and guidance from the co-leader.

Principles of teaching such as clear communication, use of diverse teaching methods, and personalization are often used as criteria to measure teacher effectiveness (Table 18–9).

Health-Related Educational Materials

PRINT MATERIALS

Problems of Low Literacy

Learners often need to have the teaching experience supplemented with print materials. Print materials can serve to reinforce teaching and provide reminders about new behaviors after the learner has left the educational setting. Unfortunately the problem of illiteracy is prevalent in the United States. Studies of reading abilities indicate that approximately 50% of health care clients have difficulty reading educational materials written at the fifth-grade level (Doak et al., 1985).

A study of clients at public health clinics revealed that most of the clients had a sixth-grade reading comprehension level. Also there was a gap of more than 5 years between the client reading level and the comprehension levels required to use the educational materials (Davis et al., 1990). The materials tended to be written at an 11th grade reading level or above.

Research by Streiff (1986) revealed that client-reported years of education is not always an indicator of reading ability. The average difference in reported and actual reading levels was 3.1 grades, with a wide variation among individuals. Streiff proposes that the clients' reading abilities actually be tested in the health care setting before health teaching is initiated.

If testing reading abilities is not possible, the work of Burmeister (1978) can be applied by the community health nurse. The nurse should be aware of the educational demographics of the community or target group for education. Assuming the group has gone to school, it is likely that one third of the learners will read within 1 or 2 years of their reported grade level. It is possible that one third of the group will read at *2 years below* reported grade level. The nurse should plan to use materials that are readable at this lowered reading level.

The range of reading achievement among high school graduates ranges from grades 6 to 17 or more (Burmeister, 1978). For an adult group of reported high school graduates, selected materials should be readable at the sixth grade level.

Low literacy does not only indicate a client's lack of reading ability, but also affects his or her ability to understand verbal instructions. Often when patients are questioned about understanding, they will indicate that they do understand, even if they do not. Sometimes, when confronted with a fast-paced educational program, low-literacy clients will withdraw from the situation, appearing to have low motivation to participate (Doak et al., 1985). Patients with low reading and comprehension skills and limited vocabulary are not able to express what is not understood, and therefore may choose to attempt to conceal their illiteracy.

Predicting Readability of Materials

The readability of existing health education materials has been studied extensively. The analysis of written educational materials used in public clinics by Davis and others (1990) revealed that the educational materials were written at the 11th to 14th grade levels. A similar analysis in an ambulatory care setting found that all educational materials exceeded the 6th grade reading level, and were written at up to the 15th grade level (Streiff, 1986).

The challenge for nurses preparing health education programs is to select or create print materials that can be understood by the learners. The nurse should remember that, although some individuals in the group may have advanced literacy, it is easier for a good reader to read down than for a low-literacy learner to read up.

Existing print materials can be analyzed for actual readability of the text. Readability formulas, such as the SMOG readability formula (McLaughlin, 1969), Fry readability graph (Fry, 1977), or Flesch readability graph (Flesch, 1949) are useful in determining the appropriateness of health education materials. The SMOG readability formula has been chosen for inclusion in this text because of its ease in use. The SMOG formula can be used for print materials with varying lengths, including pamphlets with fewer than 30 sentences. The nurse should practice the use of the SMOG formula until it becomes a natural part of his or her practice (Table 18–10).

Selection of Materials

In addition to readability other factors should be considered when choosing print material. These selection factors include analysis of the content, format, and appropriateness of the print material for the target group.

Content. The content of the print material should be assessed to determine that the information is accurate, is up to date, and presents all of the information a learner needs to know to change behavior. The nurse should discern whether there is too much unnecessary information that might confuse the learner. (Remember, print materials are a supplement, not a substitute for education.) The material should be organized in a logical manner and should answer all of the questions it raises. Resources for more information should be included.

Format. The nurse should assess the format of the print material. The type and size of print are important, especially when working with groups whose visual acuity may be decreased, such as the elderly. Although the use of all capital letters appears larger and more clear, it actually makes the print more difficult to read. Because capital letters do not vary in size and shape, it is difficult for the eye to differentiate between letters. Many recommend using bold print to highlight important aspects and to use upper and lower case letters in the text.

It is easier for the eye to read materials with a right margin that is "ragged," that is, lines of varying lengths, than to read materials with lines that are all the same length. Headings should be used for paragraphs. Each paragraph should present one idea and be about four sentences long. There should be enough space between paragraphs or sections of the print material so it does not appear crowded. Use of white space is pleasing to the eye and can also be used for emphasis.

A consideration particular to health-related materials is the inclusion of medical jargon and abbreviations. Even though the nurse understands the terms, the general public needs definitions of words that are not in everyday use (Weinrich and Boyd, 1992; Allensworth and Luther, 1986).

Selection of Materials for Target Groups. The selection of print materials appropriate for ethnic and cultural groups is of particular concern to the community health nurse. The assistance of a member of the target group is useful in selecting materials that avoid offending the community. Photographs or sketches of people should represent the ethnicity of the community. For example a booklet on new baby care with photographs of only white middle-class families is not likely to be effective in a community of low-income black single mothers.

The nurse must determine whether resources or commodities mentioned in the material are readily available in the community. For example a nutrition pamphlet emphasizing fresh fruits and vegetables is not useful if these foods are too expensive or not available in the community. A better choice of pamphlet might be one that compares the nutritional values of affordable and available frozen and canned foods.

NONPRINT MATERIALS

Purpose of Audiovisual Materials

Nonprint materials, often called audiovisuals (AVs), can take a variety of forms including a simple diagram or picture, audiotape, record, film, slides, transparencies, videotape, or radio, television, or computer-assisted learning (CAL) programs. Audiovisuals enhance learning through clarification and reinforcement and provide the convenience and cost-effectiveness of being used over and over without use of the nurse's time. Audiovisual materials can often be adjusted to the learner's own pace to meet individual learning needs.

Audiovisuals are used to provide experiences that might not be possible otherwise (Narrow, 1979). These include bringing an expert into the community via videotape, transporting the learner to a new community and culture, or allowing the learner to experience a life event—such as what happens during a heart attack—without actually being there.

TABLE 18–10

The SMOG Readability Formula

To calculate the SMOG reading grade level, begin with the entire written work that is being assessed and follow these four steps:

1. Count off 10 consecutive sentences near the beginning, in the middle, and near the end of the text.
2. From this sample of 30 sentences, circle all of the words containing three or more syllables (polysyllabic), including repetitions of the same word, and total the number of words circled.
3. Estimate the square root of the total number of polysyllabic words counted. This is done by finding the nearest perfect square and taking its square root.
4. Finally add a constant of 3 to the square root. This number gives the SMOG grade, or the reading grade level that a person must have achieved if he or she is to fully understand the text being assessed.

A few additional guidelines will help to clarify these directions:

a. A sentence is defined as a string of words punctuated with a period (.), an exclamation point (!), or a question mark (?).
b. Hyphenated words are considered as one word.
c. Numbers that are written out should also be considered, and if they are in numerical form in the text, they should be pronounced to determine whether they are polysyllabic.
d. Proper nouns, if polysyllabic, should also be counted.
e. Abbreviations should be read as unabbreviated to determine if they are polysyllabic.

Not all pamphlets, fact sheets, or other printed materials contain 30 sentences. To test a text that has fewer than 30 sentences:

1. Count all of the polysyllabic words in the text.
2. Count the number of sentences.
3. Find the average number of polysyllabic words per sentence as follows:

$$\text{Average} = \frac{\text{Total No. of polysyllabic words}}{\text{Total No. of sentences}}$$

4. Multiply that average by the number of sentences short of 30.
5. Add that figure to the total number of polysyllabic words.
6. Find the square root of the number you obtained in step 5, and add the constant of 3.

From: McLaughlin, G. H. (1969). SMOG grading: A new readability formula. *Journal of Reading, 12,* 639–646.

Perhaps the quickest way to administer the SMOG grading test is to use the SMOG conversion table. Simply count the number of polysyllabic words in your chain of 30 sentences and look up the approximate grade level on the following chart.

SMOG Conversion Table

Total Polysyllabic Word Counts	*Approximate Grade Level (±1.5)*
0–2	4
3–6	5
7–12	6
13–20	7
21–30	8
31–42	9
43–56	10
57–72	11
73–90	12
91–110	13
111–132	14
133–156	15
157–182	16
183–210	17
211–240	18

SMOG conversion table developed by Harold C. McGraw, Office of Educational Research, Baltimore County Schools, Towson, Maryland.

Selection of Audiovisual Materials

The nurse should preview the audiovisual aid and determine whether it is necessary to meet the learning objectives. All audiovisuals cost money. With current trends to limit health costs, the nurse is required to consider the cost of renting or purchasing the audiovisual aid.

The nurse also needs to consider the cost of nursing time. For example a videocassette about dietary fat and cholesterol may be expensive in both staff time and production costs. The nurse could easily teach the same information using less expensive charts or pictures. However if a learning objective is for each learner to plan low-fat meals for a week, keeping within the family budget, the investment in a CAL program could save nursing time. Instead of the nurse working with each learner individually, the learner would receive corrections and positive reinforcement from the computer.

TABLE 18–10

The SMOG Readability Formula *Continued*

Using the SMOG Readability Formula

CHILDREN AND ALCOHOL

Parents who are clear about not wanting their children to use illicit drugs may find it harder to be tough about alcohol. After all, alcohol is legal for adults, many parents drink, and alcohol is a part of some religious observances. As a result, we may view alcohol as a less dangerous substance than other drugs. The facts say otherwise.

> 4.6 million teenagers have a drinking problem.

> 4 percent of high school seniors drink alcohol every day.

> Alcohol related accidents are the leading cause of death among young people 15 to 24 years of age.

> About half of all youthful deaths in drowning, fires, suicide, and homicide are alcohol related.

> Young people who use alcohol at an early age are more likely to use alcohol heavily and to have alcohol related problems; they are also more likely to abuse other drugs and to get into trouble with the law.

> Young people whose body weight is lower than that of adults reach a higher blood alcohol concentration level than adults and show greater effects for longer periods of time.

$$\frac{\text{Total No. of polysyllabic words}}{\text{Total No. of sentences}} = \frac{28}{10} = 2.8 \times (30 - 10) = 56$$

56 + polysyllabic words (28) = 84

Nearest square root of 84 = 9

9 + constant 3 = 12th grade level

From U.S. Department of Education. (1990). *Growing up drug free: A parent's guide to prevention* (publication No. 269–883: QL Z). Washington, DC: U.S. Government Printing Office.

The nurse should determine the appropriateness of the audiovisual aid based on the reading and comprehension abilities of the target group. An audiotape or television program is not useful if the language is too difficult for the group to comprehend. The inclusion of spoken medical jargon is often a problem.

Lack of reading ability also affects the ability of the learner to understand pictures and diagrams. The nurse should assess pictures and captions for clarity. An important consideration for low-literacy learners is that the visual material should have a very limited objective, and the caption should be comprehensible to low-literacy readers (Doak et al., 1985).

Use of Audiovisual Materials

Use of audiovisual materials also depends on the equipment available. Nurses should practice using the equipment. When practicing the nurse should move about the room to be sure the audiovisual material can be seen and heard. Use of audiovisual equipment is not difficult, but the nurse should feel comfortable using it. The nurse should be able to solve such problems as burned-out light bulbs and upside-down slides. It is essential to remember to bring an extra light bulb and an extension cord to the presentation. Some of the advantages, disadvantages, and uses of audiovisual aids are listed in Table 18–11.

SOURCES OF EDUCATIONAL MATERIALS

Community health nurses who prepare educational programs need to locate sources for educational materials. The first place to start is your own agency. Virtually all community health agencies keep resource manuals, often compiled by the nurses themselves. Resources may be distributors of educational materials or other community agencies. Often businesses and agencies are able to supply

TABLE 18–11
Use of Audiovisual Teaching Aids

Overhead Transparencies

Advantages

1. Simple to plan and design
2. Does not usually require darkened room
3. Can be prepared by variety of simple, inexpensive methods
4. Simple-to-operate projector; presentation rate controlled by instructor
5. Can present information in a systematic, developmental sequence
6. Allows presenter to face audience, either sitting or standing
7. Color can be used for emphasis
8. Useful with large groups; provides more informality than slides
9. Can lessen dependency on notes
10. Can provide audience involvement

Disadvantages

1. Bulky projector
2. Projector often noisy; can be distracting to audience or interfere with view of screen
3. Tendency to disregard legibility requirements
4. "Keystoning" (distortion of picture) can occur

Flip Charts

Advantages

1. Very inexpensive
2. Simple to plan and prepare
3. Provides degree of informality
4. Useful for small to medium-sized groups in informal settings
5. Requires no special skill or training
6. Can be used in dynamic manner with audience involvement and feedback
7. Can be used to lessen dependency on notes for presentation

Disadvantages

1. Less dynamic and more limited in presenting information
2. Cannot be seen in large rooms
3. Impractical portability and storage
4. Difficult to change and resequence

Slides

Advantages

1. Colorful, realistic reproductions of original subjects
2. Easily revised and updated
3. Easily handled, stored, and rearranged for various uses
4. Useful for large groups and auditorium presentations
5. Remote control capability
6. Easily portable and compatible with universally available equipment
7. Can reduce dependency on notes

Disadvantages

1. Requires skill in photography or support personnel for preparation
2. Can get out of sequence
3. Tendency to put too much information on one slide because of ease of photography
4. If the slide can be read by holding 1 to 2 inches away, then information is legible; if not, then it is illegible
5. Requires darkened room

TABLE 18–11
Use of Audiovisual Teaching Aids *Continued*

Videotape

Advantages

1. Provides motion and color
2. Audience is accustomed to video viewing
3. Allows for easy replay
4. Equipment generally available
5. Can combine still and moving images
6. Picture and sound synchronized
7. Usually feasible to do some local production of reasonably high quality
8. Very useful with small groups
9. Tapes are portable and easy to store
10. Tape is reusable

Disadvantages

1. Resolution may not be appropriate for images with fine detail
2. Color may not be accurate
3. Requires trained support personnel for good production
4. Generally not suitable for large groups or auditorium presentations unless several monitors are used

Motion Pictures

Advantages

1. Provides motion with excellent color representation
2. Can combine still and moving images
3. Can be projected for large groups and auditorium presentations
4. Good image definition

Disadvantages

1. Expensive to produce
2. Requires careful planning and production skill
3. Film cannot be reused
4. Usually requires assistance (projectionist) to use in presentation

From Kemp, J. E. (1980). *Planning and producing audio-visual materials* (4th ed.). New York: Harper & Row.

or can suggest how to obtain materials. Another source to consider in your own agency is the educational services department. Most large community health agencies employ at least one person to coordinate health education.

Time on the telephone can bring great results. A telephone directory of community services is often on a bookshelf in your own agency. This volume is usually published annually by the state or local government. Do not overlook the regular telephone book as a resource for finding educational materials. There may be listings in the front of the book of governmental or private agencies that offer health services. Other places to look in the telephone book are in the government section or under health services or health care.

A special note for the nurse using the telephone is to create a personal resource telephone book. When a call is productive, make a brief note of the agency telephone number, services and materials available, and the name of the contact person. Networking, or the contacting of colleagues, is an invaluable tool for all aspects of nursing care delivery.

There are opportunities to locate educational materials from private sources. Businesses in the community such as pharmaceutical companies or manufacturers of medical devices sometimes supply materials. Businesses are usually very eager to supply the nurse educator with pamphlets and samples for the educational group. Often these materials are beautifully illustrated with photographs of people using specific products, and free samples such as diapers or coupons are sometimes provided. The nurse should review the materials for appropriateness before use. A free disposable diaper is a nice bonus, but will be used and discarded. The most appropriate pamphlet will last much longer.

Finally the nurse should visit the community library and the local video store. The library usually keeps catalogues of community resources. Many libraries and video stores loan videotapes with health information at minimal or no cost. Again review of these materials is needed before recommending them to the learners.

Some specific sources of health education information are listed in Table 18–12. This list is not meant to be exhaustive, but can be used as a starting point for nurses planning health education in the community.

PREPARING YOUR OWN TEACHING AIDS

If nurses cannot find appropriate teaching materials, they can design some. An advantage to designing teaching aids is the ability to make the teaching aid specific to the community. Nurses who teach and then make an audiotape for reinforcement enhance learning by the familiarity of their voice. Likewise videotapes, slides, or photographs with familiar faces and surroundings from the community can be an advantage. The nurse may choose to rewrite teaching aids that are too difficult for the target group to read, or to supplement existing materials with culture-specific information. Creating teaching aids can also be cost effective. Principles for assessment of print and audiovisual materials apply when designing teaching aids.

It is the rare individual who never says to herself or himself, I wish I could find . . . , or I wish I had saved . . . . Narrow (1979) has described an excellent method for the community health nurse to develop a resource file. Suggestions include cutting and saving articles and pictures in newspapers, magazines, pamphlets, or old books, being careful to note the source of each. These materials do not have to be from professional publications. A simple picture with an easy-to-read caption found in a lay magazine can be effective. Materials that cannot be cut out can be duplicated. With these clippings the nurse should develop a filing system; categorization can be by disease, by nursing diagnoses, or by health-related topic. Narrow (1979) suggests that all of these clippings should be filed about once per month and the file reviewed to discard information that is out of date. Using this file when looking for an educational aid or when the need exists to create your own educational aid will save time and energy.

TABLE 18–12

Sources of Health Education Materials

Education and Resource Locator Guides
American Hospital Association. (1985). *Patient educator's resource guide: Organizational and print resources for program development.* Chicago. 840 N. Lake Shore Dr. Chicago, IL 60611 (312) 280–6000 Order Processing Department: 1–800–AHA–2626
Guide to Locating Patient Education Audio-visual Materials. (1989). Reference Section, Public Services Division, National Library of Medicine, U.S. Department of Health and Human Services, Public Health Service, National Institutes of Health. St. Louis: Health Sciences Communications Association.
Frank, C. (Ed.). (1990). *Patient Education Sourcebook Volume 2.* St. Louis: Health Sciences Communications Association. 6105 Lindell Blvd. St. Louis, MO 63112 (no telephone orders)
Wasserman, P., & Grefsheim, S. (Eds.). (1987). *Encyclopedia of Health Information Sources.* Detroit: Gale Research Company. Book Tower 835 Penobscot Bldg. Detroit, MI 48226–4094
Weiner, D. J. (Ed.). (1991). *The Video Source Book,* (12th ed.). New York: Gale Research Company. Book Tower 835 Penobscot Bldg. Detroit, MI 48226–4094 1–800–877–4253
Health-Oriented National Organizations
American Cancer Society Audiovisual Program Assistant 19 W. 56th St. New York, NY 10019 (212) 320–3333
American Dental Association Bureau of Audiovisual Services 211 E. Chicago Ave. Chicago, IL 60611 (312) 440–2500 Sales: (800) 947–4746
American Health Foundation 320 E. 43rd St. New York, NY 10017–4849 (212) 953–1900
American Heart Association 7320 Greenville Ave. Dallas, TX 75231–4599 (214) 373–6300

Continued

TABLE 18–12

Sources of Health Education Materials *Continued*

Health-Oriented National Organizations *(continued)*

American Lung Association
1740 Broadway
New York, NY 10019–4373
(212) 315–8700
American Red Cross
431 18th St. N.W.
Washington, DC 20006
(202) 737–8300
Association for the Care of Children's Health
3615 Wisconsin Ave. N.W.
Washington, DC 20016
Health Insurance Association of America
1025 Connecticut Ave. N.W.
Suite 1200
Washington, DC 20036–5405
(202) 223–7780
National Dairy Council
111 N. Canal St.
Chicago, IL 60606
National Health Council
1730 M St. N.W.
Suite 500
Washington, DC 20036
(202) 785–3910

Selected Federal Government Clearinghouses

National Clearinghouse for *ALCOHOL AND DRUG* Information
P.O. Box 2345
Rockville, MD 20852
(301) 468–2600
Clearinghouse on *CHILD ABUSE AND NEGLECT* Information
P.O. Box 1182
Washington, DC 20013–1182
(703) 385–7565
(800) 394–3366
National *CHOLESTEROL* Education Program Information Center
P.O. Box 30105
Bethesda, MD 20814–0105
(301) 251–1222
(301) 951–3260
National *DIABETES* Information Center
Box NDIC
9000 Rockville Pike
Bethesda, MD 20892
(301) 468–2162
FOOD AND NUTRITION Information Center
National Agricultural Library, Room 304
Beltsville, MD 20705–2351
(301) 504–5719
National HEALTH INFORMATION Clearinghouse
P.O. Box 1133
Washington, DC 20013
Center for HEALTH PROMOTION AND EDUCATION
Centers for Disease Control and Prevention
1600 Clifton Rd., NE
Atlanta, GA 30333
National *HIGH BLOOD PRESSURE* Education Program Information Center
P.O. Box 30105
Bethesda, MD 20814–0105
(301) 251–1222

TABLE 18–12

Sources of Health Education Materials *Continued*

Selected Federal Government Clearinghouses *(continued)*

Office of *MINORITY HEALTH* Resource Center
P.O. Box 37337
Washington, DC 20013–7337
(800) 444–6472
(301) 587–1983
Clearinghouse for *OCCUPATIONAL SAFETY* and Health Information
Technical Information Branch
4676 Columbia Pkwy.
Cincinnati, OH 45226–1988
(800) 35-NIOSH
President's Council on *PHSYICAL FITNESS* and Sports
701 Pennsylvania Ave. N.W.
Suite 250
Washington, DC 20004
(202) 272–3421
Consumer *PRODUCT SAFETY* Commission
5401 Westbard Ave.
Bethesda, MD 20816–1469
(301) 504–0800
Office on *SMOKING* and Health
Technical Information Center Park Building, Room 1–16
5600 Fishers Ln.
Rockville, MD 20857

Principles of Teaching

We can now consider the teaching principles that the nurse can use throughout the health education process. The nurse can think of these principles as an umbrella covering the entire teaching-learning process. A little bit of coverage can make the experience more comfortable for the nurse and the learners (Fig. 18–2).

PHYSICAL ENVIRONMENT

Location of the meeting is the initial consideration. A convenient location prevents transportation problems that prohibit attendance. Often health education occurs in health centers or in public facilities such as schools, libraries, or fire halls. In areas with public transportation these places are generally accessible during the day, but may not be as accessible during the evening, especially if bus routes change after business hours. In rural areas or areas with no public transportation educational programs may be offered in conjunction with other events such as church meetings.

Another consideration is the safety of the neighborhood and available lighting if the educational session is held in the evening. It may be possible for the nurse to make some security arrangements at the facility if problems exist. Encouraging participants to "come with a friend" is another good suggestion to promote safety.

The nurse should preview the physical environment to assess the size of the room and ensure adequate seating for

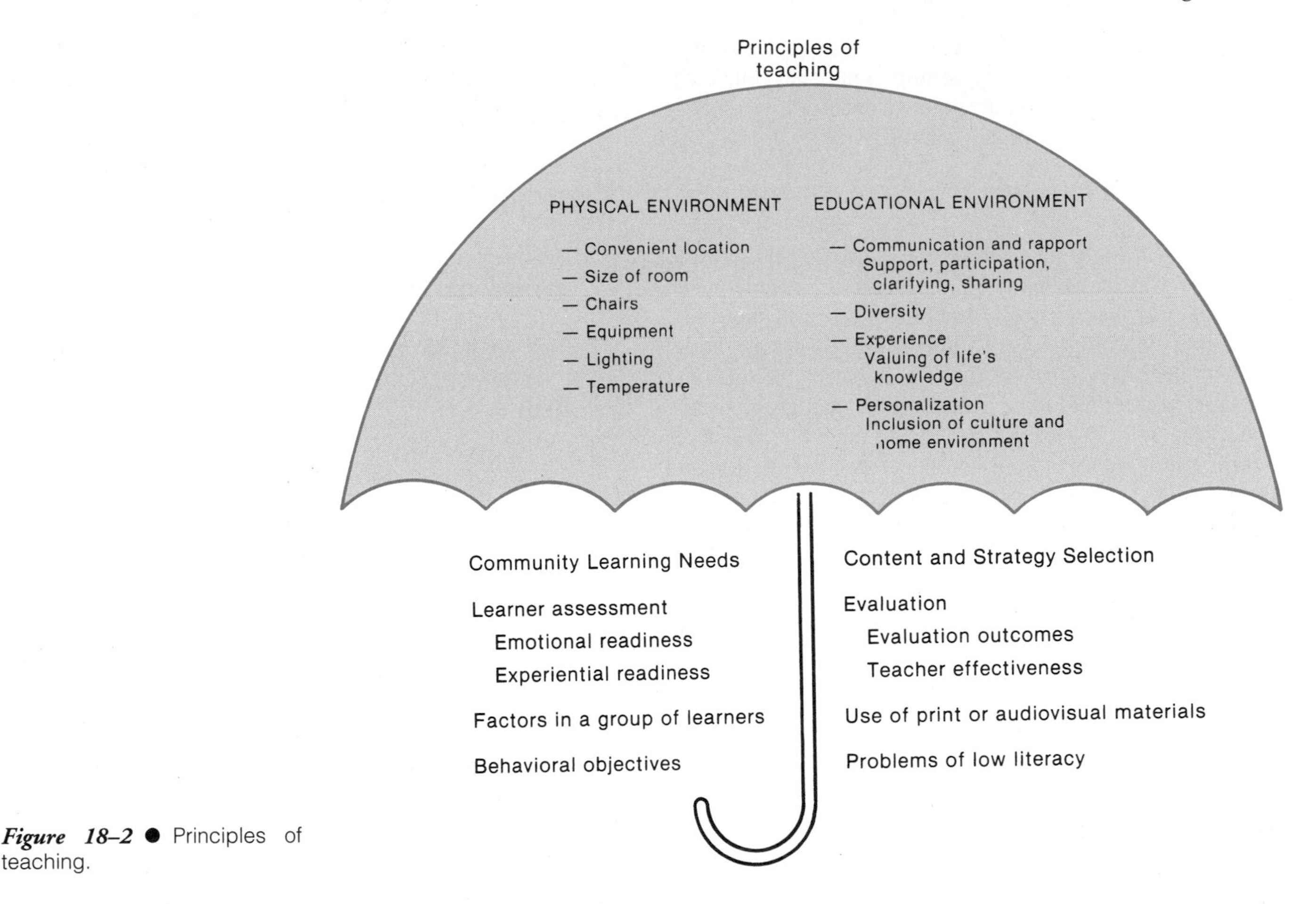

Figure 18–2 ● Principles of teaching.

the number of people expected. The nurse should arrange seating to suit the educational plan before the group arrives. If small group discussion is planned, chairs around a circular table is ideal. For larger groups just a circle of chairs is appropriate. If lecture and demonstration are planned, chairs in a semicircle allow everyone to see the demonstration. With very large groups use of several semicircular rows is still effective if the chairs are not directly behind one another. If a large group breaks into smaller groups after a lecture, the nurse can ask the group to take a few minutes to rearrange their seats for small group time.

Two comfort factors are the lighting and temperature of the room. The ability to adjust the lighting is particularly important when using slides or television. The nurse should practice lighting adjustments before the group arrives. Temperature is important because learners who are too cold or too warm may have difficulty concentrating.

EDUCATIONAL ENVIRONMENT

In addition to assessing and altering the physical environment, the nurse should adjust the educational environment to promote the optimal learning experience. Using the following principles the nurse can improve the response of the participants to the educational program.

Communication and Rapport

Learning should be a shared experience. The nurse's communication skills and ability to develop rapport with the learners enhance education. When the nurse offers some initial information about credentials and experience it increases the group's confidence in the nurse as a resource. The nurse should encourage group participation and communicate willingness to support the learners until objectives are met. The nurse may want to increase the learners' comfort by assuring the freedom to ask questions and make mistakes within the group.

The nurse needs to be flexible. Even when a lecture is planned the nurse needs to allow time for audience participation, especially with adult learners who expect to share. The nurse needs to develop the ability to reinforce and clarify health information for the group. Rapport is enhanced as the nurse values member contributions to the group.

The nurse might not be able to answer all discussion questions. A candid statement such as, "I don't know the answer to that, but I can look for it," or "Let me tell you some of the resources we could both use to find the answer," supports the learner's needs and creates a climate of shared responsibility for learning. This also reinforces for adult learners that it is acceptable to ask for help and use community resources to meet learning needs.

Diversity

The nurse should plan the health education program to provide a variety of learning experiences. Based on the assessment of learner needs teaching strategies should be matched to learning styles. Some people learn by doing, some by hearing, others by reading. A variety of teaching strategies will retain learner interest and meet group needs. The opportunity to choose a strategy to meet the objectives also meets the needs of adult learners for self-direction and control over the learning environment.

Experience

Each learner brings his or her experiences, positive or negative, into the educational setting. The nurse needs to consider individual experiences when planning the content and strategies for health education. Listening carefully to the experiences of the group gives the nurse the needed information. The learner who has had a negative experience with health education could be reluctant to participate. In this situation it is particularly important for the nurse to develop rapport and clearly assess learner needs.

Personalization

Learners will have differences in age, gender, experience, socioeconomic status, culture, and other factors. The use of cultural examples in the content can be useful for personalization. Learning can also be personalized with the use of individual learning contracts.

Another way to personalize teaching is to ask the learners how they will apply the knowledge at home. Sharing application ideas in the group provides reinforcement of content and also stimulates learning by encouraging others to try new ideas.

KEY IDEAS

1. Delivery of health education is an increasingly important role of the community health nurse. The current public and professional emphasis on health and wellness provides the perfect opportunity for community health nurses to use their teaching skills.
2. Promotion of a healthy lifestyle through health education is a vital aspect of community health nursing.
3. To plan and implement health education programs the nurse must have an awareness of the teaching-learning process and how it can be applied in a variety of community settings with individuals, families, and groups.
4. Assessment of the community and the learners is necessary before the content and strategies for health education are planned.
5. Behavioral objectives are a useful tool for planning and evaluating learning experiences.
6. Content and strategies of the educational program should be tailored to the needs of the community or group.
7. Print and audiovisual materials need to be carefully analyzed prior to use.
8. A variety of teaching techniques, personalized instruction, and interpersonal support promote lifestyle changes.
9. Principles of teaching can be used to enhance the teaching-learning process.

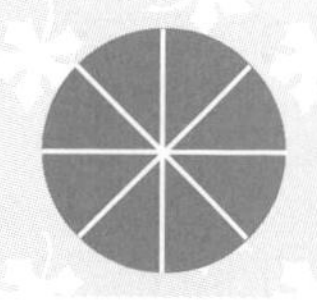

CASE STUDY: *Planning a Health Education Program*

Ginny is a community health nurse who has spent most of her career working in ambulatory care clinics. She decided she needed a change and moved to a new community. She quickly found a challenging job as an occupational health nurse in an electronics plant. Part of the job description for her new job includes planning and implementing health education programs.

After spending a few months in her new office Ginny has begun to see some trends in the type of assistance and individuals who are seeking it. Many of them are young men, 25 to 35 years old, who request blood pressure checkups. Most of the men have normal blood pressure and Ginny is not sure why they continue to come to her office. Ginny enjoys talking and begins to conduct informal assessments on the workers as they come to see her. Many of them have young families to support and fear losing their jobs. Some talk with her about the inability to cope with problems at home and the inability to sleep at night. Few of them perform any regular cardiovascular exercise, and when she sees them in the cafeteria, Ginny observes them eating high-fat foods with little nutritional value. When their weight and height are assessed more than two thirds of the men are found to be overweight. Ginny wants to begin her health teaching programs, but cannot decide what content to include. She is not sure whether she needs to do any more assessment of the group, as she may already have more health teaching to do than she can handle.

Where should Ginny begin? Is her needs assessment complete? How should she prioritize the content of the teaching program? Does she know enough about the learners to plan teaching strategies? Will anyone be interested in participating in a health education program?

Teaching Plan

Needs Assessment and Learning Diagnosis

Ginny recognizes the need for health education on cardiovascular health, diet, and stress reduction. She also recognizes the importance of continuing the establishment of rapport. To begin her health education series Ginny plans to combine a continued needs assessment with a brief health teaching session.

The needs assessment will help Ginny clarify the priorities of the learning needs. A brief teaching will help to establish rapport and identify herself as a resource to the workers.

The health teaching will be "You Are Too Busy to Exercise." Ginny has chosen exercise because daily exercise can positively affect each of the identified health problems.

Ginny makes sure that the health education session is held at a convenient time, and that all workers are given paid time to attend if they desire. The needs assessment is accomplished by briefly sharing her observations, and requesting a show of hands to indicate interest in the cardiovascular health topics. Ginny is also open to discussion and suggestions for future topics, and writes these on the overhead.

Constructing the Lesson Plans

Overall Goal. The learners will participate in daily physical activities that promote health and well-being.

Behavioral Objectives (Samples)

1. Ninety-eight percent of the learners will determine two times during the work day when they could walk instead of using the elevator or shuttle bus.
2. Ninety-eight percent of the learners will select two enjoyable physical activities that can be integrated into the family lifestyle.
3. Sixty percent of the learners will engage in physical activity for 30 minutes three times during the week.
4. Ninety percent of the learners will explore their feelings about starting an exercise program.

Content

- Health benefits of a regular exercise program
- Safety considerations for beginners, e.g., existing health problems
- Examples of how to fit exercise into daily life
- Popular family activities that promote exercise and family togetherness
- How to choose an activity program that you will continue
- Examples of common excuses for not exercising
- Benefits of support from others
- List of community resources for low-cost activities

Teaching Strategies

- Lecture
- Small group discussion for generation of more ideas and examples
- Use of overhead projector for listing of group ideas
- Use of "buddy system" to offer support
- Role playing of the sedentary worker and his or her support buddy offering encouragement
- Continued intervention by giving each participant a hang-tag for his or her rear-view mirror with a reminder to park far away and walk to work
- Provision of pamphlets and brochures from community groups that offer organized activities

Evaluation Methods and Results

- "Game-show" style questions were used to evaluate objectives 1 and 2; all of the participants were able to meet the objectives during the class.
- Objective 4 was measured by observing the participants verbally sharing ideas in class and in small groups. All of the participants were able to meet this objective.
- To evaluate objective 3 participants were asked to report their exercise patterns at 1 month. Seventy percent of the participants reported increasing exercise to 30 minutes three times per week.

Additional Evaluation

- Evaluation of teacher effectiveness was accomplished by using an evaluation tool (see Table 18–9).
- Evaluation of the need for additional health education sessions was based on requests to repeat the session by workers who could not attend and on attendance at subsequent sessions.

GUIDELINES FOR LEARNING

① Select a teaching aid such as a booklet or pamphlet that you have used in the past for health education of a family or group. Analyze the teaching aid for readability, content, and format. Noting your results, will you use the material again or look for different material?

② Talk with a community health nurse about some completed group health education sessions. Did the nurse consider the education to be successful? What criteria were used to measure success? What would the nurse do differently if she or he were repeating the program? Was the nurse reimbursed specifically for teaching or was it considered part of the job?

③ Working with a peer group, develop a health education plan for implementation either with actual clients or with a group of peers. Videotape the implementation of the program. With the group review the videotape and offer constructive suggestions to one another on the improvement of your teaching techniques.

④ Participate as a learner in a nurse-coordinated health education group in your community. How did you choose the group that you attended? Were your learning needs met? Did you experience a change in behavior? What made the experience a positive or a negative one?

REFERENCES

Allensworth, D., & Luther, C. (1986). Evaluating printed materials. *Nurse Educator, 11* (2), 18–22.

American Nurses' Association (ANA). (1986). *ANA standards of community health nursing practice.* Washington, DC: Author.

ANA. (1991). *ANA standards of nursing practice.* Washington, DC: Author.

ANA. (1980). *Nursing: A social policy statement.* Washington, DC: Author.

Atwood, H., & Ellis, J. (1971). Concept of need: An analysis for adult education. *Adult Leadership, 19,* 210–212.

Bille, D. (1981). *Practical approaches to patient teaching.* Boston: Little, Brown.

Bloom, B. S. (Ed.). (1956). *Taxonomy of educational objectives: The classification of educational goals.* New York: David McKay.

Burmeister, L. (1978). *Reading strategies for middle and secondary school teachers.* Reading, MA: Addison-Wesley.

Davis, T., Crouch, M., Wills, G., Miller, S., & Abdehou, D. (1990). The gap between patient reading comprehension and the readability of patient education materials. *The Journal of Family Practice, 31* (5), 533–538.

De Muth, J. S. (1989). Patient teaching in the ambulatory setting. *Nursing Clinics of North America, 24*(3), 645–655.

de Tornay, R., & Thompson, M. A. (1982). *Strategies for teaching nursing* (2nd ed.). New York: John Wiley & Sons.

Doak, C., Doak, L., & Root, J. (1985). *Teaching patients with low literacy skills.* Philadelphia: J. B. Lippincott.

Flesch, R. (1949). *The art of readable writing.* New York: Harper & Row.

Fry, E. (1977). Fry's readability graph: Clarification, validity, and extension to level 17. *Journal of Reading, 21,* 242–252.

Gessner, B. A. (1989). Adult education: The cornerstone of patient teaching. *Nursing Clinics of North America, 24*(3), 589–595.

Green, L., Kreuter, M., Deeds, S., & Partridge, K. (1980). *Health education planning: A diagnostic approach.* Palo Alto, CA: Mayfield Publishing.

Grolund, N. E. (1970). *Stating behavioral objectives for classroom instruction.* New York: Macmillan.

Janosik, E. H., & Phipps, L. B. (1982). *Life cycle group work in nursing.* Monterey, CA: Wadsworth.

Joyce, B., & Weil, M. (1980). *Models of teaching* (2nd ed.). Englewood Cliffs, NJ: Prentice-Hall.

Kaufman, M., Hawkins, J. W., Higgins, L. P., & Friedman, A. H. (Eds.). (1988). *Dictionary of American nursing biography.* Westport CT: Greenwood Press.

Kemp, J. E. (1980). *Planning and producing audio-visual materials.* New York: Harper & Row.

Lindeman, C. A. (1988). Nursing research in patient education. *Annual Review of Nursing Research, 6,* 29–60.

McLaughlin, G. H. (1969). SMOG grading: A new readability formula. *Journal of Reading, 12,* 639–646.

Narrow, B. W. (1979). *Patient teaching in nursing practice.* New York: John Wiley & Sons.

Oberst, M. (1989). Perspectives on research in patient teaching. *Nursing Clinics of North America, 24*(3), 621–628.

Rankin, S., & Duffy, K. (1983). *Patient education: Issues, principles, and guidelines.* Philadelphia: J.B. Lippincott.

Redman, B. K. (1984). *The process of patient education,* (5th ed.). St. Louis: Mosby.

Redman, B. K. (1988). *The process of patient education* (6th ed.). St. Louis: Mosby–Year Book.

Rosenstock, I. M. (1974). Historical origins of the health belief model. In M. Becker (Ed.). *The health belief model and personal behavior.* Thorofare, NJ: Slack.

Smith, C. E. (1989). Overview of patient education. *Nursing Clinics of North America, 24*(3), 583–587.

Spadero, D. C. (1983). Assessing readability of patient information materials. *Pediatric Nursing, 9*(4), 274–287.

Spellbring, A. M. (1991). Nursing's role in health promotion. *Nursing Clinics of North America, 26*(4), 805–814.

Streiff, L. (1986). Can clients understand our instructions?. *IMAGE: Journal of Nursing Scholarship, 18*(2), 48–52.

Stromborg, M., & Cohen, R. (1991). Evaluating written patient education materials. *Seminars in Oncology Nursing, 7*(2), 125–134.

U.S. Department of Health and Human Services (1990). *Healthy people 2000: National health promotion and disease prevention objectives. Summary report.* Washington, DC: U.S. Government Printing Office.

Weinrich, S., & Boyd, M. (1992). Education in the elderly: Adapting and evaluating teaching tools. *Journal of Gerontological Nursing, 18,*(1) 15–20.

BIBLIOGRAPHY

Maraldo, P. J., & Solomon, S. B. (1987). Nursing's window of opportunity. *IMAGE: Journal of Nursing Scholarship, 19,* 83–86.

Rankin, S., & Stallings, K. (1990). *Patient education: Issues, principles, practices* (2nd ed.). Philadelphia: J. B. Lippincott.

SUGGESTED READINGS

Dixon, E., & Park, R. (1990). Do patients understand written health information? *Nursing Outlook, 38*(6), 278–281.

Evans, L. K. (1980). Health education from a group perspective. *Topics in Clinical Nursing, 2*(2), 45–48.

Miller, A. (1985). When is the time ripe for teaching? *American Journal of Nursing, 85* (7), 801–803.

Rice, M., & Valdivia, L. (1991). A simple guide for design, use, and evaluation of educational materials. *Health Education Quarterly, 18*(1), 80–85.

Unit V

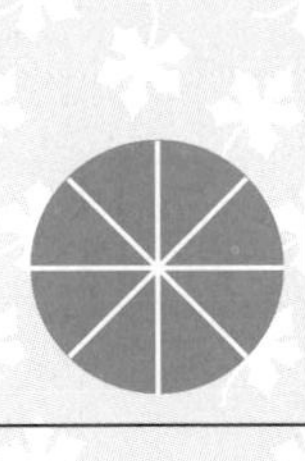

Contemporary Problems in Community Health Nursing

19
Communicable Diseases

20
Family Violence

21
Common Addictions

22
Teenage Pregnancy

23
Homelessness in America

24
Environmental Issues: At Home, at Work, and in the Community

Chapter 19

Communicable Diseases

Linda K. Matocha

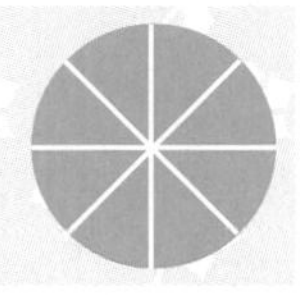

Continued

Focus Questions

What methods have been used historically to safeguard populations against communicable diseases?

What are the elements of a communicable disease, and how do they interact?

How do boards of health demonstrate responsibilities for controlling the spread of communicable diseases?

Why are the concepts of epidemiology appropriate to use for prevention and control of communicable diseases?

What are the implications for the nursing process in caring for individuals and families with communicable diseases?

Where can nurses and patients obtain information about support resources for coping with communicable diseases?

Historical Perspective

Communicable diseases occur in every country, in every urban and rural area, and in every neighborhood from the very rich to the very poor. Nurses who provide quality care in combating communicable diseases must have a basic understanding of epidemiology, infection control, microbiology, medicine, public health, and nursing. Furthermore, the community nurse must have knowledge of the legal system, which mandates prevention and control of communicable diseases locally, nationally, and worldwide. Nurses must also have knowledge of effective support systems that can be used by individuals, families, and communities. Much of this understanding and knowledge can be acquired when the community nurse studies the effects of communicable diseases from a historical perspective.

DISEASE CONTROL: BIBLICAL TIMES THROUGH THE 1900S

Communicable diseases such as smallpox and leprosy were reported even before the birth of Christ. In fact, leprosy was mentioned in the book of Leviticus in the Bible. An early written account of an epidemic recorded a plague in the Byzantine Empire about 550 A.D. (Aronson, 1978). Plague raged intermittently throughout Europe and China during the 13th and 14th centuries, decimating the population.

During the 14th century physicians first formulated a theory that attempted to explain the communicable disease process. That first theory contained some elements of truth, as follows:

1. Disease spreads through contact with an infected person or article or through environmental factors such as putrid air caused by decaying bodies, waste, garbage, and stagnant water.
2. Poorly nourished and unsanitary individuals are at risk of contracting infection.

In addition to identifying factors that bore some relation to the infectious process, the theory also declared that weather conditions and a person's moral life influenced disease spread (Risse, 1988).

The Venetians developed quarantine measures in an effort to control the spread of plague in 1656. Ships were inspected and, if infection was found, quarantined. Overland trade was suspended to keep infected people and goods from entering Venice. Public gatherings were not allowed, and schools were closed. Streets were cleaned. The sick were confined—forcibly, if necessary—to "pest houses." These measures had only limited success, as more than 10,000 citizens died from plague (Risse, 1988). Currently quarantine, sanitary precautions, and travel restrictions remain part of the arsenal used in communicable disease control.

During the 19th century the vector's role in disease transmission was still unknown (Table 19–1). Scientists developed the theory of miasma in an effort to explain the indirect transmission of disease. Communicable diseases were caused by "bad" air and an environment responsible for the spontaneous generation of infectious agents. Although this theory was not totally correct, it led to the initiation of public health control measures. Some of these (e.g., elimination of garbage, refuse, and animal remains; draining of stagnant water) often resulted in less disease because the breeding places of organisms were destroyed.

The cholera epidemic in Europe during the 1800s forced a reexamination of the prevailing theory of disease spread. Cholera spread too rapidly to be blamed on the slow development of putrid air, and it infected people who were "morally just" and lived in clean, sanitary conditions. In 1839 Theodor Schwann proposed the cell as the basic unit of life, stimulating scientists to research factors that could affect the cell. By 1900, 21 microorganisms had been identified and linked to specific diseases, including diphtheria, tuberculosis, pneumonia, and typhoid fever (Dowling, 1977). Jacob Henle developed the criteria used to link an organism to a specific disease. He maintained that to determine cause and effect, an organism must first be identified, then isolated, and finally used to generate the disease.

With the identification of disease-specific organisms, the science of microbiology was born. At last the components of a communicable disease were known. Sanitary regulation of the environment and isolation of infected individuals were accepted as strategies useful in reducing the effects of some communicable diseases. These control measures were widely enforced. Streets were cleaned, the throwing of garbage into rivers and streets was discouraged, standing water was drained, and infected individuals were isolated.

Communicable disease control measures in the United States were enacted a little later than those in the European community. Most immigrants to America were farmers and tradesmen, not scientists, and they had little understanding of how disease spread. Furthermore, in the colonies people lived farther apart, so the sanitation precautions considered beneficial in Europe were not thought to be necessary. After the colonies experienced several smallpox epidemics brought with new immigrants from Europe, they instituted communicable disease controls. By the mid-1800s laws governing quarantine were in place. In Boston ships in

TABLE 19–1

Communicable Disease Terminology

Agent: Any microorganism that can cause the infection. It may be a bacterium, virus, fungus, or parasite.
Antigenic variations: Different antigens of an organism resulting in the inability of an antigen to stimulate antibody response.
Antimicrobial agent: A substance that kills or inhibits the growth of an infectious organism.
Artificial immunity: Immunity induced by man-made vaccines or immunoglobins.
Biological agent: A substance made from a live disease-producing organism, used to kill or inhibit the growth of an infectious organism.
Carrier: A person who serves as a support for an agent and yet does not exhibit signs or symptoms of the disease. This person may infect others and can be a carrier for a short or long period of time.
Endogenous infection: An infection that lives within the host; symptoms result when the healthy balance between the host and agent are disrupted.
Exogenous infection: Infection is transmitted from outside the host.
Host: An animal or human that can sustain the life of an infectious agent.
Infective dose: The number of organisms required to cause infection in a host.
Invasiveness: The ability of the organism to enter the host and disseminate through the tissues.
Morbidity: The disease rate usually expressed as prevalence of disease. It can also be expressed as a ratio of the number infected with a disease to the total number in a population.
Mortality: The death rate from a disease. It can also be expressed as ratio of the number died from a disease to the number infected with the disease.
Natural immunity: The immunity achieved when an animal or human is infected with an organism and antigenic response occurs naturally within the body.
Nosocomial: An infection acquired during care, not the reason for seeking care; usually related to infectious agents in the care environment.
Pandemic: An epidemic occurring around the world.
Pathogenicity: The proficiency of the organism to generate the disease; usually described in terms of the organism's virulence and invasiveness.
Period of infectivity: The period of time when the source is contagious.
Reservoir: The site where the agent (organism) is naturally found. A carrier can serve as a reservoir.
Resistance: The ability of an organism to remain unaffected when exposed to an infectious agent.
Source: The place where the agent is transferred from a host or reservoir through direct or indirect transmission by a vehicle; the immediate place from which an organism is transmitted.
Vector: A carrier for infections; usually an insect but can be an animal.
Vehicle: An inanimate object that transmits infectious organisms.
Virulence: The severity of the disease produced by the organism; usually described in terms of morbidity, mortality, and communicability of the disease.

which infection was found were required to fly a red flag, and red flags were put on houses with infected family members. Citizens were encouraged to avoid contact with people in "red flag" households. As in Europe, this method of control was not totally effective.

In 1869 the first state health department was established in Massachusetts; other states soon followed. By 1901 all but five states had some type of board of health. The Massachusetts health department controlled communicable diseases through regulation of sanitary conditions and by building water and sewage systems. As boards of health developed they began to realize the importance of accurate statistics in tracking and controlling communicable diseases. Statistics provided a way to identify trends, incidence, and effective treatment.

Communicable disease control at the federal level was almost nonexistent until the 1800s. The Fifth Congress of the United States passed an act in 1798 designed to furnish health assistance for seamen. In 1872 the Marine Hospital Service, the forerunner of the Public Health Service, and the American Public Health Association were founded. The American Public Health Association provided a forum for physicians and other public health workers to set standards of care. In 1878 the Quarantine Act was passed, granting the federal government the power to impose quarantine. In 1912 the Marine Hospital Service officially became the Public Health Service (PHS), and states were held responsible for reporting statistics to the federal government via the PHS (Mullan, 1989).

Federal support for research assistance in communicable disease control led to several important actions. In 1930, the Ransdell Act established the National Institute of Health (NIH), which continues to be the major source of research for the U.S. Public Health Service. In 1946 the Communicable Disease Center, currently known as the Centers for Disease Control and Prevention (CDC), was established. CDC's original mandate was for infectious disease control. Over the years, however, its scope has expanded to include an emphasis on noninfectious diseases and environmental issues. The CDC is responsible for collecting morbidity and mortality statistics on reportable infectious diseases.

The 1970s was a decade of health reform and legislation. The needs of migrant workers were supported, and vaccines were made available to the poor. The funding for the NIH was increased, and a national effort began to decrease the incidence of cancer, heart attacks and strokes. In the 1980s the important role of the PHS was underscored by the advent of human immunodeficiency virus (HIV) infection. The need for HIV prevention and education efforts, the issue of confidential or anonymous testing and counseling, the need for contact tracing and notification, and the care of infected individuals in hospitals and in the community have served to emphasize the need for a public health response to communicable diseases.

ROLE OF THE NURSE IN COMMUNICABLE DISEASE CONTROL

Historically nursing has been an integral part of disease control. Individuals with communicable diseases have always needed reliable nursing care. Initially nursing was provided by members of religious orders, who were often the only help available during epidemics. In 1883 communicable disease nursing was based primarily on the premise of preventing disease spread through cleanliness and fresh air. Aronson (1978) recalls the safety precautions for nurses making home visits:

> Before leaving the patient's house, the nurse was required to wash her hands with carbolic soap and rinse her mouth with a fresh potassium permanganate solution. It was very important for the nurse . . . to do the disinfection because . . . people were very slow to learn. . . . (p. 15).

In addition to caring for the sick, teaching hygiene to families was a major responsibility of community nurses and is still a primary focus in the current control of communicable disease today.

ISSUES OF POPULATION SAFETY VERSUS INDIVIDUAL RIGHTS

Throughout history governments and public health officials have struggled with the problem of balancing individual rights with the right of the community to be protected from infection. As a general rule, the safety of populations has taken precedence over individual rights. To reduce the risk of exposure in populations, individual rights have been curtailed or revoked. For example:

- Lepers were forced to wear bells or special colors to warn others of their passing.
- Lepers were quarantined in separate communities.
- Cities required individuals to dispose of their sewage in approved privies.
- People who polluted water sources were imprisoned.
- Plague victims were isolated in their homes or removed to central "infected houses."
- During epidemics, the names of infected individuals were published.

The same strategies were used in other epidemics, including the measles epidemics early in this century. Failure to comply with regulations was punished by civil penalties such as fines or by more drastic measures such as imprisonment or execution (Risse, 1988).

In the United States, similar isolation techniques were followed, often at the expense of individual rights or property:

- In 1888 the Marine Hospital Service quarantined yellow fever victims in a camp close to the Florida border.
- In 1900 the citizens of Chinatown in San Francisco were driven from their homes to quarantine camps, and some homes and businesses were set afire during a plague epidemic.
- In the 1914 and 1919 polio epidemics, physicians and nurses made house-to-house searches to identify all infected persons. Infected children were removed to hospitals, and the rest of the family was quarantined until noninfectious. Parents could not leave their home to bury their child if the child died in the hospital.
- During World War I prostitutes were confined in central locations and treated to reduce the spread of venereal disease epidemics.
- During that same war the first widespread immunization program mandated that children be vaccinated against typhoid (Risse, 1988).

Today the issue of individual rights versus community protection is an ongoing concern. Workplace safety is one important issue. Carriers of hepatitis A are restricted from certain jobs such as food handling. The CDC recommends that HIV-infected health care workers be selectively assigned to duties so as not to place other health care workers or patients at risk. The CDC recommends that persons at risk for HIV infection not give blood and that they change risky sexual and intravenous drug practices.

An important area in which individual rights clash with public safety is the right of people to continue to knowingly place others at risk. Two salient contemporary examples of this problem are the following:

1. What should be done with a tuberculosis patient who refuses to follow the treatment regimen?
2. What should be done with an HIV-infected individual who continues to share needles or engage in unprotected sex after diagnosis?

Some states have laws to enforce treatment of tuberculosis to protect the public. Most public health practitioners prefer to enroll the patient in the treatment regimen by using education, encouragement, and careful monitoring of compliance. However, if these measures fail, individuals may be restrained in hospitals or institutions for a course of therapy until they are no longer infectious and the disease is contained (see Ethics Box I).

The problem of HIV-infected persons who continue risky behaviors is more difficult. How would you go about monitoring what people are doing in their private lives? Should you even try? Health care workers have been struggling with this dilemma for quite some time. Unlike tuberculosis, HIV and the acquired immunodeficiency syndrome (AIDS) have no cure. If you were to confine these patients, for how long would you do so? For life? At the present time only a few AIDS patients have been confined against their will because of their refusal to protect others against infection.

Epidemiology Applied to Communicable Disease Control

Epidemiology began as the study of communicable diseases affecting large populations (see Chapter 11). While the scope of epidemiology has expanded to include noncommunicable diseases and other health-related issues, epidemiological principles are still the backbone of communicable disease control.

Ethics Box I

Gail A. DeLuca Havens, M.S., R.N., C.N.A.

Tension between Individual and Societal Rights

Codes of ethics can be thought of as moral codes. Moral commitments "to uphold the values and special moral obligations" (American Nurses' Association [ANA], 1985, p. i), such as maintaining competency in practice, are expressed in the ANA Code for Nurses and made by individuals when they become nurses. The fundamental concept underlying the Code for Nurses is respect for persons. Certain principles growing out of this concept guide nurses' decision making. These include fostering self-determination, doing good, avoiding harm, being truthful, respecting privileged information, keeping promises, and treating people fairly. In their moral decision-making hierarchy, Beauchamp and Childress (1989) refer to principles and rules as action guides. Principles are the more global and basic conceptions that justify the rules.

When considering ethical principles, it is important to remember that individuals are *interdependent* members of a community. The nurse will encounter situations when the tension between individual liberty and the need to preserve the health and well-being of the community creates an ethical dilemma in practice. For instance, the nurse promises, as expressed by the principle of fidelity in the ANA Code, to maintain patient confidentiality. However, such a promise is not absolute when innocent parties are in direct jeopardy (ANA, 1985) (e.g., threatened with being killed). This particular kind of dilemma is made even more troublesome for the nurse who is attempting to deal with two opposing or contradictory promises. For example, the implicit promise of the nurse to maintain patient confidentiality, as expressed in the ANA Code, may contradict the nurse's obligation to obey a law that requires reporting a particular situation (Veatch and Fry, 1987). The nurse also has an ethical responsibility to respect the client and promote self-determination. Consider the following situation.

Kay is a community health nurse who has been employed by a home health agency for more than 10 years. Several of her clients live in a homeless shelter and have been referred to her agency for follow-up tuberculosis treatment after hospital discharge. Today she is making her first visit to Paolo, a 33-year-old Hispanic man discharged after hospitalized treatment for acute, infectious tuberculosis. Kay explains that her agency, along with the city's health department, helps persons with tuberculosis continue to take their medication as prescribed until they are cured.

Kay asks Paolo how he is feeling this morning. He replies that he is tired; he didn't sleep well this first night in a place not familiar to him. After she completes Paolo's admission history and physical examination, Kay tells him that she, or a nurse substituting for her, will be visiting Paolo daily for 2 weeks to observe him taking his medication and then twice weekly for at least 6 months. Paolo protests that he is not a child and that he can be depended on to take his medication as prescribed. Kay explains that the current standard of care is that everyone in the community being treated for tuberculosis receives directly observed medication therapy. It will help him remember to continue to take medication as prescribed, particularly when he begins to feel better. Stopping the medication makes the treatment he received in the hospital ineffective. Stopping medication often results in tuberculosis becoming infectious again. In addition, not completing treatment increases the likelihood that he will develop a type of tuberculosis that is resistant to medication therapy (Bayer et al., 1993). He could feel very ill again. The city has an obligation to protect its residents from becoming infected with tuberculosis. Kay tells Paolo that she will be communicating with the health department because they are the ones who referred him to her.

Paolo agrees, reluctantly, to cooperate in therapy. He asks how long it will take to be cured. Kay knows that the response to therapy varies, but most persons can be cured within 3 to 18 months (Bayer et al., 1993). Kay explains that 6 months of medication has been prescribed to cure his tuberculosis. Before Kay leaves, Paolo takes his first dose of medication, and they establish a schedule for his observed daily self-administration.

Continued

Paolo's treatment continues as planned over the next several months. He gains strength and eventually finds a job. Returning to work requires that his medication regimen be modified. Paolo has no trouble adapting it to his more demanding schedule. Several weeks pass with this new arrangement until, one evening, Paolo does not appear. Kay leaves a message for him to call her, but does not hear from him. When Paolo fails to appear again the following evening, Kay returns to the shelter. Eventually, Kay learns that Paolo has not been complying with his prescribed medication regimen. He does not deny it and tells Kay that, because he has has been taking medication for more than 3 months and feels better, he believes that he is cured of his tuberculosis and no longer needs therapy.

How should Kay respond? Should she respect Paolo's right to self-determination by not interfering with the decisions he has made? What if Paolo were to be harmed by this noninterference? What if others were to be harmed? Does Kay's obligation to Paolo to maintain confidentiality remain even when his behavior might compromise the health and well-being of others? Under what circumstances might a nurse place the health and well-being of members of a community before those of an individual client?

In this situation, because Paolo is an adult who is responsible for his own health, Kay could simply disregard the fact that Paolo has not been complying with his prescribed medication regimen. However, she would not be helping Paolo to protect himself or others.

Another strategy that Kay might employ would be to engage Paolo in problem solving to further explore his reasons for not complying with the medication regimen. Uncovering reasons for noncompliance often results in identifying ways to avoid it. One of the strategies recommended in directly observed therapy is for the nurse to adopt a nonjudgmental attitude toward clients, acknowledging that individuals often will not be 100% compliant with medication regimens. Kay could acknowledge that because he is feeling better, it is understandable that Paolo is not taking his medication as prescribed. However, she also ought to remind him that he places himself at great risk for getting very sick again and developing drug-resistant tuberculosis by not following his medication regimen. This course of action might also be an opportunity to foster Paolo's self-determination, to maintain the confidential nature of his care, and to strengthen the patient–nurse relationship.

However, adopting this strategy does jeopardize Paolo's health and the health of the people with whom Paolo comes in contact. Kay does not know whether Paolo's tuberculosis is infectious. Kay initiates tuberculosis screening for the people with whom Paolo has been in contact and creates an opportunity for Paolo to have his tuberculosis reevaluated. This action ought to diminish the potential for harm from active tuberculosis to Paolo and to others with whom he has been in contact. Because Kay's authority has been delegated by the health department, she can communicate with the health department without legally violating confidentiality.

Kay is aware that many states require quarantine of individuals who do not successfully complete a medication regimen for tuberculosis. To protect the public, a community health nurse can recommend that formal action be taken to ensure that a person complies with treatment. In this instance, quarantine means that persons can be hospitalized or incarcerated for treatment of tuberculosis against their will.

As a third strategy, Kay can follow the established protocol to initiate quarantine, reporting Paolo's lack of compliance with medication therapy to the appropriate people. However, it breaches the confidential nature of the client–nurse relationship and compromises the trust and mutual respect that have been established between Paolo and Kay. The ANA Code alerts nurses to the reality of suspending individual rights, but warns that this condition ought "to be tolerated as briefly as possible" (p. 3). Usually a nurse does not select the third alternative until the second alternative has proven ineffective.

How might Paolo be affected by this experience? How might Kay be affected by this experience? Which alternative would you choose?

References

American Nurses' Association. (1985). *Code for nurses with interpretive statements.* Kansas City, MO: Author.

Bayer, R., Dubler, N. N., & Landesman, S. L. (1993). The dual epidemics of tuberculosis and AIDS: Ethical and policy issues in screening and treatment. *American Journal of Public Health, 83*(5), 649–654.

Beauchamp, T. L., & Childress, J. F. (1989). *Principles of biomedical ethics* (3rd ed.). New York: Oxford University Press.

Veatch, R. M., & Fry, S. T. (1987). *Case studies in nursing ethics.* Philadelphia: J. B. Lippincott.

EPIDEMIOLOGICAL PRINCIPLES AND METHODS

Prevention of communicable diseases begins with knowledge about the links in the chain of infection. The relationships and interactions among the infectious agent, the host, and the environment (i.e., the epidemiological triangle) are important. Communicable disease control depends on discovering the weak link in the triangle and developing measures that attack and reduce or eliminate that threat. Control efforts include prevention activities as well as measures to reduce the seriousness of an illness as measured by severity, the length of time ill, the cost of treatment, the short- and long-term effects, and the risk of death.

COMMUNICABLE DISEASE INVESTIGATION

In accordance with epidemiological principles, communicable disease investigation involves five steps: identify the disease, isolate the causative agent, determine the method of transmission, establish the susceptibility of the populations at risk, and estimate the impact on the population. With this knowledge public health officials can plan an effective intervention program. The community health nurse contributes to the investigation effort at every level. The nurse in direct patient care may be the first to identify the onset of a communicable disease, to determine new victims and their relationship to known victims (contact cases), and to discover patterns in the spread of the communicable disease. The role of the community health nurse has broadened beyond direct care. Nurses are currently involved with other health care professionals in population-focused investigation and intervention program design.

CAUSATIVE AGENT

Factors associated with the disease include pathogenicity, infective dose, physical characteristics, organism specificity, and antigenic variations (Brachman, 1989b). Pathogenicity encompasses invasiveness and virulence, terms used to assess the strength of the agent on victims. Highly virulent organisms cause greater morbidity and mortality. For example, some influenza viruses are more virulent than others. Although similar, the symptoms of influenza A are usually more severe and last longer than the symptoms of influenza C (Betts and Douglas, 1990). The degree of invasiveness is important, because highly invasive organisms have an opportunity to affect more body systems. For example, the bacterium causing gonorrhea is usually confined to the genitourinary region. However, the spirochete that causes syphilis invades many different tissues, including the brain, resulting in more diverse symptoms.

The amount of agent needed to produce illness varies. Some agents are highly infectious, while others are less so. For example, a disease such as chickenpox is highly infectious. Many people become infected even when exposed to relatively small amounts of chickenpox virus. Agents that are less infectious, such as tuberculosis, require host exposure to larger numbers of tuberculosis bacilli for longer periods to increase the likelihood of transmitting disease.

Transmission ability is also influenced by the agent's host requirements (agent specificity) and its ability to vary its genetic structure (mutate). Some agents are very particular about hosts. For example, the smallpox virus can infect only humans. Those agents that are limited in the hosts they can infect are considered very agent specific.

The ability of some agents to alter their genetic structure also poses problems for control efforts, as different strains may make treatment less effective. For example, many variations of gonorrhea are resistant to penicillin. In recent years tuberculosis has become difficult to treat because of strains resistant to traditional drug therapy (Centers for Disease Control and Prevention [CDC] 1993b).

MEANS OF TRANSMISSION

The frequency of transmission of an infectious disease is dependent on the opportunities present for organism transport from its source to a new host. Transmission can occur through direct or indirect contact (Fig. 19–1). Direct contact includes direct, physical contact with an infected individual or animal or carrier, or with large droplets (>5 μm) that travel very short distances (<1 m). Indirect contact involves passive transmission by something other than the source. This is usually an object that has been in direct contact with the source (e.g., contaminated water, air, dust,

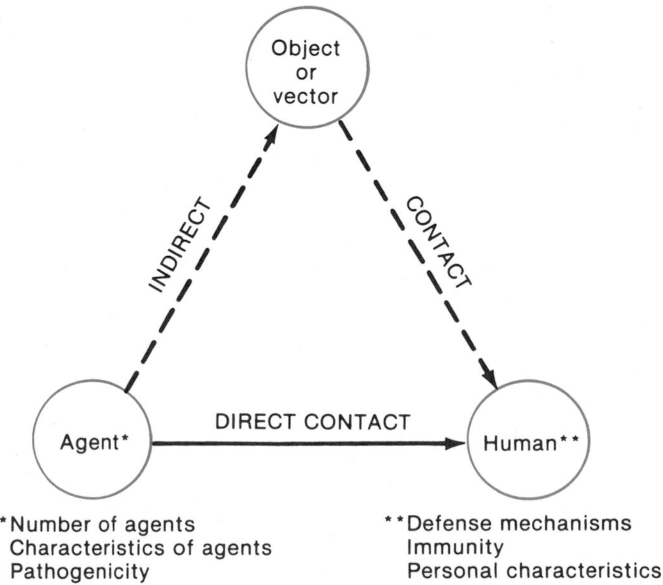

Figure 19–1 ● Transmission of communicable disease.

dressings, instruments, body secretions, small droplets traveling longer distances, or vectors). For example, *Salmonella* bacteria can be transmitted directly (through person-to-person contact by the oral–fecal route) or indirectly (by way of food contaminated with infected feces). Knowledge about transmission methods allows community health nurses to reduce the risk of transmission to communities through health education and supervision of good aseptic technique.

CHARACTERISTICS OF THE HOST

Individuals possess nonspecific defense mechanisms to combat or impede transmission of communicable diseases. These include tears, skin, mucus, saliva, and the cilia (hairs) in the nose. Nose hair, for example, traps organisms transmitted by breathing and reduces an agent's chance of reaching a vulnerable body site. Even when defense mechanisms are compromised, health care professionals can assist in reducing the chance of infection. For example, *Staphyloccus* bacteria enter the body through a break in the skin barrier. Even when a wound breaks the skin barrier, good aseptic technique will reduce the risk of staphylococcal infection.

Immunity, either natural or artificially created, is another host characteristic useful in combating communicable disease. The immune system can halt symptoms by stopping the infection process before symptoms develop. Immunity is one example of primary prevention. Natural immunity occurs when the individual has been infected with the disease and develops an immunity from the body's antigen antibody response to the infection. Before the advent of vaccines, mothers deliberately exposed their children to others with mumps or measles, purposely infecting them. This was done because it was widely believed at the time that young children would be less seriously ill than they would be if infected as an adolescent or adult.

Artificial immunity is developed through vaccination rather than through exposure to a communicable disease. Artificial immunity can be active or passive. Active immunity is a result of vaccination with live, killed, or attenuated organisms or a toxoid of the agent. Live vaccines usually last for long periods but may not be advisable for certain individuals. For example, pregnant women and immunocompromised individuals should not be vaccinated with live antigen (e.g., polio vaccine). The shorter acting vaccines using toxoid or attenuated, absorbed, and killed toxins (e.g., tetanus toxoid), need boosters to keep antibody levels high enough to be effective. These can be used by most people.

Passive immunity can also be used to prevent infection. This type of immunity is derived from either antitoxins or antibodies, such as those transmitted from a mother to a fetus (immunoglobulin). This immunization is temporary and will have to be repeated with each exposure. An additional fact to remember is that immunoglobulin should not be given with live vaccines of measles, mumps, or rubella, as the expected antibody response is decreased when they are given together.

ENVIRONMENT

The environment also affects the mode of transmission. Altering the environment to reduce conditions that favor the spread of infectious agents is a very effective means of communicable disease control. Temperature, humidity, radiation, pressure, and ventilation can all be used to decrease the transmission of infectious diseases. For example, organisms that thrive in heat can be exposed to cold, those that grow best in humidity can be controlled in a climate with little humidity, and so on.

Crowding, famine, and the mobility of people increase the possibility of spreading infections. Crowding is a problem because it provides agents with many potential victims rather than just a few. In a famine, humans are weakened by poor nutrition and other health problems and are less able to resist an infectious disease. Such an environment provides an agent with many more susceptible hosts than would be the case in a well-fed population. Finally, mobility increases the likelihood that agents are carried to other environments. The most obvious way to combat such a spread is quarantine. Countries routinely close borders when threatened by severe communicable diseases. During the 1950s, before the polio vaccine was available, the primary method of reducing the spread of polio was home quarantine.

AGENT/HOST/ENVIRONMENT AND FAVORABLE CONDITIONS

A basic knowledge of the impact of environment, host, agent, and the interrelated features in disease transmission is essential for community health nurses. Nurses must have the skill to assess households and communities for favorable environments, susceptible hosts, and likelihood of viable agents. In addition, they must have the expertise to advise or provide families and communities with the strategies necessary to make the environment less habitable, reduce host susceptibility, and reduce or eliminate the agent source. In some instances interventions can be directed at only one factor; in others, all three may be altered to improve community resistance to infection. For example, HIV can be transmitted by needles contaminated with HIV-infected blood. A weak bleach solution will kill the virus, altering the environment and reducing the risk to a potential host (Fig. 19–2). HIV can also be transmitted by sexual contact with an HIV-infected person. Using barrier method precautions during sexual contact (dental dam, condoms, or nonoxynol-9 spermicidal jelly) will contain and/or kill the virus. Diseases spread through contaminated water or food are controlled by boiling or treating the water (chlorination) and by storing, preparing, and serving foods

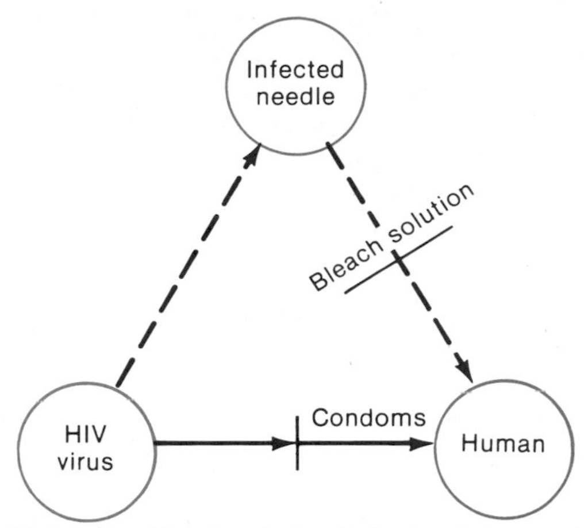

Figure 19–2 ● Breaking the chain of infection in human immunodeficiency virus (HIV) and acquired immunodeficiency syndrome.

using sanitary techniques. Insects can be eliminated, and animals can be killed or treated to reduce the spread of infection. For example, meats, poultry, vegetables, and fruits are inspected for infestation and approved only when they are free from contaminants and safe for human consumption.

RESEARCH ON COMMUNICABLE DISEASES

The first methodical studies on communicable disease were done in 1913. In these studies scientists explored the effects of water quality and pollution, and the resulting information helped in the design of community interventions to control the spread of disease through contaminated water. Surveys and contact investigation strategies were refined. In Maryland studies of pellagra and influenza served as the prototype for current research strategies. Presently there are several organizations committed to researching the characteristics and transmission patterns of communicable diseases.

Research Organizations

The two most important research centers devoted to the study of the incidence of communicable diseases, treatment for diseases, and trends in diseases are the Centers for Disease Control and Prevention (CDC) and the World Health Organization (WHO). In the United States the CDC, based in Atlanta, receives reports from local and state health departments and publishes a yearly summary of communicable diseases in the *Morbidity and Mortality Weekly Report.* Whenever there is an unusual outbreak of disease, the CDC sends scientific teams to the location of the outbreak to assist local authorities. The CDC is equipped with modern computer and telecommunication technologies to track data and coordinate monitoring efforts.

WHO supervises research efforts worldwide. Founded in 1948, it is a specialized organization within the United Nations that operates autonomously. The organization's goal is to achieve the highest possible health status for all people of the world. WHO has been involved in the research of communicable diseases since its inception and monitored the smallpox epidemic and vaccination efforts; in fact, smallpox eradication is credited to the coordinated effort of WHO (Neff, 1990). Worldwide immunizations efforts are currently being coordinated by WHO.

In 1983 the 30th World Health Assembly generated a health research strategy to provide health services to all the countries of the world by the year 2000 (WHO, 1986). To reach that goal a strategy was devised that examined the following four questions:

1. How does the disease start?
2. In the light of knowledge of its origin, how can disease be prevented or, where this is not possible, managed in other ways?
3. What kind of research is needed to prevent or manage disease?
4. What is the role of WHO within the total research framework? (pp. 7–8)

WHO has a broader vision than most organizations. It is pledged to support rapid worldwide progress in acquiring adequate nutrition, uncontaminated water, suitable sewage facilities, contraception, and immunization against communicable diseases.

The research thrust of WHO is the adaptation of solutions from one part of the world to similar situations in other areas. Researchers will continue to study interventions in health care. Successful interventions will be adapted for different cultures, and unsuccessful interventions will be discarded. When WHO's goal is met, health services will be available in every country, and the rates of communicable diseases will be dramatically reduced. Community health nurses are an integral part of WHO's intervention and research initiatives. It is the health practitioners, many of them nurses, who work on site who are able to provide accurate, realistic, reliable data to assist this mighty effort.

HIGH-RISK POPULATIONS

Community health nurses understand that there are high-risk populations that need special attention for prevention through treatment and recovery. Schimpff (1990) calls these individuals "compromised hosts," which he defines as "an individual who has one or more defects in the body's natural defense mechanisms, defects sufficiently significant that the individual is rendered predisposed to severe, often life-threatening infection" (p. 2258).

The age, sex, genetic differences, and general well-being of the host can contribute to or decrease the resistance to infectious diseases. Generally infants, young children, and elderly individuals who are undernourished, do not get enough sleep, or have a chronic illness have a lower resistance to infection. Community health nurses who understand these factors can develop nursing strategies to increase resistance and generate more efficient defense mechanisms in patients at particular risk.

From the very beginning of the study of communicable diseases, the very young and the elderly have been recognized as being at greater risk for developing infectious diseases. The severity of illness in these groups is also greater. Preschool children are at risk because they spend a lot of time in groups and do not have fully developed immune systems.

Many elderly have diminished immunity from underlying medical problems or an impaired nutritional status (Miller, 1990). Their skin is fragile and easily broken, and they may have been exposed for longer periods to environmental hazards. Consequently, they are at increased risk for urinary tract infections, infectious diarrhea, and upper respiratory infections such as tuberculosis and pneumonia.

Immunosuppressed patients are also at risk for contracting communicable diseases. People undergoing immunosuppressive therapy after bone marrow or organ transplantation or therapy for acute lymphocytic leukemia do not have an intact immune system. They risk infection from multiple diseases. Other conditions that may cause a defect in the cellular immunity of a person are Hodgkin's disease and HIV infection. Cancerous conditions such as acute leukemia, myeloma, hairy cell leukemia, and brain tumors predispose patients to reduced resistance to diseases. Patients with spinal cord injuries are susceptible to urinary tract infections and skin infections. Persons who have undergone a splenectomy are at risk because they have a diminished ability to produce antibodies and clear bacteria from the bloodstream. Without these functions, adults and children are at risk for pneumonia, influenza, and meningitis.

Intravenous drug abusers are at risk because drug abuse can directly cause infection. Persons who use parenteral drugs are generally infected through contamination of the needle and syringe. An infected needle left by one person and "shared" by another will transmit infection. Dobkin (1989) reports that more than one fourth of drug abusers admitted to hospitals are admitted for treatment of infections. Both HIV and hepatitis B can be transmitted in this way. Infected needle sites are common and are caused by frequent use of dirty needles.

There are indirect causes for the increase of infections in intravenous drug abusers as well. Many drug abusers are poorly nourished, live in substandard conditions with poor sanitation, and are more often exposed to others who carry communicable diseases (Schwartz and Gillmore, 1990).

Health care workers are also considered a risk group because their work environment places them in proximity to numerous infectious organisms. Hepatitis B and HIV infection can both be transmitted when health care workers are exposed to blood, semen, or vaginal secretions. The resurgence of tuberculosis and other drug-resistant infections is another occupational hazard for health care workers. Patients come to health care facilities with these infections, and it may take some time before the infection is confirmed or treatment is effective. During this time health care workers are unknowingly at risk. Correct and consistent infection control measures are absolutely necessary to provide optimal protection both in inpatient and community settings (CDC, 1990). Community health nurses should be especially vigilant to maintain safe technique during home visits (CDC, 1988).

Trends in Communicable Diseases

The study of diseases over time provides valuable information for public health planners. Trends are studied so that community health needs can be anticipated and intervention strategies preplanned. Trends are also useful in examining the impact of intervention programs. If programs are effective and efficient, they can be used again and again with modifications that consider physical, psychological, sociological, and economic changes in the population. There are several ways to examine trends in communicable diseases. Brachman (1989a) indicates that variations in frequency can be examined for regular trends or episodic occurrence. Regular trends include expected seasonal and yearly variations. For example, hay fever occurs during the fall and spring seasons, and upper respiratory infections are common in the winter. An episodic occurrence is a sudden change in the rate of transmission or an epidemic. For example, a large number of community residents may suddenly contract food poisoning, or a measles epidemic may hit the entire country.

Trends can also be observed over longer periods of time. At the beginning of this chapter a historical review provided evidence of change in the characteristics, spread, and treatment of communicable diseases over centuries. A more detailed examination of United States data presents a clear picture of communicable disease trends since the 1950s (Table 19–2). As public health measures become more effective in controlling certain communicable diseases, other diseases, new diseases, or mutant strains of known diseases become more prominent.

SUCCESSES IN COMMUNICABLE DISEASE CONTROL

Public health practices have initiated community protection measures such as providing safer environmental conditions and treatment and immunization programs as soon as they become available. Water quality regulations, sewage regulations, and food-handling regulations have

TABLE 19–2

Frequency of Notifiable Diseases over Time

Disease	Number of Cases							
	1930	1940	1950	1960	1970	1980	1990	1992
AIDS	NA	NA	NA	NA	NA	NA	41,595	42,978
Legionellosis	NA	NA	NA	NA	NA	475	1,370	1,289
Measles (rubeola)	419,465	291,162	319,124	441,703	47,351	13,506	27,786	9,804
Mumps	NA	NA	NA	NA	104,953	8,576	5,292	2,460
Pertussis	166,914	183,866	120,718	14,809	4,249	1,730	4,570	2,791
Poliomyelitis	9,220	9,804	33,300	3,190	33	9	7	0
Rabies, animal	3,002	7,210	7,901	3,567	3,224	6,421	4,826	7,844
Rabies, human	59	41	18	2	3	0	1	86
Rheumatic fever	NA	NA	NA	9,022	3,227	432	108	127*
Rubella (German measles)	NA	NA	NA	NA	56,552	3,904	1,125	148
Smallpox	48,907	2,795		Last Documented Case in the United States 1949				
Syphilis	213,309	472,900	217,558	122,538	91,382	68,832	134,255	34,547
Tuberculosis	124,940	102,984	121,742	55,494	37,137	27,749	25,701	24,073
Typhoid fever	27,201	9,809	2,484	816	346	510	552	382

Data from Centers for Disease Control and Prevention. (1979). *Annual summary;* (1990). *Summary of notifiable diseases;* (1992). *Annual summary.* Atlanta: Author.
*Represents 1991 data; 1992 data not available.
AIDS = Acquired immunodeficiency syndrome; NA = not available.

decreased the incidence of enteric diseases. Currently water is chlorinated, milk is pasteurized, preservatives are added to foods, and safe sewage plants are built. The result is that the number of cases of anthrax, diphtheria, malaria, typhoid, and other similarly spread diseases has greatly diminished (Table 19–2).

Antibiotics help reduce the spread of communicable diseases (e.g., rheumatic fever, tuberculosis, and syphilis) by lessening the time during which infected persons are contagious. By the end of the 1950s, the incidence of tuberculosis and syphilis was significantly reduced. The impact on rheumatic fever is not as apparent because that disease was not reportable until after 1950.

Smallpox inoculation eradicated smallpox from North America in 1950. Much later, the program was successful worldwide, and smallpox vaccination is no longer needed. Rabies is controlled by vaccination of potential animal carriers and of humans at greatest risk (e.g., animal control personnel). Although it is not feasible to inoculate every animal, a large segment of potential domestic animal carriers have been vaccinated. This strategy effectively reduces the human rabies cases to a mere handful each year. Immunization programs have dramatically decreased the incidence of childhood diseases such as measles, mumps, pertussis, polio, and rubella. In 1977, a national campaign, The Childhood Immunization Initiative, resulted in massive immunizations of young children.

COMMUNICABLE DISEASES OF CONCERN

Although there have been significant successes in communicable disease control since the 1940s, a number of diseases have created concern within the public health community. There has been a resurgence in the incidence of preventable childhood illnesses (e.g., measles), tuberculosis, sexually transmitted diseases, and hepatitis and the emergence of new diseases, the most prominent of which is HIV infection (Table 19–2). The *Healthy People 2000 objectives* have targeted all of these communicable diseases for special attention to significantly reduce their impact on the American people (Table 19–3).

Measles. The resurgence of certain communicable diseases has been the result of lapses in control measures and diminished effect of vaccine over time. When immunization efforts were relaxed in the 1980s, young people became more susceptible. The most apparent proof of these lapsed immunization practices was the increase in measles cases in the late 1980s and early 1990s. Between 1989 and 1991, 55,000 new cases were reported, and 132 people died. The Department of Health and Human Services estimates treatment costs for these cases at more than $165 million (Shalala, 1993). Currently there is renewed emphasis on childhood immunization in the public health arena. In 1993 President Clinton announced the National Immunization Campaign, designed to provide access to immunizations for every child in the country. Investigations of the resurgence of measles in high school and college populations have revealed that the vaccine did not provide lifetime immunity. A booster dose is now recommended for continued protection against measles.

Drug-Resistant Diseases. One trend of special concern to public health practitioners is the increase in drug-resistant strains of organisms causing communicable diseases. After

TABLE 19–3

Healthy People 2000 Objectives: Health Status

1. Confine the annual incidence of diagnosed AIDS cases to no more than 98,000. (Baseline: An estimated 44,000 to 50,000 diagnosed in 1989.)
2. Confine the prevalence of HIV infection to no more than 800 per 100,000 people. (Baseline: An etimated 400 per 100,000 in 1989.)
3. Reduce gonorrhea to an incidence of no more than 225 cases per 100,000 people. (Baseline: 300 per 100,000 in 1989.)
4. Reduce *Chlamydia* infections to no more than 170 cases per 100,000 people. (Baseline: 215 per 100,000 in 1988.)
5. Reduce primary and secondary syphilis to an incidence of no more than 10 cases per 100,000 people. (Baseline: 18.2 per 100,000 in 1989.)
6. Reduce genital herpes and genital warts to 142,000 and 385,000 cases, respectively, each year. (Baseline: 167,000 and 451,000, respectively, in 1988.)
7. Reduce the incidence of pelvic inflammatory disease to no more than 250 cases per 100,000 women age 15 through 44. (Baseline: 311 per 100,000 in 1988.)
8. Reduce sexually transmitted hepatitis B infection to no more than 30,500 cases annually. (Baseline: 58,300 in 1988.)
9. Reduce indigenous cases of vaccine-preventable diseases as follows:

Disease	1988 Baseline	2000 Target
Measles	3058	0
Rubella	225	0
Mumps	4866	0
Pertussis	3450	1000

10. Reduce epidemic-related pneumonia and influenza deaths among people age 65 and older to no more than 7.3 per 100,000 people. (Baseline: Average of 9.1 per 100,000 during the period from 1980 through 1987.)
11. Reduce viral hepatitis as follows:

	1987 Baseline (per 100,000)	2000 Target (per 100,000)
Hepatitis B	63.5	40
Hepatitis A	31	23
Hepatitis C	18.3	13.7

12. Reduce incidence of tuberculosis to no more than 3.5 cases per 100,000 people. (Baseline: 9.1 per 100,000 in 1988.)

From USDHHS. (1990). *Healthy people 2000: National health promotion and disease prevention objectives* (Publication No. (PHS) 91-50213). Washington, DC: U.S. Government Printing Office.

years of successful treatment, gonorrhea, tuberculosis, and syphilis are on the rise. These increases are the result of less success with standard antibiotic therapies. Drug-resistant strains of communicable disease are a special concern not only because they are more complicated to treat, but also because the delay in control increases the risk of infection for all, including health care workers. Community health nurses must be alert to screen high-risk groups (Table 19–4), aware of current treatments, and able to identify the signs of drug resistance in patients.

Tuberculosis. Nearly one third of the world's population is infected with tuberculosis. It is the leading infectious cause of death in the entire world, causing more than 2.5 million deaths each year (Kochi, 1991). In the United States effective treatment and case-finding produced dramatic results. By the 1980s fewer than 30,000 new cases were reported each year. In the mid 1980s, however, the downward trend halted. Each year the number of cases that occur is larger than would have been expected if the trend had continued to decline. Reichman (1993) attributes the resurgence of tuberculosis to changes in health priorities, a reduction in available funds for programs, and an upsurge in susceptible risk groups. Programs that provided supervised administration and incentives for compliance with the medication regimen were eliminated (Brudney and Dobkin, 1991). Without these control measures, multidrug-resistant strains developed as tuberculosis patients became less compliant with their drug therapy. These strains are a public health concern because they require longer, more costly treatment, which is less successful. Multidrug-resistant tuberculosis is often fatal; the cure rate is only 50% (Pearson et al., 1992).

Coupled with the advent of multidrug-resistant strains has been an upsurge in at-risk populations. The poor and others in crowded living arrangements (e.g., prisons and homeless shelters) and persons who are immunosuppressed are always at risk for developing tuberculosis in the presence of the organism. HIV-infected individuals are at special risk; there has been a dramatic increase in the

TABLE 19–4

Groups at Greater Risk for Contracting Disease

Tuberculosis
HIV-positive individuals
Prisoners and homeless persons
Poor urban individuals
Minorities (American Indians and Alaska Natives, Asians, Pacific Islanders, blacks, Hispanics)
Health care workers
Sexually Transmitted Diseases
Adolescents
Young adults
Persons with multiple sex partners
Drug-related, prostitutes
Prostitutes
Minority groups (blacks and Hispanics)
Hepatitis
Persons with poor personal hygiene or living in poor conditions (overcrowding, unsanitary conditions)
Persons who emigrate from areas where HBV is common (Africa, Asia, South America)
Travelers to areas where hepatitis is endemic
Intravenous drug users
Persons with multiple sex partners
Alaska Natives
Health care workers
HIV
Persons with multiple sex partners
Intravenous drug users
Prostitutes
Minority groups (blacks and Hispanics)
Bisexual and homosexual males

Compiled from Bayer, R., Dubler, N. N., & Landesman, S. L. (1993). The dual epidemic of tuberculosis and AIDS: Ethical and policy issues in screening and treatment. *American Journal of Public Health, 83*(5), 649–654; Schwartz, P., & Gillmore, M. R. (1990). Sociological perspectives on human sexuality. In K. K. Holmes, P. A. Mardh, P. F. Sparling, & P. J. Weisner (Eds.), *Sexually transmitted diseases* (pp. 45–53). New York: McGraw-Hill; and USDHHS. (1990). *Healthy people 2000: National health promotion and disease prevention objectives* (Publication No. (PHS) 91-50213). Washington, DC: U. S. Government Printing Office.
HBV = Hepatitis B virus; HIV = human immunodeficiency virus.

number of persons with the dual diagnosis of HIV and tuberculosis (Bayer et al., 1993).

Sexually Transmitted Diseases. The incidence of sexually transmitted disease (STD) is estimated at approximately 12 million cases per year. According to the American Public Health Association (APHA) (1993a), the STD problem in the United States is much greater than in any other industrialized country. The two most common problems are *Chlamydia* and human papillomavirus (HPV) infection, which are not reportable communicable diseases. There are approximately 4 million new cases of *Chlamydia* and 1 million new cases of HPV each year. The cost of treatment is high and is compounded when drug-resistant strains develop. The cost of care for *Chlamydia* alone is approximately $2 billion per year (APHA, 1993a). Both syphilis and gonorrhea have developed drug-resistant strains, requiring more prolonged and costly treatment. Some STDs (e.g., herpes) have no cure and require lifelong monitoring to control. The rise in STDs is related to the development of drug-resistant strains and the increased incidence of sexual activity in certain aggregates within the population. Those at greater risk include adolescents and young adults, drug addicts, persons with multiple sex partners, and prostitutes (Schwartz and Gillmore, 1990). The greatest risk is to individuals who engage in unprotected sexual activity. Teenagers are particularly vulnerable because they tend to ignore the consequences of unprotected sex (Boland, 1991). Prostitutes who have unprotected sex have the highest risk of transmitting and acquiring an STD (Plummer and Nugugi, 1990). Public health efforts to reduce STD should stress primary prevention to reduce the incidence of STDs *and* the long-term effects associated with certain STDs (e.g., chronic illness, sterility, and cancer).

Hepatitis. There are several types of hepatitis (A; B; non–A, non–B; and delta), all caused by different viruses. Hepatitis can be transmitted by fecal–oral contamination, sexual intercourse, or injections. Hepatitis is a reportable disease but is very underreported. The CDC estimates that approximately 300,000 people are infected with hepatitis B each year, but only about 22,000 cases are reported (CDC, 1992a).

Hepatitis A and hepatitis B are the two most common forms of hepatitis. Hepatitis A virus (HAV) is transmitted by the fecal–oral route, so nonhygienic living conditions place people at risk. Some HAV outbreaks have been traced to infected food handlers serving the public (e.g., in restaurants). Sanitary control measures reduce the spread of HAV.

Hepatitis B virus (HBV) is passed from one person to another through blood and body fluids shared through sexual relations, needles, toothbrushes, and razors (CDC, 1992a). The increase in HBV is largely due to needle sharing and sexual relations with infected persons. Groups at particular risk include those with multiple sex partners, intravenous drug users, travelers to and emigrants from HBV-endemic countries, health care workers and others exposed to blood and blood products in their work (e.g., police and institutional staff), hemophiliacs, and men who engage in homosexual intercourse. Since the mid-1980s homosexual men and health care workers have reduced their risk. Homosexual men are employing safer sex practices, and health care workers are more careful to use universal precautions.

Hepatitis-infected individuals can become chronic carriers for life. The greatest risk for acquiring carrier status is in the very young. Ninety percent of infants infected with HBV at birth will become carriers, whereas the risk for young adults is less than 10% (CDC, 1992a).

Human Immunodeficiency Virus. More than 1 million Americans are infected with HIV, and close to 400,000 have been diagnosed with AIDS (Roper et al., 1993). By the end of 1993 more than 300,000 people have died from AIDS. Because AIDS-related care is long term and extensive, the cost of treatment is high. The annual cost of care is estimated at $13 billion (U.S. Department of Health and Human Services [USDHHS], 1990). Currently, there is no cure for AIDS, but some treatments have increased the time people survive with the disease.

Because AIDS is a disease that weakens an individual's body defense system, people with AIDS experience many different symptoms or conditions. For diagnostic purposes the CDC has developed a listing of conditions that are diagnostic of AIDS (Table 19–5). A number of communicable diseases are among these, including candidiasis, herpes, tuberculosis, and pneumonia.

The groups at special risk for acquiring HIV infection are similar to those at risk for HBV infection. Most diagnosed AIDS patients are male (75%) and homosexual or bisexual (66%). Among newly diagnosed AIDS cases, the most rapid growth is among intravenous drug abusers, women, infants born to infected women, and teenagers ("Sex Overtakes Drug Use," 1993). Approximately 20% to 35% of infants born to infected mothers become HIV positive. Adolescent AIDS cases increased 77% between 1990 and 1992 (House Select Committee, 1992). Blacks and Hispanics are at greater risk than whites (USDHHS, 1990). HIV rates among Hispanics vary depending on the country of origin. Cubans and Puerto Ricans are at greater risk than Mexican Americans (Diaz et al., 1993). AIDS prevention strategies must be geared toward all who engage in risky behaviors.

There is a long time delay between HIV infection and the development of AIDS; in fact, the average latency period is 11 years (Hein, 1993). Because of this time delay, aggregates among the more recently determined high-risk groups are often unaware of or dismiss their danger. Because many of their compatriots do not have noticeable symptoms, it is easier to ignore the problem. Public education campaigns should be directed toward increasing awareness of the problem.

TABLE 19–5

Conditions Included in the 1993 AIDS Surveillance Case Definition

Conditions
Candidiasis of bronchi, trachea, or lungs
Candidiasis, esophageal
Cervical cancer, invasive*
Coccidioidomycosis, disseminated or extrapulmonary
Cryptococcosis, extrapulmonary
Cryptosporidiosis, chronic intestinal (>1 month's duration)
Cytomegalovirus disease (other than liver, spleen, or nodes)
Cytomegalovirus retinitis (with loss of vision)
Encephalopathy, HIV-related
Herpes simplex: chronic ulcer(s) (>1 month's duration); or bronchitis, pneumonitis, or esophagitis
Histoplasmosis, disseminated or extrapulmonary
Isosporiasis, chronic intestinal (>1 month's duration)
Kaposi's sarcoma
Lymphoma, Burkitt's (or equivalent term)
Lymphoma, immunoblastic (or equivalent term)
Lymphoma, primary, of brain
Mycobacterium avium complex or *Mycobacterium kansasii,* disseminated or extrapulmonary
Mycobacterium tuberculosis, any site (pulmonary* or extrapulmonary)
Mycobacterium, other species or unidentified species, disseminated or extrapulmonary
Pneumocystis carinii pneumonia
Pneumonia, recurrent*
Progressive multifocal leukoencephalopathy
Salmonella septicemia, recurrent
Toxoplasmosis of brain
Wasting syndrome owing to HIV

From CDC. (1993c). 1993 Revised Classification system for HIV infection and expanded surveillance case definition for AIDS among adolescents and adults. *Morbidity and Mortality Weekly Report, 41*(RR-17); 1–19.

*Added in the 1993 expansion of the AIDS surveillance case definition.

AIDS = Acquired immunodeficiency syndrome; HIV = human immunodeficiency virus.

INFLUENCE OF MODERN LIFESTYLE AND TECHNOLOGY

Some current trends in communicable diseases can be attributed to modernization and new technology. Industrialization and the crowding of large numbers of people into the relatively small space of a city provide fertile ground for the increase of certain diseases. Crowding threatens sanitary and other environmental conditions. In hard economic times more families become homeless as a result of increases in unemployment and a reduction in affordable housing. These families are forced to move in with relatives, producing more crowded conditions, or they move to housing that is affordable but frequently less safe, with environmental hazards and more crime.

The greater mobility of individuals and groups has facilitated the transmission of diseases that would not otherwise cross natural boundaries, such as oceans or mountains. Each year more and more people travel to other countries for leisure and business. The spread of HIV infection can be traced to international and intracountry travel. For example, within Africa the incidence of HIV infection is heavily concentrated along travel routes (rivers and roads) from one country to another. HIV has also been traced to transoceanic travel as travelers infected elsewhere return to their home countries (Risse, 1988).

Even modern medical interventions increase the possibility of rapidly transmitting communicable diseases. Hickman catheters threaded into the jugular vein to provide easy access for drug administration and diagnostic procedures, central venous pressure catheters, and other intravenous lines provide a route whereby infectious organisms can enter a human. Intubations, intracranial pressure monitors, and respiratory nebulizers are all sources of nosocomial infections. Nosocomial infections may account for 15% of hospital deaths directly related to infections acquired in the hospital. Although nosocomial infections are not required to be reported under the National Notifiable Disease Surveillance System (NNDSS), one "new" disease so mandated is legionellosis. Legionellosis flourishes as a result of new technology, thriving in damp, moist areas such as heating and air conditioning ventilation systems. Legionellosis was first identified during an epidemiological investigation of an outbreak of illness among veterans attending an American Legion Convention in the early 1980s. There have been periodic outbreaks ever since, although careful maintenance of ventilation systems reduces the probability of infection.

Role of Boards of Health

LEGISLATIVE MANDATE

Local boards of health are charged with maintaining the health of the community. To do this, they provide direct services to individuals, gather data from these individuals and families, collate the data, report the data to state and local agencies, and maintain records for research purposes. They make rules and regulations at the local level and are expected to carry out the legislative mandates of both the state and federal governments. The costs for carrying out the mandates are usually shared by all three levels of government. Through the CDC the federal government offers financial assistance for many programs seeking to control infectious diseases. For example, in 1989 the CDC funded 63 separate projects on STDs (Cates and Toomey, 1990).

ENVIRONMENTAL CONTROL

The primary responsibility for environmental oversight and prevention of associated health problems rests with the health department. Bennett and Searl (1982) list some of the responsibilities related to water, food, and sewage controls. The water supply is protected by chlorinating and fluoridating municipal water supplies, testing private and public drinking water for contaminates, regulating the digging of wells, and limiting or restricting construction in watershed districts. The health department protects food supplies through surveillance of restaurants, grocery stores, and markets. They check for proper food storage, preparation, and service and monitor the health of those serving and preparing the food. If there is any food processing or packaging plants within the jurisdiction, these are scrutinized as well. Sewage disposal and treatment are controlled. Public swimming pools and beaches are inspected frequently to ascertain the safety of water and facilities. Most local boards of health either have direct control or work closely with the public agency that mandates construction codes for public and private buildings.

REPORTABLE DISEASES OVERSIGHT

The CDC tracks national statistics and trends on communicable diseases through the NNDSS, which maintains regular surveillance of all mandatory reportable diseases, as well as of other diseases of interest or concern (Table 19–6). The CDC also issues guidelines and recommendations on the prevention and treatment of specific diseases. An excellent source for this information is the *Morbidity and Mortality Weekly Report* published by the CDC. This publication is a valuable resource for community health nurses, as it provides information on specific diseases and public health problems and supplies epidemiological data on reportable diseases as well as other communicable diseases and public health concerns such as *Chlamydia* and adolescent homicide.

State public health departments have the legal responsibility for controlling communicable diseases and reporting notifiable communicable diseases to the CDC. Figure 19–3 is an example of the type of information the CDC asks states to supply on reportable communicable diseases. The state health departments issue reporting directions and treatment recommendations to local health departments. Local health departments, in turn, gather information about communicable diseases from health care providers in their region. Direct diagnosis and treatment, counseling, contact tracing, and follow-up are done by local health departments. Community health nurses perform many of these services.

In addition to collecting information on all notifiable communicable diseases, states may investigate other health concerns at their discretion. Throughout the U.S. approximately 87 diseases are reportable through the health department surveillance systems. Surveillance data are necessary, for they help the CDC and individual states to decide which health concerns should have priority. They also yield information that can be useful when designing and implementing health care prevention and promotion programs.

Many communicable diseases have seasonal fluctuations or uneven geographical distributions or selected risk groups. Others have cycles when they are more or less severe. Surveillance data reveal these trends. Appropriate strategies can then be planned to prevent or reduce the impact of these diseases. Surveillance also assists in identifying the most effective control methods. For example, the CDC was able to identify a resurgence of measles among teenagers and young adults. On investigation, researchers decided the combined measles-mumps-rubella vaccine was less long acting than previously thought. New immunization standards were developed to include a booster dose around age 11 or 12 years.

IMMUNIZATIONS AND VACCINES

Immunization is the most effective primary prevention method for controlling communicable diseases in popula-

TABLE 19–6

National Notifiable Diseases Surveillance System List of All Notifiable Diseases

Surveillance Mandatory		
AIDS	Hansen's disease	Rabies (animal)
Amoebiasis	Hepatitis A	Rabies (human)
Anthrax	Hepatitis B	Rheumatic fever
Aseptic meningitis	Hepatitis (non-A, non-B)	Rocky Mountain spotted fever
Botulism (infant)	Hepatitis (unspecified)	Rubella
Botulism (wound)	Legionellosis	Salmonellosis
Botulism (unspecified)	Leptospirosis	Shigellosis
Brucellosis	Lyme disease	Syphilis (all stages)
Chancroid	Lymphogranuloma venereum	Syphilis (primary and secondary)
Cholera	Malaria	Syphilis (congenital)
Diphtheria	Meningococcal infections	Toxic shock syndrome
Encephalitis (post-chickenpox)	Mumps	Trichinosis
Encephalitis (post-mumps)	Pertussis	Tuberculosis
Encephalitis (post-other)	Plague	Tularemia
Encephalitis (primary)	Poliomyelitis (paralytic)	Typhoid fever
Gonorrhea	Psittascosis	Yellow fever
Granuloma inguinale		

Surveillance Maintained but not Mandatory	
Campylobacter infection	*Listeria monocytogenes* (listeriosis)
Chlamydia trachomatis infection	Mucopurulent cervicitis
Dengue fever	Nongonococcal urethritis
Genital herpes simplex virus infection	Pelvic inflammatory disease
Genital warts	Reye's syndrome
Giardiasis	Spinal cord injury
Haemophilus influenzae (invasive disease)	Varicella
Kawasaki syndrome	All other unusual outbreaks

TABLE 19–7

Recommended Schedule for Routine Active Vaccination of Infants and Children

Vaccine	At Birth (Before Hospital Discharge)	1–2 mo	2 mo*	4 mo	5 mo	6–18 mo	12–15 mo	15 mo	4–6 yr (Before School Entry)
Diphtheria-tetanus-pertussis†			DTP	DTP	DTP			DTaP/DTP‡	DTaP/DTP
Polio, live oral			OPV	OPV	OPV§				OPV
Measles-mumps-rubella							MMR		MMR‖
Haemophilus influenzae type b conjugate									
HbOC/PRP-T†,¶			Hib	Hib	Hib		Hib**		
PRP-OMP¶			Hib	Hib			Hib**		
Hepatitis B††									
Option 1	HepB	HepB‡‡				HepB‡‡			
Option 2		HepB‡‡		HepB‡‡		HepB‡‡			

From CDC. (1994). General recommendations for immunization. *Morbidity and Mortality Weekly Report, 43*(RR-1), 9.

*Can be administered as early as 6 wk of age.

†Two DTP and Hib combination vaccines are available (DTP/HbOC [TETRAMUNE]; and PRP-T [ActHIB, OmniHIB] that can be reconstituted with DTP vaccine produced by Connaught).

‡This dose of DTP can be administered as early as 12 mo of age provided that the interval since the previous dose of DTP is at least 6 mo. *Diphtheria and tetanus toxoids and acellular pertussis vaccine (DTaP) is currently recommended only for use as the fourth and/or fifth doses of the DTP series among children aged 15 mo through 6 yr (before the seventh birthday).* Some experts prefer to administer these vaccines at 18 mo of age.

§The American Academy of Pediatrics (AAP) recommends this dose of vaccine at 6–18 mo of age.

‖The AAP recommends that two doses of MMR should be administered by 12 yr of age with the second dose being administered preferentially at entry to middle school or junior high school.

¶HbOC: [HibTITER] (Lederle Praxis), PRP-T: [ActHIB; OmniHIB] (Pasteur Merieux), PRP-OMP: [PedvaxHIB] (Merck, Sharp, and Dohme). A DTP/Hib combination vaccine can be used in place of HbOC/PRP-T.

**After the primary infant Hib conjugate vaccine series is completed, any of the licensed Hib conjugate vaccines may be used as a booster dose at age 12–15 mo.

††For use among infants born to HBsAg-negative mothers. The first dose should be administered during the newborn period, preferably before hospital discharge, but no later than age 2 mo. Premature infants of HBsAg-negative mothers should receive the first dose of the hepatitis B vaccine series at the time of hospital discharge or when the other routine childhood vaccines are initiated. (All infants born to HBsAg-positive mothers should receive immunoprophylaxis for hepatitis B as soon as possible after birth.)

‡‡Hepatitis B vaccine can be administered simultaneously at the same visit with DTP (or DTaP), OPV, Hib, and/or MMR.

Form Approved
OMB NO 0920-0009
EXPIRATION DATE 9-86

PERTUSSIS REPORT

Patient	Name (last, first, M.I.)		Hospital Record No.
	Address	City	Zip
Reporting Physician Nurse/Hosp/ Clinic	Name		Telephone
	Address	City	Zip

ID Assigned by CDC (1-10) (11-16)

PERTUSSIS REPORT

Definitions on Back

State Case Number ________

Enter appropriate code, number, or date.

DEMOGRAPHICS

Date of Birth	Age at onset of illness	Sex	County	State	Zip of Case
Mo. Day Yr. (17-22)	(23-24) mos. (if < 2 years old) (25-26) yrs. (if ≥ 2 years old)	1 Male 2 Female 9 Unknown (27)	(28-30)	(31-32)	(33-37)

VACCINE HISTORY

Number of DTP doses prior to onset of illness (Enter 9 if unknown) (38)

Date of last DTP prior to onset of illness Mo. Day Yr. (39-44)

CLINICAL SYMPTOMS AND SIGNS

Any cough?	Earliest cough onset date	Paroxysmal/spasmodic cough	Onset date	Duration of any cough (days)	Any coughing at last interview?
1 Yes 2 No 9 Unknown (45)	Mo. Day Yr. (46-51)	1 Yes 2 No 9 Unknown (52)	Mo. Day Yr. (53-58)	(59-60)	1 Yes 2 No 9 Unknown (61)

Whoop	Apnea	Cyanosis	Vomiting	Cold-like symptoms
1 Yes 2 No 9 Unknown (62)	1 Yes 2 No 9 Unknown (63)	1 Yes 2 No 9 Unknown (64)	1 Yes 2 No 9 Unknown (65)	1 Yes 2 No 9 Unknown (66)

Hospitalized	Number of days hospitalized	Number of physicians visits (excluding visits during hospitalizatoin) (Leave blank if unknown)	Outcome	Date of last interview
1 Yes 2 No 9 Unknown (67)	(68-70)	(71-72)	1 Case survived 2 Case died 9 Unknown (73)	Mo. Day Yr. (74-79)

COMPLICATIONS

Chest x-ray for pneumonia	Generalized or focal seizures	Acute encephalopathy
1 Positive 2 Negative 3 Not done 9 Unknown (80)	1 Yes 2 No 9 Unknown (81)	1 Yes 2 No 9 Unknown (82)

TREATMENT

Was antibiotic given?
1 Yes
2 No
9 Unknown
(83)

If yes, please complete antibiotic information.

What antibiotic did the patient receive first? (84)
1 Erythromycin
2 Ampicillin/Amoxicillin
3 Other ________

Date started Mo. Day Yr. (85-90)

Actual number of days taken (91-92)

What antibiotic did the patient receive second? (93)
1 Erythromycin
2 Ampicillin/Amoxicillin
3 Other ________

Date started Mo. Day Yr. (94-99)

Actual number of days taken (100-101)

LABORATORY

Tests for *Bordetella pertussis:*

Test	Date specimen taken	Results	Laboratory
DFA	Mo. Day Yr. (102-107)	1 Positive 2 Negative 3 Not done 9 Unknown (108)	1 State 2 Other 9 unknown (109)
Culture	Mo. Day Yr. (110-115)	1 Positive 2 Negative 3 Not done 9 Unknown (116)	1 State 2 Other 9 unknown (117)

Date Form Completed:	Form Completed By:	Date Form Completed:	Telephone:
Mo. Day Yr. (118-123)	________	Mo. Day Yr. (124-129)	(Area Code) ________

ATTN: Surveillance, Investigations and Research Branch
Division of Immunization
Center for Prevention Services
Centers for Disease Control
Atlanta, Georgia 30333

This report is authorized by law (Public Health Service Act, 42 USC 241) and is recommended by the Conference of State and Territorial Epidemiologists. While your response is voluntary, your cooperation is necessary for the understanding and control of the disease.

CDC 71 14A REV 11-83

Figure 19–3 ● Pertussis report. (Courtesy of Centers for Disease Control and Prevention, Atlanta.)

TABLE 19–8

Immunization Recommendations for Adults and Older Children

Tetanus: Booster every 10 years through life span
HIB *(Haemophilus influenzae type B)*
- All people 65 or older
- Adults and children with long-term heart or lung problems, kidney disease, cystic fibrosis, chronic metabolic disease, anemia, severe asthma, cancer, and immunological disorders such as HIV infection
- Residents of nursing homes and other institutions of any age if they have serious long-term health problems
- Medical staff in health care facilities, both community and inpatient
- Family members and others who provide care to high-risk persons

Hepatitis B
- Adults at increased risk as a result of occupational, social, family, environmental, or illness-related exposure to hepatitis B virus, including:
  - Homosexual males
  - Intravenous drug users
  - Heterosexual persons with multiple partners or with other sexually transmitted diseases
  - Household and sexual contacts of hepatitis B carriers
  - Workers in health care–related and public safety occupations with risk of exposure to blood
  - Residents and staff of institutions for the developmentally disabled
  - Hemodialysis patients
  - Hemophiliacs and other patients with blood disorders
  - Morticians and their assistants
  - Inmates in long-term correctional facilities

From CDC. (1991). Update on adult immunizations. *Morbidity and Mortality Weekly Report,* 40(RR-12), 94.

tions. Unfortunately, however, vaccines are not presently available for all communicable diseases. Immunization is important not only for children, but also for elderly, chronically ill, and other individuals at increased risk (e.g., health care workers). Tables 19–7, 19–8, and 19–9 provide a list of recommended immunizations, suggested target groups, and contraindications to administration.

State and local health departments provide immunization clinics and free immunizations to select populations, and oversee vaccine distribution and safety. Local health departments have the responsibility to report specific vaccine-related information to the U.S. Department of Health and Human Services in compliance with the Child Injury Act. All health care providers who give a vaccine must record the serial number of the vial, the name of the company, and any adverse reactions to the vaccine. If the vaccine is privately purchased, the report goes through the local board of health to the Food and Drug Administration; if it is publicly purchased, reporting is done directly to the CDC.

In the early 1980s a number of severe reactions (i.e., psychomotor limitations and paralysis) to the pertussis vaccine generated concern that parents were not receiving adequate information about the risks associated with vaccines. As a result, in 1986 Congress passed the National Childhood Vaccine Injury Act, or Child Injury Act. This law requires a parent's signature testifying that he or she has been informed and established (1) a reporting system for tracking all vaccine doses and (2) a fund to assist children with adverse reactions to the vaccine. To receive compensation for vaccine reactions, the affected person must have an injury of at least 6 months' duration and at least $1000 in expenses directly related to the injury. A sample of the application form to receive compensation is provided in Figure 19–4.

PROTECTION OF INTERNATIONAL TRAVELERS

Local boards of health serve the public by acting as a conduit of information on health-related matters for international travelers. They are a source of information on the immunizations required by other countries and strategies to protect a traveler's health while in another country. Most of the travel-related information is supplied to local and state units by the Office of Overseas Travel at the CDC. Available information includes water and food safety, sanitary conditions, and the sanctions or penalties for illegal drug use. Travelers receive information on the steps necessary to ensure that they are in compliance with the laws regulating legal medication use in foreign countries. In most countries travelers must carry documentation on prescription drugs. Community health nurses in local health departments can assist travelers to collect information pertinent to their travel plans.

Nursing Care in the Control of Communicable Diseases

Community health nurses may focus their energies on population groups or on individuals and family members. In either case, their ultimate goal is the same: protecting populations from the spread of communicable diseases. To be effective, community health nurses must be familiar with basic information about communicable diseases, including causative organism, incubation period, mode of transmission, symptoms, protective measures, and the necessary treatments. This information is critical to planning care aimed at preventing transmission of infectious diseases or ameliorating the symptoms of those who have acquired the disease. Basic information about specific diseases is given in Table 19–10. The diseases are arranged according to five general routes of infection: respiratory, integumentary, gastrointestinal, bloodborne, and sexually transmitted. Some diseases can be transmitted through more than one route. For example, HIV and hepatitis are discussed under bloodborne disease, but both are also transmitted through sexual contact, and hepatitis can be

TABLE 19–9

Guide to Contraindications and Precautions to Vaccinations*

True Contraindications and Precautions	Not True (Vaccine May Be Administered)
General for all vaccines (DTP/DTaP, OPV, IPV, MMR, HIB, HBV)	
Contraindications Anaphylactic reaction to a vaccine contraindicates further doses of that vaccine Anaphylactic reaction to a vaccine constituent contraindicates the use of vaccines containing that substance Moderate or severe illnesses with or without a fever	Mild to moderate local reaction (soreness, redness, swelling) following a dose of an injectable antigen Mild acute illness with or without low-grade fever Current antimicrobial therapy Convalescent phase of illnesses Prematurity (same dosage and indications as for normal, full-term infants) Recent exposure to an infectious disease History of penicillin or other nonspecific allergies or family history of such allergies
DTP/DTaP	
Contraindications Encephalopathy within 7 days of administration of previous dose of DTP **Precautions†** Fever of ≥40.5°C (105°F) within 4 hr after vaccination with a previous dose of DTP Collapse or shocklike state (hypotonic-hyperresponsive episode) within 48 hr of receiving a previous dose of DTP Seizures within 3 days of receiving a previous dose of DTP§ Persistent, inconsolable crying lasting ≥3 hr within 48 hr of receiving a previous dose of DTP	Temperature of $<$40.5 C (105 F) following a previous dose of DTP Family history of convulsions‡ Family history of sudden infant death syndrome Family history of an adverse event following DTP administration
OPV§	
Contraindications Infection with HIV or a household contact with HIV Known altered immunodeficiency (hematological and solid tumors; congenital immunodeficiency; and long-term immunosuppressive therapy) Immunodeficient household contact **Precaution†** Pregnancy	Breast-feeding Current antimicrobial therapy Diarrhea
IPV	
Contraindication Anaphylactic reaction to neomycin or streptomycin **Precaution†** Pregnancy	
MMR§	
Contraindications Anaphylactic reactions to egg ingestion and to neomycin‖ Pregnancy Known altered immunodeficiency (hematological and solid tumors; congenital immunodeficiency; and long-term immunosuppressive therapy) **Precaution†** Recent (within 3 mo) immune globulin administration	Tuberculosis or positive skin test Simultaneous tuberculosis skin testing¶ Breast-feeding Pregnancy of mother of recipient Immunodeficient family member or household contact Infection with HIV Nonanaphylactic reactions to eggs or neomycin

Continued

TABLE 19–9

Guide to Contraindications and Precautions to Vaccinations* *Continued*

True Contraindications and Precautions	Not True (Vaccine May Be Administered)
HIB	
None identified	
HBV	
None identified	Pregnancy

From Centers for Disease Control. (1993) Guide to contraindications and precautions to vaccinations. *Morbidity and Mortality Weekly Report 42*(RR-5), 12–13.

*This information is based on the recommendations of the Advisory Committee on Immunization Practices (ACIP) and those of the Committee on Infectious Diseases (Red Book Committee) of the American Academy of Pediatrics (AAP) as of October 1992. Sometimes these recommendations vary from those contained in the manufacturer's package inserts. For more detailed information, providers should consult the published recommendations of the ACIP, AAP, American Association of Family Practice Physicians, and the manufacturer's package inserts.

†The events or conditions listed as precautions, although not contraindications, should be carefully reviewed. The benefits and risks of administering a specific vaccine to an individual under the circumstances should be considered. If the risks are believed to outweigh the benefits, the vaccination should be withheld; if the benefits are believed to outweigh the risks (for example, during an outbreak or foreign travel), the vaccination should be administered. Whether and when to administer DTP to children with proven or suspected underlying neurological disorders should be decided on an individual basis. It is prudent on theoretical grounds to avoid vaccinating pregnant women. However, if immediate protection against poliomyelitis is needed, OPV, not IPV, is recommended.

‡For children with a personal or family (siblings or parents) history of convulsions, acetaminophen should be considered before DTP is administered and thereafter every 4 hours for 24 hours.

§There is a theoretical risk that the administration of multiple live virus vaccines (OPV and MMR) within 30 days of one another if not administered on the same day will result in a suboptimal immune response. There are no data to substantiate this lack of response.

||Persons with a history of anaphylactic reactions following egg ingestion should be vaccinated only with extreme caution. Protocols that have been developed for vaccinating such persons should be consulted (J Pediatr 1983;102:196–9; J Pediatr 1988;113:504–6).

¶Measles vaccination may temporarily suppress tuberculin reactivity. If testing cannot be done the day of MMR vaccination the test should be postponed for 4 to 6 weeks.

DTP = Diphtheria-tetanus toxoid and pertussis vaccine; DTaP = diphtheria and tetanus toxoids and acellular pertussis vaccine; OPV = oral poliovirus vaccine; IPV = inactivated poliovirus vaccine; MMR = measles-mumps-rubella vaccine; HIB = *Haemophilus-influenzae* type b vaccine; HBV = hepatitis B vaccine.

transmitted through the fecal–oral (gastrointestinal) route as well.

PRIMARY PREVENTION

The major thrust of community health in controlling communicable diseases is primary prevention. Community health nurses play a vital role in eliminating or reducing the spread of disease through immunization administration, prophylactic measures, and health education. Health teaching efforts are geared toward risk reduction (e.g., increasing public awareness of risky behavior, eliminating or reducing the risk of personal behaviors, and providing information for caregivers on methods to isolate and destroy bacterial/viral agents and self-protection techniques).

Immunizations

Vaccines, when available, are the most effective way to control contagious diseases. Immunizations are available for measles, mumps, rubella, diphtheria, pertussis, tetanus, polio, influenza, and hepatitis B. Research continues on the development of vaccines for chickenpox, HIV, herpes virus, and cytomegalovirus. Rabies vaccine is only selectively available to persons at high risk because of costs and side effects. Although a tuberculosis vaccine is available, it is not in common use in the United States because the rate of infection has been low and the vaccine is only moderately effective. In conjunction with the *Healthy People 2000* objectives, community health nurses should strive to increase immunization rates among all designated target groups by expanding education programs on the need for immunization, identifying and targeting risk groups, and improving access to immunization through public and privately financed efforts.

Community health nurses educate parents of children as well as other susceptible individuals about the importance of immunizations and supply immunizations through clinic facilities (Table 19–11). When reviewing individual records, nurses should be especially diligent to ensure that vaccinations for all clients are up to date. Nurses should be aware that persons at high risk who are immunized against hepatitis B virus should be checked in 1 year for adequate antibody response. Revaccination is necessary for individuals who have few or no antibodies at that time.

Elderly individuals need an immunization program that is different from that used for children and younger adults. By age 65 years most older Americans have developed an immunity to measles (rubeola) and diphtheria, but they need to maintain their polio, tetanus, influenza, hepatitis, and pneumococcal vaccine protection (CDC, 1991). Influenza vaccines are modified each year to accommodate new strains. Unless elderly and chronically ill persons are revaccinated yearly, they may not be protected from the most recent form of influenza. Elderly individuals are at risk for tetanus because few were vaccinated as children. The laws mandating childhood diphtheria, pertussis, and tetanus immunizations were not in effect when these

VACCINE ADMINISTRATION RECORD

The doctor or clinic may keep this record in your medical file or your child's medical file. They will record what vaccine was given, when the vaccine was given, the name of the company that made the vaccine, the vaccine's special lot number, the signature and the title of the person who gave the vaccine, and the address where the vaccine was given.

"I have read or have had explained to me the information in this pamphlet about measles, mumps, and rubella diseases and MMR, Measles-Rubella, Measles, Mumps, and Rubella vaccines. I have had a chance to ask questions that were answered to my satisfaction. I believe I understand the benefits and risks of the MMR, measles, mumps, and rubella vaccines and ask that the vaccine checked below be given to me or to the person named below for whom I am authorized to make this request."

Vaccine to be given: MMR ☐ Measles and Rubella ☐ Measles ☐ Mumps ☐ Rubella ☐

Information about person to receive vaccine (Please print.)				
Name: Last First Middle Initial			Birthdate	Age
Address: Street	City	County	State	Zip
Signature of person to receive vaccine or person authorized to make the request (parent or guardian): X			Date:	

MMR#10/15/91

For Clinic/Office Use

Clinic/Office Address: ______________________

Date Vaccine Administered: ______________________

Vaccine Manufacturer: ______________________

Vaccine Lot Number: ______________________

Site of Injection: ______________________

Signature of Vaccine Administrator: ______________________

Title of Vaccine Administrator: ______________________

Figure 19–4 ● Vaccine administration record. (From Centers for Disease Control and Prevention. (1991). *Measles, mumps, and rubella: What you need to know.* U.S. Department of Health and Human Services publication No. B31656. Atlanta: Author.)

individuals were children. More than half of the cases of tetanus during the period from 1982 through 1986 occurred in persons over the age of 60 (Hinman, Orenstein, Bart, and Preblud, 1989). Community health nurses should be especially vigilant to search for outdated or nonexistent immunizations in elderly individuals and other risk groups.

All clients should be well informed of the risks associated with each vaccine they receive. Every health care provider who administers immunizations should be aware of the responsibility to provide this information to the client or, in the case of children, to the parents.

There are important considerations for the nurse to remember when screening patients before administering the vaccine. Assess the person's health status. Ask if the individual has been ill recently or under a physician's care; for a female, if she might be pregnant; and if the individual has had previous reactions to medications or foods. There are a number of situations in which immunizations should not be given or should be delayed. These include the following:

1. Any child who experiences seizures after an initial dose of a vaccine series (e.g., diphtheria-pertussis-tetanus) should not continue to receive the additional doses in the series.
2. Patients with chronic renal disease should probably not receive immunizations, because the ability to clear medication from the body is compromised.

TABLE 19–10

Communicable Diseases, Community Health Concerns, and Treatment

Disease (Causative Agent)	Symptoms	Mode of Transmission	Complications and Community Health Concerns	Specific Treatment (if any)
Respiratory route				
Chickenpox (Varicella zoster virus)	Incubation period, 12–21 days. Low-grade fever, listlessness. Lesions within 2–4 days. Rash has three phases: raised spots, fluid-filled vesicles, and scabs. Rash itches and is found over entire body, including mucous membranes such as mouth.	Very contagious (person-to-person direct contact or contact with airborne droplet). Vesicles are contagious, scabs are not. Communicable 2 days before to 6 days after vesicles appear. Primarily affects children.	Grandparents and older adults should avoid caring for children because they may develop shingles.	Immunosuppressed persons should be treated with gamma globulin. Vaccine in development.
Diphtheria (*Corynebacterium* diphtheria)	Flulike symptoms with sore throat, fever, and involvement of adenoids and larynx with potential respiratory distress. Characterized by formation of yellow/white membranes on tonsils and pharyngeal walls.	Person-to-person direct contact or contact with airborne droplet. Usually affects children under 15 years but may affect adults.	Asymptomatic carrier state possible; should be treated with antibiotics.	Antitoxin immediately on diagnosis and antibiotics (e.g., penicillin and/or erythromycin). Isolate until three negative throat cultures.
Pertussis or whooping cough (*Haemophilus pertussis* bacteria)	Incubation period, 7–10 days. Characteristic cough is nonproductive with quick expiratory phase followed by inspiratory "whoop." Pneumonia and ear infections may be present. Small scleral and conjunctival hemorrhages can occur owing to severe coughing. Convulsions may occur.	Person-to-person direct contact or droplet spread. Very contagious. Affects females more than males. Infants younger than 1 year are severely affected.	Incidence has increased in recent years because of lower immunization rates and concern about side effects of vaccine. Severity of illness and risk of death far surpass the risks from vaccination.	Antibiotics. Hospitalization with oxygen support and nasotracheal suctioning may be necessary.
German measles/rubella (rubella virus)	Incubation period, 14–21 days. Mild in adults and young children, with a macular rash on scalp, body, and limbs lasting 1 to 3 days. Severe in early fetal development and can result in congenital malformations and death; late fetal infection carries risk of birth defects. Conditions associated with fetal infections include low birth weight, deafness, cataracts, glaucoma, heart disease, and mental retardation.	Person-to-person direct contact or droplet spread. Communicable 4 days before to 4 days after rash appears. Highly contagious. Common in children 5 to 10 years of age.	Women of childbearing years should be immunized before pregnancy. Vaccine is live, so it must not be given to pregnant women. Reinfections can occur but are rare.	None

Continued

TABLE 19–10

Communicable Diseases, Community Health Concerns, and Treatment *Continued*

Disease (Causative Agent)	Symptoms	Mode of Transmission	Complications and Community Health Concerns	Specific Treatment (if any)
Measles/rubeola (rubeola/virus)	Incubation period, 7–21 days. Rash, usually starting on the face and spreading to body, lasting 6 days. Koplik spots in mouth that are bluish white and very fine. Coldlike symptoms and cough. Lasts 4–5 days.	Person-to-person direct contact with saliva or droplets. Common disease of childhood. More common in poorly immunized populations and in teens owing to inadequate vaccine in the 1970s and early 1980s.	Complications are pneumonia and encephalitis. No congenital malformations, but can cause spontaneous abortion and prematurity. Children who are HIV positive and asymptomatic should be considered for the vaccine because the illness could be fatal. Persons allergic to eggs may have severe reactions to vaccine.	None
Mumps (mumps virus)	Incubation period, 14–26 days. Low-grade fever, headache, earache, pain and swelling of parotid glands (unilateral or bilateral). Swelling lasts about a week. Early fetal infections can result in spontaneous abortion.	Person-to-person direct contact with saliva or droplet. More commonly a childhood disease. Communicable 6 days before to 9 days after swelling.	Infrequent complications are encephalitis and meningitis. Orchitis occurs in males who have reached puberty, but sterility is rare. Potential for spontaneous abortion if woman is infected in early pregnancy. Persons allergic to eggs may have severe reactions to vaccine.	None
Tuberculosis *(Mycobacterium tuberculosis)*	Low-grade fever, listlessness, night sweats, respiratory congestion, cough, hemoptysis. Sites other than the lungs may be infected; if so, symptoms will be specific to the site. (Other sites include meninges, joints, bladder, and lymphatic system.)	Inhalation from droplet containing bacteria. Risk factors include poverty, poor health, and age. Very young and very old are most susceptible.	Infection with the bacteria produces disease in approximately 10% of cases in the United States. Mantoux test is used to screen for infection and disease. Incidence is on the rise owing to increased incidence in HIV patients and rise of drug-resistant strains of tuberculosis.	Multiple drug therapy with three to six drugs for 6 to 12 months for persons with the disease. Persons infected are treated prophylactically with one medication for up to 6 months. Drug-resistant individuals may need a variety and mix of drugs over time to ensure appropriate treatment.
Influenza (influenza type A or B virus, or potentially a third [Type C] virus)	Respiratory symptoms such as runny nose or cough. May be accompanied by headache and fever. Sometimes may be accompanied by gastrointestinal symptoms such as nausea and vomiting.	Inhalation from droplet spread. Very infectious.	Rapid antigenic variation makes it difficult for the host to develop immune response. Influenza causes more pandemics than any other organism. Complications include pneumonia, croup, Reye's syndrome, toxic shock syndrome, myocarditis, and myocardial infarction.	None. Yearly vaccination recommended for susceptible individuals (i.e., elderly and chronically ill persons). Vaccine must be reconfigured each year to meet the specific characteristics of the current strain.

Continued

TABLE 19–10

Communicable Diseases, Community Health Concerns, and Treatment *Continued*

Disease (Causative Agent)	Symptoms	Mode of Transmission	Complications and Community Health Concerns	Specific Treatment (if any)
Integumentary route				
Pediculosis (parasitic lice)	Incubation period, 2 weeks. Lice and eggs may be present in scalp hair or pubic hair or on the body. Itching and other signs of skin irritation, such as a rash or swollen glands, may be present.	Direct contact or indirect transfer of adult lice, nits, or eggs via body contact, or contact with personal items that are infected with the parasites.	Nuisance disease; not easily transmitted from person to person.	Hair and pubic lice are treated with medicated shampoos such as Kwell in several applications. Nits (eggs) should be removed from scalp hair with a fine-toothed comb. Body lice are eliminated by dusting clothes with 1% malathion powder and washing all affected garments in very hot water.
Impetigo (group A streptococcal or staphylococcal bacteria)	Incubation period, 4–10 days. Skin blisters usually found in the corners of the mouth or near edge of nose. Blisters break and form yellow crusts that resolve with little or no scarring; blisters may be itchy, and scatching may occur. Fever, malaise, and headache may be present.	Direct contact with lesions or secretions. Very contagious. Scratching spreads the disease to other areas of the body or other persons. Communicable as long as lesions persist.	Most common in hot, humid climates. Very contagious and problematic in children. Infected children should be kept from school until completely healed.	Penicillin and/or erythromycin and topical antibiotics to treat skin eruptions.
Rabies (rabies virus)	Three phases: prodromal, neurological, and coma. Prodromal: wound heals and symptoms of minor infection are present lasting 2–10 days; these include fever, headache, chills, sore throat, and pain at site of bite. Neurological: lasts up to 7 days and includes hallucinations, stiffness, disorientation, and seizures. Coma: death may occur if treatment is not given.	Transmitted through bites from an infected animal.	Treatment is difficult, and fatality rate is high. Prevention is the main community health thrust. Domestic animals should be immunized and populations educated to avoid wild (e.g., fox, raccoon) or unknown animals.	Rabies vaccine. Hospitalization with isolation.
Scabies (parasitic mite)	Incubation period, 2–6 wk; reinfections in 1–4 days. Skin rash, scratching may occur. Burrows on skin look like gray/white tracts; lesions may be evident around wrists and belt line.	Direct contact. Transmitted by mites that burrow under skin and lay eggs. Clothing and other personal items may hold mites or eggs. Communicable as long as eggs or mites are alive.	Concerns similar to those for pediculosis.	Hot bath, vigorous body scrub followed by application of 5% solution of benzyl benzoate or Kwell. Application should be repeated in approximately 1 wk. Bedding and clothing must be thoroughly cleaned.

Continued

TABLE 19–10

Communicable Diseases, Community Health Concerns, and Treatment *Continued*

Disease (Causative Agent)	Symptoms	Mode of Transmission	Complications and Community Health Concerns	Specific Treatment (if any)
Gastrointestinal route				
Candidiasis (*Candida* fungus)	Depend on site of infection. Gastrointestinal infection produces diarrhea and may be accompanied by cramping. Vaginal infections have vaginal symptoms.	Highly infectious. Found on skin and under finger- and toenails and may be passed to gastrointestinal tract by hand-to-mouth transmission. Vaginal infection common in females, easily transferred to males during sexual contact.	Infants can be infected during vaginal delivery	Multiple oral and topical drugs depending on site of infection, including nystatin, clotrimazole, and amphotericin B.
Salmonellosis (several types of *Salmonella* bacteria)	Incubation period, 6–72 hr. Sudden onset of acute gastroenteritis with abdominal cramps, diarrhea, nausea, and sometimes vomiting and dehydration. Headache and fever are present. Stools are loose for days after acute episode.	Direct via person-to-person oral–fecal contact or indirectly by ingestion of food contaminated with feces containing *Salmonella.* Communicable during entire period of infection, which may be as long as a year or more.	Infections most frequent from July to November with warm weather. Uncooked eggs and meats are major harborer of bacteria. Carriers continue to excrete organisms in stool for more than 1 year after symptoms disappear. Drug-resistant strains becoming more common.	Antibiotics for severe symptoms. Carriers treated with ampicillin.
Polio (strains of poliovirus)	Incubation period, 7–14 days or longer. Muscle weakness progressing to paralysis. May affect any muscle group, including limbs and respiratory muscles. Pain may accompany muscle weakness. There is little or no loss of sensation despite paralysis.	Direct contact of virus with mouth.	Humans are the only natural host and reservoir of the virus. Localized outbreaks in the U.S. are usually in unvaccinated or undervaccinated communities. Some recurring muscular weakness has been recently seen in persons who recovered from the illness years ago.	None.
Shigellosis (variety of bacterial agents)	Incubation period, 1–7 days. Diarrhea, fever, and nausea. Can progress to toxemia, vomiting, and tenesmus. Blood, mucus, and pus may be found in stool.	Person-to-person by fecal–oral route or, more rarely, from contaminated water. Communicable as long as organism is present, which may be a month or more. Infants and young children are more often infected because of poor hygiene.	Most contagious condition caused by bacteria. Seasonal; more common in warm weather.	Antibiotics for severe symptoms.
Intestinal parasites (roundworms and pinworms)	Abdominal pain; blood stools or diarrhea may be present. Occasional nausea and vomiting.	Transmitted via ingestion of eggs of the worms, either directly via hands and fingernails or through food and water containing eggs.	Diagnosis of pinworms made by application of cellophane tape to anal area early in the morning to confirm eggs.	Treat with mebendazole until stools are clear of parasites.

Continued

TABLE 19–10

Communicable Diseases, Community Health Concerns, and Treatment *Continued*

Disease (Causative Agent)	Symptoms	Mode of Transmission	Complications and Community Health Concerns	Specific Treatment (if any)
Toxoplasmosis (Protozoa)	Most persons have no symptoms or only mild symptoms, including enlarged lymph nodes, fever, night sweats, sore throat, or rash. Immunosuppressed persons, including HIV-positive individuals, may develop toxoplasmic encephalitis; hemiparesis, seizures, visual complications, mental disorientation, and listlessness. Fetal infection may result in spontaneous abortion, stillbirth, or varied complications after birth, including blindness, encephalitis, hydrocephalus, and anemia.	Contact with the protozoa via uncooked or undercooked meat or via airborne contact from the feces of cats.	Health education related to proper preparation of meats and care of cat litter is important. Toxoplasmosis screening should be done on pregnant women.	Immunosuppressed individuals are treated with a variety of drugs for up to 4–6 wk after symptoms resolve; infected pregnant women are also treated.
Hepatitis A (hepatitis A virus)	Incubation period, 15–30 days. Rapid onset of flulike symptoms, nausea and vomiting, abdominal cramps, jaundice; may also be asymptomatic. Long period of recovery (1–3 mo).	Person-to-person by oral–fecal route. Very contagious and spreads rapidly. Also may be spread indirectly if virus is present in milk, undercooked shellfish, or contaminated water.	Common in daycare centers, homosexuals, and illicit intravenous drug users.	Immune serum globulin can be administered if exposed individuals are identified.
Serum route				
Hepatitis B (hepatitis B virus)	Incubation period, 1–6 mo. General flulike symptoms or no symptoms. Liver deterioration, if present, is noted by markedly enlarged liver, dark urine, light stool, jaundiced eyes and skin, skin eruptions. Symptoms last 4–6 wk.	Exposure to infected blood (e.g., through sexual activity and intravenous drug paraphernalia). In health care workers exposure to infected blood is often via accidental needle puncture.	Complications include chronic hepatitis, cirrhosis, liver cancer, and death. Persons who need frequent blood transfusions are at increased risk. Health care workers are at increased risk to exposure. Chronic carriers can transmit disease to others; drug users are at risk for carrier status.	Vaccination for at-risk populations is recommended.

Continued

TABLE 19–10

Communicable Diseases, Community Health Concerns, and Treatment *Continued*

Disease (Causative Agent)	Symptoms	Mode of Transmission	Complications and Community Health Concerns	Specific Treatment (if any)
Human immunodeficiency virus (HIV)	Incubation period, potentially 10 yr or more. Flulike symptoms may or may not be noted immediately after infection. Symptoms of immune compromise including opportunistic infections and cancers that allow for the diagnosis of AIDS (i.e., Kaposi's sarcoma, *Pneumocystis carinii* pneumonia, toxoplasmosis, candidiasis, cryptococcus, cytomegalovirus, herpes simplex, and others). Eventual outcome is death.	Exchange of secretions and semen during sexual intercourse; parenteral exposure of blood and blood products from mother to fetus; breast milk.	Testing for HIV infection is confidential. Persons positive for HIV infection may be asymptomatic for years, which is problematic because they may unknowingly engage in risky behavior putting others at risk. Health teaching about safe sexual and personal habits is a concerted community health effort to control spread. HIV screening requires retesting at intervals after possible infection because the virus is not immediately detectable. There is a window period of approximately 1–12 wk after infection when test results may be negative. People must be encouraged to retest as needed to ensure accurate testing results.	Treatment depends on specific presenting opportunistic illness or disease. Azidothymidine (AZT), didanosine (DDI), and dideoxycytidine (DDC) appear to slow the spread of the virus; AZT is particularly toxic and cannot be tolerated by many. Research continues in an attempt to find an effective treatment; at present none exists. Efforts at vaccine development continue.
Sexually transmitted route				
Herpes (herpes simplex virus; HSV 1, oral; HSV 2, genital)	Incubation period, 2 wk. Lesions at site of infection are fluid filled and rupture and ulcers form scabs. Lesions may or may not be painful. Virus stays dormant in body, and successive eruptions occur commonly as a result of stress or other illnesses. HSV 2 symptoms may include fever and other flulike symptoms. In women, vaginal discharge, painful intercourse, and painful urination may be present.	Direct contact with oral and genital secretions. HSV 1 and HSV 2 viruses have recently been found in genital and oral sites previously thought to be exclusive to one or the other.	Complications include increased risk of cervical cancer. Infants exposed through birth canal may experience blindness, brain damage, or death. Recurrence in infected individuals places new sexual partners at risk. Protection of sexual partners during infectious periods should be stressed; condom use is important.	Incurable; acyclovir is given to treat existing cases and suppress recurrent episodes.

Continued

TABLE 19–10

Communicable Diseases, Community Health Concerns, and Treatment *Continued*

Disease (Causative Agent)	Symptoms	Mode of Transmission	Complications and Community Health Concerns	Specific Treatment (if any)
Cytomegalovirus (CMV)	Incubation period varies. If symptomatic, resembles mononucleosis; adults are mostly asymptomatic. Virus remains in body for life. Fetal infections can result in congenital anomalies, including mental retardation, deafness, jaundice, chorioretinitis, hydrocephaly, and epilepsy. Symptoms in newborns may not be immediately evident at birth but usually present during the first 6 months.	Transmitted through blood transfusions, organ transplants, breast milk, from children's urine and respiratory tract, and through sexual contact with semen and vaginal secretions.	Immunosuppressed individuals are at risk for frequent infectious episodes.	Ganciclovir is used to treat retinal CMV but is not successful against gastrointestinal, respiratory, and systemic CMV. Vaccine development is experimental and minimally useful to date.
Venereal warts (papillomavirus)	Condylomata warts, which may or may not be painful. Infants may develop respiratory symptoms.	Close contact with warts; may also be sexually transmitted. Passed to infants during passage through the birth canal.	Most serious complication is the link between the disease and malignancies of the cervix and genital tract.	Cryotherapy, laser therapy, or podophyllin in tincture of benzoin compound to remove or destroy warts.
Gonorrhea (*Neisseria gonorrhoeae*)	Incubation period, 2–30 days. Frequently asymptomatic, especially in men. Symptoms: women—pain, heavy purulent vaginal discharge, pain in the genital and pelvic area; men—discharge from penis, pain on urination, urinary frequency.	Primarily sexual contact. Can be transmitted to mucous membranes other than genitalia.	Complications include arthritis, blood, meningeal and heart infections, and sterility. In women, pelvic inflammatory disease; in men, narrowing of the urethra and swelling of the testicles. Children born during an active case may contact ophthalmia neonatorum, leading to blindness. Incidence is alarmingly high and most prevalent in young adults, 15–35 yr old. *Chlamydia* is frequently present with gonorrhea.	One-time dose of ceftriaxone, cefixime, ciprofloxacin or ofloxacin. Antibiotics appropriate to treat for *Chlamydia* and trichomoniasis are often prescribed simultaneously. Test of cure in 4–7 days after treatment ends to ensure treatment effectiveness is especially important, because drug-resistant strains are becoming more frequent.
Chlamydia (*Chlamydia* bacteria)	Incubation period, 1–3 wk. Symptoms consist of other infections such as nongonococcal urethritis, pelvic inflammatory disease, inflammation of cervix, and conjunctivitis. In infants, as a result of vaginal delivery: eye infections and pneumonia.	Primarily sexual contact but infections can occur in other areas of the body if contact is made with the bacteria.	Complications in women include pelvic inflammatory disease and cervical dysplasia; in men, prostatitis and epididymitis occur. Frequently occurs with other sexually transmitted diseases. This is the most frequently occurring sexually transmitted disease.	Doxycycline, azithromycin, tetracycline or erythromycin. Test of cure in 4–7 days after treatment is completed.

Continued

TABLE 19–10

Communicable Diseases, Community Health Concerns, and Treatment *Continued*

Disease (Causative Agent)	Symptoms	Mode of Transmission	Complications and Community Health Concerns	Specific Treatment (if any)
Syphilis *(Treponema pallidum)*	Incubation period, first stage, 10–90 days. Disease has three stages if left untreated. First stage: canker sore at site of infection (genital, rectum, lips); sore is usually painless. Second stage: occurs 3–6 wk later; generalized flulike symptoms and may have body rash, sores, inflamed eyes. Third stage: starts when disease becomes dormant, which may last years. Symptoms may recur, including blindness, deaf- ness, brain damage, paralysis, heart disease, and death.	Sexual contact	Incidence is increasing, especially among young adults. Complications of untreated syphilis include blindness, deafness, brain damage, paralysis, heart disease, and death.	Large-dose intramuscular penicillin; if individual is allergic to penicillin, oral tetracycline or doxycycline is given. Patients must be rescreened at 3, 6, and 12 months because some infections are resistant to treatment. Drug-related strains are becoming problematic.
Pelvic inflammatory disease (gonorrhea, *Chlamydia, Trichomonas* bacteria, and other organisms)	Abnormal vaginal discharge, severe abdominal/pelvic pain and tenderness, painful intercourse, irregular vaginal bleeding, chills, fever, and nausea and vomiting. Can be fatal.	Infections caused by sexually transmitted disease that spread to the upper genital tract of women.	Most common complication is sterility. Others include chronic abdominal pain; chronic infection of fallopian tubes, uterus, and ovaries; ectopic pregnancies.	Oral antibiotics, outpatient care; if no substantial improvement within 72 hours, hospitalization is necessary. Antibiotics should be specific for the particular organism causing the infection.
Trichomoniasis (protozoa *Trichomonas vaginalis*)	Incubation period, 1–6 wk. Men usually asymptomatic but can have slight, clear penile discharge and itch on urination. Women have thin yellow/green/gray vaginal discharge with odor and burning, redness, itching of genitalia; may have frequency of urination.	Sexual contact with exchange of body fluids.	Sexual partners must be treated at the same time, even though men are commonly asymptomatic.	Metronidazole (Flagyl, Protostat, or Metryl) given orally for 7–10 days. Vinegar douche may alleviate vaginal symptoms.

3. Tuberculin test results may be incorrect if given simultaneously with live virus vaccine. Tuberculin testing should be scheduled before administering any live vaccine or at least 30 days after vaccine administration.

Community health nurses must provide health teaching at the time of immunization. The nurse should encourage the patient to remain for at least 15 to 20 minutes after vaccine administration to ensure that there will not be a reaction. Epinephrine should be kept available so that it can be administered to reduce the effects of a reaction, if any.

Documentation is very important. Every patient should be given a written record of the immunizations he or she has received, when these were administered, and possible reactions. Clinic or organization records must be comprehensive to comply with the National Vaccine Injury Compensation Act.

Prophylactic Measures

Prophylactic measures are aimed at reducing the risk of illness to those already exposed to a communicable disease.

TABLE 19–11

HEALTHY PEOPLE 2000

Healthy People 2000 Objectives—Primary Prevention: Immunizations

1. Increase immunization levels as follows:
   Basic immunization series among children under age 2: at least 90%. (Baseline: 70% to 80%, estimated in 1989.)
   Basic immunization series among children in licensed child care facilities and in kindergarten through postsecondary educational institutions: at least 95%. (Baseline: For licensed child care, 94%; for children entering school for the 1987–1988 school year, 97%.)
   Pneumococcal pneumonia influenza immunization among institutionalized chronically ill or older people: at least 80%.
   Pneumococcal pneumonia and influenza immunization among noninstitutionalized, high-risk populations, as defined by the Immunizations Practices Advisory Committee: at least 60%. (Baseline: 10% estimated pneumococcal vaccine, 20% influenza vaccine in 1985.)
   Hepatitis B immunization among high-risk populations, including infants of surface antigen–positive mothers: at least 90%; occupationally exposed workers: at least 90%; intravenous drug users in drug treatment programs: at least 50%; homosexual men, at least 50%.
2. Expand immunization laws for schools, preschools, and day-care settings to all states for all antigens. (Baseline: Nine states and the District of Columbia in 1990.)
3. Increase to at least 90% the proportion of primary care providers who provide information and counseling about immunizations and offer immunizations as appropriate for their patients.
4. Improve the financing and delivery of immunizations for children and adults so that there is no financial barrier to receiving recommended immunizations. (Baseline: Financial coverage for immunizations was included in 45% of employment-based conventional insurance plans; in 62% of plans with preferred provider organizations; and in 98% of health maintenance organization plans in 1989; Medicaid covered basic immunizations for eligible children, and Medicare covered pneumococcal immunization for eligible older adults in 1990.)
5. Increase to at least 90% the proportion of public health departments that provide adult immunization for influenza, pneumococcal disease, hepatitis B, tetanus, and diphtheria.

From USDHHS. (1990). *Healthy people 2000: National health promotion and disease prevention objectives* (DHHS Publication No. (PHS) 91-50213). Washington, DC: U.S. Government Printing Office.

Chemoprophylactic efforts include administration of vaccines, vaccine booster doses, or other medication. Not all communicable diseases have applicable prophylactic measures. Community health nurses should know which diseases have risk reduction medication so that they can direct those exposed for appropriate treatment. Table 19–12 lists selected prophylactic recommendations for specific communicable diseases.

TABLE 19–12

Prophylactic Treatment Available for Communicable Diseases

Measles, diphtheria, or tetanus: Vaccination or booster dose, based on immunization history.

Diphtheria: Antibiotic therapy for nonimmunized and immunized persons with positive nose and throat cultures.

Pertussis: Children with an incomplete immunization series are given a booster dose. In addition, all exposed close contacts receive erythromycin for 2 weeks.

Haemophilus influenzae type B: All persons in nonimmunized exposed households with children under 4 years of age are given rifampin.

Tuberculosis: Isoniazid for 3 to 6 months. Other medication may be recommended because of increasing risk of exposure to drug-resistant strains.

Syphilis: Penicillin; recommended dosage identical to treatment dose for disease.

Ophthalmia Neonatorum: Gonorrhea: 1% silver nitrate or erythromycin ophthalmic ointment to both eyes of all newborns. *Chlamydia:* erythromycin ophthalmic ointment to both eyes of all newborns.

Hepatitis B: Immune globulin followed with hepatitis vaccine.

Data from Benenson, A. S. (Ed.). (1990). *Control of communicable disease in man.* Washington, DC: American Public Health Association; and United States Preventive Service Task Force. (1989). *Guide to clinical preventive services.* Baltimore: Williams & Wilkins.

Sanitation

Community health nurses must be aware of the sanitary conditions of the environment in which they and their patients live, work, and play. Some homes do not have running water or adequate sewage; community health nurses may practice in neighborhoods where this is considered normal. Other community health nurses are called into neighborhoods during a disaster when sanitation methods have been suspended temporarily. For example, during riots and after hurricanes, entire neighborhoods may be without adequate, safe sanitation resources. Accurate assessment is imperative so that nurses can develop appropriate objectives and nursing strategies when there is no adequate source of safe water, safe waste disposal, or safe food preparation and storage.

Employment

There is an additional need for nurses to be aware of health codes in employment situations. States and the federal government have established employment regulations that attempt to safeguard workers, and knowledge of the regulations affecting local employers is important. Nurses must play an integral role in educational, research, and practice efforts to develop and enforce those regulations.

Health care workers themselves may be at risk. Nurses, police officers, firefighters, paramedics, ambulance personnel, morticians, and those in other similar professions are at risk for most communicable diseases, including tuberculosis, tetanus, typhoid, hepatitis B, HIV, and diphtheria. Many agencies require employees to receive immunizations and specialized education to protect them from communicable diseases. The Occupational Safety and Health Association has directed that employees be provided with safety measures to help protect them from bloodborne pathogens (Bureau of National Affairs, 1992). The Occupational Safety and Health Agency (OSHA) requires that employers provide health workers with yearly in-service education on infectious disease control.

Travel

Community health nurses are frequently called on to advise clients traveling to other countries about protection from infectious diseases. Nurses should remind clients about changes in climate, hygiene, safe food preparation, water purity, and sewage management. Simple rules such as eating only fruits or vegetables that can be peeled and using bottled water for drinking and brushing the teeth are very effective preventive measures. Caution about diseases endemic to the region and disease-specific safety precautions should be provided to travelers.

Information on mandatory immunizations is available from local health departments and the CDC. Community nurses should remind travelers to allow enough time to receive all the necessary immunizations (6 months may be needed). Many immunizations cannot be given together, and some (e.g., hepatitis) require a series of inoculations over a set time to provide maximum protection.

Community Support Programs and Services

Community health nurses have a proud, rich heritage of participating in community support programs and services. Nurses play an integral role in planning and implementing strategies to improve the health of the nation (USDHHS, 1990). Many of the *Healthy People 2000* health objectives can be addressed through primary prevention efforts. Nurses independently design or collaborate with others in devising prevention programs aimed at improving environmental conditions and reducing the spread of communicable diseases. Community health nurses also participate in specific strategies to decrease the incidence of HIV infection, sexually transmitted diseases, and other infectious diseases (Table 19–13). They can educate the community on the importance of being tested for HIV and hepatitis B; they can instruct individuals and families on methods of preventing and transmitting sexually transmitted diseases; they can enlighten communities on the importance of immunizations in children, adults, and elderly individuals; and they can take part in community efforts to improve sanitation measures.

PREVENTION RELATED TO MODE OF TRANSMISSION

Health education on preventive measures can be taught to family members and significant others at risk or in direct contact with infected persons. Community health nurses can tailor general precautions to the specific route of transmission.

Respiratory Route. Action should be geared toward reducing the risk of contact with droplets to eliminate spread. In light of the risk that pneumonia, tuberculosis, and other respiratory conditions pose to those exposed, containing respiratory secretions is vital. Affected persons should be instructed to sneeze and cough into tissues and dispose of them in a receptacle. Although most pathogens die when exposed to heat, light, and air, frequent hand washing will further reduce the threat of passing viable organisms from the hand to other persons.

Integumentary Route. Reducing the spread of parasites to uninfected persons depends on personal hygiene habits. Hats, combs, brushes, and other personal items should never be shared. Parasitic spread is especially difficult to control in children, hence the recurring outbreaks of head lice in elementary schools. Scrupulous bathing and hand washing with hot water and soap reduce the potential transfer of eggs, viruses, and bacteria. When close personal contact encourages spread, sexual contact should be avoided with the infected individual until he or she is free of parasites.

Clothing and bed linens should be washed in very hot water. Sharing clothing and bedding with infected individuals should be avoided. Scabies and lice can also be killed by sealing infected linens or personal items in plastic bags for 2 weeks.

Gastrointestinal Route. Prevention is geared toward reducing the chance of transferring pathological organisms to the mouth and digestive tract. Meticulous hand washing after toileting or changing infant diapers and before working with food products is imperative. Fingernails should be kept short and the area under the nails cleaned regularly to eliminate this potential reservoir. For those organisms that thrive in stool, isolation and careful disposal of infected stool and clean bathroom facilities are important.

Proper storage and refrigeration of foods as well as effective food preparation and handling are crucial. Fastidious cleaning of equipment used in food preparation is essential, both in homes and institutions. Chemical treatment of the water supply, proper disposal of garbage, and sanitation of sewage complete the efforts at reducing pathogenic organisms.

Serum Route. Efforts are directed toward reducing the risk of exposure to infected blood and blood products.

TABLE 19–13

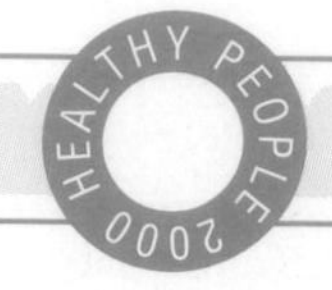

Healthy People 2000 Objectives—Reduce Risk for STDs and HIV

Education and Counseling

1. Increase to at least 75% the proportion of primary care and mental health care providers who provide age-appropriate counseling on the prevention of HIV and other sexually transmitted diseases. (Baseline: 10% of physicians regularly assessed the sexual behaviors of their patients in 1987.)
   (*Note:* Primary care providers include physicians, nurses, nurse practitioners, and physician assistants.)
2. Increase to at least 95% the proportion of schools that have age-appropriate HIV education curricula for students in 4th through 12th grade, preferably as part of a quality school health education. (Baseline: 66% of school districts required HIV education but only 5% required HIV education in each school year for 7th through 12th graders in 1989.)
3. Provide HIV education for students and staff in at least 90% of colleges and universities.
4. Increase to at least 90% the proportion of cities with populations over 100,000 that have outreach programs to contact drug abusers (particularly intravenous drug abusers) to deliver HIV risk reduction messages.
5. Increase to at least 50% the proportion of family planning clinics, maternal and child health clinics, sexually transmitted disease (STD) clinics, tuberculosis clinics, drug treatment centers, and primary care clinics that screen, diagnose, treat, counsel, and provide (or refer for) partner notification services for HIV infection and STDs (gonorrhea, syphilis, and *Chlamydia*). (Baseline: 40% of family planning clinics provided such services for bacterial STDs in 1989.)
6. Include instruction on STD transmission prevention in the curricula of all middle and secondary schools, preferably as part of a quality school health education. (Baseline: 95% of schools reported offering at least one class on STDs as part of their standard curriculum in 1988.)

Behavior Change

1. Reduce the proportion of adolescents who have engaged in sexual intercourse by age 15 to no more than 15% and by age 17 no more than 40%. (Baseline: In 1988 27% of girls and 33% of boys had had sexual intercourse by age 15; 50% of girls and 66% of boys had had sexual intercourse by age 17.)
2. Increase to at least 50% the proportion of sexually active, unmarried people who used a condom at last sexual intercourse. (Baseline: In 1988 19% of sexually active, unmarried women aged 15 through 44 reported that their partners used a condom at last sexual intercourse.)

Special Population Targets		
Use of Condoms	*1988 Baseline*	*2000 Target*
By partners of sexually active young women age 15–19	26%	60%
By sexually active young men age 15–19	57%	75%
By intravenous drug users	—	60%

3. Increase to at least 50% the estimated proportion of intravenous drug users not in treatment who use only uncontaminated drug paraphernalia ("works"). (Baseline: 25% to 35% of opiate abusers in 1989.)

Screening Programs

1. Reduce to no more than 1 per 250,000 units of blood and blood components the risk of transfusion-transmitted HIV infection. (Baseline: 1 per 40,000 to 150,000 units in 1989.)
2. Increase to at least 80% the proportion of HIV-infected people who have been tested for HIV infection. (Baseline: An estimated 15% of approximately 1 million HIV-infected people had been tested at publicly funded clinics in 1989.)
3. Increase to at least 90% the proportion of local health departments that have ongoing programs for actively identifying cases of tuberculosis and latent infection in populations at high risk for tuberculosis.

From USDHHS. (1990). *Healthy people 2000: National health promotion and disease prevention objectives* (DHHS Publication No. (PHS) 91-50213). Washington, DC: U.S. Government Printing Office.

Infected persons should be monitored for adequate control of body secretions, including blood and semen. Because sexual contact affords the opportunity for exposure to contaminated blood, such contact should be discontinued or barrier protection used. Needle exchange programs are a newer effort aimed at reducing the risk of infection among users of illicit intravenous drugs. Users are given sterile needles in exchange for used ones. Needle exchange programs are controversial, because many fear it will encourage the use of illicit drugs. A federal review of needle exchange programs in the United States, Canada, and Europe found that they are effective in reducing the spread of HIV infection and have not resulted in an increase in drug abuse ("Needle exchanges," 1993). The city government of Baltimore has launched a pilot program to provide clean needles to drug addicts; public health officers estimate that about 25% of all drug addicts in the city are infected with HIV.

Meticulous screening of the blood supply is important to reduce risk to patients who must be transfused or maintained on blood products. Efforts to improve the safety of the blood supply continue. One measure of success is the reduction in HBV and HIV infections among individuals who must receive blood or blood products. Vaccination for hepatitis B is recommended for all risk groups, including patients who must receive blood products on a long-term basis, as well as health care personnel and policemen. Community health nurses should be careful to identify every individual at risk and encourage immunization.

Health care workers must practice universal precautions at all times. Working outside the hospital setting should not lull community health nurses to be less vigilant in using appropriate precautions. Trotter (1992) has an especially useful guide for teaching safety precautions to HIV patients and their families (Table 19–14).

Sexually Transmitted Route. Essentially, precautions involve reducing sexually risky behavior. Efforts include abstaining from sexual intercourse, reducing the number of sex partners, using barrier contraception during intercourse and foreplay, and avoiding sexual activity with infected persons who have not been treated or have not completed treatment. Community health nurses should concentrate their efforts at public education in these areas. Health teaching should be aimed at populations at special risk.

The majority of HIV infection is sexually transmitted (Roper et al., 1993). At the present time, the homosexual population has made considerable progress in reducing the spread of HIV, primarily through the use of safer sexual practices and behavioral changes (Catania et al., 1992). Fineberg (1988) has predicted that consistent use of condoms could prevent approximately half of all sexually transmitted HIV infection. Condom use would have the added benefit of reducing the incidence of other STDs as well.

Targeting teens and women, the two fastest growing risk groups, is vital. Approximately half of U.S. teenagers engage in unprotected sexual intercourse (CDC, 1992b). This fact is especially troublesome because current information indicates that the spread of HIV in adolescents is primarily through heterosexual activity, not intravenous drug use (Hein, 1993). When planning programs for adolescents, community health nurses should try to provide a reality-based experience by encouraging clients to delay sexual activity and to act responsibly when engaging in such activity, and by providing access to or information on resources for condoms. Whenever possible, the use of teenage speakers who are infected with HIV is a powerful tool for communicating the realities of ignoring the problem (Hein, 1993).

Women who engage in heterosexual activity are another group at increased risk for STD and HIV infection. Kost and Forrest (1992) report that only 20% of sexually active American women have male partners who use condoms, and even then such use is only intermittent. Condom use appears to be linked to socioeconomic status rather than race. Poor women of all races are less likely to have male partners who use condoms. For those women who are reluctant to insist on condom use or whose partners refuse to wear condoms, the new female condom is a decided advantage (Gollub and Stein, 1993). In 1993, the Food and Drug Administration recommended female condoms for both contraceptive use and STD prevention. Nurses can provide women with information on the availability and use of female condoms, which are now available.

SECONDARY PREVENTION

The second level of prevention includes measures directed at early detection of disease. Efforts are directed toward early treatment to ensure treatment effectiveness and to minimize the spread of disease within the population (Table 19–15). Secondary prevention activities include antibiotic drug therapy, contact tracing, and follow-up of those infected or exposed. The community health nurse's role in secondary prevention includes identification of cases (screening and case-finding); validation of illness; administration or observation of medication administration; and provision of education, oversight, and support of caregivers.

Screening Programs

Screening programs are designed to evaluate large numbers of people for possible infection. This early detection of disease or the carrier state can reduce complications and diminish further transmission of disease in a community. One early example is the screening of immigrants on Ellis Island between 1890 and 1920. More than 20 million people were evaluated by the Marine Hospital Service for signs and symptoms of disease. Those who were found to be infected with a communicable disease (typhus, cholera, plague, smallpox, and yellow fever) were denied entry into the United States until they were no longer infected.

Screening for communicable disease involves interviewing, obtaining a physical assessment, collecting laboratory samples, and performing other diagnostic tests. Screening programs for communicable diseases are most often cost effective when the screening procedure is relatively quick and inexpensive and the communicable disease is highly infectious or has the potential to inflict very serious harm on the population. Screening may be done as part of employment (e.g., tuberculosis and hepatitis) or school enrollment (e.g., college requirements for measles titer). More frequently, screening is targeted at special risk groups; for example, studies show people often have more than one STD at the same time. Gonorrhea and *Chlamydia* or HIV and other STDs are seen simultaneously (Otten et al., 1993). Nurse practi-

TABLE 19–14

Guidelines for People with AIDS Living in the Community

As you know, the AIDS patient is immunosuppressed and is at risk for many opportunistic infections. Therefore, the following guidelines are suggested for health education to patients and family members to safeguard both the AIDS patient and household members:

Personal Cleanliness/Personal Articles

1. Handwashing after use of toilet or contact with body fluids is important.
2. Do not share thermometers, razors, razor blades, toothbrushes, douche or enema equipment, or any equipment contaminated with body secretions.

Kitchens and Bathrooms

Kitchens and bathrooms may be shared. Good household cleaning practices will prevent the spread of infection.

1. Eating utensils used by all household members must be washed with *hot* water and soap. Dishes should air dry rather than be dried with a towel.
2. Kitchen counters should be cleaned with scouring powder or weak bleach solution.
3. Refrigerators should be cleaned regularly with soap and water to control molds.
4. Kitchen floor should be mopped weekly or more often, if necessary. Dispose of mop water by pouring down toilet and disinfecting toilet with bleach solution.
5. Toilet, bathtub, shower, and bathroom floor should be cleaned with a freshly prepared solution of one part liquid bleach to 9 parts water. If the patient spills urine or has watery diarrhea that splashes onto the toilet seat, the seat must be wiped off after each spill and then cleaned with the 1:9 bleach solution.
6. Sponges used to clean floors or body fluid spills should be cleaned by soaking them for 5 minutes in a bleach solution (1 part bleach to 9 parts water). When at all possible, *use paper towels* rather than sponges because they can be disposed of and do not harbor microorganisms that are dangerous to immunosuppressed clients.

Food Preparation

People with AIDS can safely cook for others. They should follow the usual practices for safe food preparation. Because their immune system is altered, they are at risk for food poisoning and should be very aware of safe food preparation and food storage.

1. Wash hands thoroughly before food preparation.
2. Do not lick fingers or mixing spoon while cooking.
3. Avoid unpasteurized milk to reduce risk of *Salmonella* exposure; thoroughly wash uncooked chicken; do not use cracked eggs.

Laundry and Linens

1. Clothing or linen soiled with body fluids should be stored separately in a plastic bag and should be washed separately in a washing machine using *hot* water and detergent, and bleach. Liquid Lysol can be used for colored laundry. (Wear disposable gloves when touching the soiled clothes or linen.) Linens not soiled by body fluids may be handled in the usual manner without special precautions.
2. Used towels and washcloths should not be shared by household members. However, they can safely be used by others after they have been washed using the laundering procedure as above.

Preventing Cross-Infection

1. Wear gloves when handling body fluids, linens, or other objects contaminated with body fluids. (People with exudative lesions or weeping dermatitis should refrain from caring for the patient until the condition resolves.)
2. Disposable gowns or aprons may be worn to protect clothing from becoming soiled with body fluids.
3. Caregivers with a cold or flu should wear a mask when in close personal contact with the person with AIDS to protect the patient, as AIDS patients are very susceptible to opportunistic infections.
4. Ensure good ventilation in the living quarters.

Trash Disposal

1. Body wastes such as urine, feces, blood should be flushed down the toilet.
2. Discard dressings, diapers, Chux, or any materials soiled with body fluids and secretions in a plastic bag. Pour in a 1:9 bleach/water solution until soiled contents are soaked. Place sealed bag into another plastic bag, seal again, and place in regular trash.
3. Sharps should be discarded in a special sharps container provided by a home care agency. Transport container back to agency for incineration when container is three-fourths full. If no sharps container is available, use a metal coffee can or a puncture-proof plastic container to discard needles and sharps. When container is three-fourths full, transport it to the incinerator *or* pour 1:9 bleach/water solution over needles. Seal container, place it in a plastic trash bag and discard it in the trash.

Sexual Practices

1. Precautions must be taken to prevent the sharing of body secretions; therefore, information about "safe sex" practices should be provided to the patient and families. Pamphlets and counseling are available.

Pets

Pets can be a source of potential infection to the immunosuppressed patient. Therefore, the following guidelines are provided regarding the care of pets and their habitats:

1. Clean bird cages wearing gloves and mask, as birds can spread psittacosis.
2. Clean cat litter boxes wearing gloves and mask to prevent toxoplasmosis.
3. Change water in tropical fish tanks wearing gloves and mask to prevent *mycobacterium* infection.

TABLE 19–15

Healthy People 2000 Objectives—Secondary Prevention for Communicable Diseases

1. Increase to at least 50% the estimated proportion of all intravenous drug abusers who are in drug abuse treatment programs. (Baseline: An estimated 11% of opiate abusers were in treatment in 1989.)
2. Increase to at least 50% the proportion of clinics that screen, diagnose, treat, counsel, and provide (or refer for) partner notification services for HIV infection and bacterial sexually transmitted diseases. (Baseline: 40% of family planning clinics only provided such services in 1989.)
3. Increase to at least 90% the proportion of primary care providers treating patients with sexually transmitted disease who correctly manage cases, as measured by their use of appropriate types and amounts of therapy. (Baseline: 70% in 1988.)
4. Increase to at least 90% the proportion of primary care providers who provide information and counseling about and offer appropriate immunizations to their patients.
5. Increase to at least 85% the proportion of people found to have tuberculosis infection who completed courses of preventive therapy. (Baseline: Survey of health departments found that 66.3% completed treatment in 1987.)

From USDHHS. (1990). *Healthy people 2000: National health promotion and disease prevention objectives* (DHHS Publication No. (PHS) 91-50231). Washington, DC: U.S. Government Printing Office.

tioners, community health nurses, and others who provide care should be aware of the need to screen for other STDs at the time a person seeks treatment. All tuberculosis patients should be screened for HIV, and all HIV patients should be screened for tuberculosis.

For most communicable diseases, screening is done for both public protection and early treatment. Because HIV infection has no cure, screening programs for this communicable disease are more controversial. Opponents argue that there is no need for screening, because once identified, infected individuals may be discriminated against in employment opportunities, health insurance plans, and other areas. Others argue there is much to be gained by early identification of HIV infection. Otten et al. (1993) state that HIV screening is done for four reasons:

- To promote behavior changes,
- To provide entry into clinical care,
- To provide information for partner notification and education, and
- To protect the blood supply.

Screening does increase population protection by reducing the risk to close contacts. HIV screening will not facilitate a cure, but it does allow HIV-infected individuals the opportunity to seek supportive care earlier, thus increasing their quality of life. The CDC suggests that hospitals and clinics with large numbers of HIV/AIDS cases should routinely test for infection (APHA, 1993b). Screening would still be voluntary and confidential and should include a pretest and posttest counseling session. Patients who test positive would be referred for further services, but all patients would be counseled about risky behaviors and safer sex practices. Health professionals who need resources for counseling and teaching HIV/AIDS patients can call a special toll-free telephone number provided by the U.S. Public Health Service and listed in the community resources at the end of the chapter (Table 19–16).

Anonymous, Blind, or Confidential Testing. In addition to routine testing, people can be screened for communicable diseases in anonymous, blind, or confidential programs. These three methods are normally used when screening for communicable diseases that carry a degree of public censure or stigma. Blind screening involves testing samples drawn for other purposes and stripped of identification (e.g., hospitalized patients who have blood drawn for routine admission blood work). The purpose is to get an accurate estimate of communicable disease in the population. Bayer (1993) reports that blind studies can provide valuable information about patterns. However, blind studies do not allow for treatment, because samples are not traceable to the person who provided the sample.

Anonymous testing allows people to register under an identifier code or number, while confidential testing registers people by name. In both cases, test results are available only to the client. Anonymous testing is offered as a strategy to increase people's willingness to come for testing. Goldbaum et al. (1993) report that anonymous testing may increase the number of persons willing to be tested for HIV, but further research is indicated.

Screening procedures for HIV/AIDS have been altered to better achieve a decrease in risky behavior. Formerly, anonymous and confidential testing results were supplied over the telephone. Currently, however, most programs require those tested to pick up the results in person, even when negative, to provide an additional opportunity to counsel clients on risk factors, risky behaviors, and safer sex precautions. Community health nurses and others involved in HIV screening programs should counsel clients about the issues listed in Table 19–17. People may become depressed on learning of their HIV-positive status. Cleary et al. (1993) found that up to one third of HIV-positive patients in their study reported depression. It is very important for community health nurses to refer newly diagnosed HIV-positive individuals for counseling and support services.

Case-Finding and Contact Tracing. Case-finding interviews designed to identify contacts of infected individuals are often also the responsibility of the community health nurse (Poulin et al., 1992). The purpose of case-finding is to identify every case of disease and to provide swift

TABLE 19–16

Community Resources

American Academy of Pediatrics
141 Northwest Point Blvd.
P.O. Box 927
Elk Grove Village, IL 60009–0927

The Report of the Committee on Infectious Diseases of the American Academy of Pediatricians gives immunization recommendations and other information.

American College of Obstetricians and Gynecologists
Resource Center
409 12th St. S.W.
Washington, DC 20024

Technical bulletins contain information including the recommended immunizations for pregnant women

Sexually Transmitted Diseases (journal)
American Venereal Disease Association
Box 385
University of Virginia Hospital
Charlottesville, VA 22908

Control of Communicable Diseases in Man (manual)
American Public Health Association
1015 15th St. N.W.
Washington, DC 20005

Division of Immunization
Centers for Disease Control and Prevention
Atlanta, GA 30333

Division of Quarantine
Centers for Disease Control and Prevention
Atlanta, GA 30333

Boards of health/health departments

City, county, and state departments of health provide information on screening, immunizations, incidence, and treatment recommendations. Refer to the telephone directory.

TABLE 19–16

Community Resources *Continued*

Guide for Adult Immunization (journal)
American College of Physicians
Division of Scientific Activities
Health and Public Policy
4200 Pine St.
Philadelphia, PA 19104

Health Information for International Travel (journal)
Superintendent of Documents
U.S. Government Printing Office
Washington, DC 20402

National Vaccine Injury Compensation Program
Health Resources and Services Administration
Parklawn Bldg., Room 7-90
5600 Fishers Lane
Rockville, MD 20857

Morbidity and Mortality Weekly Report (journal)
Subscription Information:
Superintendent of Documents
U.S. Government Printing Office
Washington, DC 20402

WHO Publications Centre, U.S.A.
49 Sheridan Ave.
Albany, NY

American Public Health Association *Special Initiatives on AIDS* Series
- Report 1: Casual contact and the risk of HIV
- Report 2: Contact tracing and partner notification
- Report 3: Illicit drug use and HIV infection
- Report 4: HIV antibody testing
- Report 5: Public health implications of PCP prophylaxis
- Report 6: Pediatric HIV infection
- Report 7: Public health implications of early intervention in HIV disease
- Report 8: Women and HIV disease
- Report 9: Tuberculosis and HIV disease

Each report is $3.50 per copy for APHA members, $5.00 per copy for nonmembers. Orders must be prepaid. Order from APHA, Publication Sales, Dept. 5037, Washington, DC 20061–5037.

Public Health Service AIDs Hotline
1–800–342–AIDS (for general public)
1–800–933–3413 (for health professionals only; 10:30 A.M. to 8 P.M.)

treatment for new cases. Searching for potential victims begins by identifying individuals with the most intimate contact (level 1) and proceeding to less intimate contacts (level 2 and 3) (Fig. 19–5). For most communicable diseases, there is no need to proceed to level 2 if no cases are discovered in the level 1 contacts. For example, when screening a school for head lice, the nurse would first screen the grade in which the contact case was found and any grades that contain family members of that child. If these grades are free of lice, there is little purpose in screening the rest of the school. In light of the current cost-cutting imperative, nurses should consider the cost-effectiveness of health screening and save resources for necessary services.

All sexual partners should be identified when performing contact tracing for STDs and HIV. Sometimes people will have multiple sex partners whom they consider casual acquaintances rather than close partners. For contact tracing, all sexual partners are level 1 contacts. Case-finding requires patience and sensitivity on the part of the investigator. Some communicable diseases, particularly STDs and HIV infection, may be a source of embarrassment for the victims. If the nurse is not accepting and caring during the interviews, clients may not cooperate, thereby reducing the chance of locating potential victims. Table 19–18 provides a number of "golden rules" that interviewers may find useful when conducting contact tracing interviews.

TABLE 19–17

Counseling Topics in HIV Screening Programs

Pretest

Routes of transmission
Client risk behaviors
Risk reduction education

Posttest

If negative: Give results; review risk reduction education; provide referrals

If positive: Give results; review potential impact of infection on health status; provide information to reduce risk of infection in others; provide emotional support, referrals, treatment for concurrent treatable diseases (STDs), and contact tracing.

Specimen Collection

Community health nurses are often expected to obtain specimens from clients, prepare the specimens for transport to the laboratory, and receive the results. Accurate laboratory results are dependent on correct collection, storage, and transport of specimens. The nurse should take care to follow laboratory directions exactly (e.g., refrigerate the sample if so directed). In addition, nurses need to be safety conscious, as specimen collection can be very dangerous if the nurse is careless. All nurses must consistently follow appropriate infection control measures, including universal precautions (see Chapter 29).

Test results take time, and community health nurses should be familiar with the usual time frame for each test. Bacterial cultures are usually available in a short time because most grow in hours. *Mycobacterium* organisms (i.e., tuberculosis) may take weeks to grow, so culture results may take a long time. The patient and family members will be anxious to learn the results as soon as possible, and informing them of the expected arrival time will help reduce some of their anxiety.

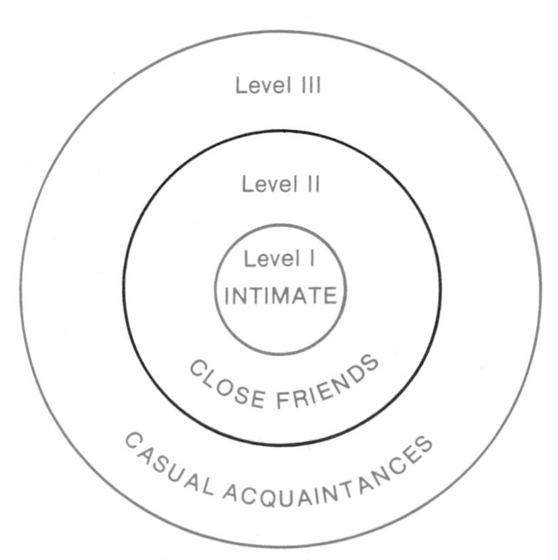

Figure 19–5 ● Case-finding priority contacts.

TABLE 19–18

Golden Rules of Interviewing

1. Initial contact should be with a named source, not other household members.
2. If you must leave a telephone message, provide no information other than name and telephone number.
3. Emphasize client confidentiality related to test results and other services.
4. Allow the contact a choice of interview location and time.
5. In cases involving drugs do not ask for drug sources or specific drugs.
6. When tracing, interviewees are not to be given the name of the initial contact, no matter how insistent they might become.
7. Incomplete information should be recorded because it may help with later contact tracing.
8. It is possible to be flexible, informal, and supportive and still get all the information required in the survey.
9. Cooperation may be encouraged by explaining the risks; adopting a "you help us, we will help you" attitude; and leaving a business card with people reluctant to name contacts at first interview.
10. Respect all contacts.

Modified from Poulin, C., Gyorkos, T. W., MacPhee, J., Cann, B., & Bickerton, J. (1992). Contact-tracing among injection drug users in a rural area. *Canadian Journal of Public Health, 83*(2), 106–108.

Laboratories require accurate information accompanying the specimen to assist in the identification of the infectious agent. The nurse can aid the process by supplying detail on signs, symptoms, and patient activities and lifestyle patterns as clues to assist in the laboratory investigation.

Comfort Measures

Most communicable diseases are treated at home, not in the hospital. In addition to care and treatment regimens applicable to specific diseases, there are general symptomatic comfort and care measures that the nurse can teach to caregivers.

In general, rest, adequate nutrition and hydration, and fever control are important. Bed rest may be necessary, especially with childhood diseases and hepatitis. Adequate hydration is essential and may be problematic in children and the elderly. The nurse should instruct caregivers to be alert for signs of poor hydration (e.g., poor skin turgor and depressed fontanelles in infants). Intravenous fluid replacement may be necessary, especially if gastrointestinal upsets are severe, as may be the case in salmonellosis or shigellosis.

Aspirin or acetaminophen can be used to reduce fever. However, aspirin should be avoided in children because of the link to Reye's syndrome. High fevers are common in children and may require water sponge baths for cooling.

Skin disruptions such as blisters and body rashes require scrupulous hygiene to reduce the risk of infection.

Scratching can exacerbate the problem and in certain conditions may spread the disease. Some relief from itching may be gained by bathing in tepid water with cornstarch or oatmeal. Children can sleep with cotton gloves to reduce the risk of scratching in their sleep. Genital eruptions from STDs should be kept clean and as dry as possible. A hair dryer on a mild heat setting can be used to ensure that wet skin and skin folds are completely dry. Loose clothing and cotton underwear can help to speed healing.

Compliance with prescribed medication is essential. Failure to follow through with the complete medication regimen is thought to be one important reason for the increasing numbers of drug-resistant organisms. Compliance can be particularly problematic when therapy is long term as in tuberculosis, in which patients are required to be on medication long after symptoms have resolved. Nurses can play a vital role by helping patients understand the importance of maintaining drug treatment and by providing oversight to validate and support compliance.

Documenting resolution of a disease is the important last step in treating the illness. *Test of cure* is the term used to indicate that a treated individual has had repeated laboratory tests and is no longer contagious or is free of the disease. This is particularly important in diseases that can linger or relapse if not completely eliminated in an individual (e.g., diphtheria, gonorrhea, and *Chlamydia*).

Legal Enforcement

It is imperative that nurses become knowledgeable not only about agency regulations for control of communicable diseases but also about state statutes and regulations and enforcement. Some regulations give the nurse an enforcement responsibility. For example, nurses must report the incidence of communicable disease or a violation of sanitary codes. States have different regulations concerning enforcement provisions, so nurses must explore the rules of the state in which they practice.

The law does allow public health officials to compel individuals to comply with treatment if noncompliance endangers the general public. Tuberculosis care is one example. Public health officers have the authority to require compliance with treatment and the legal means to ensure compliance through forced institutionalization if all other methods fail. Incarceration is a viable but last-choice option. Community health nurses are involved in monitoring compliance through directly observed medication administration. When patients are not compliant, nurses may be called on to initiate legal action for confinement or to serve as a witness during the court proceedings. Public health laws require that patients be afforded due rights, including counsel and a hearing when constraint measures are indicated (Bayer et al., 1993).

Exclusion from School

Children who have symptoms that may be due to a communicable disease should be kept home from school. Chickenpox is extremely contagious, especially before eruption of skin lesions, and there is no proven effective vaccine. Nurses should be aware of any children complaining of sore throats or other "cold" symptoms that may indicate respiratory transmission. Parents should be encouraged to keep those children at home. If there are resulting skin eruptions, parents should notify the school nurse or daycare personnel so that other parents can be informed that their child has been exposed. Nurses have an added responsibility to teach children about hand washing, using tissues frequently, disposing of those tissues, and other wellness behaviors that reduce the chance of respiratory infection. Children with chickenpox may return to school when the vesicles have dried as scabs.

Children are also at risk for rapid infections caused by pests and organisms transmitted through the integumentary route. Lice and scabies can infect children in daycare centers, classrooms, and summer camps rapidly. Nurses should examine all other children and adults when infection is suspected. Parents and guardians will have to be notified about the infections so that they can initiate treatment efforts. If the child has come in contact with linens or clothing, then dry cleaning and laundering in extremely hot water are necessary. Nurses can teach children not to share brushes and combs and can teach teachers and daycare workers to observe children for frequent scratching and scratch marks. The earlier the infestation can be detected, the easier it will be to prevent further spread and provide effective treatment.

TERTIARY PREVENTION

Tertiary prevention that is concerned with rehabilitation of lingering dysfunctions after illness is not as frequently addressed in community nursing, because most communicable diseases resolve swiftly, resulting in few long-term rehabilitative needs. Several important exceptions are hepatitis, HIV infection, and some STDs, which produce long-term needs that can be classified as tertiary prevention needs. A number of STDs (e.g., herpes) have no cure and require lifelong vigilance. Others (e.g., those with gonorrhea and human papillomavirus) can develop complications, especially reproductive problems such as impaired fertility, sterility, or uterine cancer.

Conclusion

Opportunities exist for the expansion of community health nurses' responsibilities in the control of communicable diseases. Nursing and society have too long depended on environmental and medical science to prevent and cure infectious diseases. The advent of a new contagion (HIV), the antigenic variations in the older known contagions, and the continuing presence of preventable diseases have revealed that humanity and science do not have the means of completely controlling or preventing contagious diseases. The science of nursing must be ready to provide strategies for disease prevention and health promotion. Nurses must give care to infected individuals and their families to promote higher levels of wellness. In addition, community health nurses can explore factors that affect human health behaviors, lifestyles, and participation in activities that reduce exposure to communicable diseases.

KEY IDEAS

1. Knowledge of the characteristics of specific infectious agents, their modes of transmission, and the susceptibility of human hosts help identify ways to prevent the transmission of communicable diseases.
2. Many communicable diseases have been reduced in the United States since the 1940s as a result of environmental sanitation, immunization, antibiotic treatment, and lifestyle changes. Renewed emphasis is being placed on immunizations to prevent communicable diseases of childhood.
3. Sexually transmitted diseases and infections from hepatitis B and HIV are rising. Multidrug-resistant forms of tuberculosis are emerging as a new concern.
4. Health care workers, including community health nurses, are at greater risk than the general public for contracting bloodborne pathogens. Use of universal precautions is essential.
5. All levels of government have some responsibility for the prevention and control of communicable diseases to protect the health of the public. The right of the public to be protected may take precedence over an individual's right to refuse treatment.
6. At the federal level, the Centers for Disease Control and Prevention collects information on reportable diseases, conducts research, and recommends appropriate prevention and treatment protocols. State and local health departments have responsibility for environmental control, identifying and reporting communicable diseases, ensuring the availability of immunizations, and seeing that communicable diseases are treated when medically possible. Each state has its own laws governing communicable disease control.
7. Many of the *Healthy People 2000* objectives address the reduction of communicable diseases. Populations are targeted for interventions based on the epidemiology of specific communicable diseases. Community health nurses independently and in collaboration with others devise programs for communicable disease prevention.
8. Community health nurses are key health care providers in the prevention and control of communicable diseases.
9. Primary prevention includes teaching about ways to minimize the risk of communicable diseases, including the importance of immunizations. Community health nurses should be diligent to ensure that all individuals are current on their immunizations.
10. In secondary prevention, community health nurses screen those who may be infected and assist those with communicable diseases to access appropriate medical treatment, follow the treatment regimen, and prevent the spread of disease to others. CHNs conduct contact tracing as one way of case-finding.
11. Nursing case management is important for persons who are carriers of communicable diseases, such as hepatitis B, and for those with chronic infections such as HIV.

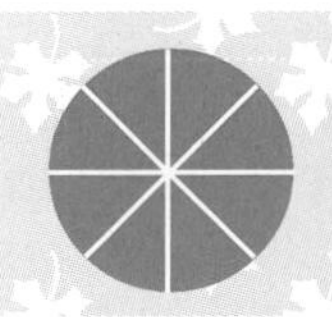

APPLYING THE NURSING PROCESS: *A Client at Risk for AIDS and STDs*

Ms. Roberts enters the health department STD clinic, where the community health nurse proceeds with the intake interview. The care at the clinic is based on the concept of case management. Personnel consist of a nurse, physician, social worker, and family planning counselor who work as a team and have weekly meetings to review cases.

During the interview Ms. Roberts tells the nurse that she is a 33-year-old unmarried woman with a suspicion that she might have been exposed to the AIDS virus. Ms. Roberts shares that she is currently sharing her apartment with her partner, Mr. Thomas. Ms. Roberts fears that she was exposed to HIV when she was 26 years old by sharing needles with a group of friends who were intravenous drug abusers. She also had multiple sex partners during this same period, and did not use condoms. There is no pertinent past medical or familial history. Ms. Roberts states she has not used intravenous drugs for more than 5 years. Furthermore, she assures the CHN that she has not had sexual contact with anyone except Mr. Thomas for 6 months.

Ms. Roberts also states she thinks she might be pregnant. She is feeling tired all the time and has lost some weight. She has been vomiting in the morning and has noticed a yellow cervical discharge. The nurse questions Ms. Roberts and finds out that her last menstrual period was 4 weeks earlier. Her vital signs are assessed and are found to be within normal limits. Ms. Roberts states that she really would like to be pregnant. She really loves Mr. Thomas, and they have talked about having a baby in the near future. The community health nurse begins to counsel Ms. Roberts about HIV testing according to the clinic protocol. After the counseling session, the nurse questions Ms. Roberts and is convinced that she fully understands about the enzyme-linked immunosorbent assay (ELISA) and Western blot tests. Ms. Roberts also understands that the results are fairly reliable, but there is some error associated with each test. Furthermore, the tests indicate only that she has been exposed to the virus. The community health nurse takes the blood sample, marks it, and sends it to be tested. Ms. Roberts is told that the results will not be given over the telephone.

The nurse next goes with Ms. Roberts to see the clinic physician, who examines Ms. Roberts and performs a pregnancy test. During the vaginal examination the physician notes that there is a thick yellow cervical discharge. A sample of the secretion is obtained and sent to the laboratory. The nurse tells Ms. Roberts that she will be called on the telephone when the result of this test is returned to the clinic. The nurse then begins to educate Ms. Roberts about the routes of transmission of HIV and STDs and about safer sex practices. She counsels Ms. Roberts to encourage Mr. Thomas to use a condom with nonoxynol-9 spermicide.

The pregnancy test comes back positive. The nurse must decide whether to call and tell Ms. Roberts immediately or to wait until the HIV test results come back. If she tells her about the pregnancy test without the HIV test results, Ms. Roberts may become elated about the pregnancy, only to be immediately disappointed by the HIV test result later. The nurse discusses the problem with health care team members, who recommend that Ms. Roberts be told of the pregnancy so that she can internalize this information before she learns about her HIV status.

When the nurse calls Ms. Roberts she is very excited about the pregnancy and states she cannot wait to tell Mr. Thomas. She agrees to call the maternity clinic and make an appointment.

One week later the result of the cervical secretions culture returns, and it is positive for gonorrhea. The nurse calls Ms. Roberts so Mr. Thomas can be tested and treatment for gonorrhea can begin as soon as possible. The couple comes to the STD clinic and both are treated with penicillin.

Three days later the results from the HIV tests come back positive. The nurse telephones Ms. Roberts and asks her to come to the clinic for the results.

Assessment

- Conduct family assessment.
- Assess for denial, anxiety, fear, anger, sadness, or depression related to HIV status.
- Assess family and social supports.
- Assess knowledge of both partners regarding STD and HIV/AIDS, including prevention of transmission.
- Assess attitude toward pregnancy.
- Assess the need for primary medical care services for treatment of HIV.

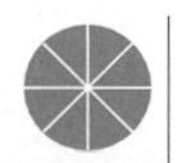

Nursing Diagnosis	Goal	Interventions
Fear related to possible HIV infection	The client will learn of her HIV status.	Counsel the client about HIV testing, protocol, confidentiality, and how results are reported. Review risk factors for HIV infection/AIDS.
High risk for infection, STD	The client will receive appropriate diagnosis and treatment for STD.	Arrange for a vaginal smear. Provide appropriate treatment for gonorrhea as prescribed after diagnosis. Review prescribed medication therapy with the client. Arrange for retest after completion of the medication regimen.
Grieving related to positive HIV test result	The client will express acceptance of her HIV-positive status.	Encourage the client to express her emotions related to the positive test result. Provide the telephone number of a counseling service and/or arrange for immediate counseling, depending on the client's emotional state. Provide a crisis hotline telephone number for after-hours counseling, if needed. Assess the client's available support services. Refer the client to an HIV/AIDS support group. Arrange for referral for assessment of HIV infection and ongoing care for HIV-related problems with a specialty clinic or physician.
High risk for infection transmission	The client and partner will express plans to use condoms to prevent infection transmission	Screen the client for possible intimate contacts and notify partners. Arrange for testing of contacts. Arrange for treatment of contacts who test positive for STD. Arrange for counseling of contacts who test positive for HIV.

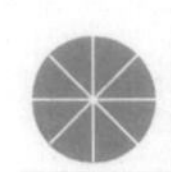

Nursing Diagnosis	Goal	Interventions
Knowledge deficit, physiological changes of pregnancy, STDs, and HIV infection/AIDS	The client and partner will base their decisions on accurate information.	Arrange referral to an obstetric clinic for the client; discuss the risk of HIV transmission to the fetus. Assess the client's and partner's knowledge of STDs; provide accurate information, and correct any misconceptions. Assess the client's and partner's knowledge of HIV/AIDS; provide accurate information and correct any misconceptions; specifically, provide information on safer sex practices.

Evaluation

Ms. Roberts comes to the clinic that afternoon and is told the tests indicate she is positive for HIV. Ms. Roberts is devastated. She does not know what to do. She is too upset to hear much of what the nurse has to say about what the future might be for her and the baby. Ms. Roberts discusses her fears and her feelings of shame. The nurse stays with Ms. Roberts until she is calmer and makes another appointment to discuss future plans. Ms. Roberts is invited to telephone to ask questions and discuss her concerns. The nurse also gives a telephone number of the local AIDS program office and pamphlets about HIV infection. Ms. Roberts is asked to try to remember her sexual contacts and her IV drug partners. Ms. Roberts knows she must go home and tell Mr. Thomas that he has been exposed to HIV, and that their baby may be infected. The nurse requests that Mr. Thomas telephone the clinic.

Mr. Thomas telephones the clinic the next day and makes an appointment to be tested for HIV the following week. His tests come back negative. The couple decide to have the baby based on the information that between 20% and 65% of infants from infected mothers are infected with HIV (Neal et al., 1990). They have contacted the AIDS office and the maternity clinic. Both agencies have given them information and have been supportive.

The future may be uncertain, but the couple is developing a professional support system. They have not yet told their families, but they are discussing how it can best be done. They thank the nurse and the clinic staff for their help. They continue to be seen at the STD clinic until the gonorrhea infections in both have been cured. In collaboration with staff in the health department maternity clinic and AIDS program, the nurse will use a case management approach to continue to provide support to Ms. Roberts, Mr. Thomas, and their baby.

GUIDELINES FOR LEARNING

1. Develop a position paper on the following debatable issue: Should individual rights be compromised to control the spread of communicable diseases for the good of society?
2. Survey the role of boards of health in your community and state to determine how communicable diseases are prevented and controlled. What services do the boards provide?
3. Develop an educational program for pregnant adolescents to inform them about communicable diseases.
4. Explore the legal statutes in your state pertaining to control of communicable diseases.
5. Investigate the immunization criteria used in your state.
6. If possible, make arrangements through a clinical instructor to visit an STD clinic in your area, and spend the day observing and assisting in nursing responsibilities.
7. Note three diseases with distinctive trends in incidence (see Table 19–2). Determine the reasons for the changes in incidence.

REFERENCES

American Public Health Association (APHA). (1993a). *Action alert.* July 27. Washington, DC: Author.

APHA. (1993b). CDC pushes ahead with routine AIDS testing. *The Nation's Health, April,* 2.

Aronson, S. P. (1978). *Communicable disease in nursing.* New York: Medical Examining Publishing

Bayer, R. (1993). The ethics of blinded HIV surveillance testing. *American Journal of Public Health, 83*(5), 496–497.

Bayer, R., Dubler, N. N., & Landesman, S. L. (1993). The dual epidemic of tuberculosis and AIDS: Ethical and policy issues in screening and treatment. *American Journal of Public Health, 83*(5), 649–654.

Benenson, A. S. (Ed.). (1990). *Control of communicable disease in man.* Washington, DC: American Public Health Association.

Bennett, L. C., & Searl, S. (1982). *Communicable disease handbook.* New York: John Wiley & Sons.

Betts, R. F., & Douglas, Jr., R. G. (1990). Influenza virus. In G. L. Mandell, R. G. Douglas, & J. E. Bennett (Eds.). *Principles and practices of infectious diseases* (3rd ed.) (pp. 1306–1325). New York: Churchill Livingstone.

Boland, M. G. (1991). The child with HIV infection. In J. D. Durham, & F. L. Cohen (Eds.). *The person with AIDS: Nursing perspectives* (pp. 316–347). New York: Springer.

Brachman, P. S. (1989a). Principles and methods. In G. L. Mandell, R. C. Douglas, & J. E. Bennett (Eds.). *Principles and practices of infectious diseases* (3rd ed.) (pp. 147–155). New York: Churchill Livingstone..

Brachman, P. S. (1989b). Transmission and principles of control. In G. L. Mandell, R. G. Douglas, & T. E. Bennett (Eds.). *Principles and practices of infectious diseases* (3rd ed.) (pp. 155–158). New York: Churchill Livingstone.

Brudney, K., & Dobkin, J. (1991). Resurgent tuberculosis in New York City: Human immunodeficiency virus, homelessness, and the decline of tuberculosis control programs. *American Review of Respiratory Diseases, 144,* 745–749.

Bureau of National Affairs. (1992). Bloodborne pathogens. *Occupational Safety and Health Reporter,* Sec. 1910.1030(c)(2)(i), 41–46.

Catania, J. A., Coates, T. H., & Kegeles, S. (1992). Condom use in multi-ethnic neighborhoods of San Francisco: The population-based AMWN (AIDS in Multi-Ethnic Neighborhoods) Study. *American Journal of Public Health, 82*(2), 284–287.

Cates, W., & Toomey, K. E. (1990). Sexually transmitted diseases: Overview of the situation. *Primary Care, 17*(1), 1–27.

Centers for Disease Control and Prevention (CDC). (1988). *Guidelines for prevention of transmission of human immunodeficiency virus and hepatitis b virus to health-care and public-safety workers.* A response to P.L. 100-607: The Health Omnibus Programs Extension Act of 1988.

CDC. (1990). Guidelines for preventing the transmission of tuberculosis in health-care settings, with special focus on HIV-related issues. *Morbidity and Mortality Weekly Report, 39*(RR-17).

CDC. (1991). Update on adult immunization. *Morbidity and Mortality Weekly Report, 40*(RR-12), 1–94.

CDC. (1992a). Important information about hepatitis B, hepatitis B vaccine, and hepatitis B immune globulin. In *Hepatitis B: 5/27/92.* Washington, DC: CDC, U.S. Department of Health and Human Services.

CDC. (1992b). Selected behaviors that increase risk for HIV infection among high school students—US, 1990. *Morbidity and Mortality Weekly Report, 41,* 231–240.

CDC. (1993a). Contraindications and precautions to vaccinations. *Morbidity and Mortality Weekly Report, 42*(RR-5), 12–13.

CDC. (1993b). Initial therapy for tuberculosis in the era of multidrug resistance: Recommendations of the Advisory Council for the Elimination of Tuberculosis. *Morbidity and Mortality Weekly Report, 42*(RR-7), 1–8.

CDC. (1993c). 1993 Revised classification system for HIV infection and expanded surveillance case definition for AIDS among adolescents and adults. *Morbidity and Mortality Weekly Report, 41*(RR-17), 1–19.

CDC. (1994). General recommendations on immunization. *Morbidity and Mortality Weekly Report 43*(RR–1), 9.

Cleary, N., VanDevanter, T., Rogers, T. F., Singer, E., Shipton-Levy, M., Steilne, A., Stuart, A., Avorn, J., & Pindyck, J. (1993). Depressive symptoms in blood donors notified of HIV infection. *American Journal of Public Health, 83*(4), 534–539.

Diaz, T., Buehler, J., Castro, K., & Ward, J. (1993). AIDS trends among Hispanics in the United States. *American Journal of Public Health, 83*(4), 504–509.

Dobkin, J. F. (1990). Infections in parenteral drug abusers. In G. L. Mandell, R. G. Douglas, & J. E. Bennett (Eds.), *Principles and practices of infectious diseases* (3rd ed.) (pp. 2276–2280). New York: Churchill Livingstone.

Dowling, H. F. (1977). *Fighting infection: Conquests of the twentieth century.* Cambridge, MA: Harvard University Press.

Fineberg, H. V. (1988). Education to prevent AIDS: Prospects and obstacles. *Science, 239,* 592–596.

Goldbaum, G., Pearlman, T., Wood, R., & Krueger, L. (1993). Differences between anonymous and confidential registrants for HIV testing—Seattle, 1986–1992. *Morbidity and Mortality Weekly Report, 42*(3), 53–56.

Gollub, E. L., & Stein, Z. A. (1993). Commentary: The new female condom—item 1 on a women's AIDS prevention agenda. *American Journal of Public Health, 83*(5), 498–500.

Hein, K. (1993). "Getting real" about HIV in adolescents. *American Journal of Public Health, 83*(4), 492–494.

Hinman, A. R., Orenstein, W. A., Bart, K. J., & Preblud, S. R. (1989). Immunization. In G. L. Mandell, R. G. Douglas, & J. E. Bennett (Eds.). *Principles and practices of infectious diseases* (3rd ed.) (pp. 2320–2334). New York: Churchill Livingstone.

House Select Committee on Children, Youth and Families. (1992). *A decade of denial: Teens and AIDS in America.* Washington, DC: U.S. Government Printing Office.

Kochi, A. (1991). The global tuberculosis situation and the new control strategy of the World Health Organization. *Tubercle, 72,* 1–6.

Kost, K., & Forrest, J. D. (1992). American women's sexual behavior and exposure to risk of sexually transmitted diseases. *Family Planning Perspectives, 24,* 244–254.

Miller, C. A. (1990). *Nursing care of older adults: Theory and practice.* Glenview, IL: Scott, Foresman, and Co.

Mullan, F. (1989). *Plagues and politics: The story of the United States Public Health Service.* New York: Basic Books.

Neal, A., Baulos, R., & Holt, E. (1990). Transmission of HIV-1 infections from mothers to infants in Haiti. *Journal of the American Medical Association, 264*(16), 2088–2092.

Needle exchanges found to be effective. (1993, October 1). *Baltimore Sun,* p. 23A.

Neff, J. M. (1990). Variola (smallpox) and monkey viruses. In G. L. Mandell, R. G. Douglas, and J. E. Bennett (Eds.). *Principles and practices of infectious diseases* (3rd ed.) (pp. 1137–1138). New York: Churchill Livingstone.

Otten, M., Lardi, A., Wroten, J., Witte, J., & Peterman, T. (1993). Changes in sexually transmitted disease rates after HIV testing and posttest counseling, Miami, 1988 to 1989. *American Journal of Public Health, 82*(4), 529–533.

Pearson, M. I., Jereb, J. A., & Frieden, T. R. (1992). Nosocomial transmission of multidrug-resistant mycobacterium tuberculosis: A risk to patients and health care workers. *Annals of Internal Medicine, 117,* 191–196.

Plummer, F. A., & Nugugi, E. N. (1990). Prostitutes and their clients in the epidemiology and control of sexually transmitted diseases. In K. K. Holmes, P. A. Mardh, P. F., Sparling, & P. J. Weisner (Eds.). *Sexually transmitted diseases* (pp. 71–76). New York: McGraw-Hill.

Poulin, C., Gyorkos, T. W., MacPhee, J., Cann, B., & Bickerton, J. (1992).

Contact-tracing among injection drug users in a rural area. *Canadian Journal of Public Health, 83*(2), 106–108.

Reichman, L. B. (1993). Fear, embarrassment, and relief: The tuberculosis epidemic. *American Journal of Public Health, 83*(5), 639–641.

Risse, G. B. (1988). Epidemics and history: Ecological perspectives and social responses. In E. Fee & D. M. Fox (Eds.). *AIDS: The burdens of history* (pp. 36–66). Berkeley: University of California Press.

Roper, W. L., Peterson, H. B., & Curran, J. W. (1993). Commentary: Condoms and HIV/STD prevention—clarifying the message. *American Journal of Public Health, 83*(4), 501–503.

Schimpff, S. C. (1990). Infections in the compromised host—an overview. In G. L. Mandell, R. G. Douglas, & J. E. Bennett (Eds.). *Principles and practices of infectious diseases* (3rd ed.) (pp. 2258–2265). New York: Churchill Livingstone.

Schwartz, P., & Gillmore, M. R. (1990). Sociological perspectives on human sexuality. In K. K. Holmes, P. A. Mardh, P. F. Sparling, & P. J. Weisner (Eds.). *Sexually transmitted diseases* (pp. 45–53). New York: McGraw-Hill Information Services.

Sex overtakes drug use as source of women's AIDS. (1993, July 23). *Washington Post,* p. 12.

Shalala, D. E. (1993). The future of health care reform in America. *Phi Kappa Phi Journal, 53*(3), 10–11.

Trotter, J. (1992). *Guidelines for people with AIDS living in the community*. Unpublished manuscript.

U.S. Department of Health and Human Services (USDHHS). (1990). *Healthy People 2000: National health promotion and disease prevention objectives* (Publication No. (PHS) 91-50213). (1990). Washington, DC: U.S. Government Printing Office.

U.S. Preventive Service Task Force. (1989). *Guide to clinical preventive services.* Baltimore: Williams & Wilkins.

Wing, K. R. (1985). *The law and the public's health.* Ann Arbor, MI: Health Administration Press.

World Health Organization. (1986). *Health research strategy for health for all by the year 2000.* Subcommittee report to the Advisory Committee on Health Research. Geneva, Switzerland: Author.

BIBLIOGRAPHY

American Academy of Pediatrics. (1988). *Report of the Committee on Infectious Diseases* (21st ed.). Committee on Infectious Diseases, American Academy of Pediatrics, Elk Grove Village: IL.

Baker, D. A. (1989). *Clinical management of sexually transmitted diseases.* New York: IntraMed Communications.

Bartlett, J. (1990). *Pocketbook of infectious disease therapy.* Baltimore: Williams & Wilkins.

Bergquist, L. M. (1984). *Changing patterns of infectious disease.* Philadelphia: Lea & Febiger.

Centers for Disease Control (CDC). (1988). Condoms for prevention of sexually transmitted diseases. *Morbidity and Mortality Weekly Report, 37*(9), 133–137.

CDC. (1989). Guidelines for prevention of transmission of human immunodeficiency virus and hepatitis B virus to health-care and public-safety workers. *Morbidity and Mortality Weekly Report, 38*(S-6), 1–37.

CDC. (1989). Recommendations of the immunization practices advisory committee: General recommendation on immunization. *Morbidity and Mortality Weekly Report, 38(13),* 205–214; 219–227.

CDC. (1989). Sexually transmitted diseases: Treatment guidelines. *Morbidity and Mortality Weekly Report, 38*(S-8), 1–38.

CDC. (1990). Update on hepatitis B prevention. *Morbidity and Mortality Weekly Report, 36,* 353–366.

Chorba, T. L., Berkelman, R. L., Safford, S. K., Gibbs, N. P., & Hull, H. F. (1990). Mandatory reporting of infectious diseases by clinicians. *Morbidity and Mortality Weekly Report, 39*(RR-9), 1–28.

Cockburn, A. (1963). *The evolution and eradication of infectious diseases.* Baltimore: The Johns Hopkins Press.

Covington, T. R. (1987). *Sex care: The complete guide to safe and healthy sex.* New York: Pocket Books.

Cutler, J. C., & Arnold, R. C. (1988). Venereal disease control by health departments in the past: Lessons for the present. *American Journal of Public Health, 78*(4), 372–376.

Fee, E., & Fox, D. M. (1988). *AIDS: The burdens of history.* Berkeley: University of California Press.

Holmes, K. K., Mardh, P. A., Sparling, P. F., Wiesner, P. J., Cates, W., Lemon, S. M., & Stamm, W. E. (1990). *Sexually transmitted diseases.* New York: McGraw-Hill.

Ibrahim, M. A. (1985). *Epidemiology and health policy.* Rockville, MD: Aspen.

Last, J. M. (1987). *Public health and human ecology.* Norwalk, CT: Appleton & Lange.

Mandell, G. L., Douglas, R. G., & Bennett, J. E. (Eds.). (1990). *Principles and practice of infectious diseases* (3rd ed.). New York: Churchill Livingstone.

Sharp, N. (1992). Tuberculosis is back. *Nursing Management, 23*(5), 28–32.

West, K. H. (1987). *Infectious disease handbook for emergency personnel.* Philadelphia: J. B. Lippincott.

Winslow, C. E. A., Smillie, W. G., Doull, J. A., Gordon, J. E., & Top, F. H. (1952). *The history of American epidemiology.* St. Louis: Mosby.

World Health Organization. (1985). *Control of sexually transmitted diseases.* Geneva, Switzerland: Author.

SUGGESTED READINGS

Benenson, A. S. (Ed.). (1990). *Control of communicable disease in man.* Washington, DC: American Public Health Association.

Mandell, G. L., Douglas, R. G., & Bennett, J. E. (Eds.). (1990). *Principles and practice of infectious diseases* (3rd ed.). New York: Churchill Livingstone.

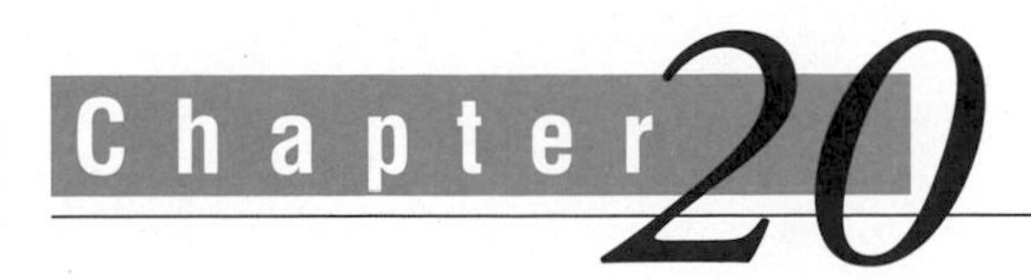

Violence: A Social and Family Problem

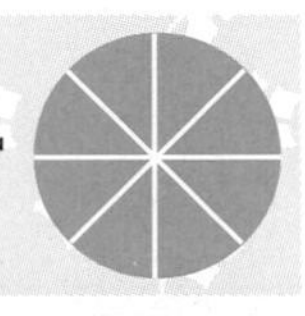

Frances A. Maurer

Continued

Focus Questions

What are some of the factors that contribute to family violence?

What criteria are useful in assessing for possible abusive or neglectful situations?

What are the responsibilities of the community health nurse as a health professional in abusive situations?

What community resources are available to prevent abuse and to assist the victims and perpetrators in abusive situations?

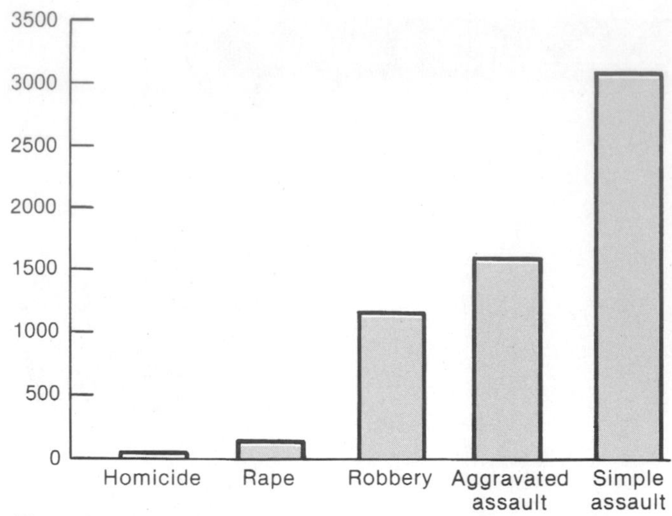

Figure 20–1 ● Violent acts during 1991 (in thousands). (Data from U.S. Department of Justice. (1991). *Criminal victimization in the U.S.* Washington, DC: Author.)

Violence is an emotional issue that generates enormous public concern in the United States. On a daily basis local and national news reports are replete with examples of violent actions and their tragic consequences. In fact violence has become so commonplace that it is unusual to find anyone who has not been exposed either by personal experience or by acquaintance with a victim. Expressions of concern for personal safety and security are coupled with increasing public anger at the limitations people must impose on their personal lives to reduce the risk of harm. In some communities violence is so prevalent that residents are desensitized. Anger has been replaced by resignation. Community members feel powerless to stop it and instead concentrate on efforts to ensure their safety and that of their family members.

Extent of the Problem

- A violent crime occurs in the United States every 17 seconds.
- Suicide is the eighth leading cause of death.
- Homicide is the tenth leading cause of death.
- One hundred eight of every 1000 women are raped each year.
- Homicide is the second leading cause of death in persons 15 to 24 years old.
- Homicide is the leading cause of death in young black males.*

According to the Federal Bureau of Investigation (FBI) violent behavior is on the rise nationwide; it has increased 45% in less than 10 years (Fig. 20–1). The U.S. Surgeon General has identified violent behavior and exposure to violent acts as one of the nation's most important health concerns (Novello et al., 1992). Adolescents and young adults are at especially high risk of being a victim or a perpetrator of violence, and minority young are at an exceptional risk. About half the arrests for violent crimes are of people 25 years or younger. Young black males are especially vulnerable; they are eight times more likely to be murdered than are their white male counterparts.

As a nation America appears more inclined toward violent behavior than other developed countries. Both the incidence of violent crimes and the murder rate are higher here than in comparable populations in Europe and Canada (Fingerhut and Kleinman, 1990). A clear, definitive explanation for this disparity is not available, although the difference in gun regulations is cited as a contributing factor (Koop and Lundberg, 1992).

The Causes of Violence: Societal, Individual, and Family Factors

Efforts to develop an encompassing explanation for violent behavior have not been successful (Lidz et al., 1993). Studies have identified certain factors that place individuals at greater risk for engaging in violence (Table 20–1). However not everyone to whom these risk factors apply behaves violently. To date there is no accurate method to predict which individuals at risk will actually engage in violent behavior. An individual's use of violence seems to be influenced by a variety of factors both external (family, society, and other environmental conditions) and internal (innate personality characteristics).

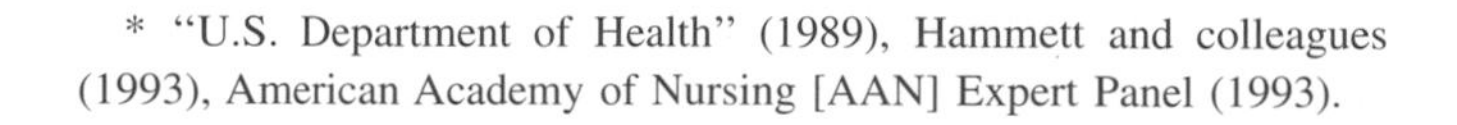

* "U.S. Department of Health" (1989), Hammett and colleagues (1993), American Academy of Nursing [AAN] Expert Panel (1993).

TABLE 20–1

Factors Associated with Risk of Violence

Factors Associated with Risk of Violence
Sociological
Low socioeconomic status
Involvement with gangs
Drug dealing
Access to guns
Media exposure to violence
Community exposure to violence
Developmental/Psychological
Alcohol or drug abuse
Rigid sex role expectations
Peer pressure, especially for adolescents
Poor impulse control
History of mental health problems
High individual stress level
Manual laborer, unemployed, or employed part-time
Younger than 30 years
Family
History of intergenerational abuse
Social isolation
Parents verbally threaten children
High levels of family stress
Two or more children

EXPOSURE AND SOCIAL CONDITIONING

Violence flourishes when force is considered an acceptable strategy in the problem-solving process. Generalized exposure to violence seems to reduce the individual's inhibitions toward aggressive actions. In American culture aggressive actions are applauded in sports, movies, and television (Zuckerman and Zuckerman, 1985; Centerwell, 1989). At sporting events the audiences seem to encourage and even expect athletes to engage in excessive force in competition. Hockey is an especially salient example of violence: many hockey injuries occur during time-outs or after the referee has interrupted play. Television and movies expose audiences to ever-increasing violence, which is justified as necessary heroics.

Viewing of violence has been linked to aggression among children and selected adult populations (Surgeon General's Scientific Advisory Committee, 1972; Katz, 1980; Centerwell, 1992). Women are a common target of media violence. Gelles and Straus (1988) report that men who have been exposed to violent pornography are less inclined to consider coercive sexual encounters as rape. One survey of adult videos found that a third involved themes of violence and degradation (Duncan, 1991). Personal exposure to violence increases the individual risk of engaging in violent behavior (Fitzpatrick and Boldizar, 1993). Adolescents are particularly vulnerable and are exposed to increasing violence at school and in the community (Gainer et al., 1993).

- According to the FBI for the 10 years ending in 1991 the incidence of adolescent crime increased 24% for rapes, 47% for assaults, and 92% for homicides.
- The Centers for Disease Control and Prevention (CDC) estimate that 20% of high school students bring weapons to school.
- The CDC estimates that 3 million cases of violence occur in schools each year.*

Adolescents are at risk because they are self-conscious and want to belong. At the stage in life when peer group influence is strongest, many see their peers use physical assault as a solution to conflict. Schools must deal with fighting and weapons on a daily basis. An alarming number of adolescents know victims of or have witnessed assaults, rapes, or other life-threatening events. Inner-city youth have the greatest exposure risk (Gladstein et al., 1992).

GANGS AND VIOLENCE

The very real risk of personal injury is one of the reasons gangs are flourishing in some communities. Gangs can provide a sense of stability and family for many adolescents with unstable family situations. Interviews with gang members in the Los Angeles area provide four reasons for joining gangs: (1) peer pressure, (2) protection, (3) companionship, and (4) excitement (Hochhaus and Sousa, 1988).

Some gangs are nonviolent and provide a positive support network for adolescents. Many engage in criminal acts and contribute to the increase in violent crime in their communities. They traffic in drugs and engage in drug-related assaults and homicides (Johnson, 1990). They are involved in intergang disputes and other types of aggravated assault and battery as well as criminal acts against personal property (Speigel, 1986; Agopian, 1989). Individual gang members may oppose violence, but peer pressure forces their participation in violent and illegal activities (Hochhaus and Sousa, 1988). Peer pressure and the threat of retaliation make it difficult for individuals to leave gangs.

The majority of interventions aimed at gangs and gang activity have been directed by social activists, psychologists, and sociologists. Primary prevention efforts include teaching constructive conflict resolution and violence prevention, providing alternative social activities, and offering education and training programs (Bell and Jenkins, 1991). Some experts suggest that prevention efforts need to include communities at risk and to address the underlying social and economic problems that contribute to violent activity (Huff, 1989).

Nurses and other health professionals have engaged in few gang-related interventions. They are, however, involved in violence and substance abuse reduction interventions directed at individuals, adolescent groups, and

* Roberts and Quillian (1992); "Physical fighting among" (1992).

families. Some of these efforts are presented later in the discussion of child abuse.

GUNS AND VIOLENCE

The manufacturing and licensing of guns are more lenient in the United States than in other developed countries (Fingerhut and Kleinman, 1990). Guns are clearly associated with violent behavior and are the most frequently used weapon in homicides, violent assaults, and other crimes (Hammett et al., 1993). A major effort is under way to limit the variety and accessibility of guns to the general public through state and federal laws (Hagland, 1992). Opponents of gun control, such as the National Rifle Association, argue that criminal assault and injury will continue despite gun control, and that assailants will simply switch to other weapons. Proponents argue that stricter gun control laws will help to bring murder and injury rates in line with those of other nations (Koop and Lundberg, 1992). Other weapons require greater physical effort and afford most victims a longer reaction time in which to avoid or reduce personal injury. The American Nurses' Association (ANA) supported the Brady Bill, a federal effort that called for a mandatory waiting period for handgun purchase. The American Association of Nurses (AAN) Expert Panel on Violence recommends that nursing firmly support making handguns illegal (AAN Expert Panel, 1993).

STRESS LEVELS

The inability to handle stressful situations or exposure to an increasing number of stressors is associated with violent behavior (Roberts and Quillian, 1992; Hammond and Yung, 1993; Else et al., 1993). Some individuals may cope well with minor incidents but find a series of stressful incidents hard to handle. For example the higher the level of stress within the family the greater the risk of child abuse. Gelles and Straus (1990) reported that one third of all families that experienced 10 or more life stresses in 1 year reported at least one episode of violence against a child in the home. This rate is a hundredfold greater than the rate in families that reported only one life stress in the same time frame.

SOCIOECONOMIC STATUS

Poverty is the single factor most strongly associated with violence. Individuals are at greater risk of engaging in violent acts and of being the victims of violent acts if they are poor (Fitzpatrick and Boldizar, 1993). Research indicates that risk increases as the poverty level rises and as the median income and job availability within a community decrease (Huff, 1989). Poverty increases stress to families and communities by heightening concerns about the ability to secure a safe environment in which to live, the ability to earn an adequate salary, and the ability to provide the necessities of life for self and family members. Poverty lowers self-esteem and expectations for future success and fosters social alienation (Thompson and Norris, 1992). People who feel isolated from the mainstream of society find it harder to identify with middle-class values. Some find it easier to justify the use of violence and criminal conduct to secure money and other desirable goods (Earls, 1991).

SUBSTANCE ABUSE

Studies indicate that excessive use of drugs and alcohol is positively correlated with the incidence of violent behavior both inside and outside the family (Potter-Efron and Potter-Efron, 1990; Famularo et al., 1992). Alcohol and drug use is highly correlated with aggravated assault, homicide, and suicide (Lester, 1993; Giannini et al., 1993). The upsurge of violent behavior in juveniles is especially troublesome. According to the FBI the increases are directly attributable to the increases in the sale and distribution of heroin and cocaine. Kingery and colleagues (1992) report that adolescents who use drugs and alcohol are more likely to fight and risk assault and injury than non–drug-using peers.

INDIVIDUAL PERSONALITY

There is a weak correlation between mental illness, psychosis, and abuse (Straus, 1980). A number of personality characteristics are also weakly linked with violence. These include depression, immaturity, impulsiveness, and borderline and antisocial traits (Gelles and Cornell, 1990; Else et al., 1993). As is true of persons with the other identified risk factors, most individuals with mental illness and the personality traits described are not violent or abusive. To date research has not been able to devise a common personality profile for abusers.

FAMILY STRUCTURE AND SOCIAL SUPPORT NETWORK

The cohesiveness of the family unit has an impact on violent behavior (Mollerstron et al., 1982). Seventy percent of juvenile crime offenders, including violent offenders, come from single-parent homes. Although no definitive reason for this phenomenon has been found, single-parent households are at greater risk of experiencing multiple stressors and poverty. One fifth of all children in the United States live in households at or below the poverty level, most in female-headed households. These families get little economic relief in child support from the fathers (Children's Defense Fund [CDF], 1992). Other stressors include difficulty with supervision of children, little or no relief from parenting responsibilities, poor housing and related problems, and the demands of work on time and energy.

Since 1950 the percentage of single-parent households has tripled, increasing the risk of poverty for children and adolescents.

Social support networks tend to reduce the risk of violence in the family and the community. Families uninvolved in the life of the community are not likely to be concerned about their neighbors. Families who move frequently are less likely to have regular contact with their own parents, relatives, neighbors, and friends. They generally do not engage in social or recreational activities (Garbino and Gilliam, 1980). In times of crisis they have few resources to help reduce anxiety and stress and are less likely to be influenced by community standards of behavior.

The Impact of Violence on the Community

Abusive behavior within the family has an impact on the entire community, economically and emotionally. The family unit is the first place in which acceptable social behavior is learned. Violence within the family unit increases the probability that an individual will resort to violence as a coping mechanism, first with family members, then with peers, acquaintances, and strangers. Children from abusive situations are more likely to engage in violent activity such as fighting with other children and adults at home or school or in other settings. They are more likely to engage in illegal activities such as stealing, destruction of private property, and dealing and abusing drugs. They are at greater risk of arrest. Interviews with inmates at adolescent and adult correctional facilities indicate the majority (75% to 90%) of inmates come from violence-prone families (Carr, 1977; Widom, 1989).

Although community health nurses may encounter violence and violence-related concerns in a number of situations, their most frequent professional contact is with individuals and families in clinics and home environments. For this reason the remainder of this chapter concentrates on family violence and the nursing role in prevention and intervention with the family unit.

Violence within the Family Unit

Family violence involves the direct use of force, emotional battering, or neglect by a family member against another. It may be directed against a child, a spouse or partner, or an elder parent. In 1990 there were more than 6 million cases of family violence in the United States: 2,508,000 cases of child abuse, 3 to 4 million cases of spouse or partner abuse, and 700,000 to 1.5 million cases of elder abuse (Daro and McCurdy, 1991; *"Policy Statement"* 1993; AAN expert panel, 1993).

It is very difficult to determine with certainty the actual prevalence of family violence. Many cases go unreported, and most are not criminally prosecuted. Family violence researchers use data from both small and national samples to estimate the extent of the problem. Whenever possible national survey data and projections were used in this chapter as they are more representative of the general population.

GENERATIONAL PATTERNS OF COPING

Families differ in their effectiveness as a system. Effective families are able to promote the growth and development of members and maintain cohesiveness as an identifiable unit. Effective families are not necessarily free from problems, but they have developed effective coping skills that enable them to deal with problems appropriately as they arise.

Learning to be a responsible family member is not a natural instinct. Humans have minimal preparation for parenthood and therefore tend to repeat patterns learned in the family of origin. Patterns of family interaction are passed from one generation to another, and if the family has been ineffective in handling stress, frustration, and anger, the next generation is liable to respond in like manner.

The pattern of intergenerational abuse has been widely documented. Abused children are more likely to be abusive in later relationships, including those with their own children and spouses (Egeland et al., 1987; Bergman and Brismar, 1992). Children who are witnesses to the abuse of other family members are at greater risk of becoming victims or of participating in abusive adult relationships (Nadelson and Sauzier, 1986).

REASONS FOR CONTINUATION OF FAMILY VIOLENCE

Gelles and Straus (1988) contend that people abuse family members because they suffer few or no repercussions. Social attitudes, the private nature of family violence, and the structural inequalities in family relationships combine to create a climate in which violence is acceptable. Parental use of physical punishment is considered appropriate and is widely practiced. In one survey three of four respondents felt that slapping a 12-year-old child was good, normal discipline, and one in three felt that hitting a spouse was normal and useful behavior (Straus et al., 1980). Longitudinal surveys indicate that these attitudes have not altered appreciably (Gelles and Cornell, 1990). Violent acts against family members usually go unpunished, though similar actions against other people would be criminally prosecuted. One source estimates that only 1 in 100,000 abusive family members faces arrest for family violence (Senate Committee on Labor and Human Resources, 1990).

Privacy of the Family Is Sacrosanct

There is a reluctance to breach family privacy. Neighbors, other family members, and authority figures such as teachers, health professionals, police, and prosecutors are often unwilling to intervene because family issues are considered private matters (Jecker, 1993). The structure of modern family living arrangements also works to ensure the privacy of family violence. Since the late 1800s family size has decreased, and larger-group multigenerational family living arrangements have sharply declined (Laslett, 1973). As a result there are fewer family members to assert social controls and stop family violence.

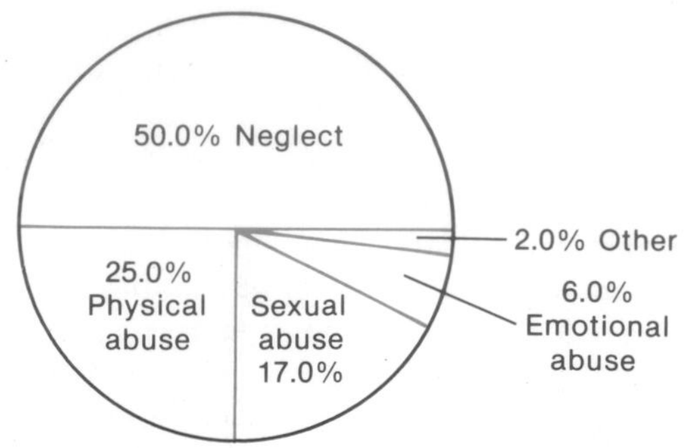

Figure 20–2 ● Types of child abuse and neglect. (Data from Children's Defense Fund. (1992). *The state of America's children*. Washington, DC: Author.)

Inequality of Family Members

By custom and law power within the family is unequally distributed. Historically women and children were considered property, and had few rights under the law. Children could be sold into slavery, loaned to work for wages collected by the father, or bartered into marriage without legal recourse. In fact today it is very difficult for minor children to establish rights independent of their parents. Weitzman (1981) notes that according to common law, husbands were considered as heads of households and wives were subordinate. Since the late 1900s women have slowly acquired the right to personal assets and property independent of a spouse on a state-by-state basis. It was 1929 before women in the United States were granted the right to vote nationwide. In English Common Law (the underpinnings of the U.S. judiciary system) physical punishment of a wife was permissible as long as the stick used was no larger in diameter than a man's thumb, hence the *rule of thumb* (Dickstein and Nadelson, 1986). One Pennsylvania town still had a law in 1970 that allowed wife-beating at certain times and days (Williams-White, 1986). Despite the repeal of most such laws the social inequality among family members persists, creating a climate in which violence persists.

Rewards of Intimate Violence

There are a number of positive aspects to the use of violence. There is the reward of releasing anger and frustration. The family member who is targeted may be the direct cause of the anger or may serve as a substitute for someone else. Anger is frequently displaced toward family members because they are more vulnerable. In other words a person cannot hit the boss, but they can go home and hit their spouse.

There are power, control, and self-esteem rewards in the use of force. Force is one way of exerting control; the controller's reward is getting his or her own way. Most abusers have low levels of self-esteem. Power and control enhance self-esteem, thus further rewarding the abuser. For abusive individuals, control at home acts to buttress egos that are wounded or damaged by events outside the home and serves to enhance or allay personal anxiety.

Child Abuse and Neglect

- Twenty-five of every 1000 children are abused or neglected each year.
- One in every 5 to 10 girls and 1 in every 10 to 50 boys is sexually abused during childhood or adolescence.
- Homicide is the leading cause of death in children 6 weeks to 2 years old.*

Since the early 1980s the number of reported cases of child abuse and neglect has increased 212% according to the American Humane Association (Starr et al., 1990). The increase has coincided with a vigorous effort to publicize child abuse as a major health issue and to influence public opinion to oppose the acceptance of violence against children. It has been difficult to determine whether the increase in reported cases is an actual gain in the abuse rate or a reflection of an increased willingness to report suspected cases. Some child care experts argue that recognition of the extent of the problem, coupled with an awareness of professional and personal responsibilities to protect children, may have led to the increase in reporting suspected cases (NCCAN, 1988; Starr et al., 1990).

Whatever the reason for the increase the rise in reported cases has been dramatic. Figures 20–2 and 20–3 illustrate types and trends of abuse. Approximately 40% of reported cases are substantiated and found to merit legal action. The remaining 60% are unsubstantiated, requiring no action. This does not necessarily mean the reported incident did not occur, merely that there is not enough evidence to warrant action.

* National Center for Child Abuse and Neglect (NCCAN) (1988); AAN Expert Panel (1993); "Policy Statement" (1993).

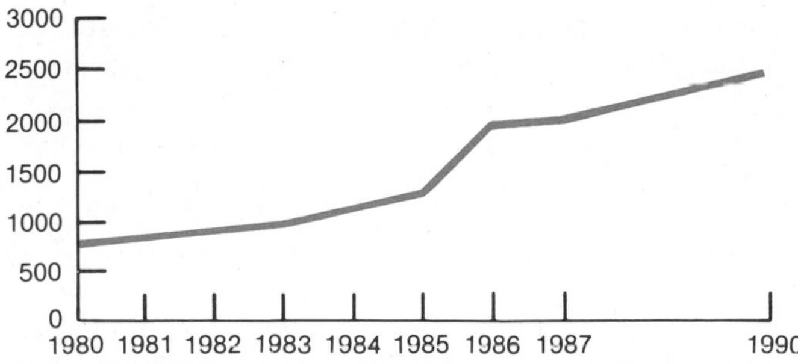

Figure 20–3 ● Trends in child abuse cases (in thousands) for selected years. (Data from American Association for Protecting Children: *Highlights of the official child neglect and abuse report.* (1992). Denver: American Humane Association; and Children's Defense Fund: *The state of America's children.* (1992). Washington, DC: Author.)

FACTORS ASSOCIATED WITH ABUSE AND NEGLECT

A number of factors associated with families involved in child abuse should be addressed in an assessment. These include parental responsibility, precipitating circumstances, and special characteristics of abused children and abusive parents.

A Family Responsibility

Child abuse and neglect are a family phenomenon. All adult members of the household are involved and are responsible or culpable for the abuse. Although one adult may be the actual perpetrator, other adults who remain passive and do not take action to protect the child are also liable.

Patterned Abuse

Physical assaults are rarely isolated instances; abuse is usually ongoing. In most cases a repetitive pattern of assaultive behavior is identified, rather than a single attack. In one study a history of previous abuse was noted in 20% of confirmed cases and 22% had multiple injuries. In almost all cases of child death there is evidence of previous abuse, and in half a prior report of abuse or neglect had been filed with the state's child protective agency (Sabotta and Davis, 1992). It must be noted that children do die from a first incident of abuse, but more often they have been exposed to repeated episodes.

Special Victim

Sometimes abuse is inflicted on all of the children in a family unit; in others one child is singled out or targeted to receive more or all of the abusive attention. A child who is considered different is at special risk of abuse (e.g., a special-needs child with physical or emotional handicaps or a child with behavioral problems). It is important to note that other siblings in the family, though spared the immediate punishment, are also affected by the abuse. Removal of a targeted child does not guarantee a solution to the problem. Another child in the household usually becomes the next target.

Abusive Parents and Caretakers

Statistics of *reported* cases show individuals who are poor, young, and black and who have little education are more frequent abusers (American Association for Protecting Children [AAPC], 1990). Experts caution that reported case data are biased (NCCAN, 1988). Poverty seems to be the only clear risk factor of the four. Parental education is a poor predictor. Family studies show the rate of abusive incidents is relatively stable across educational levels, with a slightly lower risk for parents with an eighth grade or lower education (Wolfner and Gelles, 1993).

Social expectations about race and poverty may influence who is reported as abusive. Turbett and O'Toole (1986) reported on a blind study in which physicians and nurses reviewed children's medical records to identify suspected abuse. Cases were more frequently labeled "suspicious" when parents were black or poor, even when the injuries and explanations were similar.

Blacks are at greater risk for *reported* abuse. National family surveys do not show black families to be at greater risk (Gelles and Cornell, 1990). The discrepancy between reported cases and family survey data may be explained by reporting bias and the greater number of black families who are poor. In fact black family culture may provide supports to reduce risks for abusive situations. Blacks and Hispanics tend to have greater extended family involvement and to use family networks for emotional, financial, and child-rearing support. These characteristics may offset the stressors of higher unemployment and less socioeconomic power.

Children encounter violence from caretakers other than parents. Daycare providers (especially unlicensed providers), family friends, and neighbors may also abuse children (CDF, 1992; Kelley et al., 1993).

It is often easier for middle- and upper-income persons to avoid detection and reporting to social service. The children of financially stable families are usually cared for by family physicians rather than by emergency room personnel, who are more socialized to suspect and report abuse. Affluent parents are also able to "doctor shop." They can afford to seek care from a variety of sources, which reduces risk of detection, because it is harder to identify a pattern of injuries requiring medical care.

Women vs. Men as Abusers

Statistically women tend to abuse more frequently than men, perhaps because they are more often the primary child-care providers. Women abusers are more likely to engage in moderately abusive behavior. There is no gender difference when the abuse is severe (Wolfner and Gelles, 1993). Males are the likely perpetrators in child sexual abuse. Fathers and father figures in the home are most frequently implicated in sexual abuse cases, with stepfathers being five to eight times more likely to engage in incestuous relationships than birth fathers (Russell, 1984; Margolin, 1992).

TYPES OF ABUSE

Physical Abuse

Physical abuse has dramatic consequences for some victims.

- Approximately 1 in every 5 children who are identified as abused is seriously injured, and some die of maltreatment.
- Almost 1400 children died as a result of child abuse in 1991.
- Ninety percent of fatalities occur in children between the ages of 0 to 5 years; half of those are in infants.
- Every year 1000 children die from suspicious accidents.*

Suspicious accidents are those in which the health care providers and/or the investigating officers are not convinced that the injuries sustained were caused in the manner reported, but evidence is insufficient to prove otherwise.

* CDF (1992); McClain et al. (1993).

> "For example a 14-month-old died from massive internal injuries. The child's caretaker explained that the injuries occurred when he accidentally kicked the child while he was sleeping and she fell into a fan."

Physical abuse is quite simply the infliction of physical harm upon a child. The Conflict Tactic Scale classifies physical abuse as moderate or severe. Table 20–2 provides examples of moderate and severe actions as well as some injuries that may be indicative of child abuse. Since abuse is often not an isolated incident, evidence of past injuries may be present when a child is brought for treatment. The explanation for old or healing injuries should be carefully explored.

Sexual Abuse

It is important to note that sexual abuse against children can be committed by strangers, acquaintances, or trusted leaders of the community, as well as by family members. In approximately 90% of cases the perpetrator is a family member or acquaintance (Conte and Berliner, 1981). Sexual assault of a child by a parent or close relative is called *incest.*

Sexual abuse is defined as any action in which the child is used as an object to meet adult sexual needs and desires.

TABLE 20–2

Selected Examples of Physically Abusive Actions and Injuries

Physically Abusive Actions	
Mild/moderate	*Severe*
Push	Kick
Throw something	Bite
Grab	Hit with fist
Spank with bare hand	Spank with an object
	Try to hit with an object
	Beat up
	Threaten with a weapon
	Use a weapon

Physical Injuries Presented in Child Abuse Cases		
Type	*Very Suspicious*	*Inconclusive, Investigate*
Physical	Immersion burns Whiplash syndrome in infants Cauliflower ears Spiral fractures of upper extremities X-ray evidence of healed or healing fractures with no history of treatment Identifiable marks on body, such as handprint, belt buckle, human bites, shoe print, cigarette burns	Subdural hematoma Fractured skull Injuries to face, black eye, loose or missing teeth, fractured jaw Fractures of extremities Inexplicable scars Chest or abdominal injuries, inconsistent with reason for trauma
Sexual	Report of sexual conduct with adolescents or adults Evidence child posed for pornography Sexually transmitted diseases Enlarged/stretched vaginal opening	Repeated urinary tract infection with negative urine cultures Genital itching or discharge, lacerations, bruises, or injury to genitals

This includes actions that are assaultive and violent as well as sexual exploitation of a nonviolent type. Sexual contact ranges from petting to actual intercourse, including mutual masturbation or fondling and caressing of the genitals. Sexual exploitation includes the use of children to stimulate others or the posing of children for sexually explicit pornography. Some families may allow 12- to 15-year-old girls to date young adult males (older than 18 years).

> "In one family when the 12-year-old became pregnant and the father of the baby wanted to care for the infant, the girl's family retaliated by charging him with statutory rape. Prior to this disagreement his actions had been sanctioned by family members."

Immediate detection is difficult, and public sensitization to the significance of the problem is a recent development. Adult victims report that their efforts as children to seek adult help were rebuffed. Many cases come to light years after the assault occurred. A number of American celebrities including a former Miss America, Marilyn Van Derbur, and Oprah Winfrey have joined in the national publicity effort to inform children of their rights and stress adult responsibility in reporting suspicions to the appropriate authorities.

Emotional Abuse

Emotional abuse is usually more difficult to discern and document. The actual number of cases are, again, hard to pinpoint, although experts suggest that cases of emotional abuse occur much more frequently than cases of physical abuse.

Emotional abuse is an ongoing, substantive effort, rather than an isolated instance. It involves words or actions that depreciate the victim's self-worth and can be nonverbal as well as verbal. The perpetrator directs efforts toward convincing the victim that he or she is worthless, stupid, repulsive, crazy, unwanted, or unloved. Children subjected to constant criticism will eventually believe that they are "bad." The child frequently reacts to this type of abuse by holding in or not expressing feelings to avoid additional abuse. Repressed feelings usually present through other outlets. Table 20–3 reviews behaviors and symptoms common in abusive and neglectful situations. As with sexual abuse, problems may not become evident until adult life.

NEGLECT

Neglect can be either physical or emotional or a combination of the two. The distinguishing feature of neglect is omission (a failure to act). Commitment of an action (commission) is the distinguishing feature of abuse. In general child neglect does not progress to child abuse, although the two may co-exist (American Association for Protection of Children [AAPC], 1986).

Physical neglect involves the failure to provide adequate food, clothing, and shelter, which are the basic necessities to maintain physical well-being. Negligent behavior would include failure to ensure a child is adequately clothed for the weather (e.g., summer shorts or no outerwear during a snowstorm) or failure to protect against accidental injury (e.g., allowing children to play on a window ledge with no safeguard against falls).

Emotional neglect involves the failure to foster feelings of love, belonging, and recognition in the child. The child receives little attention, and opportunities that would enhance feelings of self-esteem, belonging, and self-efficacy are not provided or are blocked. In some instances there is a combination of emotional and physical neglect resulting in outright "ignoring" of the child. Nonorganic "failure to thrive" in infants is often the result of a combination of physical and emotional neglect (Daro, 1988). It is important to note that not all cases of "failure to thrive" are the result of neglect; there are biological (organic) reasons some babies do not do well.

TABLE 20–3

Selected Behaviors to Assess in Child Abuse and Neglect

Selected Behaviors to Assess in Child Abuse and Neglect
Behaviors of Abusive Parents
Do not volunteer information or are vague about cause of child's illness or injury
Tell contradictory stories or parents tell contradictory stories to explain injury
Delay getting medical attention for child
Respond inappropriately to child during treatment, such as ignoring, offering no comfort, or showing no concern, or conversely, showing overinvolvement with attention
Have record of "hospital shopping" or using different facilities for treatment of child
Blame siblings or babysitters without substantiation or place blame on child's clumsiness
Behavior of Abused Child
Accepts injury as punishment
Tells several stories of how injury occurs, which may appear rehearsed
Gives story inconsistent with observed injuries
If confronted, often defends parent or refuses to cooperate with investigation
Has psychosomatic complaints with no obvious organic cause
Emotional abuse should be ruled out with withdrawn children, overeaters, truants, and runaways
Behavior of Neglected Child
Vacant or frozen affect
Does not cry, even if situation warrants
May be wary of physical contact, or crave physical contact with virtual strangers
Has delayed development, physically, emotionally, cognitively
Poor grooming of body, hair, and clothes on a regular basis
Behavior related to lack of supervision, including poor school performance and attendance
Pregnancy in young females in both abuse and neglect situations

Although it is sometimes blatantly apparent, neglect is usually more insidious and often requires astute observation to pinpoint. Neglect is a pattern of regular omission to provide care rather than a single instance of negligence. When being interviewed by the community health nurse neighbors or relatives in neglect cases will frequently recall that they felt uneasy about a situation, but did not have enough reason to report the parent or caretaker to the appropriate authorities. They often wondered whether their interpretation of an incident or incidents was too harsh on the parent.

Substance abuse and addiction are frequently implicated in parental failure to provide an adequately nurturing environment. In some regions of the country judicial action charging neglect and/or abuse has been attempted against alcohol- and drug-addicted pregnant women who are placing the fetus in medically compromising situations. Support for this type of action is mixed; many feel that treatment rather than punishment of the individual is a more appropriate reaction to the problem.

IMPACT OF CHILD ABUSE LAWS

As a result of national concern the federal government enacted the Child Abuse Prevention and Treatment Act in 1974. This law defined child abuse and neglect and established the National Center on Child Abuse and Neglect (NCCAN), which has funded some research and demonstration projects and collected national survey data on the incidence and prevalence of child abuse and neglect.

Child abuse and neglect are crimes in all 50 states. These laws emerged from the moral concerns of protecting the vulnerable and promoting nurturing families (see Ethics Box II). These laws serve to provide protection for abused and neglected children, but some problems remain. Each state has different criteria and procedures for reporting suspected cases. The majority of cases that are prosecuted involve physical injury. The emotional aspect of abuse is not clearly addressed in most laws and has been difficult to prosecute in practice. Physical neglect of a persistent nature with severe consequences is more likely to incur legal prosecution than are subtler forms of physical and emotional neglect.

In neglect an adult's recognition that his or her actions have adverse consequences to the child is usually a legal requirement to show intent. Economic, emotional, and mental health factors may cloud the issue.

> "A child was seen for an ear infection. An antibiotic was prescribed but the prescription was never filled. The child developed complications and was hospitalized."

Does this constitute deliberate neglect? Some of the issues the law would examine before deciding to prosecute include parental understanding of the risks of withholding medication, ability to pay for the prescription, and finally intent. Was the decision not to provide medication deliberate or the result of multiple stressors and poor coping skills?

Even when parents are prosecuted and found guilty, problems with legal oversight occur. Significant delays in taking the case through the court system mean that an average wait of 5 years is not unusual (Bishop et al., 1992). The delay allows children to be exposed to additional risk, even when substantial injuries have been documented. Effective supervision of families and children by designated agencies is a problem that is primarily related to funding (Murphy et al., 1992). Since the mid-1970s social service agencies have simultaneously experienced escalations in caseloads and reductions in budgets.

As an alternative to parental punishment, jail time, and dissolution of the family, family preservation programs are popular. Preservation programs stress intensive intervention with all family members and stringent supervision. The intent is to keep families together rather than to place children in foster care. Where there has been adequate support in terms of monies and personnel such programs have been successful (Hutchinson, 1993). Family preservation programs have also experienced funding cuts, which hamper their ability to provide services to at-risk families.

LONG-TERM CONSEQUENCES

Children who are abused or mistreated are at increased risk for learning disorders, mental retardation, and developmental delays, including language, speech, and gross motor activities. Research indicates that intelligence level as measured by IQ tests is also affected. Abused and neglected children average lower IQ scores than children with similar characteristics who have not been abused (Starr, 1988; Gelles and Cornell, 1990; Groves et al., 1993).

Initiating mutually satisfying interpersonal relationships with peers and adults is difficult for mistreated children. Their social skills and self-concept suffer. They have difficulty setting limits or boundaries with others. Classmates may describe them as socially withdrawn or as troublemakers. They tend to feel most comfortable with children from similar dysfunctional situations, and less comfortable with children from functional family structures. This pattern continues into adulthood, placing them at risk for selecting similarly mistreated marital partners (Herman, 1986).

The long-term effect of incest is not clearly known; however recent data suggest that the results are devastating to both males and females. A disproportionate number of clients in psychiatric facilities report a family history of sexual abuse (Carmen, 1986). Other victims report lifelong difficulty in maintaining healthy adult relationships—especially with members of the opposite sex—and problems with sexual dysfunction (Herman, 1986). There is some evidence to suggest that prostitution and promiscuous

Ethics Box 11

Gail A. DeLuca Havens, M.S., R.N., C.N.A.

Protecting the Vulnerable

"Victoria has become so introverted since the beginning of the school year. Her school work is suffering terribly. She rarely engages in conversations or in play with classmates and her absences have increased significantly. I know something is troubling her, but she has not shared anything with me when we have had the opportunity to talk. I came to see you today in the hope that, as our school nurse, you might be able to find out what is troubling her."

In response to the third grade teacher's plea, Melissa, the community health nurse for the four Central City elementary schools, establishes a rapport with Victoria over the next several weeks. Today Melissa asks Victoria why she was absent from school all of last week. Tearfully Victoria describes the beating she received from her mother a week ago. She hadn't cleaned up the kitchen to her mother's satisfaction. Her mother had hit her so hard that it hurt to walk. She described her urine as having looked "like blood," as well. Melissa learns that Victoria has been receiving beatings from her mother since her father left the family last summer. Melissa has a sister and a brother, both younger than she. Melissa does not believe that they have been hurt by their mother.

This situation presents questions regarding the rights of children vs. the rights of parents. When does a child cease to be the biological offspring of two individuals and become, instead, a member of society with all of the rights, duties, and responsibilities accorded such individuals? Parents in our society are permitted a great deal of latitude in raising their children. To a great extent the process of child-rearing is defined by the prevailing cultural norms of the particular family unit. It is presumed that the safety and well-being of the child will be preserved within that family unit. As in Victoria's situation, however, when a question of child abuse arises it becomes necessary to question the scope of parental authority. Child abuse is contrary to the societal norms that set the standards for moral parental behavior. A child has the right to be protected from harm. Being a parent, however, does not make one incapable of inflicting harm to one's child. Under what circumstances do others have a duty to protect children from their parents? Are there limits to parental authority or do parents have inviolate rights to exercise their discretion in raising their children? What obligations, if any, do others have to the abuser?

Melissa believes that she is obliged to protect Victoria from further harm. She is also concerned for the future safety and well-being of Victoria's siblings.

Finally she is concerned about the changes in Victoria's mother's behavior and the underlying problems. Melissa is also aware that the law requires her to report any suspected cases of child abuse to the local child protection agency caseworker.

Melissa considers the courses of action that she perceives are options in this situation. She can ask Victoria's mother to come to school to discuss the child's problems in school with her. This might offer a means to reveal to Victoria's mother the harm she is doing to her daughter. It also might provide a catalyst for her to seek counseling and support. This action might serve to diminish the harm to Victoria, if her mother appears for the meeting. However she has not kept appointments scheduled in the past by Victoria's teacher. If Victoria's mother does meet with Melissa the concern remains that she will be angry at the nurse's interference in her private life and retaliate by becoming even more abusive of Victoria.

The other course of action that Melissa is obliged to take is to report Victoria's story and past behavior observed in school to the child protection agency that serves the neighborhood in which Victoria and her family live. This action has the advantage of involving individuals in the case who have expertise and accountability in this type of family problem. It is an action that will better serve the interests of Victoria, her siblings, and her mother. The short-term consequences of the action revolve around the issue of trust, as Victoria confided in Melissa as the school nurse, not necessarily intending that others would become involved in the situation. Again there is the fear of possible reprisal by Victoria's mother. Another consequence is the possibility of Victoria being placed in a foster home.

The nurse's primary moral concern in this situation is the protection of Victoria from further harm. Nonmaleficence, or avoiding harm, is one of the fundamental principles that guide nurses' clinical decision

Continued

making (American Nurses' Association, 1985). Beauchamp and Childress (1989) state that "Refraining from aiding another person, by not providing a good or by not preventing or removing a harm, can be devastating in its consequences, and as morally wrong as inflicting a harm." Even though Melissa is not harming Victoria directly, having knowledge of the harm she is experiencing and choosing not to intervene carries with it the same moral force as direct harm. There is an equally compelling moral principle operating here, however. By acting to protect Victoria from harm Melissa acknowledges that the child is a distinct member of society, and that she is not defined solely by her mother's identity. In essence, by her actions Melissa acknowledges Victoria's autonomy, her independence as a person with particular needs and rights, and her separate identity.

A second moral concern is that Victoria be a member of a safe, nurturing family unit. To protect her from further abuse and to ensure that her family becomes a safe haven for Victoria, it is necessary that her mother's needs be attended to. Melissa is aware that people usually attribute responsibility for an abusive incident to the parent (Sykes et al., 1987). However, a characteristic that is common to abusing parents is a history of having been abused themselves (Kuhn & Ross, 1985). Victoria's mother must be "reparented" to effectively intervene in the child abuse cycle (Hunka et al., 1985). As Melissa intervenes in this case she acknowledges her professional and moral commitment to assist both Victoria and her mother.

References

American Nurses' Association. (1985). *Code for nurses with interpretive statements.* Kansas City, MO: Author.

Beauchamp, T. L., & Childress, J. F. (1989). *Principles of biomedical ethics* (3rd ed.) (p. 122). New York: Oxford University Press.

Hunka, C., O'Toole, A., & O'Toole, R. (1985). Self-help therapy in parents anonymous. *Journal of Psychosocial Nursing, 23*(7), 24–32.

Kuhn, J., & Ross, M. (1985). Primary prevention of child abuse. *MCN: American Journal of Maternal Child Nursing, 10,* 198.

Sykes, M. K., Hodges, M. C., Broome, M., & Threatt, B. J. (1987). Nurses' knowledge of child abuse and nurses' attitudes toward parental participation in the abused child's care. *Journal of Pediatric Nursing, 2*(6), 412–417.

sexual activity are more prevalent in adults who were sexually assaulted as children.

Spouse or Partner Abuse

According to national crime statistics, battering is the single most common cause of injury to women, far exceeding accidental injuries and injuries received from other criminal activity.

- One in every 3 women is assaulted by her husband or male companion at least once during the relationship.
- Thirty of every 1000 women are severely physically abused by a male partner each year.
- Spouse abuse is the leading cause of injury for women.*

Police report that 30% to 50% of their cases are investigations of domestic violence (Berrios and Grady, 1991). One survey of hospitals in Boston found that 70% of all assault victims admitted to the emergency room were women attacked at home. Battery of the female partner is often accompanied by physical or sexual abuse of the children (Nadelson and Sauzier, 1986; AAN Expert Panel, 1993). Whenever and wherever women seek care for injuries, health providers should be aware of the probable risks to children in the household.

Injuries sustained in violent episodes are significant. A study by Berrios and Grady (1991) indicated that 25% of abused women required hospitalization and 13% required major surgical treatment. The vast majority of victims requiring treatment had previous experiences with abuse. Women are at increased risk during pregnancy; it is not uncommon for a woman to report that a first episode of abuse occurred during pregnancy. Recent surveys of battered women report that 30% to 60% were abused during pregnancy and about 50% had needed medical care for a previous incident (Helton et al., 1987; McFarlane et al., 1992).

DEFINITION

Spouse abuse entails verbal and physical attacks by one marital partner against the other. Abuse can occur between unmarried partners as well, but is called *spouse abuse* in this chapter.

Physical assault ranges in degree from slapping to murder. Physical attacks almost always occur in a family climate in which the abusive spouse invests considerable energy verbally deriding the partner. Derogatory actions are aimed at reducing the victim's self-esteem and identity. A common theme of verbal criticism is the victim's inability to perform usual duties and activities in an effective and efficient manner. Verbal abuse serves a dual purpose: it convinces the victim that he or she deserves harsh treatment, and it serves to reinforce the abuser's

* Barber-Madden et al., 1988; Grisso et al., 1991.

belief that his or her actions are justified, even required, to ensure that the spouse acts appropriately.

Ninety-five percent of all abusers are male, although some male advocacy groups dispute that figure (Jones, 1980; Gelles and Straus, 1988). There is legitimacy to the claim that some men may not report abuse for fear of ridicule, but the overwhelming evidence indicates that males are the usual aggressors. Data suggest that women do hit male partners, often in self-defense after men strike first. Men are seldom seriously hurt. In those instances in which men and women engage in physical assault, the greater physical damage is caused by the male assailant (Gelles and Cornell, 1990). For this reason the remainder of the discussion about spousal abuse refers to women as victims and men as abusers.

An alarming new trend is the rise in violent behavior between dating couples, especially teenagers. Levy (1991) reports that approximately 25% of teenagers say they have experienced physical violence in relationships. The characteristics and risk factors for victims and offenders in dating violence are similar to those at risk for spousal violence (Tontodonato and Crew, 1992).

CHARACTERISTICS OF ABUSERS AND VICTIMS

A number of important factors are associated with spouse abuse: socioeconomic status, education, occupation, and personality traits.

Socioeconomic Status

The relationship between socioeconomic status and spouse abuse is similar to that for child abuse. *Reported* cases indicate that families at or below the poverty level are at a five times greater risk. National family surveys indicate that socioeconomic status is a risk factor, but that abuse is prevalent at all income levels. The real incidence of abuse among families with college educations and higher socioeconomic status may be hidden. The social sanctions against abuse are greater in these groups. Both victims and abusers experience similar reactions such as withdrawal or distancing from friends and acquaintances who know of or have witnessed abusive incidents. Experts suggest that this leads to vigorous efforts to hide abusive incidents from public scrutiny (Justice, 1992).

Education Level and Occupation

The impact of education and occupation on spousal assault is not definitive, but is entwined with a variety of other factors that affect risk. Women with some college education are at less risk, perhaps because they have more financial independence. Abusers are more often skilled or semi-skilled workers, compared with other occupations, and unemployed or partially employed. These groups may experience greater financial and role-related stress.

Personality Traits

Abusers characteristically are emotionally dependent and very egocentric. They have poor social skills, explosive tempers, limited tolerance of frustration, and a need for instant gratification. They have a need to exert power and control over a partner and use a variety of methods to do so. Figure 20–4 illustrates the relationship between physical and sexual assault and other types of intimidating and controlling behavior.

Battered partners tend to be unsure or unable to identify their own ego needs. They tend to sublimate their own needs to those with whom they are involved, including partner, children, parents, and friends. They are usually economically and emotionally dependent on their partner. Battered women generally subscribe to the belief that the responsibility for making a relationship work is women's work, and to admit to battering would be to acknowledge failure in that role (Williams-White, 1986). Abused individuals also subscribe to the belief that acceptance of violent behavior will eventually lead to long-term resolution of family problems. An example follows.

> "Justine is unmarried but lives with Tom, the father of her three children. She had been sexually assaulted by both her father and her stepfather. She entered the relationship with Tom to leave home. She has completed the ninth grade and has never been employed. Tom is employed as a maintenance worker. He is extremely jealous and controlling of her relationships with others. On weekends he drinks alcohol with his brothers at home. They spend most of their time criticizing Justine, belittling her lack of education and her housekeeping skills. Tom and his brothers believe that a woman's role is subservient to a man's."

CYCLICAL PHASES OF ABUSE

There is a classic cyclical pattern common to most domestic violence episodes. Walker (1979) identified three general phases of the abuse cycle: (1) the tension-building phase, (2) the battering phase, and (3) the apologetic phase (Fig. 20–5). In the tension-building phase the batterer's levels of frustration, anger, and belittlement of the victim escalate. The victim attempts to placate the abusive individual by being attentive, nurturing, and self-deprecating.

Despite attempts to calm the situation, the tension escalates. During the battering phase the abuser vents his rage by physically punishing the victim. As soon as the anger is dissipated the abuser moves to the apologetic phase during which he is very contrite and loving. He assures the victim that the episode will not be repeated. This is often

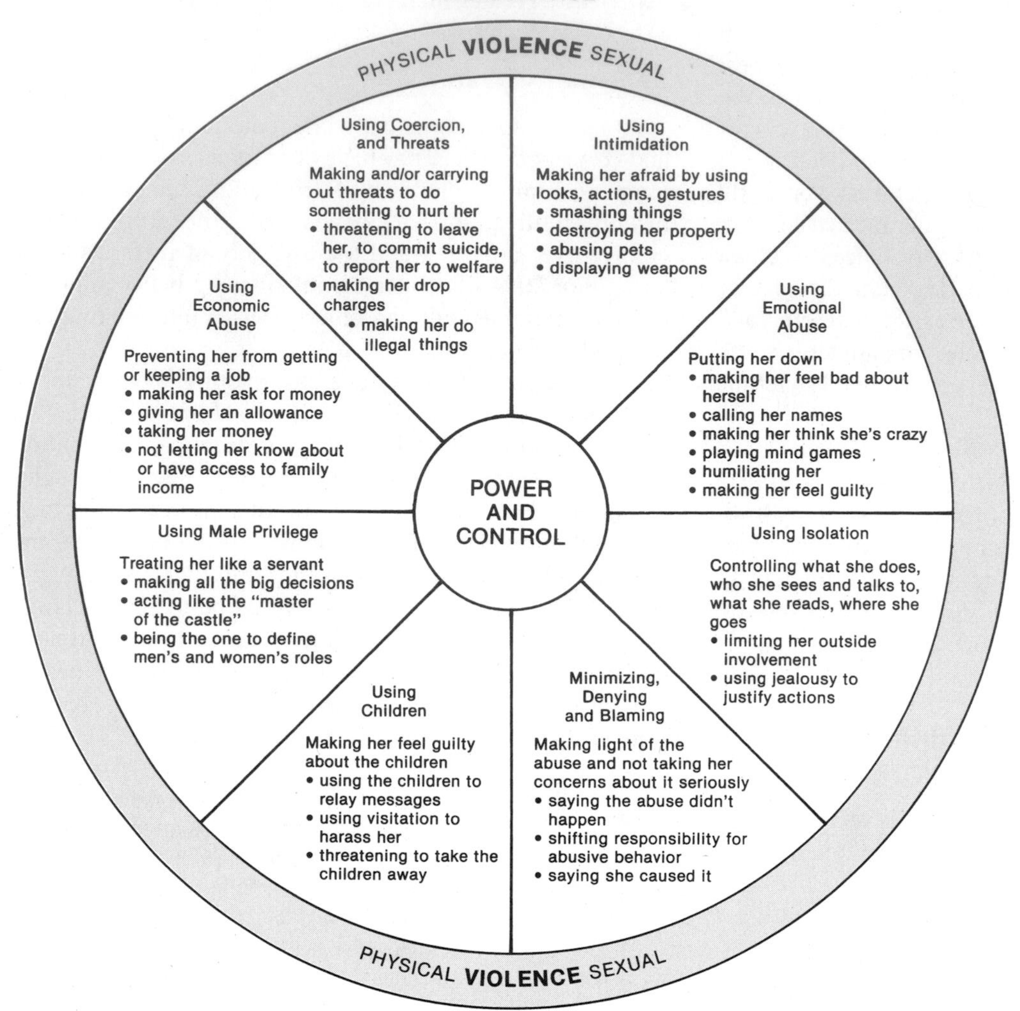

Figure 20–4 ● Relationship of violence to use of power and control. (Redrawn from Domestic Abuse Intervention Project, Duluth, Minnesota.)

referred to as "the honeymoon phase." The offender may bring gifts of candy, flowers, or clothes. He will make an effort to please in other ways, such as helping with housework or planning activities that are sure to please family members.

Unlike in spouse abuse, the apologetic phase is not as evident in child abuse. The abuser feels his or her actions were appropriate, acceptable discipline and therefore an apology is unwarranted.

Battery phase
CYCLE OF ABUSE
Escalating tension phase
Apologetic phase

Figure 20–5 ● Cycle of abuse. (Data from Walker L. E. (1979). *The battered woman.* New York: Harper & Row.)

VICTIM BLAMING

Although the batterer attempts to please, he refuses to acknowledge blame for the abuse. He will explain that the victim's behavior was the root cause of the assault. The abuser's sincerity, coupled with the victim's willingness to accept most or sole responsibility for "fixing" problems and maintaining the relationship, lead to the victim's acceptance of blame for abusive behavior. If only I had not gotten him mad, or I know he hates me to fold his socks that way are illustrative of victim comments in explaining abusive behavior.

WHY SPOUSES STAY

One of the most difficult things to accept is the battered spouse's continued reluctance to end the relationship. The most frequently heard comment is, Why doesn't she just leave? Women stay for a variety of realistic and unrealistic reasons, the most frequent of which are:

- She hopes her husband will reform.
- She feels there is no place to go.
- Children make it difficult to leave, both for financial reasons and because it is harder to find alternative living arrangements.
- She has financial problems: she is unemployed or has no money.
- She is afraid of living alone.
- She is emotionally dependent on the abusive spouse.
- She believes that divorce is shameful.
- She fears reprisal from her husband.

All reasons except shame related to divorce were true in Justine's case.

Many battered women fear reprisals from their partner if they choose to leave. Their concern is very real. The latest crime statistics indicate that women are more likely to experience a battering episode if they leave or attempt to leave the relationship. Abusive partners often go to great lengths to bully or terrorize a partner who has left. For this reason shelters for battered women often do not publish their address. In rural areas it is much more difficult to "hide" the shelter from the abuser.

LEGAL EFFORTS TO COMBAT SPOUSE ABUSE

Legal efforts to combat spouse abuse are limited and inconsistent. The courts are usually lenient when dealing with family violence cases. Penalties for abusive partners are not consistent with penalties imposed on individuals convicted of similar offenses against strangers, friends, or acquaintances. There is a tendency to consider the relationship as a mitigating factor that provides some rationale for the perpetrator's behavior. The news is full of reports of women who have secured restraining orders that were subsequently violated by abusers, sometimes with tragic results to the women or to their children.

Congress has introduced legislation intended to make stalking a federal offense. This legislation would benefit some spouse abuse victims who are separated or divorced from their spouses. Some states have initiated stalking laws for their jurisdictions. It remains to be seen whether these laws will be effective and whether they will be applied equally to spouses and to other stalkers.

Police officers have been reluctant to get involved in domestic violence situations (Hirschel and Hutchinson, 1992; Dunford, 1992). They cite the transitory nature of the complaint and risk of personal harm as the most common reasons for this position. Law enforcement officers are frustrated by the number of cases of abused partners who file charges and then do not follow through with the complaint, allowing the batterer to go free. Police see this as wasted effort on their part. Domestic violence complaints are personally dangerous, precipitating one of the most frequent situations in which physical injuries are sustained by law enforcement officers (Gelles and Cornell, 1990). Though legitimate, such concerns do not justify limited, delayed, or no response to reports of violent episodes. Greater public concern, changing attitudes in law enforcement, and successful lawsuits for poor or delayed police response have helped to change the way that police and communities respond to abusive family members.

Evidence suggests that abusers will control their behavior in response to social pressure (Lore and Schultz, 1993). A number of states and municipalities have developed a comprehensive approach aimed at reducing the number of repeat offenders. These programs include mandatory arrest, followed by counseling and, in some instances, jail time, even for first offenders. The intent is to penalize the offender and address his offensive behavior. Experts note that the only way to break the cycle of violence is to treat the offender in addition to the victim (Gelles and Cornell, 1990). Early evaluation of mandatory arrest and counseling programs seems to suggest that they are more successful than past efforts (Randall, 1991).

The ultimate decision to stay in an abusive situation or to leave is the victim's. Leaving a relationship is a difficult decision; many choose to stay. Andresen (1985) reported that 55% of women at one shelter had returned to their partners by 2 months after leaving the shelter. Health professionals must work hard to accept the situation when a spouse decides to stay. The emphasis should be on maintaining an accepting, supportive relationship with the victim. Over time it may be possible to see positive results from sustained support.

Nursing Care in Abusive Situations: Child or Spouse Abuse

Community health nurses see children and families in a wide variety of settings and community organizations. They are in a key position to identify and intervene in problematic cases. Their long-term relationship with clients and families allows them the opportunity to provide ongoing monitoring of at-risk families. Nursing efforts should be directed at ensuring safety, emotional support, and advocacy for abuse victims, as well as primary prevention aimed at reducing risk and eliminating the intergenerational transmission of violence.

ASSESSMENT TO IDENTIFY SUSPICIOUS CASES

The community health nurse should always be alert to possible abuse or neglect situations. Some of the risk factors for abuse in families were identified earlier in the chapter (see Table 20–1). This is essential information for nursing practice. Moldanado (1991) cautions that accurate documentation by the nurse of assessment risk, anticipatory guidance, and physical condition is essential.

Physical and Sexual Abuse

Any unexplainable injury is suspicious; ask for an explanation. Be accessible and open to parental concerns. Be nonjudgmental and allow the parent to ventilate his or her feelings. Sometimes parents are concerned enough about their behavior to seek the nurse's opinion. They may attempt to justify their behavior or the behavior of another caregiver by presenting a list of complaints about the child. From conversation and observation the nurse will be able to identify areas for intervention.

In spouse abuse, victims may be ashamed or reluctant to volunteer information, but most will explain if asked. A direct but measured question, for example, Your injuries could have been caused by someone hurting you. Has someone? is often effective. McFarlane et al. (1991) found that adding five abuse-related questions to a nursing history form prompted women to relate their experiences.

The type of injury and the circumstances under which it occurred should be evaluated. Question whether the explanation of cause is consistent with the type of injury found. Serious injuries in children deserve special vigilance. Certain trauma is particularly suggestive of physical or sexual abuse (see Table 20–2). Most injuries are not so easily classified as resulting from abuse. Children are very active, sometimes clumsy, and not often safety-conscious. Bruising is common. Nurses must be sensitive to subtle signs of abuse or neglect. Do not readily dismiss an observed incident or reports by friends or neighbors, even if no observable injuries are present.

Emotional Abuse

Assessing for emotional abuse is more problematic. Gelles and Cornell (1990) report that emotional abuse is frequently overlooked by health professionals. Community health nurses are in a position to observe family dynamics and interactions more frequently than are other professionals. Consistent tension, anger, or demeaning remarks are cause for concern.

Frequent episodes of yelling, cursing, or derogatory remarks aimed at the child are indicative of emotional abuse. Some children react to a nonsupportive and hostile environment by displaying behavioral problems at home or school. Some develop somatic complaints. If there is no obvious explanation for such behavior in a child, consider the possibility of abuse. Increased stress may also result in numerous physical complaints for physically or emotionally abused spouses. A number of studies indicated that abused women have a greater number of physical concerns and seek medical care more frequently than do women who are not abused (McLeer et al., 1989). Sometimes the only signs of abuse are emotional and stress-related. Table 20–4 lists common health and behavioral indicators the nurse can use to screen for abuse. When a client is often anxious or ill with no obvious biological cause, the nurse should explore the possibility of abuse.

TABLE 20–4

Emotional and Physical Problems Associated with Violence Victimization

Physical
Atypical chest pain
Asthma
Recurrent headaches
Somatic complaints with no identifiable cause
Eating disorders and other gastrointestinal tract complaints
Emotional
Anxiety, panic attacks
Depression
Drug overdose
Forgetfulness
Hopelessness/helplessness/suicide attempts
Guilt
Inability to solve problems or make decisions
Low self-esteem
Sleep disturbances

More often than not the nurse is faced with situations that are not clearly abusive or neglectful and finds making a decision about contacting local authorities very difficult.

> "Jim is a 7-year-old boy whose school reports that he is often tardy, comes wearing dirty clothes, and is doing poorly academically. The community health nurse is visiting his mother and new sister for well-baby visits. Jim's mother says that she is exhausted caring for the infant and is doing the best she can."

Is Jim being neglected? Does the nurse have enough evidence to warrant contacting protective service? Are the conditions in the home different from those in which many poor people live in your area? The nurse might want to look closely at issues such as (1) whether Jim has enough to eat, (2) whether he is adequately clothed for the weather, (3) whether he has missed school altogether and if so, how much? Most of the time, single episodes do not exist as clear evidence of abuse or neglect. Frequently the accumulation of concerns, circumstances, and observations points toward abuse or neglect.

In making decisions about case reporting, the community health nurse must examine the impact of personal values and expectations on the assessment of the situation. It should be clear that the reasons for suspecting abuse or neglect are not just a difference in personal values.

> "During a home visit with Joan D. the community health nurse finds Joan and her three children (18 months and 3 and 4 years old) still in sleepwear at 2 P.M. They are having a breakfast of hamburgers,

chips, and soda. Ms. D. explains they just got out of bed because they all were up late last night watching videotapes. The community health nurse is personally upset that Joan's children are up late at night and are not eating the usual breakfast-type foods. ”

In this instance the community health nurse and the family have different sleep-wake patterns and dietary habits. Although the nurse may feel that the mother demonstrates neglectful behavior, the situation as presented does not justify her feelings. If the children are adequately fed and given sufficient sleep time, the mother is not neglectful.

LEGAL RESPONSIBILITIES OF THE COMMUNITY HEALTH NURSE

Most states specifically mandate health professionals, including nurses, as one of the group of designated professionals who are required to report child abuse. Neighbors, friends, or relatives of the child may also take action but are not clearly enjoined to do so by law. The law requires that all *suspected* cases be reported, but does not expect health professionals to determine the validity of the claim. It is up to the local authorities (social welfare and/or legal) to conduct an investigation and to make that determination.

The procedure used to report abuse varies from state to state. Most states require a report to either the department of social services or the police. The procedure for investigating reported cases also varies among states. Table 20–5 illustrates a common procedure in some states.

TABLE 20–5

Typical Procedure for Notification and Investigation of Child Abuse and Neglect Cases

Actions Taken by Community Health Nurse

Identify suspected case abuse/neglect

Verbally report to
1. Child protection agency
   or
2. Local law enforcement

Send written report to child protection agency within 48 hours of initiating complaint and send a copy to the state's attorney's office

Actions Taken by Designated Child Protection Agency

Prompt investigation within 24 hours if abuse, usually longer—perhaps as much as 5 days—if neglect

Completed investigation within 10 days and report of findings to state's attorney's office

Dispensation of case
1. No evidence found
2. Inconclusive, file kept open
3. Evidence exists, action taken

Possible actions include
1. Mandated supervision in home
2. Conditions imposed on parents to continue custody (e.g., attend parenting classes, drug rehabilitation)
3. Temporary removal of children to foster care or other relatives' homes
4. Permanent removal of child from home
5. Court action to cease parental rights to clear for adoption

Exemptions from Liability

One very real concern in reporting suspected cases is the possibility of a legal suit should the investigation not result in charges against the parent or caregiver. In every state the law protects health care professionals from legal action if the charges are unproved. The threat of legal action against an individual who reports suspicions can have an impact on the willingness to report. It is hoped that protection offered by law will encourage those who have concerns to feel more comfortable about reporting such incidents to the appropriate parties.

The Nurse's Legal Responsibility in Spouse Abuse

There are no state laws that require health professionals to report spouse abuse. The law assumes that adults are capable of such reporting themselves. Laws in every state provide civil or criminal penalties, or both, for abusers in family situations. Some states mandate social agencies to provide service to violent families and some specify the duties of police and the courts in domestic violence. The nurse should be aware of the legal remedies for victims and, if necessary, advise them of their rights.

ENSURING THE SAFETY OF THE ABUSE VICTIM

Once the nurse has confirmed a suspected abusive situation, the priority is to ensure the safety of the victim or victims. Potential for injury is the number one concern. Efforts should be directed toward eliminating potential harm or reducing the risk of continued assault by removing the woman or children, or both, from the abuser as soon as possible. Families may choose to stay with relatives or friends or use the services of a shelter. There are more than 1200 shelters and safe houses in this country that offer temporary lodging to women and children. Shelters are often overcrowded. Studies show that approximately 40% of those seeking shelter have to be turned away because of space limitations (AAN Expert Panel, 1993).

The police or state agency that investigates child abuse is authorized to remove a child who is in imminent danger of injury or additional injuries. In the majority of child abuse cases there is no *immediate* danger, and the child remains in the home. In situations of spouse abuse in which children are not at risk, the victim is the sole decision-maker. Women may choose to stay, which may be difficult for the nurse and others to accept.

CRISIS INTERVENTION/ ANTICIPATORY GUIDANCE

For any *reported* cases of child abuse or neglect an investigation is mandatory. Investigation by authorities is usually very upsetting to families, and is an added stressor to those who originally precipitated the situation under investigation. Nursing actions should be directed toward prioritizing and addressing the immediate needs of family members. Rather than work alone the nurse usually works with a number of other professionals; these may be colleagues from the nurse's workplace or from a variety of other agencies depending on the state structure for addressing abuse or neglect situations. For example a social worker, school guidance counselor, school pupil personnel worker, psychologist, home aide, addiction counselor, and nurse might all be involved in the intervention plan. The team develops a plan with multiple interventions, including safeguarding at-risk members and helping the abusive member to develop coping skills. Coping skill counseling would include conflict resolution, communication skills, and techniques to improve self-control and parenting skills. The community health nurse is particularly effective in educating and supporting the parenting needs of abusive parents (Reuter, 1988).

In spouse abuse, especially if the victim chooses to remain in the abusive situation, the nurse may be the woman's only resource. The nurse can provide emotional support and allow the woman to ventilate her feelings. Some of the more common reactions women experience include helplessness, shame, embarrassment, guilt, anger, and fear of further abuse. The community health nurse should make sure a plan has been mapped out and resources identified in case circumstances dictate that the woman should leave.

MONITORING OF ONGOING CASES

Monitoring confirmed cases of child abuse or neglect usually falls under the jurisdiction of a designated state or local social service agency and the courts. Community health nurses could be involved with providing health care services. In that capacity the nurse should monitor the health and welfare of abused members and, if necessary, make more referrals to protective service. In cases in which no legal action is taken the community health nurse may be the only professional to have regular contact with family members, which makes vigilant monitoring for recurrent problems especially important.

REFERRAL TO COMMUNITY RESOURCES

Communities offer a variety of resources to victims of family violence. The community health nurse should not wait for a crisis to explore the community's resources; he or she is in the position to identify appropriate community resources applicable to families before, during, or after abuse has occurred. Table 20–6 provides examples of some community resources for families dealing with child or spouse abuse. They are only a sample listing. Nurses must be familiar with the specific resources available within the community to ensure speedy referrals.

Community health nurses can address the health needs of women and children living in shelters. Stress-related and other health issues need to be considered. Most shelter staff members are not trained to provide health care services. Hollenkamp and Attala (1986) have reported on a volunteer effort by community nurses in a local shelter that provides assessment, screening, referral, and health education. Community health nurses can become involved in similar efforts in their communities and can advocate for provision of paid nursing staff in shelters.

PRIMARY PREVENTION

The single most effective way to deter violence against children and spouses is to make efforts to reduce the possibility of violent acts. Primary prevention measures should include public education efforts to transform attitudes about child and spousal violence as well as to identify and assist individuals at risk.

Intervention with Families at Risk

Intensive support and anticipatory guidance for families at risk has been successful in reducing family violence. Risk factors for potential abuse are identical to the risk factors identified for actual abusive situations. Health teaching and support for persons at risk are effective ways that community health nurses can intervene before risk becomes reality (Ryan, 1989).

Child Abuse and Neglect

Community health nurses traditionally provide parental education about growth and development and stress effective parenting skills in their care to families. Browne (1989) suggests that screening should include at least three nurse checks in the first 9 months of life. The first screening should include assessment for the risk factors associated with abuse and neglect. The next visit should explore parents' perceptions of their child and specific family stressors. The third visit should review infant behaviors and attachment. Reviewing developmental milestones, such as motor and cognitive abilities of infants and children, helps parents to recognize age-appropriate behavior. The nurse can validate realistic expectations for the child with the parent and dispel unrealistic ones. Abusive parents often have unrealistic expectations of age-appropriate behavior for children (Gelles and Cornell, 1990).

“A 6-month-old girl is admitted to the hospital for injuries sustained in a beating. The parent said that the baby was not cooperating with toilet training and needed to be disciplined. 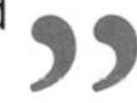

Parent-Child Interactions

Discipline is another area for intervention. By observing parent-child interplay the nurse can get a good idea about parenting technique and bonding. A key indicator of parental risk for neglectful behavior is poor maternal-infant bonding. If bonding appears weak the nurse can work on increasing attachment and parental confidence in the role of caretaker. The nurse should encourage the parent to be consistent in setting limits and should explore alternatives to hitting as a means of discipline. The community health nurse can act as a role model by demonstrating appropriate limit-setting behavior when he or she interacts with the child.

Access to positive role models is crucial for at risk

TABLE 20–6

Community Resources for Child Abuse

Community Resources for Child Abuse
Local
Department of social services: operates child protective service and foster care program
Big Brother and Big Sister Programs: afford opportunity for children to have supportive relationship with adults
Home care assistance program: offers parents opportunity to have parenting and organizational role models in the home who also provide emotional support and informal counseling
Perinatal classes: provide prospective parents with information and parental skills prior to delivery
Family preservation programs: offer intensive support and counsel to maintain family unit
Foster Grandparent Program: provides low-income elders (older than 60 years) with stipend to assist abused, disadvantaged, and handicapped children with counsel, educational, and emotional support
YWCA: offers variety of family support programs, varies with area
Regional or National
National Committee for Prevention of Child Abuse 322 S. Michigan Ave., Ste. 950 Chicago, IL 60604 312–663–3520
National Runaway Switchboard 1–800–621–4000 Personnel available 24 hours/7 days per week
Agency Information and Referral Service 1–800–621–3860: 24-hour national confidential crisis intervention for adolescents
National Council on Child Abuse and Family Violence 1050 Connecticut Ave. N.W., Ste. 300 Washington, DC 20036 202–429–6695
Community Resources for Battered Spouse
Local
Department of social service: emergency financial assistance including Aid to Families with Dependent Children (AFDC), Food Stamps, emergency shelter funding
Local legal assistance: provides restraining order against abusive spouses
Local legal defense fund: provides legal assistance for women with little or no income
YWCA: provides a variety of programs, including support groups
Crisis telephone line: offers immediate assistance and advice as well as counsel during crisis
Shelters: offer temporary shelter for battered spouse and children
Regional and National
National Coalition Against Domestic Violence 1500 Massachusetts Ave. N.W., Ste. 35 Washington, DC 20005 202–293–8260 1–800–333–SAFE
Emerge: A Men's Counseling Service on Domestic Violence 25 Huntington Ave., Rm. 324 Boston, MA 02126
Shelter Aid Hotline 1–800–333–SAFE
Battered Women's Shelters: YWCA Salvation Army
National Alcohol and Drug Helpline offers referrals 1–800–821–4357

Continued

TABLE 20–6

Community Resources for Child Abuse *Continued*

Commmunty Resources for Elderly

Local

Meals programs such as Meals on Wheels: offers meals delivered to the home at least 5 days/week, free of charge, asks for contribution.
Senior centers: offer classes, films, cultural pursuits, group activities, dance, exercise, assistance with forms for Internal Revenue Service, Medicare, and Medicaid (for more active adults). Most programs offer transportation services.
Senior daycare: provides custodial and nursing care to seniors who have needs but are mobile enough to go to a set location. Provides relief for family caregivers, allows elder to stay in home longer, as family members may work and leave elder at daycare. Usually on a sliding scale for fee for service. Most often offers pick-up by transportation.
Senior companion programs: offer part-time work to low-income seniors (60 years and older) to assist frail elderly in their home with friendly visits, shopping, and emotional support.
State or local office on aging: provides information on a variety of elderly resources, consumer information, and education. National Institute on Aging will provide a list of offices if you have difficulty finding a listing in the telephone directory.

Regional or National Programs

American Association of Retired Persons (AARP)
1909 K St. N.W.
Washington, DC 20049
202–872–4700

National Council of Senior Citizens
925 15th St. N.W.
Washington, DC 20005
202–347–8800

National Institute on Aging Information Center
2209 Distribution Circle
Silver Spring, MD 20910

Older Women's League
1325 G. St. N.W.
Washington, DC 20001
202–783–6686

Specialty organizations for specific medical conditions can often offer support, information, referrals, and medical resources. Examples are:
- Alzheimer's Disease and Related Disorders Association
- American Cancer Society
- Arthritis Foundation
- National Osteoporosis Foundation
- American Heart Association
- American Diabetic Association

Home Monitoring Devices for Emergencies

Lifeline Systems, Inc. 1–800–451–0525
American Medical Alert 516–536–5850

Home Health Services, Potential Sources

Local visiting nurses association
Nonprofit social service agencies in your area
Hospital-based home health agencies
Homemaker home health aide services

families. Community health nurses need to advocate for programs that provide regular contact and support. Neergaard (1990) recommends foster grandmother programs. This program matches volunteer older women with young, at-risk mothers and has proved to be a successful intervention effort. Social support programs such as this can be expanded to include abusive as well as at-risk parents.

Violence Interventions in School-Age Children

As children grow their horizons expand and their exposure to violence increases. The community health nurse can assist parents to recognize and counteract some of these influences. Roberts and Quillian (1992) have integrated the topic of violence into a general health teaching tool that nurses can use periodically with parents. The list of health teaching issues in Table 20–7 includes many of these suggestions.

Spouse Abuse Intervention

Individual intervention should be geared toward identifying partners at risk in relationships. The nurse can help couples work on effective communication, decision-making, conflict resolution, and setting personal limits on

TABLE 20–7

Nurse/Parent Guide to Anticipatory Violence Counseling with Children

- Periodically review television and movie-viewing habits; encourage limits on viewing time and types of shows
- Stress the influence of peer pressure and recognize that it increases with age of the child
- For elementary school children
  - Teach coping techniques to avoid fights in school and neighborhood (e.g., walk away from situation)
  - Review stranger danger and good touch/bad touch safety issues
- For children 10 to 11 years old
  - Teach the danger of alcohol and drugs; start no later than 10 years of age
  - Identify high-risk situations in which drinking, drugs, or other problems are most likely to occur and role-play how to avoid or get out of them
- For children 13 to 19 years old
  - Review tobacco, alcohol, and drug use and the social and health consequences of each
  - Reinforce the correlations between substance abuse and accidents
  - Explore exposure to school violence
  - Reinforce previous teaching related to avoidance of violent situations

Data from Roberts, C., & Quillian, J. (1992). Preventing violence through primary care intervention. *Nurse Practitioner, 17*(8), 62–64, 67–70.

conduct. The nurse can help to validate what is appropriate and inappropriate conduct for a partner. Assisting a potential victim to identify and set limits on intrusive or threatening behavior is effective.

“During a clinic appointment the community health nurse notices that Carol M.'s boyfriend repeatedly makes derogatory comments about her personality, her intelligence, and her physical appearance. Carol seems upset. During a conversation the nurse determines that Carol is hurt by her boyfriend's comments and validates with Carol that the comments are hurtful. Carol and the nurse explore ways in which Carol can set limits on her boyfriend's abusive remarks. During subsequent visits, the nurse will monitor and encourage Carol in her efforts. If the boyfriend's behavior remains the same, the nurse should explore other options, such as ascertaining Carol's feelings on leaving the relationship, and encourage supportive relationships.”

Community Efforts at Primary Prevention

The community health nurse can develop and assist with the delivery of community education and support programs aimed at reducing child abuse. The nurse can organize parent support groups and parenting classes. Civic groups are open to guest speakers. The nurse can use these forums to educate about child and spouse abuse and the impact of exposure to violence on children.

Part of the role of the community health nurse includes working for the health of communities as well as that of individuals and families. In that role nurses should become more politically active to work toward a healthy community. Some of the ways the nurse can address child abuse and violence in the community include (1) advocating for inclusion of conflict resolution techniques in school curricula; (2) working with community groups to develop programs geared toward reducing violence exposure and improving safety for communities at risk; and (3) lobbying the state legislators to increase funding for programs that supply economic, health, and other support services to low-income at-risk communities.

Spouse abuse prevention should include public education designed to transform attitudes about spousal violence. Media awareness programs are designed to meet several goals:

- Assist women to recognize their legal rights in abusive situations.
- Enhance public awareness that spousal violence requires legal intervention and is not just a private matter between partners.
- Recognize the need for improving the uneven application of legal restraints and prosecution of violent partners.
- Encourage efforts designed to assist with behavioral changes in battering and battered individuals.
- Discourage "victim blaming" dialogue in public and private discussions about spousal violence.
- Enhance public understanding of the need for *long-term* programs to support both victim and abuser to improve the chances of success.

Working to prevent or ameliorate child and spouse abuse should be a commitment for every community health nurse. Taylor and co-workers (1992) warn that change takes a long time. The community health nurse cannot expect to see substantive change in a week or a month; rather the nurse must be prepared for a sustained long-term effort.

Elder Abuse

- It is estimated that 700,000 to 1.5 million cases of elder abuse occur each year (U.S. House Select Committee on Aging, 1990; AAN Expert Panel, 1993).
- One in every 20 elder Americans is physically abused (Pillemer and Finkelhor, 1988).

Elder abuse has received less media attention than child or spouse abuse; nevertheless it is a serious problem. A majority of elder abuse is related to caregiving. As the elderly population increases more people are involved in caring for older adults, and we can expect an increase in the number of abusive incidents.

The elderly run the risk of abuse at the hands of professionals, family members, and other caregivers. Elders in nursing homes run the greatest risk of abuse. Only about 5% of the elderly population live in institutional facilities; the other 95% live independently or in association with family members or other caretakers (Baldwin, 1990). Because the vast majority of elderly persons live outside of nursing homes most cases of abuse are found in community settings, though the risk of abuse is higher for nursing home residents.

For the elderly living in community settings risk is directly correlated to certain characteristics of their living arrangements. Elder abuse is more common if the older adult lives with family members. Elders who live independently are at less risk (Asley and Fulmer, 1988; Capezuti, 1990). A particular problem in gathering elder abuse data is the reluctance of elderly and caregivers to report suspected cases. Surveys of service agencies, health professionals, and the elderly indicate that approximately 84% of cases or suspected cases are not reported (Goldstein, 1986). Elderly persons do not report because they or their spouses may be afraid of the caretakers, ashamed of the problem, or have limited alternatives for living arrangements. Health professionals do not report incidents out of ignorance of the problem, ignorance of their legal responsibilities in suspected cases, and lack of knowledge about or failure to adequately assess at-risk situations, and because of a very real concern that an alternative living arrangement may be less tolerable than the current one.

DEFINITION

Elder abuse is defined as maltreatment of older persons (usually older than 65 years). Abusive and neglectful actions are included in the definition of elder abuse. Abuse can be physical, emotional, or financial. Failure to provide adequate care and comfort for seniors who are under the community health nurse's care would be considered neglect. Financial exploitation of vulnerable elders is a growing problem, recently identified as the single most common form of elder abuse. Miller (1990) lists six different forms of abuse, including self-neglect or abuse. Some elderly persons are unable or unwilling to provide themselves with adequate food, clothing, or shelter, or may actually engage in self-injurious behavior. Self-abuse and self-neglect are usually associated with depression and other mental health problems.

FACTORS ASSOCIATED WITH ABUSIVE FAMILY MEMBERS

Elder abuse is found in all socioeconomic groups and at all educational levels. The most common abuser is the elder person's spouse. Other frequent elder abusers are daughters, sons, other family members, or paid caregivers. Studies find the abuser to be the spouse in 65% of cases and the children in approximately 23% to 30% of cases (Pillemer and Finkelhor, 1988). Early studies seemed to show that women abused more often than men (Goldstein, 1986). More recent surveys indicate that both sexes are equally abusive or that men are slightly more abusive (Gelles and Cornell, 1990).

The single most important factor in elder abuse is the elder member's loss of independence. When an elderly member of the family becomes dependent on others for care, the risk of abuse rises. Financially dependent elderly with few monetary resources are at risk because they have limited options for alternative living arrangements. The greater the physical dependence, the greater the elder's risk. Confusion, incontinence, frailty, or severe physical and mental disabilities demand enormous amounts of time, energy, and patience from caregivers. Caregivers frequently have many other obligations. Families who have caregiving responsibilities for two generations, their parents and children, are termed *sandwich generation* caregivers. For these individuals the burden of work, children, and caring for an elderly parent can be overwhelming. If there is only a single caregiver, or one who receives little relief from other family or community members, the feelings of frustration and resentment are compounded.

There are few substantial data to support other risk factors for elder abuse. Some studies show a slight relationship between other types of family violence (e.g., child abuse); others report no substantial evidence of intergenerational abuse (Johnson et al., 1985; Pillemer and Suiter, 1988). There is no compelling evidence that substance abuse plays a role in elder abuse, although a few studies show an increased risk when caregivers are substance abusers (Goldstein, 1986; Heckheimer, 1989). As a result, elder abuse does not fit well with the family violence framework for child and spouse abuse (Philips, 1988). Nurses need to consider elder abuse in conjunction with caregiver issues and stressors.

NURSING CARE FOR ELDERS AND CAREGIVERS

Community health nurses are involved in primary, secondary, and tertiary prevention efforts for elders and caregivers. Four major areas in which nurses play an important role in addressing elder abuse are (1) identification of suspected cases; (2) reduction of risk and maintenance of independence; (3) oversight, supervision, and encouragement of caregivers; and (4) development of support groups for caretakers.

Identification of Suspected Cases

Early identification of at-risk situations is important. To that end the nurse should become proficient at identifying potential or probable abusive or neglectful situations. Clearly any unexplained bruises or injuries should be assessed and evaluated. Elders do tend to bruise more easily than younger adults, but explanations that do not ring true and repeated incidences of bruising should arouse suspicion. Reporting and documenting injuries are an important part of the nursing process.

"The nurse makes an initial home visit with Mr. S., a 75-year-old man who lives alone. He has been referred for home health care after being discharged from the hospital with left-sided hemiparesis from a recent cardiovascular accident. The nurse finds Mr. S. alone, sitting in a chair in his bedroom. His clothes are soiled with urine. He says his son looks in on him all the time, but cannot remember when he was there last. A table by his chair holds a carton of sour milk, a box of dry cereal, and some crackers, but no telephone. The nurse is unable to contact the son and Mr. S. cannot supply the names of other family members to contact."

Overmedication is a particular concern that can hamper physical activity, reduce the quality of life, and be potentially life threatening. Overmedication can be inadvertent or deliberate. Sometimes caretakers consider the use of medication to be humane, a way to control behavior and allow the elderly to remain in a familiar environment. A caregiver might use his or her own medications, such as sedatives or painkillers, to keep the older adult sedated or inactive. Under no circumstances should overmedication be condoned.

The nurse needs to be aware of prescribed medication dosages and alert for deliberate or inadvertent overmedication. Miller (1990) suggests the nurse review medications at every home or clinic visit. The existing supply should be checked and tallied to see whether the remaining medication matches what would be expected if someone were taking the medication as prescribed. An oversupply indicates noncompliance or undermedication; too few pills may indicate overmedication. Use of other medication sources by caregivers can be difficult to discern. A groggy, disoriented, or stuporous elderly person may be overmedicated, especially if there is no obvious organic cause for the condition. Inexplicable episodes of clumsiness or falls in an otherwise adequately ambulatory adult are also cause for concern.

The Nurse as Threat or Advocate

It may be difficult for the nurse to decide whether there is sufficient reason to suspect abuse. Caregivers and the elderly might be reluctant to share information or to answer questions. The nurse may be viewed as a threat rather than an asset, especially if the family or elder person fears removal from the home.

"Mrs. E. is a 67-year-old woman with Parkinson's disease. She is recently widowed. Although she can walk with a walker, she requires help with activities of daily living (ADL) and needs assistance to travel outside the home. On a monthly home check the nurse finds that Mrs. E.'s much younger stepsister, Mrs. T. (42 years old) and her husband have moved in to help. Since the nurse's last visit the furniture has been replaced with modern black lacquer pieces and she has a new car. Mrs. E. tells the nurse that she misses her old furniture, but her brother-in-law did not like it. A new car has been bought with Mrs. E.'s funds and is driven by Mrs. T. Mrs. T. gave the old car to her son because Mrs. E. "did not need it any more." Mrs. E. tells the nurse she is afraid that she does not have much money left in her bank account, but begs the nurse not to do anything about it because she wants to stay in her home."

Mrs. E.'s concern about institutionalization is valid. Gelles and Cornell (1990) report that in one study of elder abuse cases almost half were resolved by placing the elderly person in a nursing home.

The overriding principle guiding the nurse's decision should be the safety and well-being of the elder client. The two examples provided are not uncommon situations encountered by the community health nurse. If reasonable evidence of abuse is present, the nurse should report the circumstances and let the designated authorities do a thorough review.

Legal Responsibilities of the Nurse

Most states have laws that require the reporting of elder abuse. State definitions of elder abuse vary; some do not include neglect and very few include financial exploitation. The specific agency to which the nurse reports varies according to the state involved but is usually the state's social service agency (adult protective services) or an independent senior service agency (office on aging). As with child abuse, the nurse will have to state the circumstances that have led to the belief that a problem exists, the name of the individual, the address, and the name of the caregiver if it is known.

Autonomy vs. Safety

One of the most difficult issues in elder care is what to do when an older adult chooses to remain in a difficult situation. In cases in which immediate danger to life is present, the state may act and mandate action to safeguard the individual.

"An elderly couple, 68-year-old Marie and 79-year-old Ryan M., were forcibly removed from their home and placed in a nursing home. Mr. M. was blind, diabetic, and had numerous open wounds on both legs. Mrs. M. was confused, and frequently disoriented. Their home reeked of urine. The couple had not paid their electric, telephone, and water bills for over a year. They had no water because of unrepaired plumbing problems. They were malnourished and seldom shopped for food, although money was available. Mr. M. was prescribed insulin injections, but the couple seldom remembered to administer them. Both vigorously resisted institutionalization. Six months after placement, both are still adamant that they want to return home. ”

Usually the state only acts in extreme cases of mental incompetence or physical incapacity. For the most part the law recognizes an adult's right to self-determination. Community health nurses frequently come in contact with elders who choose to remain in abusive or neglectful situations. In situations in which the law concurs, accepting the personal right of elders may be one of the most difficult situations a nurse can face. Whenever possible the first efforts to address elder care issues should be accomplished by good resource management rather than legal intervention.

Reducing Risk through Community Resources

Because maintaining financial and physical independence is the single most important factor in reducing elder abuse, a thorough knowledge of the community resources available for elders is important. Table 20–6 provides a sampling of community resources available to the community health nurse who is planning elder care. Chapter 27 also provides resource materials.

Most metropolitan communities offer a variety of home-related services to assist independent living. These include home repair services, home maintenance services, fuel assistance programs, home visiting programs, daily telephone call programs, meal delivery services, and medically related services such as home aides, registered nurses, physical therapy, and physician visit services.

Transportation to and from appointments may be the only assistance needed to maintain autonomy. The ability to get to medical appointments, go shopping for groceries, and other important services can make the difference between living alone and having to seek other living arrangements. Most communities offer transportation services, although some may be limited in the locations served and the distances covered. Some have strict criteria for the elders they will transport: elders may be required to be independently mobile and not depend on a walker, cane, or wheelchair.

Another important service that can be found occasionally is grocery shopping to order, with delivery services to the home. Supermarket chains have marketed this service for persons who are too busy to do their own shopping, but it is certainly useful for elderly persons who are handicapped by lack of transportation or by physical needs. In rural areas the nurse may need to help create informal networks of friends and volunteers to address the variety of needs.

Assistance to Caregivers

According to Janz (1990) nurses act as counselors and resource directors to assist families at risk for elder abuse. Counseling families to recognize caregiver stress and its impact on both the elder and the caregiver is essential. Baldwin (1990) provides a list of 10 steps that are useful in stress reduction for caregivers and advises that the nurse teach the family about a variety of stress-reduction techniques and assist family members in selecting those best suited to meet their needs.

The nurse should also serve as a resource person and advise the elder and caregiver of community resources that are available to assist with care and support.

A few community services are designed to assist caretaker families, including those who have had a history of abusive episodes, to understand and address the stresses that occur in elder care. These services are usually available to any caregiver. Crisis hotlines are equipped to handle situations related to elder care and elder abuse. Classes in family dynamics help to explore the stressors in multigenerational families and identify effective coping methods. Counseling services are available and are frequently mandated for those found guilty of abuse. Support services for caregivers, including group meetings, allow members to support each other and to provide helpful strategies to assist with everyday problems.

A variety of types of respite care are available. Adult daycare offers families or caregivers the opportunity to place the elder member in a supervised structured setting during the day while the caregivers are at work. This relieves families of the anxiety of leaving a parent at home unsupervised or of finding suitable custodial care. Some facilities have begun to offer weekend programs so that family members can do their home maintenance chores or recreation activities with some measure of comfort. Another form of respite care involves providing care services for elderly family members on a 24-hour basis for certain periods to allow caregivers a break from their duties. These programs can provide care for weekends or longer time frames to allow family members to take a vacation or short rest periods. Not all communities offer respite services.

The Nurse's Role in Community Education and Advocacy

Community health nurses should become involved in exploring service options for elderly individuals and in educating the general public in the problems of older individuals and their caregivers. These goals can be partly accomplished by designing and delivering educational programs to community groups and organizations, or by advocating for legislation designed to assist elder independence and elder caregivers whenever possible. Public understanding about the aging process and safeguards to

TABLE 20–8

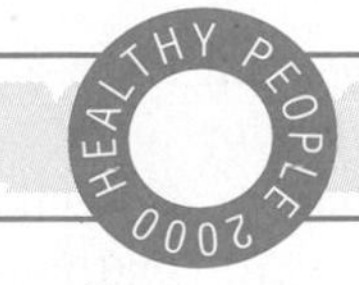

Violence-Related National Health Objectives for the Year 2000

Societal Violence

Health Status Objectives

Reduce suicides to no more than 10.5 per 100,000 persons (now 11.7). Special at-risk groups with higher rates include young males (20–43 years) and older white males (65 years and older).
Reduce homicide to no more than 7.2 per 100,000 persons (now 8.5). Special at-risk groups include young males, especially young black males.
Reduce weapon-related violent deaths (guns and knives) to no more than 12.6 per 100,000 persons (now 14.9).
Reduce assault injuries to no more than 10 per 1000 persons (now 11.1).
Reduce rape and attempted rape of women to no more than 107 per 100,000 persons (now 120).

Risk Reduction Objectives

Reduce by 20% the incidence of physical fighting among adolescents.
Reduce by 20% the incidence of weapon carrying by adolescents age 14 to 17 years.
Reduce by 20% the proportion of weapons that are inappropriately stored and dangerously available.

Service and Protection Objectives

Increase by at least 50% the proportion of elementary and secondary schools that teach nonviolent conflict resolution.
Extend coordinated, comprehensive violence prevention programs to at least 80% of local jurisdictions with populations over 100,000.

Child, Spouse, and Elder Abuse

Health Status Objectives

Reduce to less than 25.2 per 1000 children the rising incidence of maltreatment (now 25.2).
Reduce physical abuse of women by male partners to no more than 27 per 1000 couples (now 30).

Service and Protection Objectives

Extend protocols for routinely identifying, treating, and properly referring suicide attempts, victims of sexual assault, and victims of spouse, elder, and child abuse to at least 90% of hospital emergency departments (not specifically mentioned are community-related health professionals, who should also become more proficient).
Increase to at least 30 the number of states in which at least 50% of children identified as physically or sexually abused receive physical and mental evalution with appropriate follow-up as a means of breaking the intergenerational cycle of abuse.
Reduce to less than 10% the proportion of battered women and their children turned away from emergency housing owing to lack of space (now 40%).

From U.S. Department of Health and Human Services. (1992). *Healthy people 2000: National health promotion and disease prevention objectives.* Washington, DC: Government Printing Office.

ensure a safe and secure environment for the senior members of our communities will go a long way toward reducing the problems of elder abuse.

Conclusion

Community health nursing is in a unique position to address the health needs related to violent behavior. The very nature of community nursing directs community health nurses toward establishing long-term relationships with individuals, families, and communities. The problems that occur as a result of violence are not readily solved. Community health nurses have the knowledge, perseverance, and sensitivity to assist clients in coping with the many concerns and health needs associated with violent behavior. Focusing on community needs as outlined in *Healthy People 2000* is an excellent starting point (Table 20–8).

KEY IDEAS

1. Violence is a major public health concern.
2. Violent behavior is the result of the complex relationship of many issues and is influenced by sociological, environmental, and individual factors.
3. Certain individual and group characteristics place people at risk of being victims or perpetrators of abusive behavior, but not all persons with risk factors become victims or abusers.
4. Women, children, and older adults are at special risk for family violence, because society has been

reluctant to breach the family structure and dictate behavior.

5. There is mounting evidence that education, social pressure, and mandatory punishment for abusive behavior are effective.
6. Primary prevention is the single most important method of preventing violent behavior among family members and society at large.
7. Behavioral and social changes needed to mitigate violent activity or risk of victimization are long-term activities.
8. Community health nurses are uniquely qualified and well situated to work with victims and abusers and in primary prevention efforts with individuals and community groups.

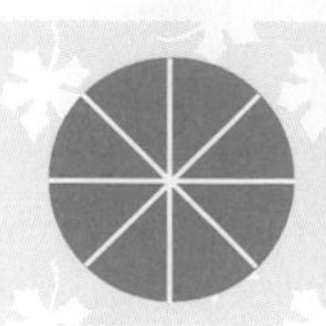

APPLYING THE NURSING PROCESS: *A Violent Family*

Ms. Jones, a community health nurse, has been asked to do a home assessment on the Charles family. When Ms. Jones visits Mrs. Charles she finds a 20-year-old woman living at home with three children, ages 3 and 2 years and 7 months. Mrs. Charles is attempting to correct the 3-year-old by threatening to beat her with a belt if she doesn't stop pulling her sister's arm. The home is unkempt and cluttered, with dried food and several days' worth of dishes piled in the sink. The children are in their nightwear and are just eating breakfast at noon. During the conversation that follows, Mrs. Charles shares her concerns about money and her anxiety about having to care for the children by herself. She relates that Mr. Charles has been ordered by the court to remain outside the home and undergo therapy, because he has been found to be responsible for a broken arm suffered by the 2 year old. She also tells the nurse that she has visited social services for an application for financial assistance, but that she has not completed the application. Mrs. Charles has about $20 and 2 days' supply of food left in the house.

Assessment

- Financial resources
- Food supply
- Status of financial assistance (AFDC) application
- Integrity of home environment with respect to safety and adequacy
- Existence of health conditions requiring immediate medical attention
- Available social support network for family
- Mr. Charles's compliance with court order, degree of family interaction with him, and safety concerns related to that interaction
- Parenting skills of Mrs. Charles
- Immunization status of children

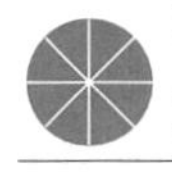

Nursing Diagnosis	Goals	Interventions
Ineffective family coping related to insufficient financial resources	The family's financial situation will improve	Review the client's Aid to Families with Dependent Children (AFDC) application, and help the client complete the form appropriately as necessary Arrange for emergency food assistance, including an AFDC emergency grant for food and funds for living expenses

		Review and help the client contact other potential sources of financial assistance, such as church organizations and social service agencies
Altered parenting as evidenced by ineffective limit-setting and of threats of physical abuse	The client will demonstrate improved parenting skills	Review the client's typical disciplinary practices; help her recognize which practices are successful and which are unsuccessful Acknowledge any frustration that the client expresses Explore the client's own experience with her parents' disciplinary practices when she was a child; elicit her feelings, both positive and negative, about these practices Teach the client about normal growth and development milestones for her children's age levels Help the client identify effective age-appropriate discipline strategies Reinforce effective discipline efforts
Ineffective individual coping related to multiple stressors	The client will exhibit improved coping skills	Review the client's available sources of support, such as other family members, friends, and neighbors Provide a list of available community resources, such as Parents Anonymous, other support groups, and counselors Arrange for a home aide worker to assist with organizational skills and provide emotional support Provide guidance and encouragement in developing problem-solving and decision-making skills; if appropriate, draft a contract or a written plan with achievable, mutually agreed-on goals for the client to accomplish between visits

Evaluation

During the initial home visit the nurse determines that the family's food supply is sufficient to last 1 week. Mrs. Charles and the nurse complete the forms for AFDC support and the nurse arranges for

Continued

same-day transportation to social services for Mrs. Charles so she can apply for emergency funds and food and submit her paperwork for monthly AFDC support.

As the nurse helps Mrs. Charles to address some of her immediate needs, the client is more willing to share other pieces of information. The nurse learns that Mrs. Charles is behind in her rent and that the landlord has given her an eviction notice. Mr. Charles has been visiting the house periodically (two or three times a week). He usually shows up to spend the night when he can't find another place to stay, and his visits usually include a demand for money from Mrs. Charles. She tells the nurse she has been getting $50/week from her mother, but has given at least half to Mr. Charles because "she does not want to deal with telling him no." Mrs. Charles does not feel that she or other family members are in danger from her husband; she reports that he has been demanding but "has not lifted a finger to anyone since the judge told him to stop beating on us."

The family does have some support from Mrs. Charles's mother and one sister who live nearby. Her mother agreed to babysit while Mrs. Charles went to social services that afternoon. Both her mother and her sister have offered to babysit the children and to transport Mrs. Charles, but she does not like to ask them for much because they are always pressuring her to "get rid of that bum you married."

Assessment of the living environment finds the family living in a two-bedroom apartment in substandard condition, with a clogged bathtub, dripping sink faucet, multiple worn areas in the flooring that exposes rotting wooden floors, and inadequate heat throughout the apartment. Three space heaters, which are a safety hazard, are located in both bedrooms and the living room. Mrs. Charles indicates that she has complained about the problems on numerous occasions, but that the landlord has not fixed them. She would be willing to move if more adequate shelter arrangements could be found.

At the end of the visit the nurse decides that the family needs biweekly visits until food, shelter, and funds are in place and adequate, with weekly visits for several months to help Mrs. Charles focus on learning to use available community resources, ensure healthful conditions for family members, and improve parenting skills.

GUIDELINES FOR LEARNING

1. Follow several reported family abuse cases in the newspaper to their conclusion in the court system. Review the life experiences of the individuals involved, both abusers and abused, and try to understand the family dynamics of each case.
2. Become familiar with attempts to change laws related to abuse: What are the proposed new dimensions? Why were they proposed? What are the positions of advocates and opponents of the new law? Determine your position on the effort.
3. Consult with fellow students and health professionals about their experiences with abusive situations: How were the situations resolved? Were the individuals involved satisfied that the victims were adequately protected? What would you do under similar circumstances?
4. Explore community resources that might be valuable references for children, spouses, or elders in need. Review the funding of such resources. Are they adequate to meet the needs as identified by the agency personnel and persons assisted?
5. Review state and local funding for abuse support programs. Correspond with your local state representative to determine his or her position on funding priorities for abusive resources.
6. Discover whether your community has respite care for caregivers. If none is available, what actions could you take to encourage the community to provide such a resource?
7. Reflect on the meaning of family violence to you. What experiences with social, intimate, or family violence have you had? How do your experiences and background affect your reaction to violent situations and victims of family violence?

REFERENCES

American Academy of Nursing (AAN) Expert Panel. (1993). AAN working paper: Violence as a nursing priority: Policy implications. *Nursing Outlook, 41*(2), 83–92.

American Association for Protecting Children (AAPC). (1986). *Highlights of the official child neglect and abuse report, 1984.* Denver: American Humane Association.

AAPC. (1990). *Highlights of the official child neglect and abuse report, 1988.* Denver: American Humane Association.

Agopian, M. W. (1989). Targeting juvenile gang offenders for community service. *Community Alternatives International Journal of Family Care, 1*(1), 99–108.

Andresen, P. A. (1985). The prevention and treatment of spouse abuse: A community health perspective. *Journal of Community Health Nursing, 2,* 181–190.

Asley, J., & Fulmer, T. (1988). No simple way to determine elder abuse. *Gerontological Nursing, 9,* 286–288.

Baldwin, B. (1990, July-August). Family caregiving: Trends and forecasts. *Geriatric Nursing,* 172–174.

Barber-Madden, R., Cohn, A. H., & Schloesser, P. (1988, Summer). Prevention of child abuse: A public health agenda. *Public Health Policy,* 167–176.

Bell, C. C., & Jenkins, E. J. (1991). Traumatic stress and children. Third National Conference: Health care for the poor and underserved "children at risk" (1991, Nashville, Tennessee). *Journal of Health Care for the Poor and Underserved, 2*(1), 175–185.

Bergman, B. K., & Brismar, B. G. (1992). Can family violence be prevented? A psychosocial study of male batterers and battered wives. *Public Health, 106*(1), 45–52.

Berrios, D. C., & Grady, D. (1991). Domestic violence: Risk factors and outcomes. *Western Journal of Medicine, 166*(2), 133–136.

Bishop, S. J., Murphy, J. M., Jellinek, J. S., Quinn, D., & Poitrast, F. G. (1992). Protecting seriously mistreated children—Time delays in a court sample. *Child Abuse and Neglect, 16*(4), 465–474.

Brayden, R. M., Altemeier, W. A., Dietrich, M. S., Tucher, D. D., Christensen, M. J., McLaughlin, F. J., & Sherrod, K. E. (1993). A prospective study of secondary prevention of child maltreatment. *Journal of Pediatrics, 122,* 511–516.

Browne, K. (1989). The health visitor's role in screening for child abuse. *Health Visitor, 62*(9), 275–277.

Capezuti, L. (1990). Commentary on the debate over dependency as a relevant predisposing factor in elder abuse and neglect. *Journal of Elder Abuse and Neglect, 2*(1, 2), 63–65.

Carmen, E. (1986). Family violence and the victim-to-patient process. In L. J. Dickstein & C. C. Nadelson (Eds.). *Family violence: Emerging issues of a national crisis.* Washington, DC: American Psychological Press.

Carr, A. (1977). *Some preliminary findings on the association between child maltreatment and juvenile misconduct in 8 New York counties: Report to the Administration for Children, Youth, and Families* (National Commission on Child Abuse and Neglect). Washington, DC: U.S. Government Printing Office.

Centerwell, B. S. (1989). Exposure to television as a risk factor for violence. *American Journal of Epidemiology, 129,* 643–652.

Centerwell, B. S. (1992). Television and violence: The scale of the problem and where to go from here. *Journal of the American Medical Association, 267,* 3059–3063.

Children's Defense Fund. (1992). *The state of America's children.* Washington, DC: Author.

Conte, J. R., & Berliner, L. (1981). Sexual abuse of children: Implications for practice social casework. *Journal of Contemporary Social Work, 62,* 601–606.

Daro, D. (1988). *Confronting child abuse.* New York: The Free Press.

Daro, D., & McCurdy, K. (1991). *Current trends in child abuse reporting and fatalities: The results of the 1990 annual 50 state survey.* Chicago: National Committee for Prevention of Child Abuse.

Dickstein, L. J., & Nadelson, C. C. (Eds.). (1986). *Family violence: Emerging issues of a national crisis.* Washington, DC: American Psychological Press.

Duncan, D. F. (1991). Violence and degradation as themes in "adult" videos. *Psychological Reports, 69*(1), 239–240.

Dunford, F. W. (1992). The measurement of recidivism in cases of spouse assault. *Journal of Criminal Law and Criminology, 83*(1), 120–136.

Earls, F. (1991). Not fear, nor quarantine, but science: Preparation for a decade of research to advance knowledge about causes and control of violence in youths. *Journal of Adolescent Health, 12,* 619–629.

Egeland, B., Jacobvitz, D., & Papatola, K. (1987). Intergenerational continuity of abuse. In R. Gelles & J. Lancaster (Eds.). *Child abuse and neglect: Biosocial dimensions.* New York: Aldine Gruyter.

Else, L. T., Wonderlich, S. A., Beatty, W. W., Christie, D. W., & Stanton, R. D. (1993). Personality characteristics of men who physically abuse women. *Hospital and Community Psychiatry, 44*(1), 54–58.

Famularo, R., Kinscherff, R., & Fentron, T. (1992). Parental substance abuse and the nature of child maltreatment. *Child Abuse and Neglect, 16,* 475–483.

Fingerhut, L. A., & Kleinman, J. C. (1990). International and interstate comparison of homicide among young males. *Journal of the American Medical Association, 263,* 3292–3295.

Fitzpatrick, K. M., & Boldizar, J. P. (1993). The prevalence and consequences of exposure to violence among African-American youth. *Journal of the American Academy of Child and Adolescent Psychiatry, 32,* 424–430.

Gainer, P. S., Webster, D. W., & Champion, H. R. (1993). A youth violence prevention program. Description and preliminary evaluation. *Archives of Surgery, 128,* 303–308.

Garbino, J., & Gilliam, G. (1980). *Understanding abusive families.* Lexington, MA: Lexington Press.

Gelles, R. J., & Cornell, C. P. (1990). *Intimate violence in families* (2nd ed.). London: Sage Publications.

Gelles, R. J., & Straus, M. A. (1988). *The definitive study of the causes and consequences of abuse in the American family.* New York: Simon and Schuster.

Giannini, A. J., Miller, N. S., Loiselle, R. H., & Turner, C. E. (1993). Cocaine-associated violence and the relationship to route of administration. *Journal of Substance Abuse Treatment, 10*(1), 67–69.

Gladstein, J., Rusonis, E. J., & Heald, F. P. (1992). A comparison of inner-city and upper-middle class youths' exposure to violence. *Journal of Adolescent Health, 13,* 275–280.

Goldstein, M. Z. (1986). Elder neglect, abuse, and exploitation. In L. J. Dickstein & C. C. Nadelson (Eds.). *Family violence: Emerging issues of a national crisis.* Washington, DC: American Psychological Press.

Grisso, J. A., Wishner, A. R., Schwarz, D. F., Weene, B. A., Holme, J. H., & Sutton, R. L. (1991). A population-based study of injuries in inner-city women. *American Journal of Epidemiology, 134,* 59–68.

Groves, B. M., Zuckerman, B., Marans, S., & Cohen, D. J. (1993). Silent victims. Children who witness violence. *Journal of the American Medical Association, 269,* 262–264.

Hagland, M. M. (1992). Jim Brady speaks out on handgun violence. *Hospitals, 66*(21), 66.

Hammett, M., Powell, K. E., O'Carroll, P. W., & Clanton, S. T. (1993). Homicide surveillance—United States, 1979–1988. *Morbidity and Mortality Weekly Reports, 41*(No. SS–3), 1–34.

Hammond, W. R., & Yung, B. (1993). Psychology's role in the public health response to assaultive violence among young African-American men. *American Psychologist, 48*(2), 142–154.

Heckheimer, E. F. (1989). *Health promotion of the elderly in the community.* Philadelphia: W.B. Saunders.

Helton, A., McFarlane, J., & Anderson, E. (1987). Battered and pregnant: A prevalence study. *American Journal of Public Health, 77,* 1337–1339.

Herman, J. (1986). Recognition and treatment of incestuous families. In L. J. Dickstein & C. C. Nadelson (Eds.). *Family violence: Emerging issues of a national crisis.* Washington, DC: American Psychological Press.

Hirschel, J. D., & Hutchinson, I. W. (1992). Female spouse abuse and the police response—The Charlotte, North Carolina experiment. *Journal of Criminal Law and Criminology, 83*(1), 73–119.

Hochhaus, C., & Sousa, F. (1987–88). Why children belong to gangs: A comparison of expectations and reality. *High School Journal, 71*(2), 74–77.

Hollenkamp, M., & Attala, J. (1986). Meeting health needs in a crisis shelter: A challenge to nurses in the community. *Journal of Community Health Nursing, 3*(4), 201–209.

Huff, C. R. (1989). Youth gangs and public policy. *Crime and Delinquency, 35,* 524–537.

Hutchinson, E. D. (1993). Mandatory reporting laws: Child protective case finding gone awry? *Social Work: Journal of the National Association of Social Workers, 38*(1), 56–63.

Janz, M. (1990). Clues to elder abuse. *Geriatric Nursing, 11,* 220–222.

Jecker, N. S. (1993). Privacy beliefs and the violent family. Extending the ethical argument for physician intervention. *Journal of the American Medical Association, 269,* 776–780.

Johnson, E. M. (1990). Chemical dependency and black America: The government responds. *Journal of National Black Nurses' Association, 4*(2), 47–56.

Johnson, T., O'Brien, J., & Hudson, M. F. (1985). *Elder neglect and abuse: An annotated bibliography.* Westport, CT: Greenwood Press.

Jones, A. (1980). *Women who kill.* New York: Holt, Reinhart, and Winston.

Justice, B. (1992). Suffering in silence and the fear of social stigma: Survivors of violence. *National League for Nursing* (Publication No. 15-2461), 269–289.

Katz, L. (1980). *T.V. and kids violence: Position statement on media violence in childrens' lives, adopted by National Association for Education of Young People.* Washington, DC: NAEYP.

Kelley, S. J., Brant, R., & Waterman, J. (1993). Sexual abuse of children in day care centers. *Child Abuse and Neglect, 17*(1), 71–89.

Kingery, P. M., Pruitt, B. E., & Hurley, R. S. (1992). Violence and illegal drug use among adolescents: Evidence from the U.S. National Adolescent Student Health Survey. *International Journal of the Addictions, 27,* 1445–1464.

Koop, C. E., & Lundberg, G. D. (1992). Violence in America: A public health emergency: Time to bite the bullet. *Journal of the American Medical Association, 267,* 3075–3076.

Laslett, B. (1973). The family as a public and private institution: A historical perspective. *Journal of Marriage and the Family, 35*(3), 480–494.

Lester, D. (1993). Restricting the availability of alcohol and rates of personal violence (suicide and homocide). *Drugs and Alcohol Dependence, 31*(3), 215–217.

Levy, B. (1991). *Dating violence: Young women in danger.* Seattle: Seal Press-Feminist.

Lidz, C. W., Mulvey, E. P., & Gardner, W. (1993). The accuracy of predictions of violence to others. *Journal of the American Medical Association, 269,* 1007–1011.

Lore, R. K., & Schultz, L. A. (1993). Control of human aggression. A comparative perspective. *American Psychologist, 48*(1), 16–25.

Margolin, L. (1992). Child abuse by mothers' boyfriends—Why the overrepresentation? *Child Abuse and Neglect, 16,* 541–551.

McClain, P. W., Sacks, J. J., Froehlke, R. G., & Ewigman, B. E. (1993). Estimates of fatal child abuse and neglect, United States, 1979 through 1988. *Pediatrics, 91,* 338–343.

McFarlane, J., Christoffel, K., Bateman, L., Miller, V., & Bullock, L. (1991). Assessing for abuse: Self-report versus nurse interview. *Public Health Nursing, 8,* 245–250.

McFarlane, J., Parker, B., Socken, K., & Bullock, L. (1992). Assessing for abuse during pregnancy: Severity and frequency of injuries and associated entry into prenatal care. *Journal of the American Medical Association, 267,* 3176–3178.

McLeer, V. S., Anwar, R. A. H., Herman, S., & Maquilling, K. (1989). Education is not enough: A systems failure in protecting women. *Annals of Emergency Medicine, 18,* 651–653.

Miller, C. (1990). *Nursing care of older adults: Theory and practice.* Glenview, IL: Scott Foresman.

Moldanado, S. A. (1991). Documentation of client encounters by public health nurses at a county health department. *Journal of Community Health Nursing, 8*(3), 171–178.

Mollerstron, W. W., Patcher, M. A., & Milner, J. S. (1992). Family functioning and child abuse potential. *Journal of Clinical Psychology, 48,* 445–454.

Murphy, J. M., Bishop, S. J., Jellinek, M. S., Quinn, D., & Poitrast, F. G. (1992). What happens after the care and protection petition: Reabuse in a court sample. *Child Abuse and Neglect, 16,* 485–493.

Nadelson, C. C., & Sauzier, M. (1986). Intervention programs for individual victims and their families. In L. J. Dickstein & C. C. Nadelson (Eds.). *Family violence: Emerging issues of a national crisis.* Washington, DC: American Psychological Press.

National Center for Child Abuse and Neglect. (1988). *Study findings: National study of the incidence and severity of child abuse and neglect* (DHHS Publication No. OHDS81–30325). Washington, DC: U.S. Government Printing Office.

Neergaard, J. A. (1990). A proposal for a foster grandmother program to prevent child abuse. *Public Health Reports, 105*(1), 89–98.

Novello, A. C., Shosky, J., & Froehlke, R. (1992). From the Surgeon General, US Public Health Service. *Journal of the American Medical Association, 267,* 3007.

Philips, L. R. (1988). The fit of elder abuse with the family violence paradigm, and the implications of a paradigm shift for clinical practice. *Public Health Nursing, 5,* 222–229.

Physical fighting among high school students—United States, 1990. (1992). *Morbidity and Mortality Weekly Report, 41*(6), 92–94.

Pillemer, K., & Finkelhor, D. (1988). The prevalence of elder abuse: A random sample survey. *The Gerontologist, 28*(1), 51–57.

Pillemer, K., & Suiter J. (1988). Elder abuse. In V. B. Hasselt, R. L. Morrison, A. S. Bellack, & M. Hersen (Eds.). *Handbook of family violence.* New York: Plenum Press.

Policy statement: Domestic violence. (1993). *American Journal of Public Health, 83*(3), 458–462.

Potter-Efron, R. T., & Potter-Efron, P. S. (1990). *Aggression, family violence, and chemical dependency.* New York: Haworth Press.

Randall, T. (1991). Duluth takes a firm stand against domestic violence: Mandates abuser arrest, education. *Journal of the American Medical Association, 266,* 1180–1184.

Reuter, M. M. (1988). Parenting needs of abusing parents: Development of a tool for evaluation of a parent education program. *Journal of Community Health Nursing, 5*(2), 129–140.

Roberts, C., Quillian, J. (1992). Preventing violence through primary care intervention. *Nurse Practitioner, 17*(8), 62–64, 67–70.

Russell, D. E. H. (1984). The prevalence and seriousness of incestuous abuse: Stepfathers vs. biological fathers. *Child Abuse and Neglect, 8*(1), 15–22.

Ryan, J. M. (1989). Child abuse and the community health nurse. *Home Healthcare Nurse, 7*(2), 23–26.

Sabotta, E. E., Davis, R. L. (1992). Fatality after report to a child abuse registry in Washington State, 1973–1986. *Child Abuse and Neglect, 16*(5), 627–635.

Senate Committee on Labor and Human Resources. (1990). *Domestic violence: Terrorism in the home.* 101st Congress, 2nd Session, Senate Hearing 101–897.

Speigel, I. A. (1986). The violent gang problem in Chicago: A local community approach. *Social Service Review, 60*(1), 94–131.

Starr, R. H. (1988). Physical abuse of children. In V. B. Van Hasselt, R. L. Morrison, A. S. Bellack, & M. Hersen (Eds.). *Handbook of family violence.* New York: Plenum Press.

Starr, R. H., Dubowitz, H., & Bush, B. A. (1990). The epidemiology of child maltreatment. In R. T. Ammerman & M. Hersen (Eds.). *Children at risk: An evaluation of factors contributing to child abuse and neglect.* New York: Plenum Press.

Straus, M. A. (1980). The marriage license as a hitting license: Evidence from popular culture, law, and social science. In M. A. Straus & G. T. Hotaling (Eds.). *The social cause of husband-wife violence.* Minneapolis: University of Minnesota Press.

Straus, M., Gelles, R. J., & Steinmetz, S. K. (1980). *Behind closed doors: Violence in the American family.* Garden City, NJ: Anchor.

Surgeon General's Scientific Advisory Committee on Television and Growing Up. (1972). *The impact of televised violence.* Washington, DC: U.S. Government Printing Office.

Taylor, W., Fulmer, T., Helton, A., & Cross, P. O. (1992). Nurses battle family violence: Breaking the cycle of violence takes time and caring. *American Nurse, 24*(4), 1, 7–8.

Thompson, M. P., & Norris, F. H. (1992). Crime, social status and alienation. *American Journal of Community Psychology, 20*(1), 97–119.

Tontodonato, P., Crew, B. K. (1992). Dating violence, social learning theory, and gender: A multivariate analysis. *Violence and Victims, 7*(1), 3–14.

Turbett, P., & O'Toole, R. (1986). *Physicians' recognition of child abuse.* Paper presented at the American Sociological Association Annual Meeting, New York.

U.S. Department of Health and Human Services education about adult domestic violence in U.S. and Canadian medical schools–1987-88. (1989). *Morbidity and Mortality Weekly Report, 38*(2), 17–19.

U.S. House Select Committee on Aging. (1990, May). *Elder abuse: A decade of shame and inaction.* Hearing before the House Select Committee on Aging. 101st Congress, 2nd Session.

Walker, L. E. (1979). *The battered woman.* New York: Harper and Row.

Weitzman, L. J. (1981). *The marriage contract: Spouses, lovers and the law.* New York: The Free Press.

Widom, C. S. (1989). The cycle of violence. *Science, 244,* 160–166.

Williams-White, D. (1986). Self help and advocacy: An alternative approach to helping battered women. In L. J. Dickstein & C. C. Nadelson (Eds.). *Family violence: Emerging issues of a national crisis.* Washington, DC: American Psychological Press.

Wolfner, G. G., & Gelles, R. J. (1993). A profile of violence toward children: A national study. *Child Abuse and Neglect, 17*(2), 197–212.

Yegides, B. L. (1992). Family violence: Contemporary research findings and practice issues. *Community Mental Health Journal, 28,* 519–530.

Zuckerman, D. M., & Zuckerman, B. S. (1985). Television's impact on children. *Pediatrics, 75,* 233–240.

BIBLIOGRAPHY

Ammeran, R. T., & Hersen, J. (Eds.). (1992). *Assessment of family violence: A clinical and legal sourcebook.* New York: Wiley.

Dickstein, L. J., & Nadelson, C. C. (1989). *Family violence: Emerging issues of a national crisis.* Washington, DC: American Psychological Press.

Gelles, R. J., & Cornell, C. P. (1990). *Intimate violence in families* (2nd ed.). Newbury Park, CA: Sage Publications.

Hutchings, N. (1988). *The violent family: Victimization of women, children and elders.* New York: Human Sciences Press.

Kashani, J. H., Daniel, A. E., Kandoy, A. C., & Holcomb, W. R. (1992). Family violence: Impact on children. *Journal of the American Academy of Child and Adolescent Psychiatry 31*(2), 181–189.

Kempe, C. H., & Helfer, R. E. (1980). *The battered child* (3rd ed.). Chicago: The University of Chicago Press.

Pavcza, G. J., Cohen, D., Eisdorfer, C., Freels, S., Semla, T., Ashford, J. W., Hirschman, R., Luchins, D., & Levy, P. (1992). Severe family violence and Alzheimer's disease: Prevalence and risk factors. *Gerontologist, 32,* 493–497.

SUGGESTED READINGS

Barber-Madden, R., Cohn, A. H., & Schlosser, F. (1988). Prevention of child abuse: A public health agenda. *Journal of Public Health Policy, 9*(2), 167–176.

Bullock, L. F., Bendella, J. A., McFarlane, J. (1989). Breaking the cycle of abuse: How nurses can intervene. *Journal of Psychosocial Nursing and Mental Health Services, 27*(8), 11–13.

Fedders, C. (1987). *Shattered dreams.* New York: Harper and Row.

Kjervik, D. K. (1990). Legal and ethical issues: Ethical dilemmas of battered women. *Journal of Professional Nursing, 6,* 163.

Marshall, E., Buckner, E., & Powell, K. (1991). Evaluation of a teen parent program designed to reduce child abuse and neglect and to strengthen families. *Journal of Child and Adolescent Psychiatric and Mental Health Nursing, 4,* 98–100.

Neergaard, J. A. (1990). A proposal for a foster grandmother intervention program to prevent child abuse. *Public Health Reports, 105*(1), 89–93.

Randall, T. (1991). Duluth takes firm stance against domestic violence: Mandates abuser arrest, education. *Journal of the American Medical Association, 266,* 1180–1184.

Reuter, M. M. (1988). Parenting needs of abusing parents: Development of a tool for evaluation of a parent education class. *Journal of Community Health Nursing, 6,* 128–140.

Rind, P. (1992). Teens and toddlers aim to reduce child abuse among adolescent parents. *Family Planning Perspectives, 4*(1), 37–40.

Rosenberg, J. L., & Henley, M. A. (Eds.). (1991). *Violence in America: A public health approach.* New York: Oxford University Press.

Suditud, C., & Mock, D. (1988). Interrupting the cycle of child abuse. *American Journal of Maternal Child Nursing, 13,* 196–199.

Chapter 21

Common Addictions

Mary Ann Walsh Eells

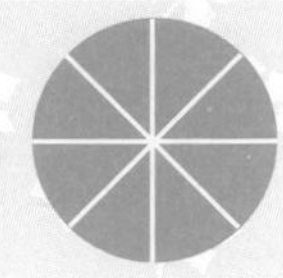

Focus Questions

Abuse and addictions: When do behaviors of excess go beyond one's ability to "just say no"?

What are some common myths and attitudes about addiction: facts vs. feelings?

What do we really know about addictions: Are they genetically determined or affected by powerful environmental forces, including the family?

How can community health nurses help to prevent addictions?

What behavior patterns alert the nurse to the presence of addiction and suggest specific interventions?

How can community health nurses assist individuals and families recovering from addictions?

What resources for problems of addiction exist in the community currently and how is this picture changing?

What Is the Problem?

Babylon has been a gold cup in the Lord's hand to make all the earth drunk; the nations have drunk of her wine, and that has made them mad.

JEREMIAH 25:15–16

This and other passages in the Old Testament offer significant lessons by characterizing the high costs exacted by indiscriminate use of alcohol. Even then the price was high for individuals, and families, and nations. The abuse of alcohol was described as draining the strength, weakening the physical defenses, and making individuals physically ill. As well as causing personal injury and death, alcohol abuse incited violence and led to impaired judgment, memory, and reasoning. Degradation of the human spirit, apathy, irresponsibility, shame, and corruption were other possible outcomes that were deplored.

Although science has documented these consequences today, the abuse of alcohol and other drugs continues to present the same, and even larger, problems. Modern transportation and communication have facilitated market penetration efforts and extended the reach of drug lords and drug dealers into urban, suburban, and rural U.S. communities. Problems of addiction comprise the greatest health and social problem of our time, placing enormous burdens on the economy and particularly on the health care industry. In addition to direct costs, addictions account for as much as 50% of other health care costs by fueling many medical and psychiatric problems. Closely linked to patterns of substance abuse are quickly increasing rates of sexually transmitted diseases among women and teenagers, including human immunodeficiency virus (HIV) infection. Complications of substance abuse also include cancer, diabetes, and cardiovascular problems; auto injuries and fatalities; assaults, homicides, and other crimes; behavioral and learning problems; and the abuse of children (who may later initiate another destructive cycle with their own children). The problems of addiction affect everyone in the country, though the negative impact falls most heavily on the vulnerable populations that are least able and least likely to help themselves.

Since the mid-1980s most health care resources have been spent on acute inpatient treatment of addicted individuals. Comparatively little has been expected of the public health field and community health nursing as regards addiction. Problems of addiction have become public health problems of such magnitude that the field can no longer deny that all community health nurses must be prepared to address them.

This chapter provides a broad and comprehensive overview of problems of addiction, highlights the most prevalent addictions and the most serious complications—including associated family problems, and presents effective nursing interventions that the community health nurse may utilize.

WHAT IS ABUSE AND WHAT IS ADDICTION?

The meanings of *abuse* and *addiction* are undergoing change with advances in science. All the addictions appear to be part of a larger constellation of related disorders, thought to be clustered around some underlying defect, mechanism, or multifactored cause that is yet to be discovered. Many of the repetitive behaviors with addictions involve multiple brain reward regions and neurotransmitters that also regulate normal consumptive behaviors necessary to survival, such as eating and drinking (Hyman and Nestler, 1993). Scientists are involved in a widely publicized search for genes that predispose persons to alcoholism and other addictions by regulating brain function (Blum and Payne, 1991; Bower, 1992).

Numerous environmental conditions, such as physical and psychological trauma, are also significantly powerful factors that play a part in the expression of all psychiatric disorders, including addictions (Hyman and Nestler, 1993). Genetic vulnerability and environmental factors interact to produce addiction; yet addiction can apparently be induced without genetic vulnerability through abuse of a psychoactive substance. The best-documented genetic etiology occurs with the concurrent presence of intense substance dependence and another psychiatric disorder (Pickens, 1983).

Though not well documented, a common clinical observation is that when an addictive substance is stopped, the addicted individual becomes caught up in what is now being called a *process addiction* (e.g., compulsive overeating or exercise). The individual may also become newly addicted to a second drug or substance, such as nicotine. These observations have led scientists to suspect a common underlying factor that affects all compulsive and addictive behaviors. The category of *substance addictions* involves the abuse of ingested alcohol, illicit drugs, prescription drugs, nicotine, caffeine, and inhalants. *Substance addictions* involve the abusive ingestion of a psychoactive drug, whereas *process addictions* are characterized by compulsive behaviors (e.g., gambling, sex, overeating, exercise, and workaholism). Unlike substance addictions the newly described process addictions are not yet formally recognized by psychiatry and therefore are not included in the revised third edition of the *Diagnostic and Statistical Manual of Mental Disorders* (DSM-III-R) (American Psychiatric Association [APA], 1987). However most professionals in the field of addiction find themselves attempting to help individuals with these so-called disorders.

Substance addictions and their associated problems are the primary focus of this chapter; however community health nurses should also have a beginning knowledge of the process addictions, as they present further problems for many persons recovering from substance dependence.

Distinguishing between the labels of *abuse* and *addiction* has presented long-standing difficulties due to the lack of scientific knowledge. It is helpful to think of both abuse and addiction as existing along a continuum. For example in the United States the majority of youngsters and teenagers undergo a period of experimentation with alcohol and other drugs. During this period of growth and development some even abuse the substances to a point at which their lives or the lives of others may be endangered or affected. This type of *abuse* constitutes a repeated, maladaptive, inappropriate pattern of use that negatively affects health. Most young people easily relinquish these patterns of substance abuse as they become involved in careers and/or marriages that are incompatible with continuing heavy substance use.

A subset of individuals, however, continues to abuse psychoactive substances despite the life changes introduced by marriages and careers. At some point they cross over the line into addiction. Such individuals are perhaps helpless to do otherwise in the face of an inborn vulnerability that, according to researchers, seems to account for a significant metabolic change at the cell level during every substance use. Despite its heavy physical and social costs, true addiction takes away the possibility of individual control, to the point at which "just saying no" is an impossibility.

Definitions of addiction are continually being refined as the science of addiction advances. Generally, *addiction* or psychoactive substance dependence, as defined in DSM-III-R, is a pattern of pathological, compulsive use of a psychoactive substance that could involve physiological dependence (APA, 1987). Social, psychological, physical, and occupational conesquences are included. The new DSM-IV, currently under revision, is likely to include a somewhat narrower definition of substance dependence with more emphasis on the manifestations of physiological dependence and less emphasis on psychosocial aspects (APA, 1992).

TABLE 21–1

Common Central Nervous System Effects of Stimulant and Depressant Drugs of Abuse

Stimulants*	Depressants†
Most body functions increased	Most body functions decreased
Increases blood pressure	Decreases blood pressure
Increases heart and pulse rate	Decreases heart and pulse rate
Slows digestive system action	Speeds digestive system
Produces hyperglycemia	Produces hypoglycemia
Facilitates air intake	Hinders air intake
"Fight or flight" mechanisms	Produces relaxation, calmness
Handwriting larger	Handwriting smaller
Time seems to pass slowly	Time seems to pass quickly, person feels under time pressure
Metabolic rate increases	Metabolic rate decreases
Body temperature increased	Body temperature reduced
Pupils dilate (mydriasis)	No mydriasis

*Includes cocaine, amphetamines, caffeine, nicotine, and amphetamine-like hallucinogens (e.g., LSD, PCP, and marijuana).

†Includes alcohol, barbiturates, tranquilizers, and benzodiazepines (e.g., Xanax, Librium, Halcyon).

Substance Addictions

Most agree that making a diagnosis of a true substance addiction depends on the presence of two cardinal signs, which make the diagnosis obligatory. These are (1) *tolerance* and (2) withdrawal symptoms, which constitute *physical dependence* (or *tissue dependence*) on the substance. *Tolerance*, or the capacity to ingest more of the substance than other persons without showing impaired function, can be discerned in very early addiction. In our country recognizing tolerance is blocked by the cultural myth that a man should be able to "hold his liquor." The consequence is that signs of tolerance that could lead to early intervention are often overlooked, and the addiction progresses. A late-developing symptom of chronic addiction is a reduced tolerance for high blood levels of alcohol or other drugs, which develops when the diseased liver can no longer process the ingested substance as efficiently.

The other cardinal sign of substance addiction, *physical dependence*, is shown by the nervous system effects that occur with addiction. Many substances of abuse commonly fall into one of two major categories: central nervous system depressants and stimulants. For example alcohol is a depressant drug, and has a dose-dependent effect on blood pressure and pulse rate (Table 21–1). However when the blood alcohol level declines, nervous system activity rebounds. The opposite set of symptoms then appears, including increases in blood pressure and pulse rate. An interesting parallel occurs with cocaine addiction and withdrawal. Abuse of cocaine has dose-dependent stimulant effects (see Table 21–1). The smoking of "crack," a purer form of cocaine, greatly intensifies the stimulant effects and sympathetic nervous system activity increases greatly, sometimes to the point of cardiac arrest. Conversely as blood levels decline, very intense depressant withdrawal symptoms are precipitated, which tends to trigger repetitive use.

Stimulant effects occur with any cocaine use, though in high doses these effects become exaggerated. Acute cocaine intoxication can also include behavioral symptoms of psychomotor activation, euphoria, grandiosity, impaired judgment, impulsiveness, hypersexuality, hypervigilance, and compulsivity (Chychula and Okore, 1990). As binges lengthen, euphoria lessens and is replaced by anxiety, hyperactivity, irritability, panic, paranoid feelings, and feelings of impending doom.

Extreme depressant effects (see Table 21–1) occur rapidly when the supply of cocaine is exhausted and the individual "crashes" (i.e., begins detoxifying from the drug). As withdrawal continues a short, relatively calm, almost normal period sets in. However cocaine craving and negative feelings increase strongly as withdrawal continues, which trigger efforts to find more cocaine. If abstinence continues for a prolonged period (months), cravings decrease somewhat, but they can still be stimulated by environmental conditions reminiscent of previous usage. The implication is that recovery from significant cocaine dependence is highly problematic, and pharmacological remedies are being sought to facilitate the process of recovery from cocaine addiction.

The information presented in Table 21–1 is useful in determining the type of drug ingested, identifying the state of withdrawal symptoms, and deciding on specific treatment for detoxification (withdrawal). In treating detoxification symptoms, drugs from the same category are used to "bring down" (or detoxify) the client by attenuating withdrawal symptoms. For example in inpatient settings chlordiazepoxide hydrochloride (Librium) in decreasing doses is often used to modulate the withdrawal symptoms that occur with declining levels of blood alcohol.

It is interesting to note that the severity of withdrawal symptoms involving sympathetic nervous system hyperactivity can be modulated effectively by careful nursing, counseling, and supportive care (Institute of Medicine, 1990), instead of by administration of pharmacological agents. Such treatment of withdrawal is more apt to occur in outpatient settings. An alcoholic in withdrawal who is experiencing excitatory (stimulant) effects (see Table 21–1) can be isolated in a quiet room and calmed by nursing care that includes frequent checks of vital signs; linen changes as necessitated by diaphoresis; offer of bedpan, meals, and fluid; care of immediate needs and support during and following vomiting; offer of words of reassurance; and reality orientation to time, place, and person.

A reliable tool, the Clinical Institute Withdrawal Assessment for Alcohol (CIWA), can be used to monitor closely the severity of withdrawal symptoms involving sympathetic nervous system activity (Foy et al., 1988; Sellers and Naranjo, 1985). Use of the tool provides a structured method of delivering nursing interventions and tracking client symptoms. Withdrawal symptoms are self-limited; they occur mostly during the first 2 days of withdrawal and end within 3 to 7 days. Mild withdrawal is characterized by anxiety, irritability, hand tremor, sweating, nausea, vomiting, diarrhea, sleep disturbance, and rapid heartbeat. Pulse rate and blood pressure levels should gradually decrease; increasing pulse rates and blood pressure within the first 24 hours signal the onset of seizures and require medical treatment.

Only a small percentage of persons experience more serious withdrawal symptoms, with 1% to 3% experiencing seizures or delirium tremens (profound confusion, hyperactivity, and hallucinations), usually by the second or third day of withdrawal. Concurrent physical illnesses, recent and prolonged heavy alcohol intake, and previous episodes of withdrawal tend to produce more severe withdrawal that requires medical treatment.

In addition to physical symptoms, impaired occupational, social, and family functioning inevitably occurs in the lives of addicted individuals. The DSM-III-R includes symptoms of dependence related to such psychosocial patterns (APA, 1987). These are as follows: (1) presence of symptoms of intoxication or withdrawal when fulfillment of major role obligations is expected (work, school, homemaking, child care); (2) giving up or reduction of important social, occupational, or recreational activities because of substance use; and (3) continued use despite family arguments about it. Although these broadly described psychosocial symptoms are difficult to assess comprehensively, attempts have been made to do so in research tools such as the Addiction Severity Index (McLellan et al., 1980; 1985). Addiction treatment facilities often design their own psychosocial assessment tools for in-house use. The recent trend (APA, 1991) has been to narrow the assessment to emphasize physical symptoms, thereby diminishing the importance of psychosocial factors.

Community health nurses are often the first to see patterns indicative of addiction; therefore they are important case-finders. Families with addictions exhibit characteristic dysfunctional family patterns (Eells, 1986). One pattern involves the labeling or blaming of an individual as being the source of the family problem when, in fact, the entire family system is severely dysfunctional. The adolescent who smokes marijuana at school is often the index case in a dysfunctional family with other alcohol and drug problems. Non-addicted family members frequently present as overfunctioners; their overresponsible behaviors are linked to the irresponsible behaviors exhibited by the addicted family member. The overresponsible family members are eager and willing to work on the family dysfunction with community health nurses. As the family work progresses, the overresponsible individuals are able to stop taking on responsibilities belonging to the addicted family member, and he or she is then more easily recruited into treatment (see Secondary Prevention in this chapter).

Process Addictions

Addictions to certain processes (e.g., exercise) were only recently recognized; they are not as well researched as substance addictions and are still controversial in concept. However, the clinical information about many of these process addictions is broad and substantial, and substance addiction–oriented interventions have been used effectively with them. Like substance abuse addictions, the process addictions appear to have cross-addiction potential (individuals may switch from one to another). Addictions to food, exercise, gambling, spending money, work, sex, and romantic love fall in the category of process addictions.

Clinical observation of such syndromes precedes data gained through research, and this is the case presently with most of the process addictions. Nevertheless treatment using a substance addiction model has been quite effective with process addictions to gambling, sex, and food.

There has been less success in treating the entangled and destructive relationships between addicted partners and their significant others. These relationships are very intense, all-consuming, compulsive, enduring, and destructive for both partners. For example such relationships often trigger relapses for the substance abuser. Health professionals often feel helpless in dealing with persons, many of whom are women, who are caught up in such relationships. Conventional mental health therapies have been used with this particular population.

Although criticized by some as a fad, the recognition of addictive patterns in relationships (i.e., "addiction" to another person) and the characterization of these as *co-dependence* has moved the addictions field forward in both understanding and treating addiction. The co-dependence concept is easily comprehended and understood by those whose loved ones are experiencing problems of addiction, and it created a needed avenue for recruitment into treatment for those non-addicted individuals living with addicted partners or family members. Such persons often experience numerous psychosocial and physical problems from carrying the burdens of child-care and employment, and coping with the underfunctioning and addicted family member. The co-dependence movement has also triggered the creation of numerous self-help groups (Co-dependents Anonymous, or CODA) throughout the United States. Finally participation in CODA has been instrumental in bringing into treatment many co-dependent individuals who develop addictions to psychoactive substances as well.

An outstanding theoretical and clinical book that includes a conceptual framework for co-dependence as a process addiction deserves mention here (Mellody et al., 1989). The book is an example of how the astute clinical observations of a nurse clinician (Mellody) can describe an unexplored area for which clinical research is required. Mellody constructed a comprehensive theory for co-dependence problems that occur with addictions, usually in the addict's significant others.

Mellody defined co-dependence as a developmental problem resulting from dysfunctional childhood experiences (e.g., child abuse). Also implicated were the sense of self and relationships with others including a Higher Power. The Higher Power concept, important to recovery from problems of addiction, involves the acceptance of a force or spiritual power greater than the self.

Mellody described five core symptoms of co-dependence: (1) difficulty experiencing appropriate levels of self-esteem by feeling either worth less than others or set apart from and superior to others; (2) difficulty in setting functional boundaries or limits with others (this also involves not taking responsibility for one's own thinking, feelings, and behavior); (3) difficulty in owning or acknowledging one's own reality (how one looks, thinks, feels, and behaves); (4) inability to be "political" with one's reality (i.e., a lack of sensitivity to one's impact on others); and (5) difficulty in acknowledging and meeting one's own wants and needs (this can involve being too dependent or too independent of others, being needless and wantless, or getting basic needs and wants confused).

Interestingly, most co-dependents have a varying combination of the five core symptoms. For example a co-dependent living with an addicted partner may (1) feel worthless, (2) allow unwanted physical touching, (3) feel responsible for the feelings and actions of the addict, (4) inflict one's feelings on other family members, such as children, insensitively, and (5) consistently neglect personal needs.

An example of the relationship between co-dependence and substance addiction involved Mary, whose husband Dan was addicted to "speedballs" (heroin and cocaine combined and used intravenously). Mary, a superresponsible person, was nevertheless overly dependent on Dan. She overvalued Dan's every word and deed, was extremely emotionally overreactive to his behavior, suffered great shame and psychic pain emotionally, and was completely focused on taking care of Dan and his addiction to the exclusion of her own needs and those of their child. Her self-esteem was very low, she could not set boundaries with Dan regarding acceptable and nonacceptable behaviors, and she lacked any personal goals or direction. Totally consumed by Dan's illness, she gave too much time, attention, and value to Dan. She felt she gave Dan unconditional love and assumed it would cure his problem; she expected unconditional love from him in return for her devotion. Dan, of course, consumed by his addiction, was unable to care for himself appropriately, let alone attend to Mary's needs.

A master's level nurse, by focusing on the definition of co-dependence and its core symptoms, helped Mary apply Mellody's suggested clinical exercises. Mary began to define a self and personal goals, set boundaries with Dan, and require that he enter treatment. Today Mary is functioning well in all aspects of her life, including the care of their teenage son, while Dan pursues treatment and a predictably long recovery period for his heroin and cocaine addictions.

Addictive Eating Patterns

Another registered nurse, Flood (1989), presented information on eating disorders utilizing a substance addictions model. Like alcoholism and other drug addictions eating disorders are true addictions; they are chronic and progressive and have definite signs and symptoms. Flood included anorexia nervosa and bulimia nervosa in this category. Her model also suggests a continuum, with milder syndromes of compulsive overeating at one end and the more severe problems of anorexia and bulimia at the other.

Neurobiologists believe the same areas of the brain and the reward pathways involved in normal appetite and pleasure are involved with substance dependence and process addictions, such as food addictions (Blum and Payne, 1991). This explains what could be a unique problem with overcoming food addiction, in that the individual must use these brain structures and processes to continue eating. There is therefore no opportunity for these used brain patterns to become extinguished. In fact they continue to be stimulated with even the biological necessity of normal eating, which may in turn trigger out-of-control eating patterns. Unfortunately abstinence from the substance of abuse is impossible for food addicts, so abstinence is redefined as following a structured food plan.

Love and Sex Addiction

Many individuals seem to exhibit addictive patterns in love and sex relationships. These process addictions exhibit the same patterns of compulsive use, interference with life functioning, and even altered physiological states that are associated with substance addictions. In fact process addictions frequently occur in the same individuals who are substance addicted and/or in their significant others.

Love and sex addiction are similar in that they can involve being overly focused on a partner or another individual and on the relationship with that person. Too much time and value is assigned to the other and obsessive plans are compulsively acted out. Extremely intense positive and negative feelings and unrealistic expectations occur with these activities. In both love and sex addiction, neglecting to care for oneself and the inability to act in one's own best interests occur.

Love addiction is similar to co-dependence, described earlier, but is characterized by intensity and a romantic overfocus on an intimate partner or spouse. Co-dependence can involve an overfocus on any individual. The partners that love addicts choose are generally individuals who engage in substantial distancing from the relationship and is often an addicted individual. Together they engage in a pattern of mutual emotional abuse, with no true intimacy, though it often appears superficially that the love addict suffers most.

Mellody provided a detailed description of the recovery process from love addiction along with related self-help measures (Mellody et al., 1992). A summary of the characteristics of recovered individuals would include the ability to value themselves, set boundaries with others, accurately perceive their own realities, sensitively express their own thinking and feeling, and care for their own wants and needs. Names of therapists in the United States and in other countries who have been trained by Mellody can be obtained by contacting her.

Community health nurses can intervene earlier if they recognize the existence of patterns of love and sex addiction. Long before there is helpful contact with other health professionals, community nurses encounter combinations of both sets of symptoms (central nervous system symptoms of addiction and related relationship patterns) as they interact with clients in clinics or in the home setting.

Defeating Attitudes and Myths

Denial of a problem is the greatest deterrent to solving that problem, and so it is with addictions. By now most health professionals have heard that the existence of denial is a hallmark of addiction problems. Few can appreciate the strength of that denial without working directly with addicted clients and their families for some period. Denial with addiction can include outright denial that an addiction problem exists as well as the minimization of symptoms of addiction and its related physical complications and psychosocial consequences.

Professional attitudes and myths that constitute a pattern of denial among health professionals are operating today in the field of public health. These may prove an even greater deterrent to overcoming problems of addiction in the community than the denial patterns of clients. It may help to list the defeatist attitudes and myths held by some health professionals along with the facts of addiction.

Myth 1. Only Those Working in the Field of Addictions can Treat Addictions Problems. Millions of people are addicted and countless others are affected by their addictions, though not addicted themselves. This is simply too large a burden for only addictions specialists to undertake, who numbered only 44,098 persons in the last available survey of treatment facilities (National Institute on Alcohol Abuse and Alcoholism [NIAAA], 1983). Federal initiatives have attempted to redress this problem through the education of health professionals including physicians, nurses, social workers, and psychologists. Interventions by health professionals could expand efforts to control addictions in that primary, secondary, and tertiary preventions can be instituted at the first point of contact with the health care system and in other organizations in which these professionals work.

Myth 2. Family Intervention with Addictions can Be Used Effectively Only by Family Therapists. Again the group of available, trained personnel educated as family therapists is insufficient to address the widespread problems of family dysfunction related to problems of addiction. Although their numbers remain undocumented, there are but a handful of academic programs teaching family therapy in the United States, and many counselors acquire beginning knowledge by attending short-term workshops. Community health nurses have traditionally dealt with family systems, which constitute one of the major systems targeted by them for nursing interventions. Community nurses can learn to apply effectively the recently promulgated family systems theory concepts to help families. In fact the newer concepts coming from the family systems field are being taught in many nursing education programs, and nurses can utilize this knowledge with problems of addiction in families. Minuchin demonstrated that lay community people can be trained to understand and effectively apply family systems theory principles (Minuchin et al., 1967). This introduces another possibility: that the community health nurse may be able to teach, coach, and supervise others to utilize family systems theory with families involved in problems of addiction.

Myth 3: It Takes a Recovering Addict to Treat Individuals with Problems of Addiction. It does not take having cancer, schizophrenia, or a fractured pelvis to professionally care for groups of clients with these conditions. Neither does it take a recovering addict to care for addicts. Again, the population of individuals available to intervene is insufficient to address the task, even if every recovering person could be pressed into service. Known and effective strategies for intervention can be taught and learned by community health nurses as well as many other professionals.

Myth 4: The Only Way to Have an Impact on the General Population Is to Educate People about Addiction. Some believe the only available intervention for problems of addiction is more community education. However education cannot be the only modality used to overcome community problems with addiction. Education is costly and education of the general public takes longer, costs more, and may not be as effective as other workable interventions. Educative efforts should be used where most cost-effective, for example in the preparation of health professionals whose knowledge is used over a lifetime career. Some effective educative efforts with the general public have occurred through the media.

Alternative interventions for problems of addiction include the focused teaching of new behaviors to family members. However already existing community resources, such as self-help recovery groups, may be even more effective. Referral to 12-step recovery groups, such as Al-Anon, initiate and augment the long-term education of family members about addiction that the community health nurse need not undertake alone.

The family systems interventions mentioned previously are critical to ongoing recovery and the prevention of relapse to addiction. Without family intervention, addicts treated in costly inpatient programs return to the family, only to relapse when family dynamics supportive to the addictive process continue.

Myth 5: Community Health Nurses Should Not Take an Active Role in Intervening with Problems of Addiction: They Should Simply Refer Clients to Those in the Addictions Field. It is no longer possible to overlook the widespread prevalence of addictions and their associated morbidity, which affects hundreds of thousands of people in communities. All nurses must prepare themselves to respond to the challenges addictions present.

Long before the addicted individual is treated (and many never reach a treatment facility), the addict's family suffers from psychological, social, and physical problems; spiritual deficits; and lack of hope. These individuals deserve the attention of community health nurses. Many of these individuals already constitute a major part of the community health nurse's caseload. Yet without the knowledge of addictions, community health nurses will fail to recognize or assess problems of addiction.

It is interesting that many of the skills needed to intervene with addictions are also needed for other conditions that community health nurses address every day in practice. Nurses are learning to address family dynamics that impinge on their nursing interventions, often rendering them ineffective. The best planned teaching is of little use to a client if the family interactions are persistently chaotic. Community health nurses can intervene to quiet this chaos, teach family members of addicts about addiction and its associated family patterns, and encourage them to engage in self-care while attending to other more conventional health care needs. Attending to family intervention shortens the time required to recruit the addicted family member into treatment and tends to relieve physical and emotional symptoms among all family members.

Myth 6: The Client Must "Hit Bottom" or Ask for Help Before Being Helped with Problems of Addiction. The addicted client is caught up in an addictive pattern, which includes a skewed physiology and disturbed brain function, that does not permit recognition of the need for help. Dealing with addicted clients can be compared to caring for anesthetized persons still in the recovery room after major surgery. The addict is unable to help himself.

The most effective way to recruit an addicted person into treatment involves mobilizing those around him to become instrumental in requiring treatment and in making the necessary arrangements. Virtually all those who enter treatment for addiction do so in response to outside pressure. The family system is more powerful than any given family member. An outside authority may sometimes have influence; for example individuals have occasionally stopped abusing substances after physicians have told them they must or they will die from their physical conditions. Similarly, employers can exert pressure by threatening job loss because of poor performance due to addictions. However addicted individuals can often find other physicians or employers who will overlook their symptoms of addiction. The lasting constant in the addict's life, his family, can exert an effective, continuing pressure for treatment and recovery. The methods of intervention involving the family are discussed in the section on Secondary Prevention.

When addicts are fortunate enough to have people who care about them sufficiently to require them to enter treatment, the social and physical consequences of addiction can be aborted at an early stage. Otherwise the worst outcomes may be realized, including life-threatening physical illness, incarceration, institutionalization for chronic mental illness brought about by irreversible brain damage, or death. As obvious as it is to the outside observer that an addict has "hit bottom," it too often goes unrealized by the addicted person until serious consequences have occurred.

Where Is the Problem?

By most conservative estimates more than 12 million Americans have significant problems with alcohol, as documented by careful epidemiological studies using accepted diagnostic criteria. Similarly about 21 million Americans have tried cocaine and nearly 3 million of them use the drug regularly. More than 1 out of 5 adult Americans continue their addiction to nicotine by smoking tobacco. The epidemiology of other associated types of problems, such as gambling addictions, and the extent of family problems related to addictions has not yet been documented. Many of the *Healthy People 2000* objectives address substance abuse (Table 21–2).

INCIDENCE AND PREVALENCE: EPIDEMIOLOGICAL STUDIES

Prevalence of Alcohol and Other Drug Abuse

Major epidemiological studies were conducted by the National Institute of Mental Health to estimate the prevalence (number of existing cases) and incidence (number of new cases) of psychiatric and substance abuse disorders in the U.S. population (Myers, et al., 1984; Ross et al., 1988). These studies are usually referred to as the epidemiologic catchment area, or ECA, studies. Catchment areas are circumscribed areas of the United States in which individuals residing in households, group homes, and long-term institutions were evaluated. The ECA studies were conducted with well-trained researchers on a carefully drawn household sample of as many as 20,000 individuals who were representative of all citizens of the United States, with the current diagnostic criteria. Such large and comprehensive studies are costly and therefore rare, but are invaluable for identifying special populations with specific health needs and for planning appropriate community health services.

Study results were reported on lifetime prevalence, or estimates of the proportion of individuals who ever have experienced particular psychiatric diagnoses (Myers et al., 1984; Robins et al., 1984). The most common diagnoses in decreasing order of prevalence were (1) alcohol abuse and dependence, (2) phobia, (3) major depressive episode, and (4) drug abuse and dependence.

Six-month prevalence rates showed alcoholism to be the most common disorder for men of all ages, with drug abuse and dependence being the second most common problem in men aged 18 to 24 years. Among women of the same age group the most common diagnoses were depression and phobias, followed by drug abuse and drug dependence.

It is worth noting that alcoholism is by far the most common disorder, despite the tendency of many to abuse multiple drugs, and is still the most researched and written about of all substance dependencies.

Prevalence of Dual Diagnoses

Clients with co-existing substance abuse and mental illness (dual diagnoses) pose a major challenge to professionals working in the community. Such clients generally have a poorer treatment outcome and a more complicated withdrawal and recovery and are overrepresented in certain special disadvantaged populations (e.g., the homeless). In addition treatment is problematic because both types of treatment agencies—mental health and substance abuse—may each reject the client on the basis of the other diagnosis. Research to improve the assessment and treatment of problems that co-exist with substance dependence is sorely needed, because dual diagnoses are very common.

The ECA data provide a starting point for assessing the lifetime prevalence of some co-morbidities (NIAAA, 1991a). Based on the ECA data, alcoholics were 21 times more likely than nonalcoholics to also have a diagnosis of antisocial personality disorder (Regier et al., 1990). This figure is most likely inflated due to the fact there is overlap in symptoms for the two diagnoses because alcohol intoxication diminishes inhibitions and increases antisocial behaviors. Nevertheless individuals with both diagnoses tend to have an earlier age at onset and a more rapid and serious course of illness.

The NIAAA report mentions the odds for other psychiatric disorders among alcoholics. Alcoholics are more likely than the general population to have drug abuse (3.9 times); mania (6.2 times); and schizophrenia (4.0 times).

Another "dual diagnosis" is the simultaneous occurrence of two or more substance dependence disorders. Alcoholics are more likely than nonalcoholics to also use cocaine (35 times); sedatives (17 times); opioids (13 times); hallucinogens (12 times), and marijuana (6 times).

Ross and co-workers (1988) evaluated the lifetime and current prevalence of mental disorders in 501 patients seeking treatment for alcohol and other drug problems. Their findings indicated that 78% of their subjects had a

TABLE 21–2

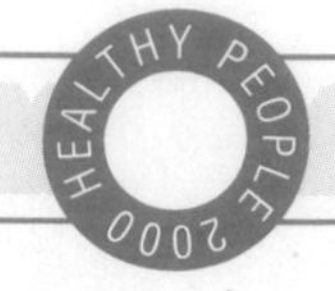

Healthy People 2000 Objectives Regarding Addictions

Health Status Objectives

1. Reduce deaths caused by alcohol-related motor vehicle crashes to no more than 8.5 per 100,000 population (baseline: 9.7 per 100,000 in 1987).

Special Population Targets		
Alcohol-Related Motor Vehicle Crash Deaths (per 100,000)	**1987 Baseline**	**2000 Target**
American Indian/Alaskan Native men	52.5	44.8
Persons aged 15–24 years	21.5	18.0

2. Reduce cirrhosis deaths to no more than 6 per 100,000 population (age-adjusted baseline: 9.1 per 100,000 in 1987).

Special Population Targets		
Cirrhosis Deaths	**1987 Baseline**	**2000 Target**
Black men	22.0	12.0
American Indians/Alaska Natives	25.9	13.0

3. Reduce drug-related deaths to no more than 3 per 100,000 population (age-adjusted baseline: 3.8 per 100,000 in 1987).

Risk Reduction Objectives

4. Reduce the proportion of young persons who have used alcohol, marijuana, and cocaine in the past month, as follows:

Substance/Age (Years)	1988 Baseline (%)	2000 Target (%)
Alcohol/12–17	25.2	12.6
Alcohol/18–20	57.9	29.0
Marijuana/12–17	6.4	3.2
Marijuana/18–25	15.5	7.8
Cocaine/12–17	1.1	0.6
Cocaine/18–25	4.5	2.3

5. Reduce the proportion of high school seniors and college students engaging in recent occasions of heavy drinking of alcoholic beverages to no more than 28% of high school seniors and 32% of college students (baseline: 33% of high school seniors and 41.7% of college students in 1989).
   Note: Recent heavy drinking is defined as having 5 or more drinks on one occasion in the previous 2-week period as monitored by self-reports.
6. Increase the proportion of high school seniors who perceive social disapproval associated with the heavy use of alcohol, occasional use of marijuana, and experimentation with cocaine, as follows:

Behavior Disapproved Of	1989 Baseline (%)	2000 Target (%)
Heavy use of alcohol	56.4	70
Occasional use of marijuana	71.1	85
Trying cocaine once or twice	88.9	95

Note: Heavy drinking is defined as having five or more drinks once or twice each weekend.

Services and Protection Objectives

7. Establish and monitor in 50 states comprehensive plans to ensure access to alcohol and drug treatment programs for persons traditionally underserved.
8. Provide to children in all school districts and private schools primary and secondary school educational programs on alcohol and other drugs, preferably as part of quality school health education (baseline: 63% provided some instruction, 39% provided counseling, and 23% referred students for clinical assessments in 1987).
9. Extend adoption of alcohol and drug policies for the work environment to at least 60% of worksites with 50 or more employees.
10. Extend to 50 states administrative driver's license suspension/revocation laws or programs of equal effectiveness for persons who are determined to have been driving under the influence of intoxicants (baseline: 28 states and District of Columbia in 1990).

TABLE 21–2

Healthy People 2000 Objectives Regarding Addictions–Continued

HEALTHY PEOPLE 2000

Services and Protection Objectives *Continued*

11. Increase to 50 the number of states that have enacted and enforce policies, beyond those in existence in 1989, to reduce access to alcoholic beverages by minors.
12. Increase to at least 20 the number of states that have enacted statutes to restrict promotion of alcoholic beverages that is focused principally on young audiences.
13. Extend to 50 states legal blood alcohol concentration tolerance levels of .04% for motor vehicle drivers aged 21 years and older and .00% for those younger than age 21 years (baseline: 0 states in 1990).
14. Increase to at least 75% the proportion of primary care providers who screen for alcohol and other drug use problems and provide counseling and referral as needed.

From U.S. DHHS. (1990). *Healthy People 2000: National Health Promotion and Disease Prevention Objectives—Summary report.* Washington, DC: Government Printing Office.

lifetime psychiatric disorder in addition to a substance abuse diagnosis, and 65% of them had a current psychiatric disorder. Those abusing both alcohol and other drugs exhibited the most psychiatric impairment; conversely, those with psychiatric disorders had more severe problems with substance abuse. The most common psychiatric disorders were antisocial personality disorder, phobias, psychosexual dysfunction, major depression, and dysthymia (chronic mild depressive syndrome).

Yet another type of dual diagnosis, substance dependence with co-occurring medical conditions, should be mentioned. Diseases that are strongly linked to alcohol consumption, not all of which are reversible with abstinence from alcohol, include liver disease, pancreatitis, malabsorption of nutrients, alcohol cardiomyopathy, brain damage and adult dementia, failure of reproductive function, and cancers of the mouth, larynx, and esophagus (NIAAA, 1991a).

Implications for nursing services in the community are enormous. First, alcohol abuse and dependence is the most prevalent diagnosis for all mental disorders in the United States, as shown by the aforementioned epidemiological studies (Myers et al., 1984; Robins et al., 1984). The already-heavy economic burden for treatment of substance abuse is increased with coexisting disorders. These combined factors, only recently substantiated by epidemiological data, impose a high level of need for professional care by community workers, including nurses. It may be safe to venture a guess that the majority of clients already seen by community health nurses either have addictions (and/or mental disorders) or are family members whose health and well-being are affected by those addictions. The message is clear. In the future, community health nurses should be expected to assume an even greater role in the prevention and treatment of problems of addiction as they relate to mental disorders. For example community nurses will be expected to differentiate between the dual problems of substance dependence and psychiatric disorders and make appropriate referrals. As knowledge about dual diagnoses advances, updating the education for community nurses who have ongoing contact with this special population becomes crucial.

Enhanced information about dual diagnoses, including neuroscience data, is already being taught in a few U.S. schools of nursing that have been federally funded by NIAAA for the purpose of integrating addictions nursing into undergraduate and graduate curricula. The Ohio State University and New York University Schools of Nursing have published well-developed and comprehensive content modules for courses at the undergraduate and the graduate levels (Burns et al., 1991; Naegle, 1991). Although this program funding is no longer available to support similar endeavors, other federal programs are available and new initiatives can be expected to reinstitute these needed federal programs.

Prevalence of Substance Abuse Among Registered Nurses

Many researchers have attempted to estimate the prevalence of substance abuse among nurses. Bissell and Haberman (1984) hypothesized that 40,000 nurses were addicted to alcohol alone in the United States. Research-based studies have described patterns of addiction and correlate family, personal, and professional characteristics of nurses with problems of addiction (Haack and Harford, 1984; Sullivan, 1987a, 1987b). However there appeared to be a lower rate of substance addiction among nurses than was projected. Conclusive findings were obtained by examining a large sample of nurses included in prior epidemiological studies (Trinkhoff et al., 1991). The actual incidence of alcohol abuse was lower than that of the general population. Nevertheless it is important to identify even small subpopulations of nurses with problems of substance dependence for the following reasons: the possible negative consequences for clients of the addicted nurse, the need for associated disciplinary action by state boards of nursing (Sullivan, 1990), and the need for treatment of the addicted nurse.

For nurses and women generally some researchers have found a strong link between psychological symptoms of depression that preceded the substance abuse. Sullivan (1987a, 1987b) reported that 64% reported current or depressive symptoms that preceded the abuse. To be confident of the validity of these suggestive findings with a small sample of nurses, further research is being conducted with a larger sample that is representative of nurses in the United States.

Studies of substance abuse among nurses are likely to continue to provide useful insights about addictions in women generally. Studies of problems of addiction among women, only available in the past decade, show that addiction is also related to employment and unemployment patterns, the loss of family roles, and the occurrence of adverse life situations such as health problems (Institute of Medicine, 1990).

DEMOGRAPHICS

Some of the research on the demographic parameters related to addiction are unfortunately limited by the lack of random samples. Because addicted individuals are available for study only when they appear for treatment, convenience samples are more frequently reported in the literature. Nevertheless findings from these studies are interesting and have implications for further research.

Distribution by Age

Evidence from the previously cited epidemiological studies (Myers et al., 1984; Robins et al., 1984), also documented that for all age groups, alcohol abuse/dependence was by far the most common of all mental disorders, ranging from a 15.7% to 17.4% prevalence in six major geographic areas in the United States. The study sites included both urban and suburban areas.

Usually addictions are thought to be problems of youth or adulthood, but not of old age. Boyd (1991) summarized the research results on substance abuse occurring in the elderly population, especially citing studies by Bienenfeld (1987) and Atkinson (1984). Taken together the findings documented that about 10% of the elderly population had a history of alcohol-related problems and that certain subgroups had a higher rate of alcohol problems (20% of nursing home residents and as many as 60% of elderly men admitted to acute care settings). Data from the NIAAA also demonstrated higher rates of alcohol dependence among elderly individuals who were widowers, single, having difficulty with the police, and living in poorer socioeconomic areas (Secretary of the Department of Health and Human Services, 1990).

Reports may underestimate the true rate of substance abuse among the elderly because the data do not include the potential danger of drug interactions. This population group takes large amounts of prescription drugs and over-the-counter drugs for chronic problems. Neither do the available reports include data about the use and abuse of illicit stimulants and depressants. Such use is often thought to be minimal in this age group because many addicts die before they reach old age. Finally clinical observations show that by middle age most surviving addicts are "burned out" from abusing drugs and have stopped using them at the same time that other problems, such as dementia, have increased.

The ECA data clearly showed that younger age groups are most affected by alcohol and other drug abuse (Robins et al., 1984). For the age group of 18- to 24-year-olds, alcohol and drug abuse/dependence was by far the most common of all mental health disorders, affecting 11% to 17.5% of this group and varying according to the specific geographic site studied.

Under the auspices of the Substance Abuse and Mental Health Services Administration (SAMHSA) ongoing national surveys help to track the fluctuations in alcohol and other drug use as an aid to intervention and program planning. The National High School Senior Survey on Drug Abuse is an annual survey conducted by the National Institute on Drug Abuse (NIDA, 1991). It was expanded in 1991 to include 8th and 10th graders. The preliminary 1992 findings show continued declines in cocaine and other drug use among high school seniors (SAMHSA, 1993). In 1992, 40.7% used an illicit drug at least once at some point in their lifetime; 27.9% reported binge drinking in the 2 weeks before the survey; and 17.2% reported daily smoking of cigarettes.

Eighth graders showed higher rates of licit (e.g., alcohol and tobacco) and illicit drug use than they did in 1991. In 1992, 2.9% had ever used cocaine; 13.4% reported binge drinking in the 2 weeks before survey; and 7% reported daily smoking of cigarettes.

These findings clearly imply that the measures to combat drug abuse must continue. Special populations in the community, mentioned previously, are in need of prevention and intervention efforts by community health nurses.

The extent to which high-intensity drug use exists in the community is monitored quarterly in the nation by the Drug Abuse Warning Network (DAWN), Office of Applied Studies, SAMHSA. DAWN collects information on patients seeking hospital emergency room treatment related to abuse of drugs and includes reportable episodes for nonmedical use of a legal drug (including suicide attempts) and any use of an illegal drug. In highlights from the third quarter of 1992 by DAWN, estimates show 13,400 heroin-related emergencies, the highest level since estimates were first available from DAWN in early 1988 (SAMHSA, 1993). There were 30,900 cocaine-related episodes, little changed from previous reports; however, a 30% increase in cocaine episodes and 42% increase in heroin episodes occurred in the 35 years and older group.

Distribution by Race

Small research studies have had intriguing results and shown a diverse picture of substance dependence by race. Robyak and associates (1989) reported significantly different drinking practices in comparison groups of black and white men who were hospitalized alcoholics. White male alcoholics reported greater daily alcohol consumption than black male alcoholics. Black men reported alcohol use as a means of improving mental functioning; white males more often reported alcohol use as a means of relieving psychological distress.

The epidemiological data (Robins et al., 1984) on lifetime prevalence rates showed a varying picture of racial differences for alcohol, dependent on geographic site studied. The lifetime prevalence rate in Baltimore for blacks was 14.6%, and for others the rate was 13.2%. In St. Louis, the lifetime prevalence rate for others was greater (16%) than that for blacks (14.7%). Overall the lifetime prevalence rates for alcohol abuse were similar for blacks and others. The data also showed no significant differences in drug abuse/dependence in these two populations, contrary to current stereotypes that blacks are more involved in drug abuse.

Other racial minority groups, notably American Indians and Alaskan Natives, have well-documented and high mortality rates that are alcohol related (NIAAA, 1990). Suicide, homicide, alcoholic cirrhosis of the liver, and unintentional injuries are among the 10 leading causes of death among this population and higher than the general population. However it is impossible to generalize about drinking and drug abuse patterns for all American Indian tribal groups because there is great diversity, with some tribes being mostly abstinent. Finally although consumption of alcohol is generally low among American Indian women, they are very susceptible to alcohol-related problems and account for nearly half of the cirrhosis deaths in this population.

Hispanics exhibit great cultural diversity in patterns of alcohol use, with international comparisons showing male and female Spanish nationals to be heavier users of alcohol than American Hispanics or Mexicans (NIAAA, 1990). Hispanics in the United States with origins in Mexico, Puerto Rico, Cuba, and other Latin American countries show significant differences by gender, with Hispanic men exhibiting a high intake mostly in their young adult years and Hispanic women exhibiting a very low intake of alcohol. Hispanic men have a higher prevalence of alcohol-related problems than either black or white Americans, which has led to an effort to identify at-risk Hispanic adolescents for prevention efforts.

Distribution by Gender

Researchers have identified two familial subtypes of alcoholism, which have different implications for substance dependence in women (NIAAA, 1990). The first, type I alcoholism, occurred in both male and female biological relatives; it was a milder form of the disease, was associated with a later onset of abusive drinking (age 26 years or after), and was associated with little criminality. Type II alcoholism occurred almost exclusively in male biological relatives, was associated with an early onset of problem drinking and more severe consequences, and was associated with both physical conditions and high levels of criminal activity. Type II alcoholism was unaffected by environmental influences whereas type I alcoholism was more vulnerable to environmental conditions. Environmental influences such as low socioeconomic conditions and rural backgrounds were correlated with increased severe drinking in the type I population.

The clinical usefulness of these findings was unexplored. However it is useful for community health nurses to know that the early onset of major alcohol problems in males, before age 26 years, indicates a more intense pattern of substance dependence that therefore is much more difficult to interrupt. Conversely type I alcoholism, which is more open to the influence of environmental conditions, is more treatable by changing the environmental conditions.

Epidemiological data on the lifetime prevalence of substance abuse by gender shows interesting differences between men and women (Robins et al., 1984). Only 4.2% to 4.8% of female groups sampled had alcohol abuse and alcohol dependence problems, compared with 19.1% to 28.9% of males. This trend was repeated in the data for drug abuse and dependence, with males experiencing rates ranging from 6.5% to 7.4% and females, 3.8% to 5.1%. Although the percentage of affected females was smaller, those who do experience substance dependence problems are the target of public health interventions during their childbearing years to prevent complications in the children. The most frequent psychiatric disorder for men was alcohol abuse and dependence, leading to the conclusion that this disorder constitutes an ongoing and major public health problem for men.

Distribution by Socioeconomic Level

Distribution data of the lifetime prevalence of substance dependence were available by educational level and type of geographic area, though not by socioeconomic level (Myers et al., 1984; Robins et al., 1984). Homeless populations may not have been adequately represented. Nevertheless the most prevalent disorder (alcohol abuse) was found 9.5% of the time in college graduates, as compared with a rate of 12.2% in those not graduating from college. Alcohol abuse and dependence are frequent among the homeless with other prevalence estimates ranging from 20% to 45% of the total (NIAAA, 1990). They also exhibited high rates of dual diagnoses. Taken together study findings show that more substance dependence is found in those at poorer socioeconomic levels. There are several implications. It might be predicted that this population will bring to treatment the fewest resources, will require longer—and therefore more expensive—treatment for dual diagnoses, and will therefore exhibit a poorer success rate with treatment (Booth et al., 1991). It is also important to remember that type I alcoholism is associated with environmental conditions such as poverty and, therefore, is partially treatable by changing environmental conditions.

Risk Profiles for Children and Families

Pihl and colleagues (1990) summarized the literature on inherited predisposition to alcoholism in sons of male alcoholics. They found that certain word descriptors were frequently applied to the behavior of male and female children of alcoholics during childhood: conduct-disorder, impulsivity, hyperactivity, and attention-deficit disorder (inability to sustain attention necessary for routine tasks). These findings held up when data were controlled for the influence of environment and during longitudinal studies. The children of alcoholics performed more poorly in school, suffered certain cognitive deficits, and completed fewer years of school. The behaviors tended to continue into adulthood (Silver, 1992).

Reduced amplitude for a certain brain wave pattern (called the *P300 brain wave*), which integrates brain activity occurring in the right and left brain hemispheres, has been found in alcoholics and sons of alcoholics. It is associated with the ability to attend to one's surroundings and to perform tasks that require sustained attention. It is also thought to be related to the aforementioned pattern of attention-deficit disorder.

Such findings bring hope to the future prevention and treatment of substance dependence. If a measurable biological marker predictive of problems with addiction later in life could be identified, prevention could occur and pharmacological remedies could be identified; perhaps then there would be no need for crude and dangerous self-medication with alcohol and other drugs.

Pihl and colleagues (1990) also pointed to the many findings on the families of children of alcoholics: their families tended to be severely disrupted, and interpersonal relationships were either impoverished or filled with conflict. The authors called for further efforts to systematically collect family data. They also pointed to the fact that the existence of alcoholism in men of at least two close generations places children at increased risk for addiction.

Years of clinical observation by the author of this chapter lead to mention of another characteristic that is typical of addicts' families. When genogram information is completed for at least three generations, a striking pattern emerges. Various combinations of both substance and process addictions are frequently present in the same individual. This further supports the notion of the existence of a single or of several closely related mechanisms that underlie all addictions. It is also strong support for encouraging the participation of all family members in 12-step self-help groups to begin to address all addictions problems that exist in the family system. As family members learn about the problems of addiction and healthy recovery patterns, future addictions may be prevented. Because both blatant and hidden addictive patterns coexist in such families, appropriate intervention involving the entire family may prove to be the single most cost-effective weapon against addictions, because it addresses multiple problems. It would be interesting to test this idea by comparing the overall incidence of addictions in two groups of families, one in which all family members receive intervention and a second in which only the active addict receives treatment.

TRENDS

Trends in alcohol and drug use and dependence are continually monitored by means of several national efforts now housed under Substance Abuse and Mental Health Services Administration (SAMHSA). In 1992 SAMHSA was reorganized and brought together National Institute on Alcohol and Alcohol Abuse (NIAAA), National Institute on Drug Abuse (NIDA), and the National Institute on Mental Health (NIMH).

The national surveys under SAMHSA include several on alcohol and drug problems. The National Drug and Alcoholism Treatment Unit Surveys (NDATUS) have monitored the increased number of individuals being treated for alcoholism between 1974 and 1992 (SAMHSA, 1993). This increase may represent better data through increased reporting, more available resources, or improved access to treatment. Similar conditions have affected the reported cases of drug abuse. A new client data system (CDS), soon to produce analyzed data with a client focus, is the national repository for information on clients admitted to state-funded units for the treatment of alcohol and drug abuse. Early data on alcohol and drug abuse analyzed by the CDS showed only 30% of the total number admitted to treatment units used alcohol alone, 27% used another drug alone, and 44% of the total used both alcohol and other drugs.

The previously mentioned DAWN, which monitors problems with alcohol and other drugs in hospital emergency room patients, helps to indicate early changes in illicit street drug use, the latest trend being increases in heroin use. The National Household Survey on Drug Abuse alerts the nation to shifts in household use of illicit drugs.

Over time, fluctuations occur as fads in certain drugs of abuse sweep the nation. Recent shifts have occurred in figures for cocaine abuse, for example. Although the incidence has not risen, heavier usage is now reported in certain subgroups. The view has come to be accepted that the abuse of alcohol and other drugs will always be present in our society, and that fluctuations occur, at times reaching epidemic proportions for certain drugs.

A few years ago alarming increases in drug use were documented for the adolescent population; however these figures have stabilized or even declined, whereas figures for alcohol abuse are once again on the rise for teenagers. Of most concern is the fact that children in ever-younger age groups are experimenting with both drugs (hallucinogens and marijuana) and alcohol, which gives some urgency to arguments for earlier prevention efforts. Another concern is the rising incidence of all drug use among young women who are just entering their childbearing years. Anti-drug programs are generally based on these trends and seek to prevent drug abuse behaviors that pose special health or social problems.

Case-finding efforts are on the rise with regard to the so-called process addictions, as knowledge about these disorders has made possible a new treatment option. However existing treatment resources in most U.S. communities are quite limited for the process addictions of gambling, sex and love, food, and exercise. No significant studies have yet revealed the true incidence of these disorders; however small studies show the process addictions to be more widespread in the population than previously thought.

At least partly owing to the recovery movement, more attention in recent years has been directed toward adult children of alcoholics, and the consequences of neglect and abuse from their parents have emerged more clearly. A significant correlation has been documented between genetics and the neurological sensitivities created by early childhood trauma and, during later addiction, the neurologically related *kindling phenomenon* (when low doses of abused drugs kindle complications of addictions, such as cardiac arrest and seizures).

A further trend is that child abuse has been categorized more specifically into emotional, verbal, physical, sexual, and spiritual types of abuse (Mellody et al., 1989). The associated poor parenting skills in families with addiction are being highlighted and more easily assessed. Many adults who were abused as children in families with addictions are working through these issues of abuse in therapy and demonstrating that deep childhood wounds can be healed. Clinical experience with this population is revealing how profound and far-reaching are the effects of child abuse. As this problem is receiving more attention and scientific substantiation, a strong call is being heard to improve poor parenting skills. Community health nurses are in key positions to apply this developing knowledge through assessment and case-finding and to implement effective interventions (see Chapter 20).

Effects of Problems of Addiction

The widespread and significant effects of substance abuse/addictions and process addictions have led some to call our culture an "addicted society." Without question the total effects of addiction impinge on all citizens, either directly or indirectly, through economic costs alone. Some of the social and human costs are outlined in the following pages.

EFFECTS ON INDIVIDUALS AND FAMILY MEMBERS

Fetal Alcohol Syndrome

Fetal alcohol syndrome (FAS) is a pattern of abnormalities found in children born to alcoholic mothers. The NIAAA (1991b) summary on this syndrome pointed out the following facts: alcohol ingested during pregnancy is directly and acutely toxic to the fetus; malnutrition does not play a part in the etiology of FAS; and FAS does not occur in the absence of alcohol ingestion. The criteria for defining FAS were standardized by the Fetal Alcohol Study Group of the Research Society on Alcoholism (Rosett, 1980) and modifications were made in 1989 by Sokol and Clarren (1989). The present criteria include (1) prenatal and/or postnatal growth retardation with weight and/or length below the 10th percentile; (2) central nervous system involvement, including neurological abnormalities, developmental delays, behavioral dysfunction, intellectual impairment, and skull or brain malformations; and (3) a characteristic face with short palpebral fissures (eye openings), a thin upper lip, and an elongated, flattened midface and philtrum (the groove in the midline of the upper lip) (Fig. 21–1). It should be noted that it is difficult

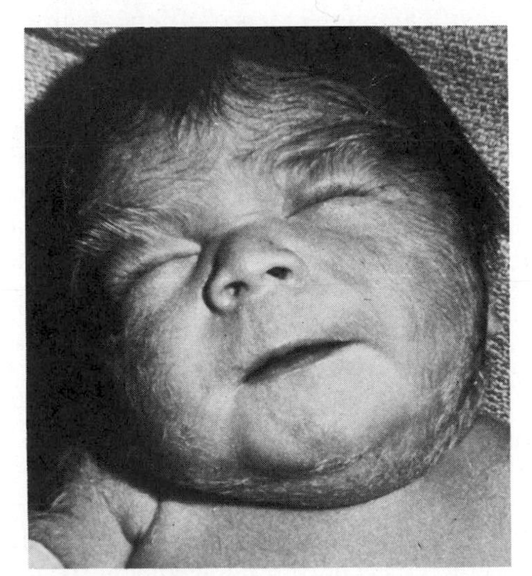

Figure 21–1 ● Fetal alcohol syndrome. Note the long smooth philtrum and the small midface. (From Jones KL, & Smith DW: Recognition of the fetal alcohol syndrome in early infancy. *Lancet* 2:999, 1973.)

to detect FAS during the neonatal period because the facial features associated with the syndrome are difficult to recognize and the central nervous system dysfunction may not be identified until several years after birth.

Learning deficits, learning problems, attention and memory deficits, and speech and hearing impairment are the most debilitating symptoms of FAS, and these often persist into adulthood. Long-term care needs include supervised and/or residential care for mental retardation.

Ernhart and colleagues (1987) found a trend toward increasing head and facial abnormalities with increasing embryonic alcohol exposure. Even at the lowest reported levels of alcohol intake, there was an effect, so that a clear threshold (minimum amount of alcohol to produce an effect) could not be defined.

Community health nurses and other workers have performed admirably in recent years by educating pregnant and other women of childbearing age to the dangers of alcohol intake during pregnancy. However, the necessity of this intervention occurs anew with each generation of young women.

Infants of Cocaine-Addicted Mothers

Fetal exposure to maternal cocaine ingestion has been associated with similarly compromised growth, development, and neurobehavioral problems. Additional problems occur with cocaine abuse, however, including congenital malformations and serious complications of pregnancy such as abruptio placentae and intracranial hemorrhage.

The short half-life of cocaine is well known for encouraging a pattern of intense binge use (Chychula and Okore, 1990). In pregnant women the resulting tachycardia and hypertension reduce blood available to the fetus and usher in a host of consequences (Chasnoff et al., 1985). There are significantly higher rates of complications of pregnancy, with a high incidence of fetal distress in labor and higher perinatal complication rates.

During the first 4 months of life, cocaine-exposed infants continue to experience an abstinence syndrome and exhibit abnormal behaviors, including rapid mood changes and tremulousness. Children exposed to cocaine in utero have great difficulty in bonding. Though emotionally labile they are difficult to soothe, hold, and cuddle, which further hampers positive interactions with their drug-abusing mothers and makes them vulnerable to future parental abuse and neglect. A hypothetical description of what "nursery life" must be like for these infants includes the constant experience of what must seem a hostile environment, laden with intensely unsettling stimuli of touching and sounds that produce frightful spasms in the infant's hyperactive nervous system. Community health nurses are teaching women of childbearing age about the dangers of cocaine use during pregnancy. They also assist mothers to care for and bond with their cocaine-exposed infants.

Infants born to heroin- and methadone-addicted or marijuana-abusing mothers experience similar complications of pregnancy, withdrawal symptoms after birth, and compromised growth and development patterns. Longitudinal research is sorely needed on the development and life course of these children to better inform clinical interventions.

Children and Other Family Members

Attending a meeting of Adult Children of Alcoholics (ACA or ACOA self-help groups), based on the 12-step program of Alcoholics Anonymous, will clearly illustrate to health professionals the amount of damage still present in adults who grew up in families with addiction. The family members exhibit problems of low self-esteem, inability to set realistic and effective interpersonal boundaries, and difficulty in meeting their own needs for self-care. Tolerance of inappropriate behavior from others, unmet dependence needs, and numbed feelings and memories are also consequences that continue to complicate their lives and relationships as adults.

Understanding co-dependence issues can also be gained through attendance at other self-help meetings of Al-Anon and Co-dependents Anonymous (CODA), groups for those with an addicted loved one. Co-dependents exhibit overfocus on their addicted partners, unrealistic expectations of others, perfectionism, unmet dependency needs, lack of self-care, and deep associated psychic pain.

Other problems including physical and mental illnesses, such as depression and other addictions, are found frequently in family members who live with the identified addicted individual. It is especially important to assess, diagnose, and appropriately refer children who are most likely to experience neglect and abuse and are least able to help themselves.

Unfortunately arrest of the active addiction and abstinence do not result in immediate or substantial improvements in the problems experienced by family members as a result of the addiction. A long recovery period from addiction and all of its sequelae is needed and is likely to take place over a period of years (Eells, 1991). Long recoveries underline the importance of continuing assessment, ongoing family intervention, and appropriate referrals when necessary for emotional and physical problems. When recovery is complicated by personality deficits or emotional disorders in recovering adults, an even longer healing period and effective interventions are needed. The community health nurse can assist such families by encouraging active participation in self-help groups, by helping to establish social support systems (especially with extended family members alienated during the period of active addiction), and by intervening to bring into balance dysfunctional family patterns (see Chapter 10).

Pathophysiological Effects of Addiction in Women

Numerous studies show that women, especially those addicted to alcohol, have more rapid development of physiological damage than do men. Recent studies show that the stomach linings of alcoholic women lack the enzyme alcohol dehydrogenase, though it is present in alcoholic men. The result is that pure alcohol is rapidly distributed in higher doses through the bloodstream in women, creating opportunities for toxic levels of blood alcohol to damage tissue and organs. The enzyme causes the first metabolic breakdown in alcohol in the stomach for men, lessening both the amounts of pure alcohol released quickly into the bloodstream and the chances for organ damage.

The ingestion of alcohol during pregnancy is associated with spontaneous abortion and FAS. Furthermore, ingestion of even moderate doses of alcohol over time has been shown to be related to increased risks for all types of reproductive system cancers for women.

Family Dysfunction

Family dysfunction and appropriate interventions have been addressed comprehensively in Chapters 8 and 10 of this book and in many other publications (Eells, 1986, 1989, 1991). Although space here does not permit a full elaboration of the family dynamics associated with addiction, key points are summarized in Table 21–3. The importance of knowing how to intervene to change dysfunctional patterns in families with problems of addiction cannot be stressed enough.

As shown in Table 21–3, the most important family system problem with addiction is probably the strong tendency for the family to reorganize and exclude the addicted individual (often a parent). The parent subsystem is left in a weaker position as the result. The spousal/parental subsystem may be further weakened by a too strong alliance between one of the partners and that partner's parent or other extended family member. Another pattern that materially weakens the spousal/parental subsystem is overcloseness between a grandparent and one or more of their children. The inevitable result is weak parental authority with this child while the stronger grandparent pattern also permits parents to underfunction in their parental role. Inner city families with problems of addiction often exhibit this very picture, with a strong grandparent caring for the grandchild and a weak drug-addicted parent. The weak parent and the grandchild are both treated as children by the grandparent. Too often the weak parent then introduces the child to street life, including drug abuse and prostitution. When the natural hierarchy of the different generations is interrupted by disturbed patterns, serious dysfunctions—often including addictions—appear in some or all of the family members.

TABLE 21–3

Common Family Patterns Occurring with Problems of Addiction

Dysfunctional Family Pattern	Typical Behaviors
Family reorganizes	Addicted one is excluded from the overcloseness of the remaining family members.
Weak parental platform	Spouses in conflict, divided as how to parent their children.
"Triangulation" of children	Nonaddicted parent overly close to a special child; addict may be the child or opposite spouse.
Overfunctioning	Nonaddicted parent and/or child attempt to compensate by being responsible, overachieving.
Pursuing/distancing	Cycles of pursuing and distancing in interactions between spouses, alternating with drug use.
"Triangulation" of extended family members	One spouse closer to extended family member than to partner.
Cross-generational triangle(s)	Grandparent is overly close to one or more grandchild and parental authority with that child is thereby compromised.
Multigenerational patterns	Above patterns repeated from generation to generation.

Parents in these families, whether or not they are addicted, usually "triangle in" (or are overly close to) special children. If a non-addicted parent is present, that parent is closer to the children as a general rule. Children triangled into the parental relationship, caught up in a pattern of overcloseness to one parent and distance from the other parent, cannot attend to their normal developmental tasks. They grow up either overfunctioning and overachieving—therefore acting as parents to their own parents—or significantly underfunctioning, therefore becoming unsuccessful, inadequate adults.

Addictions, Sexually Transmitted Diseases, and HIV

Although needle sharing by intravenous (IV) drug users facilitates the transmission of HIV infection and other bloodborne diseases, sexual practices also play an important role (see Ethics Box III). High-risk sexual practices are fueled by the abuse of mood-altering licit or illicit drugs, due to their effects on brain function. Higher cortical functions involving judgment, cognition, and perception are compromised, precautions are not taken, and riskier sex behaviors take place.

Furthermore, drug abusers and their partners often share a history of abuse as children in their dysfunctional families

Ethics Box III

Gail A. DeLuca Havens, M.S., R.N., C.N.A.

Conflict Among Community Values

Tom sits and listens to the rancor and divisiveness being expressed by some of the city's residents at a forum called to discuss the implementation of the needle exchange program within the city next month. He feels a momentary twinge of regret for having brought the issue to this point. Tom is a community health nurse and clinical director of the municipally operated community-based health care center with the largest caseload of human immunodeficiency virus (HIV)-infected clients in the city. He understands that the critical nature of the near-epidemic proportions of the incidence of acquired immunodeficiency syndrome (AIDS) in the community requires proven interventions if the spread of HIV is to be controlled. Unfortunately a needle exchange program, although shown to be a very effective deterrent to the spread of the virus, comes with a large price tag: polarization of community residents because of the moral questions it raises. It's Tom's turn to speak.

"I'm pleased to see so many of our city's residents participating in the forums about the needle exchange program. I understand that the program is very controversial. It is viewed by many as sending a message that this city condones drug addiction. It is feared to contribute to an increase in drug addiction. And from a practical viewpoint, it was in direct violation of one of our city ordinances, namely, the prohibition against possession of intravenous injection paraphernalia. As a point of information, the law has been amended to allow an exception such as this.

"I understand that for many of you this program represents a degradation of the prevailing moral norms that exist in this city. You are afraid that clean needles will encourage drug abuse. A well-conceived needle exchange program, however, includes more than the exchange of contaminated equipment for clean needles and syringes. The cornerstone of such a program is the educational focus on a drug-free existence. Unfortunately, in some metropolitan areas of the United States, drug users who decide to "break the habit" do not have immediate access to counseling and support, but instead, are placed on waiting lists for drug-free instruction and rehabilitation. It has been reported that, perhaps, a million addicts have wanted treatment that was not available. Some have remained on waiting lists for 8 months or longer [Anderson, 1991]. We are fortunate in our city in that we believe we have the necessary resources dedicated to the drug treatment component of the needle exchange program to ensure that anyone wishing to enroll in the program will have immediate access.

"Needle exchange programs have been found to be very effective interventions, with some programs 100% effective against the increase of HIV infection. In countries outside of the United States, needle exchange options have met with extraordinary success in terms of preventing or slowing HIV infection among intravenous (IV) drug users [Anderson, 1991]. This success has occurred with no increase in drug abuse. I believe that if we fail to initiate such a program in our city, where the incidence of AIDS is significantly higher than the national average within cities of comparable size, we will be guilty of the greater moral harm. For not only do we deny noninfected drug users in our city the means to maintain their HIV-free status, we also prevent them from participating in drug-free educational opportunities that have the potential to empower them to break their drug habit. I ask you to understand that by *not* initiating this program, we condemn some fellow citizens to death through the uncontrolled spread of HIV. I am here this evening to respond to your questions and to ask for your cooperation and support as we prepare to begin the needle exchange program in our city next month."

The moral issues that are present in this case exist because of differences in fundamental perspectives over what ought to be societal priorities for health care in the face of the growing numbers of HIV-positive people in the United States. It is estimated that the sharing of drug paraphernalia and sexual intercourse are associated with approximately 95% of all reported cases of AIDS (Ginzburg, 1989). One million individuals in this country have a positive HIV status (Roper et al., 1993).

Historically needle exchange programs in this country have been regarded as symbolic endorsements of illegal drug use and a perceived major threat to the integrity of our societal norms. They have been characterized as an "affront to our social order" (Anderson, 1991).

In addressing this dilemma several fundamental questions might be posed. What obligations does society have to its individual members? And are they obligations that apply to every member of society? Do the benefits to individual members of a society to be derived from a needle exchange program outweigh the harm to society, collectively, that is inherent in such a program? Which harm is the community willing to tolerate: the potential for harm to the community's moral norms by condoning illegal drug use and by creating a situation that might precipitate drug use or the certain harm that will befall drug users who are exposed to HIV infection through needle sharing?

When we speak the language of obligations, we are implying that corresponding rights exist. Certain obligations fall to a society to ensure that the rights of its individual members are met. But individual rights were not conceived as having infinite dimensions. Rather they are defined by the rules and norms imposed on them by society. It is the existence of prevailing norms of a society and its general moral code that frequently precipitate a moral dilemma. City residents are being asked to support a program that contradicts the prevailing moral norm. Furthermore, to compound the moral tension, they are being asked to support a program for individuals living at the edges of society, namely drug abusers. Do the nature of the situation and the characteristics of the individuals who will benefit from a needle exchange program limit society's obligation?

One approach to the resolution of this dilemma would be for the residents of the city to refuse to condone and support a needle exchange program, rationalizing that they have no obligation to support individuals' drug habits. An alternate approach of the city's residents would be, considering the positive empirical evidence, to support the needle exchange program, thereby fulfilling a societal obligation to its individual members, regardless of lifestyle. Also, the city would be protecting the public through the control of communicable disease.

Finally, where do the nurse's moral and professional obligations lie in this situation? The American Nurses' Association (ANA) Code for Nurses was modified substantially in 1985 so that the obligations of its members to individual members of society are expressed by the corresponding rights of clients. That is, the client has a right to nursing care that "transcends all national, ethnic, racial, religious, cultural, political, educational, economic, developmental, personality, role, and sexual differences" (ANA, 1985, p. 3). Furthermore, "the provision of high quality nursing care is not limited by personal attitudes or beliefs" (ANA, 1985, p. 3). Accordingly, the nurse's practice ought to include nonjudgmental care and advocacy that respects the uniqueness of the clients and supports the clients' right to care.

Tom has chosen this approach. What would you have done?

References

American Nurses' Association. (1985). *Code for nurses with interpretive statements.* Kansas City, MO: Author.

Anderson, W. (1991). The New York needle trial: The politics of public health in the age of AIDS. *American Journal of Public Health, 81,* 1506–1517.

Ginzburg, H. M. (1989). Needle exchange programs: A medical or a policy dilemma? *American Journal of Public Health, 79,* 1350–1351.

Roper, W. L., Peterson, H. B., & Curran, J. W. (1993). Commentary: Condoms and HIV/STD prevention-clarifying the message. *American Journal of Public Health, 83,* 501–503.

of origin. Resulting low self-esteem and poor ability to set interpersonal boundaries does not result in the personal assertiveness that is necessary for self-care and safe sexual practices.

The combination of developmental lack in self-care and substance abuse by women or their partners often results in unsafe sex practices. Such practices result in the spreading of sexually transmitted diseases including the recent increase in the heterosexual transmission of HIV infection to women.

COSTS OF PROBLEMS OF ADDICTION

It is impossible to measure comprehensively some of the social costs of addiction, which include family disruption and suffering of all family members (including the addicted individual). However it is possible to measure the economic burdens brought about by problems of addiction, as discussed in the following section.

Economic Costs

Addictions. Rice et al. (1990) published a comprehensive update on the total economic costs of alcohol and other drug abuse and mental illness in the United States. The economic impact to the nation included direct treatment costs and indirect costs consisting of lost earnings due to lower productivity, premature death, physical complications, and related costs. The estimated magnitude of these combined disorders was staggering, with 1985 costs amounting to $218.1 billion and 1988 estimates projected at $273.3 billion. In 1985 the cost of alcohol abuse alone was $70.3 billion; other drug abuse, $44.1 billion; and mental illness, $103.7 billion. As mentioned previously there is considerable overlap in these three populations, which highlights the importance of identification, assessment, and treatment for persons with dual diagnoses of substance dependence and mental illness.

Problems Associated with Addictions. Direct and indirect costs of care for intravenous drug users with HIV infection were estimated at $967 million (Rice et al., 1990). Estimated costs of FAS were $1.6 billion. This included early care for the children and later supervised or residential care for retarded persons with FAS, regardless of age. Finally, abuse of alcohol and other drugs is a major health problem among the homeless. Rice and colleagues cited many small studies of estimates of the homeless population and their high incidence of addictions problems.

The NIAAA report underscored findings and observations of Rice and co-workers, stated that the figures could be underestimated, and provided a further summary of the following points: (1) many costs cannot be measured directly, (2) estimates provide an idea of the dimensions of the problem and, (3) alcohol involvement often goes unreported in hospitals (NIAAA, 1990).

Other Costs: Impaired Driving

Figures available from the U.S. Department of Transportation (Office of Substance Abuse Prevention, 1991b) show the adverse consequences of impaired driving (defined as driving under the influence of alcohol or other drugs) to include the following: (1) one motor vehicle fatality occurs every 23 minutes, (2) automobile crashes were the leading cause of death for persons age 5 to 34 years and, (3) 78% of fatally injured drivers 25 years or older were intoxicated.

Alcohol is not the only drug to impair the ability to drive motor vehicles. Abuse of any mood-altering drug has this potential, as does use of therapeutic doses of many common over-the-counter drugs, such as antihistamines, and prescription drugs.

The national health promotion objectives, detailed in the publication *Healthy People 2000,* advocate for lower blood alcohol levels (BAC) of 0.04% for drivers 21 years and older and 0.00% for drivers younger than 21 years. States that have adopted lower legal BACs for drivers younger than 21 years have already demonstrated decreased fatalities among this age group (USDHHS, 1991).

Impairment occurs not only in the ability to operate motor vehicles but also to operate heavy transportation vehicles, including airplanes. Crash results are costly in human lives and are reported by the national news media. The resulting public pressure has led to efforts at control through drug testing programs, employee assistance programs, and stricter regulation for airline pilots and other transportation vehicle operators.

Other adverse consequences also arise as the result of alcohol and drug abuse. The economic cost is difficult to assess, but social costs mount for accidental drownings, falls, fires and burns, suicides, crime and violence, and child and spouse abuse. Surely human costs heavily outweigh the economic costs outlined here.

The Role of the Community Health Nurse

Great needs exist among individuals, families, and aggregates for nursing care by community health nurses with preparation in the area of addictions. New and exciting opportunities have emerged for their participation in roles in a variety of community settings as the emphasis shifts from acute inpatient care to care in community settings. Approaches to care have become more comprehensive with an emphasis on prevention of substance abuse problems with special populations or groups with special health care needs who have been underserved. Whether a community health nurse is a novice or an expert, learning to apply the rapidly developing knowledge about addictions is facilitated by reading and having adequate reference tools at hand. Table 21–4 lists primary, secondary and tertiary levels of intervention.

PRIMARY PREVENTION

The benefits of health promotion and disease prevention include improved health, reduced medical costs and loss of time from school and work, and greatly improved quality of life for individuals, family members, and the community. With current and developing knowledge about addictions, future generations have the hope of being addiction free. Prevention is advancing on many fronts owing to the work of government and other agencies, private groups such as

TABLE 21–4

Substance Abuse Interventions by Levels of Prevention

Primary Prevention
REDUCE AVAILABILITY OF ALCOHOL TO YOUTH
Advocate enforcement of restriction of sale of alcohol to minors
Advocate substance-free recreation centers and programs
Advocate decreased blood alcohol levels related to driving
IMPROVE SOCIAL CONDITIONS TO REDUCE SITUATIONAL STRESSORS
Support improved economic standards for the poor
Advocate for daycare and supervised after-school programs for children
SUPPORT FAMILIES DURING TIMES OF STRESS
Strengthen support for unemployed families
STRENGTHEN PARENTING
Teach parenting classes that focus on nurturance, safety, age-appropriate discipline, age-appropriate play and learning, and fostering self-esteem, self-efficacy, and self-control in children
STRENGTHEN INTRAPERSONAL AND SOCIAL RESILIENCE FACTORS IN CHILDREN
Advocate school, church, and community curricula that foster self-esteem, self-efficacy, health, decision-making, and self-control
Secondary Prevention
Case-finding: screening and recruitment into treatment
Refer substance abusers and family members
Strengthen support systems
Advocate insurance coverage for treatment and counseling
Advocate workplace substance programs
Tertiary Prevention
Refer to support programs during recovery
Monitor for depression and refer as needed
Advocate substance-free living and leisure environments for those in recovery

Compiled by Smith, C: University of Maryland.

Mothers Against Drunk Driving (MADD), and individual health professionals.

The community health nurse can act in a variety of roles. He or she can be an *educator* by continually enhancing knowledge about problems of addiction and sharing it widely with numerous populations. There is a great need to educate community members, employers, nurses and other health professionals, and family members. Education in the schools about the effects of alcohol and other drugs on driving is an outstanding example of a prevention effort that has paid off in a decreased number of teenage fatalities in motor vehicle crashes.

Other examples include *health promotion* through helping individuals to find alternatives to mood-altering drugs, smoking, and the process addictions mentioned previously. Satisfying alternatives are found in productive relationships, including healthy family relationships; goal-directed activities; social support for oneself and toward others; participation in altruistic activities; and in one's lifelong adventures in growing and developing as an individual.

With regard to *health promotion* for communities, the Office of Substance Abuse Prevention (OSAP) has excellent technical resources to help community nurses shift from a more conventional service delivery model to a "community empowerment system," which is being utilized for community prevention efforts (OSAP, 1991a). The intervention skills of the community health nurse related to advocacy and collaboration are quite advantageous in the application of community empowerment models.

Many helpful resources are published by OSAP and are available through the National Clearinghouse for Alcohol and Drug Information. The preceding citation alone contains literally thousands of hints, suggestions, activities, and helpful strategies. For example, information on leadership structures show these vary according to ethnic group. In the African-American communities, community leaders should be identified and involved. The preferred point of intervention among Hispanics is the family. The variation among American Indians will be chiefly tribal, usually with community action initiated by a small group of interested and committed people. In each community the nurse's ability to assess community systems will be challenged; creativity is needed to adapt prevention efforts to the local system.

SECONDARY PREVENTION

The early diagnosis and treatment of addictions is desperately needed. Community health nurses can be truly effective *advocates* for the family afflicted by addictions when comprehensive assessment skills permit early recognition and treatment. Early detection and treatment can prevent diseases of addiction from progressing. Primary health care providers are in the best position to provide these services. *Advocacy* here is strengthened also by the knowledge and utilization of family systems intervention.

Based on a comprehensive assessment of the addicted individual, as well as an assessment of dysfunction in the family system and the unmet needs of other family members, community health nurses can *collaborate* with family members who are willing to work on these problems.

Community health nurses can and should function as *case managers* by monitoring and coordinating resources and services during all stages of addiction: the evolution of the addiction and family dysfunction, the acute crisis stage of active addiction, and the prolonged period of recovery for all family members (Willenbring et al., 1991). Nurses who are knowledgeable about addictions can coordinate and, what is more important, integrate resources.

With problems of addiction it is essential that community health nurses take on a strong *teaching and counseling* role. Clients and families need to learn about the disease concept of addictions; the predictable symptoms and relapses over the course of illness and recovery; the management of symptoms; medical and other complications of addictions; as well as how to lessen the effects of addiction on all family members through strengthening family functioning. Through their knowledge of community resources for addiction, community health nurses can counsel family members on locating appropriate community resources, such as 12-step self-help groups, and interacting with them to secure assistance. More nursing efforts involving *collaboration* may be directed toward other family members and community resources than toward the addict during the stages of active addiction. Direct nurse intervention with the addict during periods of relapse require knowledge of relapse management, family intervention, and *collaboration* with members of self-help groups and/or *referral* to addictions specialists.

Assessment and Recruitment into Treatment

The DSM-III-R (APA, 1987) is an excellent reference. It lists diagnostic criteria for problems of substance dependence, including a range of symptoms indicative of dependence on the substance, intoxication, and symptoms of withdrawal.

Recruiting individuals into treatment usually requires some leverage and is usually most effective when the power of the family system, a partner or parent, an employer, the school system, or the legal system is enlisted. Direct attempts to educate the addict may seem futile in the short run. However during recovery clients often mention that they did hear the information, but they were unable to act on it by seeking treatment. The inability of the addicted individual to help himself or herself into treatment during active addiction is characteristic. Instead what is required is the intervention of an individual (or system) outside oneself for recruitment into treatment. The beliefs that an addict has to "hit bottom" before entering treatment, has to want treatment, or has to act on his or her own to get help are false beliefs. The addict is caught up in the powerful grip of addiction. Only later, in recovery, will he or she develop the capacity to help himself or herself.

Neither can the nonaddicted family members assess the need for treatment and actively seek it without help. Someone else, most often a health professional, must help plan and structure a session during which they confront the addicted family member. During such a planned confrontation critical information is shared with the addict by family members. This includes what the other family members have observed about the addictive symptoms, the personal impact each has experienced, the impact of symptoms on job performance and the worry this creates for family members, the future implications of the addiction for the health of all family members, the current needs for treatment of the addiction, and the discussion of what treatment is available and what treatment has been planned.

It is important to fully prepare nonaddicted family members in advance of such confrontations by asking them to verbalize whatever addictive symptoms they have noticed and the impact the addiction has had on them. Advance preparation also involves their attendance at open meetings of Alcoholics Anonymous (AA), Narcotics Anonymous or the self-help group appropriate to the addiction. They also need to attend in advance meetings of Al-Anon or Al-Ateen, to begin to understand the impact of addiction on them as well as to begin to mobilize needed social support from others who have lived through similar situations involving addiction. Family members are also encouraged to visit a recommended treatment facility that they have helped to choose because of its recommended quality or convenient geographic location. Reading published materials about addiction is also very helpful to family members, and these are readily available in bookstores, libraries, and addiction treatment offices.

The actual confrontation includes the helping professional, family members who actually conduct the meeting, and, of course, the addicted family member. It is advisable to exclude children too young to understand the purpose of the meeting and employers who are unsympathetic to the problems of addiction. The most senior family member should begin with a statement of his or her observations and the effects of the addiction that he or she has experienced personally. The last person to speak is the most junior family member. Having contacted treatment facilities for this purpose, the professional can contribute details about the current availability of treatment; however even this contribution may not be needed by a well-prepared family group.

The session ends with a firm family statement by the most senior member requiring the addicted family member to enter and fully participate in treatment, which includes attendance at AA or another self-help group if appropriate. The members will have been prepared in advance to deal with denial of the need for treatment or procrastination by the addict by calmly proceeding to help the person decide which personal belongings to bring if inpatient treatment is in order and discussing transportation arrangements, which local meetings the addict will attend first, and whether other family members will accompany the addict.

Coaching Family Members

It is extremely important to communicate to family members that there is cause for hope, that the addicted member can be treated, and that they need never be alone in coping with the addiction problems. They also need to hear that the problem is neither their nor the addict's fault, but that it is the responsibility of each to actively engage in treatment and self-help. Immediate needs of the family also include information about the addiction, community resources available to them, and the types of treatment available. It helps them to know the physiological nervous system effects of the drug of abuse and the opposite symptoms that can be expected during periods of withdrawal.

Bcforc thc addicted individual is recruited into treatment family members can educate themselves about addiction and at the same time increase their social supports in several ways. The locale they live in undoubtedly has its own alcohol and drug abuse program and can provide very useful materials, advice, and assistance. Family members can also attend one or more sessions of AA or Narcotics Anonymous (NA). It is inspiring to see other addicts in recovery and to hear their stories. Some will share their telephone numbers and will be ready to give assistance to family members.

Perhaps most important, family members must be taught that they too have developed problems associated with living with the addiction. They can benefit greatly from regularly attending Al-Anon meetings, both as an aid to their own recovery and as a way to mobilize social support. Al-Anon members will suggest that they seek out a "sponsor," a person experienced in recovering from living with an addict, who can be of immense assistance to the family member who is new to Al-Anon.

One of the most symptom-relieving interventions available is the simple construction of a family genogram or diagram (information on this method is found in Chapter 9). Not only are intense feelings alleviated, but an excellent relationship with the family members can be established by this means. Clients must always be cared for within the context of their unique family situations. Gathering a family history in this way helps the community health nurse to appreciate the nuclear and extended family situation, is an aid to planning care, and is essential to planning family interventions.

Screening and Assessment Tools

Table 21–5 summarizes suggested methods and tools for various problems related to addiction including screening; identification of medical problems; diagnosis of alcohol, drug, and mental illness; and family dysfunction. The utilization of appropriate screening techniques to identify those at high risk for substance dependence and associated medical complications is critical. Currently available laboratory tests for detecting the biochemical markers of heavy drinking are not as sensitive as self-report screening instruments, although the latter can be complicated by denial (Sokol et al., 1989).

The CAGE questionnaire is a brief, four-item screening instrument named for the symptoms it detects (Mayfield et al., 1974; Ewing, 1984). The questions are:

1. Have you ever felt you should ***C***ut down on your drinking?
2. Have people ***A***nnoyed you by criticizing your drinking?
3. Have you ever felt bad or ***G***uilty about your drinking?
4. Have you ever had a drink first thing in the morning (***E***yeopener) to steady your nerves or to get over a hangover?

TABLE 21–5

Assessment and Screening Methods and Tools for Addiction

Purpose	Content Measured	Sample Method/Tool
Screening	Is an alcohol problem present?	CAGE tool*
		T-ACE†
	Are associated medical problems present?	Alcohol Use Disorders Identification Test (AUDIT)‡
Problem assessment		
I	Level of alcohol use	Quantity-frequency
	Pattern of use	Time-line life history
	History of use	Life history of use
II	Signs and symptoms for formal diagnosis	DSM-III-R
III	Consequences of use	Michigan Alcoholism Screening Test (MAST) or short-form (SMAST)§
Clinical treatment	Medical	Addiction Severity Index (ASI)‖
	Psychiatric	
	Alcohol and drug use	
	Consequences of use	
Family	Dysfunction patterns	Genogram
	Family support	

*Mayfield et al., 1974; Ewing, 1984; Bush et al., 1987.
†Sokol and Clarren, 1989.
‡Babor et al., 1989.
§Hedlund and Vieweg, 1984; Selzer, 1971; Selzer et al., 1975.
‖McLellan et al., 1980; McLellan et al., 1985.

TABLE 21–6
Short Michigan Alcoholism Screening Test (SMAST)

1. Do you feel you are a normal drinker? (By normal we mean you drink less than or as much as most other people.) (No)
2. Does your wife, husband, a parent, or other near relative ever worry or complain about your drinking? (Yes)
3. Do you ever feel guilty about your drinking? (Yes)
4. Do friends or relatives think you are a normal drinker? (No)
5. Are you able to stop drinking when you want to? (No)
6. Have you ever attended a meeting of Alcoholics Anonymous? (Yes)
7. Has drinking ever created problems between you and your wife, husband, a parent, or other near relative? (Yes)
8. Have you ever gotten into trouble at work because of drinking? (Yes)
9. Have you ever neglected your obligations, your family, or your work for 2 or more days in a row because you were drinking? (Yes)
10. Have you ever gone to anyone for help about your drinking? (Yes)
11. Have you ever been in a hospital because of drinking? (Yes)
12. Have you ever been arrested for drunken driving, driving while intoxicated, or driving under the influence of alcoholic beverages? (Yes)
13. Have you ever been arrested, even for a few hours, because of other drunken behavior? (Yes)

Possible scores: 0–13
Alcoholism-indicating responses in parentheses—assign one point each.
0–1 points—nonalcoholic
2 points—possibly alcoholic
3 points or more—alcoholic
"Yes" response to questions 6, 10, or 11—alchoholic

From Selzer, M.L., Vinokur, A., van Rooijen, L. (1975). A self-administered short Michigan Alcoholism Screening Test (SMAST). *Journal of Studies on Alcohol 36*(1): 117–126. Used with permission. Copyright 1975 Rutgers University Center of Alcohol Studies, New Brunswick, NJ.

More than one positive response is strong indication that an alcohol problem exists, and one positive response should arouse strong suspicion of a drinking problem.

The Michigan Alcoholism Screening Test (MAST) is a formal, face-to-face, pencil-and-paper interview questionnaire comprising 25 items; it has been shortened to the 13-item short MAST (SMAST) questionnaire (Selzer, 1971; Selzer et al., 1975) (Table 21–6).

Sokol and others developed a brief, simple questionnaire to help circumvent denial and underreporting of heavy drinking by pregnant women (Sokol et al., 1989). The NIAAA report summarized the following information about the instrument (NIAAA, 1991c). The instrument, referred to as T-ACE correctly identified a percentage (69%) of "risk drinkers" (defined as those consuming 1 oz of absolute alcohol per day, equivalent to two standard drinks). The performance of the T-ACE was better than other widely accepted standard instruments, such as the MAST and CAGE. The key feature of the brief test is a tolerance ("T") question, "How many drinks does it take to make you feel 'high'?" Two or more drinks are a measure of tolerance, which is a cardinal sign of alcoholism. Since laypersons are usually unaware of the true meaning of tolerance, the question is less likely to trigger denial of an alcohol problem.

Since the T-ACE is a general test, further validation may prove it to be a useful screening test with other populations of problem drinkers. The remaining three questions include annoyance with criticism ("A"), cutting down (drinking) ("C"), and eyeopeners ("E"), or early morning drinks.

The drug abuse screening test (DAST) is helpful in screening for nonalcohol substance abuse (Table 21–7).

TERTIARY PREVENTION

Factors Preventing Relapse

Pettinati and co-workers (1982) documented that when alcoholics consistently attend AA meetings they exhibit lower rates of relapse, a higher level of occupational and interpersonal performance, and a lower incidence of complicating psychiatric diagnoses. Positive social supports, living in a family setting, adequate socioeconomic resources, and the lack of a family history of alcoholism and drug abuse have also been associated with better chances at recovery for all addictions.

Pettinati and colleagues also found marked symptoms of certain mental disorders in alcoholics, depression being the most common. In some groups of alcoholics studied, the mental disorders complicated recovery and were associated with relapse. Today most researchers believe that earlier and more adequate assessment of co-morbid mental disorders in conjunction with appropriate treatment could decrease the incidence of relapse in these groups. The group that fared the worst in the study had psychotic or psychopathic symptoms (see a psychiatric nursing text for information about these and other mental disorders mentioned).

Alcoholics Anonymous groups teach that relapse is the rule with addictions and that more severe alcohol depen-

TABLE 21–7

Drug Abuse Screening Test (DAST)

Instructions: The following questions concern information about your involvement and abuse of drugs. Drug abuse refers to (1) the use of prescribed or over-the-counter drugs in excess of the directions and (2) any nonmedical use of drugs. Carefully read each statement and decide whether your answer is yes or no, then circle the appropriate response on the separate answer sheet.

1. Have you used drugs other than those required for medical reasons?
2. Have you abused prescription drugs?
3. Do you abuse more than one drug at a time?
*4. Can you get through the week without using drugs (other than those required for medical reasons)?
*5. Are you always able to stop using drugs when you want to?
6. Do you abuse drugs on a continuous basis?
*7. Do you try to limit your drug use to certain situations?
8. Have you had "blackouts" or "flashbacks" as a result of drug use?
9. Do you ever feel bad about your drug use?
10. Does your spouse (or parents) ever complain about your involvement with drugs?
11. Do your friends or relatives know or suspect you abuse drugs?
12. Has drug abuse ever created problems between you and your spouse?
13. Has any family member ever sought help for problems related to your drug use?
14. Have you ever lost friends because of your use of drugs?
15. Have you ever neglected your family or missed work because of your use of drugs?
16. Have you ever been in trouble at work because of drug abuse?
17. Have you ever lost a job because of drug abuse?
18. Have you gotten into fights when under the influence of drugs?
19. Have you ever been arrested because of unusual behavior while under the influence of drugs?
20. Have you ever been arrested while driving under the influence of drugs?
21. Have you engaged in illegal activities in order to obtain drugs?
22. Have you ever been arrested for possession of illegal drugs?
23. Have you ever experienced withdrawal symptoms as a result of heavy drug intake?
24. Have you had medical problems as a result of your drug use (e.g., memory loss, hepatitis, convulsions, bleeding)?
25. Have you ever gone to anyone for help with a drug problem?
26. Have you ever been in a hospital for medical problems related to your drug use?
27. Have you ever been involved in a treatment program specifically related to drug use?
28. Have you been treated as an outpatient for problems related to drug abuse?

Possible scores: 0 to 28. A score of 6 or above is considered a positive screening for drug abuse. The higher the score, the greater the likelihood that the problem is severe.

From Skinner, H. A. (1982). The drug abuse screening test. *Addictive Behaviors, 7*(4), 363. With permission from Pergamon Press Ltd., Headington Hill Hall, Oxford, England.

*Items 4, 5, and 7 are scored in the "no" or false direction.

dence tends to be a key factor. By the time they enter treatment most addicted individuals have experienced many unsuccessful attempts to abstain from the addictive substance or process. Such episodes could be expected to continue and are, in fact, rather typical of early sobriety. Those who are newly sober should be taught that relapse is common in early recovery; they should be encouraged to quickly resume attendance at AA meetings after relapse if it occurs and discuss the relapse with fellow members. Their social support is instrumental in avoiding further and sustained relapses.

DeSoto and associates (1985) provided some data that may help to explain the frequency of relapse among recovering alcoholics in AA. Participants in the study exhibited a very high level of emotional symptoms. When newly abstinent, their symptoms were at about the same high level experienced by newly admitted psychiatric inpatients. Symptoms declined somewhat during the first 5 years of sobriety, though they were still at a high level, and thereafter symptoms dramatically diminished. However even 15 years later the level of emotional symptoms was higher than the norm.

Severe problems occur with relapse prevention of drug abuse problems, particularly with "crack" cocaine. Cravings for cocaine can be evoked when the addict is in the same environment in which the drug was abused, when talking with friends who participated in drug taking, and even by contact with clothing worn during a period of use. Changing one's circle of friends, avoiding environments that pose dangerous temptations, and making other changes to decrease the stimulatory effect of these factors is essential in avoiding further cocaine use. New drugs to control cocaine craving, a major problem during recovery, are being tested for approval.

Other approaches to relapse have been identified. These include formal programs proposed by individual authors and incorporated into some inpatient treatment programs. They are not used widely and are in development stages; therefore they are not included in this chapter.

Community Resources

The most commonly utilized community resources are outlined in this section. The reader is referred Table 21–8 for other resources.

DETOXIFICATION AND TREATMENT

Medical detoxification is available in most hospitals and is beginning to be available at some outpatient treatment centers for substance dependence. The approach is chiefly pharmacological. Drugs from the same stimulant or depressant category are often utilized for this purpose. An AA method used before special inpatient units were available was to simply give the individual some of the alcohol or other drug he abused to alleviate severe withdrawal symptoms.

A danger with detoxification is nervous system complications, particularly seizures during withdrawal from

TABLE 21–8

Other Resources and Publications for Addictions

1. *Alcohol Alert.* Published quarterly. Disseminates important clinically related research findings to health professionals, each bulletin focusing on a central theme. Free. National Institute on Alcohol Abuse and Alcoholism, Office of Scientific Affairs, Scientific Communications Branch, Room 16C–14 Parklawn Bldg, 5600 Fishers Lane, Rockville, MD 20857.
2. *Alcohol Health and Research World.* Quarterly. Peer-reviewed current research information in readable format. $11/year. Superintendent of Documents, U.S. Government Printing Office, Washington, DC 20402–9371. Telephone: (202) 783–3238. FAX: (202) 275–0019.
3. *The Prevention Pipeline.* Bimonthly information service offering current, comprehensive information on the prevention of alcohol and other drug problems. $20/year. National Clearinghouse for Alcohol and Drug Information, Department PP, P.O. Box 2345, Rockville, MD 20847–2345.
4. *SAMHSA News.* Substance Abuse and Mental Health Services Administration. Quarterly, current information on substance abuse treatment and prevention, mental health problems. $11/year. Superintendent of Documents, P.O. Box 371954, Pittsburgh, PA 15250–7954.
5. *NIDA Research Monograph Series.* Excellent publications devoted to a single topic, often based on technical review sessions held on-site at NIDA. Numbered in order of publication date. Single copies free for monographs No. 71 through 121 (1987 to present) from the National Clearinghouse for Alcohol and Drug Information (NCADI), P.O. Box 2345, Rockville, MD 20852. Telephone: (301) 468–2600 and 1–800–729–6686.
6. *National Clearinghouse for Alcohol and Drug Information (NCADI)* is the government unit for the wide dissemination of numerous publications and other comprehensive aids on problems of alcohol and other drug abuse, most of which are free. Contains a library and conducts literature reviews for public use. P.O. Box 2345, Rockville, MD 20852. Telephone: (301) 468–2600 and 1–800–729–6686.
7. *National Nurses Society on Addictions.* A national professional nurses' organization. 5700 Old Orchard Road, Skokie, IL 60877.

alcohol and cardiovascular complications with high doses of cocaine. The tendency to experience seizure can be medically estimated by knowing the approximate last dose of alcohol ingested and the time from the last dose until withdrawal occurs in a predictable way over time. As the blood alcohol level drops, sympathetic motor activity is stepped up, blood pressure and pulse rate increase, and seizures occur. An increasing pulse rate and blood pressure are warning signs. Though seizures are rare, they are more likely to occur with very high doses of alcohol, pointing to the need for a history of consumption of alcohol during an intake history. Seizures are, of course, a medical emergency.

12-STEP PROGRAMS

A gap of at least 20 years occurred between the emergence of the disease concept of alcoholism and adequate, available professional help in the health care system. In the meantime AA was the only readily available source of help for families and addicted individuals. Alcoholics Anonymous responded (and continues to respond) to this challenge admirably; it depends on the resources of its members—recovering alcoholics—to help the suffering alcoholic and his family. The AA philosophy and inspirational stories of personal recovery are found in the *Big Book* (AA, 1976).

Group meetings of AA can be held wherever two alcoholics are willing to meet, and are found all over the United States and the world. Meetings can be readily located by calling the AA telephone number in a given geographic location. Nurses are encouraged to attend open meetings but cannot attend "closed" meetings, which only members may attend. Alcoholics Anonymous provides fellowship, social support, constructive suggestions, methods that have proved effective over years, sponsorship of the new member by an older member, and a suggested program of hope for the recovering individual. Participation is strictly voluntary and the only requirement for membership is a desire to stop drinking.

Narcotics Anonymous (NA), Gamblers Anonymous (GA), Sex and Love Addicts Anonymous (SLA), Overeaters Anonymous (OA), and Co-dependents' Anonymous (CODA) are other self-help groups that have spun off from the AA movement.

SELF-HELP GROUPS AND PROGRAMS FOR SPOUSES AND CO-DEPENDENTS

Other 12-step programs modeled on AA include the Al-Anon groups (Al-Anon, Al-Ateen, and Al-Atot). Partners and spouses living with a beloved addict can find substantial help, support, and suggestions in dealing with active addiction and early recovery of the addict in these groups. There is an emphasis on self-focus, taking responsibility for self, "detaching with love" from the addictive behaviors by not being overly involved with them, and finding self-direction. Variations of Al-Anon groups exist for other process and substance addictions, such as Gam-Anon, for relatives and friends of individuals addicted to gambling.

The new co-dependence movement and CODA has created yet another type of 12-step self-help group for partners. Whereas Al-Anon groups encourage self-focus, these groups are likely to focus on relationships with others by incorporating the new language of the co-dependence movement. Principles often mentioned include learning to establish personal boundaries in relationships, meeting one's own wants and needs in a relationship, and being able to sensitively express feelings and thoughts to one's partner. It is interesting to note that individuals with a history of substance dependence who are well along in their recovery often attend CODA meetings. Removal of the addiction problem helps co-dependent relationship problems to surface.

SELF-HELP GROUPS AND PROGRAMS FOR ADULT CHILDREN OF ALCOHOLICS

Al-Anon affiliated groups of adult children of alcoholics (ACOAs) are a new development in the substance abuse field. Their growth was stimulated by the written accounts of a few pioneer authors who described the experiences of growing up in an addicted family and who suggested steps toward recovery (Wegscheider, 1981; Woititz, 1983). The ACOA groups, which follow the AA model, have grown rapidly in number in the United States. As with most 12-step groups interested community professionals give frequent workshops on the issues faced by ACOAs.

Funding Issues and Access to Care

Much controversy about what to do about addictions continues to exist. A movement advocating compassionate treatment over punishment of drunkenness began in the 1930s, and the self-help group of AA was established in 1935. Jellinek (1960), a physician, published a "disease concept of alcoholism" which profoundly affected the development of the field. Basically, the disease model views addiction as a progressive, chronic disease that is treatable primarily through abstinence. Participation in the 12-step program of AA is compatible with this approach. Although the disease model influenced psychoanalytic and other models used for treatment, no other conceptual framework to date has either superseded it or proved more effective.

Adherents to the disease model have prevailed in the field of treatment for addictions. Public drunkenness was finally decriminalized on a national scale through the Uniform Alcoholism Treatment and Prevention Act of 1974, bringing treatment under the aegis of health care. A system of care eventually developed that consisted largely of 28-day inpatient programs, but they were not a part of the traditional health care system, as health care practitioners had little training in addictions. The programs have been funded primarily through state and local taxes as well as health insurance programs, but the efficacy of these treatment centers as the major treatment modality for addictions is being questioned strongly (Peele, 1990).

The movement of the entire health care system to using more outpatient care is also having an effect. The inpatient treatment centers, which expanded rapidly in the past decade, are now contracting in size and number, and many are closing due to economic difficulties. The burden of clients needing treatment is now thrown back on the more conventional system of self-help groups, jails, social service agencies, hospitals, and, recently, homeless shelters. Numerous studies have shown that a very high proportion of admissions to hospitals are of persons with substance abuse problems, though hospital personnel are not trained to manage these problems.

As in the rest of the health care system, the most important recent development to have an impact was the advent of managed care (medical case management). Although originally designed to coordinate and mobilize health care resources to meet the needs of clients, its effects on the addictions field have been chaotic. Providers see it as primarily a cost-savings effort that limits access and results in many poor clinical decisions made by nonproviders. Critics believe that a well-developed treatment system already in place was profoundly compromised with the advent of managed care. The proliferation of managed care companies and their cost-cutting approaches have introduced as much chaos into treatment for addictions as they have into other sectors of the health care system.

The financing of treatment for process addictions has been nonexistent because these problems are not listed in medical diagnostic manuals. When inpatient treatment is needed urgently, the client's problem is given the label of a formal psychiatric diagnosis and treated under this label. This has been problematic, however, since the appropriate psychiatric diagnosis is often that of personality disorder. Personality disorders are usually thought to be developmental problems and therefore are not reimbursable under many health insurance plans.

INSURANCE COVERAGE

The picture for financing the needed treatment for addictions with regard to Medicaid and Medicare is similar to that for other disease conditions mentioned elsewhere in this text.

Until recently, private insurance funded the stay of many clients in 28-day inpatient treatment programs. With benefits recently being cut back by numerous employers, even the best private insurance has curtailed subsequent treatment stays. The result is that even clients most responsive to inpatient treatment may not receive it.

At present the group of clients with the best access to care are veterans of the armed services. Veterans Administration hospitals accept veterans with addiction problems after other resources are exhausted and provide treatment, including long-term care needed for many drug addictions. No treatment is available for the still controversial category of process addictions; however provision is made for outpatient treatment in some VA settings by labeling and treating the associated personality disorder mentioned previously. In addition many with process addictions also suffer from substance dependence (e.g., gamblers often abuse alcohol and other drugs), so that treatment for the substance dependence can occur as inpatient care and the client can then seek self-help groups appropriate to the process addiction once he or she is discharged from the hospital.

KEY IDEAS

1. Alcohol abuse and dependence is the foremost mental disorder in the United States. Drug abuse and dependence is fourth.
2. Men, the poor, and the homeless have higher prevalence rates of substance abuse and addiction than does the overall population. Blacks and whites in the United States have similar rates of alcohol abuse.
3. Alcohol-related motor vehicle deaths are extremely high among American Indian and Alaskan Native men.
4. Persons with dual diagnoses of substance abuse and another mental illness or alcohol abuse and drug abuse are increasing in number. They are more seriously ill than those with a single diagnosis.
5. Substance abuse is a repeated, maladaptive, inappropriate pattern of use of alcohol and other drugs that negatively affects health.
6. Addiction or psychoactive substance dependence is a pattern of pathological, compulsive use of a psychoactive substance that can involve physiological dependence (APA, 1987). The two cardinal signs of substance addiction are tolerance and withdrawal.
7. Research continues to explore genetic predispositions to addictions. Although controversial, clinical syndromes are being described for process addictions, such as addictions to gambling, spending and debt, work, and sex.
8. Unhealthy patterns of relationships often exist between those addicted to substances and their loved ones. Co-dependence refers to the intrapersonal and interpersonal problems often experienced by nonaddicted individuals who are in relationships with addicted individuals.
9. Substance abuse affects all family members, not just the abuser or addict.
10. It is not true that addicts "must hit bottom" before they obtain treatment. However, denial and disturbed brain functioning in addiction often prevents the addicted person from recognizing his or her problem. Outside pressure from significant others is usually necessary to encourage the addict to seek care.
11. Community health nurses are important casefinders because they are often the first to see patterns of addiction.
12. Family members of the addict often may be ready to seek help before the addict.
13. Community health nurses need to recognize early signs of addictions to teach family members about addiction, teach new behaviors to family members, refer family members to self-help recovery groups, and encourage family members to confront the addict to seek care.
14. Primary prevention activities in the *Healthy People 2000* objectives are targeted toward adolescents and young adults. Interventions include school prevention programs, environmental changes (such as reduced advertising and access to alcohol, and reductions in legal blood alcohol concentrations to 0.00% for drivers younger than 21 years.
15. Seconday prevention efforts include more screening for alcohol and drug problems, stronger penalties for driving while intoxicated, and increasing access to alcohol and drug treatment programs.
16. Recovery from substance addiction occurs over years and usually involves some relapses. A strong support system, including 12-step programs and self-help groups for family members, are important.
17. Community health nurses are front-line health professionals who are able to assist those with addictions and their families.

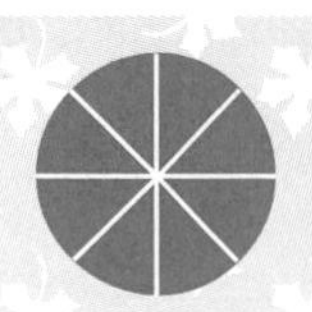

APPLYING THE NURSING PROCESS: *An Alcoholic Client*

Dan is a successful 45-year-old salesman who owns his own business. He lives with his wife and his 18-year-old son. His problems with alcoholism have been developing insidiously since he began to drink at the age of 21 years. Heavy drinking ensued a few years later. Although his family members complain about his drinking, he denies he has a problem with alcohol. Dan has experienced some impairment of his ability to perceive distance from objects; a few days ago his car collided with another car while he was driving and Dan was arrested for driving under the influence. He has also had episodes of memory loss associated with drinking more heavily than usual. His beverage preference is beer, and he can easily consume two six-packs of beer in an average evening of drinking.

Dan's wife Jan has tried everything to get Dan to quit drinking and is embittered over his lack of cooperation, absences from home to drink, deteriorating work performance, failure to help around the house, and constant conflicts between him and their teenage son. Jan presents as a martyr in her situation who overfunctions and tries her best to selflessly care for her family but obviously neglects her own needs. She appears sad and dejected.

The community health nurse became involved in this family through a physician referral that was associated with Dan's discharge from the local hospital; he had had a second serious episode of gastric bleeding secondary to long-standing gastrointestinal problems and heavy alcohol intake.

Assessment

1. Assess the extent to which Dan uses alcohol and other drugs.
2. Complete a biopsychosocial assessment of Dan and his family. Assess the adequacy of self-care activities.
3. Assess Dan and family members for signs and symptoms of emotional problems and addictive patterns (including process addictions).
4. Complete a family genogram of at least three generations and identify dysfunctional patterns.
5. Assess the extent of the family's resources and social support to sustain the individual/family through an acute episode of Dan's illness.
6. Assess the community resources available to the individual/family.

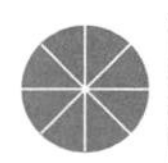

Nursing Diagnosis	Goals	Interventions
Ineffective family coping related to father's alcohol addiction	The family will obtain information about available alcohol treatment and social support services. Family members will express their thoughts and feelings about coping with the father's alcoholism. Family members will identify strengths and weaknesses in their coping patterns and demonstrate improved coping behaviors and better family interactions.	Assist the family in identifying and securing needed treatment and support services for the father, such as Alcoholics Anonymous, and inpatient detoxification and outpatient alcoholism treatment centers. Assist family to explore insurance coverage for Dan's care and family counseling. Refer Dan to mental health services for evaluation of depression and potential self-harm. Assist family to identify how they would like to see family members function and interact. Teach family members about addiction, withdrawal, and recovery.
Self-concept disturbance, mother and son, related to living with an alcoholic father	The mother and son will express their thoughts and feelings about how the father's alcoholism has affected them personally.	Assist the mother in identifying useful family support services, such as Al-Anon.

Continued

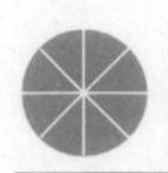

Nursing Diagnosis	Goals	Interventions
	The mother and son will identify their strengths and weaknesses in coping with the father's alcoholism, and identify coping skills that they wish to strengthen.	
Spiritual distress related to crisis of the father's alcoholism	Family members will express reduced feelings of hopelessness, discouragement, and despair and an increased sense of hope and purpose.	Explore with family members the meaning the experience has for them. Refer the family to individual and/or family counseling, including a religious or spiritual advisor, if appropriate. Present the idea that recovery is possible.

Evaluation

Evaluation of the effectiveness of the community health nurse's interventions may be based on the following:

- Appropriate detoxification and treatment for Dan's alcoholism.
- Family reports of hopefulness.
- Satisfaction with and utilization of available community resources for alcoholism and family problems of addiction.
- The capacity to maintain self-focus and recovery for each individual family member.
- Awareness and use of relapse prevention methods by family.
- Family acceptance of necessity of a long recovery period.
- Decreased conflict between Dan and his son.
- Increased participation by Dan in family activities.
- Family members' expressions of satisfaction with improved family functioning and spiritual supports available to them, a sense of meaning and purpose to their lives, both previous and subsequent to Dan's treatment.

GUIDELINES FOR LEARNING

1. Read a daily newspaper and make note of the news reports on motor vehicle accidents, episodes of domestic quarrels or public violence, and legal problems that involve alcohol or other drugs. What major changes in society would have to occur to decrease or eliminate such incidents?
2. Have a dialogue with a friend or relative and encourage him or her to share with you his or her life experiences with alcohol or other drugs. Empathize nonjudgmentally with positive and negative feelings as this information is shared with you. In what way do these experiences influence the kind of choices the person makes today and his or her beliefs about the use of alcohol or other drugs?
3. Attend an open meeting of AA after telephoning the local office to locate a meeting convenient for you. Note members' positive and negative feelings as they share their stories of substance abuse and recovery. Note how their experiences influence the kind of choices they make today, what they believe about the use of alcohol/drugs, and how they value life today. How has this experience changed your previous perceptions, beliefs, and values concerning addictions?
4. Reflect in writing on your personal experiences with alcohol and/or other drugs. When first using these substances, what were your initial physiological reactions? What were your feelings and thoughts about the experience? If you abstained from using substances, reflect on that experience. Reflect on changes in the pattern of your personal experiences over the years with alcohol and/or other drugs. Have your subjective, physiological, cognitive, and emotional perceptions changed from

your very first experience? Would you like to change any patterns in the future?

⑤ Look at your collection of family photographs. Recall and record experiences with alcohol/other drugs you either observed or heard about with various relatives. Compare your experiences with theirs and note similarities or differences. Share your thoughts and feelings with an understanding family member, friend, or significant other.

⑥ Review your personal knowledge and experience with colleagues who abuse alcohol or other drugs. Contact the State Board of Nursing to identify policies and procedures related to impaired professionals. Reflect on the information you obtain. Is there anything you would like to change based on your experiences and observations? Share your thoughts and feelings with a nurse colleague.

⑦ Record your understanding of symptoms of co-dependence before attending a meeting of Co-dependents Anonymous. After the meeting give some thought to the belief of some that many nurses exhibit co-dependent behaviors. Compare your experiences with the experiences of those attending the CODA meeting. Do any similarities or differences exist? Share your thoughts with a trusted nurse colleague.

REFERENCES

Alcoholics Anonymous. (1976). *Alcoholics anonymous* (3rd Ed.). New York: Author.

American Psychiatric Association. (1987). *Diagnostic and statistical manual of mental disorders, revised* (3rd ed.). Washington, DC: Author.

American Psychiatric Association. (1991). *DSM-IV options book: Work in progress.* Washington, DC: Author.

Atkinson, R. M. (1984). Substance use and abuse in later life. In: R. M. Atkinson (Ed.). *Alcohol and drug abuse in old age* (pp. 2–21). Washington, DC: American Psychiatric Press.

Babor, T. F., de la Fuente, J. R., Saunders, J., & Grant. (1989). *AUDIT: The Alcohol Use Disorders Identification Test: Guidelines for use in primary health care.* Geneva, Switzerland: World Health Organization.

Bienenfeld, D. (1987). Alcoholism in the elderly. *American Family Physician, 36*(2), 163–169.

Bissell, L., & Haberman, P. W. (1984). *Alcoholism and the professions.* New York: Oxford University Press.

Blum, K., & Payne, J. E. (1991). *Alcohol and the addictive brain.* New York: The Free Press.

Blume, S. B. (1989). Dual diagnosis: Psychoactive substance abuse dependence and the personality disorders. *Journal of Psychoactive Drugs, 21*(2): 139–144.

Booth, B. M., Yates, W. R., Petty, F., & Brown, K. (1991). Patient factors predicting early alcohol-related readmissions for alcoholics: Role of alcoholism severity and psychiatric co-morbidity. *Journal of Studies on Alcohol, 52*(1), 37–43.

Bower, B. (1992). Abusive inheritance. *Science News, 142*(20), 332–333.

Boyd, M. (1991). Substance abuse in the aging. In E. G. Bennett & D. Woolf (Eds.). *Substance abuse: Pharmacologic, developmental and clinical perspectives* (2nd ed.) (pp. 171–184). Albany, NY: Delmar Publishers.

Burns, E. M., Thompson, A., & Ciccone, J. K. (Eds.). (1991). *An addictions curriculum: For nurses and other helping professionals.* Columbus, OH: Ohio State University School of Nursing.

Bush, G., Shaw, S., & Cleary, P. (1987). Screening for alcohol abuse using the CAGE questionnaire. *American Journal of Medicine, 82*, 231–235.

Chasnoff, I. J., Burns, W. J., Schnoll, S. H., & Burns, K. A. (1985). Cocaine use in pregnancy. *The New England Journal of Medicine, 313*, 666–669.

Centers for Disease Control and Prevention. (1991). Progress towards achieving the 1990 national objectives for the misuse of alcohol and drugs. *Morbidity and Mortality Weekly Report, 39*, 256–258.

Chychula, N. M., & Okore, C. (1990). The cocaine epidemic: A comprehensive review of use, abuse and dependence. *Nurse Practitioner, 15*(7), 31–39.

Cloninger C. R., Bohman, M., & Siqvardsson, S. (1981). Inheritance to abuse: Cross-fostering analysis of adopted men. *Archives of General Psychiatry, 38*, 861–868.

DeSoto, C., O'Donnell, W., Allred, L., & Lopes, E. (1985). Symptomatology in alcoholics in various stages of abstinence. *Alcoholism: Clinical and Experimental Research, 9*(6), 505–512.

Eells, M. A. W. (1986). Interventions with alcoholics and their families. *Nursing Clinics of North America, 21*(3), 493–504.

Eells, M. A. W. (1989). *Case studies in home health: Problem families, problem agencies.* Baltimore, MD: Williams & Wilkins.

Eells, M. A. W. (1991a). Family therapy. In E. G. Bennett & D. Woolf (Eds.). *Substance abuse* (2nd ed.) (pp. 267–279). Albany, NY: Delmar Publishers.

Ernhart, C. B., Sokol, R. J., Martier, S., Moron, P., Nadler, D., Ager, J. W., & Wolf, A. (1987). Alcohol teratogenicity in the human: A detailed assessment of specificity, critical period, and threshold. *American Journal of Obstetrics and Gynecology, 156*, 33–39.

Ewing, J. A. (1984). Detecting alcoholism, the CAGE questionnaire. *Journal of the American Medical Association. 252*, 1905–1907.

Flood, M. (1989). Addictive eating disorders. *Nursing Clinics of North America, 24*(1), 45–52.

Foy, A., Mareh, S., & Drinkwater, V. (1988). Use of an objective clinical scale in the assessment and management of alcohol withdrawal in a large general hospital. *Alcoholism, 12*, 360–364.

Haack, M., & Harford, T. (1984). Drinking patterns among student nurses. *International Journal of the Addictions, 19*, 577–583.

Hedlund, J. L., & Vieweg, B. W. (1984). The Michigan Alcoholism Screening Test (MAST): A comprehensive review. *Journal of Operational Psychiatry, 15*, 55–64.

Hyman, S. E., & Nestler, E. J. (1993). *The molecular foundations of psychiatry.* Washington, DC: American Psychiatric Press.

Institute of Medicine. (1990). *Broadening the base for treatment of alcohol problems.* Washington, DC: National Academy Press.

Jellinek, E. M. (1960). *The disease concept of alcoholism.* New Haven, CT: Yale University Press.

Kimmel, W. A. (1992). *Need, demand and problem assessment for substance abuse services* (Technical Assistance Publication Series No. 3; DHHS Publication No. (ADM)92-1741). Washington, DC: U.S. Government Printing Office.

Krulewitch, C. J., & Herman, A. A. (1991). *Substance abuse and pregnancy: A comprehensive bibliography.* Washington, DC: National Institute of Child Health and Human Development.

Marley, R. J., Witkin, J. M., & Goldberg, S. R. (1991). Genetic differences in the development of cocaine-kindled seizures. In *Problems of drug dependence* (Research Monograph No. 105). Rockville, MD: National Institute of Drug Abuse.

Mayfield, D. G., McLeod, G., & Hall, P. (1974). The CAGE questionnaire: Validation of a new alcoholism screening instrument. *American Journal of Psychiatry, 131*, 1121–1123.

McLellan, A. T., Luborsky, L., Woody, G. E., & O'Brien, C. P. (1980).

An improved diagnostic evaluation instrument for substance abuse patients: The Addiction Severity Index. *Journal of Nervous and Mental Diseases, 168,* 26–33.

McLellan, A. T., Luborsky, L., Cacciola, J., Griffith, J., McGahan, P., & O'Brien, C. P. (1985). *Guide to the Addiction Severity Index.* Washington, DC: U.S. Government Printing Office.

Mellody, P. (with Miller, A. W., & Miller, J. K.). (1989). *Facing codependence: What it is, where it came from and how it sabotages your life.* San Francisco: Harper.

Mellody, P. (with Miller, A. W., & Miller, J. K.). (1992). *Facing love addiction: Giving yourself the power to change the way you love—The love connection to codependence.* San Francisco: Harper.

Minuchin, S., Montalvo, B., Guerney, B. H. L., Rosman, B. L., & Schumer, F. (1967). *Families of the slums.* New York: Basic Books.

Myers, J. K., Weissman, M. M., Tischler, G. L., Holzer, G. E., Leaf, P. J., Orvaschel, H., Anthony, J. C., Boyd, J. H., Burke, J. D., Kramer, M., & Stoltzman, R. (1984). Six-month prevalence of psychiatric disorders in three communities: 1980 to 1982. *Archives of General Psychiatry, 41,* 959–967.

Naegle, M. A. (Ed.). (1991). *Substance abuse in nursing* (vol. 1–3). New York: National League For Nursing.

National Institute on Alcohol Abuse and Alcoholism. (1991a). Alcoholism and co-occurring disorders. *Alcohol Alert,* No. 14 (PH302), 1–4.

National Institute on Alcohol Abuse and Alcoholism. (1991b). Fetal alcohol syndrome. *Alcohol Alert,* No. 13 (PH297), 1–4.

National Institute on Alcohol Abuse and Alcoholism. (1983). *National drug and alcoholism treatment utilization survey* (executive report). Rockville, MD: Author.

National Institute on Drug Abuse. (1990). *National Drug and Alcoholism Treatment Unit Survey (NDATUS) 1990: Main findings report.* Rockville, MD: National Clearinghouse for Alcohol and Drug Information.

National Institute on Drug Abuse. (1991). *National Household Survey on Drug Abuse: 1990 findings* (DHHS Publication No. (ADM)91–1732). Washington, DC: U.S. Government Printing Office.

National Institute on Drug Abuse. (1992). *Socioeconomic and demographic correlates of drug and alcohol use: Findings from the 1988 and 1990 National Household Surveys on Drug Abuse* (DHHS Publication No. (ADM) 92–1906). Rockville, MD: Author.

Office of Substance Abuse Prevention. (1991a). *The future by design: A community framework for preventing alcohol and other drug problems through a systems approach* (DHHS Publication No. (ADM)91-1760). Washington, DC: U.S. Government Printing Office.

Office of Substance Abuse Prevention. (1991b). *Prevention resource guide: Impaired driving* (DHHS Publication No. (ADM-91)1876). Washington, DC: U.S. Government Printing Office. (Also distributed by National Clearinghouse for Alcohol and Drug Information, P.O. Box 2345, Rockville, MD 20852, 1–800–729–6686.)

Office of Substance Abuse Prevention. (1991c, October). *Prevention resource guide: Women* (DHHS Publication No. (ADM-91)1877). Washington, DC: U.S. Government Printing Office. (Also distributed by NCADI, P.O. Box 2345, Rockville, MD 20852, 1–800–729–6686.)

Peele, S. (1990). Why and by whom the American alcoholism industry is under seige. *Journal of Psychoactive Drugs, 22*(1), 1–13.

Pettinati, H., Sugarman, A. A., & Maurer, H. (1982). Four year MMPI changes in abstinent and drinking alcoholics. *Alcoholism: Clinical and Experimental Research, 6*(4): 487–494.

Phibbs, C. S., Bateman, D. A., & Schwartz, R. M. (1991). The neonatal costs of maternal cocaine use. *Journal of the American Medical Association, 266,* 1521–1526.

Pickens, R. (moderator). (1993). *Genetics and drug abuse panel.* Presented at the National Institute on Drug Abuse. 2nd National Conference on Drug Abuse Research and Practice, July 14–17, 1993, Washington, DC, Renaissance Hotel.

Pihl, R. O., Peterson, J., & Finn, P. (1990). Inherited predisposition to alcoholism: Characteristics of sons of male alcoholics. *Journal of Abnormal Psychology, 99,* 291–301.

Regier, D. A., Farmer, M. E., Rae, D. S., Locke, B. Z., Keith, S. J., Judd, L. L., & Goodwin, F. K. (1990). Comorbidity of mental disorders with alcohol and other drug abuse. *Journal of the American Medical Association, 264,* 2511–2518.

Rice, D. P., Kelman, S., Miller, L. S., & Dunmeyer, S. (1990). *The economic costs of alcohol and drug abuse and mental illness: 1985. Report submitted to the Office of Financing and Coverage Policy of the Alcohol, Drug Abuse, and Mental Health Administration, U.S. Department of Health and Human Services.* (DHHS Publication No. (ADM) 90-1694). Washington, DC: U.S. Government Printing Office.

Roberts, S. J. (1988). Social support and helpseeking: A review of the literature. *Advances in Nursing Science, 10,* 1–11.

Robins, L. N., Helzer, J. E., Weissman, M. M., Orvaschel, H., Gruenberg, E., Burke, J. D., & Regier, D. A. (1984). Lifetime prevalence of specific psychiatric disorders in three sites. *Archives of General Psychiatry, 41,* 949–958.

Robyak, J. E., Byers, P. H., & Prange, M. E. (1989). Patterns of alcohol abuse among Black and White alcoholics. *International Journal of the Addictions, 24*(7), 715–724.

Rosett, H. L. (1980). A clinical perspective of the fetal alcohol syndrome. *Alcoholism: Clinical and Experimental Research, 4*(2): 119–122.

Ross, H. E., Glaser, F. B., & Germanson, T. (1988). The prevalence of psychiatric disorders in patients with alcohol and other drug problems. *Archives of General Psychiatry, 45,* 1023–1031.

Secretary of the Department of Health and Human Services. (1991a). *Drug abuse and drug abuse research. The Third Triennial Report to Congress from the Secretary, Department of Health and Human Services* (DHHS Publication No. (ADM)91-1704). Washington, DC: U.S. Government Printing Office.

Secretary of the Department of Health and Human Services. (1990). *Alcohol and health. Seventh Special Report to the U.S. Congress, from the Secretary of Health and Human Services* (DHHS Publication No. (ADM)91-1656). Washington, DC: U.S. Government Printing Office.

Sellers, E. M., & Naranjo, C. A. (1985). Strategies for improving the treatment of alcohol withdrawal. In E. M. Sellers & C. A. Naranjo (Eds.). *Research advances in psychopharmacological treatments for alcoholism* (pp. 157–168). Amsterdam: Excerpta Medica.

Selzer, M. L. (1971). The Michigan alcoholism screening test: The quest for a new diagnostic instrument. *American Journal of Psychiatry, 127,* 1653–1658.

Selzer, M. L., Vinokur, A., & van Rooijen, L. A. (1975). A self-administered Short Michigan Alcoholism Screening Test (SMAST). *Journal of Studies on Alcohol, 36,* 117–126.

Silver, L. (1992). Diagnosis of attention-deficit hyperactivity disorder in adult life. *Child and Adolescent Psychiatric Clinics of North America, 1,* 325–334.

Sokol, R. J., & Clarren, S. K. (1989). Guidelines for use of terminology describing the impact of prenatal alcohol on the offspring. *Alcoholism: Clinical and Experimental Research, 13,* 597–598.

Sokol, R. J., Martier, S. S., & Ager, J. W. (1989). The T-ACE questions: Practical prenatal detection of risk-drinking. *American Journal of Obstetrics and Gynecology, 160,* 863–870.

Stoffelmayr, B. E., Benishek, L. A., Humphreys, K., Lee, J. A., & Mavis, B. E. (1989). Substance abuse prognosis with an additional psychiatric diagnosis: Understanding the relationship. *Journal of Psychoactive Drugs, 21,* 145–152.

Substance Abuse and Mental Health Services Administration (SAMHSA). (1993). News briefs: Surveys. *SAMHSA News, 1*(2): 16, 19.

Sullivan, E. J. (1987a). A descriptive study of nurses recovering from chemical dependency. *Archives of Psychiatric Nursing, 1,* 194–200.

Sullivan, E. J. (1987b). Comparison of chemically dependent and nondependent nurses on familial, personal and professional characteristics. *Journal of Studies on Alcohol, 48,* 563–568.

Sullivan, E. J. (1990). Drug use and disciplinary actions among 300 nurses. *The International Journal of the Addictions, 25,* 375–391.

Trinkhoff, A., Eaton, W. W., & Anthony, J. C. (1991). The prevalence of

substance abuse among registered nurses. *Nursing Research, 40*(3), 172–175.
U.S. Department of Health and Human Services. (1991). *Healthy people 2000: National health promotion and disease objectives.* Washington, DC: U.S. Government Printing Office.
U.S. Public Health Service. (1990). *Healthy people 2000: National health promotion and disease prevention objectives* (summary report—prepublication copy). (DHHS Publication No. (PHS) 91-50213). Washington, DC: U.S. Government Printing Office.
Wegscheider, S. (1981). *Another chance: Hope and help for alcoholic families.* Palo Alto, CA: Science & Behavior Books.
Willenbring, M. L., Ridgely, M. S., Stinchfield, R., & Rose, M. (1991). *Application of case management in alcohol and drug dependence: Matching techniques and populations* (DHHS Publication No. (ADM) 91-1766). Washington, DC: Alcohol, Drug Abuse and Mental Health Administration.
Woititz, J. G. (1983). *Adult children of alcoholics.* Pompano Beach, FL: Health Communications.

SUGGESTED READINGS

Barton, J. A. (1991). Parental adaptations to adolescent drug abuse: An ethnographic study of role formulation in response to courtesy stigma. *Public Health Nursing, 8*(1), 39–45.
Captain, C. (1989). Family recovery from alcoholism: Mediating family factors. *Nursing Clinics of North America, 24*(1), 55–67.
Cutezo, E. A., & Dellasega, C. (1992). Substance abuse in the homebound elderly: A casefinding approach. *Home Healthcare Nurse, 10*(1), 19–23.
Dumas, L. (1992). Assessing the cocaine-addicted mother: Guidelines for the initial visit. *Home Healthcare Nurse, 10*(1), 12–18.
Edelstein, S. B., Kropenske, V. L., Faber-Brook, S. E., & Struning, M. (1990). Innovations in family and community health. A model program for enhancing services to chemically dependent infants. *Family and Community Health, 12*(4), 82–86.
Eells, M. A. W. (1991b). Strategies for promotion of avoiding harmful substances. *Nursing Clinics of North America, 26*, 915–927.
Finley, B. (1989). The role of the psychiatric nurse in a community substance abuse prevention program. *Nursing Clinics of North America, 24*(1), 121–136.
Kurtz, E. (1982). Why A.A. works. *Journal of Studies on Alcohol, 43*, 38–80.
Magilvy, J. K. (1987). Health of adolescents: Research in school health. *Issues in Comprehensive Pediatric Nursing, 10*(5/6), 291–302.
Nuckols, C. C., & Greeson, J. (1989). Cocaine addiction: Assessment and intervention. *Nursing Clinics of North America, 24*, 33–43.
Rieder, B. A. (1990). Perinatal substance abuse and public health nursing intervention. *Children Today, 19*(4), 33–35.
Saylor, C., Lippa, B., & Lee, G. (1991). Drug-exposed infants at home: Strategies and supports. *Public Health Nursing, 8*(1), 33–38.
Staff, A. (1991). Substance abuse: The dracpackers . . . mobile team to visit clients. *Nursing Times, 87*(4), 29–31.
von Windeguth, B. J., & Urbano, M. T. (1989). Cocaine-abusing mothers and their infants: A new morbidity brings challenges for nursing care. *Journal of Community Health Nursing, 6*(3), 147–153.
Wenders, P. (1987). *The hyperactive child, adolescent and adult.* New York: Oxford University Press.
Zerwekh, J. V. (1991). At the expense of their souls . . . clients' substance abuse and violence are threatening the nurses' own physical and emotional well-being. *Nursing Outlook, 39*(2), 58–61.

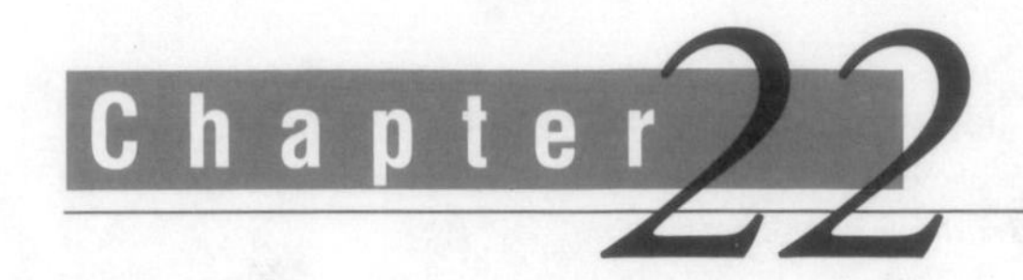

Teenage Pregnancy

Frances A. Maurer

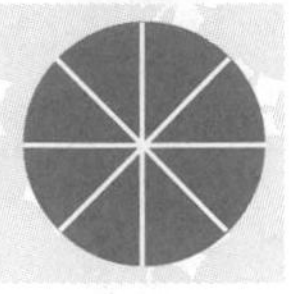

Continued

Focus Questions

What are some of the reasons teenagers become pregnant?

What are some of the factors associated with increased risk of pregnancy for young girls?

What are some of the social costs of teenage pregnancy?

What are some of the personal costs associated with early parenting for adolescents and their infants?

How can community health nurses act to reduce the risks of teenage pregnancy?

What are your responsibilities as a health professional visiting an at-risk family?

What community programs are available to assist teenage parents and their children?

Teenage pregnancy is a major public health problem in this country. The United States leads nearly all other developed nations in its teenage pregnancy, abortion, and childbearing rates. According to researchers (Trussell, 1988; Henshaw and Vort, 1989; *Statistical Abstracts of the United States,* 1992; "Number of U.S. pregnancies," 1993):

- More than 1 million teenagers become pregnant each year.
- More than 500,000 children are born to mothers under the age of 19 each year.
- One of every 10 adolescent girls becomes pregnant.
- One of every 20 adolescent girls gives birth.
- Five of every 6 teenage pregnancies are unintended.
- Pregnant teenagers are more likely to drop out of high school, live in poverty, and have limited occupational choices than girls who do not become pregnant during the teenage years.

Teenage pregnancy has far-reaching effects. Adolescents and their infants experience many problems. They are at greater risk for serious medical complications, low birth weights, and poorer outcomes than older women and their infants (Haiek and Lederman, 1989; Levy et al., 1992). Teenagers who become pregnant jeopardize their educational progression and endanger their future expectations (Auterman, 1991). Children born to adolescent mothers are at greater risk of poverty. Family members and significant others are also affected, as they are called on to provide physical, emotional, and financial support while burdened with their own responsibilities (May, 1992).

Social Implications of Teenage Pregnancy

Teenage pregnancy has both short- and long-term effects on the national economy. Public funds, so ultimately all taxpayers, pay for a significant amount of the care and consequences associated with teen pregnancy.

It is difficult to determine the exact costs of teenage pregnancy and adolescent motherhood, but some costs can be identified. A majority of the public assistance program Aid to Families with Dependent Children (AFDC) is distributed to women who become parents during their teenage years (McAnarney and Greydanus, 1989). These costs are just the tip of the iceberg. Additional costs of teenage pregnancy include (1) medical care for pregnant adolescents without private health insurance and (2) the higher costs of medical care for their infants, who are at greater risk for medical complications and death (Auterman, 1991).

ROLE IN THE POVERTY CYCLE

Families headed by young females are seven times as likely to be poor as other families (Auterman, 1991). There are approximately 600,000 families with children five or under headed by mothers age 14 to 24. Most (66%) live below the poverty line (Children's Defense Fund [CDF], 1991). Teenage pregnancy is viewed as the hub of the poverty cycle in the United States, because teenage mothers are likely to rear children who repeat the cycle. In one study, 82% of pregnant girls 15 years or under had been born to teenage mothers (Wilkerson, 1991).

COSTS OF SOCIAL PROGRAMS

Public programs assume a significant share of routine prenatal and perinatal care for young women and their infants and most of the cost of extended hospitalization and follow-up care required for low-birth-weight infants. However, young mothers and their families affect social welfare programs in ways other than medical costs. The need of young mothers to care for infants and children and their relatively low educational levels limit their ability to sustain and hold jobs providing a living wage. As a result, adolescent women and their dependent children are at greater risk of needing and remaining on welfare programs

Ethics Box IV

Gail A. DeLuca Havens, M.S., R.N., C.N.A.

Distributing Community Resources Fairly

"It seems like coercion to me," states Eileen. "Like we are being vindictive and punishing a teenager for getting pregnant and electing to carry the baby to term. Teenagers are babies themselves in many respects. This doesn't solve the problem, it hides it, so the community doesn't have to confront the underlying reasons for the high incidence of teenage pregnancy that prevail here. This proposed regulation is nothing more than a cop-out."

Cynthia disagrees. "In this day and age, getting pregnant is a choice. If a teenager with no means of financial support chooses to get pregnant, especially when she already has one child, then she should expect to have to decide whether she wishes to practice birth control in the future or have the aid for her dependents decreased if she has additional children. We can't afford to keep supporting all these young mothers and their babies in this city, particularly when so many of our other health and social services are significantly underfunded. Consider the dollars we spend per capita on programs for the learning disabled in our city, for example. Or the percentage of the city's budget allocated to programs for the elderly. Both are significantly underfunded in comparison to the dollars spent for similar programs in cities of comparable size throughout the state."

On the way home, Eileen and Cynthia continue the debate over the Department of Social Services' proposed regulation requiring that females in the community younger than 18 years who are receiving Aid to Families with Dependent Children (AFDC) must show evidence of practicing birth control to continue the aid. The proposal includes free birth control counseling and products as well. Eileen and Cynthia are both community health clinical nurses employed by the community. Eileen practices in the Pediatric Service and Cynthia in the Council on Aging's Geriatric Intervention Program. They have just attended the last of the public hearings sponsored by a joint task force created by the Departments of Health and Social Services and the school board to hear opinions from members of the health care professions and from members of the community at large regarding the proposal, which is intended to address the problem of teenage pregnancy in the community. Now the task force will deliberate the issue and make recommendations to the departments and the board. If you were a member of the task force, how would you go about the decision-making process? What would be your decision? Why?

The problem appears to be just distribution of resources. The community has a finite budget allocated for multiple social services that serve many different populations. It is being argued that a disproportionate amount of the community's social services budget is being spent on aid to the dependent children of teenage mothers. A plan intended to ensure a more equitable distribution of social service resources across the community's populations has been proposed as a solution. Theoretically, limiting the number of people covered by the AFDC program ought to make a greater percentage of the city's budget available for other, underserved social services programs. The plan's defenders believe that although the solution does not include all the choices a teenage mother might be accustomed to, it does offer reasonable options considering the overall needs of the community. Detractors of the plan argue that it violates the autonomy of teenage mothers in the community because it coerces them into not becoming pregnant to have the means they need to care for the children they presently have. Coercion has been characterized as an extreme form of influence that entirely compromises one's autonomy (Beauchamp and Childress, 1989).

If the proposal is adopted, it would be a step toward a more equitable distribution of resources, and thus, if planning has been accurate, it ought to have some short- and long-term effects on the social services programs for the community. A plan such as this is grounded in the ethical theory of utilitarianism, which seeks to maximize the positive consequences of an action by achieving the greatest good for the greatest number (Beauchamp and Childress, 1989). Services in need of resources ought to be targeted, monitored, and measured to see if they do indeed benefit. Adopting the proposal has the potential to jeopardize the health and well-being of a population of children already at risk—namely, the children of teenage mothers. If teenage females continue to have children, their ability to care for those children already dependent on them will be diminished owing to a lack of resources. The short-term consequences might be a rising incidence of children who fail to thrive, are afflicted by disease, or are disabled with developmental and psychological problems. The long-term consequences might be a generation of children who would overburden the community's social services. Such an action would contradict the ethical principle of nonmaleficence (i.e., avoiding harm), contained in the Code For Nurses (American Nurses' Association, 1985). In addition it would go against the value of promoting autonomy and self-determination through the achievement of health and well-being, as expressed by the Code.

Not adopting the proposal is an alternative. However, this changes nothing for the community and for its teenage mothers. Another alternative to be considered is one that attempts to address the issue of teenage pregnancy in the community by seeking ways to discover the underlying causes of the increased incidence of teenage pregnancy. One strategy that has been successfully introduced in a growing number of communities is school-based clinics. Decreased fertility rates, decreased pregnancy rates, and later sexual activity are evidence of the success of school-based clinics. Outcomes directly attributable to school-based clinics include improvements in students' health, lowered birth rates, increased use of contraceptives, and improvements in school attendance (Heller, 1988).

References

American Nurses' Association. (1985). *Code for nurses with interpretive statements.* Kansas City, MO: Author.

Beauchamp, T. L., & Childress, J. F. (1989). *Principles of biomedical ethics* (3rd ed.). New York: Oxford University Press.

Heller, R. G. (1988). School-based clinics: Impact on teenage pregnancy prevention. *Pediatric Nursing, 14*(2), 103–106.

for longer periods of time than are other welfare applicants (Auterman, 1991).

Approximately one half of all families receiving AFDC are families of women who gave birth as adolescents (Burt, 1986). The cost of such assistance to the country is difficult to determine. Approximately 60% of AFDC payments go to single women who became mothers during their teenage years (Zill et al., 1991). For 1990 that percentage represented $12.5 billion of the $21.2 billion spent for AFDC (see Ethics Box IV).

Efforts to combat teenage pregnancy have been sporadic and have met with only partial success. Failure to vigorously address the problems of adolescent pregnancy, teenage mothers, and their children reduces the possibility of successful medical and life outcomes for both the teenagers and their children. Nurses, especially community health nurses, have many opportunities to meet adolescents, as their practice arena includes school health, family planning, home health, pediatric and obstetrical clinics, and a variety of child and adolescent screening programs. Community health nurses have a unique opportunity to affect teenage pregnancy rates and reduce the health risks for both the pregnant adolescent and her infant (Baisch et al., 1988; Oda, 1991).

For the community health nurse to provide quality care for pregnant adolescents, it is important to understand the scope of the problem, needs, concerns, and health issues that affect pregnant teenagers. In some parts of the world, particularly developing countries, adolescent pregnancy is common and expected, not problematic. In developed countries, however, there are social and medical benefits to delaying childbirth and child rearing. Early pregnancy is discouraged in young women. Despite these efforts, however, adolescent pregnancy remains a problem in most of the developed world.

Comparison of Pregnancy-Related Problems in Developed Countries

Sexual activity among teenagers is commonplace in all developed countries (Alan Guttmacher Institute [AGI], 1986). Although the levels of teenage sexual activity are similar, developed countries differ in the ways they deal with sex education and sexually active teens. Experts suggest that the United States' methods are not as effective as those used by other developed countries, as evidenced by significantly higher rates of teenage pregnancy, birth, and abortion (AGI, 1986; Davis, 1989).

DIFFERENCES IN TEENAGE SEXUAL BEHAVIOR

An Alan Guttmacher Institute study (1986) shows little difference in sexual experience or age of initial sexual intercourse among teenagers in developed countries. There are, however, differences in contraceptive behaviors. Teenagers in the United States are less likely to be aware of contraceptive methods, to know or to explore how to

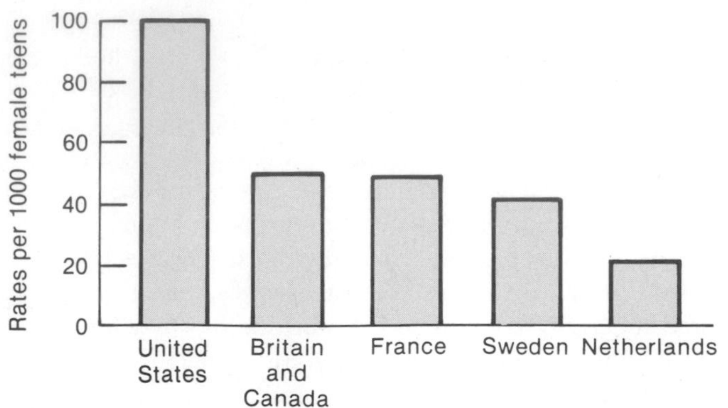

Figure 22–1 ● Adolescent pregnancy rates per 1000 female teenagers in five countries. (From Alan Guttmacher Institute: *Teenage pregnancy in industrialized countries.* New Haven, Conn, Yale University Press, 1986.)

obtain and use contraceptives, and to initiate action to protect themselves from unwanted pregnancies either before or just after their first sexual experience (Davis, 1989). The reason for such sexually risky behavior is at least partially the result of how sexuality and sexual behaviors are addressed in the United States.

In other developed countries, information about sexual intercourse and birth control is regularly provided to teenagers. Government-sponsored sex education programs in the school systems are common. Programs include health teaching on contraceptive methods, encouragement of responsible sexual activity, and easy access to contraceptives. Service is generally provided in a nonjudgmental fashion. In contrast, with some exceptions, the United States has provided little information on contraceptives, and contraception is not an important element of most school-based sex education programs (Perkins, 1991). The United States has also been ambivalent about providing contraceptive services to teenagers. In some instances federal or state funding for clinics serving large numbers of young disadvantaged females has been reduced or discontinued. Some federal programs have actively attempted to restrict rather than increase access to reproductive services (Senderowitz, 1992). Parental permission requirements and abstinence only programs are two methods supported at the federal level.

Community health nurses providing care to sexually active and pregnant teenagers believe a balanced approach is best. A strategy that encourages abstinence, delayed initiation to sexual activity, and responsible contraception for those who choose to be sexually active is a more comprehensive approach.

PREGNANCY RATE COMPARISONS AMONG SELECTED COUNTRIES

The United States leads most developed nations in the rate of teenage pregnancy. A study of 37 countries conducted by the Alan Guttmacher Institute (1986) reported that the United States had a higher pregnancy rate than almost every industrialized nation, and this rate was two or more times greater than those of the five most comparable countries (Fig. 22–1).

Teenagers appear to run a greater risk of pregnancy at an earlier age in the United States compared with other countries. Figure 22–2 reports the available data for teenagers 14 and 15 years of age in six developed countries. The United States leads all the others, with an early pregnancy rate three times greater than its neighbor, Canada.

ABORTION RATES IN DEVELOPED COUNTRIES

As with pregnancy rates, the abortion rate is higher in the United States than in five comparable countries (Table 22–1). The significantly higher U.S. rates are influenced in large measure by the higher pregnancy rates in this country. Although it is true that the abortion rate (per 1000 females) is highest in the United States, the actual choice of abortion as an outcome of pregnancy is a common choice in all six countries. Once they are pregnant, many teenagers choose abortion with some choice variation among countries. In

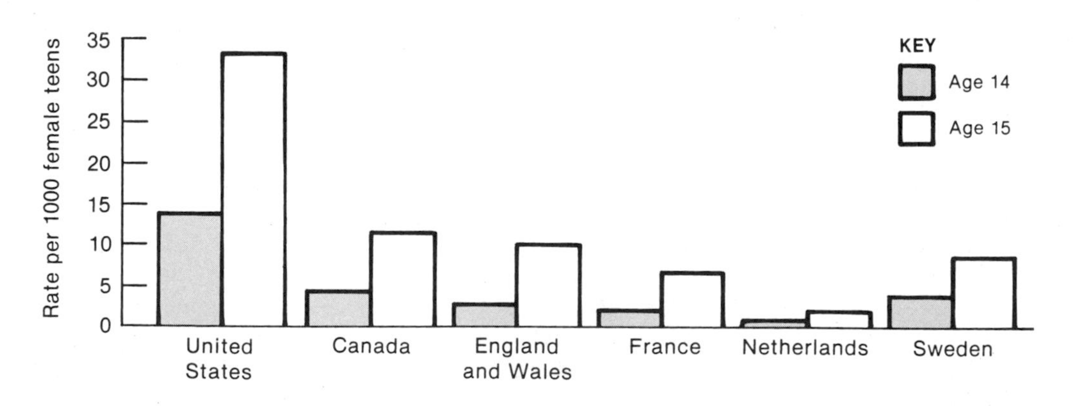

Figure 22–2 ● Adolescent pregnancy rates per 1000 female teenagers by ages 14 and 15 years in six countries. (From Alan Guttmacher Institute: *Teenage pregnancy in industrialized countries.* New Haven, Conn., Yale University Press, 1986.)

TABLE 22–1

Abortion Data by Country, Ages 15–19

Country	Abortion Rate per 1000 Women	Abortion Percentage of Total Pregnancies in Age Group
United States	43.3	45
Canada	26.4	41
England and Wales	16.8	37
France	22.9	42
Netherlands	5.3	37
Sweden	20.1	58

From Alan Guttmacher Institute. (1986). *Teenage pregnancy: The problem that hasn't gone away.* New York: Alan Guttmacher Institute.

fact, teenagers in Sweden have the highest abortion rate followed by that of teenagers in the U.S.

Sexual Activity, Teenage Pregnancy, and Births in the United States

Sexual intercourse, especially unprotected intercourse, invites the risk of pregnancy. Sexual activity among teenagers is at an all-time high ("Number of U.S. pregnancies," 1993).

SEXUAL ACTIVITY AMONG TEENAGERS

Currently it is the exception rather than the norm for teenagers to abstain from sex. The level of recurrent sexual activity for persons age 13 to 19 years increased rapidly during the 1970s and has remained relatively stable at 46% since 1980 (AGI, 1981; Pittman and Adams, 1988; Forrest and Fordyce, 1988).

Sexual intercourse increases with age in adolescents. Between the ages of 15 and 17 years, 50% of males and 33% of females are sexually active. By age 19 years, 80% of males and 70% of females report experiencing intercourse (Zelnik and Kantner, 1978; *Morbidity and Mortality Weekly Report [MMWR],* 1992). The mean age at first intercourse has remained relatively stable, at 16.1 years, since the mid-1970s (Dryfoos, 1982; U.S. Department of Health and Human Services [USDHHS], 1990).

Research suggests that the single most important influence on a teenager's decision to begin sexual activity is the attitudes and behaviors of peers (Zelnik and Shah, 1983; Hayes, 1987). Before 1980, race, socioeconomic status, type of neighborhood and dwelling, and religion were significantly related to age at first intercourse. Although many of these differences are still valid, they are diminishing in significance (Plotnick, 1992).

There is some difference in the onset of sexual behavior among races. Blacks are sexually active at an earlier age, but white youths are rapidly catching up (Moore et al., 1986; Perkins, 1991). The average age at initial sexual experience is 16.4 for white females and 15.5 for black females (AGI, 1981; Perkins, 1991). Hispanics generally begin sexual activity later than blacks but earlier than whites.

Regular religious participation slightly reduces sexual activity, although one survey reports that age at initial sexual activity in Methodist teenagers was similar to that in teenagers in general (AGI, 1981; Studer and Thornton, 1987).

Academic standing, maternal education level, and community expectations also influence the adolescent's decision-making process related to sexual activity. Students who are academically motivated and progressing well in school generally delay sexual activity (Mott and Marsiglio, 1985). Marsiglio and Mott (1986) report that the higher the mother's education level, the longer a female teenager will delay first intercourse. An explanation for the delay may be that the girl's long-term educational expectations are similar to the mother's, and therefore, she delays gratification.

Common opinion links single-parent families, poor parental communication on sexual matters, and school-based sex education with early sexual activity. However, studies have produced no clear evidence linking family composition or poor parental communication with age at first sexual intercourse (Perkins, 1991). Most studies find no relationship or only very weak correlations between school-based sex education and a teenager's decision to initiate sexual activity. There is some evidence to suggest that such education does encourage sexually active teenagers to use contraceptives (Marsiglio and Mott, 1986; Perkins, 1991).

PREGNANCY RATES AND OUTCOMES

Between 1973 and 1984 the pregnancy rate increased 20% from 82.1 to 109 per 1000 population (AGI, 1986; Hayes, 1987). The actual number of pregnancies increased through 1978 and has since declined (Fig. 22–3). Since the mid-1980s the rate of pregnancy among U.S. teenagers has remained relatively stable, although the actual number of teenage pregnancies has declined because of a smaller population of young people. The teenage cohort (ages 13 to 19) represents a smaller percentage of the entire population than in 1970, and with fewer young people, fewer become pregnant, even though the rate at which they become pregnant has only slightly diminished since the 1970s (Marchbanks, 1991).

From the mid-1970s to the mid-1980s, the birth rate also declined. The most dramatic reason was the presence of abortion as an alternative to delivery among adolescents.

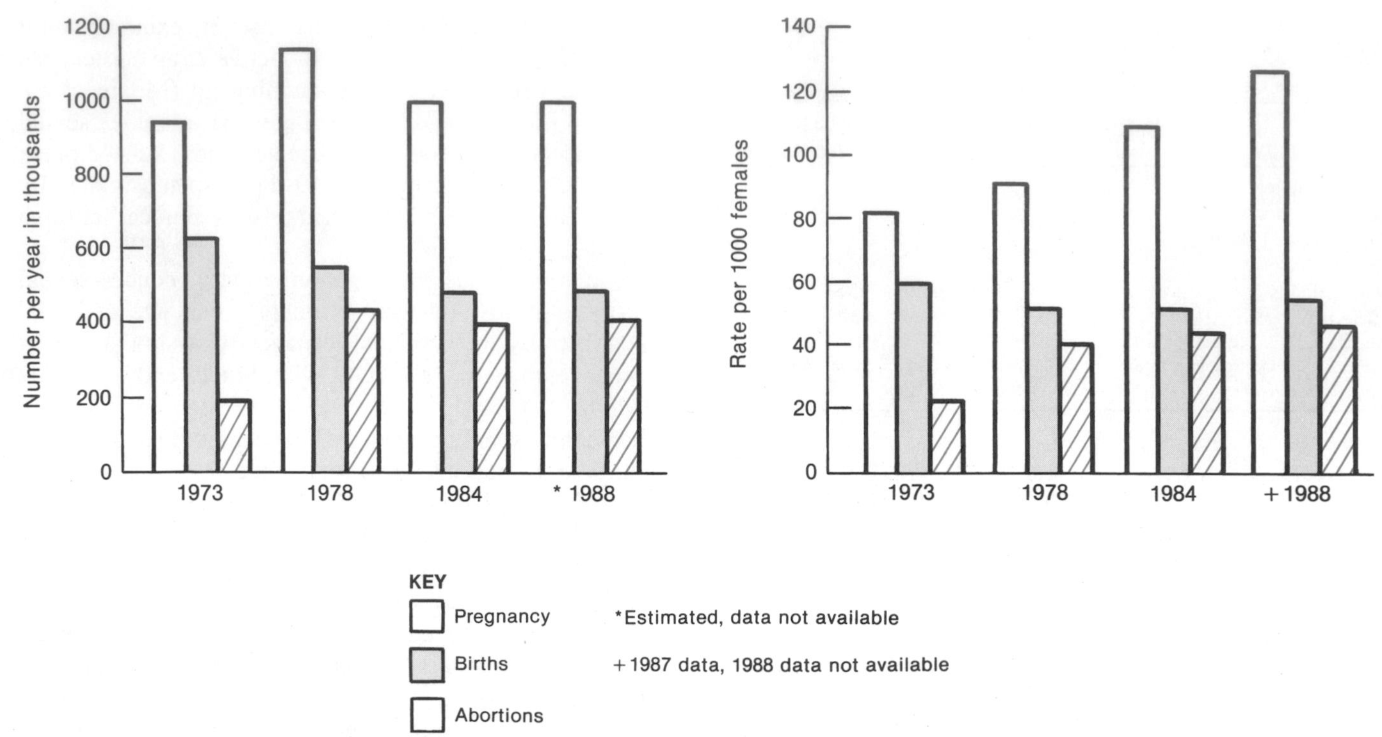

Figure 22–3 ● Pregnancies, births, and abortions for selected years in U.S. adolescents aged 19 years or younger. *Left,* Number per year. *Right,* Rate per 1000 females. (Data from Alan Guttmacher Institute: Teenage Pregnancy in Industrialized Countries. New Haven, Conn, Yale University Press, 1986; Forrest JD, Singh S: The sexual and reproductive behavior of American women, 1982–1988. Fam Plann Perspect 22:206–214, 1990; National Center for Health Statistics: Trends in Teenage Childbearing, United States, 1970–1981. Washington, D.C., U.S. Department of Health and Human Services, publication No. (PHS)84–1919, 1984; and National Research Council's Panel on Adolescent Pregnancy and Childbearing: Risking the Future: Adolescent Sexuality, Pregnancy, and Childbearing. Washington, DC, National Academy Press, 1987.)

Figure 22–3 shows the relationship between the abortion rate and the birth rate. In 1973 almost 60% of teenage pregnancies resulted in live births, 23% resulted in abortion, and the remainder were miscarriages. A little more than 10 years later, fewer than half of teenage pregnancies resulted in a live birth, while another 40% were aborted (Hayes, 1987). The trend among pregnant teenagers indicates that abortion is considered a viable alternative for many. Abortion rates have risen most sharply among younger teenagers. In teenagers 15 and younger, abortion is the most common choice (1.4 abortions for every live birth) (Auterman, 1991).

PREGNANCY PLANNING

Most teenagers who have infants are unmarried, and most of their pregnancies were unplanned (AGI, 1986). Fewer than one fourth of teenage pregnancies are preplanned. This is true for both married and single teenagers, although married teenagers, as might be expected, have a higher rate of planned pregnancies (Dryfoos, 1982). Among unwed teenagers, 80% of pregnancies and two thirds of births are reported to be unintended. One particularly important consequence of the increasing number of out-of-wedlock pregnancies has been the increasing number of teenage mothers and their children who experience financial hardship (CDF, 1991).

MARITAL STATUS, PREGNANCY, AND BIRTHS

The incidence of unwed pregnancy and births has been rising since the mid-1960s. The National Center for Health Statistics (1984) reported a 34% increase in the number of births to unwed teenagers between 1970 and 1981. Marriage used to be a common response to pregnancy. Today, however, fewer teenagers are choosing marriage as an alternative than in the 1960s and 1970s. Barrett and Robinson (1985) report that only 10% of unwed pregnancies currently result in marriage. Furthermore, although only 4% of teenagers are married, accidental pregnancy is still the main reason for marriage. By 1978 60% of births to married teenagers were the result of premarital conception (Zelnik and Kantner, 1978).

RACIAL DIFFERENCES IN PREGNANCY AND ADOLESCENT BIRTHS

A common public perception is that most pregnancies and births to teenagers occur in racial minorities. This is simply not true. White teenagers account for the largest percentage of pregnancies and births each year (68%), followed by blacks and Hispanics (Pittman and Adams, 1988). Black and Hispanic teenagers do have a greater rate of adolescent pregnancy, but because they are fewer in number, the overwhelming majority of teenage births are to white mothers.

Although birth rates for unwed black teenagers decreased 14% between 1970 and 1980, black teenagers are still at greater risk for pregnancy out of wedlock than white teenagers. Pregnancy rates for unwed white teenagers actually increased 15% between 1970 and 1981 (AGI, 1986).

Unwed mothers continue a trend toward keeping their infants, rather than place them for adoption. By 1980, the vast majority (96%) did so (AGI, 1981). As a result, there is a greater demand for adoptions than there are infants placed for adoption. Black teenagers continue to keep their infants at a slightly higher rate than white teenagers.

Reasons for Pregnancy Among Adolescents

With advances in birth control, increased sexual activity does not necessarily mean an increase risk of pregnancy. Why, then, are teenage pregnancy rates so high? There is no single, clear-cut reason. Teenagers get pregnant for a variety of reasons. Any effort at reducing the rate of adolescent pregnancy must begin with a clear understanding of the conscious or unconscious reasons for and motives that affect teenage pregnancy. Several factors are correlated with pregnancy in the teenage population (Table 22–2).

HORMONAL CHANGES, AWAKENING SEXUAL AWARENESS, AND PEER PRESSURE

Adolescence is a time of heightened sexual awareness in young men and women, a time when physical changes prompt a reevaluation of body image and an increase in self-consciousness. During adolescence, curiosity about sex, sexual functioning, and reproduction are common. Young teenagers experiment with sexual activity and increasing degrees of physical intimacy.

The age at first menses is correlated with the beginning of sexual activity in women, and earlier menarche is associated with earlier onset of intercourse (Soefer et al., 1985). Improvements in nutritional status and health care are considered to be responsible for a change in the average age of menarche in the United States. Currently, menarche occurs at an average age of 12.6 years (Bullough, 1981). As a result, an increased number of young girls are physically mature yet not emotionally ready to deal with the demands of young adulthood, including sexual issues.

With this increase in sexual awareness, peers exert considerable pressure to conform or "get with it." Additional influences come from sexually provocative materials that are extensively used in advertising, television, movies, videos, and music, particularly music aimed at the teenage audience (Davis, 1989). Educators, social workers, and health professionals have expressed concern about the influence of extensive exposure to sexually explicit messages that imply indiscriminant sexual activity is the norm (National Institute of Mental Health, 1982; Sachs, 1986; AGI, 1986).

Adolescence is a period of heightened sexual awareness, curiosity, and experimentation. Hormonal changes appear to correlate with increased intercourse. The younger age at first menses, coupled with the proclivity of sexually explicit messages in the media and peer pressure, provides an atmosphere conducive to sexual activity.

TABLE 22–2

Factors Associated with Teenage Pregnancy

Factors Associated with Teenage Pregnancy
Physical maturation
Curiosity
Peer pressure
Sexually explicit media message
Inaccurate knowledge related to sexuality and contraceptives
Increased public acceptance of unmarried mothers
Poor contraceptive practices
Bid for independence
Need for love and acceptance
Present rather than future orientation

INACCURATE OR LACK OF KNOWLEDGE ABOUT SEX AND CONCEPTION

The increase in sexual activity among teenagers has not been accompanied by increased knowledge about sexual function, procreation, or birth control. Studies indicate that teenagers remain woefully ignorant about conception and the menstrual cycle (Darabi et al., 1982; Davis and Harris, 1982; Landrey et al., 1986). For example, many adolescents believe that a woman cannot get pregnant during her first intercourse or without an orgasm (Landry et al., 1986), but in fact, 20% conceive during their first sexual experience, and 50% conceive within the first 6 months of sexual activity (Zabin et al., 1979).

Misunderstandings abound related to risk periods and timing, including periods of susceptibility during the menstrual cycle, age-related susceptibility, and timing of male ejaculation (Pletsch and Leslie, 1988). Common misconceptions include the following:

- "I won't get pregnant if my boyfriend withdraws before he comes (ejaculates)."

- "You cannot get pregnant if your menstrual period is not regular yet, or if you are real young, even if you have a regular period."
- "You will not get pregnant the first time you have sex."
- "You will not get pregnant if you do not have sex regularly."
- "You cannot get pregnant if you have sex __ days after you have your period."

Although these misconceptions are not exclusive to adolescents, lack of access to reliable information compounds teenagers' misconceptions. Studies indicate that peers are the most common source for information about sex and contraceptives (Zelnik, 1979; Amonker, 1980; Thornburg, 1981). Literature and parents are distant second and third resources for sexual information, followed by schools, ministers, and health professionals. It is clear that unless community health nurses and other health professionals make an effort to provide information, few teenagers will actively seek out a nurse or other professional as a resource.

MISUSE OR NONUSE OF CONTRACEPTIVES

Teenagers also lack accurate knowledge about specific birth control methods and the correct use of contraceptives (Pollack, 1992). Studies indicate that most teenagers are not familiar with a diaphragm or intrauterine device (Amonker, 1980). Those who are often have misconceptions and may believe, for example, that the string from an IUD hangs outside the labia, that the pill causes cancer (Stammer, 1985) or makes the user fat, and that condoms get in the way or reduce feeling during intercourse. Interviews with teenagers by community health nurses provide evidence that teenagers are not correctly using birth control. Common statements include the following:

- "I take the pill whenever my boyfriend and I have sex, every single time."
- "If I miss the pill by accident, I will take all the ones I have missed, sometimes 4 or 5 days' worth. It's not a big deal; I'm very careful."
- "I always use the foam. If my boyfriend and I are going to make love, I put it in at the beginning of our date. I never miss."
- "My mother told me to douche after every time we make love, and I do."

Community health nurses should carefully explore a teenager's knowledge base and correct any misconceptions about birth control methods. This is the important first step in providing teenagers with clear, accurate directions regarding the use of birth control.

Even when provided with accurate information about birth control methods, teenagers do not use birth control on a regular basis. Several studies (AGI, 1981; Zelnick and Kantner, 1979; Kisker, 1985; Howard and McCabe, 1992) indicate the following common reasons given by teenagers for irregular use or nonuse of birth control:

- A belief that pregnancy is not possible at the time of intercourse.
- Unprepared to have intercourse at that time.
- Unwilling to appear to partner to be prepared to have sex.
- Lack of knowledge about methods or where birth control materials could be obtained.
- A belief that contraceptive use is wrong or dangerous.
- A belief that birth control methods are too difficult or unpleasant.
- The partner objects to the use of birth control.

The number of teenagers who use birth control has increased since the mid-1980s. It is clear that some teenagers are beginning to recognize the importance of contraceptive use. According to the Youth Risk Behavior Survey, 80% of sexually active high school students reported using contraceptives during sexual intercourse (*MMWR,* 1992). However, the survey did not explore the regularity and accuracy of contraceptive use and contained some disturbing information. Fewer than half of the teenagers used condoms, and many reported using withdrawal as a birth control method. Other studies show that approximately half of sexually active teenagers consistently use birth control (CDF, 1989). Regular effective contraceptive use increases with age during the teenage years (Whitley and Schofield, 1986).

Adolescents often have intercourse without discussing contraception with their partner. Many report that it is difficult to discuss this issue, especially with a new partner. They feel awkward and fear appearing immature or unsophisticated (Kisker, 1985). Some feel that talking about or using contraception will cause them to lose their partner. Girls report that male partners complain when asked to use condoms.

Several factors associated with the distribution and appropriateness of contraceptive methods contribute to ineffective use or nonuse among teenagers. First there is the problem of access as noted earlier by those interviewed. The most effective birth control methods (intrauterine device or birth control pills) require appointments and examinations by health care professionals. This often is not easy or possible for teenagers, who are not knowledgeable about the health care delivery system. Cost is an issue, and most have never sought care without their parents' permission. Most major cities have family planning clinics serving adolescents, but in smaller cities and rural areas, accessible services for teenagers are harder to find. Public funding for adolescent reproductive services has been reduced. Teenagers reluctant to ask for parental cooperation or permission in seeking contraceptive services have very limited choices when public funding is inaccessible or reduced.

Currently the federal government has expressed renewed interest in improving health care for children and young adults. Support for sex education, accurate birth control information, and improved access and funding for birth control services should be incorporated into any comprehensive adolescent health program.

The limited access to certain types of birth control and the difficulty of matching teenagers with an appropriate and acceptable contraceptive method increases the risk of pregnancy in this population. Teenagers engage in sexual behavior on an irregular, sporadic basis (Hayes, 1987). Only 30% of sexually active teenagers have intercourse three or more times a month (Zelnick, 1983). In adults with similar sexual practices, barrier contraceptives (sponge, diaphragm, spermicide, or condom) would be the appropriate choice; all except the diaphragm are available without a prescription. However, teenagers are not reliable contraceptive users, and many health care professionals believe that the best contraceptive choices are ones that do not rely on planning or application at intercourse (e.g., birth control pills, intrauterine device, or the levonorgestrel implant [Norplant] system). Unfortunately, these methods are also the most costly ones and require medical prescription and follow-up.

DESTIGMATIZATION OF ILLEGITIMACY

Social norms have changed since the 1970s, and currently illegitimacy is not as uncommon or as unacceptable as in the past (Humenick et al., 1991). Formerly pregnancy out of wedlock resulted in severe social censure, especially for women. Options for girls who were pregnant were limited. Generally, they were not allowed to continue in school. Usually they married the father of the child or gave the infant up for adoption (Braithwaite and Taylor, 1992). Abortion became a legal option in the United States after 1973 with the Supreme Court's decision in favor of abortion.

Currently, if the infant is carried to term, the teenager usually keeps the child. Marriage and adoption are no longer considered the best solutions. Indeed, statistics seem to indicate that teenage marriages are not the most successful solution, as approximately three of every five teenage couples are separated or divorced within the first 6 years (Furstenberg, 1979; Morrison and Jensen, 1982; Furstenberg and Brooks-Gunn, 1985).

Unwed motherhood is common. The Children's Defense Fund (1989) reports that 60% of teenage births are to unwed mothers. By comparison, in 1960 only 15% of adolescent mothers were unwed. Pregnant teenagers are encouraged to stay in school and complete their education, and many young girls choose to remain single. A lessening of the stigma associated with illegitimacy and the high failure rate associated with young marriages are two of the most important reasons for the change.

EFFORTS AT INDEPENDENCE

Adolescence is a turbulent period. The teenager must contend not only with sexual changes and feelings, but also with a wide variety of conflicting emotions and developmental tasks. This is a period of increasing independence, a period in which children complete the task of separation from their parents and further develop their own identity. It is a time of uncertainty and conflict, a time of exploration.

As the child explores and develops, many conflicts arise with parents and other authority figures. Attempts at independence, if severely restricted, may lead to "acting out" behaviors. Pregnancy can be one means of acting out; others include running away, poor school performance, and substance abuse. This is not to suggest that every female teenager whose independence is curbed will become pregnant. However, research strongly suggests that pregnancy can be an outcome for some who perceive themselves as being severely restricted by their parents. Interviews with 14- and 15-year-old girls reveal that spite is a powerful motivating force for some girls (Black and DeBlassie, 1985). Some studies indicate that there are significant mother–daughter or parent–child conflicts in a portion of the pregnant adolescent population (Bulcholz and Gol, 1986).

A NEED TO FEEL SPECIAL, LOVED, AND WANTED

Pregnancy may also result from a need to be nurtured or loved or to feel special. Teenagers who do not have particularly successful life experiences or who consistently fail develop a poor self-image. If their need for nurturing and self-esteem is not met in other ways, they may be particularly vulnerable to or at risk for pregnancy. Pregnancy can make a person feel special. The teenager receives extra attention from family, peers, and acquaintances (Ktsanes, 1980). For the first time she may be on "center stage" in the family unit. Some girls become pregnant because they expect the infant to meet their need for love and attention (Fisher, 1984). In this way they will have someone to give them unconditional love.

The need for love and attention may also be the motivating force in providing sexual favors. Girls may feel pressured into sexual relations with boys because they fear losing their boyfriend if they do not comply. Intercourse may be a means of ensuring a continued, exclusive, caring relationship (Davis, 1980). This is particularly important to teenagers who do not feel needed or cared for within the family unit. Pregnancy may represent an additional tie to the boyfriend, another means of ensuring that the relationship will continue.

In general, pregnancy as a strategy to compensate for unmet needs, to enhance self-esteem, or to assert independence is not particularly beneficial or successful. Parenting provides ample opportunity for failures, which are not helpful to a teenager already faced with repeated failures in her life experience. An infant cannot meet all the nurturing expectations of the adolescent; in fact, an infant has significant nurturing and attention needs of its own.

Although pregnancy can become a stimulus for positive growth in an adolescent, generally the results are more negative than positive. Pregnancy places additional burdens on teenagers, who are already attempting to cope with the normal maturational crisis of adolescence (Bulcholz and Gol, 1986).

LACK OF FUTURE-ORIENTED REASONING IN ADOLESCENTS

Because engaging in sexual intercourse need not result in pregnancy, why do so many teens fail to use or only intermittently use contraceptives? Cognitive development may play a particularly relevant role in the explanation. Adolescence is a period of developmental transition from concrete to abstract reasoning. Studies suggest that some pregnancies may result because the adolescent has not completed this transition and is not able to use abstract reasoning.

Teenagers generally live in the present; future planning is minimal. This concentration on the present may partially explain why some do not seek contraceptive services even though they are sexually active (Bulcholz and Gol, 1986). Teenagers who are oriented to the present and just beginning to develop abstract reasoning are often unable to consider the future consequences of their current sexual activity (Sachs, 1986).

Adolescents who engaged in risk behavior despite information and a source of birth control were found to be limited in their ability to identify all potential alternatives and consequences of their action (Rogel et al., 1979). Teenagers do not feel personally vulnerable. They reason that pregnancy or sexually transmitted disease will happen only to others, so sexual intercourse does not entail personal risk (Perkins, 1991). On the other hand, teenagers who inaccurately believe they are pregnant are more inclined to use regular birth control after their pregnancy scare (Kisker, 1985).

As adolescents become more developmentally mature and more proficient at identifying psychosocial costs, their use of contraceptives increases (Cvetkovich et al., 1975; Cvetkovich and Grote, 1981). Older girls are more likely to use birth control, and there is an age-related correlation between first intercourse and use of contraceptives. In other words, the older the teenager is during her first sexual experience, the more likely she will be to use contraceptives (Zelnick and Shah, 1983).

Knowledge of the motives and reasoning of sexually active teenagers helps the community health nurse identify teenagers at particular risk for pregnancy. It is important information for nurses who are responsible for planning and implementing care for adolescent populations.

Consequences of Early Pregnancy for Teenagers and Infants

As previously noted, there are medical, emotional, and economic consequences to pregnancy and early motherhood. The most important problems for adolescents and their offspring are outlined in the sections that follow.

PHYSICAL CONSEQUENCES FOR THE MOTHER

During maturation, rapid growth patterns place considerable demands on the body. Pregnancy places additional demands on a body already experiencing dramatic changes. In general, adolescents experience greater health problems with pregnancy than do women over 20 years of age. The consequences are especially severe to the youngest adolescents (12 to 15 years of age) (Levy et al., 1992). Older teenagers (16 to 19 years old) are not as likely to experience serious difficulties.

Teenagers are at greater risk for developing pregnancy-induced hypertension and toxemia (AGI, 1981). The incidence of hypertension ranges from 10% to 35%, which is higher than in any other age group, including women over 34 years of age. When good, consistent prenatal care is administered to teenagers, the risk of pregnancy-induced hypertension is lessened (Sacher and Neuhoff, 1982; Leppert et al., 1986).

Teenagers are at increased risk for anemia, nutritional deficiencies, and urinary tract infections (Brisbane, 1980; Bulcholz and Gol, 1986). Studies indicate that 10% to 40% of pregnant teens are anemic, a condition exacerbated by the poor nutritional status of most teenagers (Haiek and Lederman, 1989; Schneck et al., 1990).

Young girls are more likely to deliver prematurely, experience rapid or prolonged labor, develop abruptio placentae, or have fetal or maternal infections (Sacher and Neuhoff, 1982; Davidson and Fukushima, 1985; Dryfoos, 1985; Mott, 1986). Although some early studies suggested that teenagers are more prone to cesarean section deliveries, current research indicates that this is incorrect (Davidson and Fukushima, 1985; Leppert et al., 1985).

Although pregnancy-related mortality rates are generally low in the United States, the young are at greater risk than those in other age categories. As with medical complications, the greatest risk is to very young teenagers. Girls 16 years or younger are five times more likely to die as a result of pregnancy than are women 20 to 24 (Sacher and Neuhoff, 1982; Black and DeBlassie, 1985).

PHYSICAL CONSEQUENCES FOR THE NEWBORN

Infants born to teenagers are also at risk: Stillbirths are twice as common, and the mortality rate is two to four times greater during the first year of life for infants born of adolescent mothers (Sacher and Neuhoff, 1982; Black and DeBlassie, 1985). Child abuse and neglect are more common among young mothers (Marshall et al., 1991). Some studies suggest that these infants are at risk for lower IQ levels, a problem usually attributed to the mother's poor nutritional status and lack of prenatal care prior to delivery (Black and DeBlassie, 1985).

Prematurity (birth weight under 5.5 lb [2500 gm]) is a significant risk, almost 40% higher than for women 20 to 24 years old (AGI, 1981; Levy et al., 1992). Low birth weight is associated with higher rates of infant mortality, birth injuries, neurological defects, and mental retardation. Among teenagers, low birth weight is a greater risk if the mother is not physically mature (Frisancho et al., 1985). Birth weights increase with the age of the mother, but all teenagers are at greater risk for having low-birth-weight infants than those in other age groups (Loris et al., 1985).

LESS PRENATAL CARE

Many pregnant teenagers delay seeking prenatal care or do not receive regular care (Geronimus, 1986; Pomeranz et al., 1991). Only one in every five teenagers initiates care during the first trimester. The same teenagers at greatest risk for pregnancy—those from poor families—are also at greatest risk for poor prenatal care (Miller and Stokes, 1985). In general, this group tends to be more illness- than prevention-oriented in their health practices. Delays in seeking prenatal care may also be influenced by denial of the pregnancy and an orientation toward concrete, present-centered reasoning.

Regular prenatal care has been found to reduce the risks inherent in early pregnancy, even though complication rates remain above those in other age groups (Leppert et al., 1986; Nelson, 1989). Short gestation, low birth weight, and neonatal mortality have all been reduced with regular prenatal care (Geronimus, 1986). Porterfield and Harris (1985) reported that nine prenatal visits reduced the risk of pregnancy-induced hypertension, toxemia, and abrupt or prolonged labor in the adolescent population.

Home visits by community health nurses to adolescents during pregnancy and after birth improved pregnancy outcomes and infant health status and delayed repeat pregnancies for the adolescent mother (Olds et al., 1986a, 1986b, 1988).

PSYCHOSOCIAL CONSEQUENCES

Pregnancy can be a psychological crisis that disrupts the adolescent's momentum toward independence. It represents an abrupt transition to adulthood. The pregnant teenager must learn to relate to the unborn child and to function as a parent while struggling to solidify her own identity, a daunting task.

A pregnant girl or young mother may become socially isolated because friends do not have the same interests. If her family is not supportive or pleased about the pregnancy, there may be additional stress. In one study, unmarried pregnant teenagers experienced more self-doubt, uncertainty, loneliness, and helplessness than their nonpregnant peers (Lieberman, 1980). Giblin and colleagues (1986) reported that pregnant adolescents more often are overweight and complain of headaches, nervousness, and feelings of depression or sadness.

Teenage mothers frequently lack the emotional and social supports available to older mothers. Stress and isolation increase after delivery, when the adolescent must cope with demands of the infant, and interactions with peers become limited. Stress may culminate in child abuse or suicide, especially in unwed teenagers (Baldwin, 1976).

EDUCATIONAL AND ECONOMIC CONSEQUENCES

Pregnancy and child rearing are often the reasons adolescents drop out of school, and the younger the teenager at the time of pregnancy, the greater the danger that she will not complete high school. For example, after becoming pregnant, only 20% of girls age 17 years or younger will complete high school, and only 60% will complete eighth grade (Morrison and Jensen, 1982; Furstenberg et al., 1987).

Lack of education hampers the mother's prospects in the job market. The income of young mothers is only half that of women who delay childbearing until after age 20 years (Black and DeBlassie, 1985). Families headed by teenage mothers are seven times more likely to be below the poverty level and are more likely to have had welfare assistance (Wallace et al., 1982; Leibowitz et al., 1986; Burt, 1986).

Pregnancy Effects on Family Dynamics

Pregnancy affects both the individual teenager and the members of her family. Pregnancy represents added economic and emotional pressure, and all too often it is a burden that the family is not equipped to deal with. In some cases grandparents become the infant's primary caregiver. As such, their usual pattern or routine may be drastically changed.

> One grandmother commented, "My husband and I worked all our lives so that we could travel in our retirement. Instead, we are taking care of our grandson so my daughter can finish high school. And then what?"

Siblings and other family members can become resentful. Siblings may feel they have to compete for attention, and when the infant arrives, both siblings and other household members may have less privacy and may be forced to share sleeping space to accommodate the new arrival. Sometimes the extended family shares or assumes the economic costs of caring for the pregnant teenager and her child.

Adolescent Fathers

Adolescent males share the responsibility for a large percentage of unplanned teenage pregnancies each year (AGI, 1981). Little attention has been focused on teenage fathers. For the most part, they are perceived as self-centered and uncaring, concerned with "scoring" (having intercourse) rather than the potential consequences of sexual activity. Several studies have found that teenage males feel that it is acceptable to lie to a girl to "score" (Sorenson, 1973; Vadies and Hale, 1977).

There is a renewed interest in fathers and the role fathers play in child rearing. The experiences of adolescent fathers are being studied, and evidence suggests that they are affected by the pregnancy. Most are ill prepared to assume the role of fatherhood, and few relish the opportunity. Adolescent fathers report feeling frightened and disturbed by the responsibilities and neglected in the decision-making process, although few abandon the mother during pregnancy (Vinovskis, 1986).

Fathers generally are available to the pregnant teenager prior to delivery, but their relationship with the mother and infant weakens over time. Studies indicate that 50% to 84% are still involved at delivery, but by the time an infant is 1 year of age, only half still visit on a regular basis. By the time the child is 5 years old, only a handful have regular contact with their child (Furstenberg, 1979; Vas et al., 1983). A later study performed by Westney and co-workers (1986) reported that two thirds of fathers have some contact 2 years after delivery, and half have some contact for 3 years.

Before delivery, most unwed fathers plan to contribute financially to the support of the mother and the child, but only a few follow through (Barret and Robinson, 1982). One reason is that many have few economic resources (Westney et al., 1986). Teenage fathers, like teenage mothers, have monetary and educational problems. Although more teenage fathers than mothers complete high school, almost half drop out, which leaves them open to the same economic difficulties as teenage mothers (Barret and Robinson 1985; Dearden et al., 1992).

Before the 1970s adolescent fathers had few legal rights. Since then, the courts have established rights related to custody and notification of adoption proceedings, and in some instances the right to be notified before an abortion. Along with more legal recognition has come increased pressure to contribute economically to the welfare of the child. Both state and federal governments have enacted procedures aimed at increasing the financial contribution of absentee fathers; these have met with some success (Smoller and Ooms, 1987).

If a parent has been ordered by a court to pay child support and fails to do so, the parent may be held in contempt of court. Income may be garnished by the federal government and paid to the proper state for distribution to the family. Federal law also allows states to establish similar programs and use a variety of enforcement powers to recover child support monies.

The health care system has devoted most of its attention to caring for the adolescent mother, and the adolescent father has been largely ignored. Much work must be done to address adolescent male health, sexuality, and role in teenage pregnancy. The following initiatives appear promising:

- Primary prevention stressing male responsibilities in birth control
- Secondary prevention geared toward increasing adolescent fathers' role in pregnancy and child care
- Tertiary prevention directed at improving parenting skills and supporting lifestyle changes (e.g., education, job training) that increase the possibility of financial stability and independence

Nursing Role in Teenage Pregnancy

It is apparent that pregnancy during the teenage years presents some unique risks and special needs for the teenager, her pregnancy, and her infant. The best choice for most young girls is to delay pregnancy until they are physically and emotionally mature. For this reason, primary prevention is a crucial component of any intervention program. However, if young girls become pregnant, it is imperative that they receive adequate prenatal care coupled with long-term postpartum follow-up to ensure a healthy outcome for both mother and child.

A comprehensive intervention program should address all prevention levels: primary, secondary, and tertiary. Perrin (1992) recommends that all programs include the "4 M's": managing, mending, mentoring, and modeling. Community health nurses, because of their expertise in assessment, health teaching, and program development, are well suited to this task. Their accessibility to adolescent populations places them in a pivotal position to play a significant role in the delivery of care before sexual activity and contraception, during pregnancy, and during long-term follow-up with the parents and child.

Secondary Prevention: The Case of Pregnant Teenagers

National health objectives for maternal and infant health are listed in Table 22–3. When a teenager becomes pregnant, care is directed toward providing a satisfactory and healthy outcome. The critical elements of any program are as follows:

- Early detection
- Pregnancy resolution services
- Prenatal health care
- Childbirth education
- Parenting education

EARLY DETECTION

Early detection provides a longer time to decide what to do about the pregnancy and a longer period of prenatal care if the adolescent decides to continue the pregnancy. Community health nurses can facilitate early detection by considering the possibility of pregnancy during the initial assessment of physical complaints by female adolescents. Fatigue, appetite loss, nausea and vomiting, weight loss, or missed menstrual periods coupled with a history of sexual activity and inadequate birth control, are indicative symptoms.

Sensitive but direct questioning is important. The nurse's demeanor and attitude during an interview can facilitate or hamper the assessment process. The community health nurse must be accepting of the teenager or else the teenager will be reluctant to share information, ask questions, and express concerns. It is not uncommon for teenagers to deny or attempt to hide their pregnancy. If the nurse is brusque or abrupt, it is unlikely the teenager will feel comfortable seeking or volunteering information of an intimate nature.

Previous experience with nurses and other health care providers has an impact on a teenager's willingness to seek care when in need. Allen (1980) reports that the most important reason for delaying care among teenagers is nonuse of the health care system for medical needs. Nonuse was often related to past negative experiences with health care providers. Young children and teenagers are astute observers, and the community health nurse can act as an advocate for the system by taking care to ensure that young clients are always treated with respect and dignity.

PREGNANCY RESOLUTION SERVICES

Once pregnancy is confirmed, the teenager faces an important decision. The American College of Obstetrics and Gynecology, Planned Parenthood, the American Nurses' Association, and numerous other professional health care organizations take the position that a comprehensive program should include all possible pregnancy options: abortion, adoption, and keeping the baby.

TABLE 22–3

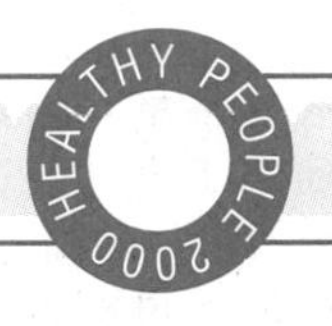

Healthy People 2000: Maternal and Infant Health

Health Status Objectives

Reduce infant mortality to no more than 7 deaths per 1000 births (31% reduction; blacks to 11 deaths per 1000 births)

Risk Reduction Objectives

Reduce low birth weight to no more than 5% of live births (28% decrease; blacks to no more than 9% of live births)

Reduce severe complications of pregnancy to no more than 15 per 100 deliveries (currently 22 per 100)

Increase abstinence from tobacco use by pregnant women to at least 90% and increase abstinence from alcohol, cocaine, and marijuana by pregnant women by at least 20% (currently 75% for tobacco; no statistics available on drugs)

Service and Protection Objectives

Increase first trimester prenatal care to at least 90% of live births (18% increase)

Increase to at least 60% the proportion of primary care providers who provide age-appropriate preconception care and counseling (no current baseline)

Increase to at least 90% the proportion of women and infants who receive risk-appropriate care (no current baseline)

Increase to at least 90% the proportion of infants age 18 months and younger who receive recommended primary care services at the appropriate intervals (no current baseline).

From U.S. Department of Health and Human Services. (1990). *Healthy people 2000: National health objectives* (DHHS Publication No. (PHS) 91-50213). Washington, DC: U.S. Government Printing Office.

Abortion

Adolescents choose abortion more frequently than adults and wait longer to do so. Almost 40% of all adolescent pregnancies are terminated by abortion (CDF, 1986). Melton and Russo (1987) report that teenagers have late abortions (after 12 weeks' gestation) twice as often as adult women.

Abortion is a controversial issue. Both supporters and opponents are vocal and strident. Since 1980 abortion opponents have attempted to reduce access to and availability of abortion services. Efforts were concentrated at the federal level and were aimed at reducing funding and tightening regulations for programs receiving public money. Federal funding for Medicaid abortion services was eliminated. Any state that wanted to continue funding had to assume all the costs for abortion services. Some states chose to continue funding, while others chose not to do so. Because many pregnant teenagers are served by publicly supported programs, their access to abortion services was directly affected by the changes.

Federal regulations in the 1980s imposed restrictions on health professionals involved in counseling adolescents. Counselors, including nurses, were banned from listing abortion as an option, from exploring teenagers' personal perceptions of the advantages and disadvantages of the procedure, and from providing referrals for abortion services (Bullis, 1992). The American Public Health Association joined with professional nursing organizations and most other major professional health care organizations in opposition to this ruling. President Clinton rescinded this order when he took office in 1993.

Currently restrictive efforts are primarily targeted at the states in an attempt to change the legal criteria for abortion services (e.g., parental notification and waiting periods) (Wilmoth, 1992). Melton and Russo (1987) report that these restrictions are costly, cause embarrassment to the adolescent, and merely delay rather than prevent abortions. The Supreme Court has upheld some but not all of the state initiatives on parental notification and waiting periods (Bullis, 1992). In general, state initiatives that allow teenagers an alternative to parental notification or do not impose an "undue burden" in waiting time have been upheld; the remainder have not.

It is difficult to determine whether abortion restrictions have had an impact on teenage abortion. There has been no appreciable change in the rate of teenagers seeking abortion services. The unresolved question is whether abortion rates would have been higher without the legal and financial obstacles. Stevens and associates (1992) report that limited access to Medicaid funding increases the hardships for low-income women who choose the abortion option.

For many health care providers, including community health nurses, the abortion issue was their first personal experience with practice limitations. For some, it produced a personal ethical crisis. As one nurse related in reference to the "gag rule":

> I had to decide whether to follow my professional commitment to provide comprehensive counseling to pregnant teens or to follow federal regulations.

A few health care providers agreed with the restrictions, some disagreed but followed them, some found ways to circumvent them, and some completely disregarded them. Most public health nurses involved in family planning services favor accessible abortion as a pregnancy resolution option (Oakley et al., 1990).

Adoption

Adoption is a less controversial but infrequent choice for teenagers. Only 1 in 20 pregnant teenagers chooses this option. White teenagers are more likely to relinquish their infants for adoption than are black teenagers (Hayes, 1987). Teenagers who choose adoption are older, farther along in their schooling, and are more future oriented with respect to educational goals than are teenagers who keep their infants (McLaughlin et al., 1988).

Along with efforts to restrict abortion during the 1980s, there was a federal effort directed by the Office of Adolescent Pregnancy Programs to encourage the adoption option among pregnant teenagers. Research studies were funded that were intended to improve the likelihood of adoption and to identify factors that influenced the adoption choice. The results have been inconclusive; no appreciable change has occurred in the adoption rate among the targeted groups (Nichols, 1991).

Adolescents appear satisfied with their pregnancy decisions. Despite assertions that teenagers who choose abortion or adoption suffer negative psychologic consequences, no evidence supports this position (Wilmoth, 1992). In general, teenagers feel they made the best personal choice at the time. Most are satisfied with their decision, although adoption choosers are slightly less satisfied than others (McLaughlin et al., 1988).

PRENATAL HEALTH CARE

Once a teenager decides to continue the pregnancy, effort is directed toward ensuring a healthy outcome for the mother and infant. Early initiation and regular continuance of prenatal care significantly reduce the risk for both adolescents and their infants (Saller and Crenshaw, 1987; American Nurses' Association [ANA], 1987).

Prenatal Programs Available To Teenagers

Three types of programs offer prenatal care to adolescents: clinic programs, private medical services, and school-based prenatal programs. The choice of program depends on the accessibility and the financial circumstances of the teenager and her family.

Private practice care is provided by physicians in single or group practice or associated with a health maintenance organization. Usually these services are available only to people who are covered by a medical insurance plan or can afford to pay. Most family insurance plans limit coverage to children under 18 years of age, although some plans will provide coverage until age 21 or 23 if the child is a full-time college student. Parents may be surprised to find that their child is not insured and unprepared to meet the expenses of pregnancy when their child is not a full-time student.

For families without insurance or the financial resources to pay for prenatal care, there are several options. One option is medical assistance. With a Medicaid or medical assistance card, prenatal and other services are paid for by a combination of state and federal funds. Teenagers who qualify for Medicaid benefits have some choice in their prenatal care provider, but private physicians and health maintenance organizations may limit the number of Medicaid clients they accept. The pregnant adolescent and her family may have to approach a number of service providers before being accepted by one. In these circumstances, community nurses act as a resource by providing the family with a list of practitioners willing to accept Medicaid patients.

Prenatal and obstetrical clinics associated with publicly funded hospitals accept medical assistance clients. They also offer sliding-fee programs for people with limited financial means who do not qualify for Medicaid. Other sources of prenatal clinic care are state and county health departments. Some hospitals and health departments operate satellite clinics in low-income neighborhoods with high rates of adolescent pregnancy. Because socioeconomic status has been associated with a greater number of potential complications, clinics serving low-income teenagers expect to experience a larger number of clients requiring intense supervision. The community health nurse can identify pregnant teenagers, refer them for medical care, and provide home visits to personalize education.

Prenatal care services that prove successful in getting teenagers to utilize and comply with the overall program of care are those that provide an accepting, caring atmosphere and work to reduce obstacles to beginning or continuing care. The best results have been in comprehensive community-based programs with a heavy outreach and educational emphasis, using multidisciplinary health care teams, especially community health nurse involvement, and home visits (Goldberg et al., 1986). The community health nurse acts as the broker or case manager of prenatal care and sees that clients are provided with needed services. The nurse is the team member who spends the most time with the adolescent, providing most of the health screening assessments, counseling, and education for pregnant clients.

School-based prenatal services are offered in conjunction with other school-run clinic services or in separate schools designed for the exclusive use of pregnant teenagers (Washburn, 1989; Oda, 1991). School-based prenatal services also employ a comprehensive approach to care and are usually found in large school districts with high rates of adolescent pregnancy. Generally they are not readily available in smaller school districts and rural areas. Prenatal school programs generally result in a high degree of compliance with appointments and the care regimen, a reduction in the number of complications, and a secondary benefit of increased school attendance both before and after delivery (Schmitter, 1984; Miller, 1984).

Special Needs of Pregnant Adolescents

A standard obstetrics text should serve as the basis for formulating a comprehensive plan of care. However, there are some special concerns that the community health nurse must consider when planning prenatal care for pregnant teenagers. As previously noted, adolescent mothers and their infants are at greater risk for serious medical problems than older mothers and their infants. Age alone is not the problem. The risk associated with early pregnancy has been correlated with factors such as lower socioeconomic status, poor prenatal care, inadequate nutrition, and unhealthy lifestyle practices (Isbner and Wright, 1987). When care is taken to reduce the associated risks, teenage pregnancy is less problematic.

Nichols (1991) states that the essential components of a prenatal program to reduce low-birth-weight infants should include the following:

- Ongoing risk assessment
- Individual care and case management
- Nutrition counseling
- Health education aimed at reducing poor health habits
- Stress reduction
- Social support services

In addition, any good prenatal program should include preparation for labor and delivery, introduction to newborn care, and exploration of birth control options for postdelivery use. Table 22–4 provides more detail on specific health issues related to nutrition and health habits in teenagers.

Support Systems

During pregnancy the expectant teenager looks for emotional, financial, and physical support from family members. The community health nurse and other caregivers must be alert when assessing the degree of support available from family and others. Adolescent pregnancy is often associated with or precipitates a family crisis. Some families may be unable or unwilling to provide support. If

TABLE 22–4

Nutrition and Health Habits of Special Interest in Adolescent Pregnancy

Nutritional Oversight

Pregnancy places additional demands on growing bodies. Pay careful attention to weight gain, diet adequacy, and compliance with prenatal vitamin supplements. Adolescents can recall the basic food groups and recommended servings for adequate nutritional intake. However, basic knowledge does not constitute compliance with nutritional demands. A more accurate picture is established by monitoring weight and reviewing a 24- to 72-hour diet recall. It is harder for the teenager to spontaneously fabricate a nutritionally sound diet than recite the components of a sound diet.

Some prenatal programs provide referral and consultation with a registered dietitian. A nutritionist can tailor nutritional information to specific needs (e.g., ethnic, religious, or vegetarian preferences). Specifically tailored dietary pamphlets are available from the U.S. Department of Agriculture or the American Dietetic Association.

The Women, Infants, and Children (WIC) supplemental food program is available for pregnant teenagers and their infants. Studies indicate that the program has been especially effective in reducing the risk of low birth weight and improving the chance of full-term delivery for teenagers and single women (Hayes, 1987).

Teenagers in need of drastic dietary modifications often respond best to gradual changes. Nutritional contracts between the community health nurse and the teenager can provide for gradual additions or deletions. For example, three glasses of milk per day can be added to a diet very poor in calcium and dairy products during one clinic visit, and certain junk foods can be reduced or eliminated at the next visit. This will eventually result in a more nutritionally sound diet. Incremental adjustments with positive reinforcement are successful because they give the adolescent reachable, realistic goals while reaffirming her partnership in the effort.

Body Image

For most teenagers body image is inexplicably linked to self-esteem. The teenage years are a time of heightened concern with appearance and attractiveness. Teenage girls are very concerned about their weight, and pregnancy brings a change in shape and weight. Young women may have underlying eating disorders such as bulimia or anorexia. Some teenagers want to conceal their pregnancy because they are ashamed, afraid, or feel less attractive to their partner. Nurses should assess the adolescent's attitude toward the weight gain and bodily changes associated with her pregnancy.

Watch for attempts to conceal poor weight gain (i.e., with large, sloppy clothing or a refusal to wear maternity clothing). If there is no financial or fashion explanation for such behavior, consider pregnancy adjustment difficulty. Counseling is appropriate. It is especially important that pregnant adolescents with eating disorders receive immediate treatment to reduce fetal risk.

Education on appropriate weight gains and normal body changes during and after the pregnancy help allay anxiety. A review of the "normal" weight loss that can be expected immediately after delivery and during the initial postpartum period will also prepare the teenager for the most likely results. Stressing good nutrition as a means of benefiting the fetus as well as controlling excessive weight gain would be one way to link a healthy diet intake to the teenager's interest in her figure.

Stress Associated with Pregnancy

Clothing and general appearance provide clues to general well-being in addition to those associated with concealment or weight concerns. An unkempt appearance (beyond the current fashion trends) and inattention to body hygiene may signal self-esteem difficulties and depression. Serious mental health issues always require follow-up. If the nurse can determine that the attitudinal change is associated with pregnancy, it is likely to be an outward sign of conflict related to the pregnancy. A realization of the eminent arrival of parenthood can precipitate a crisis. The teenager must struggle with the infant's effect on her, her partner, and her family's future. The first sign of this crisis may be disheveled appearance, poor hygiene, multiple days absent from school, or inattentiveness to school work and performance.

Sexual Activity and Risk of Sexually Transmitted Diseases

Although sexually active, teenagers often do not have accurate information concerning reproductive biology, disease transmission, or effective birth control practices. They are hesitant to ask questions or engage in dialogue on sex-related subjects with health care professionals and other adults. Prenatal care providers must assume the responsibility for incorporating health teaching in this area. Issues to address include an assessment of the teenager's knowledge of the process of procreation; information related to continued sexual activity during pregnancy; clear explanations of the need for abstinence when medical conditions warrant; and a review of the risks related to sexually transmitted diseases (STDs).

Pregnant adolescents are at high risk for a concurrent STD. Studies indicate that 40% to 50% of all pregnant teenagers have an STD, usually *Chlamydia*, gonorrhea, syphilis, or trichomoniasis (Pomeranz et al., 1991; Oh et al., 1993). If the teenager has an STD, there are a number of important areas to stress:

- Clear instructions regarding the treatment regimen, the importance of compliance, and complications associated with an untreated STD
- Health teaching about STDs in general, stressing risky behavior and safer sex precautions
- Regular monitoring during prenatal visits to ensure problem resolution (Oh et al., 1993)

Sexually active teenagers are often too embarrassed to speak freely about sexual matters with partners. They often do not know their partners' history with respect to other contacts or STDs. Along with misinformation or misconceptions about transmission routes and the likelihood of infection, sexual ignorance contributes the probability of reinfection. The community health nurse who can establish a good rapport with prenatal teenagers improves the likelihood that this information will be accepted and applied. At the very least, the nurse should help the adolescent to reduce risky sexual practices. Teenagers with a history of multiple partners or who tolerate a partner's multiple sexual contacts require long-term monitoring and counsel. The use or toleration of multiple partners is often indicative of serious personal difficulties. The nurse's goal should be establishing a relationship that encourages and supports long-term counseling.

TABLE 22–4

Nutrition and Health Habits of Special Interest in Adolescent Pregnancy *Continued*

Cigarette Smoking and Use of Other Drugs

Cigarette smoking or drug or alcohol use will increase the risk of complications in the adolescent and her infant. Public health professionals are concerned that cigarette use is increasing in adolescent girls while decreasing in most other groups. Smoking is associated with lower birth weights in infants.

The National Longitudinal Youth Survey reported on the association between drugs and adolescent pregnancy. The results showed that adolescent females who use illicit drugs are four times more likely to become pregnant than those who do not (Mensch and Kandel, 1992). Accurate assessment of the type of substance, amount, and regularity of use is crucial. Any harmful substances should be discouraged. Teenagers tend to separate cause and effect as well as "tune out" information provided by adults. For this reason it is important to present information in a factual manner without embellishment.

Any substance assessment should include the use of prescription and over-the-counter medications. Drugs used to treat common adolescent problems, such as acne and allergies, or over-the-counter medications such as aspirin or weight control pills might be overlooked by teenagers when providing a drug history.

Rest and Activity Schedules

Teenagers may continue with a reasonably active schedule when there are no serious problems. Adolescents should be reminded that short periods of rest are important. Extensive activity with little rest or sleep time, or extremely vigorous activities and sports should be curtailed for the duration of the pregnancy. The community health nurse should review the teenager's normal activity schedule at several intervals during the prenatal program to ensure that these activities fall within normal limits or within the recommended range if restrictions apply.

Teenagers in school can be excused from gym class by a physician's note. If gym consists of relatively mild exercises or noncontact sports, then the mother can attend for most of the pregnancy. Sometimes, the adolescent is embarrassed to go to the gym even when physical activity is not particularly strenuous. Healthy physical activity should be encouraged, but not at the risk of emotional stress.

this is the case, the teenager will need help identifying, assessing, and selecting other possible support sources.

There are a number of potential sources: other relatives, the father of the infant and his family, church organizations, other community groups, and clubs and organizations in which the teenager has participated. The state social services agency can provide financial support and medical services (Medicaid). If the teenager is separated from her family, social services can arrange financial assistance for housing or, for younger teenagers, foster care.

Pregnancy for adolescents often accompanies other personal problems or emotional issues. Problems that began before the pregnancy usually last long after the pregnancy is resolved, including poor school performance or attendance, few close personal relationships, multiproblem family situations, and unemployment. Adolescents in such circumstances often have diminished self-esteem. Failure to address related problems and issues in a supportive, caring atmosphere is equivalent to providing only partial care to the pregnant adolescent. Persistent home visitation by the community health nurse is one way to provide long-term support. Olds and associates (1988) report that adolescent mothers visited by community health nurses had better employment records, fewer pregnancies, and delayed a second pregnancy longer than adolescents who did not receive home visits.

The Adolescent Father

Secondary prevention efforts aim to improve parental participation in prenatal care, childbirth preparation, and parenting activities ("Pregnancy program targets teen fathers," 1991). Such programs are intended to improve the quality and duration of the father–child relationship. Community health nurses can assist in these efforts by encouraging the father's participation in prenatal visits.

Most fathers are curious and interested in the process of gestation and delivery but are uncomfortable asking questions and hesitant in interacting with adult health care providers. The community health nurse can invite the father to prenatal classes, encourage questions and participation in prenatal visits, and acknowledge the father's role as a partner in the birth process. Fathers can be encouraged, but not forced, into participating in the delivery process.

CHILDBIRTH EDUCATION

Teenagers are likely to get information about labor and delivery from their peers; much of this may be erroneous. Community health nurses can assess the teenager's knowledge base, correct misconceptions, and reinforce valid information. If the adolescent's mother or other relative is involved, the nurse should include her or him in the dialogue. The mother's knowledge base may be incorrect or outdated if it consists solely of her own personal experiences. Including the mother in the interview allows the nurse to correct misinformation, acknowledge the mother's contribution to her daughter's care, and facilitate the mother's cooperation with the prenatal and postpartum programs.

The delivery of a child usually represents a pregnant adolescent's first experience with hospitalization. Most hospitals or birthing centers provide tours and orientation prior to delivery. Whenever possible, teenagers should be encouraged to attend an orientation program. Most facilities allow a support person to remain with the teenager during delivery. The nurse might have to help the teenager choose her support person, especially if a number of persons are available. This decision should be made as soon as possible. If the teenager has opted for natural childbirth classes, the person who will support her in labor should attend classes with her if at all possible.

Delivery care costs may be separate from prenatal services, especially if prenatal care is provided by a private physician. Teenagers with private health insurance or medical assistance are covered or can afford delivery costs. Hospital-based or health department prenatal clinics usually have reduced fee programs for teenagers or families with financial hardships. Most teenagers, because they are on a limited budget, can qualify. Community health nurses providing prenatal care are aware of the financial resources available within their communities and can refer teenagers and families for the necessary financial help. Social workers in prenatal clinics or the hospital can be useful in providing this assistance.

PARENTING EDUCATION

Postpartum Care

Postdelivery care varies widely in scope and duration of services. All prenatal programs provide a postpartum check for the mother. A well-baby check is included in most services, although a private obstetrical practice may rely on the mother to make her own arrangements for all infant care. The most extensive postpartum care is delivered in community programs that rely heavily on nurses. These programs usually include the following:

- Health assessment of both mother and infant
- Newborn care education and supervision
- Parental education on growth and development and parenting skills
- Review of role adjustments and available supports
- Sex education and birth control information

One valuable component of these programs is the emphasis on regular contact with the new mother, starting the first week after delivery. Studies show that regular nurse visits reduce anxiety and increase infant health as measured by fewer accidents and emergency department visits than in infants not visited (Olds et al., 1986a, 1986b). Mothers experience many concerns or problems prior to the first scheduled clinic or physician visit. Earlier contacts allow the teenager and nurse to address these issues and reduce anxiety. Contact need not always be in person; some care can be provided by telephone monitoring of the new mother.

Health Status of the New Mother. At a minimum, the new mother should have a 6-week postpartum examination. Some community health programs start home visits at about 2 weeks postpartum. The physical assessment should focus on the standard postpartum areas as well as on specific concerns of the adolescent. Consistent with teenagers' concern about body image, frequent questions about weight loss and figure restoration include the following:

- "How long will it take me to lose all the weight?"
- "Why is my figure different even though I'm back to my normal weight?"
- "When is it safe to diet?"
- "When can I start an exercise or diet program to lose weight?"

Role Adjustment and Emotional Support

Adjusting to the role of parent during adolescence is particularly difficult. Conflict is not unexpected. The adolescent mother needs support as she attempts to integrate her new responsibilities into her daily routine. The teenager may be juggling school and infant care. Fatigue and stress are common and can be exacerbated if she attempts to resume her social activities in addition to her other obligations. The first task, and one that may best be accomplished on a home visit, is to assess the support systems available to the teenage mother. If the adolescent is involved in a comprehensive prenatal–postpartum program, then health care professionals have already assessed available support. If not, the nurse should look at the immediate family, other relatives, significant others, and the father of the infant and his family. Even if support systems are adequate, the family may need some help in understanding and supporting the adolescent as a maturing individual.

A common problem in families is role conflict. Family members may expect the teenager to instantly become an adult and mother, or the opposite, to remain a child and allow her parents to assume all the responsibilities for her infant. Neither situation is especially healthy for the adolescent or infant. Ideally, both parents should be encouraged to continue developing as individuals (for example, to continue their education, participate in some social activities, and explore relationships with peers) and at the same time increase their proficiency and confidence in parenting.

When support is minimal or lacking, the community health nurse may be able to refer the teenager to other possible resources, such as parenting programs, cooperative daycare, or programs that pair the new mother with an older adolescent mother with a successful experience. One such program, the Nike-Footed Health Worker Project (Perino, 1992) pairs older teenagers trained to provide support and guidance with younger teenagers in an effort to improve parenting skills.

Adequate support is an important concern, because adolescent mothers have higher rates of child abuse and neglect (Elster et al., 1983). Adequate physical and emotional support, along with health teaching and realistic expectations for their children, successfully reduces the incidence of abuse and neglect in at-risk mothers (Marshall et al., 1991; Olds et al., 1986) (see Chapter 20).

Health Status of the Newborn

In addition to the usual newborn assessment, the community health nurse should look for signs of adequate maternal–infant bonding. Evidence of attachment includes calling a child by its given name, cuddling, talking to the infant, and demonstrating an interest in infant care and development. Sometimes teenagers demonstrate difficulty in bonding simply because they have had no previous experience with infants and are afraid to do anything. Sometimes another person has assumed the role of caregiver and the teenager becomes an observer rather than caregiver. Bonding can be evaluated in clinic situations, but home visits allow the nurse a more accurate picture of the nature and the scope of the teen–infant relationship, as the nurse can observe for a longer time and evaluate the interaction among the infant, teenager, and other caregivers. When another person assumes most of the responsibilities for infant care, the nurse should explore the adolescent's wishes. The teenager may want to care for her infant and may simply require encouragement, demonstration, and supervision to become confident in infant care. The nurse may have to suggest that family members help by supporting the teenager as she attempts to establish a relationship with her child.

Health Teaching Regarding Newborn Care

Most prenatal care includes basic information about child care, although the extent of the content varies. Adolescents will have had more formalized classroom instruction if they participate in a school-based prenatal program. Even if the teenager has received extensive preparation, she will usually need health teaching reinforced after delivery. The most common topics teenagers identify for review and reinforcement are listed in Table 22–5.

Because teenagers are usually present oriented, they frequently do not pay attention to information that has no immediate relevance. Then the infant arrives and problems develop. It is very frightening to be in the position of caring for a tiny infant and be presented with a crisis.

- "My (1-week-old) baby won't eat, I've tried everything: formula, toast, and oatmeal!"

TABLE 22–5

Suggested Health Teaching Topics and Content for Teenage Mothers

Positioning and handling of infant
Nutrition (Breast-/bottle-feeding technique, feeding schedule, dietary recommendations for the first 6 months, and vitamin and iron supplements)
Hygiene (Skin care and bathing, care of diaper rash, nail care, and umbilical and circumcision care)
Elimination (Diapering and frequency of changes, bowel movements [frequency and appearance], constipation, and recognition of problems)
Growth and development (Normal growth and development, chart of developmental milestones, and suggested techniques to encourage development)
Immunization schedule (Recommended schedule, rationale for administration, possible side effects)
Recognition of illness (Behaviors that signal distress or discomfort, thermometer reading and normal vs. abnormal readings, common symptoms [e.g., upper respiratory infection, dehydration, and diarrhea]), teenager's health coverage and selection of a clinic or private physician

- "My baby won't stop crying; he cries for a solid hour and then starts again!"
- "My baby won't stop having bowel movements. They are so runny, and now he has little pink dots all over his behind."

Under these circumstances, the teenage mother becomes very receptive to reviewing and discussing child care issues. Community health nurses should take advantage of the adolescent's concern to teach healthy infant care and distinguish between normal and abnormal infant behavior.

An important point to remember is that people vary in child care custom and practices. Child care techniques common to a culture or family tradition need not be discouraged or eliminated if they do no harm. For example, some families swaddle (tightly wrap) infants, whereas others do not; some introduce solid foods early, others do not; some use an umbilical band, others do not; some pierce the infant's ears, others do not. When the nurse comes in contact with child care practices contrary to the agency's standard protocol or teaching plan, or to her or his own personal habits or values, the practices should be evaluated in terms of harmfulness. Any health care professional who discourages or disapproves of practices posing no harm runs an unnecessary risk of altering or alienating the family–provider relationship. An important question to ask is, "Is this care issue worth jeopardizing my ability to continue to provide health care to this mother and her infant?" If the answer is "no," then clearly you are better off not running the risk.

Sexual Activity and Contraceptive Use

Ideally, contraception should be addressed as part of the prenatal program. The adolescent must decide if she will continue sexual activity and must be honest with the nurse about her decision. Sometimes the mother is no longer involved with the father of the infant and announce that she does not intend to be sexually active or to have another child. These girls should be helped to explore the risks involved if they change their minds without adequate protection. The community health nurse can help the adolescent select the most appropriate form of contraception from several alternatives. Once an adolescent has been pregnant, she risks repeating the situation. Fifteen percent of teenagers are pregnant again within 1 year, and 30% are pregnant again by the end of 2 years (AGI, 1981).

Even if there is no immediate need, contraception should be reviewed. If the adolescent has already used birth control, it is helpful to identify the method, how it was used, and the reason for discontinuance. Such a review helps the nurse to determine whether contraception was used properly and to correct any misconceptions or faulty technique. Make sure that the teenager is aware of community resources (family planning clinics) where she may be supplied with contraceptives.

Primary Prevention

National health objectives for family planning are listed in Table 22–6. Approximately 55% of teenagers in the United States are sexually active and thus at risk for pregnancy (MMWR, 1992). At least 48% of females and 61% of males in the teenage population are at risk of becoming a parent. Clearly one of the most important tasks in reducing teenage pregnancy is to intervene with at-risk groups. Although teenagers from low-socioeconomic-status households and those with less education are at greatest risk, pregnancy is a significant factor for all teenage groups. Interventions should be targeted to all.

Primary prevention of teenage pregnancy has three focuses:

1. To delay or stop participation in sexual activity
2. To provide access to contraceptives
3. To strengthen future life goals

Most experts believe that a comprehensive primary prevention program should include sex education, family life education, family planning, and some form of life planning program that stresses identification of future goals and steps to those goals (Furstenberg, 1980). Most of the available primary prevention programs address one or two but not all aspects of a comprehensive program.

EDUCATION PROGRAMS

Three of the elements of a comprehensive prevention program are addressed in educational initiatives. A good program will include all three: sex, family life, and contraceptive education. Most educational efforts are school based. Sex education is provided by some private schools and by public schools in approximately 70% of the states (Norr, 1991). These programs receive limited funding, and in most, student access is limited. A typical sex education effort consists of fewer than 10 class periods scattered throughout a student's 12 years of education.

TABLE 22–6

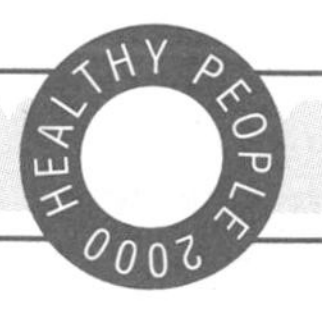

Healthy People 2000: Family Planning

Health Status Objectives

Reduce teenage pregnancies to no more than 50 per 1000 girls aged 17 and younger (30% decrease; black adolescents to 120 per 1000 [current baseline, 186]; Hispanic adolescents to 105 per 1000 [current baseline, 158])

Reduce unintended pregnancies to no more than 30% of pregnancies (46% decrease; black women to 40% [current, 78%])

Risk Reduction Objectives

Reduce the proportion of adolescents who have engaged in intercourse to no more than 15% by age 15 and 40% by age 17 (current baseline, 27% girls and 33% boys age 15; 50% girls and 66% boys by age 17)

Increase to at least 90% the proportion of sexually active unmarried young who use contraception (current baseline, 78% at most recent intercourse; 63% at first intercourse among young women age 15 to 19)

Service and Protection Objectives

Increase to at least 85% the proportion of people ages 10 through 18 who have discussed human sexuality, including values, with parents and/or have received information through another parentally endorsed source such as school (current baseline, 66%).

From U.S. Department of Health and Human Services. (1990). *Healthy people 2000: National health objectives* (DHHS Publication No. (PHS) 91-50213). Washington, DC: U.S. Government Printing Office.

Sex and Contraception Content

Sex education contains, at the very least, information about the anatomy and physiology of reproduction in males and females. Beyond this narrow focus, there is little agreement and much controversy over appropriate content for sex education classes. A good sex education program encourages self-esteem and responsible decision making in addition to containing specific information on sexual matters.

Some programs include information on sexual orientation, sexually transmitted diseases, and contraceptives. These topics are the most contentious and engender public debate and opposition by parents or community groups. When faced with protest, school districts are reluctant to go against parental wishes. Thirty percent of states discourage or prohibit pregnancy prevention content (Kenney et al., 1989). School districts are also reluctant to improve or add to existing content because it might generate renewed public interest and opposition. Teachers feel constrained by community opposition, and some stick to a prepared script rather than risk discussion and exploration of sexual topics (Forrest and Silverman, 1989).

The majority of public opinion appears to support sex education with content aimed at reducing teenage pregnancies (Schubot and Schmidt, 1989). Opponents are often well organized and very vocal. The Surgeon General of the United States has made clear the intention to upgrade sex education content, including contraceptive information, and to improve teenagers' access to contraceptive services.

The best way to reduce concern and increase community support of sex education is to expand the content to address community concerns wherever possible. Although a comprehensive sex education curriculum cannot ignore contraceptive information, there are legitimate issues related to abstinence, the advantages of delayed sexual activity, and the medical risks of teenage sexual conduct (e.g., sexually transmitted diseases) that should be addressed. A program that provides such an approach is comprehensive and has the additional advantage of increasing community support. One such program in South Carolina has successfully reduced the pregnancy rate by 50% in just 5 years (Vincent et al., 1987). A description of this program and samples of other innovative primary and tertiary prevention efforts appear in Table 22–7.

Family Life Programs

Family life programs offer information on family systems and the interactions and influences of such systems among family members. Topics include marriage, divorce, separation, and birth. Most family life programs are offered at the junior or senior high school level as an elective course, which means they do not reach many teenagers and can not target those at greatest risk. Family life programs utilize a variety of teaching techniques, including simula-

TABLE 22–7

Community Resources

Adolescent Pregnancy Programs
Office of Population Affairs
U.S. Public Health Service
West Bldg.
5600 Fishers Lane
Rockville, MD 20857
(301) 594-4004
Funds research and demonstration projects

Children's Defense Fund
122 C Street, N.W.
Washington, DC 20001
(202) 628–8787
Provides statistics about children's issues. Advocates for policy changes favorable to children. Funds some projects related to child welfare.

Goodwill Industries of America, Inc.
9200 Wisconsin Avenue
Bethesda, MD 20814
(301) 530–6500
Local Goodwill stores are a good resource for used clothing and furniture for poor families.

March of Dimes Birth Defects Foundation
1275 Mamaroneck Avenue
White Plains, NY 10605
(914) 428–7100
Funds research for serious child health problems.

National Commission to Prevent Infant Mortality (Congressional Commission)
330 C. St., S.W., Room 2014
Washington, DC 20201
(202) 205–8364

Planned Parenthood Federation of America, Inc.
810 7th Avenue
New York, NY 10019
(212) 541–7800
Provides effective birth control services for all, including the financially disadvantaged. Works at the national level to influence legislation concerning reproduction.

Salvation Army
120 West 14th St.
New York, NY 10011
(212) 541–7800
Local Salvation Army stores are a good resource for used clothing, furniture, and infant equipment for poor families. Many provide additional services locally to needy families.

Women, Infants, and Children Program
Information Officer
Food and Nutrition Program
U.S. Dept. of Agriculture
Alexandria, VA 22302
(703) 305–2276
Provides supplemental food and infant formula for qualified pregnant women and their infants. Local distribution is handled by local area health departments or other agencies. For your local distribution agency or further information, contact the Department of Agriculture address above.

tion and game playing, which helps concrete thinkers consider the rigors as well as the delights of parenting. One popular technique requires students to assume full time personal responsibility for the welfare of a raw egg for 1 week. Students must ensure that the egg is always in the presence of a responsible person and comes to no harm. They are then graded on how well they accomplish the task.

Role of the Nurse in Education

In some school systems with school nurses, the nurse is involved in both sex and family life education. If family life courses are not available in the school system or are not reaching at-risk teenagers, nurses may consider implementing a program with their community agency's support or in conjunction with other community organizations such as the Young Men's or Young Women's Christian Association.

Community health nurses can provide factual sex education to teenagers in class as they provide other health services. Most sex education teachers have little training in sex education (Forrest and Silverman, 1989). For many, sex education is not their primary focus. They may have been "drafted" because they teach science or have a free class period. Nurses are effective sex educators because they are equipped to provide sexual content in a factual and nonsensational approach. They are also proficient at encouraging and guiding client discussion, characteristics helpful in addressing sex education with teenagers.

CONTRACEPTIVE SERVICES

Access to and regular use of birth control is the goal of contraceptive services for adolescents. Family planning clinics and private physicians are one source; school-based clinics are a more recent effort. Table 22–8 provides examples of several school-based contraceptive programs.

Community health nurses can encourage clinic attendance, promote access to contraception, and provide referrals to appropriate contraceptive services when counseling individuals or teaching sex education classes. The

TABLE 22–8

Selected Examples of Prevention Programs

Prevention	Program	Description
Primary Prevention	**South Carolina Community Approach**	University-organized project that emphasizes delaying sexual activity for adolescents, provides information on contraception, and promotes consistent contraceptive use for the sexually active teenager. Program includes consultation with community leaders; training of sex education teachers; mini-courses for parents, church, and community leaders; implementation of sex education in all grades; use of radio to announce abstinence and contraceptive messages. *Results:* drop in teenage pregnancy rate from 54% to 25% in 5 years (Vincent, Clearie, and Schluchter, 1987).
Primary Prevention	**Durham, North Carolina**	Similar to the South Carolina project. Involves parents and adolescents in education, role modeling for adolescents, special programs targeting adolescent males. Developed in conjunction with the Young Women's Christian Association, a local college, and a coalition of community groups (Frazier, 1987).
Primary Prevention	**School-based Clinics**	Minneapolis-St. Paul has clinics in junior and senior high schools. These provide family planning, contraceptives, education, and follow-up to increase effectiveness of contraceptive use. Results were positive when compared with clinics that did not offer such intensive care (Edwards, Steinman, Arnold, and Hakanson, 1980).
Primary Prevention	**School-based Clinics**	Johns Hopkins established clinics near schools in Baltimore. Education, counseling, and contraceptives were involved. Intended population was at-risk teens (low-income junior and senior high school students). When compared with control schools (with no services), students had better knowledge and later age at first intercourse, used contraceptives sooner after the start of sexual activity, and had lower pregnancy rates (Zabin, Hardy, Streett, and King, 1984; Zabin, Hirsch, Smith, Streett, and Hardy, 1986; Zabin, Hardy, Smith, and Hirsch, 1986).
Secondary Prevention	**School-based Care**	*Mother-Infant Care Program, St. Paul, MN.* Included infant daycare. Mothers continued before and after delivery. Dropout rate decreased from 45% to 10% (Edwards, Steinman, and Hakanson, 1977).
Secondary Prevention	**School-based Care**	*Adolescent Obstetric Clinic, Medical University of South Carolina.* Developed a similar program but did not include child care. Dropout rate was reduced by 15% (Piechnik and Corbett, 1985).
Secondary Prevention	**School-based Care**	*Young Mothers Educational Development, Syracuse, NY.* Special program for pregnant and young mothers; included daycare. Reported that 68% returned to school after delivery; the majority improved their school performance (Murdock, 1968).
Tertiary Prevention	*Frank Porter Graham Child Development Center.*	Designed for socially disadvantaged parents. Educational daycare from 3 months of age, free medical care, and transportation to center. No formal parental education. Experimental group had fewer pregnancies and their children performed better (educationally) than controls (Campbell, Breitmayer, and Ramey, 1986).
Tertiary Prevention	*Project Redirection.*	Large intervention in four cities; services included employment training, peer group sessions, mentor relationship with an older woman role model for 12 months. Teenagers had fewer repeat pregnancies and stayed longer in school after birth than control groups. There was no difference in employment status between the groups (Polit and Kahn, 1985).
Tertiary Prevention	*Teen Father Collaboration.*	Multiple services offered to adolescent fathers for a period of 2 years. Many different agencies involved, so services were not standardized. Most offered parenting skills training, vocational and job placement, counseling, family planning. No control group. Half returned and completed school; increased employment; most used available counseling services (Sander and Rosen, 1987).

nurse must emphasize the importance of contraceptive use by *all* sexually active adolescents.

The key to compliance with birth control methods in teenagers is a regular, continued attendance at a clinic site (Shea et al., 1984). Any clinic program should provide regular contact and monitor compliance; school-based programs have been particularly successful in this effort (Norr, 1991). The most successful teenagers are those who are persistent and conscientious with birth control from the beginning. Studies show that adolescents who still practice accurate contraception 4 months after starting will continue effective use for 1 to 3 years or longer (Litt and Glader, 1987). Community health nurses are adept at monitoring compliance and encouraging cooperation with adolescents. Nathanson and Becker (1985) found that nurses provided clear, directed, and parent-like (but not authoritarian) guidance that improved compliance.

LIFE OPTIONS PROGRAMS

Life options programs attempt to expand an adolescent's future goals and expectations by improving educational and employment prospects. Because future-oriented, goal-directed adolescents are less likely to become pregnant, the expected result is a reduction in the rate of teenage pregnancies.

Programs may be school or community based and target especially risky populations such as low-income teens (Edelman and Pittman, 1986). Efforts are directed toward reducing social factors associated with increased pregnancy rates (Dryfoos, 1984). Life option programs offer a variety of structures and strategies, including the following:

- One-on-one mentoring and role modeling with successful adults
- Community service participation
- Remedial education
- Tutoring services
- Counseling both professional and peer groups
- Self-worth enhancement techniques
- Exposure to new experiences (e.g., concerts, museums, and travel) to expand life options

These are relatively new programs intended to provide long-term intensive support to targeted teenagers. The results take years to achieve. Norr (1991) suggests that public enthusiasm and funding are minimal because these programs are hard to evaluate and costly and cannot provide speedy results. However, long-term evaluation is needed.

Tertiary Prevention

Tertiary prevention is rehabilitative. With respect to teenage pregnancy, prevention aims to improve the chances of self-sufficiency for adolescent mothers and fathers while ensuring a healthy, supportive environment for their children. None of the interventions are unique to tertiary prevention, aside from those aimed at enhancing child welfare.

Preventing or delaying another pregnancy is a priority. Statistics show that teenagers (both boys and girls) who are parents run a significant risk of having another child while they are still teenagers (Klerman et al., 1982; CDF, 1988). The same strategies employed in primary prevention to avoid pregnancy can be used to prevent repeat pregnancy. Accurate information, accessible contraceptive services, regular clinic visits, and monitored compliance with contraceptive use have been effective in reducing the incidence of a second or third pregnancy in adolescent parents.

Parenting support, ideally started during and immediately after delivery, is continued long term, sometimes for 2 or 3 years. Parenting classes, individual counseling, and peer support groups are all successful interventions (Jones, 1991). Home visits by community health nurses and trained community parent aids provide young mothers and fathers (when present) with encouragement and monitoring.

School-based infant and child care programs are beneficial to young mothers and their children. They increase the likelihood that the mother will complete high school while providing support and guidance for her parenting efforts (Jones, 1991). Infants and children are ensured quality child care, educational companionship, and a "head start" on learning opportunities (Jones, 1991).

A number of innovative interventions have combined strategies into comprehensive support programs (see Table 22–8). Sex education, birth control support, life options steps, parenting support, and child care services have all been promising, although Jones (1991) believes program evaluations need to be longer term with better controls. Evaluation efforts have been short term, with little follow-up beyond 2 to 3 years. Flick (1991) believes this is shortsighted, as the lifestyle changes such programs hope to impact are long term, and benefits may accrue to parents and children beyond the scope of the project. She suggests that programs extend their follow-up to 10 or 15 years. Parenting support and child care services hold particular promise. Flick cites an example of a preschool program that followed children to age 19. This program showed little short-term effect, but by age 19 the preschool group was more educated, less involved in crime and less welfare dependent than a matched cohort (Berruta-Clement et al., 1984).

Conclusion

Teenage pregnancy is a significant problem in the United States. It places adolescent parents and their children at great risk for poverty, poor education, and limited life options. It will remain so as long as society does not vigorously attack the root causes that affect at-risk adolescents.

Nurses, particularly community health nurses, are well suited to address the issues of adolescent pregnancy. Their professional roles in schools, clinics, screening programs, health departments, and community outreach centers provide access to at-risk populations. They have the opportunity, sensitivity, and commitment to work to achieve positive outcomes for adolescents and their children.

Beyond the scope of care to individuals, community health nurses are sensitive to the community in which they practice. Community health nurses are uniquely equipped to assess communities, identify needs and special risk groups, and formulate solutions. Nurses have an obligation to meet the special needs of pregnant adolescents through participating in program design and development, organizing community support, and advocating for policy changes and funding. There is no easy, simple solution to teenage pregnancy. A protracted, balanced, and relentless effort is needed, as a half-hearted, piecemeal approach has negative consequences. The benefits of a comprehensive, committed approach include a more promising future.

KEY IDEAS

1. In the United States an adolescent female's risk of pregnancy is 10% (100 of every 1000 young women), which is significantly higher than in other developed countries.
2. The majority of pregnant teenagers are white. However black and Hispanic teenagers are at greater risk of becoming pregnant and receiving poor prenatal care because of higher poverty rates.
3. There is no single cause of teenage pregnancies; instead, a combination of social and personal factors are responsible.
4. Adolescents who have children are more likely to discontinue education, need public assistance, continue on public assistance for a longer period, and have a poor work history over time than are adolescents who postpone childbearing.
5. Teenage pregnancy follows a generational pattern: Teenage mothers are more likely to have children who also become pregnant during adolescence.
6. Pregnant teenagers and their infants are at greater risk of medical complications (e.g., hypertension, toxemia, anemia, low birth weight, stillbirth, and infant mortality) than older women and their infants.
7. The impact of fatherhood on teenage boys and inclusion of fathers in the maternity and postpartum experience is a relatively new phenomenon.
8. Primary prevention programs that include sex education, contraceptive information, and access to contraceptive services have been found to delay sexual activity and increase contraceptive use in sexually active teenagers.
9. Secondary prevention programs that include early initiation of adequate, regular prenatal care have been documented to reduce medical complications and improve the health status of both pregnant teenagers and their newborn infants.
10. Tertiary prevention programs that provide a variety of support services for new mothers and their infants reduce health risks for both mother and child and increase the chances that the mother will continue her education.
11. Community health nurses have an enormous opportunity to affect the teenage pregnancy rate and improve the status of adolescent mothers and their children.

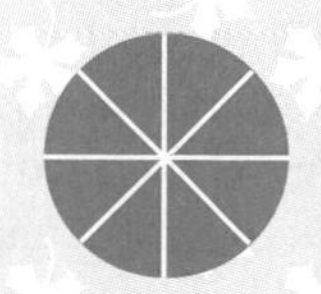

APPLYING THE NURSING PROCESS: *A Pregnant Adolescent*

Ann Jones is a 16-year-old white girl who comes to the family planning clinic for a pregnancy test. She is 5 months pregnant. She tells the community health nurse that she delayed coming to the clinic because she was afraid her mother would talk her into an abortion. In the initial interview the nurse learns that Ann:

- Is happy she is pregnant and wants to keep her infant
- Feels fine
- Does not need maternity clothes because "I am watching my weight and have not gained *one* pound yet"

- Is not sure she can continue to live with her mother because her mother is "mad I got knocked up and is not talking to me right now"
- Is one grade behind but is doing "okay" in school

She also tells the nurse that the father of the infant, Bob, is a sophomore in high school, lives with his parents, and is willing to help with finances. Bob works 15 hours per week at a fast-food restaurant after school. His parents are not yet aware that Ann is pregnant, but Bob thinks they will be very angry with both him and Ann.

Assessment

- Compare actual weight gain with expected weight gain for 20 weeks of pregnancy
- Review dietary intake
- Ascertain what financial assets and health insurance, if any, are available to client
- Determine presence of risk factors associated with poor maternal and infant outcomes
- Ascertain client's knowledge level related to pregnancy, childbirth, and child care

Additional areas for further assessment include:

1. Progress and satisfaction with school, including expected schedule for graduation.
2. Experience with birth control, birth control plans after delivery, and accuracy of sexual knowledge.
3. Experience with child care, accuracy of information, skill level, and education related to deficient areas.
4. Health teaching on growth and development.
5. Community support referrals or resources to provide ongoing support after delivery.

Planning

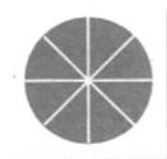

Nursing Diagnoses	Nursing Goals	Nursing Actions
1. Alteration in nutrition less than body requirement related to lack of knowledge and body image concerns.	Adequate dietary intake for a pregnant woman. Normal weight gain during pregnancy.	Accurately assess weight and height. Perform routine prenatal blood tests. Provide prenatal vitamins and instructions. Educate client regarding normal weight gain and relationship to good infant outcome. Perform 72-hour diet recall. Arrange for nutritional consultation with registered dietitian. Arrange for weekly monitoring of weight status.
2. Inadequate support systems related to parental disapproval, age, and earning power of father of the infant.	Immediate adequate financial and emotional support. Assist client to begin future planning for herself and infant.	Determine if Ann can or cannot live at home. Consult with social worker to explore financial assistance eligibility. Review potential support (emotional and financial) (e.g., older independent siblings, other relatives). Request mother to accompany Ann on next clinic visit.

Continued

		Follow up with home visit to gather additional information related to mother–daughter relationship. Arrange for a joint clinic visit to assess Bob's willingness to provide emotional support and his parents' opinion of the pregnancy.
3. Potential for hypertension, anemia, and preeclampsia related to young maternal age and delay in initiation of prenatal care. 4. Potential infant risk for low birth weight and prematurity related to poor prenatal care.	(For both diagnoses 3 and 4): Reduce potential for maternal complications. Reduce potential for poor infant outcomes at delivery.	(For both diagnoses 3 and 4): Arrange for immediate physical assessment by nurse midwife or obstetrician. Complete nursing assessment related to new prenatal client, including health habits, lifestyle patterns, and exposure/use of legal and illegal substances known to affect pregnancy. Perform a home visit to assess the physical environment and resources such as heat, water, food, adequacy of shelter, and potential to accommodate new infant. Develop a health teaching plan to address any health problems found by the nurse and by the physical assessments, teach normal physiological changes associated with pregnancy, and prepare for labor and delivery.

Evaluation

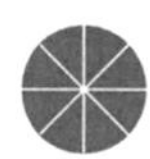

Problem 1

On her first clinic visit Ann's weight (110 lb) and height (5′5″) were recorded and her initial blood tests were performed. These tests showed she was anemic and her blood type was O+.

Her lack of weight gain was problematic. The nurse provided health teaching on normal weight gain during pregnancy (30 to 35 lb) and contracted with Ann to try to gain at least 1 lb per week for the duration of her pregnancy. The nurse also reviewed with Ann her 72-hour diet recall, which was deficient in calories, fruits and vegetables, and dairy products. The nurse and Ann jointly modified Ann's diet, increasing the amount of fruits and vegetables and adding four glasses of whole milk daily as an initial first step.

Because of Ann's late registration for prenatal care and her lack of weight gain, she was scheduled for weekly visits to the clinic for the duration of her pregnancy. The community health nurse planned these visits to monitor her progress and provide positive reinforcement. A nutritional consultation was arranged for her second clinic visit.

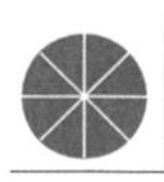

Problem 2

A social work consultation was arranged during the first clinic visit. Ann was uncertain whether she could continue living at home but planned to do so for the near future. The social worker provided her with an emergency telephone number she could call for assistance if a crisis developed in her living arrangements. Ann identified an older sister as someone she could rely on for emotional support but was not sure whether her sister could help with finances, as she was strapped for cash and living with her boyfriend.

Ann was asked to bring Bob and her mother to the clinic during the second or third visit so that the nurse and social worker could discuss Ann's concerns with both of them. Bob came for the second clinic visit, but Ann's mother refused to come to the clinic.

Bob appeared supportive of Ann but was not able to contribute much financially. His parents were very upset by the pregnancy but offered to help Ann with some financial assistance. Bob appeared interested in the progress of Ann's pregnancy; in fact, he was the one who had persuaded her to make the initial appointment.

During a home visit with Ann and her mother, the community health nurse confirmed that Ann's mother was very upset with her and was discouraging her from living at home. The mother stated, "Ann needs to assume her responsibilities as an adult, since she chose to become pregnant." Ann's older sister agreed to allow her to live with her and her boyfriend if Ann could contribute to the household expenses.

The social worker made a visit to the older sister's apartment and considered the living space adequate to accommodate Ann and her infant. She reported to clinic personnel that Ann's sister appeared to be a stable and supportive influence. The social worker assisted Ann with applications for AFDC (welfare), food stamps, and WIC (supplemental food program for women, infants, and children) and arranged for an emergency grant. Ann moved in with her sister after her third clinic visit.

Ann is now in her 27th week of pregnancy and reports that her living arrangements are satisfactory. She has acquired some infant supplies, and Bob's parents have purchased a crib and stroller.

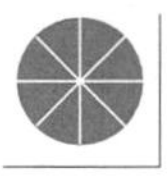

Problems 3 and 4

Ann received a physical examination by a nurse midwife during her second clinic visit. The nurse midwife found her underweight but essentially healthy, but was concerned that her fundal height was smaller than expected for 20 weeks of pregnancy. She suspected intrauterine growth retardation and ordered a sonogram. The sonogram report confirmed her suspicion but recommended a repeat sonogram in 4 weeks, with no amniocentesis at this time.

The nursing assessment indicated that Ann had some lifestyle risks. She admitted to smoking a pack of cigarettes each day and drinking beer during social dates. She denied the use of illegal drugs or marijuana. Her sleep pattern showed that she was in the habit of staying up late at night (1 to 2 A.M.) and on school nights got only 4 or 5 hours of sleep. Ann agreed to try going to sleep by midnight on school nights. The nurse counseled Ann regarding the medical concerns of smoking and drinking during pregnancy. Ann agreed to try to cut down on cigarettes and reported that she could stop drinking because "I only do it when I'm with people who drink; I don't really like the taste of beer."

After her next three clinic visits Ann had gained a total of 10 pounds. She reported that she had cut back to half a pack of cigarettes and was in bed most nights by midnight. She was having a lot more trouble with the smoking changes than with the dietary changes. The nurse and the nutritionist provided positive reinforcement for her efforts.

The community health nurse made a home visit to Ann's new apartment. She found it cluttered but clean. Ann showed her the bedroom and her infant's furniture. The bedroom was crowded with new curtains and wall decorations for the infant. Ann's sister and boyfriend arrived during the visit and spent some time talking with the nurse about expected infant care during the first 3 months. Both expressed interest in helping with the new arrival.

During the remaining clinic visits, the community health nurse plans to address the following topics with Ann:

- Signs and symptoms of true labor and who to call to assist her with the decision to go to the hospital
- What to expect during labor and delivery
- Breast- or bottle feeding
- Plans for birth control after delivery
- Review of growth and development in the infant's first year of life

After delivery Ann will be followed in the family planning clinic, and her infant will be seen for well-baby checks. The health department is participating in a parenting support program and the nurse is recommending that Ann attend that support group.

GUIDELINES FOR LEARNING

1. Identify a client who is a teenage mother in your clinical area and explore with her what she finds rewarding and difficult about her situation. Review her educational progress, her child care, and her living arrangements.
2. Discuss with adolescents their feelings toward sexual activity, perception of risks, and educational and future goals. Encourage them to share their personal experiences related to how they acquired sexual information and conversations they may have had with others regarding sexual activity or risky behavior.
3. Become familiar with a specific community's values related to sex education and contraceptive services for adolescents. Identify the proponents and opponents of these measures, their arguments, and their stated goals. Identify your own values and positions.
4. Review the sex education and family life lesson plans in your school district, if they exist. Describe the content and teaching strategies. Do you think it is adequate? When was the last time the content was changed or upgraded? What are the qualifications of the teachers? Do teachers use a prepared script? Are teachers comfortable allowing discussion and statements of views by children or adolescents in class?

REFERENCES

Alan Guttmacher Institute (AGI). (1981). *Teenage pregnancy: The problem that hasn't gone away.* New York: Author.

AGI. (1986). *Teenage pregnancy in industrialized countries.* New Haven, CT: Yale University Press.

American Nurses' Association. (1987). *Access to prenatal care: Key to prevention of low birth weight.* Kansas City, MO.

Amonker, R. G. (1980). What do teens know about the facts of life? *Journal of School Health, 50*(9), 527–530.

Auterman, M. E. (1991). Community-based secondary prevention with the pregnant adolescent. In S. S. Humenick, N. N. Wilkerson, & N. W. Paul (Eds.). *Adolescent pregnancy: Nursing perspectives on intervention.* White Plains, NY: March of Dimes Birth Defects Foundation.

Baisch, M. J., Goldberg, B. D., Fox, R. A., & Kinservik, M. A. (1988). Teen pregnancy service: Infant outcomes through two years of age. *Journal of Pediatric Nursing, 3*(5), 329–337.

Baldwin, W. H. (1976). Adolescent pregnancy and childbearing—growing concerns of Americans. *The Population Bulletin, 31*(2), 2–21.

Barrett, R. L., & Robinson, B. E. (1982). Issues and problems related to the research of teenage fathers: A critical analysis. *Journal of School Health, 52,* 596–600.

Barrett, R. L., & Robinson, B. E. (1985). The adolescent father. In S. M. Hanson & F. W. Bozett (Eds.). *Dimensions of fatherhood.* Beverly Hills, CA: Sage Publications.

Berruta-Clement, J. R., Schweinart, I. J., Barnett, W. S., Epstein, A. S., & Weikart, D. P. (Eds.). (1984). Changed lives: The effects of the Perry Preschool Program on youths through age 19. In *Monographs of the High/Scope Research Foundation* (200–203). No. 18. Ypsilanti, MI: High/Scope.

Black, C., & DeBlassie, R. R. (1985). Adolescent pregnancy: Contributing factors, consequences, treatment, and plausible solutions. *Adolescence, 20*(78), 281–290.

Braithwaite, R. L., & Taylor, S. E. (Eds.). (1992). *Health issues in the black community.* San Francisco: Jossey-Bass.

Brisbane, H. E. (1980). *The developing child* (3rd ed.). Peoria, IL: Charles A. Bennett.

Bulcholz, E. S., & Gol, B. (1986). More than playing house: A developmental perspective on the strengths in teenage motherhood. *Theory and Review,* 347–357+.

Bullis, R. K. (1992). The Supreme Court's legacy of abortion counseling: Ethics and implications. *Journal of Sex Education and Therapy, 18*(3), 186–199.

Bullough, V. L. (1981). Age at menarche: A misunderstanding. *Science, 213,* 365–366.

Burt, M. R. (1986). Estimating the public costs of teenage childbearing. *Family Planning Perspectives, 18*(5), 221–226.

Campbell, F. A., Breitmayer, B., & Ramey, C. T. (1986). Disadvantaged single teenage mothers and their children: Consequences of free educational day care. *Family Relations, 35,* 63–68.

Children's Defense Fund (CDF). (1986). *Maternal and child health data book; The health of America's children.* Washington, DC: Author.

CDF. (1988). *Teenage pregnancy: An advocate's guide to the numbers.* Washington, DC: Author.

CDF. (1989). *A vision for America's future.* Washington, DC: Author.

CDF. (1991). *Child poverty in America.* Washington, DC: Author.

Cvetkovich, G., Grote, B., Bjorseth, A., & Sarkissian, J. (1975). On the psychology of adolescent use of contraceptives. *Journal of Sexual Research, 11,* 256–270.

Cvetkovich, G., & Grote, B. (1981). Psychosocial maturity and teenage contraceptive use: An investigation of decision making and communication skills. *Population and Environment: Behavioral and Social Issues, 4*(4), 211–226.

Darabi, K. F., Jones, J., Varga, P. L., & Hourse, M. (1982). Evaluation of sex education outreach. *Adolescence, 17*(65), 57–64.

Davidson, E. C. Jr., & Fukushima, T. (1985). The age extremes for reproduction: Current implications for policy change. *America Journal of Obstetrics and Gynecology, 152*(6 pt 1), 623–626.

Davis, K. A. (1980). *A theory of teenage pregnancy in the U.S. adolescent. Pregnancy and childbearing.* Washington, DC: U.S. Department of Health and Human Services.

Davis, S. (1989). Pregnancy in adolescents. *Pediatric Clinics of North America, 36*(3), 665–680.

Davis, S. M., & Harris, M. B. (1982). Sexual knowledge, sexual interests, and sources of sexual information of rural land urban adolescents from three cultures. *Adolescence, 18*(66), 471–492.

Dearden, K., Hale, C., & Alvarez, J. (1992). The educational antecedents of teen fatherhood. *British Journal of Educational Psychology, 62*(pt 1), 139–147.

Dryfoos, J. (1982). The epidemiology of adolescent pregnancy: incidence, outcomes, and interventions. In I. R. Stuart & C. F. Wells (Eds.). *Pregnancy in adolescence: Needs, problems, and management.* New York: Von Nostrand Reinhold.

Dryfoos, J. (1984). A new strategy for preventing unintended teenage childbearing. *Family Planning Perspectives, 16*(4), 193–195.

Dryfoos, J. (1985). School-based health clinics: A new approach to preventing adolescent pregnancy? *Family Planning Perspectives, 17*(2), 70–75.

Edelman, M. W., & Pittman, K. J. (1986). Adolescent pregnancy: Black and white. *Journal of Community Health, 11*(1), 63–69.

Edwards, L. E., Steinman, M. E., Arnold, K. A., & Hakanson, E. Y. (1980). Adolescent pregnancy prevention services in high school clinics. *Family Planning Perspectives, 12*(6), 6–14.

Edwards, L. E., Steinman, M. E., & Hakanson, E. Y. (1977). An experimental comprehensive high school clinic. *American Journal of Public Health, 67*(8), 765–766.

Elster, A. E., McAnarney, A., & Lamb, M. (1983). Parental behavior of adolescent mothers. *Pediatrics, 71*(4), 494–503.

Fisher, S. M. (1984). The psychodynamics of teenage pregnancy and motherhood. In M. Sugar (Ed.). *Adolescent parenthood.* Jamaica, NY: Spectrum Publications.

Flick, L. H. (1991). A critique of community-based tertiary prevention with the adolescent parent and child. In S. S. Humenick, N. N. Wilkerson, & N. W. Paul (Eds.). *Adolescent pregnancy: Nursing perspectives on prevention.* White Plains, NY: March of Dimes Birth Defects Foundation.

Forrest, J., & Fordyce, J. (1988). U.S. women's contraceptive attitudes and practice: How have they changed in the 1980's? *Family Planning Perspective, 20*(3), 112–118.

Forrest, J., & Silverman, J. (1989). What public school teachers teach about preventing pregnancy, AIDS, and sexually transmitted diseases. *Family Planning Perspectives, 21,* 65–72.

Forrest, J. D., & Singh, S. (1990). The sexual and reproductive behavior of American women 1982–1988. *Family Planning Perspectives, 22*(5), 206–214.

Frazier, P. (1987). A local project to reduce teen pregnancy. *North Carolina Medical Journal, 48*(5), 270–271.

Frisancho, A. R., Matos, J., Leornard, W. R., & Yaroch, L. A. (1985). Developmental and nutritional determinants of pregnancy outcome among teenagers. *American Journal of Physical Anthropology, 66*(3), 247–261.

Furstenberg, F. F. (1979). The social consequences of teenage parenthood. *Family Planning Perspectives, 8,* 148–164.

Furstenberg, F. F. Jr. (1980). *The social consequences of teenage parenthood: Adolescent pregnancy and childbearing.* Washington, DC: U.S. Department of Health and Human Services.

Furstenberg, F. F. Jr., & Brooks-Gunn, J. (1985). Adolescent fertility: Causes, consequences, and remedies. In L. Aiken & D. Mechanic (Eds.). *Application of social science to clinical medicine and health policy.* New Brunswick, NJ: Rutgers University Press.

Furstenberg, F. F., Brooks-Gunn, J., & Morgan, S. P. (1987). Adolescent mothers and their children in later life. *Family Planning Perspectives, 19*(4), 142–151.

Geronimus, A. T. (1986). The effects of race, residence, and prenatal care on the relationship of maternal age to neonatal mortality. *American Journal of Public Health, 76*(12), 1412–1421.

Giblin, P. T., Poland, M. L., & Sachs, B. A. (1986). Pregnant adolescents' health information needs: Implications for health education and health seeking. *Journal of Adolescent Health Care, 7*(3), 168–172.

Goldberg, B. D., Baisch, J. J., & Fox, R. A. (1986). Teen Pregnancy Service: An interdisciplinary health care delivery system utilizing certified nurse-midwives. *Journal of Nurse Midwifery, 31*(6), 263–269.

Haiek, L., & Lederman, S. A. (1989). The relationship between maternal weight for height and term birth weight in teens and adult women. *Journal of Adolescent Health Care, 10*(1), 16–22.

Hayes, C. (Ed.). (1987). *Risking the future: Adolescent sexuality, pregnancy, and childbearing.* Vol. 1. Washington, DC: National Research Council, National Academy Press.

Henshaw, S. K., Kenney, A. M., Somberg, D., & VanDort, J. (1989). *Teenage pregnancy in the U.S.* New York: Alan Guttmacher Institute.

Henshaw, S. K., & Vort, J. V. (1989). Teenage abortion, birth, and pregnancy statistics: An update. *Family Planning Perspectives, 21,* 85–88.

Howard, M., & McCabe, J. A. (1992). An information and skills approach for younger teens: Postponing sexual involvement program. In B. C. Miller, J. T. Card, R. L. Paifoff, & J. I. Peterson (Eds.). *Preventing adolescent pregnancy.* Newbury Park, CA: Sage Publications.

Humenick, S. S., Wilkerson, N. N., & Paul, N. W. (Eds.) (1991). *Adolescent pregnancy: Nursing perspectives on intervention.*White Plains, NY: March of Dimes Birth Defects Foundation.

Isbner, F., & Wright, W. R. (1987). Comprehensive prenatal care for pregnant teens. *Journal of School Health, 57*(7), 288–297.

Jones, L. C. (1991). Community-based tertiary prevention with the adolescent parent and child. In S. S. Humenick, N. N. Wilkerson, & N. W. Paul (Eds.). *Adolescent pregnancy: Nursing perspectives on prevention.* White Plains, NY: March of Dimes Birth Defects Foundation.

Kenney, A., Guardodo, S., & Brown, L. (1989). Sex education and AIDS education in the schools: What states and large school districts are doing. *Family Planning Perspectives, 21,* 65–72.

Kisker, E. E. (1985). Teenagers talk about sex, pregnancy, and contraception. *Family Planning Perspectives, 17*(2), 83–90.

Klerman, L., Bracken, M., Jekel, J., & Braken, M. (1982). The delivery-abortion decision among adolescents. In I. Stewart & C. Wells (Eds.). *Pregnancy in adolescence: Needs, problems, and management.* New York: Van Nostrand Reinhold.

Ktsanes, B. (1980). *The teenager and the family planning experience: Adolescent pregnancy and childbearing.* Washington, DC: U.S. Department of Health and Human Services.

Ladner, J. A., & Gourdine, R. M. (1992). Adolescent pregnancy in the African-American community. In R. L. Braithwaite & S. E. Taylor (Eds.). *Health issues in the black community.* San Francisco: Jossey-Bass.

Landry, E., Bertrand, J., Cherry, F., & Rich, J. (1986). Teenage pregnancy in New Orleans: Factors that differentiate teens who deliver, abort, and successfully contracept. *Journal of Youth and Adolescence, 15,* 259–274.

Leibowitz, A., Eisen, M., & Chow, W. K. (1986). An economic model of teenage pregnancy decision making. *Demography, 23*(1), 67–77.

Leppert, P. C., Namerow, P. B., & Barker, D. (1986). Pregnancy outcomes among adolescent and older women receiving comprehensive prenatal care. *Journal of Adolescent Health Care, 7*(2), 112–117.

Leppert, P. C., Namerow, P. B., & Horowitz, E. (1985). Cesarean section deliveries among adolescent mothers enrolled in a comprehensive prenatal care program. *American Journal of Obstetrics and Gynecology, 152*(6 pt 1), 623–626.

Levy, S. R., Perhats, C., Nash-Johnson, M., & Welter, J. F. (1992). Reducing the risks in pregnant teens who are very young and those with mild mental retardation. *Mental Retardation, 30*(4), 195–203.

Lewis, B. D. (1988). An innovative health care model for management of teenage pregnancy. *Journal of the National Black Nurses' Association, 2*(2), 58–66.

Lieberman, E. J. (1980). *The psychological consequences of adolescent pregnancy and abortion: Adolescent pregnancy and childbearing.* Washington, DC: U.S. Department of Health and Human Services.

Litt, I. F., & Glader, L. (1987). Follow-up of adolescents previously studied for contraceptive compliance. *Journal of Adolescent Health Care, 8*(1), 349–351.

Lommel, L. L., & Taylor, D. (1992). Adolescent use of contraceptives. *NAACOGs Clinical Issues in Perinatal and Women's Health Nursing, 3*(2), 199–208.

Loris, P., Dewey, K. G., & Poirier-Brode, K. (1985). Weight gain and dietary intake of pregnant teenagers. *Journal of the American Dietetic Association, 85*(10), 1296–1305.

Marchbanks, P. A. (1991). A critique of community-based primary prevention of adolescent pregnancy. In S. S. Humerick, N. N. Wilkerson, & N. W. Paul (Eds.). *Adolescent pregnancy: Nursing perspectives on prevention.* White Plains, NY: March of Dimes Birth Defects Foundation.

Marshall, E., Buckner, E., & Powell, K. (1991). Evaluation of a teen parent program designed to reduce child abuse and neglect and to strengthen families. *Journal of Child Adolescent Psychiatric and Mental Health Nursing, 4*(3), 96–100.

Marsiglio, W., & Mott, F. (1986). The impact of sex education on sexual activity, contraceptive use, and premarital pregnancy among American teenagers. *Family Planning Perspective, 18*(4), 151–162.

May, K. M. (1992). Social networks and help seeking experiences of pregnant teens. *Journal of Gynecological and Neonatal Nursing, 21*(6), 497–502.

McAnarney, E. R., & Greydanus, D. E. (1989). Adolescent pregnancy and abortion. In A. D. Hofmann & D. E. Greydanus (Eds.). *Adolescent medicine.* Norwalk, CT: Appleton & Lange.

McLaughlin, S. D., Manninen, D. I., & Winges, L. D. (1988). Do adolescents who relinquish their children fare better or worse than those that raise them? *Family Planning Perspectives, 20*(20), 25–32.

Melton, G. B., & Russo, N. F. (1987). Adolescent abortion: Psychological perspectives on public policy. *American Psychologist, 42*(1), 69–72.

Mensch, B., & Kandel, D. B. (1992). Drug use as a risk factor for premarital teen pregnancy and abortion in a national sample of young white women. *Demography, 29*(3), 409–429.

Miller, C. J. (1984). Helping the pregnant adolescent remain in school: The continuing education program. In J. Robinson & B. Sachs (Eds.). *Nursing care models for adolescent families.* Kansas City, MO: American Nurses' Association.

Moore, K., Simms, M. C., & Betsey, C. (1986). *Choices and circumstances: Racial differences in adolescent sexuality and fertility.* New Brunswick, NJ: Transaction Books.

Miller, M. K., & Stokes, C. S. (1985). Teenage fertility, socioeconomic status and infant mortality. *Journal of Biosocial Science, 17*(2), 147–155.

Morbidity and Mortality Weekly Report (MMWR). (1992). Health objectives for the nation: Sexual behavior among high school students. *40*(51 & 52), 885–888.

Morrison, J. R., & Jensen, S. (1982). Teenage pregnancy: Special counseling considerations. *The Clearing House, 56*(2), 74–77.

Mott, F. L. (1986). The pace of repeated childbearing among young American mothers. *Family Planning Perspectives, 18*(1), 5–12.

Mott, F., & Marsiglio, W. (1985). Early childbearing and completion of high school. *Family Planning Perspective, 17,* 234–237.

Murdock, C. G. (1968). The unmarried mother and the school system. *American Journal of Public Health, 58*(12), 2217–2224.

Nathanson, C., & Becker, M. (1985). The influence of client-provider relationships on teenage women's subsequent use of contraception. *American Journal of Public Health, 75,* 33–38.

National Center for Health Statistics. (1984). Trends in teenage childbearing, United States, 1970–1981. *Vital and Health Statistics,* DHHS Publ. No. (PHS)84-1919. Washington, DC: Public Health Service, U.S. Government Printing Office.

National Institute of Mental Health. (1982). *Television and behavior: Ten years of scientific progress and implications for the eighties. Summary report.* Vol. 1. Washington, DC: U.S. Dept. of Health and Human Services.

National Research Council: Panel on Adolescent Pregnancy and Childbearing. (1987). *Risking the future: Adolescent sexuality, pregnancy, and childbearing.* Washington, DC: National Academy Press.

Nelson, B. A. (1989). A comprehensive program for pregnant adolescents: Parenting and prevention. *Child Welfare, 68*(1), 57–60.

Nichols, L. D. (1991). A critique of primary prevention of adolescent pregnancy. In S. S. Humenick, N. N. Wilkerson, & N. W. Paul (Eds.). *Adolescent pregnancy: Nursing perspectives on prevention.* White Plains, NY: March of Dimes Birth Defects Foundation.

Norr, K. F. (1991). Community-based primary prevention of adolescent pregnancy. In S. S. Humenick, N. N. Wilkerson, & N. W. Paul (Eds.). *Adolescent pregnancy: Nursing perspectives on prevention.* White Plains, NY: March of Dimes Defects Foundation.

Number of U.S. pregnancies reached all-time high in 1980s. (1993). *The Nation's Health, January,* 14.

Oakley, D., Swanson, J., Swenson, I., & March, S. (1990). Public health nurses and family planning. *Public Health Nursing, 7*(3), 175–180.

Oda, D. S. (1991). The invisible nursing practice. *Nursing Outlook, 39*(1), 26–29.

Oh, M. K., Cloud, G. A., Baker, S. L., Pass, M. A., Mulchahey, K., & Pass, R. F. (1993). Chlamydial infection and sexual behavior in young pregnant teenagers. *Sexually Transmitted Diseases, 20*(1), 45–50.

Olds, D. L., Henderson, C. R. Jr., Tatelbaum, R., & Chamberlin, R. (1986a). Improving the delivery of prenatal care and outcomes of pregnancy: A randomized trial of nurse home visitation. *Pediatrics, 77,* 16–28.

Olds, D. L., Henderson, C. R. Jr., Chamberlin, R., & Tatelbaum, R. (1986b). Preventing child abuse and neglect: A randomized trial of nurse home visitation. *Pediatrics, 78,* 65–78.

Olds, D. L., Henderson, C. R. Jr., Tatelbaum, R., & Chamberlin, R. (1988). Improving the life course development of socially disadvantaged mothers: A randomized trial of nurse home visitations. *American Journal of Public Health, 78,* 1436–1445.

Perino, S. S. (1992). Nike-footed health workers deal with the problems of adolescent pregnancy. *Public Health Reports, 107*(2), 208–212.

Perkins, J. L. (1991). Primary prevention of adolescent pregnancy. In S. S. Humenick, N. N. Wilkerson, & N. W. Paul (Eds.). *Adolescent pregnancy: Nursing perspectives on intervention.* White Plains, NY: March of Dimes Birth Defects Foundation.

Perrin, K. M. (1992). The 4 Ms of teen pregnancy: Managing, mending, mentoring and modeling. *International Journal of Childbirth Education, 7*(4), 29–30.

Piechnik, S. L., & Corbett, M. A. (1985). Reducing low birth weight among socioeconomically high-risk adolescent pregnancies. *Journal of Nurse Midwifery, 32,* 88–98.

Pittman, K., & Adams, G. (1988). *Teenage pregnancy: An advocate's guide to the numbers.* Washington, DC: Children's Defense Fund.

Pletsch, P. K., & Leslie, L. A. (1988). Urban adolescents: What are their health needs? *Public Health Nursing, 5*(3), 170–176.

Plotnick, R. D. (1992). The effects of attitudes on teenage premarital pregnancy and its resolution. *American Sociological Review, 57*(6), 800–811.

Polit, D. F., & Kahn, J. R. (1985). Project redirection: Evaluation of a comprehensive program for disadvantaged teenage mothers. *Family Planning Perspectives, 17*(4), 150–155.

Pollack, A. E. (1992). Teen contraception in the 1990s. *Journal of School Health, 62*(7), 288–293.

Pomeranz, A. J., Matson, S. C., & Nelson, D. B. (1991). Delay in obstetrical care in newly diagnosed teenage pregnancy. *Clinical Pediatrics, 30*(12), 661–663.

Porterfield, L., & Harris, B. (1985). Information needs of the pregnant adolescent. *Home Healthcare Nurse, 3*(6), 40–42.

Pregnancy program targets teen fathers. (1991). *Case Management Advisor, 2*(11), 167–169.

Rogel, M. J., Peterson, A. C., Pichards, M., Shelton, M., & Zeuhlke, M. (1979). *Contraceptive behavior in adolescents: A decision making perspective.* New York: American Psychiatric Association.

Sacher, I. M., & Neuhoff, S. D. (1982). Medical and psychosocial risk factors in pregnant adolescents. In I. R. Stewart & C. F. Wells (Eds.). *Pregnancy in adolescence: Needs, problems, and management.* New York: Van Nostrand Reinhold.

Sachs, B. (1986). Reproductive decisions in adolescents. *Image, 18*(2), 69–72.

Sadler, L., & Catrone, C. (1983). The adolescent parent: A dual developmental crisis. *Journal of Adolescent Health, 4*(2), 100–105.

Saller, D., & Crenshaw, M. C. (1987). Medical complications in adolescent pregnancy. *Maryland Medical Journal, 36*(11), 935–937.

Sander, J. H., & Rosen, J . L. (1987). Teenage fathers: Working with the neglected partner in adolescent childbearing. *Family Planning Perspectives, 19*(3), 107–110.

Schmitter, T. A. (1984). The Lancaster County young motherhood service. In J. Robinson & B. Sachs (Eds.). *Nursing care models for adolescent families.* Kansas City, MO: American Nurses' Association.

Schneck, M. E., Sideras, K. S., Fox, R. A., & Dupuis, L. (1990). Low-income pregnant adolescents and their infants: Dietary findings and health outcomes. *Journal of the American Dietetic Association, 90*(4), 555–558.

Schubot, D. B., & Schmidt, N. (1989). Perception of South Dakota adults concerning selected adolescent health problems. *South Dakota Journal of Medicine, 42*(6), 17–20.

Senderowitz, J. (1992). Are adolescents good candidates for RU 486 as an abortion method? *Law, Medicine, and Health Care, 20*(3), 209–214.

Shea, J., Herceg-Baron, R., & Fustenberg, F. F. Jr. (1984). Factors associated with adolescent use of family planning clinics. *American Journal of Public Health, 74*(11), 1227–1230.

Smoller, J., & Ooms, T. (1987). *Young unwed fathers: Research review, policy dilemmas, and options. Summary reports.* Washington, DC: U.S. Department of Health and Human Services, Maximus, Inc.

Soefer, E. F., Scholl, T. O., Sobel, E., Tanfer, K., & Levy, D. B. (1985). Menarche: Target age for reinforcing sex education for adolescents. *Journal of Adolescent Health, 6*(3), 196–200.

Sorenson, D. (1973). *Adolescent sexuality in contemporary America.* New York: World Press.

Stammer, A. M. (1985). Family planning at a school for pregnant girls: Development of a conceptual framework for practice. In J. E. Hall & B. R. Weaver (Eds.). *Distributive nursing practice: A systems approach to community health* (2nd ed). Philadelphia: J. B. Lippincott.

Statistical abstracts of the United States. (1992). Washington, DC: U.S. Government Printing Office.

Stevens, L. K., Register, C. A., & Sessions, D. D. (1992). The abortion decision: A qualitative choice approach. *Social Indicators Research, 27*(4), 327–344.

Studer, M., & Thornton, A. (1987). Adolescent religiosity and contraceptive use. *Journal of Marriage and Family, 49*(1), 117–128.

Thornburg, H. D. (1981). Adolescent sources of information on sex. *The Journal of School Health, 51*(4), 272–277.

Trussell, J. (1988). Teenage pregnancy in the United States. *Family Planning Perspectives, 20,* 212–272.

U.S. Department of Health and Human Services (DHHS). (1990). *Healthy people 2000: National health objectives.* DHHS Publ. No. (PHS) 91-50213. Washington, DC: U.S. Government Printing Office.

Vadies, E., & Hale, D. (1977). Attitudes of adolescent males toward abortion, contraception, and sexuality. *Social Work in Health Care, 3*(2), 169–174.

Vas, R., Smolen, P., & Miller, P. (1983). Adolescent pregnancy: Involvement of the male partner. *Journal of Adolescent Health, 4,* 246–250.

Vincent, M., Clearie, A., & Schluchter, M. (1987). Reducing adolescent pregnancy through school and community-based education. *Journal of the American Medical Association, 257,* 3382–3386.

Vinovskis, M. A. (1986). Young fathers and their children: Some historical and policy perspectives. In A. B. Elster & M. E. Lamb (Eds.). *Adolescent fatherhood.* Hillsdale, NJ: Lawrence Erlbaum Associates.

Wallace, H. W., Weeks, J., & Medina, A. (1982). Services for and needs of pregnant teenagers in large cities of the United States 1979–1980. *Public Health Reports, 97*(6), 583–588.

Washburn, D. (1989). "Mom, I'm pregnant!": The crisis in teen pregnancy. *School Nurse, 5*(1), 8–13.

Westney, O. E., Cole, O. J., & Munford, T. L. (1986). Adolescent unwed prospective fathers: Readiness for fatherhood and behaviors toward the mother and the expected infant. *Adolescence, 21*(84), 901–911.

Whitley, B., & Schofield, J. (1986). A metaanalysis of research on adolescent contraceptive use. *Population and Environment, 8*(3–4), 173–202.

Wilkerson, N. N. (1991). Family-focused secondary prevention with pregnant adolescent and adolescent father. In S. S. Humenick, N. N. Wilkerson, & N. W. Paul (Eds.). *Adolescent pregnancy: Nursing perspectives on prevention.* White Plains, NY: March of Dimes Birth Defects Foundation.

Wilmoth, G. H. (1992). Abortion, public health policy, and informed consent. *Journal of Social Issues, 48*(3), 1–17.

Zabin, L. S., Hardy, J. B., Smith, E. A., & Hirsch, M. B. (1986). Substance use and its relation to sexual activity among inner city adolescents. *Journal of Adolescent Health Care, 7,* 320.

Zabin, L. S., Hardy, J. B., Streett, R., & King, T. M. (1984). A school-, hospital-, and university-based adolescent pregnancy prevention program. *Journal of Reproductive Medicine, 29*(6), 421–426.

Zabin, L. S., Hirsch, M., Smith, E., Streett, R., & Hardy, J. (1986). Evaluation of a pregnancy prevention program for urban teenagers. *Family Planning Perspectives, 18,* 119–126.

Zabin, L. S., Kantner, J. F., & Zelnick, M. (1979). Role of adolescent pregnancy in first month of intercourse. *Family Planning Perspectives, 11,* 215–222.

Zelnick, M. (1979). Sex education and knowledge of pregnancy risk among U.S. teenage women. *Family Planning Perspectives, 11,* 355–357.

Zelnick, M. (1983). Sexual activity among adolescents: Perspectives of a decade. In E. R. McAnarney (Ed.), *Premature adolescent pregnancy and parenthood.* New York: Grune & Stratton.

Zelnick, M., & Kantner, J. F. (1978). Contraceptive patterns and premarital pregnancy among women aged 15–19 in 1976. *Family Planning Perspectives, 10*(3), 135–142.

Zelnick, M., & Kantner, J. F. (1979). Reasons for nonuse of contraception by sexually active women age 15–19. *Family Planning Perspectives, 11*(5), 289–296.

Zelnick, M., & Shah, F. K. (1983). First intercourse among young Americans. *Family Planning Perspectives, 15*(2), 64–70.

Zill, N., Moore, K. A., Nord, C. W., & Stief, T. (1991). *Welfare mothers as potential employees: A statistical profile based on national survey data.* Washington, DC: Child Trends.

SUGGESTED READINGS

Braithwaite, R. N., & Taylor, S. E. (Eds.). (1992). *Health issues in the black community.* San Francisco: Jossey-Bass.

Humenick, S. S., Wilkerson, N. N., & Paul, N. W. (Eds.). (1991). *Adolescent pregnancy: Nursing perspectives on prevention.* White Plains, NY: March of Dimes Birth Defects Foundation.

Isbner, F., & Wright, W. R. (1987). Comprehensive prenatal care for pregnant teens. *Journal of School Health, 57*(7), 288–297.

Kenney, A., Guardod, S., & Brown, L. (1989). Sex education and AIDS education in the schools: What states and large school districts are doing. *Family Planning Perspectives, 21,* 65–72.

Kisker, E. E. (1985). Teenagers talk about sex, pregnancy, and contraception. *Family Planning Perspectives, 17*(2), 83–90.

May, K. M. (1992). Social networks and help seeking experiences of pregnant teens. *Journal of Obstetrical and Gynecological Nursing, 21*(6), 497–502.

Miller, B. C., Card, J. J., Paikoff, R. L., & Peterson, J. L. (Eds.). (1992). *Preventing adolescent pregnancy: Model programs and evaluations.* Newbury Park, CA: Sage Publications.

Olds, D. L., Henderson, C. R. Jr., Tatelbaum, R., & Chamberlin, R. (1988). Improving the life course development of socially disadvantaged mothers: A randomized trial of nurse home visitations. *American Journal of Public Health, 78,* 1435–1445.

Pletsch, P. K., & Leslie, L. A. (1988). Urban adolescents: What are their health needs? *Public Health Nursing, 5*(3), 170–176.

Chapter 23

Homelessness in America

Alwilda Scholler-Jaquish

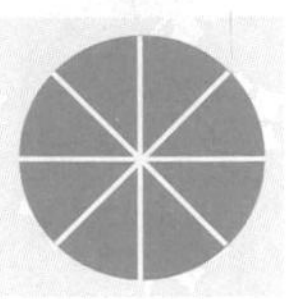

Focus Questions

How do historical perspectives relate to care of the very poor and homeless today?

How is homelessness a social, economic, political, and ethical problem?

What are the demographic differences in homelessness rates?

What predisposing factors make some people more vulnerable to homelessness than others?

How can the concept of stages of homelessness assist the community health nurse to plan interventions for homeless people?

What actions can a community health nurse take to reduce the rate of homelessness?

What can community health nurses do to relieve barriers encountered by homeless people when they attempt to obtain health care?

What actions can a community health nurse take as an advocate for the homeless?

Economic, social, and political factors have resulted in an alarming increase in the number of homeless men, women, and children. Homeless people are known by the places in which they seek refuge (e.g., street people, subway people, garage people, or dumpster people). Others live in automobiles, under bridges, and in cardboard boxes and abandoned buildings. They live not only in large cities, but also in rural areas. Homeless men, women, and children experience more health problems than the general public but often encounter multiple barriers when they attempt to obtain health care. Community health nurses find working with them daunting because of their multiple problems and the difficulty in assisting them to find help.

Homeless people include persons from all walks of life: very poor individuals, unskilled workers, farmers, housewives, social workers, health care professionals, and scientists. Some become homeless as a result of poverty or a failure of their family support systems. Others become homeless through loss of employment, abandonment, domestic violence, alcoholism, mental illness, social deviance, mental retardation, or physical illness or disability.

Definitions of Homelessness

The various definitions of homelessness reflect diverse political, social, or financial views (Table 23–1) but all definitions of homelessness include inappropriate places to sleep. Each definition contains the need for a place to stay, although the time period involved varies from overnight to 6 months.

Scope of the Problem. The 1990 United States Census tried to include homeless people. However, homeless individuals comprise a diverse population and can be difficult to count. It is estimated that 736,000 people are homeless on any given night in this country, and as many as 1.3 to 2 million individuals were homeless on at least one night during a recent year (National Alliance to End Homelessness, 1988).

History of Homelessness in the United States

Paupers were sent aboard ship with the colonists who settled America, and these colonists made an effort to care for them. However, when the burden of caring for the poor and disabled became too great, the local councils began to differentiate between the "worthy" and "unworthy" poor. Widows and orphans and others known to the settlers were worthy, whereas adult men and those unknown to the colony were unworthy. In the mid-1600s, the colonies adopted most of the tenets of an English law that limited assistance to those in need and focused responsibility on the family and the local community. Recipients of assistance included the disabled, unemployed, widows, and children, all of whom were required to meet a residency requirement before they could receive assistance. The impoverished stranger was greeted with fear and suspicion, and nonproductive men were indentured or driven from settlements (Trattner, 1984).

Paupers lived in almshouses in exchange for labor, and apprenticeships were available to poor, illegitimate, or orphaned white children. The Indians were driven off their land and ignored. Blacks were also excluded from social welfare systems and were left to the care of their masters.

TABLE 23–1

Variations in Definitions of Homelessness

Characteristics	Rivilin (1986)	Benda & Dattalo (1988)	Robertson & Cousineau (1986)	Gelberg & Linn (1988)	Stark (1987)	Bean et al. (1987)
Ability to receive personal mail	No mailing address		No mailing address			
Length of time to qualify as homeless	Cannot be sure of a place to stay for up to 30 days	No place to stay	No place to stay	Preceding night		Any length of time
Private living arrangements		Cheap hotels, rooming houses		Hotel, motel, family, or friends; less than 60 days		Hotels, motels
Public housing				Emergency shelters of any kind	Shelters	Missions, shelters
Other places used for living				Outdoors; any space not designed for shelter	Doorways, train stations, bus terminals, public parks, subways	Car, all night cafe, any public facility, tent cities, jail

Free blacks had to develop their own means of survival (e.g., housing, culture, and health care).

"Hobos," "Tramps," and "Bums." During the late 1800s the new nation became increasingly populated, and industrial centers developed in strategic areas across America. Transient labor was needed for construction, on farms, and in the major cities. "Hobos" were transient workers who traveled around the country in railroad cars looking for work. "Tramps" were transient workers or beggars who traveled on foot. "Bums" also "rode the rails," but they did not work and often robbed the hobos. Meanwhile, bums loitered in the cities and begged for money for their next drink (Hoch and Slayton, 1989).

"Skid row" is that section in urban areas where cheap hotels, diners, bars, secondhand stores, and missions provide services for the very poor and homeless. The skid row district was first described in Portland, Oregon, in 1905 (Momeni and Wiegand, 1989). Skid row populations peaked after the stock market crash in 1929 and the drought in the late 1930s created many new poor and homeless people. The skid row population overflowed into other areas of cities and did not subside until World War II, when jobs increased. Skid row areas then shrank and remained relatively small until the 1960s.

The hobos, tramps, and bums familiar in history are not found in modern society. A small group of hobos continues to ride the rails and meets once a year to celebrate a life of wandering. Each year fewer and fewer remain, as the older men die. Very few young persons join these groups of nomadic individuals.

Homelessness in its modern form appeared in the 1960s and has been related to poverty, unemployment, and inadequate housing. Although a minority of the homeless population move about the country, most homeless persons are homeless in their own home town.

SOCIAL AND POLITICAL FORCES

Since the 1940s, federal, state, and city programs have been initiated, but support has varied depending on political forces and budgetary constraints. Many argue that the government should do more for the poor, while others feel that too much has already been done. Distrust and resentment exist among wage earners who contribute through Social Security and other taxes to the cost of social welfare policies that are used for the so called unworthy poor. The strongest feelings focus on adult men who are homeless: "I have to work for a living, why don't they go get a job? I don't want my tax dollars supporting some drunk. Why don't they work hard like I do?"

In the 1980s the Reagan administration took steps to reduce Medicare, Medicaid, food stamps, housing, and other welfare programs (Stern, 1984). Millions of people lost their eligibility in the budget readjustment process (Table 23–2). New tax laws resulted in higher taxes and increased health care costs for the poor.

Societal Changes. Many jobs have disappeared as industries have moved out of major cities and relocated to rural areas or to other countries with lower labor costs. New equipment has replaced employees, and employers are using more part-time employees to reduce the costs of employee benefits. Minimum wages have remained relatively constant while prices and housing costs have continued to rise.

The widespread use of drugs has contributed to increased rates of drop-outs, teenage pregnancies, and homicides. Fewer jobs are available for unskilled workers, and persons with low levels of education have difficulty gaining entry into jobs that require semiskilled or skilled workers. Young, chronically mentally ill adults who have received minimal care are more likely to use drugs and to be involved in

TABLE 23–2

Changes in Entitlement Programs, 1980s

Title	People Affected	Changes
Aid to Families with Dependent Children (AFDC)	Women and children	Sixty percent of families lost their AFDC benefits; 500,000 low-income families were terminated from AFDC (Brown, 1989).
Social Security Act	Men	Unemployment compensation was reduced from 80% of the base rate to 25% (Brown, 1989).
Medicare/Medicaid: An Amendment to the Social Security Act	Women, children, men	Eligibility requirements for medical assistance are tied to eligibility for other benefits; 1 million persons who were disqualified from entitlement programs lost medical care also (Popp, 1988).
	Children	The Medicare/Medicaid budget was reduced by $13 billion in 2 years; 700,000 children lost Medicaid coverage due to changes in entitlements (Brown, 1989).
Food Stamp Act	Women, children	The WIC (Women, Infants and Children) and breakfast programs were cut by $1.5 million; 1 million fewer families received food stamps and another 1 million received reduced amounts of food stamps (Popp, 1988).
Supplementary Social Security Act (SSI)	Men, women	100,000 mentally ill people lost this benefit (Smith & Reeder, 1987).

violent crimes (Susser et al., 1987; Benda and Dattalo, 1988; Mangine et al., 1990).

Although many religious organizations and advocacy groups have worked to help homeless individuals, these efforts have been unable to keep pace with the growing numbers. With these increased numbers of visibly homeless men, women, and children, the general population has become afraid and has opposed spending money to help those who "should help themselves." On the city, state, and federal levels, allocations for the poor and homeless have found numerous opponents.

Rural homelessness is harder to document than urban homelessness and has not been systematically studied. A study in Ohio found that rural homeless persons were more likely to be younger, white, and married, and to have more resources such as cars, families, and places for shelter than their urban counterparts (Roth and Bean, 1986). In Missouri farming areas, the failure of banks and foreclosure of family farms and farming-related businesses have left entire households jobless and homeless (Momeni and Wiegand, 1989). The rural homeless appear to be families and individuals who have been deprived of living quarters through overcrowding in the family home, substandard housing, poverty, and depressed economic conditions (Interagency Council on Homelessness, 1990).

Low-Income Housing. The lack of low-income housing has been and continues to be a primary factor in the number of homeless families and individuals. The Housing Act of 1949 provided an incentive for the destruction of inner city dwellings under an "urban renewal" plan. During the 1950s residents of inner city ghettos were relocated to high-rise "projects" with hundreds of rental units on each site. Muggings, domestic violence, and drug-related violence make these projects almost unlivable. As a result there is an aversion among housing providers and public officials to create more "instant ghettos" consisting only of low-income people. The scarcity of public housing is related to the number of persons unable to afford a place to live (Carliner, 1987; Belcher and DiBlasio, 1990). The General Accounting Office reports that 1 million or more low-income housing units have disappeared since 1980. Other estimates of lost housing units run as high as 3.5 million (Wittman and Arch, 1987).

Before the 1980s, the federal government provided housing assistance in the form of incentives to builders, income supplements to households, financial market activities, and tax incentives. Federal and state government policies allowed for a variety of financial incentives for builders and owners of low-income housing units. In the 1970s there was an increase in construction of single-family homes. Efforts to improve substandard housing stopped, and the number of units with structural problems did not decrease during that decade. In 1983 the budget for rental assistance was cut sharply, while the number of recipients continued to increase.

Affordable housing became a critical issue in rural areas beginning in the 1950s. Modernization and mechanization lessened the need for farm labor and reduced farm employment by 45%. "Between 1940 and 1970, well over 20 million people (many of them black) were forced off the land, especially in the South, where these forces had the greatest impact" (Trattner, 1984, p. 293). These displaced people sought relief in urban areas, where there were few jobs. Homelessness was a reality in both urban and rural areas.

In 1979 the federal government was constructing 500,000 low-income housing units each year; however, by 1985, as a result of changes in governmental policy, the number was lower (Wittman and Arch, 1987). Older housing units have fallen into decay and lack adequate cooking facilities, heat, or plumbing. Median rental costs rose twice as fast as median income from 1970 to 1980. In some cases tenants pay up to 90% of their income for rental units that are unsafe for human habitation owing to rat infestation, lack of toilet facilities, or inadequate or unsafe gas and electric fixtures (Tucker, 1987).

Rent control does not cause homelessness, but it does contribute to higher rent in uncontrolled units and fewer vacancies, which are causes for homelessness. Rent control was first initiated in New York City in 1943 as an economic measure to keep the cost of rental units below the market level. The belief is that maintaining a fixed number of housing units at a low rental fee will ensure an adequate supply of low-income housing. However, landlords were unable to make a profit from the rent-controlled units, and many chose to allow the buildings to be abandoned instead of rented. The price of uncontrolled rental units then rose to offset the landlords' losses. Tucker (1987) has described the impact of rent control on reducing the construction of low-cost units, thus raising the cost of those units that remain. The burden of the high costs fell on the poorest and most vulnerable part of the population.

Demographic Characteristics

Community health nurses should be familiar with the gender, age, and racial composition of the homeless population. This information allows nurses to plan appropriate programs and interventions for the people with whom they work.

During the first half of this century, homeless persons were primarily elderly white men. There have been significant changes since the mid-1960s, reflecting a very different group of homeless people (Fig. 23–1). Although men remain the largest group of homeless people (64%), the percentage of women (21%) and teenagers and children (15%) has increased significantly. Also, the

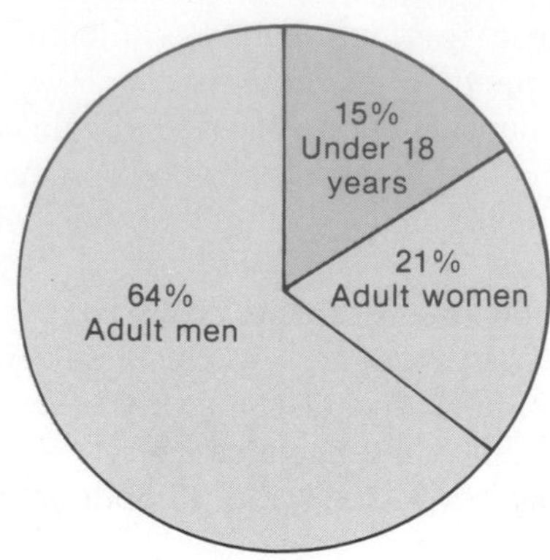

Figure 23–1 ● Percentages of men, women, and children among the homeless. (Data from Interagency Council on Homelessness. (1990). *The annual report of the Interagency Council on Homelessness.* Washington, DC: Author.)

current homeless population is much younger (First et al., 1988; Fischer et al., 1986; Robertson and Cousineau, 1986; Koegel and Burnam, 1988; Rossi and Wright, 1987) (Fig. 23–2).

Currently more than half of the homeless population is composed of blacks, Hispanics, Native Americans, and other minority groups (Fig. 23–3). These minority groups are overrepresented in the homeless population, which may be a result of poverty, unemployment, the lack of low-income housing, or racial discrimination.

STAGES OF HOMELESSNESS

There is great variation in the characteristics of homeless individuals, the length of homelessness, and the extent of disability. Therefore, the concept of stages of homelessness was designed as an intervention model (Belcher et al., 1991). Stage 1 (episodic homelessness) includes persons who are vulnerable to homelessness and may be homeless from time to time. Stage 2 (temporary homelessness) includes homeless persons who continue to identify with mainstream society. Stage 3 (chronic homelessness) includes persons for whom homelessness has become normative. This model is based on behavioral manifestations rather than length of homelessness or psychosocial problems (Table 23–3).

HOMELESS MEN

Current literature often points out the increase in homelessness among women and children. Although there is often a political and social response to these needy people, it is not uncommon to meet resistance in planning services for homeless men, who may be considered unworthy. Currently homeless men still make up the single largest and most visible subgroup of the homeless population. Since the mid-1970s there has been a significant increase in homeless men between the ages of 25 and 40 (Lindsey, 1989). The "baby boom" following World War II resulted in an overabundance of workers for a changing job market. Mental illness may account for as many as 40% of homeless people living on the street, while substance abuse accounts for approximately 30% to 33% of the population (Stark, 1987). At least 10% to 20% of homeless persons have a problem with drugs such as crack cocaine and heroin (Millburn, 1989). Many others use drugs and alcohol, including many of those who are mentally ill (Fig. 23–4).

Veterans make up at least 30% of the homeless population. A study in Los Angeles reported that the majority of homeless veterans were black, unmarried men approximately 40 years of age (Dear and Takahashi, 1990). Homelessness in black veterans appears to be related to the same social conditions that cause homelessness in nonveterans.

Dependent adult men (those who are not financially self-supporting) add strain to many families, especially when the family is already living below the poverty level

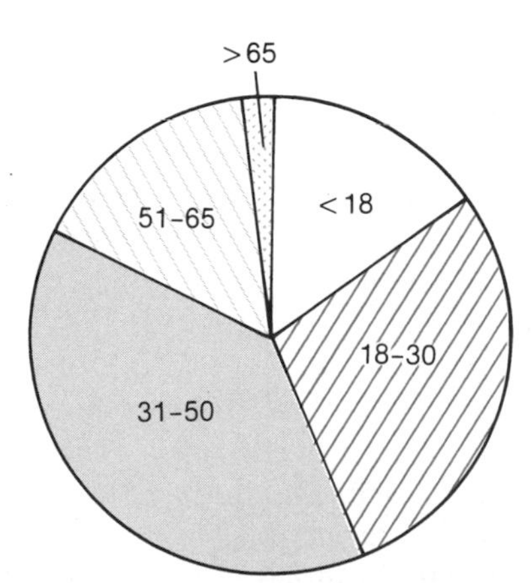

Figure 23–2 ● Age distribution of the homeless. (Data from Interagency Council on Homelessness. (1990). *The annual report of the Interagency Council on Homelessness.* Washington, DC: Author.)

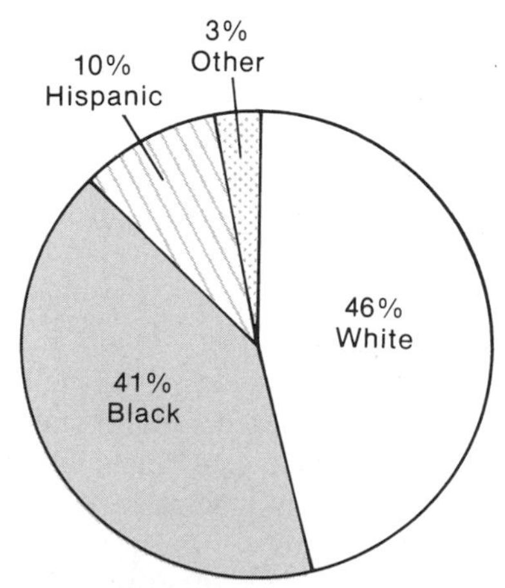

Figure 23–3 ● Racial composition of the homeless. (Data from Interagency Council on Homelessness. (1990). *The annual report of the Interagency Council on Homelessness.* Washington, DC: Author.)

TABLE 23–3

Stages of Homelessness

Stage 1: Episodic homelessness

The first stage of homelessness consists of individuals who live below or slightly above the poverty line, are socially stigmatized, and are constantly vulnerable to the harsh realities of homelessness. Their connection to a home is tenuous and may be episodic as persons move in and out of intense poverty.

Stage 2: Temporary homelessness

The second stage of homelessness consists of individuals who have recently become homeless. These individuals still identify themselves with the mainstream of their communities rather than with other homeless individuals; display symptoms of anxiety and depression; may abuse alcohol or drugs; view living on the streets or relying on shelters as an unacceptable lifestyle; and are attempting to regain a lost home, job, and social standing.

Stage 3: Chronic homelessness

The third stage of homelessness consists of individuals who have been homeless for longer periods of time. They accept their life experiences on the streets as normative, are more easily and clearly identifiable as homeless, are extremely suspicious of interacting with members of the mainstream of society, and are generally socially decompensated.

From Belcher, J. R., Scholler-Jaquish, A., & Drummond, M. (1991). Three stages of homelessness: A conceptual model for social workers in health care. *Health and Social Work, 16*(2), 87–93.

(Fig. 23–5). In addition, there are cultural expectations about the role of men in society. Dependent men are more likely than dependent women to be mentally ill, substance abusers, or involved in criminal activity (Interagency Council on Homelessness, 1990).

People who live in poverty are more at risk for temporary homelessness. Any financial emergency or job loss may result in homelessness. Some move in with family or friends for short-term living arrangements. Homeless men may develop a series of relationships with women who have lodging, move in with them, and then move out as their relationship becomes strained (Table 23–4).

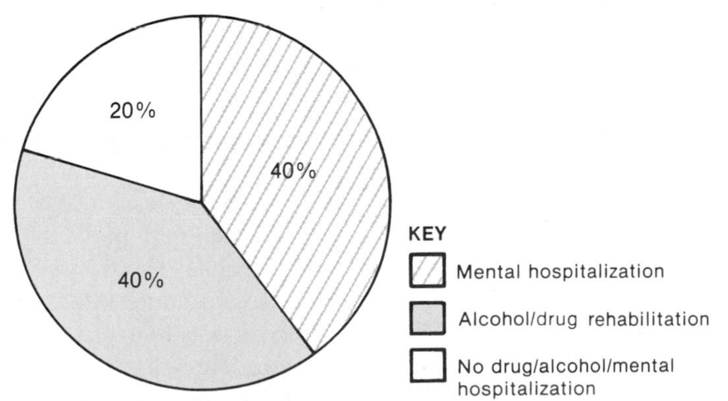

Figure 23–4 ● Prevalence of treatment for mental illness among the homeless. (Data from Interagency Council on Homelessness. (1990). *The annual report of the Interagency Council on Homelessness.* Washington, DC: Author.)

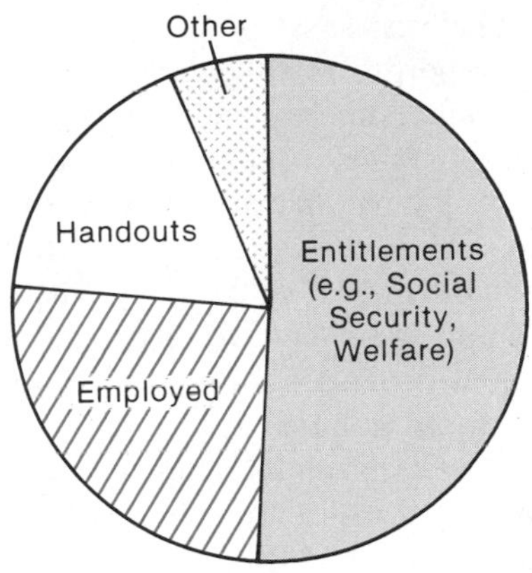

Figure 23–5 ● Sources of income among the homeless. (Data from Interagency Council on Homelessness. (1990). *The annual report of the Interagency Council on Homelessness.* Washington, DC: Author.)

TABLE 23–4

Oliver: One Homeless Man

When the community health nurse first met Oliver, he had come to the clinic wet and disheveled. He had been sleeping in a city park under a tree and was caught in a heavy rainstorm with no place to go. Oliver was 37 years old, had never been married, and had worked at odd jobs most of his life. He had completed the 10th grade in school but dropped out because it "wasn't meaningful to me then." Oliver had a psychiatric history and abused alcohol but preferred cocaine when he could get it. He did "hang out" with a group of homeless men who appeared to be near his own age. They shared their alcohol and drugs and befriended one another.

Oliver was very thin and was HIV+. The community health nurse helped Oliver get dry clothes and made an appointment for him with the infectious disease clinic and with the psychiatrist who had treated him in the past. They talked about places he could stay without exposure to the weather. Over a period of several weeks, Oliver became increasingly compliant. He began to develop a relationship with the community health nurse and followed up on his appointments because he believed that she was really interested in his well-being.

There was a significant change in Oliver's appearance. He was clean, well groomed, and appropriately dressed. Oliver went to the infectious disease clinic and started on medications; he also went to the psychiatrist, who also put him on medication. He continued to hang out with his friends. One day he came to the clinic in a very excited state and told the community health nurse that he had met a girl and he was in love. The nurse explained the necessity of using condoms when he was sexually active. Oliver said he knew how important it was, and he knew that he could hurt someone else with his disease.

Oliver stopped coming to the clinic a few weeks later. His friends told the nurse that he had moved in with his girlfriend. Over the next several months, the community health nurse asked about Oliver whenever she met one of his friends and learned that he was happy and living with his girlfriend. Almost a year later, Oliver appeared in the clinic one day. His clothing was soiled, and he appeared sad. "What happened to you, Oliver?" the community health nurse asked. "Oh, my girlfriend got tired of me and threw me out last week." Oliver was still going to the infectious disease clinic and the psychiatric clinic. Even though he was homeless again, he was remaining compliant with his medical care. The community health nurse again began to assist Oliver with his problems.

For some, homelessness becomes a long-term condition, with a few men reporting that they have been homeless for 30 to 50 years. Older homeless men are more likely to have been married at some time in their life, while many younger homeless men have never married. A study of men in New York City who were homeless for the first time (Susser et al., 1987) reported that 23% of the sample had been placed outside their home in foster care, group homes, or other special residential programs while still a child. Another 43% had run away from home, been expelled from school, or been in jail or reform school. Homeless elderly persons are faced with almost insurmountable problems in coping from day to day (Boondas, 1985).

HOMELESS WOMEN

Homeless women are not as visible and are more difficult to count than men. Estimates of their numbers range from 15 to 25 percent of the homeless population (Ropers and Boyer, 1987; Wright, 1989). There are many kinds of homeless women. One kind includes single women whose history of drug and alcohol abuse is similar to that of homeless men.

A second group includes women who have become socially and psychologically decompensated and become known as *bag ladies.* These women are alienated from the mainstream of society and use few resources. Most are white and over 40 years of age and tend to seek refuge in public buildings (Strasser, 1978) (Table 23–5). Social and psychological decompensation is a state in which the individual is so emotionally and mentally separated from society that he or she is unable to relate to others in any meaningful way. *Social decompensation* relates to the inability to interact with other human beings to communicate feelings, to make requests, or to behave in ways that are socially acceptable. *Psychological decompensation* relates to the inability to remain alert and aware of one's environment. This generally relates to the person's inability to be mentally or emotionally aware of his or her own feelings or those of others. These individuals appear to be unable to effectively make contact with others.

Another large group of women consists of mothers with dependent children in their care (Wright, 1989). Sheltered women with children numbered more than 60,000 in 1988 (Johnson and Krueger, 1989). These women tend to be young, and their rates of mental illness and substance abuse are low, although they have a higher rate of seeking treatment for addictions and mental illnesses. Homeless mothers have less education and lower employment rates, and appear to have fewer friends than other homeless persons. More than 80% of single homeless women with children are nonwhite (Interagency Council on Homelessness, 1990; Wagner and Menke, 1991).

Women are at risk for victimization and live in fear of assault and rape. One study indicates that at least 30% of homeless women of all ages reported being raped in the preceding 12 months (Breakey et al., 1989). There are fewer service facilities for women than for men, and the services tend to be of a lesser quality (Stoner, 1983).

Women with children are more likely to be found in shelters or welfare hotels. It seems that women require more stressors to become homeless, but once they become homeless, they are overwhelmed with the stress of living on the street. Women are more seriously socially and psychologically decompensated than homeless men (Bachrach, 1987). Men may become homeless after a job loss or as a result of substance abuse. However, women may move in with families and friends for months at a time. The women often stay in abusive relationships to avoid homelessness until they feel forced to move onto the streets to avoid the domestic violence. A study in Baltimore found that 41% of homeless women had a major mental illness, while another 44% demonstrated serious anxiety disorders (Breakey et al., 1989).

TABLE 23–5

Molly: A Homeless Woman

When the community health nurse visits the women's day shelter, she always speaks to Molly. Once a month she is able to persuade her to come to the examining room to talk with the nurse. Molly carries two paper shopping bags that are filled with pieces of paper, plastic, clothing, and small objects that she picks up on her daily walk. These items are important to her, and she carries the two bags wherever she goes. She avoids eye contact with the people she passes on the street. In the day shelter, she sits alone and sleeps most of the day. Showers and clothing are available for the women in the day shelter, but the staff have to be insistent to get Molly to bathe and change clothes at least once a week. Molly confides in very few people, but she does talk to the shelter staff from time to time. The women's day shelter provides a safe respite from the threats and violence on the city streets. Molly doesn't go to the night shelters because she has been beaten and raped numerous times. She remains alone and lives a solitary existence.

The community health nurse has been able to examine Molly on occasion and has learned that Molly has a large mass in her left breast. The nurse has encouraged Molly to go to a hospital for treatment but she has vigorously refused. Last month the community health nurse found a mass in Molly's right breast. The nurse continued to encourage Molly to see a physician, but if she is pressured too much, she becomes agitated and will leave the day shelter to avoid further stress. The community health nurse arranged for a female nurse practitioner to come to the clinic to examine Molly's breasts; the nurse practitioner supported the nurse's concern that Molly probably had cancer in both breasts. When the community health nurse told Molly she might have breast cancer and she might die, Molly replied, "So what. I don't care. Everyone got to die of something. Miss Nurse, don't bother me with no cancer. Just leave me alone. I'm old and I'm tired. Just leave me alone."

The community health nurse met with the shelter staff, and they agreed to continue to support Molly at the day shelter and encourage her to seek medical care. They began to talk about the need to develop a strategy in the event that Molly should need hospice care in the future.

HOMELESS TEENAGERS

Up to 500,000 teenagers leave home each year; some are runaways, while others are "throwaways." Teenagers who run away have significant psychological disturbances and a higher rate of drug abuse and contacts with the legal system than other youths. Family relationships reveal a lack of trust and security, with displacement of intense anger over small incidents (Adams et al., 1985). Studies of runaway youths have revealed a high incidence of family violence and physical abuse (Price, 1987; Powers et al., 1990).

Teenagers who run away from home for longer than 2 or 3 days tend to report a history of physical and sexual abuse at home. Incest is common among teenage girls who have fled their homes for the "safety" of the street. Teenage girls who have been sexually assaulted demonstrate more anger and more delinquent behavior, whereas teenage boys are more likely to become victimizers themselves (Swartz, 1986).

A throwaway child is one whose parents have severed all relationship with him or her. Divorce, incestuous behaviors, or scapegoating may contribute to the desertion of the child. The ultimate rejection is preceded by months and years of failed relationships. The throwaway child is usually emotionally disorganized and has low self-esteem (Hier et al., 1990).

Still other homeless youths have become separated from their families as the result of shelter policies that prohibit the admission of teenagers (Interagency Council on Homelessness, 1990). Homeless youths tend to come from dysfunctional and single-parent homes. More than half report that their parents are substance abusers (Rotherman-Borus, 1991).

Homeless youths gravitate toward neighborhoods where they are tolerated and likely to be introduced to a delinquent lifestyle, such as areas frequented by intravenous drug users and prostitutes. Risky sexual practices and drug use can lead to premature death (Rotherman-Borus, 1991). Criminal activities are common, and homeless young people often become victims of disease and violence or hardened criminals at a young age.

HOMELESS CHILDREN

Data on homelessness indicate that 15% of the total homeless population are youths under the age of 18 (Interagency Council on Homelessness, 1990). Most homeless children are preschoolers between infancy and 5 years of age. These young children may be with a single parent, usually their mother, or with intact families. Many children stay in shelters or welfare hotels, where they are subjected to distress unknown to most children. In a Massachusetts study of 151 homeless children, at least 50% were found to have severe depression, anxiety, and learning disabilities (Bassuk et al., 1986). Developmental testing of preschool children indicated that preschool homeless children exhibited significant developmental delay in all areas (Bassuk and Rosenberg, 1990). A number of health problems such as immunization delay and anemia are more severe among homeless children than other poor children. Chronic malnutrition is associated with growth delay in homeless children (Grant, 1989; Fierman et al., 1991).

Many homeless children have attended preschool programs, but only on a sporadic basis. They often have deficiencies in acquiring learning readiness and social interaction skills. School-age homeless children experience relocations and long intervals in their education. This lost school time results in academic underachievement and gaps in learning and experience. Homeless children often have difficulty finding a place to study and are isolated by other children as a result of stereotyping and labeling (Whitman et al., 1990; Wood et al., 1990). The Education for Homeless Children and Youth Project received increased federal funding in 1991 to provide opportunities for access and success in school (Jackson-Jobe, 1992).

Underimmunization or nonimmunization jeopardizes the health of homeless children, who are exposed to a wide array of environmental hazards. Crowded, chaotic environments also create conditions for conflict and violent interactions between parents and children (Molnar et al., 1990). Homeless children search for adults to nurture them and often turn to their siblings for support and nurturance. Children as young as 4 years old mimic their mother's behavior and are their mother's best friend and confidant (Bassuk and Galagher, 1990) (Table 23–6).

HOMELESS FAMILIES

An increase in homeless families has been reported in all areas of the United States. Homeless families primarily consist of one-parent families with an average of two or three young children. Two-parent families are more likely to be found in rural areas and in cities outside the major metropolitan areas. Three of four homeless families consist of a never-married mother and her children. Many of these single mothers lived with their mother or grandmother before becoming homeless. Similarly, many homeless families exhaust the resources of their families or friends before they leave or are forced out (Shinn et al., 1991). Most of the social support available to poor families is provided by other poor families.

Substandard housing, personal conflict, abuse, substance abuse, and overcrowding all contribute to family homelessness. In one study the majority of homeless female parents were in their late twenties, and about 50% of the sample consisted of minorities. Male parents averaged 34 years of age, and more than 50% were white. Usually both parents had been unemployed for more than 3 months.

TABLE 23–6

Dolly: A Homeless Child and Her Family

Portia has brought her three children to the community health clinic for immunizations. Her 6-month-old child needs immunization, and she brought her other two children along because she has no place for them to stay. The community health nurse has talked with Portia about the infant's development and notes that he is slightly below normal for his age. The nurse encourages Portia to play with the infant more often.

Tony is 3 years old and appears shy and frightened. His mother tells the community health nurse that he is afraid of the older children in the transition house where they live with other single mothers who have small children. The nurse asks about Dolly, who is almost 6 years old. When they can't find Dolly, the other nurses and Portia began to look around the clinic for her.

The community health nurse remembers that she took the children to the kitchen for cookies when they first came in the clinic. Dolly is in the kitchen and has stuffed cookies in her clothing and in a little bag she had found. When the nurse asks Dolly why she is taking so many cookies, Dolly tells the nurse in a matter-of-fact way, "Mama don't have no money today. She won't have any money until Friday. I help Mama find food when she don't have money. We need these cookies so Mama, me and Tony will have something to eat tomorrow. The baby he has milk."

When the community health nurse talks with Portia, she learns that her benefit check has been delayed for a week. In the transition house that she lives in, each family is responsible for their own food. She is receiving formula for the baby but has run out of food stamps for her and the children. The nurse asks about the soup kitchen in the area. Portia says she can't leave the children and it is too far to walk with the children. It is a dangerous place because there is drug dealing and drinking nearby.

Before the family leaves the clinic that day, the community health nurse helps Portia obtain bus tokens to another soup kitchen where other families take their children. In addition, she refers Portia to the social services worker to evaluate the amount of money and benefits that she is receiving. The community health nurse tells Dolly that they can eat some of the cookies today because her mother will have food for them tomorrow. Dolly looks at her mother, turns back to the nurse, and says, "Thank you."

Most families had left their last home as a result of job loss or eviction.

Homeless families tend to seek shelter, and women with small children receive priority for temporary housing. Two-parent families may "double up" with other families, live in tents in state parks, or live in the family car. Once homeless, families have a difficult time finding a place to live because of the lack of available housing and the substantial down payments demanded for rental units. Many families find themselves forced to choose between food and shelter. One or both parents may be employed on a full- or part-time basis, but their income is not sufficient to meet the minimal needs of their family members. Homeless families may be placed in large shelters that provide no privacy for individuals or families; the family unit is severely stressed in such an environment.

Some state and local governments use low-cost motels and hotels to house homeless families. However, the cost is extraordinary, and the living arrangements are poor. Kozol (1988) described life in a welfare hotel in New York City. These hotels provide no cooking facilities, and many are infested with cockroaches and rats.

Extrinsic Risk Factors

Many factors contribute to homelessness that are outside the control of the individual. Being aware of social and economic factors that predispose persons to become homeless can help community health nurses target those populations at risk. Community health nurses can work with others to strengthen the economic opportunities within a community, provide crisis intervention, and strengthen support systems for those who are vulnerable to homelessness.

Unemployment. Many homeless people have lost their jobs when industries relocated or technology replaced their jobs. It is hard to reenter the job market after losing a job for any reason. Homeless men under the age of 40 are likely to have never had a steady full-time job. One study suggested that there were more unemployed blacks than whites, even among higher educated individuals (First et al., 1988). Young women who are single parents or who are addicted to drugs are unlikely to have ever had a full-time job.

Underemployment. As the cost of employee benefits increased in the 1980s, businesses began to hire fewer full-time employees. Available jobs for unskilled or service workers generally pay only minimum wage, and many businesses are currently hiring part-time workers to maximize their profit. An employee who works full time at minimum wage earns an income below the poverty level. In addition, recipients of entitlement may lose their subsidies and health care benefits if they work more than a few hours a week.

Poverty. Persons living at or below the poverty level are more vulnerable and more likely to become homeless than those living above the poverty level. The 1993 poverty level for a family of four was $14,350; this represents the upper level of poverty. Between 1% and 2% of all poor people are homeless, but nearly all homeless people are poor.

Because black, Hispanic, and Native American populations are at greater risk of poverty, they are also at greater risk of homelessness. Nearly one third of all blacks live below the poverty level, a rate three times that of the white population. One of every two black children lives in poverty.

Currently 30% of the Hispanic population in the United States lives in poverty. Relatively recent significant increases in this number are due to legal and illegal immigration. Hispanics are younger than the population as a whole, and almost 90% live in urban areas (Munoz, 1988). Puerto Ricans are one of the most impoverished groups in the nation, with 40% living below the poverty level (Robertson, 1987).

In 1988, there were an estimated 1.7 million Native Americans in the United States. The National American Indian Housing Council estimates that almost one fourth of Native Americans live in dilapidated, substandard, or overcrowded housing. Many Indian families live in cars, tents, or makeshift shelters (Interagency Council on Homelessness, 1990). Native Americans live in probably the worst social and economic conditions in the nation, with an unemployment rate of 60% to 80% (Robertson, 1987).

Asians represent a small percentage of homeless individuals. However, single Asians who come to the United States without sponsorship and without a family unit tend to have homeless experiences similar to those of other minority populations (Troung, 1992).

Domestic Violence. Societal changes have made it more possible for women to escape from domestic violence. Women are more willing to flee from their homes rather than continue to expose themselves or their children to physical, sexual, or emotional violence. Domestic violence exists at all socioeconomic levels, so the threat of becoming homeless exists for middle-class women as well as for others. Domestic violence is prevalent in the history and current circumstances of homeless families (Brown, 1992) (see Chapter 20).

Evictions. For persons living in poverty, any unfortunate circumstance, such as illness, accidents, fire, job loss, or loss of transportation to work can be enough to put them at risk for eviction. Personal belongings are removed and piled outside the building. Because the primary goal is to remove the person from the premises, little care is taken with the handling or disposition of the property. For most people, an eviction is as devastating as a major fire. If the newly homeless person should leave his or her possessions, all of them may disappear before the person can return. This is a major loss and demonstrates the pain and destitution that can be experienced by homeless people. In some communities entrepreneurs collect rental information and compile a list of high-risk tenants that they sell to landlords, who then refuse to rent to anyone who has had previous problems.

Family members are sometimes evicted because of substance abuse or mental illness. The number of people who have been evicted because they have tested positive for the human immunodeficiency virus (HIV) is increasing. Persons who live at or below the poverty level face eviction if they cannot pay their monthly rent, and once evicted, few can save the security deposit, which is usually equivalent to 2 to 3 months' rent.

Deinstitutionalization. The Community Mental Health Act was passed in 1963 in response to many societal changes, including the advent of psychotropic drugs and the recognition of the effects of long-term institutionalization. This federal law was intended to establish mental health centers in local communities. However, minimal funding was provided, and the centers that were developed were insufficient for the numbers of chronically mentally ill persons who were discharged from state psychiatric institutions. As a result, mentally ill individuals went home to live in the community without appropriate treatment programs.

There were many problems associated with the deinstitutionalization process. Residents of local communities did not welcome the development of treatment programs for the chronically mentally ill in their neighborhood. Families did not know how to cope, and many mentally ill persons wandered away from home or their residential treatment program. Since deinstitutionalization began, indications have increased that the seriously mentally ill are receiving less care than they need (Aiken et al., 1986).

The deinstitutionalization components included restriction of admission to psychiatric facilities, as well as short-term hospital stays (Pepper and Ryglewicz, 1984). These policies have resulted in the gradual closure of state mental institutions. Chronically mentally ill persons are young adults who may never have been institutionalized if their behavior did not qualify them for admission under the existing guidelines. Never-institutionalized mentally ill persons have become the major concern for health care providers working with the homeless (Rossi, 1989; Wright, 1989; Eagle and Caton, 1990). Because the majority of mentally ill homeless persons pose no immediate threat to themselves or others, they often do not meet the criteria for involuntary inpatient treatment (Wright, 1989).

Fischer (1988) notes that mentally ill people are often arrested for aberrant and criminal behavior and spend time in jail or prison. Thus, local prisons are becoming like the insane asylums of the past, and neglect in a prison cell has replaced neglect in a state hospital.

Intrinsic Risk Factors

Although many social, cultural, and political factors affect homeless people, their own intrinsic ability to cope and respond to life situations also contributes to their homelessness. Mental illness, low self-esteem related to past neglect or abuse, and substance abuse are some of the intrinsic factors that predispose individuals to homelessness.

Major Mental Illness. Wide variations in mental illness among the homeless have been reported in the literature; however, there is a lack of clear information about the number of mentally ill persons who are homeless (Committee on Labor and Human Resources, 1988). The severity of symptoms has not been consistently evaluated; however, there is an indication that two thirds of mentally ill homeless persons have moderate to severe symptoms (Fischer and Breakey, 1992). The Department of Health and Human Services estimates that about one third of the homeless population suffers from severe mental illness such as schizophrenia and bipolar disorder (Interagency Council on Homelessness, 1990). Severely mentally ill persons have difficulty carrying out activities of daily living, managing themselves, engaging in interpersonal relationships, and going to work. The chances for the severely mentally ill to escape homelessness are limited because of the disruption they experience in personal judgment, motivation, and social skills (National Institute of Mental Health, 1992). Homeless, chronically mentally ill veterans are the target of national outreach programs sponsored by the Department of Veterans Affairs (Rosenheck et al., 1989).

Homeless, chronically mentally ill persons often do not seek help. They may go to soup kitchens or missions, but they are more likely to be found on steam grates and in wooded areas where they can avoid contact with health care providers. When homeless people who have major mental illnesses come to community health care clinics, community health nurses should use community resources to provide psychiatric care for them (Table 23–7).

Mood and Personality Disorders. Depression is one of the most frequent and most serious mood disorders among homeless individuals. Depression may be transient or long lasting, but it is an ever-present possibility that the community health nurse should check for with homeless clients. Suicide rates are very high among homeless persons. Nurses working in clinics that serve the homeless population should assess clients for depression and suicidal ideation. Some clients may freely tell the nurse that they are depressed; others may withhold the information unless they are asked. Consider the following scenario:

> Willie came to the walk-in health clinic in an inner city soup kitchen. It was past time to see clients, and the nurses were preparing to leave. A community health nurse asked Willie why he had come to the clinic. He said, "I'm going to kill myself today." When the nurse asked if he had a plan, he told her that he had a loaded gun under his mattress. When he left the clinic, he was going to go to his room and shoot himself in the head at 4:00 P.M. When asked why he planned to kill himself, he said he was so depressed he couldn't stand it anymore. "I'm an alcoholic. I'm all alone. I have no friends, and my family won't speak to me. I haven't had a job in over 10 years. What's the point? Life is just not worth living." The nurse told Willie that arrangements had been made for an emergency evaluation at a psychiatric hospital. He was transported to the hospital and arrived at the emergency department within an hour after he had come to the clinic.

In this situation the nurse recognized cues that indicated the client was suicidal and acted promptly to arrange for emergency psychiatric care. Although many homeless people have serious mental and emotional problems, most do not require emergency intervention. Mental disorders may precipitate homelessness or may result from the homeless experience. Two of the most severe anxiety disorders—posttraumatic stress disorder and panic disorder—may precipitate or aggravate a homeless existence. Posttraumatic stress disorder is believed to affect many Vietnam veterans. Affected individuals experience such intense stress that they develop dissociative thought processes to avoid painful memories. Many veterans remain lost to their families, friends, and themselves.

Panic disorders are severe manifestations of anxiety and are common among homeless women. Individuals may be so overwhelmed with anxiety that they are unable to take any action, or they may behave in bizarre ways in an attempt to reduce their feelings of anxiety. Homeless women are subject to physical and sexual abuse in shelters and on the streets, which may serve to exacerbate panic conditions (Breakey et al., 1989). Anxiety disorders are treatable, but many people are not aware of available resources or do not have health insurance.

The more severe personality disorders found among homeless persons include schizoaffective and schizotypal disorders. In both disorders individuals relate a long history of an inability to form meaningful relationships with others. Homeless individuals with these kinds of disorders often have never had a close friend; most have never dated, and few, if any, have ever married.

TABLE 23–7

A Successful Mental Health Referral

The community health nurse met Joe on a routine visit to a city shelter for homeless men. The shelter staff members said Joe hallucinated a lot and frightened some of the other guests. The nurse talked with Joe for some time and learned that he had been forced to leave his family home when he was 15 years old. He said his family thought he acted strange, and they didn't like him. Joe found shelter in a junk yard, where the owner befriended him. The owner allowed Joe to live in a little room behind the office. He brought Joe food and clothing so he could stay there and be on guard in case someone broke into the business. Joe had stayed there for 10 years until the owner died. It had been nearly a year since Joe had been wandering around looking for a place to stay. Before coming to the shelter he had been living in an abandoned railroad car.

He would be all right, he said, if he could just get the radio in his head to stop. The radio in his head had been with him as long as he could remember. When the community health nurse told him that she could help him control the radio in his head, he agreed to go to the psychiatric center for evaluation. Within a few days, Joe was started on antipsychotic drugs and was admitted to a halfway house. The nurse saw Joe a month later. He greeted her and said he was feeling much better because the radio in his head had stopped. The community health nurse checked on Joe from time to time. He continued to stay at the halfway house. He told the nurse, "Sometimes I don't take my medication and the radio comes back on. But when I take my medicine it goes off."

Borderline personality disorder and antisocial personality disorders are found among homeless persons who report troubled relationships with family, friends, and others. Persons with borderline personality disorder are often manipulative and have a tendency to create disharmony wherever they go. Persons with antisocial personality disorders describe a history of conflict with parental and legal authorities from an early age. These persons are more likely to have been involved in aggressive or violent actions, and many will have an extensive criminal history.

Low Self-Esteem. Homeless persons experience both acute and chronic manifestations of low self-esteem. The individual develops a sense of self from internal feelings as well as from responses from other people. Past neglect, rejection, assault, rape, or abuse contribute to low self-esteem that predisposes individuals to homelessness. Poverty has a negative impact on an individual's self-esteem, as he or she sees himself or herself as not being able to measure up to others in the environment. Poor functioning in school or dropping out of school early can be associated with low self-esteem.

Virtually everyone in society has been exposed to social norms and standards, whether from parents, school, or other persons. When the individual deviates from social standards related to substance abuse, criminal activity, unemployment, or eviction, the person experiences a loss of self-esteem. Certain conditions such as mental disorders and substance abuse have a negative effect on the individual's self-esteem.

To be homeless is to experience the most acute sense of low self-esteem. The sense exists that one does not measure up and is outside the norms of society. No matter where the person goes, to a service program, to apply for entitlements, or to apply for a job, he or she is required to say that he or she is homeless. The individual can never escape the homeless condition. Many homeless persons dress in such a way that they mingle with crowds and are not immediately recognized by others as being homeless. However, the individual recognizes that he or she is, in fact, different from those persons who leave a public event, for example, and go home at night.

When the homeless individual appears unkempt and is recognized as homeless by others, he or she is subjected to verbal abuse, stares, or total avoidance. Homeless persons speak of the alienation and pain of being shunned in public places. Eventually acute low self-esteem becomes chronic low self-esteem, from which the individual has difficulty escaping without assistance.

Chronic low self-esteem then becomes a barrier that inhibits the individual's ability to regain a positive sense of self-esteem. Chronic low self-esteem is associated with mental disorders, suicide, and chronic homelessness (Drew, 1991; Fortinash and Holoday-Worret, 1991).

Substance Abuse. As many as 70% to 80% of homeless individuals who are substance abusers are alcoholics (see Chapter 21). The number of people who are dependent on other drugs increases each year. As many as 30% of the people with substance abuse problems may also have one or more mental disorders (Fischer and Breakey, 1992).

Chronic alcoholism is a progressive, long-term, fatal disease that interferes with the individual's mental, physical, and social functioning. Koegel and Burnam (1988) conducted a study in Los Angeles of alcoholics who were homeless and compared them to a similar group of alcoholics who had stable living arrangements. The homeless alcoholics had a much longer history of disruptive behavior, including starting fights and arrests before age 15. They had a very small social support system with little, if any, contact with family members. These data suggest the importance of early recognition of and intervention in problem behavior and the need to strengthen social systems.

A review of studies of homeless populations indicates that alcoholism is six to seven times more prevalent in homeless men than in the general population; alcoholism among homeless women is 15 to 30 times more prevalent than in the general population (Fischer and Breakey, 1992). The longer a nonalcoholic person remains homeless, the more likely it is that the person will become alcohol dependent.

Drug addiction includes dependence on drugs such as cocaine, crack, heroin, and a wide variety of prescription medications and inhalants. Drug dependency involves both physical and psychological addiction, resulting in physical, emotional, and social deterioration. There is much more violence involved in drug addiction related to dealing, procurement, and use of drugs. Crimes of violence against others are more common among drug addicts, and addicts are also more prone to being the victim in drug-related activities.

The Homeless Experience

The experience of being homeless affects a person physically, psychologically, socially, and economically.

> On the personal level, home is one of those concepts most of us take so much for granted that we hardly ever pause to think about what it means. Home means family, personal space, privacy. Home means shelter, and warmth, both physical and personal. Home means favored possessions, books, records, history, memories. Home means belonging, identity, love (Jonas, 1986, p. 9).

Even though homeless persons may have lived in poverty, being uprooted means the loss of valued objects and places. They must adjust to a life situation over which they have little, if any, control. Homelessness creates "a plethora of problems and personal risks, not the least of which is a severe threat to the person's identity and sense of self" (Rivilin, 1986, p. 9). For children the loss of a home includes the loss of stability at a crucial time when they are developing a sense of themselves. A child's self-worth, personal identity, and emotional development can be seriously affected by the experience of homelessness (Rivilin, 1990).

Hygiene is a major problem for the many homeless people who have little or no access to public toilets. It is not uncommon for homeless people to partially bathe or wash articles of clothing when they have access to bathrooms. In many sleeping situations, homeless persons will not remove their clothing for fear of theft or for fear they might have to leave in a hurry. Homeless people can get fresh attire from "clothing drops" where they can obtain donated clothing, and many manage to avoid looking unkempt.

The psychological impact of homelessness can be immobilizing so that homeless people feel hopeless and powerless to change their life situation. Psychological issues include loss, loneliness, alienation, shame, fear, anxiety, low self-esteem, depression, and despair. In addition to all of this, homeless persons are made aware that they are despised and unwanted, although forced to be dependent on the goodwill of others for food, clothing, and shelter. Negative personality traits or disorders are exacerbated in this unstable lifestyle. Many have few, if any, social support systems. The very act of living requires significant effort and often leaves little time or energy for other activities.

PHYSICAL HEALTH RISKS

Homeless individuals are exposed to heat and cold, fleas, cockroaches, and rats, as well as diseases such as scabies and tuberculosis. Chronic diseases are often exacerbated because health care is not consistently obtained.

The most disconnected homeless people often refuse to leave their steam grates, cardboard boxes, or dumpsters during severe winter weather. The combination of alcohol and hypothermia seems to allow persons to survive very low core body temperatures (Weyman et al., 1974). Intoxicated persons may be unaware of their need for shelter or may be unable to reach shelter. In many cities alcoholics may be denied shelter if they are intoxicated (Dexter, 1990). Persons who survive severe exposure may experience frostbite and lose fingers, toes, hands, or feet. Every winter homeless alcoholics die from exposure to extreme cold weather.

Summer heat can result in hyperthermia and cause dehydration and heat stroke. Elderly individuals, those who are on psychotropic drugs, and those whose illnesses interfere with thermoregulatory mechanisms are at highest risk.

Poor hygiene related to bathing and not changing clothes leads to health risks and infestation. Homeless people who use shelters and missions have access to showers and clean clothing; some shelters even require showers as a condition for staying overnight. People who sleep outside or in public places have more difficulty finding places to bathe, wash underwear, and change outer clothing. Mentally ill or socially disconnected persons may rarely bathe or change their clothes. Some do not discard old articles of clothing; they just add another layer. Some people may rarely, if ever, undress, which can result in cellulitis and head and body lice. People who do not remove their shoes will have multiple problems, including toenails that assume grotesque and disabling shapes.

Life on the street is rugged and unsafe. Homeless people are aware of the dangers and know that they are subject to beatings, robberies, and rape. Persons who have cashed entitlement checks are often victimized. Many homeless persons refuse new clothes or gifts for fear that they will be subjected to physical violence.

Research designed to study the health problems of homeless persons in America reported that colds and influenza are the most common acute health problem (Brickner et al., 1985; Bowlder, 1989; Ropers and Boyer, 1987; Cuoto et al., 1985; Breakey et al., 1989). The second most common acute problem is accidents or trauma. Scabies and lice infestations not only are troublesome, but also can contribute to dangerous secondary infections. A significant portion of the homeless report having a chronic illness such as diabetes, heart disease, or peripheral vascular disease (Table 23–8).

> The medical disorders of the homeless are common illnesses, magnified by disordered living conditions, exposure to extremes of heat and cold, lack of protection from rain and snow, bizarre sleeping accommodations, and overcrowding in shelters. The stress of street life, psychiatric disorders, and sociopathic behaviors obstruct medical intervention and contribute to the chronicity of disease (Brickner et al., 1985, p. 405).

Common colds may become major problems for persons who must walk most of the day or stand and wait until the shelter doors open in the evening. The Centers for Disease Control and Prevention (1987) has published guidelines for use in controlling tuberculosis among homeless populations; these include case finding and treatment protocols. Ultraviolet lights are recommended in shelters to kill the tuberculosis bacillus. The homeless population is at risk for the acquired immunodeficiency syndrome (AIDS) because of intravenous drug use, risky sexual activity, and lack of knowledge. Nurses should use universal precautions with all homeless people. Once a homeless person has contracted HIV, the development of AIDS may be accelerated by malnutrition and repeated infections. It is not uncommon for terminally ill AIDS patients to be turned out of their homes by family and friends.

Hypertension, diabetes, respiratory illnesses, and cardiovascular diseases are the most common chronic medical problems among the homeless population (Breakey et al., 1989). Chronic alcoholics are subject to gastrointestinal disorders, esophageal hemorrhage, pancreatitis, and cirrhosis. Cancer is not generally detected until the disease is

TABLE 23–8

Physical Health Problems of the Homeless

Acute physical disorders

Upper respiratory conditions
Trauma, including major and minor injuries
Minor skin ailments
Infestations (scabies and lice)
Nutritional deficiencies

Chronic physical disorders

Alcoholism
Hypertension
Gastrointestinal disorders
Peripheral vascular disorders
Dental problems
Neurological disorders

Problems associated with pregnancy

Lack of prenatal care
Inadequate nutrition
Obstetrical complications

Physical illness in children

Upper respiratory illnesses
Minor skin ailments
Ear disorders
Gastrointestinal disorders
Trauma
Eye disorders
Lice infestations

Data from Wright, J. D., & Weber, E. (1987). *Homelessness and health.* New York: McGraw-Hill.

advanced and the person is debilitated. Health care is generally cursory, and treatment, when provided, is directed at the presenting symptoms.

Homeless women have the same illnesses as homeless men, but because they are subjected to rape, they may have more than one sexually transmitted disease. Malnutrition is a particularly difficult problem for young homeless women who are of childbearing age. Homeless pregnant women may be substance abusers and run a higher risk of acquiring and transmitting HIV to their unborn children (Christiano and Susser, 1989).

Homeless children exhibit a wide variety of physical illnesses such as asthma, anemia, diarrhea, and poor nutrition. Many homeless children are subjected to physical abuse. Immunizations may not be started, and the children may contract preventable communicable diseases. Adolescents are at an especially high risk for physical abuse and sexually transmitted diseases, including HIV (Gilliam et al., 1989).

Nursing diagnoses seen among the homeless are shown in Table 23–9.

BARRIERS TO HEALTH CARE

There are many barriers that limit the homeless person's access to health care. Health care may not be a priority and may not be considered important until the individual is ill or injured. The majority of homeless persons do not have Medicaid or health insurance, and they may be denied medical care in emergency departments or clinics. In addition, they may be denied care because they are perceived to be different or undesirable. Homeless people are often considered noncompliant because they do not carry out the prescribed medical regimen or fail to return

TABLE 23–9

Selected Nursing Diagnoses for Homeless People

Potential for injury related to unsafe environment
Altered nutrition, less than body requirements
Potential for infection related to poor nutrition
Self-care deficit: bathing and hygiene
Powerlessness related to homelessness
Ineffective coping related to substance abuse
Ineffective coping related to mental state
Ineffective family coping, compromised
Altered health maintenance
Potential for alteration in body temperature related to exposure to extreme temperatures
Hypothermia related to exposure
Hyperthermia related to exposure
Skin integrity impairment; acute or potential
Bowel elimination altered; diarrhea
Sleep pattern disturbance
Knowledge deficit related to health care needs
Sensory perceptual alterations
Thought processes, altered (acute confusion, delusions, hallucinations, suspiciousness)
Anxiety (mild, moderate, severe, extreme/panic)
Hopelessness
Powerlessness
Self-concept disturbance in self-esteem; personal identity
Family process altered
Impaired communication
Defensive coping (denial, ineffective denial)
Situational crisis
Depression
Manipulation
Impaired social interaction
Potential for self-harm; suicide
Potential for transmission of infection
Noncompliance
Social isolation
Fatigue
Fear
Spiritual distress
Fear related to continual threat of rape
Knowledge deficit related to sexually transmitted diseases
Ineffective denial related to transmission of HIV
Alteration in growth and development
Developmental and cognitive delays
Fluid volume deficit

Data from Carpenito, L. J. (1989). *Nursing diagnosis: Application to clinical practice, 1989–1990* (3rd ed.). Philadelphia: J. B. Lippincott; Cox, H. C., et al. (1989). *Clinical applications of nursing diagnosis: Adult health, child health, women's health, mental health, and home health.* Baltimore: Williams & Wilkins; and Cohen, S. M., Kenner, C. A., & Hollingsworth, A. O. (1991). *Maternal, neonatal, and women's health nursing.* Springhouse, PA: Springhouse Publishing.

Ethics Box V

Gail A. DeLuca Havens, M.S., R.N., C.N.A.

Refusing to Provide Care

The emergency department (ED) is remarkably quiet for a Friday evening. As Maureen, the Registered Nurse Manager for the evening shift, passes the doorway to the waiting room, she catches a glimpse of a dusky face and hands; a man is huddled in a corner at the far end of the room. She wonders why the person is not in one of the examining rooms being evaluated. However, before she has the opportunity to find out why this man is in the waiting room, she is called to give some assistance in calming down an 8-year-old.

Two hours later, activity has increased in the ED. Maureen is headed down the hallway adjacent to the waiting room to retrieve some supplies from a seldom-used cabinet. Her attention is drawn to the same figure in the corner of the waiting room. He doesn't seem to have moved since she noticed him earlier. There is something vaguely familiar about the huddled figure, but what draws Maureen into the waiting room and to the corner is her intuition that something is amiss here. She realizes that the person in the waiting room is experiencing respiratory distress at about the same time she recognizes the person as Horace, a homeless alcoholic who is a frequent visitor to the ED.

"Thanks for finally coming to get me, Miss Maureen. I was beginning to feel mighty poorly."

"No problem, Horace," replies Maureen, as she starts to wheel him from the waiting room into the treatment area. "What seems to be the problem?"

"Trouble breathing. When I take a deep breath it hurts right around where the doctors listen to my heart."

"How long have you been waiting to see the doctor, Horace?"

"Since one o'clock."

Maureen notes that was 8 hours ago. "Horace, did the admitting clerk register you when you arrived?"

"It seemed like she did," he replied.

Maureen situates Horace on a gurney in an examining bay and goes to retrieve his chart from the admitting clerk's area while the physician is evaluating him. Maureen is summoned back into the treatment area by a Code call. Returning, she finds that Horace has stopped breathing, and the physician is slow to respond. She notices that no one but herself seems particularly committed to responding appropriately in this emergency situation. She says, "Folks, you'd better move quickly and effectively, because if this man dies it will be your fault!"

Horace is swiftly and competently resuscitated and several minutes later is responding appropriately to verbal cues. His assessment reveals bilateral pneumonia that is compromising respiratory functions. Horace is admitted and placed on mechanical ventilation for a brief period so that he can be oxygenated properly and suctioned as needed. Horace recovers from his pneumonia and is discharged in several days without complications.

Meanwhile, Maureen questions why she didn't anticipate this kind of reaction to Horace from the ED staff. She had observed and been informed about the growing reluctance of the staff to treat Horace, yet she never considered the possibility that nurses and physicians would collectively refuse to care for a patient. What alternatives do you perceive as responses to this problem?

Over the next several days following Horace's admission, Maureen meets with each of the nurses, physicians, and support personnel on duty the evening that Horace arrested. Their anger and frustration overwhelm her at times. They no longer feel obligated to care for Horace. He doesn't care for himself, so why should they feel any moral obligation to care for him? He consumes precious resources with each almost weekly visit to the ED. Even when he agrees to be admitted to the detoxification unit, he signs himself out before he gives the treatment a chance to work. The ED care providers on duty that evening express bitter resentment at having to continue to provide services to someone who, judging from his behavior, really doesn't want to be well.

Do health care providers have a right to refuse to provide care to an individual who continuously consumes health care resources by knowingly and repeatedly placing himself or herself at risk for disease and injury? What should be Maureen's course of action? How much of the response of the center personnel is attributable to a difference between their values and Horace's values as a homeless person? A study conducted by Downing and Cobb (1990) documented that to the extent that values were synonymous with a definition of culture, cultural differences did exist between a sample of homeless men and the values of the dominant American culture.

One approach to the dilemma is to simply attribute the staff's reaction that evening as a manifestation of their job-related stress and frustration and to believe that it was a single aberrant incident that will not be repeated. However, this strategy would not acknowledge Horace's right to be treated with respect as a person. This is the fundamental principle of the Code For Nurses (American Nurses' Association, 1985), which was breached the evening in question. This strategy also does not address the underlying reason for the staff's refusal to treat Horace. Thus, there remains the potential for an incident of this nature to be repeated. The potential to inflict grave harm—namely, to act with maleficence—in the process is a real possibility as well. Finally, Maureen recalls that the ED was relatively quiet the evening of the incident involving Horace, so it is doubtful that situation-induced stress was a factor.

Maureen completes an incident report. This process will notify all appropriate nursing and medical administrative personnel who will be responsible for follow-up with the individuals involved. Still, she is left with grave concern. Nursing and medicine have a covenant with society to provide competent care to its members. Personnel are bound by the principle of fidelity to remain faithful to the trust and responsibility placed on nursing (and medicine) by society to provide care that is not limited by personal beliefs and attitudes (American Nurses' Association, 1985).

Maureen is particularly concerned about the nurses involved in this incident. Conflicting obligations of fidelity have been characterized as more pervasive and morally troubling in nursing than they are in any other area of health care. This is due primarily to the role of nursing in health care, in which an individual nurse often must choose between responsibilities to the employing institution and physicians on the one hand and responsibilities to patients on the other (Beauchamp and Childress, 1989).

Maureen decides to convene a consultant's group comprised of peers, a social worker, a representative from the institution's ethics committee, and a psychiatrist who specializes in problems professionals encounter in their practice. Her goal is to have the group meet with the ED nurses and physicians on duty the evening of the incident with Horace to engage them in ongoing dialogue and to offer continuing support for future problems of this nature.

References

American Nurses' Association. (1985). *Code for nurses with interpretive statements.* Kansas City, MO: Author.

Beauchamp, T. L., & Childress, J. F. (1989). *Principles of biomedical ethics* (3rd ed.). New York: Oxford University Press.

Downing, C. K., & Cobb, A. K. (1990). Value orientations of homeless men. *Western Journal of Nursing Research, 12,* 619–628.

to scheduled clinic visits. Unfortunately, the attitudes of health care providers can be one of the most difficult barriers for the homeless person to overcome (see Ethics Box V). Community health nurses can assist in breaking down these attitudinal barriers through case presentations and education. They can aid in the development of realistic expectations about compliance and the lack of resources available to the homeless person.

Community Health Nurse's Role in Working with Homeless People

The community health nurse working with homeless people must be a generalist in terms of health concerns. The nurse must be aware of the multiple variables that affect a homeless person's ability to cope with the stresses of living on the street. Each nurse must assume responsibility to avoid personal risk when working in environments that may be unsafe. One need not work in fear; however, psychiatric nursing principles such as setting limits, redirecting, and fostering impulse control are important skills for the nurse who works with homeless people.

Nurses must be aware of their own motives and concerns when working with homeless persons. Those who approach the homeless expecting to meet people in difficult situations will not be disappointed. However, those who approach the homeless expecting to turn their lives around may be let down. The needs of homeless people are diverse. Accomplishments are often measured in small changes, and commitment and persistence are required to continue working with individuals who may fail repeatedly in their continuing struggles (Hines, 1992). It may take many months for a homeless person to be able to trust a community health nurse. Homeless persons will quickly stop participating in a program if they sense that the nurse does not approve of them or their lives (Wright and Weber, 1987).

There are some underlying principles that will help the nurse work with homeless people. Unconditional positive regard, as described by Rogers (1980), is fundamental in working with homeless people. In essence, a nonjudgmental attitude toward clients allows persons to be who they are at that moment. The nurse must be sensitive to the reality experienced by the homeless person, which can allow for more honest communication between the individual and the nurse. Homeless people are often asked by service providers to meet expectations that may be quite unattainable. Healing relationships begin with empathic, accepting, caring, and nonjudgmental communication.

Trust has its foundation in acceptance and truth. Nurses learn to use indirect communication techniques and may be uncomfortable in using a more direct approach with the homeless person. Direct communication is not only more effective, it also allows for clearer questions and clearer responses. Direct communication includes looking at the person and speaking to the person in a clear and concise way. "When did you have your last drink?" will get a more accurate and meaningful response than, "Have you ever had a drinking problem?" Homeless persons may not respond or may make defensive responses if they feel the nurse's questions are intrusive or irrelevant. Homeless people have a tendency to be impatient and may not tolerate a complex medical history (Table 23–10).

The community health nurse must maintain a clear understanding of the reality of the world in which the nurse and the client exist. An effective nurse will provide the client with a reality that may not always be pleasant but is honest and factual. Whenever possible, the nurse should engage persons in telling their own story. If they choose not to participate, do not make an issue of it. Suggest that such information could be helpful if they are willing to share it in the future, and then focus on the essential information that is needed at that time. When communicating with clients, call them by their preferred name. It is possible to be direct and caring without being confrontational.

PROBLEM-SOLVING BEHAVIORS

Homeless individuals may never have learned effective problem-solving behaviors but instead use "street-wise" behaviors to get what they need. These behaviors include manipulation, lying, and panhandling to obtain money for food, drugs, alcohol, or a place to sleep. Each agency with which a homeless person comes into contact has its own rules and regulations. Some people find the complexity too difficult to deal with and go without services rather than be subjected to more rules, regulations, forms, and interviews. Many, if not most, homeless individuals lack an awareness of social programs, community services, or entitlements for which they may be eligible.

Homeless people often feel so overwhelmed by their daily struggle for food and shelter that they lose hope.

TABLE 23–10

Examples of Effective and Ineffective Communication with the Homeless

Ineffective Communication	Client Response	Effective Communication	Client Response
Do you have a drinking problem?	No.	About how much do you drink each day?	Six quarts of beer and a fifth of wine when I have the money.
Have you ever used drugs?	No.	Have you used cocaine or heroin today?	No. I haven't used cocaine since last week. I stay away from heroin. That's bad stuff.
When did life change for you?	Oh, I don't know. It's been a while.	How long has it been since you didn't have a regular place to live?	It was 2 years ago in January. I lost my job and my girl told me to get out.
Let me know if I can be of any help.	Okay.	Hi. I'm the nurse here. How long has it been since you had your blood pressure checked?	It's been a while. I'm supposed to be on blood pressure medicine, but I don't have any money.
Come back next Monday at 10:15 for your next appointment.	Next Monday? Well, I have to be on the other side of town for breakfast. I'll come if I can.	I am here every day from 9 A.M. to 3 P.M. I want to see your foot on Monday so that I can check your infection. It's very important. Can you make it by 3 P.M.?	I'll be here on Monday. Thank you for looking at my foot.
You missed your last appointment. You will have to wait until there is an opening in the schedule.	It was raining, and I couldn't get here on time.	I looked for you on Monday. Are you all right? Can I check your sore foot now?	It was raining, and I didn't want to get my feet wet, so I stayed where it was dry.
If drinking is a problem, why don't you go to a detox program?	I'm not ready.	You look terrible. Have you been on a drinking binge? Five or six days? When did you eat last? Can I see if there is a bed in the detox program?	I started drinking last weekend. Me and some buddies. I haven't had anything to eat and I feel real shaky. I guess I better go now. I feel real bad.

TABLE 23–11

Selected Nursing Interventions

Stage of Homelessness	Level of Prevention: *Primary Intervention*	*Secondary Intervention*	*Tertiary Intervention*
Stage 1	Improve physical environment (community, home) Provision of adequate housing Health education Sex education Drug and alcohol education Good nutrition Pregnancy and nutrition Advocacy Supporting legislation that helps the poor Increased minimum wage Child daycare Access to health care	Health screening Referral programs Case management Case finding Screening for iron, tuberculosis, HIV, hemoglobin, substance use Diagnostic services Providing treatment for acute illnesses Treating potentially life-threatening illnesses (e.g., rehydration of young children)	Control spread of disease Treatment of tuberculosis and AIDS Drug and alcohol treatment programs Treatment of mental illnesses Strengthen support systems
Stage 2	Teaching effective coping behaviors Teaching avoidance of potentially violent situations Advocacy Health education Interpersonal skills training Develop interrelationships with service providers Recommendations regarding food and handling and exposure to infectious diseases Importance of good nutrition Referrals for legal assistance	Screening for chronic illnesses Leg ulcers Drug abuse Trauma Hypertension Cancer Immunizations Monitoring psychiatric status and compliance with medical regimen Monitoring status of infectious diseases Providing on-site care in shelters and service centers	Treatment for major mental illnesses Treatment for major illnesses and injuries Detoxification programs Management of chronic illnesses Management of AIDS symptoms
Stage 3	Advocacy Outreach program Promoting legislation regarding homeless mentally ill Promoting legislation for care to homeless Locating homeless through outreach programs Multiservice programs in service sites	Case management Mobile treatment programs Monitoring changes in health status Providing access to basic nutritional needs	Protection from violence Promoting wet and dry detoxification Treatment for major illnesses Assisting persons to get into mental health programs Supervised housing Increasing independence

Effective problem-solving behaviors help clients focus on practical solutions. The nurse can help the client look at his or her problems in manageable stages, categorizing them as problems that need attention in the present, problems that can wait, and problems that will require more time or interventions. Community health nurses can help clarify the problem, help the client look for options, and provide information about resources. Some clients will need emotional support or practical assistance to accomplish the necessary solutions. The community health nurse must have access to reliable community resources.

NURSING INTERVENTIONS

Community health nurses are familiar with the concepts of primary prevention, secondary prevention, and tertiary prevention. Primary prevention includes health promotion activities, while secondary prevention includes diagnosis and treatment. Tertiary prevention is directed toward rehabilitation (Table 23–11).

The goal of care with persons in the first stage of homelessness is to prevent or at least reduce the frequency of homeless experiences, to give individuals the skills and resources to help them maintain membership in mainstream society (e.g., a job and a place to live).

In the second stage of homelessness the goal is to assist homeless persons to reduce the factors that keep them homeless and to gain the skills or ability to move into a higher level of functioning. A change in maladaptive behaviors acquired during prolonged periods of homelessness usually involves small, sequential changes toward a more stable lifestyle. Treatment of physical and emotional illnesses, including serious personality disorders and alcohol and drug problems, is essential in this stage.

Third-stage goals are to increase the amount of interaction with service providers and acceptance of at least minimal health care. This could include detoxification and treatment for chronic mental illnesses as well as for end-stage alcoholism. Supportive care and residential programs may be the highest level of functioning attainable for these persons.

Primary Prevention. Nursing interventions in primary prevention include both the individual and the community and have as their focus the prevention of homelessness. Identifying factors that contribute to family breakdown or homelessness or exacerbate homelessness are key roles of the nurse who works with individuals or families. Primary prevention within the community includes serving as an advocate and spokesperson for homeless persons and those at risk for homelessness. Nurses across the United States have responded to the needs of homeless people by planning and developing programs that provide food, shelter, and health care for homeless men, women, and children. University-based schools of nursing operate health care clinics in many states. Nursing students have opportunities to work with homeless individuals in clinics and community health settings (Anderson and Marteus, 1987; Turner, et al., 1989; Scholler-Jaquish, 1993).

Nurses who work with homeless persons not only are concerned with the individual, but also look beyond the pain and anguish they witness to the forces that have created homelessness. As advocates for homeless persons, nurses a ddress access to health care, including access to mental health and substance abuse treatment programs. In addition, they address the availability of low-income housing, welfare reform, job training, and protection from physical and sexual violence. A community health nurse can identify ways to communicate the needs of homeless persons and those at risk of homelessness to local communities and government policy makers on a state or national level.

> The American Nurses' Association has long been supportive of legislation advocating for the homeless. The national epidemic of homelessness defines a standard of health, and of caring, far lower than we as professionals will tolerate for our patients. The time for our strength and resources on behalf of the homeless is past due (Rafferty, 1989, p. 1615).

Secondary Prevention. Secondary prevention interventions include health screening, case finding, and referral programs. The community health nurse has many opportunities to prevent and detect diseases through work in community agencies or at outreach sites. In the first stage of homelessness, the nurse can be involved in screening clinics for children and prenatal programs for pregnant women. The nurse may address the care and handling of food, as well as the nutritional needs of children, pregnant women, and persons with chronic illnesses. Community health nurses can provide screening programs at service sites and test for chronic or communicable diseases.

Homeless people have difficulty gaining access to health care facilities. As a result, health care services are being provided by community health nurses in soup kitchens and shelters where the homeless can gain immediate access. Tuberculosis is an increasing problem in shelters and soup kitchens, and nurses can help prevent, detect, and treat tuberculosis (McAdam et al., 1990).

In the third stage of homelessness the nurse will be challenged to locate homeless individuals through outreach programs and mobile treatment programs. Providing access to food and basic services are important, as are protecting homeless men and women from violence. Again, health clinics located in soup kitchens and shelters are more accessible to people who use those resources.

Tertiary Prevention. Tertiary prevention interventions in the first stage of homelessness include teaching effective coping behaviors and helping persons to avoid potentially violent situations. Referral to mental health and substance abuse treatment programs are important interventions. Assisting persons with HIV to comply with their treatment plan is important as they struggle with both illness and homelessness.

In the second stage, tertiary interventions include detoxification programs, literacy and job training programs, treatment for major mental illnesses, and management of chronic illnesses.

Tertiary care in the third stage of homelessness includes nonmedical detoxification programs and assisting people to gain access to mental health programs. The numbers and kinds of problems experienced by homeless people

TABLE 23–12

Charles: Care and Respect During the Third Stage of Homelessness

Charles had been a homeless alcoholic for 40 years. He had been arrested for indecent exposure when he urinated on a public street. Charles had lived in alleys and abandoned buildings most of the time that he was not in jail for vagrancy or public intoxication. While in the city jail he had been diagnosed with cancer of the lung and prostate gland. Charles had been transferred to the state prison hospital for care. He quietly refused all treatment and escaped attention until the day his sentence was completed. The warden of the state prison then realized he had a terminally ill homeless man who needed to be discharged immediately. He sought assistance from the community health nursing department.

The community health nurse assigned to work with Charles was able to locate a geriatric foster home that was willing to accept him on a temporary basis. Despite their mutual misgivings, Charles was able to adapt to living with a family. He accepted some light household tasks, and they provided the necessary physical and emotional support that he needed. The community health nurse learned that Charles was eligible for Veterans Administration benefits and that he had worked for a railroad and was eligible for retirement benefits. The community health nurse arranged for hospice care; Charles was able to receive medical care and pay for hospice care. After living in alleys and doorways for most of his adult life, he was able to die in a caring environment. Charles was buried in a veterans cemetery with the respect and honor he had not known while he was alive.

increase over time and with age. The community health nurse will see clients with chronic illnesses such as tuberculosis, diabetes, and hypertension, as well as substance abuse and mental illness (Kinchen and Wright, 1991). The long-term effects of physical neglect, substance abuse, poor hygiene, social isolation, and psychological deterioration all affect the extent of rehabilitation that is possible. The community health nurse will assist homeless persons to enhance their ability to function at a higher level (Table 23–12).

The community health nurse who works with homeless individuals will be challenged in many ways. When resources are scarce or not available, the nurse will often have to improvise in providing care. When supplies are not available, soap, water, safety pins, and assorted items can be used to clean wounds, secure dressings, or hold supplies. One community health nurse sat down and explained to a client what she was going to use and that this was because she had nothing else on hand. When the homeless person understood that she was working with limited resources, he said, "That'll do."

TABLE 23–13

National and Community Organizations

Clearing House on Homelessness Among Mentally Ill People
8630 Fenton St.
Silver Spring, MD 20910
(301) 488-5484

Homelessness Information Exchange
1830 Connecticut Ave. NW
Washington, DC 20009
(202) 462-7551

Interagency Council on Homelessness
451 Seventh St. NW
Washington, DC 20410
(202) 708-1480

National Coalition for the Homeless
1439 Rhode Island Ave. NW
Washington, DC 20005
(202) 659-3310

National Runaway Switchboard
2210 N. Halsted St.
Chicago, IL 60614
(800) 621-4000

PUSH (People United to Save Humanity)
P.O. Box 5432
Chicago, IL 60680-9919

Salvation Army
709 Bloomfield Ave.
Verona, NJ 07044
(201) 239-0606

National Law Center for Homelessness
911 F St. NW
Suite 412
Washington, DC 20004
(202) 638-2535

Community Resources and Organizations

Community resources to serve the very poor and homeless people vary widely among states and within each state. The community health nurse must have an up-to-date list of resources (Table 23–13). More information may be available from state, city, or county governments; state and local health departments; mental health services; and the state department of social services. On a national level information is available from organizations that provide services to homeless individuals. The McKinney Homelessness Act passed in 1987 provides money to assist homeless persons through existing federal programs (General Accounting Office, 1991). The Act provides some money to shelters, soup kitchens, and health care services to provide direct services to the homeless, although a significant amount is designated for research.

KEY IDEAS

1. Homeless men, women, and children live in desolate conditions in cities, towns, and rural areas across America.
2. Many intrinsic and extrinsic factors, such as substance abuse and unemployment, contribute to homelessness.
3. Community health nurses can reduce homelessness by early intervention. The stages of homelessness intervention model can serve as a guide in assisting the community health nurse in planning nursing interventions for the homeless.
4. The community health nurse can serve as a vital link for the homeless person and foster movement toward better health and a more effective lifestyle.
5. Community health nurses can begin breaking down the barriers to health care through public and professional education. Placement of health care clinics in locations where homeless people use other services has proven to be beneficial. Outreach programs that provide food and medical services to homeless people help remove some of the barriers that homeless persons encounter.
6. Clinics or programs within an acute care hospital that serve the special needs of the homeless has also proven effective. Community networks serve to assist the client with social welfare and health care.
7. The community health nurse has a unique opportunity to identify the need for adequate low-income housing. Nurses have a responsibility to become aware of the impact that public policies have on the lives of poor and homeless individuals.

8 Community health nurses can advocate on behalf of homeless persons by writing or calling state and federal representatives with concerns related to homelessness. In addition, community health nurses can talk to professional and lay groups about issues and concerns related to the homeless. Each nurse can make a difference by sharing her or his experiences with others.

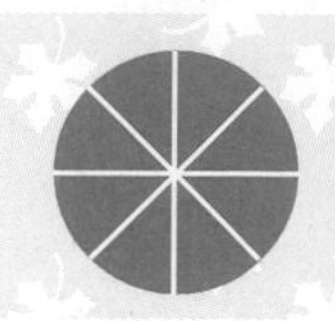

APPLYING THE NURSING PROCESS: *A Homeless Man at Risk for AIDS*

Mr. J. is a 37-year-old man who has been homeless for 2 years in a large city. He completed the 10th grade in school and has worked episodically in food service occupations. He has come to the health care clinic on several occasions for treatment of a cold or to "have my blood pressure checked." He was dependent on intravenous cocaine before he was imprisoned 5 years ago for drug-related activities. He didn't use drugs for 3 years, but since his release from prison he says he has "gotten high every chance I get. I don't have much money, so I only use cocaine about once a week. If I have a little money I may drink beer. When I don't have any money, I do without. It's too embarrassing to beg." Mr. J. has expressed interest in a drug treatment program, but there is a long waiting period for inpatient programs that accept persons without any insurance.

Mr. J. states that he is aware of behaviors that place him at risk for HIV. He carries condoms with him and states that he uses them. He is not as careful with his needles. Sometimes he forgets and borrows a friend's needle when using cocaine. Mr. J. has no steady relationships, but does stay with girlfriends for a few weeks at a time. He has a 10-year-old son whom he has not seen in 2 years. Two years ago, Mr. J. tested negative for HIV and tuberculosis. He has refused tests since that time.

Mr. J.'s blood pressure is 160/94 mm Hg. He reports that his grandmother died of a stroke 2 years ago. He has refused a complete physical examination, insisting, "What you don't know can't hurt you." On his last two visits, Mr. J. has expressed concern that anything will ever get better. He said, "This is a terrible way to live. No place to call your own. No one wants to look at me or talk to me. I just don't see the point in going on. One way or another, this has got to stop. Life hurts too much to keep going on."

During this visit Mr. J. tells the nurse that his cold doesn't seem to be getting better, saying, "I cough at night, and lately it seems that I wake up in the night sweating a lot. I don't really understand it, because the mission is pretty cold." As the nurse continues to talk with him, she learns that he has begun having diarrhea in the past week. Mr. J. asks about a change of clothes because the clothes he is wearing seem to be getting too big for him.

Based on a thorough assessment of the client, the nurse may begin to develop a mutually acceptable plan of care for Mr. J.

Assessment

1. Assess physical, psychological, social, spiritual, and environmental needs of the client.
2. Assess for the presence of depression, suicidal intentions, social isolation, ability to meet nutritional needs, self-care behaviors, and compliance with health regimen.
3. Assess the degree of family and social supports available to assist the client through prolonged homelessness (i.e., shelter, legal assistance, transportation, job training, advocacy, financial aid).
4. Assess for neglect owing to ineffective individual coping.
5. Assess the potential for injury owing to the client's lifestyle and exposure to multiple risk factors.
6. Assess the potential need for legal services.

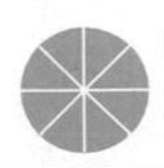

Diagnosis	Goal	Interventions
Depression as manifested by statements of hopelessness.	Client will describe an improved sense of well-being and control over his personal circumstances.	Arrange referral for psychiatric evaluation for antidepressant therapy and psychotherapy. Explore available self-help options such as psychiatric outpatient groups.
Potential for self-harm related to depression as manifested by his statement, "One way or another, this has got to stop. Life hurts too much to keep going on."	Client will verbalize a decreased level of hopelessness and despair.	Make a verbal contract with the client that he will not harm himself. Support the client through this period of distress by accepting his behavior, avoiding judgmental evaluations, and reinforcing positive statements and behaviors.
Alterations in bowel elimination as manifested by diarrhea lasting at least 1 week.	The client will report less diarrhea.	Consult with primary care provider about the use of antidiarrheal medication. Explain the effects of diarrhea on hydration.
Fluid volume deficit related to loss of body fluids, as manifested by diarrhea and night sweats.	The client will maintain adequate intake and fluid.	Increase intake of foods high in sodium and potassium. Increase daily fluid volume. Teach types of fluids to drink, such as water, soda, and hypertonic solutions.
Altered nutrition: less than body requirements as manifested by clothes that have become too big.	The client will maintain body weight.	Consult with primary provider regarding cause of weight loss. Assist the client to maintain an adequate diet with food supplements if necessary.
Alteration in health maintenance as manifested by hypertension and absence of HIV and tuberculosis testing.	The client will participate in health screening activities.	Consult with the primary care provider for a physical examination. Arrange for HIV and tuberculosis testing by primary care provider or community health agency.
Knowledge deficit related to HIV status and associated symptoms.	The client will describe the symptoms of AIDS.	Teach the client the signs and symptoms of AIDS. Assist the client to identify any signs of AIDS that he may have at this time.
Potential for transmission of infection as related to lack of knowledge about the modes of transmission of HIV.	The client will describe the ways in which HIV is transmitted and how he can use that information.	Assist the client to identify different methods for using clean needles if he continues to use cocaine (e.g., cleaning needles and syringes in bleach) and needle exchange

(Continued)

Diagnosis	Goal	Interventions
		programs where needles are available. Reinforce patient education about the use of safer sex with all sexual partners at all times.
Sleep pattern disturbance as related to night sweats.	The client will be able to sleep through the night.	Consult with primary care provider to determine cause of night sweats.
Potential for ineffective airway clearance and potential for transmission of infection.	The client will demonstrate effective coughing and increased air exchange.	Assess for contributing factors. Initiate health teaching about body positioning and secretion management. Discuss ways to avoid spread of organisms to others.
Ineffective individual coping related to substance abuse: cocaine and alcohol abuse.	The client will abstain from cocaine and alcohol use.	Assist the client to achieve abstinence through participation in Narcotics Anonymous (NA) or Alcoholics Anonymous (AA). Instill a sense of hope through helping him identify his goals for himself and exploring possibilities.
Powerlessness related to homelessness as manifested by inability to get a job.	The client will identify factors that he can control.	Assist the client to make plans for things that he can do to gain some control over his life situation (e.g., making an appointment with social services to explore the possibility of financial or housing benefits for which he may be eligible. Initiate a referral to employment or job training programs available in the community. Assist the client to identify whether a need exists for legal services.
Social isolation as manifested by exclusion from his family and perceived rejection by others.	The client will discuss ways of increasing meaningful relationships with others.	Encourage the client to talk about his feelings. Encourage the client to engage in conversations with other people in the soup kitchens and missions that he uses frequently.
Self-concept disturbance: chronic low self-esteem as manifested by denial of problems, self-neglect, and self-destructive behaviors.	The client will identify positive aspects about self.	Provide realistic positive feedback on accomplishments. Provide opportunities for positive socialization. Provide clothes that fit.

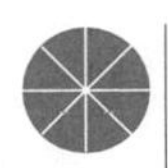

Diagnosis	Goal	Interventions
Altered sexual practices related to ineffective individual coping as manifested by short-term relationships.	The client will identify constructive coping patterns.	Assist the client to identify lifestyle changes he could make that would help him begin to develop more meaningful relationships.
Ineffective denial as related to hypertension, manifested by refusal to have a medical evaluation.	The client will identify his coping behaviors and the potential consequences.	Teach constructive problem-solving techniques. Assist the client to develop appropriate strategies.
Spiritual distress related to homelessness as manifested by questioning the meaning of life.	The client will express feelings related to his beliefs about the meaning of life.	Assist the client to begin problem-solving process and move toward new spiritual understanding. Assist the client to identify spiritual values that he acquired in the past and explore those values as important resources that he can use again.

Evaluation

The client will be instructed to return at periodic intervals to evaluate his status and compliance with medical regimen.

The community health nurse will continue to evaluate the existing problems, as well as identify any new problems that may arise. Life circumstances change for homeless people, and they do not necessarily maintain long-term relationships with one care provider. As long as the client continues to use the community health center, the community health nurse can be an important resource person for him.

Priorities for evaluation are determined by the seriousness of the client's problems.

3 Days:

- Status of diarrhea and related problems
- Level of depression and degree of risk for suicide
- Compliance in making arrangments with visits to primary provider and psychiatrist

10 to 14 Days:

- Determine if the client has been compliant with treatment and care prescribed by health care providers
- Monitor weight gain or loss
- Evaluate response to treatment
- Support positive response to care plan

4 Weeks:

- Monitor progress in relation to physical and psychiatric care plans
- Provide supportive care as needed
- Communicate with primary providers relating to recurrent problems
- Determine effectiveness of problem solving techniques
- Explore progress toward more stable living situation

GUIDELINES FOR LEARNING

① For 2 weeks clip items from newspapers and magazines concerning poverty, homelessness, and federal and state policies that will directly or indirectly affect the homeless or very poor. What are examples of inequities of access to health care? What are examples of injustices relating to health or health care based on race or income level?

② Volunteer to work in a soup kitchen or shelter for at least 4 hours. What did you feel when you first arrived? How present were you to the clients you encountered there? What was significant for you in this experience?

③ Visit an emergency department and interview staff nurses about methods of working with homeless people. Observe the patterns of interaction with clients in the waiting room or receiving ward. Do you observe differences that may not be related to the patient's condition? How do nurses respond when you ask about caring for homeless people? What are the problems they perceive, and how do they deal with them?

④ Look for a homeless person in your community. Write a description of the person and your own feelings about the person and his or her situation. How old is this homeless person? Who might this person be? Is this someone's father, brother, husband, mother, sister, or friend? How do you imagine this person became homeless? How do you feel about this person? How do you feel about yourself? Is there something that you want to do in response to this experience?

⑤ Make a list of adjectives that you hear people use to describe the homeless. What values do these words represent? How do you feel about these values? Do you share some of these values? All of them? None? What can you do to change value judgments that you disagree with in relation to providing health care to a homeless person?

REFERENCES

Adams, G. R., Gullotta, T., & Clancey, M. A. (1985). Homeless adolescents: A descriptive study of similarities and differences between runaways and throwaways. *Adolescence, 20*(79), 715–724.

Aiken, L. H., Somers, S. A., & Shore, M. F. (1986). Private foundations in health affairs: A case study of the development of a national initiative for the chronically mentally ill. *American Psychologist, 41*(11), 1290–1295.

Anderson, J. A., & Marteus, T. M. (1987). Combining community health and psychosocial nursing: A clinical experience with the homeless for generic baccalaureate students. *Journal of Nursing Education, 27*(5), 189–193.

Bachrach, L. L. (1987). Homeless women: A context for health planning. *The Millbank Quarterly, 65*(3), 371–397.

Bassuk, E. L., Rubin, L., & Lauriat, A. S. (1986). Characteristics of sheltered homeless families. *American Journal of Public Health, 76*(9), 1097–1101.

Bassuk, E. L., & Galagher, E. M. (1990). The impact of homelessness on children. In N. A. Boxill (Ed.), *Homeless children: The watchers and waiters.* New York: Haworth Press.

Bassuk, E. L. & Rosenberg, L. (1990). Psychosocial characteristics of homeless children and children with homes. *Pediatrics, 85*(3), 257–261.

Bean, G., Stefl, M., & Howe, S. (1987). Mental health and homelessness: Issues and findings. *Social Work, 32*(5), 411–416.

Belcher, J. R., & DiBlasio, F. A. (1990). *Helping the homeless: Where do we go from here?* Lexington, MA: Lexington Books.

Belcher, J. R., Scholler-Jaquish, A., & Drummond, M. (1991). Three stages of homelessness: A conceptual model for social workers in health care. *Health and Social Work, 16*(2), 87–93.

Benda, B. B., & Dattalo, P. (1988). Homelessness: Consequence of a crisis or long-term process? *Hospital and Community Psychiatry, 39*(8), 884–886.

Boondas, J. (1985). The despair of the homeless aged. *Journal of Gerontological Nursing, 11*(4), 9–14.

Bowlder, J. E. (1989). Health problems of the homeless in America. *Nurse Practitioner, 14*(7), 44, 47, 50–51.

Breakey, W. R., Fischer, P. J., Kramer, M., Nestadt, G., Romanski, A. J., Ross, A., Royall, R. M., & Stine, O. C. (1989). Health and mental health problems of homeless men and women in Baltimore. *Journal of the American Medical Association, 262*(10), 1352–1357.

Brickner, P. W., Sharer, L. K., Conanan, B., Elvy, A., & Savarese, M. (1985). *Health care of homeless people.* New York: Springer.

Brown, A. (1992). Family violence. In E. L. Bassuk & D. A. Cohen (Eds.), *Homeless families with children: Research perspectives* (pp. 37–42). Rockville, MD: Alcohol, Drug Abuse, and Mental Health Administration,

Brown, J. L. (1989). When violence has a benevolent face: The paradox of hunger in the world's wealthiest democracy. *International Journal of Health Services, 19*(2), 257–277.

Carliner, M. S. (1987). Homelessness: A housing problem? In R. D. Bingham, R. E. Green, & S. B. White (Eds.), *The homeless in contemporary society.* Newbury Park, CA: Sage Publications.

Carpenito, L. J. (1989). *Nursing diagnosis: Application to clinical practice, 1989–1990* (3rd ed.). Philadelphia: J.B. Lippincott.

Centers for Disease Control and Prevention (1987). Tuberculosis control among homeless populations. *Journal of the American Medical Association, 257*(21), 2866, 2888.

Christiano, A., & Susser, I. (1989). Knowledge and perceptions of HIV infection among homeless pregnant women. *Journal of Nurse Mid-Wifery, 34*(6), 318–322.

Cohen, S. M., Kenner, C. A., & Hollingsworth, A. O. (1991). *Maternal, Neonatal, and Women's Health Nursing.* Springhouse, PA: Springhouse Publishing.

Committee on Labor and Human Resources. (1988). *Homeless mentally ill: Problems and options in estimating numbers and trends.* Washington, DC: Author.

Cox, H. C., Hinz, M. D., Lubno, M. A., Newfield, S. A., Ridenour, N. A., & Sridaromont, K. L. (1989). *Clinical applications of nursing diagnosis: Adult health, child health, women's health, mental health, and home health.* Baltimore, MD: Williams & Wilkins.

Cuoto, R. A., Lawrence, R. P., & Lee, B. A. (1985). Health care and the homeless of Nashville: Dealing with a problem without definition. *Urban Resource, 2*(2), 17–23.

Dear, M., & Takahashi, L. (1990). *Homeless veterans in Los Angeles.* Working paper no. 30. Los Angeles, CA: Los Angeles Homeless Project, University of Southern California Department of Geography.

Dexter, R. A. (1990). Treating homeless and mentally ill substance abusers in Alaska. In M. Argeriou & D. McCarty (Eds.). *Alcoholism and drug abuse among homeless men and women* (pp. 25–30). New York: Haworth Press.

Drew, N. (1991). Combating the social isolation of chronic mental illness. *Journal of Psychosocial Nursing, 29*(6), 14–17.

Eagle, P. F., & Caton, C. L. M. (1990). Homelessness and mental illness. In C. L. M. Caton (Ed.). *Homeless in America* (pp. 59–75). New York: Oxford University Press.

Fierman, A. H., Dreyer, B. P., Quinn, L., Shulman, S., Courtlandt, C. D., & Guzzo, R. (1991). Growth delay in homeless children. *Pediatrics, 88*(5), 918–925.

First, R. J., Roth, D., & Arewa, B. D. (1988). Homelessness: Understanding the dimensions of the problem for minorities. *Social Work, March/April, 33,* 120–124.

Fischer, P. J. (1988). Criminal activity among the homeless: A study of arrests in Baltimore. *Hospital and Community Psychiatry, 39*(1), 46–51.

Fischer, P. J., & Breakey, W. R. (1992). The epidemiology of alcohol, drug and mental disorders among homeless persons. *American Psychologist, 46*(11), 1115–1128.

Fischer, P. J., Shapiro, S., Breakey, W. R., Anthony, J. C., & Kramer, M. (1986). Mental health and social characteristics of the homeless: A survey of mission users. *American Journal of Public Health, 76*(5), 519–524.

Fortinash, P. J., & Holoday-Worret, P. A. (1991). *Psychiatric Nursing Care Plans*. St. Louis: Mosby–Year Book.

Gelberg, L., & Linn, L. S. (1988). Social and physical health of homeless adults previously treated for mental health problems. *Hospital and Community Psychiatry, 39*(5), 510–516.

General Accounting Office (1991). *Homelessness: McKinney Act programs and funding through fiscal year 1990.* Washington, DC: Author.

Gilliam, A., Scott, M., & Troup, J. (1989). AIDS education and risk reduction for homeless women and children: Implications for health education. *Health Education, 20*(5), 44–47.

Grant, R. (1989). *Assessing the damage: The impact of shelter experiences on homeless young children.* Unpublished paper, New York State Office of Mental Health.

Hier, S. J., Korboot, P. J., & Schweitzer, R. D. (1990). Social adjustment and symptomatology in two types of homeless adolescents: Runaways and throwaways. *Adolescence, 25*(100), 761–771.

Hines, D. R. (1992). Presence: Discovering the artistry in relating. *Journal of Holistic Nursing, 10*(4), 294–305.

Hoch, C., & Slayton, R. A. (1989). *New homeless and old: Community and the skid row.* Philadelphia: Temple University Press.

Interagency Council on Homelessness (1990). *1990 Annual report.* Washington, DC: Author.

Jackson-Jobe, P. (1992). Conclusion: Responding to the challenge. In C. Solomon & P. Jackson-Jobe (Eds.). *Helping homeless people: Unique challenges and solutions* (pp. 101–108). Alexandria, VA: American Association of Counseling and Development.

Johnson, A. K., & Krueger, L. W. (1989). Toward a better understanding of homeless women. *Social Work, 34*(11), 537–540.

Jonas, S. (1986). On homelessness and the American way. *American Journal of Public Health, 76*(9), 1084–1086.

Kinchen, K., & Wright, J. D. (1991). Hypertension management in health care for the homeless clinics: Results from a survey. *American Journal of Public Health, 81*(11), 1163–1165.

Koegel, P., & Burnam, M. A. (1988). Alcoholism among homeless adults in the inner city of Log Angeles. *Archives on General Psychiatry, 45,* 1011–1018.

Kozol, J. (1988). *Rachel and her children: Homeless families in America.* New York: Fawcett Columbine.

Lefley, J. P. (1987). Behavioral manifestations of mental illness. In A. B. Hatfield & H. P. Lefley (Eds.). *Families of the Mentally Ill: Coping and Adaptation* (pp. 107–127). New York: Guilford Press.

Lenehan, G. P., McInnis, B. N., O'Donnell, D., & Hennessey, M. (1985). A nurses' clinic for the homeless. *American Journal of Nursing, 85*(11), 1236–1240.

Lindsey, A. M. (1989). Health care for the homeless. *Nursing Outlook, 37*(2), 78–81.

Mangine, S. J., Royse, D., Wiehe, V. R., & Neitzel, M. N. (1990). Homelessness among adults raised as foster children: A survey of drop-in center users. *Psychological Reports, 67,* 739–745.

McAdam, J. M., Brickner, P. W., Scharer, L. L., Crocco, J. A., Duff, A. E. (1990). The spectrum of tuberculosis in a New York City men's shelter clinic (1982–1988). *Chest, 94*(4), 798–805.

Millburn, N. (1989). Drug abuse among the homeless. In J. A. Momenti (Ed.), *Homeless in the United States* (Vol. 2). Westport, CT: Greenwood Press.

Molnar, J. M., Rath, W. R., & Klein, T. P. (1990). Constantly compromised: The impact of homelessness on children. *Journal of Social Issues, 46*(4), 109–124.

Momeni, J. A., & Wiegand, G. (1989). *Homelessness in the United States.* New York: Greenwood Press.

Munoz, E. (1988). Care for the Hispanic poor: A growing segment of American society. *Journal of the American Medical Association, 260,* 2711–2712.

National Alliance to End Homelessness. (1988). *Housing and Homelessness.* Washington, DC: Author.

National Institute of Mental Health. (1992). *Outcasts on Main Street: Report of the Federal Task Force on Homelessness and Severe Mental Illness.* Washington, DC: Interagency Council on Homelessness.

Pepper, B., & Ryglewicz, H. (1984). The young adult chronic patient: A new focus. In J. A. Talbott (Ed.). *The chronic mental patient: Five years later* (pp. 33–48). Orlando, FL: Grune & Stratton.

Popp, S. R. (1988). Health care for the poor: Where has all the money gone? *Journal of Nursing Administration, 18*(1), 8–12.

Powers, J. L., Echenrode, J., & Jaklitsch, B. (1990). Maltreatment among runaway and homeless youth. *Child Abuse and Neglect, 14,* 87–98.

Price, V. (1987). Runaways and homeless street youth. In Kneerin, J. (Ed.). *Homelessness: Critical issues for policy and practice.* Boston: The Boston Foundation.

Rafferty, M. (1989). Standing up for America's homeless. *American Journal of Nursing, 89*(12), 1614–1617.

Rivilin, L. G. (1986). A new look at the homeless. *Social Policy, 16*(4), 3–10.

Rivilin, L. G. (1990). Home and homelessness in the lives of children. In N. A. Boxill (Ed.). *Homeless children: The watchers and waiters* (pp. 5–18). New York: Haworth Press.

Robertson, I. (1987). *Sociology* (3rd ed.). New York: Worth.

Robertson, M. J., & Cousineau, M. R. (1986). Health status and access to health services among the urban poor. *American Journal of Public Health, 76*(5), 561–563.

Rogers, C. (1980). *A way of being.* Boston: Houghton Mifflin.

Ropers, R. H., & Boyer, R. (1987). Perceived health status among the new urban homeless. *Social Science in Medicine, 24*(8), 669–678.

Rosenheck, R., Phil, P. G. M., Leda, C., Gorcher, L., & Errera, P. (1989). *Reaching out across America: The third progress report on the Veterans Administration Homeless Chronically Ill Veterans Program.* West Haven, CT: West Haven Veterans Administration Medical Center.

Rossi, P. H. (1989). *Down and out in America: The origins of homelessness.* Chicago: University of Chicago Press.

Rossi, P. H., & Wright, J. D. (1987). The determinants of homelessness. *Health Affairs, Spring, 6*(1), 19–32.

Roth, D., & Bean, G. J. (1986). New perspectives on homelessness: Findings from a statewide epidemiological study. *Hospital and Community Psychiatry, 37*(7), 712–719.

Rotherman-Borus, M. J. (1991). Serving runaway and homeless youth. *Family and Community Health, 14*(3), 23–32.

Scholler-Jaquish, A. (1993). Health care for the homeless: RN to BSN clinical education. *Nurse Educator, 18*(5), 33–38.

Scipien, G. M., Chord, M. A., Howe, J. C., & Barnard, M. U. (1990). *Pediatric nursing care.* St. Louis: Mosby–Year Book.

Shinn, M., Knickman, J. R., & Weitzman, B. C. (1991). Social relationships and vulnerability to becoming homeless among poor families. *American Psychologist, 45*(11), 1180–1187.

Smith, E. M. (1986). A nurse-managed family health center at the University of Florida. *Journal of Nursing Education, 25*(2), 79–81.

Stark, L. (1987). A century of alcohol and homelessness: Demographics and stereotypes. *Alcohol Health and Research, Spring, 11,* 8–13.

Stern, M. J. (1984). The emergency of the homeless as a public problem. *Social Service Review, 58*(6), 291–301.

Stoner, M. R. (1983). The plight of homeless women. *The Social Service Review, 57*(12), 565–581.

Strasser, J. A. (1978). Urban transient women. *American Journal of Nursing, 78*(12), 2076–2079.

Susser, E., Struening, E. L., & Conover, S. (1987). Childhood experiences of homeless men. *American Journal of Psychiatry, 144*(12), 1599–1601.

Swartz, J. (1986). Runaways often sexually abused: Symposium. *Canadian Medical Association Journal, 134,* 944–947.

Trattner, W. I. (1984). *From poor law to welfare state: A history of social welfare in America* (3rd ed.). New York: Free Press.

Troung, L. (1992). *Why are so few Asians homeless?* Unpublished paper. National Institute of Health Minority High School Research Project, University of Maryland.

Tucker, W. (1987). Where do the homeless come from? *National Review, 39*(18), 32–43.

Turner, S. L., Bauer, G., McNair, E., McNutt, B., & Walker, W. (1989). The homeless experience: Clinic building in a community health discovery-learning project. *Public Health Nursing, 6*(2), 97–101.

Wagner, J., & Menke, E. M. (1991). Stressors and coping behaviors of homeless, poor, and low-income women. *Journal of Community Health, 8*(2), 75–84.

Weyman, A. E., Greenbaum, D. M., & Grace, W. J. (1974). Accidental hypothermia in an alcoholic population. *The American Journal of Medicine, 56,* 13–21.

Whitman, B. Y., Accardo, P., Boyert, M., & Kendagor, R. (1990). Homelessness and cognitive development in children. *Social Work, 35*(6), 516–519.

Wittman, F. D., & Arch, M. (1987). Alcohol, architecture and homelessness. *Alcohol Research and World, 11*(3), 74–79.

Wood, D. L., Valedez, B., Hayaski, T., & Shen, A. (1990). Health of homeless children and housed, poor children. *Pediatrics, 86*(6), 859–865.

Wright, J. D. (1989). *Address unknown: The homeless in America.* Hawthorne, NY: Aldine de Gruyter.

Wright, J. D., & Weber, E. (1987). *Homelessness and health.* New York: McGraw-Hill.

BIBLIOGRAPHY

Alperstein, G. (1988). Homeless children: A challenge for pediatricians. *Pediatric Clinics of North America, 35*(6), 1413–1425.

Baxter, E., & Hopper, K. (1981). *Private lives/public spaces: Homeless adults on the streets of New York City.* New York: Community Service Society.

Bowlder, J. E., & Barrell, L. M. (1987). Health needs of homeless persons. *Public Health Nursing, 4*(3), 135–140.

Bunston, T., & Breton, M. (1990). The eating patterns and problems of homeless women. *Women and Health, 16*(1), 43–61.

Burt, M. R., & Cohen, B. E. (1989). Differences among homeless single women, women with children, and single men. *Social Problems, 36*(5), 508–522.

Cohen, C. I., Teresi, J., Holmes, D., & Roth, E. (1988). The survival strategies of older homeless men. *The Gerontologist, 28*(1), 58–65.

Cohen, C. I., & Thompson, K. S. (1992). Homeless mentally ill or mentally ill homeless? *American Journal of Psychiatry, 149*(6), 816–821.

Corrigan, E. M., & Anderson, S. C. (1984). Homeless alcoholic women on skid row. *American Journal of Drug and Alcohol Abuse, 10*(4), 535–549.

Dail, P. W. (1990). The psychosocial context of homeless mothers with young children: Program and policy implications. *Child Welfare, 69*(4), 291–308.

Fischer, P. J., Shapiro, S., Breakey, W. R., Anthony, J. C., & Kramer, M. (1986). Mental health and social characteristics of the homeless: A survey of mission users. *American Journal of Public Health, 76*(5), 519–523.

Hodnicki, D. R. (1990). Homelessness: Health-care implications. *Journal of Community Health Nursing, 7*(2), 59–67.

Institute of Medicine. (1988). *Homelessness, health, and human needs.* Washington, DC: National Academy Press.

Kruks, G. (1991). Gay and lesbian homeless/street youth: Special issues and concerns. *Journal of Adolescent Health, 12,* 515–518.

Lamb, H. R. (1989). The homeless mentally ill. *The Western Journal of Medicine, 151*(3), 313.

Leshner, A. I. (1992). *Outcasts on Main Street: Report of the National Institute of Mental Health Federal Task Force on Homelessness and Mental Illness,* Washington, DC: Interagency Council on Homelessness.

Lewis, M. R., & Meyers, A. F. (1989). The growth and development status of children entering shelters in Boston. *Public Health Reports, 104*(3), 247–250.

Linn, L. S., & Gelberg, L. (1989). Priority of basic needs among homeless adults. *Social Psychiatry and Psychiatric Epidemiology, 24,* 23–29.

Lowey, E. H. (1987). Communities, obligations and health care. *Social Science in Medicine, 25*(7), 783–791.

McCausland, M. P. (1987). Deinstitutionalization of the mentally ill: Oversimplification of complex issues. *Advances in Nursing Science, 9*(3), 24–33.

Pesznecker, B. L. (1984). The poor: A population at risk. *Public Health Nursing, 1*(4), 237–249.

Scholler-Jaquish, A. (in press). Persons with chronic mental illness. In K. M. Fortinash & P. A. Holoday-Worret (Eds.). *Psychiatric and mental health nursing.* St. Louis: Mosby–Year Book.

Segal, E. A. (1991). The juvenilization of poverty in the 1980's. *Social Work, 36*(5), 454–457.

Shadish, W. R., & Lurigio, A. J. (1989). After deinstitutionalization: The present and future of long-term care policy. *Journal of Social Issues. 45*(3), 1–15.

Smith, K., & Reder, N. (1987). *Meeting basic human needs: A crisis of responsibility.* Report from the director of the Social Policy for the League of Women Voters Education Fund. Publication No. 838. Washington, DC: League of Women Voters.

Smith, L. G. (1988). Home treatment of mild, acute diarrhea and secondary dehydration of infants and small children: An educational program for parents in a shelter for the homeless. *Journal of Professional Nursing, 4*(1), 60–63.

Stephens, D., Dennis, E., Toomer, M., & Holloway, J. (1991). The diversity of case management needs for the care of homeless persons. *Public Health Report, 106*(1), 15–19.

Wood, D. (1992). *Delivering health care to homeless persons: The diagnosis and management of medical and mental health conditions.* New York: Springer Publishing.

Wright, J. D. (1990). Poor people, poor health: The health status of the homeless. *Journal of Social Issues, 46*(4), 49–64.

SUGGESTED READINGS

Boondas, J. (1985). The despair of the homeless aged. *Journal of Gerontological Nursing, 11*(4), 9–14.

Dato, C., & Rafferty, M. (1986). The homeless mentally ill. *International Nursing Review, 32*(6), 170–173.

Hilfiker, D. (1987). Unconscious on a corner. . . . *Journal of the American Medical Association, 258*(21), 3155–3156.

Kinchen, K., & Wright, J. D. (1991). Hypertension management in health care for the homeless clinics: Results from a survey. *American Journal of Public Health, 81*(9), 1163–1165.

Lenehan, G. P., McInnis, B. N., O'Donnell, D., & Hennessey, M. (1985). A nurse's clinic for the homeless. *American Journal of Nursing, 85*(11), 1237–1240.

McGrath, B. B. (1986). The social networks of terminally ill skid row residents: An analysis. *Public Health Nursing, 3*(3), 192–205.

Nymathi, A., & Shuler, P. (1989). Factors affecting prescribed medication compliance of the urban homeless adult. *Nurse Practitioner, 14*(8), 47–54.

Packett, S., Oswald, N., Bronson, S., & Kraushar, T. (1991). A problem homeless patients may not mention. *RN, 54*(11), 53–55.

Sebastian, J. G. (1985). Homelessness: A state of vulnerability. *Family and Community Health, 8*(3), 11–24.

Slavinsky, A. T. (1982 Homeless women. *Nursing Outlook, 30*(6), 358–362.

Turner, S. L., Bauer, G., McNair, E., McNutt, B., & Walker, W. (1989). The homeless experience: Clinic building in a community health discovery-learning project. *Public Health Nursing, 6*(2), 97–101.

Weis, D. (1987). Who are the working poor? *American Journal of Nursing, 87*(11), 1451–1453.

Zlotnick, C. (1987). Pediculosis corporis and the homeless. *Journal of Community Health Nursing, 4*(1), 43–48.

Chapter 24

Environmental Issues: At Home, at Work, and in the Community

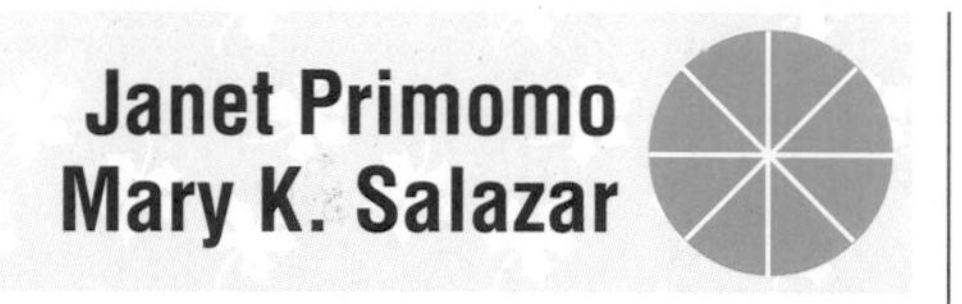
Janet Primomo
Mary K. Salazar

Focus Questions

What is meant by the term *environmental health?*

In what ways does the environment affect human health in the home, in the occupational setting, and in the community?

What are some of the key areas that are important to assess in the identification of household, occupational, or community environmental hazards?

What can community health nurses do to minimize the adverse affects of the environment on their clients' health?

What are some of the critical resources that are available to the community health nurse when working with clients in the home, in the occupational setting, and in the community?

Overview

This chapter examines the influence of the environment on the health of communities and defines the responsibilities of the community health nurse in relation to environmental health. Understanding the effects of environmental factors on health and disease requires an appreciation of the complex interplay of many factors. Social, cultural, political, economic, and physical forces interact with the psychological and physiological rhythms that form the foundation of human existence. In keeping with this assertion, this chapter examines a conceptual model of environmental health and uses this model to present an analysis and overview of factors that exist in the home, the occupational setting, and the greater community. It is hoped that the discussion in this chapter will assist the reader in recognizing the environment as an important contributor to the health and well-being of populations.

Environmental health, in the broadest sense, can be defined as the state of health that exists as a result of the forces and conditions that surround and influence human beings. Because of the dynamic nature of the environment and the community, the study of environmental health problems presents special challenges for the health professional. For example Americans tend to be on the move; their environment may regularly change and hence the environmental hazards to which they are exposed may vary. Another difficulty is that in many cases it may be months or even years after an exposure that an adverse health effect is apparent. Because of the multifactorial nature of many environmental health effects, it is often difficult to determine the precise contribution of a specific pollutant. Despite these difficulties it is essential that health professionals consider the environment in relation to the health of their clients. All too often an assessment is less than complete because environmental exposures and hazards are not included.

HISTORICAL PERSPECTIVE

Environmental health is one of humanity's oldest concerns. In prehistoric times, people often attributed disease to their gods and therefore sought to pacify these gods. As civilization developed other explanations of disease became common. Aware of the contagious nature of some diseases, the ancient Hebrews isolated persons with diseases such as leprosy as early as 1200 BC. They also prohibited the contamination of public wells.

A major shift in the understanding of the nature of disease occurred as a result of the work of the Greek physician Hippocrates around 400 BC. Hippocrates introduced the notion that diseases had natural causes and that medicine was really a science separate from the practice of religion. The Hippocratic oath professed by modern physicians concludes that the "well-being of man is influenced by all environmental factors: the quality of the air, water, and food; the winds and the topography of the land" (Dubos, 1968). A concern for public health during the years following Hippocrates is reflected by the Hebrew, Roman, and Islamic rules for personal hygiene and sanitation. The great Roman aqueducts and highly developed sewage system are testaments to their concern about the spread of disease.

While knowledge about diseases continued to accumulate, the greatest strides in the control of widespread disease did not occur until the acceptance of the germ theory in the late 19th century (Last, 1987). Because of the rapid industrial growth that occurred in American and European societies at that time, cities and towns had grown exponentially, which led to profound economic and social changes. Unsanitary conditions wreaked havoc on many communities.

Advances in scientific knowledge about the causes of disease led to the development of sewage and water purification systems in American cities, which greatly contributed to the control of some of the worst threats to long life and good health.

Environmental improvements and efforts toward the control of communicable disease continued in the 20th century with the widespread use of immunizations and the discovery of antibiotics, resulting in the virtual elimination of many previously lethal communicable diseases, such as pertussis and measles. Unfortunately, former health concerns have been replaced with a whole new set of environmental concerns resulting from the introduction of new technology and chemicals combined with lifestyle risks and stresses. The linking of environmental toxins to cancer, cholesterol accumulation to heart disease, and stress to cerebral vascular dysfunctions are just a few examples.

Social and economic aspects of the environment also contribute to contemporary health problems. Homicides and suicides, teenage pregnancy, drug abuse, and sexually transmitted diseases are among the health problems linked with social conditions that should demand the attention of health care providers. (These issues are dealt with in greater detail in other chapters.)

INVOLVEMENT OF NURSING IN ENVIRONMENTAL ISSUES

The importance of environmental health in nursing is underscored by the attention of our early leaders to the relationship between health and the physical environment. Florence Nightingale identified the environment as one of the key concepts in the nursing profession. She viewed the environment as a factor external to the patient that might influence health and illness. She recognized the role of social, political, and economic factors on the health of British soldiers in the Crimean War. Nightingale related the high infant mortality rate in London in the mid-1800s to "defective household hygiene." Nightingale identified the need for a clean environment when she outlined "five essential points in securing the health of houses." These five points included pure air, pure water, efficient drainage, cleanliness, and light (Nightingale, 1860, 1969). Nightingale's principles formed the basis of modern environmental health.

Another renowned nursing leader, Mary Breckinridge, used environmental health principles when founding the Frontier Nursing Service in Kentucky in 1925. In her description of the development of the rural health care system that she established, Breckinridge chronicled the unusual process of building a rural hospital. Critical factors that she considered in identifying a site for the hospital included the source of a clean water supply, the proper disposal of sewage, and the location for a livestock area because the nurse midwives had to use horses in the mountainous areas (Breckinridge, 1952). Although Breckinridge's goal was to establish a system of comprehensive rural health care for an underserved population, she would not have succeeded in reducing infant mortality had she not incorporated principles of environmental health into her community health practice.

In early 20th century baccalaureate nursing programs, principles of public health and community hygiene were included in the curriculum. To protect individuals from health hazards, it was clear that nurses needed a basic understanding of environmental or community hygiene to participate in community education and the development of government-sponsored interventions. Topics covered in nursing curricula included sanitation of food and water supplies, a safe system for sewage disposal, adequate housing, the control of communicable disease, community health problems in childbearing and childhood, and the organization of public health services to maintain health (Gardner, 1936).

Today nurses are challenged to address some of the same environmental problems, and many new ones, in occupational health settings and in the community at large. One of the many goals of the National Health Promotion and Disease Prevention Objectives for the Year 2000 is to minimize human exposure to toxins in the environment through the reduction or elimination of hazards; another is to decrease the number of accidental deaths (U.S. Department of Health and Human Services [USDHHS], 1990). Nurses in community health settings are working with other professionals, such as sanitarians and industrial hygienists, to help investigate and interpret environmental risks to the community. Community health nurses help to allay unnecessary fears, raise the public's awareness about environmental risks, and assist people to modify their health risks. Nurses in professional organizations, such as the American Association of Occupational Health Nurses, American Public Health Association, Nurses' Environmental Health Watch, and Nurses for the Environment (Table 24–1), acknowledge a special commitment to protecting the public's health from environmental hazards. Over the past several years the Nurses' Environmental Health Watch has worked closely with the National Student Nurses' Association to encourage students to develop and implement community health projects that focus on environmental health.

TABLE 24–1

Environmental Resources for Community Health Nurses

Professional Organizations

American Public Health Association
1015 15th St. NW
Washington, DC 20005
(202) 789–5600

Nurses for the Environment
P.O. Box 22118
Juneau, AK 99802

Nurses' Environmental Health Watch
181 Marshall St.
Duxbury, MA 02322

American Association of Occupational Health Nurses
50 Lenox Pointe
Atlanta, GA 30324
1–800–241–8014

Government Organizations

Environmental Protection Agency
Indoor Air Quality Information Clearinghouse
P.O. Box 37133
Washington, DC 20013–7133
1–800–438–4318

National Institute for Occupational Safety and Health
4676 Columbia Parkway
Cincinnati, OH 45226–1998
1–800–35–NIOSH

Other

March of Dimes Birth Defects Foundation
1275 Mamaroneck Ave.
White Plains, NY 10605
(914) 428–7100

A CONCEPTUAL MODEL OF ECOLOGICAL SYSTEMS

In environmental health, particular attention is given to the identification of both positive and negative factors in the environment that may affect human beings. The environment includes all the physical, social, cultural, political, and economic conditions that influence the life of individuals, groups, and communities. As with other areas of nursing, the focus of nurses in environmental health is to promote, maintain, and support health, and specifically to explain how the environment affects a person's well-being.

One theoretical framework that shows the various levels of systems and their interrelationships and interactions is that of ecological systems. Ecological theory has its roots in both biological and sociological sciences. Ecology is derived from the Greek word *oikos,* meaning a house or place to live. The major impetus in the development of ecology was from the biological sciences. As early as 1859 Darwin identified the "web of life" and recognized the highly complex set of interrelationships that were present between organisms and their environments. The word *ecology* was first used in 1868 by Haeckel, a German biologist. The term *human ecology* was coined in the 1920s in a sociological text in an attempt to systematically apply a basic theoretical scheme of plant and animal ecology to the study of human communities (Hawley, 1950). Cultural and sociological dimensions, as well as spatial distribution, were later included in the field of human ecology.

Ecological systems generally have several different levels (Bronfenbrenner, 1979). The simplified version in Figure 24–1 consists of two levels. The level of system closest to the human population is the microsystem. The microsystem includes the environment immediately surrounding the person (e.g., the family and the home). The macrosystem is the larger context in which the microsystem is embedded. Culture, traditions, customs, societal norms, government, economic policies, and the physical environment constitute the macrosystem. Ecological systems are involved in the process of energy and information exchange. Input in the form of energy, matter, and information pass through the boundaries of the macrosystem and microsystem. The input is processed or changed and the system releases output. Terminology used in systems theory such as *input, feedback, circulation, transformation,* and *output* help explain the actual processes that occur in the ecological system. For example the microsystem or the family of a daycare worker might be infected with *Giardia* because one of the daycare children drank contaminated water when on a hike with the parents. The child was infected with the *Giardia* organism from the macrosystem (a mountain stream). The organism then crossed the boundaries from the macrosystem to the microsystem (daycare center) and infected the worker.

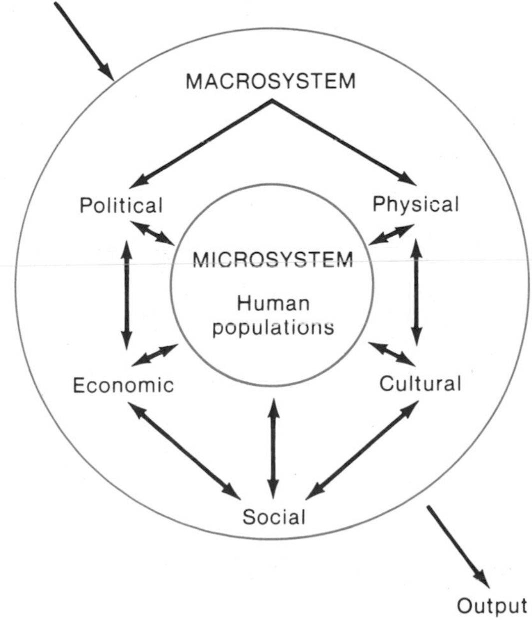

Figure 24–1 ● Simplified ecological systems model.

One of the basic principles of ecological systems theory is that everything is connected to everything. Because of the interrelationships and interactions among the different aspects of a system, change in any portion of a system might affect change in other parts of the system. In other words systems are dynamic and change is constant. The ecological systems approach is especially useful in examining complex areas that are the result of multiple factors in the environment. For example in environmental health, physical, cultural, social, political, and economic factors often interact to contribute to an environmental hazard. Later in the chapter a case example using this approach describes the role of the nurse in raising awareness about a particular environmental issue, the use of disposable diapers.

Sources of Environmental Hazards

Because of their inherent complexity, identifying the sources of environmental hazards is a major challenge for the community health nurse. By its very nature environmental health implies a public health approach to disease because environments affect many people simultaneously. Therefore epidemiology becomes an important investigational tool. It is necessary to identify which populations are most exposed to specific environmental agents (e.g., lead) and under which circumstances exposure takes place (e.g., in battery-making plants). This is not meant to imply however that health professionals should not be attentive to the effect of the environment on individuals. An assessment of the potential environmental hazards should be included in every health history. (An example of such a tool is discussed later.) The primary environments for most individuals can be divided into three broad areas: the home, the worksite, and the community. In the following sections these environments are described and epidemiological evidence suggesting possible health concerns is reviewed. Although health hazards include the many sociocultural, political, economic, and other factors inherent in any setting, the principal focus is on physical hazards (including biological and chemical factors) that exist in these environments. There is also a brief discussion of psychological hazards in the community.

ENVIRONMENTAL HAZARDS AT HOME

For many Americans the home functions as a refuge from the strains and stresses of everyday life. But how safe

TABLE 24-2

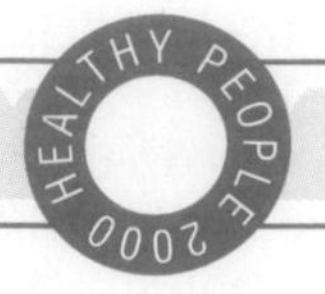

Healthy People 2000 Environmental Health Objectives

Health Status Objectives

1. Reduce asthma morbidity, as measured by a reduction in asthma hospitalizations to no more than 160 per 100,000 persons (baseline: 188 per 100,000 in 1987).

	1987 Baseline (Hospitalizations per 100,000)	Year 2000 Target
Blacks and other nonwhites	334	265
Children	284	225

2. Reduce the prevalence of serious mental retardation among school-age children to no more than 2 per 1000 children (baseline: 2.7 per 1000 children aged 10 years in 1985–1988).
3. Reduce outbreaks of waterborne disease from infectious agents and chemical poisoning to no more than 11 per year (baseline: average of 31 outbreaks per year during 1981–1988).

Average No. of Waterborne Disease Outbreaks per Year	Year 2000 Objective
13	6

4. Reduce the prevalence of blood lead levels exceeding 15 μg/dl and 25 μg/dl among children aged 6 months through 5 years to no more than 500,000 and 0, respectively (baseline: an estimated 3 million children had levels exceeding 15 μg/dl and 234,000 had levels exceeding 25 μg/dl in 1984).

Risk Reduction Objectives

5. Reduce human exposure to criteria air pollutants, as measured by an increase to at least 85% in the proportion of people who live in counties that have not exceeded any Environmental Protection Agency standard for air quality in the previous 12 months (baseline: 49.7% in 1988).

Proportion living in counties that have not exceeded criteria air pollutant standards in 1988 for:

Ozone	53.6%
Carbon monoxide	87.8%
Nitrogen dioxide	96.6%
Sulfur dioxide	99.3%
Particulates	89.4%
Lead	99.3%
Total (of any above)	49.7%

6. Increase to at least 40% the proportion of homes in which homeowners/occupants have tested for radon concentrations and have either found minimal risk or have modified homes to reduce risk to health (baseline: less than 5% of homes had been tested in 1989).
7. Reduce human exposure to toxic agents by confining total pounds of toxic agents released into the air, water, and soil each year to no more than:
   - 0.24 billion of those toxic agents included on the Department of Health and Human Services list of carcinogens (baseline: 0.32 billion pounds in 1988).
   - 2.6 billion pounds of those toxic agents included on the Agency for Toxic Substances and Disease Registry list of the most toxic chemicals (baseline: 2.62 billion pounds in 1988).
8. Reduce human exposure to solid waste–related water, air, and soil contamination, as measured by a reduction in average pounds of municipal solid waste produced per person each day to no more than 3.6 lb (baseline: 4.0 lb per person each day in 1988).
9. Increase to at least 85% the proportion of people who receive a supply of drinking water that meets the safe drinking water standards established by the Environmental Protection Agency (baseline: 74% of 58,099 community water systems serving approximately 80% of the population in 1988).
10. Reduce potential risks to human health from surface water, as measured by a decrease to no more than 15% in the proportion of assessed rivers, lakes, and estuaries that do not support beneficial uses, such as fishing and swimming (baseline: an estimated 25% of assessed rivers, lakes, and estuaries did not support designated beneficial uses in 1988).

HEALTHY PEOPLE 2000

TABLE 24–2

Healthy People 2000 Environmental Health Objectives Continued

Services and Protection Objectives

1. Perform testing for lead-based paint in at least 50% of homes built before 1950.
2. Expand to at least 35 the number of states in which at least 75% of local jurisdictions have adopted construction standards and techniques that minimize elevated indoor radon levels in those new building areas locally determined to have elevated radon levels (baseline: 1 state in 1989).
3. Increase to at least 30 the number of states requiring that prospective buyers be informed of the presence of lead-based paint and radon concentrations in all buildings offered for sale (baseline: 2 states required disclosure of lead-based paint in 1989; 1 state required disclosure of radon concentrations in 1989; 2 additional states required disclosure that radon has been found in the state and that testing is desirable in 1989).
4. Establish programs for recyclable materials and household hazardous waste in at least 75% of counties (baseline: approximately 850 programs in 41 states collected household toxic waste in 1987; extent of recycling collections unknown).
5. Establish and monitor in at least 35 states plans to define and track sentinel and environmental diseases (baseline: 0 states in 1990).

From USDHHS. (1990). *Healthy people 2000: National health promotion and disease prevention objectives. Summary report.* Washington, DC: Public Health Service.

a refuge is it? A confounding factor inherent in home hazards is their ordinariness. They are often an important part of our day-to-day existence and in many cases are unlikely to be thought of as linked with adverse health outcomes. An environmental assessment should begin by examining possible exposures in the home with attention to ordinary things that may be camouflaging underlying hazards. Key symptoms related to environmental hazards may provide clues regarding the presence of noxious substances or products. Numerous *Healthy People 2000* objectives address environmental conditions in homes (Table 24–2).

Home Safety

Every year about 20,500 Americans die as a result of accidents in their homes; another 3 million suffer disabling injuries, of which approximately 90,000 result in permanent impairment (National Safety Council, 1991, 1992). The leading cause of accidental death in the home are falls, with the majority involving persons older than 65 years. Other causes of death include poisoning from drugs, alcohol, and household chemicals (e.g., cleaning agents, gardening products); fires and burns; suffocation; drowning; and firearm accidents resulting from cleaning or playing with guns (Figure 24–2).

Despite the increase in the total U.S. population, the total number of deaths from home accidents continues to decline. The 1991 death rates from home injuries were the lowest on record (National Safety Council, 1992). Safety campaigns to modify products and teach people how to prevent accidents are effective. We must continue to educate each generation to keep rates from rising.

Falls. Falls are the major cause of accidental death; most such accidents happen to older Americans in their homes. The mortality rate for falls increases dramatically after age 74 years. While stairs are the site of about 10% of falls, the reason for falls is unspecified in almost 70% of the cases (National Safety Council, 1991). Poor lighting, loose electric cords and rugs, slippery surfaces, and clutter are thought to contribute to falls in elderly persons. Baby equipment, such as walkers, has been under scrutiny as contributing to serious falls in young children. Windows that do not have guards are hazards for small children. Nurses can provide useful information to families across the life span about the prevention of falls in the home. For example, parents should be advised never to leave a child unattended on a diaper-changing table.

Poisoning. The greatest number of documented accidental deaths in the home occur in the very young (under 4 years) and the very old (over 75 years). Poisonings are an exception to this, with more deaths and a higher death rate occurring in the 25- to 44-year-old group (National Safety Council, 1991) than any other age group. In fact deaths from poisonings in the 0- to 4-year-old group have fallen dramatically since 1958, due in part to the introduction of child-proof containers and educational campaigns such as "Mr. Yuk" (National Safety Council, 1991). Poisoning deaths include those from drugs such as cocaine, medications, mushrooms, and shellfish, in addition to commonly recognized poisons; this helps explain the higher number of deaths in the 25- to 44-year-old group. A recent study examining poisoning among older adults in Massachusetts suggested that the elderly may be at higher risk than adults in younger age groups for poisoning from prescription medications (Woolf et al., 1990). A compromising health condition, possible dementia, and failing eyesight, problems not uncommon in the elderly, may lead to an accidental overdose with tragic consequences. The findings from this study indicated that men over 70 years and women over 60 years are at greater risk of dying as a result of accidental poisoning from medications than are younger persons.

Burns. Fires and burns are the third highest cause of home deaths (National Safety Council, 1992). These deaths include fire-related injuries such as asphyxiation, falls, and trauma from falling objects. Deaths are highest among those considered to be the most dependent: the very young and very old. One of the health protection objectives in *Healthy People 2000* is to have functional smoke detectors on each floor of all residences (USDHHS, 1990). By encouraging families to install smoke detectors, nurses can help prevent burn injuries and deaths.

Drownings. Drownings are a serious cause of accidental death, with nearly 600 deaths reported in the United States in 1991 (National Safety Council, 1992). Although the majority of these deaths occur in lakes or streams, in certain parts of the country they are more likely to occur in home swimming pools (Hedberg et al., 1990). Of the documented cases of home drownings, about 50% occurred to persons under 5 years of age. An additional 4100 children under age 5 years suffered nonfatal submersions that necessitated hospital treatment in 1987 (National Safety Council, 1989).

Firearms. About 800 deaths occur annually while people are playing with or cleaning firearms (National Safety Council, 1992). The number of accidental firearm deaths and the death rate is highest for the 15- to 24-year-old group. Whereas the number of accidental firearm deaths decreased between 1953 and 1988, the firearm death rate from suicides doubled and the homicide rate tripled. The number of firearm deaths from suicides and homicides far exceeds that of home accidents, with about 33,000 deaths occurring in 1988 (National Safety Council, 1991). About 80% of these deaths are in males. Although the highest number of suicide deaths occur in the 25- to 44-year-old group, the highest rate of suicide is found in those 75 years and older. The greatest absolute number of homicide deaths occurs in persons between 25 and 44 years of age, but the death rates (homicides per 100,000) are highest for the 15- to 24-year-old group. Nurses and other health professionals are challenged to provide education about proper gun storage to minimize accidents and to address violence. Issues related to societal violence and the availability of firearms are complex and require communities to work together to reduce homicides and suicides (see Chapter 20).

Most of the accidents that occur in the home are preventable. Inadequate lighting, especially in halls, stairwells, and basements, faulty electrical appliances, broken furniture, poor placement of rugs or other items, and floors or walls in poor repair have been cited as possible factors contributing to falls, fires, and other accidental mishaps. The use of smoke detectors and safe storage of flammable materials and firearms can help to prevent accidents. Kitchens and bedrooms are the most likely sites of accidents in the home (Leeser, 1975). Accidental deaths tend to be more prevalent for families living in substandard housing because of poor construction or poor repair; however no family is immune to home hazards. Table 24–3 provides examples of the many consumer products that may cause injuries in the home.

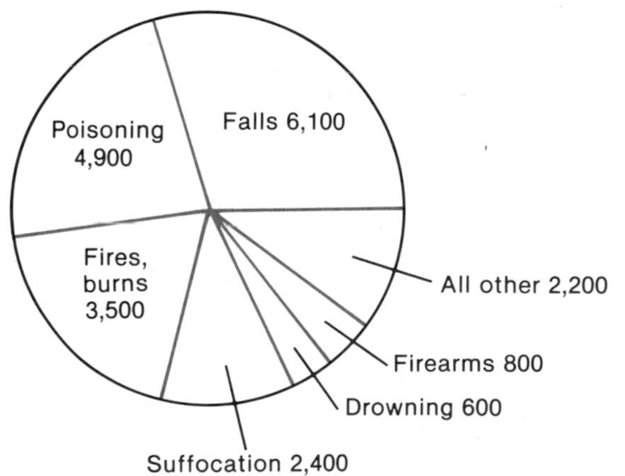

Figure 24–2 ● Number of deaths from home accidents, 1991 (total = 20,500 deaths). (Data from National Safety Council. (1992). *Accident Facts* (pp. 94–95). Itasca, IL: Author.)

Other Hazards in the Home

Garbage. Hygiene and cleanliness contribute to the maintenance of family health. A potential source of disease that is often taken for granted is the method of garbage disposal (Anderson, 1987). It has been estimated that each American produces more than 4 lb of solid waste per day, such as food scraps and paper (USDHHS, 1990). One goal of *Healthy People 2000* is to decrease this amount to less than 3.6 lb per day, thereby reducing contamination of water, air, and soil by solid waste. To maximize safety and cleanliness, garbage should be properly wrapped and garbage cans kept clean and tightly closed. Of concern in the last two decades with the increased use of disposable diapers is the improper disposal of human feces, which contains numerous enteric organisms, in garbage piles and landfills (Primomo, 1990). When handled improperly, these wastes can lead to contamination of water supplies, contribute to breeding of bacteria and virus that can be transmitted to humans via insects and rodents, and possibly serve as a reservoir for disease. Diseases that can be spread through contact with human feces include gastroenteritis, hepatitis, and polio (if live vaccines are used in immunizations). A detailed case study on the issue of disposable diaper use is provided at the end of the chapter. Hazardous wastes are discussed later in this chapter.

Radon. Radon has been of great concern in recent years. Radon is a radioactive gas that is the by-product of the decay of uranium; it occurs naturally in the soil (Loken and

TABLE 24–3

Examples of Consumer Products that Cause Injuries in the Home

Home Maintenance
- Noncaustic cleaning equipment, detergents
- Cleaning agents (except soaps)
- Drain and oven cleaners, caustics
- Miscellaneous household chemicals
- Paints, solvents, lubricants

Home Workshop Equipment
- Batteries, all types
- Hoists, lifts, jacks, etc.
- Miscellaneous workshop equipment
- Power home tools, except saws
- Power home workshop saws
- Welding, soldering, cutting tools
- Wires, cords, not specified
- Workshop manual tools

Yard and Garden Equipment
- Chain saws
- Hand garden tools
- Hatchets, axes
- Lawn, garden care equipment
- Lawn mowers, all types
- Other power lawn equipment

Packing and Containers, Household
- Cans, other containers
- Glass bottles, jars
- Paper, cardboard, plastic products

Home Furnishings, Fixtures, and Accessories
- Bathtub, shower structures
- Beds, mattresses, pillows
- Carpets, rugs
- Chairs, sofas, sofa beds
- Desks, cabinets, shelves, racks
- Electric fixtures, lamps, equipment
- Ladders, stools
- Mirrors, mirror glass
- Miscellaneous household covers, fabrics
- Other miscellaneous furniture, accessories
- Sinks, toilets
- Tables, all types

Home Structures and Construction Materials
- Cabinets or door hardware
- Ceilings, walls, panels (inside)
- Counters, counter tops
- Fences
- Glass doors, windows, panels
- Handrails, railings, banisters
- Miscellaneous construction materials
- Nails, carpet tacks, etc.
- Nonglass doors, panels
- Outside attached structures, materials
- Porches, open side floors, etc.
- Stairs, ramps, landings, floors
- Window, door sills, frames

Housewares
- Cookware pots, pans
- Cutlery, knives, unpowered
- Drinking glasses
- Miscellaneous housewares
- Scissors
- Small kitchen appliances
- Tableware and accessories

General Household Appliances
- Cooking ranges, ovens, etc.
- Irons, clothes steamers (not toys)
- Miscellaneous household appliances
- Refrigerators, freezers
- Washers, dryers

Heating, Cooling, and Ventilating Equipment
- Chimneys, fireplaces
- Fans (except stove exhaust fans)
- Heating stoves, space heaters
- Pipes, heating and plumbing
- Radiators, all

Home Communication, Entertainment, and Hobby Equipment
- Miscellaneous hobby equipment
- Pet supplies, equipment
- Sound recording, reproducing equipment
- Television sets

Personal Use Items
- Cigarettes, lighters, fuel
- Clothing, all
- Grooming devices
- Holders for personal items
- Jewelry
- Paper money, coins
- Pencils, pens, other desk supplies
- Razors, shavers, razor blades
- Sewing equipment

Sport and Recreation Equipment
- All-terrain vehicles, mopeds, minibikes
- Barbecue grills, stoves, equipment
- Bicycles, accessories
- Horseback riding equipment
- Nonpowder guns, BBs, pellets
- Playground equipment
- Skateboards
- Toboggans, sleds, snowdisks, etc.
- Trampolines

Miscellaneous Products
- Dollies, carts
- Elevators, other lifts
- Fireworks, flares
- Gasoline and diesel fuels
- Nursery equipment
- Toys

Adapted from National Safety Council. (1992). *Accident facts.* Itasca, IL: Author.

Loken, 1989). It has been estimated that up to 20,000 lung cancer deaths per year among nonsmokers are a result of radon exposure (Council on Scientific Affairs, 1987). The importance of radon as a risk is evidenced by its inclusion in the national health objectives for the year 2000. The objective is to increase to 40% the proportion of homes that are tested and found to be at little risk or found positive for radon and modified to reduce risk (USDHHS, 1990). Evidence suggests that chronic exposure to radon leads to an increase of respiratory symptoms. The risk to uranium miners has been known for several years, but the recent concern has focused on the presence of radon in homes. Investigations into the actual effects of radon exposure in homes are continuing. Certain parts of the country are more likely to have radon. Maps are available through the Environmental Protection Agency (EPA) that show areas of high concentration. The EPA is an independent agency of the federal government that has the primary responsibility for setting and enforcing standards related to environmental pollutants. A number of factors affect exposure levels to radon, including a home's construction, its ventilation properties, the presence of cracks or openings in the foundation or walls, and the occupant's living patterns. Determining the level of radon can be accomplished through the use of measuring devices that are designed for this purpose that can be obtained through private companies or government agencies. If radon exposure is suspected, clients should be referred to the EPA or to a company that has the capacity to assess the situation.

Lead. Childhood lead poisoning, one of the most common public health problems today, is preventable. Lead-based paint, including dust and chips, has long been recognized as a source of lead poisoning, particularly in young children. Other sources of lead exposure include the following: (1) contaminated soil; (2) airborne particles from steel structures, gasoline fumes, and dusts; (3) water from lead pipes or tanks; (4) food from lead containers; and (5) hobbies such as target shooting and stained glass and glazed pottery making. The government's passage of the Lead-Based Paint Poisoning Prevention Act in 1971 resulted in a lower incidence of lead poisoning from paint (Minnesota Department of Health, 1982). However recent scientific data show adverse effects from lead in young children at blood levels much lower than previously considered dangerous. Blood levels above 10 μg/dl are now considered harmful (Centers for Disease Control and Prevention [CDC], 1991). It is estimated that 3 million U.S. children have blood lead levels above 15 μg/dl (CDC, 1991). Written in 1990, the *Healthy People 2000* objectives seek to have no children with blood lead levels above 25 μg/dl and to reduce the number with levels above 15 μg/dl. Table 24–4 shows blood levels, associated symptoms, and recommended interventions for the prevention of lead poisoning.

Lead poisonings are usually associated with older, deteriorating houses. In recent years lead has been recognized as a hazard when renovating older homes. Unfortunately families renovating older homes are often unaware that lead poisoning may be a risk for their families (Marino et al., 1990). Early signs of lead poisoning include disturbances in cognition, behavior, learning, attention span, and growth and development. Colic, constipation, and upper extremity weakness are signs of chronic exposure. Continued exposure leads to central nervous system symptoms (e.g., encephalopathy) and renal and hematological effects.

Prevention of lead poisoning in young children requires community efforts to eliminate environmental exposure and to educate families about prevention. The CDC now recommends blood lead screening for all children at 9 to 12 months, then annually unless a high risk is present. Nurses working with families must have a high degree of suspicion, especially in areas where homes are older than 30 years, and encourage widespread screening for asymptomatic cases (American Academy of Pediatrics, 1987).

TABLE 24–4

Preventing Lead Poisoning: Levels, Symptoms, and Interventions

Blood Level (μg/dl)	Signs, Symptoms, Effects	Intervention
≤ 9	Transplacental transfer; minimal observable effects	Education about prevention
10–20	Developmental toxicity: growth, hearing, IQ; nerve conduction velocity	Frequent screening; education, nutrition; inspection of environment
21–44	Vitamin D metabolism; hemoglobin synthesis; mild fatigue	Medical intervention; environmental inspection and intervention
45–69	Myalgia or paresthesia; irritability, lethargy, general fatigue; gastrointestinal complaints	Medical (chelation) therapy; environmental intervention
≥ 70	Paresis or paralysis; encephalopathy: seizures, coma; colic	Medical emergency; immediate medical and environmental treatment

Formaldehyde. Formaldehyde is present in a variety of household products including carpets, draperies, shampoos, and cosmetics. As energy conservation became a high priority for American consumers in the 1980s, insulation products containing formaldehyde appeared on the market. It is also used in glues for plywood and fiberboard; thus many homes have formaldehyde in their cabinetry and furniture. The pervasive presence of formaldehyde in so many household products along with home weatherproofing that is common has resulted in an increased exposure for many persons. Because formaldehyde is primarily an allergen, the reaction of individuals is often unpredictable. The most common symptoms are eye irritation, respiratory symptoms, nausea, headache, and fatigue. Young children may have abdominal complaints. There may be an association between exposure to formaldehyde and nasal cancer.

Carbon Monoxide. Carbon monoxide is a colorless, odorless, and tasteless gas that may be emitted from the incomplete combustion of carbon materials (Minnesota Department of Health, 1982). Possible sources are improperly vented furnaces, blocked flues or chimneys, and automobile exhausts, particularly when a garage is attached to a house. Exposure to carbon monoxide may cause dizziness, headache, drowsiness, nausea, or flu-like symptoms. Continued exposure may result in unconsciousness and death. Persons who have cardiovascular or respiratory diseases are particularly vulnerable to the effects of carbon monoxide. As with formaldehyde there is an increased risk in well-insulated houses.

These are but a few examples of some of the more common environmental hazards that can be found in the home. Household products that are potentially dangerous include bleaches, drain cleaners, oven cleaners, furniture polishes, paint strippers, epoxies, paints, herbicides, and pesticides (Table 24–5). Compounding the problem is the increased insulation common in today's homes, which may prevent adequate ventilation; also exposures may be increased in confined spaces such as attics or crawl spaces. In far too many cases people tend not to recognize the potential harm that can result from these common, everyday hazards.

TABLE 24–5

Sources of Home Pollution

RADON

Colorless, odorless, radioactive gas from the natural breakdown (radioactive decay) of uranium; it is estimated that radon causes up to 20,000 lung cancer deaths per year

Sources of Radon in the Home

Soil or rock under the home; well water; building materials

ASBESTOS

Mineral fiber used extensively in building materials for insulation and as a fire-retardant; asbestos should be removed by a professional if it has deteriorated; exposure to asbestos fibers can cause irreversible and often fatal lung diseases, including cancer

Sources of Asbestos in the Home

Sprayed-on acoustical ceilings or textured paint; pipe and furnace insulation materials; floor tiles; automobile brakes and clutches

BIOLOGICAL CONTAMINANTS

Include bacteria, mold and mildew, viruses, animal dander and saliva, dust mites, and pollen; these contaminants can provide infectious diseases or allergic reactions; moisture and dust levels in the home should be kept as low as possible

Sources of Biological Contaminants in the Home

Mold and mildew; standing water or water-damaged materials; humidifiers; house plants; household pets; ventilation systems; household dust

INDOOR COMBUSTION

Produces harmful gases (carbon monoxide, nitrogen dioxide), particles, and organic compounds (benzene); health effects range from irritation to the eyes, nose, and throat, to lung cancer; ventilation of gas appliances to the outdoors will minimize risks

Sources of Combustion in the Home

Tobacco smoke; unvented kerosene or gas space heaters; unvented kitchen gas stoves; wood stoves or fireplaces; leaking exhaust flues from gas furnaces and clothes dryers; car exhaust from an attached garage

HOUSEHOLD PRODUCTS

Can contain potentially harmful organic compounds; health effects vary greatly; the elimination of household chemicals through the use of non-toxic alternatives or by using only in well-ventilated rooms or outside will minimize risks

Examples of Household Products

Cleaning products; paint supplies; stored fuels; hobby products; personal care products; mothballs; air fresheners; dry-cleaned clothes

FORMALDEHYDE

Widely used chemical that is released to the air as a colorless gas; it can cause eye, nose, throat, and respiratory system irritation, headaches, nausea, and fatigue; may be a central nervous system depressant and has been shown to cause cancer in laboratory animals; remove sources of formaldehyde from the home if health effects occur

Sources of Formaldehyde in the Home

Particleboard, plywood, and fiberboard in cabinets, furniture, subflooring, and paneling; carpeting, durable-press drapes, other textiles; urea-formaldehyde insulation; glues and adhesives

PESTICIDES

Including insecticides, termiticides, rodenticides, and fungicides—all contain organic compounds; exposure to high levels of pesticides may cause damage to the liver and the central nervous system and increase cancer risks; when possible, nonchemical methods of pest control should be used; if the use of pesticides is unavoidable they should be used strictly according to the manufacturer's directions

Sources of Pesticides in the Home

Contaminated soil or dust that is tracked in from outside; stored pesticide containers

LEAD

A long-recognized harmful environmental pollutant; fetuses, infants, and children are more vulnerable to toxic effects; if the community health nurse suspects that a home has lead paint, it should be tested

Sources of Lead in the Home

Lead-based paint that is peeling, sanded, or burned; automobile exhaust; lead in drinking water; food contaminated by lead from lead-based ceramic cookware or pottery; lead-related hobbies or occupations

Environmental Tobacco Smoke (ETS). "Cigarette smoke is the largest source of indoor air pollution" (CDC, 1993, p. 3). Since the 1960s tobacco smoking has been recognized as a cause of lung cancer and other respiratory diseases in smokers (USEPA, 1993). More recently research has shown that environmental tobacco smoke is hazardous to nonsmokers who live or work in environments occupied by smokers (CDC, 1993). Secondhand tobacco smoke has carcinogenic and toxic agents that are similar to those in mainstream smoke; tobacco smoke is classified by the EPA as a carcinogen. The CDC has developed an action guide for consumers to reduce secondhand smoke (Table 24–6).

Recent studies (CDC, 1993) of preschool children show that environmental tobacco smoke can cause respiratory tract infections such as pneumonia and bronchitis and new cases of asthma. Environmental tobacco smoke is also associated with sudden infant death syndrome (SIDS). In 1993, 9 million preschool children lived at home with at least one smoker.

Secondhand or passive smoking is a major problem in workplaces as well. Because new homes and office buildings tend to be constructed and insulated more tightly to conserve energy, toxic allergens and toxic chemicals such as environmental tobacco smoke are concentrated in indoor air (Pope et al., 1993).

Implications for Nurses

Community health nurses are in key positions to educate families about how to promote home safety and prevent accidents and hazardous exposures. Promoting health and preventing illness, sometimes referred to as primary prevention, involves educating people to eliminate hazards before exposures occur. Families should be informed about hazardous waste disposal sites and encouraged to discard their chemicals there rather than with their garbage and paper trash. Many local solid waste or environmental health divisions provide information on how to purchase and safely store and dispose of household chemicals.

Nurses play an active role in secondary prevention or screening for environmental problems. Nurses can determine hazards that may threaten the health or safety of persons in their homes. Family history should include occupations of household members; the location, age, and physical condition of the residence, school, daycare, or worksite; home remodeling activities; hobbies; use of non–lead-based ceramics for cooking or eating; source and quality of drinking water; and the health of pets. A comprehensive home assessment considers the surroundings in which the home is located (Sargis et al., 1987). For example a densely populated area or one with a high noise level (e.g., near an airport) can have untoward health effects (Salazar, 1987).

Careful observation to identify hygiene, safety, or other special needs of the family is the next step. The general state of repair of the home should be noted to determine whether any unsafe conditions are present, particularly if children or elderly persons reside there. Are sufficient lighting, adequate ventilation, and appropriate cooling and heating mechanisms available? Are smoke detectors present and in working order? Are the kitchen, bath, and laundry facilities adequate to meet the family's needs? Are any obvious sources of infectious disease evident, such as ants, flies, or rodents? Conducting a comprehensive assessment of the home environment may require several visits. The guidelines contained in Table 24–7 provide a convenient checklist for areas to consider in a home assessment.

The causes of health problems may be subtle and may require intensive investigative work on the part of the nurse. For example water contaminants may not produce a visible change in the water and some chemicals (e.g., carbon monoxide) are not easily detectable. As an example of how an environmental hazard in the home can be easily overlooked, consider a recent study that examined the toxic effects of pesticide application for fleas (Fenske et al., 1990). The findings from this study indicated that although the concentration of the pesticide (used as directed) decreased considerably in the adult breathing zone 24 hours after application, the concentration remained high in an infant's breathing zone near the floor, in part because of its concentration in the carpet or in crevices in the floor. Furthermore because infant skin may be more permeable to these chemicals, there is a higher risk for dermal absorption. It was suggested that manufacturer's instructions may not be adequate to protect young members of a household.

It is essential that we remain alert to the possible health effects of commonly used items in the home and provide

TABLE 24–6

Facts about Secondhand Smoke

Some of the key facts about secondhand tobacco smoke and its dangers are summarized below. Use them to inform your family and friends and to work for smoke-free policies in your community.

Secondhand smoke is a cause of disease, including lung cancer, in healthy nonsmokers. Each year secondhand smoke kills an estimated 3000 adult nonsmokers from lung cancer.

Secondhand smoke causes 30 times as many lung cancer deaths as all regulated air pollutants combined.

Secondhand smoke causes other respiratory problems in nonsmokers: coughing, phlegm, chest discomfort, and reduced lung function.

For many people, secondhand smoke causes reddening, itching, and watering of the eyes. About 8 of 10 nonsmokers report they are annoyed by others' cigarette smoke.

More than 4000 chemical compounds have been identified in tobacco smoke. Of these, at least 43 are known to cause cancer in humans or animals.

At high exposure levels, nicotine is a potent and potentially lethal poison. Secondhand smoke is the only source of nicotine in the air.

Nonsmokers exposed to cigarette smoke have in their body fluids significant amounts of nicotine, carbon monoxide, and other evidence of secondhand smoke.

More than 90% of Americans favor restricting or banning smoking in public places.

Forty-six states and the District of Columbia in some manner restrict smoking in public places. These laws range from limited prohibitions, such as no smoking on school buses, to comprehensive clean indoor air laws that limit or ban smoking in virtually all public places.

Adapted from Centers for Disease Control and Prevention. (1993). *It's time to stop being a passive victim.* Atlanta: Government Printing Office.

TABLE 24–7

Key Areas to Assess in the Home

Neighborhood
- Proximity to industry, highways, landfills
- Availability of basic services (health care)
- Access to grocery and clothing stores
- Transportation
- Population density (urban, suburban, rural)
- Noise

Physical Structure
- Cracks in foundation or windows
- Peeling paint
- General state of repair, including stairs

Safety Issues
- Storage for medications, cleaning supplies, chemicals
- Emergency escape route
- Smoke detectors and alarm
- Fire extinguisher
- Accident hazards appropriate to age of family members
- Locks on doors
- Outside play areas if children in the home
- Telephone

Sanitation
- Water and sewage systems
- Plumbing in bathroom and kitchen
- Food preparation, storage, and disposal
- Insects, rodents, pets
- Laundry facilities

Space
- Sleeping areas
- Privacy for members of household
- Lighting

Temperature Regulation
- Type of heat and/or air conditioning
- Ventilation
- Type of insulation

Adapted from Sargis, N., Jennrich, J., & Murray, K. (1987). Housing conditions and health: A crucial link. *Nursing and Health Care, 8*(6), 335–338.

ongoing education to families. A number of consumer resources that provide ongoing information are listed in Table 24–8. Families can be encouraged to minimize the use of household chemicals and pesticides, and to ensure safe storage when they are used. Proper ventilation should be ensured when chemicals are being used. Educating families about what to do in case of accidental poisoning is essential. Poison Control Centers are located in most major cities in the United States. Their telephone number can usually be found in the front of the yellow pages. If not, contact the local telephone operator. A well-trained Poison Control Center staff, which includes pharmacists, nurses, and physicians, is available around the clock to provide information about the prevention and treatment of poisonings.

TABLE 24–8

Resources for Consumers

Action on Smoking and Health
2013 H St. NW
Washington, DC 20006
(202) 659–4310

Americans for Nonsmokers' Rights
Suite J
2530 San Pablo Ave.
Berkeley, CA 94702
(510) 841–3032

Consumer Product Safety Commission
Look in local telephone book for listing or call 1–800–638–2772

Environmental Action
6930 Carroll Ave., Suite 600
Takoma Park, MD 20912
(301) 891–1100

Environmental Defense Fund
257 Park Ave. S
New York, NY 10010
(212) 505–2100

Environmental Protection Agency Public Information
Look in local telephone book for listing or call (202) 260–2080

Greenpeace
1436 U St. NW
Washington, DC 20009
(202) 462–1177

Group Against Smokers Pollution (GASP)
P.O. Box 632
College Park, MD 20740
(301) 459–4791

Office on Smoking and Health
Centers for Disease Control and Prevention
Mailstop K-50
4770 Buford Highway NE
Atlanta, GA 30341–3724
1–800–CDC–1311 (copies of action guide on secondhand smoke)
(404) 488–5705 (other information)

Poison Control Center
Look in local telephone book for listing or write to:
American Association of Poison Control Centers
3800 Reservoir Rd. NW
Washington, DC 20007

Sierra Club
730 Polk St.
San Francisco, CA 94109
(415) 776–2211

General Reading for Consumers

Buzzworm Magazine. (1992). *Earth journal: Environmental almanac and resource directory.* Boulder, CO: Buzzworm Books.

Caplan, R. (1992). *Our earth, ourselves.* Takoma Park, MD: Environmental Action.

Earth Works Group. (1989). *50 simple things you can do to save the earth.* Berkeley, CA: Earthworks Press.

Earth Works Group. (1991). *The next step: 50 more things you can do to save the earth.* Berkeley, CA: Earthworks Press.

Hollender, J. (1990). *How to make the world a better place.* New York: Morrow.

TABLE 24–9

Top 10 Work-Related Diseases and Injuries

1. Occupational lung diseases
2. Musculoskeletal injuries
3. Occupational cancers (except lung cancer)
4. Severe injuries and death from trauma
5. Cardiovascular disease
6. Disorders of reproduction
7. Neurotoxic disorders
8. Noise-induced hearing loss
9. Dermatological conditions
10. Psychological disorders

Adapted from Centers for Disease Control and Prevention. (1983, Jan. 21). Leading work-related diseases and injuries—United States, *Morbidity and Mortality Weekly Report,* p. 25.

ENVIRONMENTAL HAZARDS IN THE OCCUPATIONAL SETTING

Approximately 20 million work-related injuries and 390,000 new work-related diseases occur each year, affecting nearly 1 of 11 Americans (Levy and Wegman, 1988) (Table 24–9). The National Safety Council (1992) reported that almost 10,000 deaths and 1,700,000 disabling injuries were due to on-the-job accidents in 1991. It has been estimated that 100,000 persons die each year as a result of exposures to various hazards and toxins in the work setting.

A survey conducted by the National Institute of Occupational Safety and Health in the early 1970s found that 58% of workers were exposed to one or more chemical or physical hazards (Lee, 1983). Included in the sample were white collar workers, such as office workers, whose environments are generally regarded as "clean." Approximately 8000 substances were identified in that survey. More than 60,000 chemicals were used in industry in the 1980s and it is estimated that 1000 new synthetic chemicals are introduced each year (Omenn, 1986).

The losses resulting from occupational injury and illness are great. Work-related deaths and injuries cost the nation more than $63 billion in 1991 (National Safety Council, 1992). Losses occur at all levels. The employee suffers the loss of a portion of his or her wages and may be required to bear some of the expenses related to care. Additionally the employee experiences the pain and suffering related to the event. The employer may suffer from a loss of productivity, high absenteeism and turnover, and low employee morale. Society pays the extra costs involved in workers' compensation through higher costs for goods and services. Society also loses the revenue from taxes that are not being paid by an unemployed person and that person's contribution to society. These facts demonstrate the significant effect that the occupational environment can have on the health and safety of communities. The *Healthy People 2000* objectives also address occupational safety and health (Table 24–10).

History of Occupational Health in the United States

Although it is likely that occupational hazards have affected the health of communities since the first human began to work, attention to health and safety in the workplace is relatively recent. The Industrial Revolution played a major role in the development of the field of occupational health in this country and in Europe. During the 19th century, masses of Americans moved to the cities to work in the factories and sweatshops, on the railroads, or in the mines, where they were exposed to machinery, chemicals, dusts, extremes in temperatures, backbreaking chores, and other deplorable conditions. They often worked 70 to 80 hours per week and were overwhelmed with stress and fatigue; this even applied to children under 10 years of age. As concerns for health and safety grew, job safety laws slowly began to be passed. By 1900 most of the states that were industrialized had at least minimal legislation intended to protect workers.

During the early 1900s, as the industrial movement expanded, labor unrest resulted in increasing political and social awareness. The number of people who were injured or killed by machinery, the appearance of more chemicals in the workplace, and the increasing size and complexity of manufacturing operations became less and less tolerable to workers and unions. Finally in 1911 the first state workers' compensation law was passed in Wisconsin; by 1948 all of the states had a workers' compensation program. *Workers' compensation* is a liability system that provides at least partial reimbursement of lost wages and full payment for medical expenses to workers who are injured or become ill as a result of their job. Although these compensation laws have provided some relief for workers, there continue to be major deficiencies in the system. For example compensation for certain occupational diseases such as chemical sensitivity is very limited. This is largely the result of the difficulties in establishing links between the disease and the work setting. Furthermore even when he or she is compensated for injury or illness, an employee seldom recovers the full value of lost wages and expenses.

Another landmark in occupational safety and health was the passage of the Occupational Safety and Health Act (OSHAct) of 1970. The purpose of this act is "to assure as far as possible every working man and woman in the nation safe and healthful working conditions." The OSHAct created the Occupational Safety and Health Administration (OSHA) and the National Institute for Occupational Safety and Health (NIOSH). OSHA, part of the Department of Labor, establishes and enforces occupational safety and health standards. About half of the states in the nation have a state counterpart of OSHA. State law must be at least as rigorous as the federal laws. NIOSH, which is within the

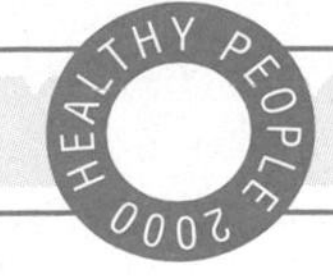

TABLE 24–10

Healthy People 2000 Occupational Safety and Health Objectives

Health Status Objectives

1. Reduce deaths from work-related injuries to no more than 4 per 100,000 full-time workers (baseline: average of 6 per 100,000 during 1983–1987).
2. Reduce work-related injuries resulting in medical treatment, lost time from work, or restricted work activity to no more than 6 cases per 100 full-time workers (baseline: 7.7 per 100 in 1987).

	1983–1987 Average Injuries per 100	Year 2000 Objective
Construction workers	14.9	10
Nursing and personal care	12.7	9
Farm workers	12.4	8
Transportation workers	8.3	6
Mine workers	8.3	6

3. Reduce cumulative trauma disorders to an incidence of no more than 60 cases per 100,000 full time workers (baseline: 100 per 100,000 in 1987).
4. Reduce occupational skin disorders or diseases to an incidence of no more than 55 per 100,000 full-time workers (baseline: average of 64 per 100,000 during 1983–1987).
5. Reduce hepatitis B infections among occupationally exposed workers to an incidence of no more than 1250 cases (baseline: an estimated 6200 cases in 1987).

Risk Reduction Objectives

6. Increase to at least 75% the proportion of worksites with 50 or more employees that mandate employee use of occupant protection systems, such as seat belts, during all work-related motor vehicle travel.
7. Reduce to no more than 15% the proportion of workers exposed to average daily noise levels that exceed 85 dB.
8. Eliminate exposures that result in workers having blood lead concentrations greater than 25 μg/dl of whole blood (baseline: 4804 workers with blood lead levels above 25 μg/dl in seven states in 1988).
9. Increase hepatitis B immunization levels to 90% among occupationally exposed workers.

Services and Protection Objectives

10. Implement occupational safety and health plans in 50 states for the identification, management, and prevention of leading work-related diseases and injuries within the state (baseline: 10 states in 1989).
11. Establish in 50 states exposure standards adequate to prevent the major occupational lung diseases to which worker populations are exposed (byssinosis, asbestosis, coal workers' pneumoconiosis, and silicosis).
12. Increase to at least 70% the proportion of worksites with 50 or more employees that have implemented programs on worker health and safety.
13. Increase to at least 50% the proportion of worksites with 50 or more employees that offer back injury prevention and rehabilitation programs (baseline: 28.6% offered back care activities in 1985).
14. Establish in 50 states either public health or labor department programs that provide consultation and assistance to small businesses to implement safety and health programs for their employees.
15. Increase to at least 75% the proportion of primary care providers who routinely elicit occupational health exposure information as part of patient history and provide relevant counseling.

From USDHHS. (1990). *Healthy people 2000: National health promotion and disease prevention objectives. Summary report.* Washington, DC: Public Health Service.

Department of Health and Human Services, was established to direct research and education efforts related to occupational diseases and injuries.

The OSHAct mandated that employers pay greater attention to health and safety concerns. A number of businesses and industries began to develop new occupational safety and health programs. Because of the recognized need for more occupational health professionals, NIOSH developed the first Educational Resource Centers (ERCs) in 1977. Through these centers, graduate-level education is provided for nurses, physicians, industrial hygienists, and safety managers; continuing education programs are developed; and research on occupational safety and health problems is conducted. There are currently 14 of these centers across the United States, at least one in each federal service region (Table 24–11).

Under the OSHAct, employers are required to adhere to specific standards. For example OSHA wrote the Hazard Communication Standard of 1986 as a result of increasing concern about employee exposure to toxic substances. It is also known as the right-to-know legislation and requires all manufacturers and distributors of hazardous chemicals to

TABLE 24–11

Educational Resource Centers Established by the National Institute for Occupational Safety and Health (NIOSH)

Alabama	University of Alabama at Birmingham; Auburn University
California	
Northern	University of California, Berkeley, Davis, and San Francisco
Southern	University of Southern California; California State University, Fullerton; University of California, Los Angeles; University of California, Irvine Consortium
Illinois	University of Illinois at Chicago
Maryland	The Johns Hopkins School of Hygiene and Public Health
Massachusetts	Harvard School of Public Health; Boston University
Michigan	University of Michigan
Minnesota	University of Minnesota; St. Paul–Ramsey Medical Center Consortium
New York/New Jersey	Mt. Sinai School of Medicine; New York University; Hunter College; City College of New York; Robert Wood Johnson Medical School Consortium
North Carolina	University of North Carolina at Chapel Hill; North Carolina State University; Duke University Consortium
Ohio	University of Cincinnati; NIOSH Division of Manpower and Training Development, Cincinnati
Texas	University of Texas; Texas A&M University Consortium
Utah	University of Utah; Utah State University Consortium
Washington	University of Washington

have material safety data sheets identifying the potential effects of the chemicals. It also requires that employees who come in contact with dangerous substances be properly trained and that employers keep a file on these employees, identifying the chemicals to which they are exposed.

In 1990, in recognition of the special needs of disabled Americans, Congress passed the Americans with Disabilities Act (ADA). Among other things, this act protects disabled Americans, including those injured on the job, from discrimination in the employment setting. If a person with a disability is qualified for a job, employers are required to make reasonable accommodations for that person. Furthermore employers may not ask questions or conduct preemployment examinations for the purpose of identifying disabilities among job applicants. Many employers are already aware of the great benefits derived by hiring persons with disabilities. Studies in companies that have hired disabled persons have repeatedly found that these individuals have low turnover, low absenteeism, and excellent performance ratings (Davies, 1989). The ADA broadens the recruiting base for employers and provides new opportunities for skilled persons who have previously been barred from the workplace.

Occupational Health Nursing

Occupational health is distinguishable as a subspecialty because of its environmental approach to disease and injury and its primary focus on prevention. The principal target of occupational health nursing practice is the aggregate of workers in the many occupational settings across the country. Occupational health nursing as an area of specialty practice was introduced in this country in the late 19th century. The first occupational health nurses were called *industrial nurses* and their primary responsibility was to care for injured workers and their families. Much of their care was provided in the home, so they often took care of other family members and taught them about general sanitation and hygiene. With the rapid expansion of industries in the early 1900s and the passage of workers' compensation laws, the demand for industrial nurses increased dramatically; their numbers grew from 38 in 1912 to 1213 in 1918 (Parker-Conrad, 1988). Occupational health services began to focus more on injuries to the workers in the work setting than on family member services in the home. The numbers of occupational health nurses continued to increase until the 1930s when the Great Depression created massive unemployment. However with the onset of World War II the demand again became strong, and by 1943 there were 11,000 nurses working in industry (Rogers, 1988). The numbers have continued to grow so that by 1992 more than 25,000 occupational health nurses were practicing in the United States (personal communication, Paul Wood, Membership Director, American Association of Occupational Health Nurses, 1992).

In 1942, in recognition of the need for a broad-based organization to meet common goals, the American Association of Industrial Nurses (AAIN) was formed as the professional association for these nurses. In 1976, in keeping with the changes that were occurring within the profession, the name was changed to the American Association of Occupational Health Nurses (AAOHN). This new term reflects the broader scope of practice of the nurse in industry today. According to 1992 figures approximately 12,500 occupational health nurses are members of AAOHN (personal communication, Paul Wood, Membership Director, AAOHN, 1992).

The certification body for occupational health nurses is called the American Board of Occupational Health Nurses (ABOHN). Registered nurses who have worked in occupational health for a minimum of 5000 hours (equivalent to 2½ full-time years) the immediate 5 years prior to applying for certification, have completed 75 units of continuing education related to occupational health and safety, and have successfully completed the board examination are qualified as certified occupational health nurses (COHN). Beginning in 1996 a baccalaureate degree will be required of applicants. As of 1992, 5326 occupational health nurses had been certified by the board.

Roles and Functions of Occupational Health Nurses. The role of the occupational health nurse has evolved and expanded in the last decade. The principal function continues to be the promotion, protection, and maintenance of the health and safety of the workers. The expanded emphasis of occupational health nursing includes wellness and lifestyle change in addition to the reduction of risks associated with environmental exposures. The practice of this specialty involves primary, secondary, and tertiary prevention. A unique body of skills and knowledge enables the occupational health nurse to provide quality nursing care and services. Special skills include training in safety hazards, disaster planning, familiarity with safety equipment, and ability to plan and implement health education programs. Special knowledge includes an understanding of the principles of safety, toxicology, epidemiology, environmental health, and industrial hygiene. (*Industrial hygiene* is a science that focuses on the identification, evaluation, and control of hazards that adversely affect workers and/or communities.) In addition occupational health nurses are required to have up-to-date knowledge of current legal standards that affect the working population.

The AAOHN has developed standards of practice that are specific to occupational health nursing. These standards provide a means for occupational health nurses to measure the quality of the service that they deliver. Current AAOHN standards cover five areas of practice: policy (philosophy, goals, and objectives for health and safety programs), staff ("professional, qualified nurse"), resources (equipment and facilities adequate for programs), nursing practice (aimed at promoting "a safe and healthful work environment"), and evaluation. The standards, which include a statement, an interpretation, and the criteria guiding the standard, are available through AAOHN (50 Lenox Pointe, Atlanta, GA 30324), or through a local organization.

The occupational health nurse is often an independent practitioner and is frequently the only health care provider in an organization. Because management may not understand the roles and functions of the occupational health nurse, she or he may need to write her or his own job description. Whereas occupational health nurses perform according to the guidelines established by the profession and by company management, she or he often determines the priorities appropriate to a situation, establishes goals and objectives, and determines the most suitable course of action. The roles of the occupational health nurse vary greatly from one setting to another. The activities of the occupational health nurse may be categorized as follows: primary care provider, counselor, advocate/liaison, administrator, educator, monitor, professional member of the health team, and researcher (Table 24–12). The occupational health nurse may function in as few as one or as many as all of these roles depending on the particular worksite.

TABLE 24–12

Responsibilities of the Occupational Health Nurse

Primary care provider: Provides care for both occupational and nonoccupational injuries and illnesses, based on a nursing assessment and diagnosis; this role includes preplacement and routine physical examinations, return-to-work assessments, and health screening

Counselor: Counsels distressed employees, identifies workplace and family stressors, and intervenes to assist with personal and emotional problems when appropriate

Advocate/liaison: Brings worker problems to the attention of management and works with management to bring about solutions

Administrator: Designs and implements comprehensive occupational health services; this area requires special skills in problem-solving, ability to communicate effectively, and ability to make independent nursing judgments

Educator: Teaches employees about good health and safety practices and motivates individuals to improve health and safety practices

Monitor: Monitors workers exposed to potentially harmful substances and monitors the worksite for potential health or safety problems

Professional member of the health team (ideally includes industrial hygienist, safety manager, and occupational physician): Collaborates with members of the team to explore and develop ways to promote the health and safety of the workers

Researcher: Systematically and continually collects data concerning the health status of the workers and the real or potential health hazards at the worksite

From Salazar, M. K., Wilkinson, W. E., & Rubadue, C. L. (1991). Occupational health nursing. In J. M. Cookfair (Ed.). *Nursing process and practice in the community,* St. Louis: Mosby–Year Book.

As with many professionals in recent years, occupational health nurses frequently are required to struggle with ethical and legal dilemmas in their practice. The struggle is often precipitated by the nurse's dual responsibilities to the employer and to the employee. It is complicated even further by his or her responsibility to the larger community. Legal and ethical problems seldom result in simple black-and-white resolutions (see Ethics Box VI). It is incumbent on occupational health nurses to keep abreast of the law and to develop lines of communications with other professionals with whom they can confer when difficult issues arise. Occupational health nurses must regularly read professional publications so that they are able to make decisions based on the latest available information.

Although there are often no easy answers, an underlying principle in these conflicts is the responsibility to know and to uphold the standards of the profession. Decision-making must be guided by commonly held and documented standards and practices as well as by the code of ethics advanced by AAOHN.* Sometimes there is a conflict between what is legal and what is ethical. It is legal, for example, for managers or supervisors to access

*To obtain a copy of the AAOHN Code of Ethics and Interpretive Statements contact: Publications, AAOHN, 50 Lenox Pointe, Atlanta, GA 30324–3176 (telephone: (404) 262–1162).

Ethics Box VI

Gail A. DeLuca Havens, M.S., R.N., C.N.A.

The Nurse as Advocate

Audrey is an occupational health nurse at a wallpaper manufacturing plant who is responsible for the on-the-job health and safety of all employees who are exposed to and/or use hazardous materials in their work. Although Audrey has practiced in this plant since 1980 she is an employee of a corporation that owns and operates a total of six similar plants. It was she who was responsible for designing, writing, and implementing the hazard communication program for the plant in 1987, thereby ensuring that the plant would be in compliance with the Occupational Safety and Health Administration (OSHA) hazard communication standard, effective in 1988.

The hazard communication program includes provisions for a material safety data sheet (MSDS) for each hazardous chemical used at the facility, labeling of hazardous chemicals, training and information for employees exposed to hazardous chemicals, and access to manufacturers' MSDSs to gain information regarding specific hazardous risks that might be required in the investigation and evaluation of any specific exposures (Mistretta and Endresen, 1992). As a result of Audrey's efforts plant employees have become aware of potential environmental hazards in the workplace and do not exceed recommended exposure times to maximum concentrations of hazardous materials. They report any unusual signs and symptoms so that Audrey can investigate potential hazardous sources in the workplace. Finally, they are alert for any changes in the work environment, e.g., poor ventilation, that might contribute to increased hazards.

This morning Audrey is meeting with Tom, the plant's general manager, to discuss the recent increase in the incidence of headaches and painful eye irritations among employees who work in one of the plant's printing areas. Audrey summarizes her findings: "Forty percent of the employees in print section E had an onset of headaches and painful eye irritations in one 24-hour period last week. In investigating, I discovered that the day before the onset of these symptoms the section had begun using a different paint pigment in one of its print runs. I reviewed the MSDS related to the pigment's ingredients and, in general, found nothing unusual. There was, however, a recommendation for use of a specific filter gauge in the ventilating system in areas in which this pigment is being used, and we are not using this filter. Employees in this section continue to experience headaches and painful eye irritation. According to the manufacturer's MSDS, no definitive long-term effects from exposure to this pigment have been confirmed. Consequently the manufacturer's MSDS does not include any warning, but only an alert that 'continued exposure to this pigment without benefit of the recommended filtration may lead to respiratory and liver problems.' "

Tom replies, "Audrey, I, too, am concerned about the physical symptoms that employees are experiencing. I have discussed the problem with the engineering personnel and with the company's corporate and legal staffs. To accommodate the recommended filtration in the plant's ventilating system we would have to make substantial modifications to the system, at an expense the company is not in a position to incur. Since no health warnings are associated with exposure to this pigment, the company will not be making any changes to the ventilating system at this time. I trust that you will continue to be responsive to employees' symptoms, so that they are alleviated as much as possible, without compromising the integrity of the company and your position in it."

As a result of the company's decision in this matter, Audrey finds herself in the midst of a dilemma precipitated by competing obligations. On the one hand she is responsible for the on-the-job health and safety of company employees, which includes fostering the well-being of employees while minimizing their exposure to harm. On the other hand as an employee herself she has a responsibility to act in the employer's best interests as well. In addition, as an employee she is concerned about continuing her employment. The potential for termination seemed a very real possibility judging from the general manager's reference to her position in the company. Her family depends on her salary and to be without it would jeopardize their well-being. In this particular case, to act in the employer's best interest it is likely that Audrey will not be able to act in the best interests of her fellow employees. In fact it is possible that she could be harming them. Should Audrey act as a "responsible" employee herself, by

(Continued)

complying with her employer's direction regarding the care of her fellow employees, or should she continue with this issue to advocate for her fellow employees?

If Audrey follows Tom's suggestion, she will avoid immediate financial expenditures for the company. This would remove a lot of the pressure, reduce her stress, and maintain the security of her position in the company and her ability to continue to support her family. As any other parent does, she has a moral obligation to attend to the safety and well-being of dependents.

However, Audrey is an occupational health nurse who "must balance the rights of the employee while working within the policies and standards set by the company" (Mistretta and Endresen, 1992, p. 400). She has a professional obligation, according to the Code for Nurses of the American Nurses' Association (ANA, 1985), and the AAOHN Code of Ethics to maintain the health, welfare, and safety of the client. The nurse is an advocate for the client. As such, she or he "must be alert to and take appropriate action regarding . . . any action on the part of others that places the rights or best interests of the client in jeopardy" (ANA, 1985, p. 6). Advocacy is regarded as a core moral concept of nursing. Accountability is regarded as another of the profession's central moral concepts. To be accountable is to be "answerable to someone for something one has done. Nurses are accountable for judgments made and actions taken in the course of nursing practice" (ANA, 1985, p. 8). Existing policies of the employing agency do not relieve the nurse of the accountability to act in clients' best interests.

In this situation, an appropriate course of action for Audrey would be to report her findings through the official channels established within her company for such actions. Reporting mechanisms should exist within an employment setting so that employees feel comfortable voicing concerns about particular problems within the work setting without fear of reprisal. Having voiced her concerns to the plant manager without a satisfactory response, Audrey should inform the next person in the chain of command, and should inform the plant manager of her action. Although it is not always easy to bring such concerns to an employer, the nurse's accountability to the workers in this plant obligates her to take action that will serve to avoid harm to them from improper ventilation.

An alternate course for Audrey would be to not pursue the reporting of employee symptoms. As OSHA has not classified the chemical as one requiring a warning, but only an alert, Audrey could rationalize this course of action as an acceptable one. It is a strategy that would also serve to preserve Audrey's standing in the company, which is extremely important to her position as family breadwinner.

Which course of action would you pursue?

References

American Nurses' Association. (1985). *Code for nurses with interpretive statements.* Kansas City, MO: Author.

Mistretta, E. F., & Endresen, L. (1992). Environmental hazards in the workplace: Legal and safety considerations. *AAOHN Journal, 40,* 398–400.

employee health records in certain instances. It is easy to imagine the potential for abuse of this privilege. The occupational health nurse has an ethical responsibility to protect the confidentiality of the employee. For this reason it is crucial that written guidelines that prevent the indiscriminate use of records be established and enforced. The AAOHN has issued a position statement and developed clear guidelines regarding the confidentiality of health information in the occupational setting (AAOHN, 1988).

Information on occupational health records may be disclosed under any of four circumstances: in life-threatening emergencies; if release is authorized in writing by the employee; for workers' compensation information; and to comply with government regulations, such as disclosure of data on occupational illnesses, injuries, and exposures (AAOHN, 1988). The AAOHN also recommends that information related to health surveillance and health examinations linked with the employee's ability to work may be disclosed to management on a need-to-know basis or to others with written employee permission. Non–work-related personal and family health information are not to be disclosed to management or regulatory agencies; such information may be released to insurance providers only with the employee's signature (AAOHN, 1988).

Because occupational hazards are the most preventable cause of disease, disability, and death, the field of occupational health "has the potential to contribute more to human welfare than any other health specialty" (Levy and Wegman, 1988). A concern of occupational health professionals is that despite the fact that most persons spend at least a third of their waking hours at work, an occupational health assessment is an often overlooked portion of a health history. Even if a person does not work, she or he is likely to live with someone who does, and that, too, can have an impact on the current state of health. Retired persons may have experienced hazardous working conditions the long-term effects of which are just showing up. One of the

Healthy People 2000 objectives for the nation is to increase to 75% the proportion of primary care providers who elicit occupational health exposures as part of their general health histories (USDHHS, 1990).

ENVIRONMENTAL HAZARDS IN THE COMMUNITY

Much attention has been focused on the environmental health of communities in recent years, in part because of shocking events at Three Mile Island and Love Canal. Three Mile Island is a nuclear power station near Harrisburg, Pennsylvania. In 1979 it was discovered that there was a leak in one of the nuclear units, which allowed the release of radioactive material into the environment. Epidemiological studies in subsequent years determined that there was an increase in the number of cases of leukemia among persons who lived near the unit (Anderson, 1987; Smith and Fisher, 1981). The national concern precipitated by this disaster was reinforced by another nuclear accident at Chernobyl in the former Soviet Union in 1986. Recent reports indicate that this area is also seeing an upsurge in cases of leukemia among children.

Love Canal is a quiet residential neighborhood in New York State that was built on an old toxic waste site. Studies conducted by the EPA (Anderson, 1987; USEPA, 1982) and by Love Canal homeowners in the 1970s revealed disease and genetic damage in residents that was probably connected to the release of toxic chemicals from this site. A number of studies revealed that the sludge at this site contained chemicals including suspected carcinogens (Anderson, 1987). Eventually many families in the Love Canal area evacuated their homes.

These three incidents barely begin to represent the problems that are likely to evolve as a result of a long history of disregard for the environment. Three Mile Island is just one of a multitude of nuclear power stations and Love Canal is just one of 50,000 toxic waste disposal sites in the United States (Anderson, 1987). It is important for local residents, professionals, and policymakers to become aware of the potentially disabling dangers that lurk in their own backyards.

The list of potential sources of hazards in our communities is ever-increasing. Determining the precise relationship between these hazards and the actual health outcome in populations poses major difficulties for epidemiologists and other scientists. All too frequently it takes many years or even decades to determine that a relationship exists. In the meantime people die from cancer, children are born with birth defects, and many people suffer a variety of respiratory problems or other chronic conditions.

There are literally thousands of potential hazards in our environments. For the sake of clarity we have classified these hazards according to their predominant characteristics. Table 24–13 lists potential sources of hazards and the toxic effects of each class. These classifications are by no means exclusive of one another; neither are they all-inclusive.

TABLE 24–13

Examples of Environmental Hazards

Agents	Examples of Harmful Effects
CHEMICAL	
Insulation (formaldehyde)	Increased respiratory allergies, chemical sensitivity
Automobile exhaust (lead)	Behavior disorders, neurological symptoms
Pesticides (polychlorinated biphenyls [PCB])	Chloracne, liver disease, headache, birth defects
INFECTIOUS	
Water supply *(Giardia lamblia)*	Diarrhea, bloating, malabsorption
Food *(Salmonella)*	Fever, nausea, watery diarrhea
Mosquito (malaria)	Chills, fever
PHYSICAL	
Physical hazards (faulty construction)	Accidential death or injury
Noise (motor vehicles, i.e., airplanes, cars, motorcycles)	Hearing problems, stress, fatigue
Radiation (radon gas)	Infertility, birth defects, leukemia
PSYCHOLOGICAL	
Natural disasters (e.g., flooding)	Hypertension
Low economic status (unemployment)	Heart disease, ulcers
Multiple role demands (working parent)	Depression, anxiety

Types of Hazards

Chemical Hazards. Chemicals come in a wide variety of forms (dusts, fumes, mists, vapors, and gases) and can affect almost every system in the body. Our surroundings are literally inundated with chemicals. Although their innovative use has improved the quality of our lives, we have also experienced the consequences of an unrelenting desire for more and better products. Love Canal is a disastrous example of the difficulty in disposing of chemicals.

One of the major challenges for health professionals is developing a full appreciation of the effect that chemicals can have on our environment. The toxic effects are frequently subtle, and persons suffering from exposures are often misdiagnosed. *Toxicology* is the science that studies the harmful effects of chemicals on humans and the ecosystems in which we live. The extent of biological damage produced by a chemical depends on two things: the amount of the exposure, or its "dose," and the "response" of the person exposed. This is called a dose-response ratio. As a general rule the higher the dose, the greater the response. However some people have hypersensitivities or hypersusceptibilities to certain chemicals and will have a response at a much lower than expected dosage.

It is impossible, within the limitations of this section, to even begin to describe the incalculable health effects that can result from exposure to the expansive array of common chemicals to which we are exposed on a regular basis. Think of the petroleum products, the solvents, the pesticides and gardening materials, the medical products, and the plastic items that are a part of your day-to-day life. Of crucial importance however is the recognition that chemical exposures may have profound effects on our communities. As health professionals it is necessary to be alert and aware so that an effective response can be mounted if it is determined that our community is at risk. It is our responsibility to participate in the education of community leaders and residents regarding these issues.

Infectious Agents. Infectious disease is considered to be environmentally transmitted when it is spread from a common source such as water, food, or animal vectors (Blumenthal, 1985). In years past many of the environmental health problems were related to infectious agents, such as typhoid, largely because of an inadequate understanding of sanitation and hygiene.

Despite the great advances in understanding microbes and hygiene, infectious disease continues to be a major public health problem in Third World countries. Although the problems are not as great in this country, they do exist. Many rural communities are not connected to safe central water systems, and municipal water supplies can be threatened through human error or the effects of old equipment. Outbreaks of foodborne diseases such as salmonellosis and hepatitis A often occur.

Vectorborne diseases may be spread by flies, mosquitoes (though rarely in this country), cockroaches, ticks, and rodents. A vectorborne disease that has captured attention recently among outdoor workers is Lyme disease, which is caused by a spirochete and transmitted by an infected tick. This disease causes fatigue, chills, and fever, which may progress to arthritis-like symptoms. A recent study examining patterns of the disease suggested that preventive behaviors, such as wearing long-sleeve shirts and long pants and self-checking for ticks may play an important part in minimizing the risk from Lyme disease (Goldstein et al., 1990).

Human feces can be a source of infectious organisms. One of the most common parasites spread in this way is roundworm, or *Ascaris lumbricoides.* About 4 million persons in this country have ascariasis (Blumenthal, 1985). It is particularly prevalent in warm areas that have poor sanitation. A not uncommon complication of an infestation (particularly in the southeastern United States) is an intestinal obstruction caused by a bolus of worms. Nurses can emphasize the importance of handwashing, safe drinking water supply, and adequate treatment for infected individuals to prevent the spread of disease. With increases in the population, the amount of human waste rapidly increases, as does the risk for these diseases.

Daycare settings are known to be a site where respiratory and enteric diseases such as giardiasis are easily transmitted among children, staff members, and families. The presence of children in diapers combined with children's natural tendency to put objects in their mouths contributes to the spread of infection. To prevent the spread of disease in daycare settings a number of interventions are recommended: (1) proper handwashing by staff members and children; (2) exclusion and/or segregation of sick children; (3) routine cleaning of play objects; (4) separation of food-handling and diaper-changing areas and staff; and (5) use of sanitary diaper-changing procedures (Holoday et al., 1990). Recommended diaper-changing procedures include having a sink and diaper pail adjacent to a separate area for diaper changing, cleaning the surface of the changing table after each child, handwashing, and using a one-piece cloth diaper system or disposable diapers. Nurses can be a resource to daycare centers by providing staff, families, and children with information on preventing illness.

Physical Agents. Accidents are a leading cause of death among persons aged 1 to 37 years (National Safety Council, 1991). Although motor vehicles are by far the single most common cause of these deaths (46,300), about 47,200 accidental deaths in 1990 were the result of non–motor vehicle causes. Many more people suffered disabling injuries. Falls, drownings, and burns were responsible for the majority of non–motor vehicle deaths, and most of these deaths were preventable. Many motor vehicle deaths would not have occurred if the victim had been wearing a seat belt, if the speed limit had been observed, or if drinking and driving had been avoided. Improperly placed items, poor or unsafe construction, and general lack of attention to safety have greatly contributed to these death statistics. Vehicle safety is addressed in *Healthy People 2000* (USDHHS, 1990). One goal is to increase the use of safety belts, inflatable safety restraints, and child safety seats to 85% from a baseline of 42% in 1988. Another goal is to increase the use of helmets from 60% to 80% of motorcyclists and from 8% to 50% of bicyclists. Nurses can participate in school, worksite, and community educational campaigns to increase the use of seat belts, child seats, and helmets.

Noise. Less tangible physical hazards that have received increasing attention in recent years include noise and radiation. Although the health effects from these factors are not as readily identifiable as other physical hazards, the long-term effects from exposure can be devastating.

Noise, although often perceived as innocuous on a day-to-day basis, has been described by some as one of the most noxious and pervasive pollutants in our modern environment (Salazar, 1987). The noise levels in our society have increased dramatically and the most obvious health effect of noise is an impairment of the ability to hear. Other problems that have been associated with noise include stress-related conditions, mental illness, social maladjustment, and pathological conditions such as atherosclerosis and heart disease.

The amount of damage incurred by exposure to noise is directly related to the frequency and intensity of the noise and the length of exposure. The OSHA standard requires that sound levels in the workplace not exceed an average of 90 dB in a 24-hour period. Yet it has been determined that sound levels of much lower intensity may cause gastrointestinal, cardiovascular, or neuroendocrine disturbances (Salazar, 1987). There is no decibel limit for sound levels in the community or in our homes. A jet engine 25 miles away has been measured at 140 dB, a jackhammer at 100 dB, and a live performance of a rock band at 110 dB.

When we become aware that someone is exposed to persistent sound our first approach should be to somehow isolate the noise, either by using sound-absorbent material or by moving the client from the source of noise. If this cannot be done it may be necessary to recommend some type of hearing protection. Our clients should be advised that the noise levels at concerts and discotheques may cause damage to the ear. Radio and cassette headsets may also contribute to increases in hearing loss if the volume is turned up too high.

Radiation. Radiation is of two types: ionizing and nonionizing. Ionizing radiation is produced when atoms disintegrate. Sources of ionizing radiation include x-ray machines, cosmic rays, uranium and other minerals, radon, nuclear power plants, television sets, and atomic fallout. Nonionizing radiation, a lower energy form of radiation, transforms energy into heat. Examples include microwaves, television and radio waves, infrared sources (e.g., welding arcs), ultraviolet rays in sunlamps or sunlight, and lasers.

Although radiation is a natural part of our environment, exposure to excessive amounts causes serious health effects. The largest source of man-made exposure to ionizing radiation is the use of x-rays. Many household products emit ionizing radiation.

In keeping with principles of toxicology, the health effects from radiation are directly related to the amount of exposure. Of greatest concern to scientists is the damage that occurs to chromosomes exposed to ionizing radiation. Excessive and prolonged exposure can cause mutagenic, carcinogenic, and teratogenic effects (Levy and Wegman, 1988). Epidemiological studies of populations exposed to high doses of radiation, such as atomic bomb survivors and patients undergoing radiation therapy, have found a much higher than expected incidence of cancer.

The effects of nonionizing radiation vary according to the source. Ultraviolet radiation causes skin cancer and is probably responsible for the increasing incidence of malignant melanoma. Infrared and ultraviolet light can cause thermal burns. Microwave radiation can cause deep thermal burns and also has been associated with impaired fertility. Lasers can cause retinal damage and severe burns. Although there has been some question about the health effects of radiation from video display terminals, conclusive evidence is lacking that they are in fact harmful. Nurses can educate communities about radiation hazards. For example school nurses can participate in primary prevention of skin cancer by teaching children to use sunscreen and to wear protective clothing.

Psychological Hazards. The last category of hazards is probably the most difficult to describe because it is more difficult to measure. There is little doubt however that psychological factors have a profound effect on the health and well-being of our communities. Stress is just as pervasive in today's environment as the other hazards mentioned. The principal difference is that it is often much easier to determine the link between physical agents and disease than it is to identify the relationship of an illness to psychological factors.

Environmentally induced stress is a natural by-product of our fast-paced society as well as a result of natural or man-made disasters (Anderson, 1987). The devices that were designed to make our lives more streamlined and efficient often succeed instead in increasing the complexity and demands of our existence. Many people find it difficult to keep up with rapidly changing technological developments and feel frustrated in their efforts to do so. The latest and greatest computer today may be obsolete by tomorrow. Persons in lower socioeconomic groups suffer even more frustration, as they seem to be falling further and further behind the mainstream of society. As the gap between rich and poor widens, the anxiety and alienation experienced by certain groups deepens. Societal stresses such as crime, poor economic conditions, changing mores, and rising unemployment affect the well-being of populations.

Many natural occurrences precipitate stress. In the last decade this country has experienced major and devastating earthquakes, floods, hurricanes, droughts, and volcanos; each has taken its toll on life and property and has added to a sense of despair. Concerns about the environment are becoming more prevalent. People have an underlying fear that our earth is being irreparably destroyed and they are overwhelmed by a sense of helplessness.

Stress is a manifestation of an effort to maintain a sense of order. As is the case with most animals, humans have the ability to adapt within certain parameters. When the psychological or physical input becomes excessive, a stress response is likely to occur. If coping mechanisms are in place, the stress can actually have positive outcomes. However if the stresses are incessant, the health of the individual or the community may be severely affected. Nurses can encourage clients and community residents to discover the underlying causes of their stress and to manage their stress. Clients may be given referrals to local mental health centers to assist in managing their stress. Families can be encouraged to prepare for natural environmental disasters such as floods and earthquakes as a means of minimizing stress. In the event of a natural disaster, the Red Cross and other community agencies can be called on to assist families (see Chapter 15).

Environmental Issues for the 21st Century

This brief overview is merely an introduction to the many environmental contaminants that threaten the health of our communities. The medium for many of these pollutants are the very things that we depend on to sustain our lives, the air we breathe, the water we drink, the food we eat, and soil that is so integral to our lives. Air, water, and soil pollution not only threaten our health but also threaten our very quality of life. Numerous objectives in *Healthy People 2000* focus on environmental pollutants and give direction to health professionals as they promote community health and prevent disease (see Table 24–2).

AIR POLLUTION

Ensuring the availability of air free of contaminants presents a unique problem for societies. Unlike other essential elements in our environment, air cannot be purified and stored so that we can release a fresh supply when the need arises. The air that surrounds us is the air that we breathe: and breathe it we must, regardless of the ultimate consequences.

The problems associated with air pollution are not new. There are some dramatic recorded incidents of acute air pollution that cost the lives of thousands of people. At least four of these have occurred in London between 1930 and 1962, and one occurred at Donora, Pennsylvania, in 1948 (Leeser, 1975). In each instance a temperature inversion occurred, which resulted in air pollution being trapped. Of course the industrial pollution was considerable to produce these dire effects. At greatest risk in such cases are those whose health is already compromised, elderly people, and debilitated persons. With the increasing incidence of chronic disease that characterizes today's populations, a greater number of people are at risk in these kinds of situations.

Air pollution is known to aggravate asthma and cardiac and chronic pulmonary diseases and to increase the susceptibility of persons with acute respiratory illnesses. Epidemiological studies suggest that it is also the cause of certain chronic degenerative diseases such as emphysema and chronic bronchitis and contributes to deaths from lung cancers and asthma. Of special concern are the risks to children growing up in a polluted environment.

The two essential types of air pollution are (Leeser, 1975): (1) the oxidizing atmosphere caused by photochemical smog and (2) the by-products of burning fossil fuels. Photochemical smog is caused by fumes emitted from automobile tailpipes. These fumes undergo a series of reactions that are catalyzed by ultraviolet light to produce irritating oxidant compounds. The burning of fossil fuels such as coal and fuel oil produces pollution from oxides of sulfur. Another pollutant released in the air is lead, again from automobile exhaust. As unleaded gas is required for all new cars, this is becoming less of a problem.

The first Clean Air Act was passed in 1963. This act provided federal monies to help states and communities combat air pollution. In 1970 this act was expanded. It set air standards for a number of chemicals known to increase the risk of illness or mortality. It specified that the EPA was to set emission standards for hazardous pollutants. As a result of growing concern about air pollution, Congress passed the Clean Air Act Amendments of 1990. These amendments broadened the original act and included specific mandates related to the control of air contaminants and to the enforcement of existing regulations. As a result of these amendments, it is now easier to ensure compliance with state and EPA air quality requirements. This is largely a result of the fact that the penalty for noncompliance has increased and that the process to impose penalties has been simplified. It is expected that the impact of these amendments will be felt well into the 21st century (Lewis, 1992).

WATER AND SOIL POLLUTION

The availability of clean, safe water is an absolute necessity in the sustenance of a healthy environment. Despite the advances that have been made in the purification of public water in the last century, water contamination remains a threat to some rural and suburban communities. Furthermore with a steadily increasing population creating more potential contaminants, there is a greater likelihood that major water supplies may be threatened in the future. The three main sources of water contamination are industrial wastes, sewage, and agricultural chemicals. Many diseases have been traced to the local water supply, including hepatitis, polio, and microbes that cause gastrointestinal diseases. At particular risk are persons who depend on well water; however contamination can occur in any water supply.

Soil serves as a receptacle for many of the pollutants that are deposited from the air or water. Radioactive matter that disperses into the environment eventually falls to the ground and settles in the soil. Human and animal excreta are often improperly disposed of. The *Ascaris* worm mentioned earlier is commonly found in the soil. Contamination of soil by hazardous waste dumps has been an ongoing and increasing problem in this century. It is estimated that at least 10,000 hazardous waste dumps in the United States pose a threat to public health (Last, 1987).

The health effects of pollution are likely to remain for many years. There have been some efforts among activists in this country to raise America's consciousness about some of these serious problems. However much remains to be done. Health professionals need to be on the frontlines in the struggle to maintain the environment. Community health nurses are in a key position to make a difference.

HAZARDOUS WASTES

Hazardous waste is defined as "any material that is of no further use and cannot be disposed of safely by allowing it to enter the environment in its original form in an uncontrolled manner" (Blumenthal, 1985). This includes infectious wastes, agricultural and industrial by-products, radioactive substances, flammable products, and chemical agents. Hospitals today are increasingly concerned not only about the volume of waste but also about the hazardous waste they produce. Hazardous waste from hospitals, medical offices, and laboratories is tightly regulated by government agencies and must be disposed of separately from regular solid waste.

Because of the potential for many health and safety problems related to waste disposal, there has been an increasing urgency in recent years to respond to this important environmental issue. There were several legislative actions in the 1960s and the 1970s that were intended to alleviate some of the problems related to hazardous waste. These include the Solid Waste Disposal Act of 1965, the Resource Recovery Act of 1970, the Resource Conservation and Recovery Act of 1976, and the Quiet Communities Act of 1978. A major government action of the 1980s was the passage in 1980 of the Comprehensive Environment Response, Compensation, and Liability Act (CERCLA), or Superfund. This act provides for an organized response to the environmental release of hazardous materials from abandoned or inactive waste sites (Blumenthal, 1985). Although government regulation is important in the effort to control the hazards posed by wastes, it is not the final solution to the problem.

Blumenthal (1985) suggests four methods of effective waste management: (1) modification of the dangerous properties of the waste so that it can be allowed to safely enter the environment; (2) storage of waste in a facility that prevents its introduction into the environment; (3) recycling; and (4) elimination of waste production. It is not uncommon to attribute many of the problems related to hazardous wastes to industries and corporations. Although industry does, indeed, play a major role in the production of waste materials, the responsibility for the associated problems belongs to all of us. As a nation we want convenient and cheap products, but we are going to have to learn how not to sacrifice the environment to satisfy this desire.

The Nurse's Responsibilities in Primary, Secondary, and Tertiary Prevention

The responsibilities of the community health nurse in relation to environmental factors include monitoring, assessing, educating, advocating, and role modeling. The levels of prevention used in public health can be applied to environmental problems as a way to understand the various points of interventions (Table 24–14).

PRIMARY PREVENTION

The activities of *primary prevention* are by far the most common and appropriate ones in the field of environmental health. The nurse can create therapeutic environments in all settings. Health promotion and illness prevention in the home, at work, and in the community are aimed at reducing the risk of exposure and illness. The focus on interventions is on the conditions that influence, produce, or predict health and illness in human beings. Nursing practice strategies are geared toward modifying the origins of the problem. Environmental factors can be manipulated through planned change to assist individuals, families, groups, and communities in promoting and maintaining

TABLE 24–14

Prevention Interventions for Environmental Safety and Health

Primary Prevention

- Advocate safer environmental design of products, automobiles, equipment, and buildings
- Teach home safety related to falls and fire prevention, especially to families with children and elderly members
- Counsel women of childbearing age regarding exposure to environmental hazards
- Advocate vehicle protection systems, such as seat belts
- Advocate use of protective devices, such as earplugs for noise
- Immunize occupationally exposed workers for hepatitis B
- Develop worksite health and safety programs
- Develop programs to prevent back injuries at work
- Support the development of exposure standards for toxins
- Support disclosure of radon and lead concentrations in homes at time of sale
- Advocate for safe air and water
- Teach avoidance of ultraviolet exposure and use of sunscreen
- Advocate for reduced waste reduction and effective waste management
- Support programs for waste reduction and recycling

Secondary Prevention

- Assess homes, schools, worksites, and communities for environmental hazards
- Routinely obtain occupational health histories for individuals, counsel about hazard reduction, and refer for diagnosis and treatment
- Screen children from 6 months to 5 years for blood lead levels
- Monitor workers for levels of chemical exposure
- Screen at-risk workers for lung disease, cancer, and hearing loss
- Participate in data collection regarding the incidence and prevalence of injury and disability in homes, schools, and worksites.

Tertiary Prevention

- Encourage limitation of activity when air pollution is high
- Support cleanup of toxic waste sites and removal of other hazards
- Provide appropriate nursing care at worksites or in the home for persons with chronic lung diseases and injury-related disabilities
- Refer homeowners to approved lead abatement resources

Compiled by Claudia Smith, University of Maryland.

health. Individuals can also be taught to use protective devices (such as bicycle helmets) and to reduce environmental hazards.

In the home environment (the microsystem level) nurses can assess for physical hazards (lead, formaldehyde, radon, chemical storage, unsafe play areas), provide education for health promotion, and facilitate and coordinate a health-promoting environment. Families should be encouraged to use community resources and obtain testing for household hazards. Nurses can also be role models for members of the community and advocate for changes in habits. For example to reduce the volume of garbage produced in the United States, nurses could incorporate "trash reduction" practices into their personal shopping habits. Buying in larger quantities or bulk, purchasing items manufactured in less packaging or recyclable packaging, or using reusable products (razors, cloth diapers) rather than disposable ones are ways to reduce household trash.

In the work setting all nurses have an opportunity to protect the environment. For example health care professionals in numerous health care settings are now using many reusable products instead of disposable ones, including cloth diapers, metal wash basins, and float-type mattress pads. Nurse managers are in strategic positions to make decisions about the types of products used and can apply the same waste reduction principles as in the home. Furthermore nurses can pressure manufacturers to reduce the packaging in many materials used in health care settings. At the community and global levels changes in policy are supported to reduce air and water pollution. Nurses can participate in public education and assist community members in interpretation of data about environmental risks.

SECONDARY PREVENTION

Activities of *secondary prevention* are equally appropriate in the home, at work, and in community settings. One of the critical roles of the nurse is to observe signs and symptoms of environmental exposures and assess all clients for environmental risks. For example a toddler living in an older building who is observed eating cracking paint or playing on a dusty floor should have a blood test to screen for lead poisoning. Farm workers who are exposed to pesticides should be screened for toxins. A thorough health history of occupational and environmental exposures is essential for all individuals. Nurses can implement health and safety classes at worksites or schools to promote health and prevent injuries and illness. For example classes in automobile safety can be arranged for young adults in schools. The early diagnosis and treatment of environmental illness, or secondary prevention, is traditionally part of the community health nurse's responsibility.

At the community or macrosystem level, nurses are involved with other health care professionals in the surveillance of health conditions that may be related to environmental and occupational exposures. For example environmental health specialists in local and state health departments play a key role in ensuring safe water, food, and air. The reporting of disease, follow-up, and intervention are all part of surveillance of environmental and occupational disease. Sources of data include health care providers, death certificates and autopsy reports, birth certificates, cancer registries, workers' compensation claims, insurance or hospital billing data, and specific environmental sampling. Nurses can participate in all the phases of data collection, analysis, interpretation, and dissemination. Nurses may be in the best position to interpret scientific findings to the community and to provide individualized and group education as needed.

TERTIARY PREVENTION

Tertiary prevention of environmental health problems occurs after the disease has been diagnosed; it is aimed at minimizing disability and maximizing functional capacity. At this level of intervention treatment strategies are used to assist the individual or community to adapt to changes resulting from the illness. For example after a nuclear accident such as that at Chernobyl, rapid evacuation of residents is imperative to minimize the exposure to radiation. Because the food and water supplies are contaminated by the radiation it is essential to obtain new sources of food and water to limit exposure. If malignancies do occur following a nuclear accident, treatment and/or palliative care, which are activities of tertiary prevention, are appropriate.

Nurses can stay informed of environmental issues by reading newspapers and joining and becoming active in consumer and health-related organizations. Being well informed is a first step in influencing the political system on environmental issues. Communicating effectively with persons in power through groups such as the American Nurses' Association, American Public Health Association, or other groups is vital. Networking with others who share the same interests is highly effective as well. Because environmental health issues have complex origins and involve many professionals, an interdisciplinary approach is most effective.

KEY IDEAS

1. The interaction of human beings with the environment continuously affects health status.
2. The environment includes physical, political, social, economic, and cultural aspects.
3. The home, the workplace (or school), and the community are important sources of environmental hazards that affect health.

4. *Healthy People 2000* objectives address prevention of home accidents, reduction of worker illnesses and injuries, and reduction of human exposure to toxic agents.
5. Hazards include chemicals, infectious agents, mechanical forces, noise, and radiation.
6. Intentional suicides and homicides exceed home accidents as causes of death. Accidental deaths from firearms have decreased because of educational programs regarding their use.
7. Falls, poisonings (including drug overdoses), and fires are the top three causes of accidental deaths in homes.
8. Persons who are physically dependent, such as preschool children and the elderly, are at highest risk of preventable home accidents.
9. Chemicals such as radon, formaldehyde, carbon monoxide, and pesticides and environmental tobacco smoke in homes contribute to respiratory illnesses.
10. Lead poisoning causes cognitive disabilities in children as well as other neurological, renal, and hematological damage.
11. Community health nurses provide education regarding safe home environments and assist families in identifying hazards that can be removed in the home.
12. Occupational health nursing is a branch of community health nursing concerned with promoting, protecting, and maintaining the health and safety of workers.
13. The most frequent work-related illnesses and injuries are lung diseases, musculoskeletal injuries, cancer, and traumatic injuries.
14. More disabling injuries occur in workplaces than in homes.
15. The Federal Hazard Communication Standard of 1986 requires employers to notify employees of exposure to toxic substances.
16. Ethical issues can face occupational health nurses as a result of competing interests of employers and employees.
17. All community health nurses need to include occupational histories when assessing the health of individuals and their families.
18. Clean air and water, as well as effective waste management, remain critical issues for the 21st century. Community health nurses can advocate for collective community action to preserve natural resources.

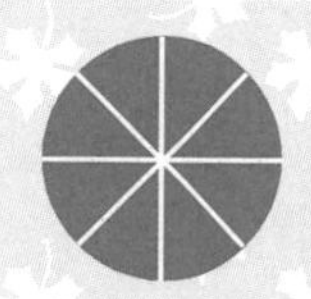

CASE STUDY
Environmental Issues Related to Disposable Diapers

From an environmental perspective the extensive use of disposable diapers has caused a great deal of concern because of the actual and potential hazards they pose to the environment. Nurses, as educators, experts, advocates, and community activists, help to protect the environment. In this case study a community education project about the environmental issues related to disposable diaper use is explored (Primomo, 1990). The community nursing process (problem assessment, analysis and diagnosis, planning, implementation, and evaluation) was used to guide the project.

Overview of Project

In 1986 nurses in the King County Nurses Association (KCNA) in Seattle began examining environmental issues as one of the association's annual health issues. An issue briefing paper was published in the KCNA's publication that focused on the solid waste crisis and what individual nurses could do to reduce waste. A task force of nurses was then formed to explore one particular area: the widespread use of disposable diapers and their contribution to the garbage crisis.

The first step taken by the task force was to *define and assess the problem*. Experts and key informants in the field of solid waste, virology, epidemiology, and infant health were interviewed. A thorough review of the literature was undertaken. Each year Americans throw away well over 16 to 18 billion disposable diapers; these make up between 2% and 4% of all solid waste. Disposable diapers account for about 80% of all diaper changes made in the United States. More than 100 different enteric pathogens are known to be excreted in human feces, including hepatitis and polio if live polio vaccine is used. Furthermore these viruses can live for months after the stool has passed from the body. Because of the volume of disposable diapers used, the amount of improperly treated feces from disposable diapers is substantial and may be polluting the ground and water near landfills. Very little data have been published on these potential hazards, but after a literature review, the task force concluded that if landfills were not properly constructed (as in some rural areas and in less developed countries), ground water and drinking water might become contaminated with excrement from disposable diapers.

Next the task force agreed that the health and environmental issues of disposable diapers had not been raised in the professional community. A position paper of the key issues served as a communication tool that was disseminated to elected officials, professionals, and interested community groups. This paper was a culmination of the efforts of the group in the *analysis and diagnosis stage* of the community health nursing process. By taking a stand and making recommendations based on a literature review, the group raised questions that had not been discussed in the scientific community. At the same time numerous environmental groups were beginning to explore ways to reduce the solid waste stream due to the closure of landfills, where about 90% of the garbage created in the United States is deposited. When the Seattle solid waste utility notified community groups of the availability of grant funds for programs aimed at reducing solid waste, KCNA was prepared to apply for funds to carry out recommendations in the position paper. The preparation of the grant application served to formalize the *planning phase* of the community nursing process.

The task force chose to focus on educating health care providers and new parents about the health and environmental issues related to disposable diaper use. The education project included the production of a professionally designed brochure in English (grade 5 reading level), Spanish, and Vietnamese. The cost, convenience, health and environmental issues, and proper method of using home-laundered diapers, diaper services, and disposable diapers were reviewed in the brochure. Brief sections on handwashing, health and safety tips, and prevention and treatment of diaper rash were included. A videotape was produced to provide another educational medium.

The *implementation phase* of the community nursing process included education programs and media publicity. The target population for the consumer education project was new parents. To reach new parents in-service education programs were conducted with the staffs of newborn nurseries and health departments and childbirth educators. These professionals could in turn educate new parents and distribute the brochure. The same material in the prochure was covered in the in-service classes. Press releases to local newspapers were used to generate interest in the project and to let the community know how to obtain the brochure. Task force members participated in radio and television news programs and responded to inquiries from newspaper reporters.

Evaluation, the final phase of the community nursing process, was conducted at various points throughout the project. Feedback from pilot testing of the brochure with a focus group of new parents provided vital information that greatly enhanced the quality of the brochure. Feedback from both the diaper service and the disposable diaper industries assisted the group in clarifying key issues. After each in-service education program responses to an evaluation questionnaire were used to improve the content of the program. Finally, on completion of the project, a process evaluation (the number of brochures produced, the number of in-service sessions) was conducted. Outcome evaluation criteria included data about diaper type used in hospitals and homes. At the beginning of the project none of the hospitals used cloth diapers. By the next year five of six area nurseries used cloth diapers. Diaper services in the area reported a 22% to 35% increase in the use of their service compared with that of the previous year.

Community Health Nurse Responsibilities

The primary responsibilities of the community health nurse in this particular environmental issue were advocacy and education of clients in the home, at work, and in the community. Primary prevention was the focus of the educational interventions. The brochure for new parents focused on the various diaper alternatives, how to deal with each alternative, diaper rash prevention, disease prevention through handwashing, and tips for baby's health and safety. Instructions that appear on the disposable diaper packages regarding how to deal with the solid fecal material in disposable diapers were reviewed. Parents were advised to empty the solid fecal material into the toilet prior to wrapping the diaper tightly and throwing it in the garbage. This common sense practice helps to minimize the potential for illness transmission from insects and rodents that can come in contact with infectious agents and spread disease.

The nurse's responsibilities included the identification of occupational groups at risk from the improper disposal of feces in the garbage. Logically, sanitation workers might come into contact with disposable diapers and therefore be at risk for several diseases. At present no studies have specifically examined this issue. Another group, diaper service workers, are also in need of health and safety information. Protective clothing, gloves, and boots should be provided. Ongoing education about hygiene practices should be conducted to reduce the potential for disease transmission to this group.

The nurse's role at the community level was again one of advocacy and education. The community health nurses educated the nursing constituency, who in turn educated new parents. The task force publicized their concern among the nursing community and broader professional groups including the American Public Health Association (1990), which later adopted a policy statement on the health and environmental hazards of disposable diapers. Articles about environmental issues and diapers were written for professional journals (Primomo et al., 1990). Members of the task force were identified as experts on diapers and public officials from around the country contacted them to obtain information. The task force built coalitions with other groups interested in solid waste issues. Thus communicating to the community at large, to government officials, and to the media to publicize the task force's position were vital elements of advocacy and education.

Application of the Ecological Systems Model

The ecological model presented at the beginning of the chapter is useful in considering the potential impact of all types of diaper products on the environment. The model is useful in identifying areas of intervention as well. Because the disposable diaper industry is a $4 billion per year business, economic issues related to their use are important considerations. Any attempt to educate consumers about alternatives to disposable diapers can be expected to meet with resistance from manufacturers (Primomo and Greenstreet, 1993). But these issues have already reached the political level in many communities and states and are unlikely to go away. The city of Seattle has an ordinance prohibiting the disposal of human excrement, including that in disposable diapers, in municipal garbage. Parents in the Seattle community have been instructed to dump the solid material into the toilet prior to throwing away the disposable diaper. Numerous states are considering various kinds of legislation to decrease the use of disposable diapers. Examples of proposed legislation include banning disposable products, levying a tax on disposable diapers because of the added financial costs that are incurred with their disposal, and creating tax breaks for diaper services. Because diapers are symbolic of the garbage crisis we face today, diapers are indeed a political issue.

Social and cultural norms of diapering methods are influenced by advertising, personal experience, information from family and friends, and recommendations from professionals. One of the goals of the diaper education project was to raise people's awareness about environmental issues related to diapers so that an informed choice about a diapering method could be made. The professional community can serve as role models on many environmental issues.

Although task force members focused primarily on the volume of garbage and infectious diseases, other environmental risks include air and water pollution produced by the manufacture of chemicals and plastics. Because about 65% of a disposable diaper is made from wood products, deforestation, global warming, and other problems are related to "disposable" products. Although the manufacture of disposable diapers uses natural resources and produces pollutants, cloth diapers require energy and water to launder, which also has a negative environmental impact.

An ecological model is useful in examining other environmental issues, including nurses' occupational exposure to chemotherapeutic agents or the use of chemical pesticides in the food supply. The community nursing process can be used to promote health and prevent illness with these and many other environmental issues.

GUIDELINES FOR LEARNING

1. Conduct further reading to compare the signs and symptoms of lead poisoning in children and adults.
2. Describe an environmental issue in your community (such as a hazardous waste site, chemical pollutants from a plastic manufacturer, or pollution from an incinerator) and the role of the community health nurse in monitoring health, raising awareness, and promoting education and advocacy.
3. Spend a day with an environmental health specialist in your local health department, an occupational health nurse, or a daycare nurse consultant, or visit community agencies such as the local poison control center. Identify the environmental hazards dealt with and the role of each professional in protecting the public from environmental hazards.
4. Use the categories outlined in the home assessment inventory in Table 24–7 and complete a home environmental assessment for a client. Outline the teaching that you consider appropriate.
5. Contact three occupational health nurses in your state. Using Table 24–12 as a guide, describe the responsibilities of each of these nurses. See whether you can identify at least one example of primary, secondary, and tertiary prevention activities in each of the settings.

REFERENCES

American Academy of Pediatrics, Committee of Environmental Hazards. (1987). Committee on Accident and Poison Prevention: Statement on childhood lead-poisoning. *Pediatrics, 79,* 457–465.

American Association of Occupational Health Nurses (AAOHN). (1988). Guidelines for confidentiality of health information. *AAOHN Journal, 36*(1), 7.

American Public Health Association (1990). Health and environmental hazards of disposable diapers (APHA policy statement No. 8910). *American Journal of Public Health, 80*(2), 230.

Anderson, R. (1987). Solid waste and public health. In M. Greenberg (Ed.). *Public health and the environment* (pp. 173–204). New York: Guilford.

Blumenthal, D. S. (1985). *Introduction to environmental health.* New York: Springer.

Breckinridge, M. (1952). *Wide neighborhoods. A story of the frontier nursing service.* New York: Harper.

Bronfenbrenner, U. (1979). *The ecology of human development.* Cambridge, MA: Harvard University Press.

Centers for Disease Control and Prevention (CDC). (1991). *Preventing lead poisoning in young children.* Atlanta: U.S. Government Printing Office.

CDC. (1993). *It's time to stop being a passive victim.* Atlanta: U.S. Government Printing Office.

Council on Scientific Affairs. (1987). Radon in homes. *Journal of the American Medical Association, 258,* 668–672.

Davies, K. (1989). A good bet? You bet! *Work: A Publication on Employment and People with Disabilities, 2*(4), 46–47.

Dubos, R. (1968). *Man, medicine, and environment.* New York: Praeger.

Fenske, R., Black, K., Elkner, K., Lee, C., Methner, M., & Soto, R. (1990). Potential exposure and health risks of infants following indoor residential pesticide application. *American Journal of Public Health, 80,* 689–693.

Gardner, M. S. (1936). *Public health nursing* (3rd ed.). New York: Macmillan.

Goldstein, M. D., Schwartz, B. S., Friedmann, C., Maccarillo, B., Borbi, M., & Tuccillo, R. (1990). Lyme disease in New Jersey outdoor workers: A statewide survey of seroprevalence and tick exposure. *American Journal of Public Health, 80,* 1225–1229.

Hawley, A. H. (1950). *Human ecology: A theory of community structure.* New York: Ronald Press.

Hedberg, K., Gunderson, P., Vargas, C., Osterholm, M., & Macdonald, K. (1990). Drowning in Minnesota, 1980–1985: A population-based study. *American Journal of Public Health, 80,* 1071–1074.

Holoday, B., Pantell, R., Lewis, C., & Gillis, C. (1990). Patterns of fecal coliform contamination in day care centers. *Public Health Nursing, 74,* 1840–1844.

Last, J. M. (1987). *Public health and human ecology.* Ontario: Appleton & Lange.

Lee, J. S. (1983, May). Environmental evaluation of the work place. *Family and Community Health,* pp. 16–23.

Leeser, I. (1975). Environmental health. In I. Leeser, C. Tuchalski, & R. Carotenuto (Eds.). *Community Health Nursing: Nursing Outline Series.* Flushing, NY: Medical Examination.

Levy, B. S., & Wegman, D. H. (1988). *Occupational health: Recognizing and preventing work-related disease* (2nd ed.). Boston: Little, Brown.

Lewis, W. (1992). Approaching 2000: A regulatory overview. *Environmental Protection, 3*(1), 32–42.

Loken, S., & Loken, T. (1989, November). Radon: Detection and treatment. *Nurse Practitioner,* pp. 45–51.

Marino, P., Landrigan, P., Graff, J., Nussbaum, A., Bayan, G., Boch, K., & Boch, S. (1990). A case report of lead poisoning during renovation of a Victorian farmhouse. *American Journal of Public Health, 80,* 1183–1185.

Minnesota Department of Health. (1982). *Assessment of health risks in the home environment.* Minneapolis: Author.

National Safety Council. (1989). *Accident facts.* 1989 Edition. Itasca, IL: Author.

National Safety Council. (1991). *Accident facts.* 1991 Edition. Itasca, IL: Author.

National Safety Council. (1992). *Accident facts.* 1992 Edition. Itasca, IL: Author.

Nightingale, F. (1969). *Notes on Nursing. What it is. What it is not.* New York: Dover (originally published in 1860 by Harrison in London).

Omenn, G. S. (1986, Summer). A framework for risk assessment for environmental chemicals. *Washington Public Health 6,* pp. 2–6.

Parker-Conrad, J. E. (1988). A century of practice in occupational health nursing. *AAOHN Journal, 36*(4), 156–161.

Pope, A., Patterson, R., & Burge, H. (Eds.). (1993). *Indoor allergens: Assessing and controlling adverse health effects.* Washington, DC: National Academy Press.

Primomo, J. (1990). Diapering decision: A community education project. *American Journal of Public Health, 80,* 743–744.

Primomo, J., Bruck, A., Greenstreet, P., Leaders, L., Pennylegion, L., Salazar, M., & Ware, A. (1990). The high environmental cost of disposable diapers. *American Journal of Maternal/Child Nursing, 15,* 279, 282, 284.

Primomo, J., & Greenstreet, P. (1993). Influencing policy on diapers: Not for babies only. *Journal of Perinatology, 13*(2), 140–143.

Rogers, B. (1988). Perspectives in occupational health nursing. *AAOHN Journal 36*(4), 151–155.

Salazar, M. K. (1987). Noise is a pollutant, too! *The Washington Nurse, 17*(5), 17.

Salazar, M. K., Wilkinson, W. E., & Rubadue, C. L. (1991). Occupational health nursing. In J. M. Cookfair (Ed.). *Nursing process and practice in the community,* St. Louis: Mosby–Year Book.

Sargis, N., Jennrich, J., & Murray, K. (1987). Housing conditions and health: A crucial link. *Nursing and Health Care, 8,* 335–338.

Smith, J., & Fisher, J. (1981). Three Mile Island: The silent disaster. *Journal of the American Medical Association, 245*(16), 1656–1659.

Taravella, S. (1990, Dec 24–31). Hospitals dispose of destructive waste practices. *Modern Health Care,* pp. 20, 26–28.

Theodorson, G. A. (1961). *Studies in human ecology.* New York: Harper & Row.

U.S. Department of Health and Human Services. (1990). *Healthy People 2000: National Health Promotion and Disease Prevention Objectives. Summary report.* Washington, DC: U.S. Government Printing Office.

U.S. Environmental Protection Agency (USEPA). (1982). *Environmental monitoring at Love Canal* (EPA 600/4–82–030a). Washington, DC: U.S. Government Printing Office.

USEPA (1993). *Respiratory health effects of passive smoking.* Washington, DC: Author.

Woolf, A., Fish, S., Azzara, C., & Dean, D. (1990). Serious poisonings among older adults: A study of hospitalization and mortality rates in Massachusetts, 1983–1985. *American Journal of Public Health, 80,* 867–869.

BIBLIOGRAPHY

Archer, D. (1989). Disease in day care. A public health problem for the entire community. *Journal of Environmental Health, 51*(3), 143–147.

Bunge, M. L. (1985). Chemical hazards in the household: What every community health nurse should know. *Journal of Community Health Nursing, 2*(1), 31–40.

Chopoorian, T. (1986). Reconceptualizing the environment. In P. Moccia (Ed.). *New approaches to theory development* (pp. 39–54). New York: National League for Nursing.

Greenberg, M. (Ed.). (1987). *Public health and the environment.* New York: Guilford Press.

Levine, A. (1982). *Love Canal: Science, politics and people.* Lexington, MA: Lexington Books.

Macinick, C., & Macinick, J. (1987). Toxic new world: What nurses can do to cope with a polluted environment. *International Nursing Review, 34*(2), 40–42.

Matthews, B. (1992). *Chemical sensitivity: A guide to coping with hypersensitivity syndrome, sick building syndrome and other environmental illnesses.* Jefferson, NC: McFarland.

Purdom, P. W. (1980). *Environmental health.* New York: Academic Press.

Rotter, K. L. (1986, Aug/Sept). Ecominnea: A strategy for teaching environmental health. *Health Education,* pp. 26–27.

Taravella, S. (1990, Dec 24–31). Hospitals dispose of destructive waste practices. *Modern Health Care,* pp. 20, 26–28.

Theodorson, G. A. (1961). *Studies in human ecology.* New York: Harper & Row.

World Health Organization. (1993). *Guidelines for drinking water quality: Volume 1, Recommendations* (2nd ed.). Geneva: Author.

SUGGESTED READINGS

Adams, R. M., Cole, J., Price, A. L., Lewis, R. C., Jr., & Cotton, W. H. (1991). Environmental health and safety in schools: An overview. *School Nurse, 7*(1), 14–18.

Gropper, E. I. (1990). Florence Nightingale: Nursing's first environmental theorist. *Nursing Forum, 25*(3), 30–33.

Iiorio, D. C. (1985, November). The agricultural worker: Occupational health's neglected client. *Occupational Health Nursing,* pp. 566–588.

Landigran, P. (1992). Commentary: Environmental disease—A preventable epidemic. *American Journal of Public Health, 82,* 941–943.

Last, J. M. (1990). Public health and the global environment. *Canadian Journal of Public Health, 81*(1), 3–4.

Lee, J. S. (1983). Environmental evaluation of the work place. *Family and Community Health, 6*(1), 16–23.

Sargis, N., Jennrich, J., & Murray, K. (1987). Housing conditions and health: A crucial link. *Nursing and Health Care, 8*(6), 335–338.

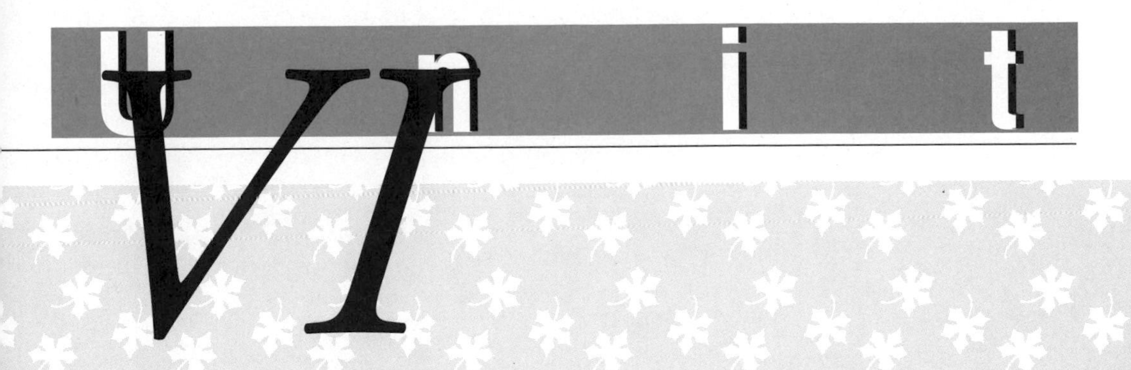

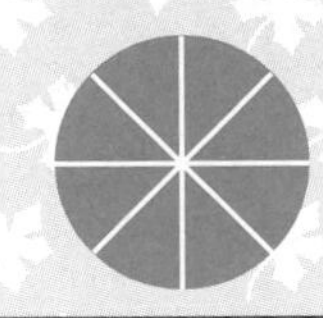

Support for Special Populations

Chapter 25

Rehabilitation Clients in the Community

Adrianne E. Avillion
Janie B. Scott

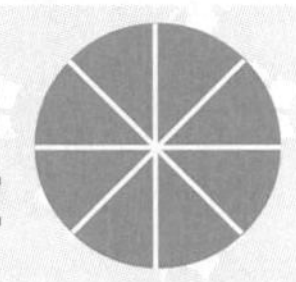

Focus Questions

What is the magnitude of disability in the United States?

What are the concepts of rehabilitation nursing?

What are some common conditions that require rehabilitation?

How does legislation affect the rehabilitation process?

What is the role of the rehabilitation nurse?

How does the rehabilitation client achieve community reintegration?

What are the responsibilities of the community health nurse in meeting the needs of rehabilitation clients?

What are community resources for individuals with disabilities?

Concept of Disability

Between 34 and 43 million people in the United States have significant, chronic disabilities (USDHHS, 1990). *Disability* is the limited ability to function physically or mentally (U.S. Department of Health and Human Services [USDHHS], 1990); the term focuses on effects rather than causes. Of those with disabilities, approximately 70% are unable to perform or have some limitation in their major life activity (play, school, work, self-care). The others are limited in their ability to perform nonmajor activities (such as climbing stairs or driving an automobile) (Fig. 25–1).

Disabilities have a variety of causes and are not evenly distributed among the population. Causes of disability include congenital defects, mental retardation, traumatic injuries, and consequences of diseases (e.g., amputation in diabetes, altered mobility related to pain from arthritis, and altered cognition in schizophrenia).

Although disability occurs in people of all ages, disability rates increase with age. However, 4 of 10 noninstitutionalized persons needing assistance with activities of daily living are under 65 years of age (LaPlante, 1988).

Disability rates are higher among the poor (USDHHS, 1990). Some reasons for this are inadequate prenatal nutrition and care, higher accident rates, less preventive care, and a higher prevalence of chronic disease among the poor. Although disability rates in the United States vary by race and ethnic group, it is important to remember that poverty is the most dominant factor (Fig. 25–2).

Many terms are associated with persons who live with disabilities. To establish a common frame of reference, several terms are defined in Table 25–1. *Impairment* relates to the organic dysfunction itself, *disability* is the difficulty to perform certain tasks because of the impairment, and *handicap* is any social disadvantage that exists because of the disability (World Health Organization [WHO], 1981).

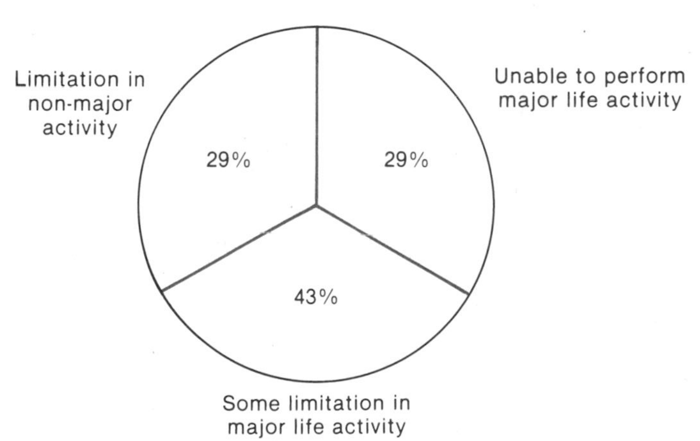

Figure 25–1 ● Intensity of disabilities (number disabled = 34 to 43 million). (Data from LaPlante M. (1988). *Data on disability from the National Health Interview Survey, 1983–1985.* Washington, DC: National Institute on Disability and Rehabilitation Research.)

RATE
RACE/ETHNICITY
Highest rate
American Indians
Blacks
Non-Hispanic whites
Hispanics
Lowest rate
Asian and Pacific Islanders

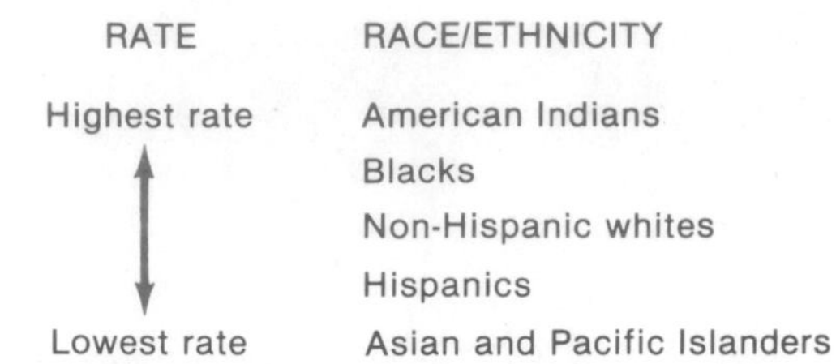

Figure 25–2 ● Rates of disabled persons in the United States by race or ethnicity. (Data from National Institute on Disability and Rehabilitation Research. (1989). *Chartbook on disability in the United States.* Washington, DC: Author.)

Not everyone who has an impairment is disabled, nor is every person with a disability handicapped. For example, an individual may be missing a fifth finger but is able to perform all desired tasks without it. This person would not have a disability. However, if this individual had been a concert pianist before the loss of the finger, such a loss would cause a disability in a major life activity (work and leisure).

The environment is the critical factor in determining the extent of an individual's handicap. Disabilities may be handicapping in one situation but not in another, depending on the factors existing in the environment. For example, consider the person with chronic obstructive pulmonary disease whose symptoms are aggravated by walking to an office on the fifth floor in a building without elevators. On arriving at work, his altered oxygenation affects his ability to concentrate. Such a person would be disabled in the major life activity of work. Furthermore, if the employer insisted that the employee must perform his job at that site, the individual would be handicapped. (Although the Americans with Disabilities Act, discussed later in the chapter, makes this employer's action illegal, such actions continue to occur.)

TABLE 25–1

Definitions

Disability: The inability to perform some key life functionings. This term is often used interchangeably with functional limitation.

Functional limitation: The result of an impairment; refers to the loss of ability to perform self-care tasks and fulfill usual social roles and normal activities.

Impairment: The residual limitation resulting from disease, injury, or a congenital defect.

Chronic illness: The irreversible presence, accumulation, or latency of disease states or impairments that involve the total human environment. Chronic illnesses have different implications for different people and are never completely cured or prevented (Lubkin, cited in Dittmar [1989]).

Handicap: The interaction of a person with a disability in the environment.

From Dittmar, S. (1989). Scope of rehabilitation. In S. Dittmar (Ed.). *Rehabilitation nursing process and application* (p. 7). St. Louis: Mosby–Year Book.

Community health nurses seek to prevent and reduce sources of handicaps, such as stereotyping, architectural barriers, and failure to accommodate those with disabilities. Such interventions are a part of rehabilitation.

Concept of Rehabilitation

HISTORICAL OVERVIEW

Rehabilitation may be defined as a dynamic process that helps a disabled person to achieve optimal physical, emotional, psychological, social, or vocational potential in order to maintain dignity, self-respect, independence, and self-fulfillment (Hickey, 1992). The mission of rehabilitation is complex. Its objectives reach beyond the rehabilitation of individual clients; they include educating all health care professionals, as well as the general public, to create a society in which individuals with disabilities have a fair chance to work, enjoy life, and live as independently as possible. Thus, rehabilitation is concerned with the quality of life.

Historically, the problems of individuals with disabilities were often treated in an indifferent fashion, without understanding, and without realization of the degree of adaptation required to successfully fulfill the activities of daily living. Indignities and isolation have long surrounded people with disabilities. Blind persons, forced to beg, and those with leprosy, shunned and ridiculed by society, illustrate the public's negative reaction to disabled individuals.

In some cultures, infants with disabilities were left to die. Because of the many superstitions and mysticism that existed during the Middle Ages, crippled, malformed, and visibly ill individuals were said to be either cursed or possessed by the Devil. This lapse into demonology lasted until the 18th century (Rosen and Fox, 1972).

Philosophical and economic factors then modified attitudes toward the disabled. As the belief in the essential worth of all individuals evolved in Western thought, those with physical and mental disabilities were more tolerated. Because of the spread and economic importance of industries in the 19th century, international legislation was passed making establishments responsible for injuries to employees. However, it was not until World War II that there was real interest in rehabilitation.

As director of the Army Air Corps Convalescent and Rehabilitation Services during World War II, Dr. Howard Rusk conceived the philosophy and concept of rehabilitation medicine. After the war, he continued his work in Bellevue Hospital in New York City. Dr. Rusk found that his efforts to rehabilitate his patients were often thwarted by the negative attitudes of health care professionals towards rehabilitation (Rusk, 1972).

Gradually, societal progress was made toward acceptance of the disabled. The World Rehabilitation Fund was founded in 1955. Its basic aim was to sponsor international projects that would help individuals with disabilities and create a better understanding of their problems. The fund also helped to train health care professionals in the rehabilitative field and increased employment opportunities for rehabilitation clients (Rusk, 1972).

Legislative efforts in recent years (discussed later) have assisted the rehabilitation movement. For example, in 1973 the Rehabilitation Act established the Architectural and Transportation Barriers Compliance Board. This board can hold public hearings, conduct investigations, and order that applicants with disabilities be recruited and hired. Section 503, Affirmative Action, deals with the regulations concerning the building of barrier-free public facilities and educational institutions (Russel, 1973).

In 1983 the American National Standards Institute published a set of standards for making buildings and facilities accessible to and usable by individuals with physical disabilities. Its specifications are recommended for adoption and enforcement by administrative authorities so that individuals with disabilities may pursue their interests, develop their talents, and exercise their skills.

Modern rehabilitation nursing emerged during World War II. As the needs and rights of individuals with disabilities became more acknowledged in society, the contributions of rehabilitation nurses were recognized as distinct and important. All nurses working with individuals with impairments, chronic diseases, and acute injuries include aspects of rehabilitation in their practice. Rehabilitation nursing is also a specialty area of nursing.

BELIEFS ABOUT REHABILITATION NURSING

"Rehabilitation nursing is the diagnosis and treatment of human responses of individuals and groups to actual or potential health problems stemming from altered functional ability and [related] altered lifestyle" (American Nurses' Association [ANA] and Association of Rehabilitation Nurses [ARN], 1988, p. 4). Community health nurses who provide rehabilitation must be skilled in providing comfort and therapy, promoting adjustment and coping, supporting adaptive capabilities, and promoting achievable independence and meaning in life (ANA and ARN, 1988).

The rehabilitation nurse functions as a teacher, caregiver, case manager, counselor, consultant, and client advocate (Mumma, 1987). These roles are practiced in collaboration with other members of the interdisciplinary rehabilitation team. The nurse practices in a partnership not only with other health care professionals, but also with the client and family.

Community health nurses work with individuals with disabilities and their families in schools, workplaces, clinics, and homes. Medicare pays for inpatient rehabilitation and home health care services for the elderly and other disabled individuals, regardless of age, who receive Social Security Disability payments. Rehabilitation services under Medicaid vary by state. Many private insurers and health maintenance organizations have instituted strict case management programs to control health care costs for those with severe disabilities (Ross, 1992). Often rehabilitation nurse specialists are the case managers for these individuals.

In the professional practice of rehabilitation nursing, the nurse must be sensitive, flexible, creative, and assertive as she or he assists clients to successfully enter or reenter a society primarily designed for able-bodied persons. Nurses must examine their own beliefs and feelings about disabilities and handicaps. Not all nurses are able to cope with the lifelong consequences of devastating illnesses or injuries such as spinal cord injuries, strokes, or muscular dystrophy. A belief in the promotion of quality of life is essential. Negative attitudes toward disability create serious obstacles to the formation of a therapeutic relationship and client adaptation.

Rehabilitation nursing should be part of all phases of recovery. For those with injuries and severe illnesses, recovery often begins with admission to the acute care facility and continues throughout community reintegration. The rehabilitation nurse must be a consistent, objective resource for the client and family as they adapt to an altered self-concept, changes in roles, and different means of fulfilling activities of daily living. In addition, the rehabilitation specialist must recognize that the ultimate outcomes of rehabilitation are dependent on interaction among the client, the rehabilitation team, and the environment (Van de Bittner, 1987).

For those whose impairment is discovered at birth or in childhood, the habilitative process begins with acknowledgement of the problem. Rehabilitation is the recovery of an ability that once existed, whereas *habilitation* is the development of abilities that never before existed in the child.

THE ENVIRONMENT AND THE REHABILITATION CLIENT

The environment has a critical impact on the rehabilitation client. Atmospheric conditions such as temperature, humidity, rain, wind, and snow can affect the signs and symptoms of many problems such as multiple sclerosis, arthritis, and chronic pain. Clients must learn to cope with such influences as they begin to reintegrate into the community. In addition physical characteristics such as steps, curbs, public transportation, and doorways can significantly hamper independent functioning.

The environment is also composed of psychosocial components. Attitudes of so-called able-bodied persons also have a profound effect on successful community reintegration. Incorrect beliefs that disabled individuals are not able to maintain jobs, attend school, or function as sexual human beings may severely inhibit or even halt the rehabilitation process. However, excessive sympathy, such as providing extra privileges, failing to hold the disabled person responsible for his or her own actions, or attributing "good" qualities to someone because he or she is disabled can be just as inhibiting. Both the physical and the psychosocial components of the environment must be structured so that individuals with disabilities have a fair chance to work, attend school, play, and live satisfying lives (see Ethics Box VII).

Myths About Disability

IMPACT ON EMPLOYMENT

Myths abound regarding the interest, motivation, and ability of individuals with disabilities to work. For example, some believe that individuals with disabilities need someone to take care of them because they do not "fit" into the workplace, and making the workplace fit them would be too costly. Others believe that disabled persons do not want to work because they receive enough income from the government. Still others believe that individuals with disabilities do not make good employees because they are unreliable, dependent, frequently absent from the job as a result of illness, and too costly to employ because of their health care costs. All of these myths and stereotypic notions are inaccurate and incorrect.

Nurses must remember that people with disabilities are people first. Abrasive personalities and behavioral characteristics may be found in any group of individuals. There are competent employees and those who demonstrate poor work habits and attitudes, regardless of the presence or absence of disability.

Studies conducted by disability organizations, the Rehabilitation Services Administration, the President's Committee on Employment of People with Disabilities, and others clearly indicate that the attendance rates of workers with disabilities are equal to or better than those of their nondisabled counterparts. Some of the barriers individuals with disabilities encounter when securing and maintaining employment include the following:

- *Lack of educational preparation.* Students with disabilities who do not plan to attend college may have little vocational preparation. These students will face unemployment, social isolation, and greater difficulties achieving integration into their communities. The U.S. Department of Education's National Institute of Disability and Rehabilitation Research declared effecting the transition of disabled students from high school to the work force to be a priority initiative (LaPlante et al., 1992).
- *Inadequate preparation in independent living skills.* Limited social, self-care, economic, or job skills may make it difficult for persons with disabilities to live independently in the community. Social and vocational supports and assistive technologies often significantly

Ethics Box VII

Gail A. DeLuca Havens, M.S., R.N., C.N.A.

Fear in the Community

Rose, a community health nurse, was delighted to learn that Mr. Wilfred had bequeathed his house to be used as a community-based mental health center. It is a lovely property but, more important, it is situated in an attractive residential neighborhood that more closely approximates the kind of environment in which the majority of clients of Waveview Village Community Mental Health Center are accustomed to living. The Waveview Village clients are currently receiving day treatment in a ramshackle house on the perimeter of the commercial district. It is a noisy and dirty area where the prevalence of drug and alcohol abusers makes it unsafe to walk the streets. Clients of Waveview Village have been teased, ridiculed, and spat on over the years by people living in the neighborhood who do not comprehend the implications of mental illness and consequently are fearful of those with mental illness.

Now, a week before the ownership of Mr. Wilfred's house is to pass to the Waveview Village Corporation, Rose is attending a special session of the zoning board called in response to a petition of people living in the neighborhood of Mr. Wilfred's house. The petition requests that the board modify the existing property use statutes to explicitly exclude community-based mental health centers from residential areas. Neighborhood residents are very agitated and fearful of having "unstable" people roaming their neighborhood. They voice concerns about personal safety, the security of personal property, and the introduction of an "undesirable element who often associate with the mentally ill," into the neighborhood.

Rose is a member of Waveview Village's board of directors. She has been asked to provide information to the zoning board about how "dangerous" clients of the Village are and whether the concerns expressed by neighborhood residents are justified. "The clients of Waveview Village are ill. As with all illnesses, whether physical or mental, a range of diagnoses will be present in the ill population. So, too, will illnesses exacerbate, or flare up. The clients who receive care at Waveview are no exception. They are well enough to stay at home at night and benefit from social connections. They come to day treatment for counseling and supervision of their medication administration.

Their care providers are committed to helping them remain in the community, provided they can clothe, feed, and shelter themselves and that there is no evident risk of harm to themselves or to others by doing so. It is the opportunity to avoid potential harm to our clients that makes Mr. Wilfred's house such an attractive setting for the Waveview Village Day Treatment Program. For those of you who are not familiar with it, the present site for the Day Treatment Program is located in an area that is not well maintained, and clients are harassed coming and going from Waveview. The opportunity to relocate the Day Treatment Program to Mr. Wilfred's house will eliminate this potential for harm to Waveview clients and will place them in an environment that is more comfortable and familiar to them. I hope that the board's decision is a favorable one for Waveview's clients."

Several days later, Rose receives a letter from the zoning board stating that they are postponing their decision to allow themselves time to become personally acquainted with some of the clients of Waveview Village. The letter asks her to arrange whatever kind of individual or group meetings she thinks would be most comfortable for the clients, while still affording the members of the zoning board the opportunity to get to know them. Usually this type of request would be rejected because it breaches client confidentiality and discriminates because of their medical diagnoses. However, a number of Waveview clients, knowing that Rose had been advocating for the Day Treatment Program to relocate to Mr. Wilfred's house, had approached her, volunteering to provide statements to the board in person. What should Rose do in this situation? Should she follow up on the clients' offers and ask them to meet with members of the zoning board, knowing that such a request will breach their confidentiality? Or should she refuse to comply with the board's request?

Community health nurses develop direct contacts with clients and their social networks, as well as relationships with mental health providers. These interfaces allow nurses to serve as natural intermediaries between the client and the larger systems of social and mental health services. Evidence of this intermediary relationship is observed in Waveview clients

(Continued)

approaching Rose to volunteer to talk with members of the zoning board, as well as in the zoning board asking Rose to arrange opportunities for them to come to know some of Waveview's clients. If Rose accepts the offers of the clients who have volunteered to meet with members of the zoning board, she will do so only after first ensuring that the clients understand that their actions will breach the confidentiality regarding their illness. She is also aware that she is contributing to that infringement. However, from a utilitarian perspective, she perceives her action to be doing the greatest possible good (Beauchamp and Childress, 1989). In that context, presuming that the zoning board decides in favor of the day treatment center, sacrificing the confidentiality of a few clients to gain access to a treatment environment that is safe and therapeutic for all may be justified.

The American Nurses' Association Code, however, clearly states that "the nurse safeguards the client's right to privacy by judiciously protecting information of a confidential nature" (American Nurses' Association, 1985, p. 1). The code recognizes that the uniqueness of individual cases can influence decisions but that all considerations are to be made "with full awareness of the need to preserve the rights and responsibilities of clients and the demands of justice. The suspension of individual rights must always be considered a deviation to be tolerated as briefly as possible" (p. 3).

On the other hand, if Rose refuses to arrange the meetings between the client–volunteers and the members of the zoning board, she will be doing so to protect the confidentiality of the client–volunteers. In this regard, Rose will be acting from a deontological perspective, the essence of which is that some actions are right (or wrong) for reasons other than their consequences (Beauchamp and Childress, 1989). However, Rose's refusal of the board's request does not actively encourage the Board to rule in favor of the day treatment program. In fact, it most likely compromises any opportunity to use Mr. Wilfred's house for the Waveview Village Day Treatment Program.

An alternative that Rose might consider is to suggest to Waveview's management staff that she work with them in arranging an open house event, inviting the residents of the neighborhood in which Mr. Wilfred's house is located to visit the present day treatment facility to see firsthand what it contains, how it is organized, and where it is located. Waveview staff, management personnel, and members of the Board of Directors would be available to discuss the philosophy, mission, and treatment goals of the Waveview Village Day Treatment Program with visitors and to answer their questions. As people become informed about a topic, they often change their opinions related to it. This strategy has the potential to diffuse the objections and resistance to relocating Waveview to Mr. Wilfred's house and to preserve the privacy of its clients.

Which course of action would you choose?

References

American Nurses' Association. (1985). *Code for nurses with interpretive statements.* Kansas City, MO: Author.

Beauchamp, T. L., & Childress, J. F. (1989). *Principles of biomedical ethics* (3rd ed.). New York: Oxford University Press.

reduce the dependence that persons with disabilities have on caregivers.

- *Feelings on the part of the individual with a disability and an employer that the individual does not "fit" into the work environment.* Discrimination in the workplace continues to exist. Individuals who sustain work-related injuries continue to quit and to be fired from their jobs because neither the employer nor the employee have information about job restructuring or worksite accommodations. The passage of the Americans with Disabilities Act in 1990 and other legislation has facilitated discussions of workers' and employers' fears and attitudes regarding individuals with disabilities in the workplace.

Potential employers have expressed concern over hiring an individual with a disability. Their fears have been based in part on the anticipation that providing worksite accommodations for this new employee may be costly. The President's Committee on Employment of People with Disabilities provides the following examples of job accommodations:

A mail carrier with a back injury could no longer carry his mailbag. A cart was purchased for $150, allowing him to keep his route.

A person who uses a wheelchair could not sit at her desk because her knees would not fit under it. The center desk drawer was removed, allowing the employee to sit and work comfortably at the desk. This simple modification cost the company and the worker nothing.

A medical technician who was deaf could not hear the buzz of a timer, which was necessary for specific laboratory tests. A $26.95 indicator light was attached.

- *A belief that supplemental incomes discourage securing employment.* When employers and others believe that individuals receiving welfare or Social Security Disability subsidies have sufficient income and are satisfied, they are not inclined to consider employment for those with disabilities. Although minimum-wage jobs still leave an individual in poverty, some individuals with disabilities may be reluctant to give up a government subsidy for a paycheck, particularly if health benefits are not included with the job.

- *People with disabilities are supposedly more unreliable in job attendance owing to frequent illness.* Some people with disabilities, as a result of their specific conditions, may be more susceptible to disability-related illnesses (e.g., urinary tract infections and skin breakdown in persons with paraplegia), but this possibility does not permit discrimination in hiring.

The number of older adults is growing, and society must include all interested individuals in the work force, even if this means changing some of the traditional rules. Perhaps older adults should not retire at 65 years of age but continue working on a reduced schedule as long as they are able. Cottage industries may serve individuals who wish to be at home with their children, as well as individuals with a disability who find commuting to and from work a hardship. Individuals with endurance problems may be encouraged to join the work force if job sharing is an option.

COMMUNITY LIVING ARRANGEMENTS

Society has fostered the myth that individuals with disabilities must be taken care of and cannot live independently. Much of the public perception has focused on individuals with developmental disabilities and those with mental illnesses living in group homes and older adults in nursing homes. Efforts are needed to assess the needs of individuals with disabilities and to project the future housing needs of all citizens.

The 1988 Fair Housing Amendments attempted to increase the access of individuals with disabilities to housing opportunities (U.S. Department of Education [USDE], 1988). Although these amendments do not cover all dwellings, multifamily housing units built after May 1991 are required to consider the needs of individuals with disabilities in accessing common building areas, kitchens, bathrooms, and environmental controls (e.g., light switches and thermostats).

A variety of living arrangements are available for individuals with disabilities, based on their income, functional status, and existing support systems. Some of these will be described later. Additional information about housing resources may be obtained by contacting an individual state's office on aging, department of housing and community development, health department, and developmental disability administration. Mental health associations, independent living centers, the federal Division of Vocational Rehabilitation (Rehabilitation Service Administration), and head injury foundations may also possess information regarding the location of specialized housing and community programs for individuals with specific disabilities.

Nursing Homes. Most nursing homes are privately run facilities for chronically ill individuals. Available services range from fully accredited rehabilitation programs to total nursing care. An individual's personal assets must be almost depleted before he or she can qualify for Medicaid, the primary payer for most nursing home residents. Older adults are typically the long-term residents in these facilities, although some younger individuals in their 20s or 30s who have spinal cord injuries, severe multiple sclerosis, or amyotrophic lateral sclerosis become residents of nursing homes because there are no other alternatives available to them in the community. The models of care that have evolved for persons with acquired immunodeficiency syndrome (AIDS) may apply here as well.

Group Homes. Group homes and supervised living quarters have been established in some communities to provide individuals with disabilities the structure and support to live outside of institutions. These living situations typically provide housing for two to four adults who may be developmentally disabled or have a head injury or a chronic mental illness.

Transitional Living. In transitional living, an individual recovering from a head injury or other condition may "try out" their independent living skills in a supportive environment. These are short-term posthospital facilities. Clients are generally expected to participate in a structured program (work, prevocational, or therapeutic activity) during the day and organize their meals and leisure activities in the evenings and on weekends. Staff are available to assist in problem solving, facilitating, socialization, and conflict negotiation.

Senior and Disabled Citizen Housing. Senior and disabled citizen housing offers individual living units designed to accommodate the needs of older adults and individuals with disabilities, regardless of age. These housing programs may offer security, social activities, and transportation to community activities and shopping.

Independent Living Apartments. Those with financial assets can purchase life-time residence and care in independent living apartments (available to single persons as well as couples). Medical, rehabilitation, and support services are offered to address specific needs. Those who ultimately require 24-hour nursing care will find it accessible in life care communities.

Support Services. Individuals with disabilities and their caregivers may take advantage of a variety of support services available within the community. The following programs are usually available for children and adults (however, eligibility requirements may vary): home health, in-home aid and personal care, respite care, Meals-on-Wheels, daycare, information and referral, and support groups (see Chapters 29 and 31).

Magnitude of Disability in the United States

TYPES OF DISABILITIES

Disability is a result of impairments that often occur because of injury or chronic disease. The National Health Interview Survey (NHIS) is a continuous, nation-wide household survey conducted by the U.S. Bureau of the Census that includes questions about disability and health. According to the 1986–1988 surveys, the five most prevalent chronic conditions causing disability are heart disease, orthopedic deformities and impairments, arthritis, asthma, and hypertension (Collins, 1993). However, greater numbers of people report having these chronic impairments and diseases than report being disabled by them (Table 25–2). Consequently, community health nursing efforts to prevent disability must address prevention and adequate treatment of these chronic conditions. Many of the Healthy People 2000 Objectives (USDHHS, 1990) specify targets for reducing the prevalence of chronic diseases and impairments (Table 25–3).

An estimated 1.5 million Americans suffer myocardial infarctions annually, and 500,000 have strokes each year (American Heart Association, 1989). According to the Task Force on Medical Rehabilitation Research (1990), one third of these individuals will be permanently disabled.

TABLE 25–2

Number of People Who Reported Impairments and Chronic Diseases, 1990

	Total No.	No. per 1000
Impairment		
Arthritis	30,833,000	125.3
Hearing impairments	23,296,000	94.7
Back injury	17,308,000	70.3
Visual impairments	7,525,000	30.6
Speech impairments	2,285,000	9.3
Paralysis (partial or complete)	1,445,000	5.9
Missing extremities (excluding toes and fingers)	1,232,000	5.0
Chronic disease		
Hypertension	7,129,000	110.2
Heart disease	9,307,000	78.5
Diabetes	6,232,000	25.3
Kidney trouble	3,061,000	12.4

Adapted from National Center for Health Statistics. (1990). *Current estimates from the National Health Interview Survey, United States, 1990.* Hyattsville, MD: U.S. Department of Health and Human Service.

About 23 million individuals have one or more chronic disorders of the musculoskeletal system (LaPlante, 1988). Included in this category are the top two leading causes of disabilities, orthopedic impairments and arthritis, which inhibit an individual's ability to work and function independently.

Some impairments and chronic diseases are associated with greater disability than others. Table 25–4 identifies chronic conditions that cause 30% or more limitation in a major activity. More than 80% of persons with mental retardation have a limitation of 30% or more. Seventy-five percent of persons with lung cancer, 70% of those with multiple sclerosis, and more than 60% of those who are blind in both eyes have a similar degree of disability.

Spinal cord and head injuries typically occur to young men between 17 and 34 years of age. Their lifelong disabilities have an impact on their own lives and on the lives of their family members. Each year in the United States about 8000 persons sustain a spinal cord injury (Carlson, 1987). A national study revealed that the majority of family members still experienced a sense of crisis 4 years after the injury (Killen, 1990). More than 2 million individuals experience traumatic head injuries each year. Approximately one in four of these individuals have residual deficits that affect their cognition and ability to live and function independently. In addition, such injuries require intensive health care resources.

The Task Force on Medical Rehabilitation Research (1990) also estimates that 5% (4 million) of those younger than 21 years of age have a developmental disability. *Developmental disabilities* are disabilities identified in individuals 21 years of age and under that are expected to continue indefinitely. Chapters 28 and 30 discuss programs that identify these children, prevent further disability, promote development and learning, and foster integration into the community.

DISABILITY BY AGE GROUP

LaPlante and Miller (1992) examined the impact of disability on basic life activities by age groups (Table 25–5). Disability rates increase with age. However, higher percentages of children, adolescents, and those over 85 receive assistance with limitations in basic life activities. Almost 25% of those with limitations in basic life activities such as dressing and food preparation do *not* receive help from others. The significance of these data substantiates the need for and importance of community health nurses as direct interventionists and case managers. Professionals who assist individuals with disabilities in community settings collaborate with the client to establish realistic goals that will foster the maintenance of independent functioning.

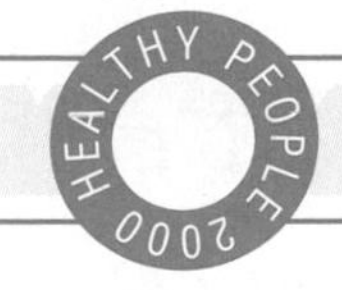

TABLE 25–3

Healthy People 2000: Objectives for the Disabled

1. Reduce to no more than 8% the proportion of people who experience a limitation in major activity owing to chronic conditions. (Baseline: 9.4% in 1988.)

Special Population Targets

Prevalence of Disability	1988 Baseline	2000 Target
Low-income people (annual family income <$10,000 in 1988)	18.9%	15%
American Indians/Alaska Natives	13.4%*	11%
Blacks	11.2%	9%

*1983–85 baseline

Note: Major activity refers to the usual activity for one's age-gender group whether it is working, keeping house, going to school, or living independently. Chronic conditions are defined as conditions that either (1) were first noticed 3 or more months previously or (2) belong to a group of conditions such as heart disease and diabetes, which are considered chronic regardless of when they begin.

2. Reduce to no more than 90 per 1000 people the proportion of all people age 65 and older who have difficulty in performing two or more personal care activities, thereby preserving independence. (Baseline: 111 per 1000 in 1984–85.)

Special Population Target

Difficulty Performing Self-Care Activities (per 1000)	1984–85 Baseline	2000 Target
People aged 85 and older	371	325

Note: Personal care activities are bathing, dressing, using the toilet, getting in and out of bed or chair, and eating.

3. Reduce to no more than 10% the proportion of people with asthma who experience activity limitation. (Baseline: Average of 19.4% during 1986–88.)
   Note: Activity limitation refers to any self-reported limitation in activity attributed to asthma.
4. Reduce activity limitation owing to chronic back conditions to a prevalence of no more than 19 per 1000 people. (Baseline: Average of 21.9 per 1000 during 1986–88.)
   Note: Chronic back conditions include intervertebral disk disorders, curvature of the back or spine, and other self-reported chronic back impairments such as permanent stiffness or deformity of the back or repeated trouble with the back. Activity limitation refers to any self-reported limitation in activity attributed to a chronic back condition.
5. Reduce significant hearing impairment to a prevalence of no more than 82 per 1000 people. (Baseline: Average of 88.9 per 1000 during 1986–88.)

Special Population Target

Hearing Impairment (per 1000)	1986–88 Baseline	2000 Target
People age 45 and older	202.5	180

Note: Hearing impairment covers the range of hearing deficits from mild loss in one ear to profound loss in both ears. Generally, an inability to hear sounds at levels softer (less intense) than 20 dB constitutes abnormal hearing. Significant hearing impairment is defined as having hearing thresholds for speech poorer than 25 dB. However, for this objective, self-reported hearing impairment (i.e., deafness in one or both ears or any trouble hearing in one or both ears) will be used as a proxy measure for significant hearing impairment.

6. Reduce significant visual impairment to a prevalence of no more than 30 per 1000 people. (Baseline: Average of 34.5 per 1000 during 1986–88.)

Special Population Target

Visual Impairment (per 1000)	1986–88 Baseline	2000 Target
People age 65 and older	87.7	70

Note: Significant visual impairment is generally defined as a permanent reduction in visual acuity and/or field of vision that is not correctable with eyeglasses or contact lenses. Severe visual impairment is defined as inability to read ordinary newsprint even with corrective lenses. For this objective, self-reported blindness in one or both eyes and other self-reported visual impairments (i.e., any trouble seeing with one or both eyes even when wearing glasses, or color blindness) will be used as a proxy measure for significant visual impairment.

Table continued on following page

TABLE 25–3

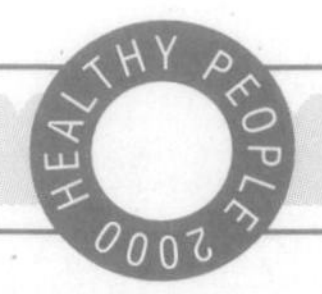

Healthy People 2000: Objectives for the Disabled Continued

7. Reduce the prevalence of serious mental retardation in school-age children to no more than 2 per 1000 children. (Baseline: 2.7 per 1000 children age 10 in 1985–88.)
   Note: Serious mental retardation is defined as an intelligence quotient (I.Q.) less than 50. This includes individuals defined by the American Association of Mental Retardation as profoundly retarded (I.Q. of 20 or less), severely retarded (I.Q. of 21–35), and moderately retarded (I.Q. of 36–50).
8. Reduce the most severe complications of diabetes as follows:

Complications Among People with Diabetes	1988 Baseline	2000 Target
End-stage renal disease (ESRD)	1.5/1000*	1.4/1000
Blindness	2.2/1000	1.4/1000
Lower extremity amputation	8.2/1000*	4.9/1000
Perinatal mortality†	5%	2%
Major congenital malformations†	8%	4%

*1987 baseline
†Among infants of women with established diabetes

Special Population Targets for ESRD

ESRD Owing to Diabetes (per 1000)	*1983–86 Baseline*	*2000 Target*
Blacks with diabetes	2.2	2
American Indians/Alaska Natives with diabetes	2.1	1.9

Special Population Target for Amputations

Lower Extremity Amputation Owing to Diabetes (per 1000)	*1984–87 Baseline*	*2000 Target*
Blacks with diabetes	10.2	6.1

Note: ESRD is defined as requiring maintenance dialysis or transplantation and is limited to ESRD owing to diabetes. Blindness refers to blindness owing to diabetic eye disease.

9. Reduce overweight to a prevalence of no more than 20% among people age 20 and older and no more than 15% among adolescents age 12 through 19. (Baseline: 26% for people age 20 through 74 in 1976–80, 24% for men and 27% for women; 15% for adolescents age 12 through 19 in 1976–80.)

Special Population Targets

Overweight Prevalence	*1976–80 Baseline*	*2000 Target*
People with disabilities	36%*	25%

*1985 baseline for people age 20–74 who report any limitation in activity owing to chronic conditions

Note: For people age 20 and older, overweight is defined as body mass index (BMI) equal to or greater than 27.8 for men and 27.3 for women. For adolescents, overweight is defined as BMI equal to or greater than 23.0 for males age 12 through 14, 24.3 for males age 15 through 17, 25.8 for males age 18 through 19, 23.4 for females age 12 through 14, 24.8 for females age 15 through 17, and 25.7 for females age 18 through 19. The values for adolescents are the age- and gender-specific 85th percentile values of the 1976–80 National Health and Nutrition Examination Survey (NHANES II), corrected for sample variation. BMI is calculated by dividing weight in kilograms by the square of height in meters. The cut points used to define overweight approximate the 120% of desirable body weight definition used in the 1990 objectives.

10. Increase to at least 40% the proportion of people with chronic and disabling conditions who receive formal patient education, including information about community and self-help resources as an integral part of the management of their condition.

Type-Specific Targets

Patient Education	*1983–84 Baseline*	*2000 Target*
People with diabetes	32% (classes) 68% (counseling)	75%
People with asthma	—	50%

TABLE 25 – 3

Healthy People 2000: Objectives for the Disabled Continued

11. Increase to at least 80% the proportion of providers of primary care for children who routinely refer or screen infants and children for impairments of vision, hearing, speech, and language and assess other developmental milestones as part of well-child care.
12. Reduce the average age at which children with significant hearing impairment are identified to no more than 12 months. (Baseline: Estimated as 24 to 30 months in 1988.)
13. Increase to at least 60% the proportion of providers of primary care for older adults who routinely evaluate people age 65 and older for urinary incontinence and impairments of vision, hearing, cognition, and functional status.
14. Increase to at least 90% the proportion of perimenopausal women who have been counseled about the benefits and risks of estrogen replacement therapy (combined with progestin, when appropriate) for prevention of osteoporosis.
15. Increase to at least 75% the proportion of worksites with 50 or more employees that have a voluntarily established policy or program for the hiring of people with disabilities. (Baseline: 37% of medium and large companies in 1986.)
    Note: Voluntarily established policies and programs for the hiring of people with disabilities are encouraged for worksites of all sizes. This objective is limited to worksites with 50 or more employees for tracking purposes.
16. Increase to 50 the number of states that have service systems for children with or at risk of chronic and disabling conditions, as required by Public Law 101-239.
    Note: Children with or at risk for chronic and disabling conditions, often referred to as children with special health care needs, include children with psychosocial as well as physical problems. This population encompasses children with a wide variety of actual or potential disabling conditions, including children with or at risk for cerebral palsy, mental retardation, sensory deprivation, developental disabilities, spinal bifida, hemophilia, other genetic disorders, and health-related educational and behavioral problems. Service systems for such children are organized networks of comprehensive, community-based, coordinated, and family-centered services.
17. Increase to at least 40 the number of states that have an effective system for recording and referring infants with cleft lips and/or palates to craniofacial anomaly teams. (Baseline: in 1988, approximately 25 states had a central recording mechanism for cleft lip and/or palate and approximately 25 states had an organized referral system to craniofacial anomaly teams.)
18. Increase to at least 95% the proportion of newborns screened by state-sponsored programs for genetic disorders and other disabling conditions and to 90% the proportion of newborns testing positive for disease who receive appropriate treatment. (Baseline: For sickle cell anemia, with 20 states reporting, approximately 33% of live births screened [57% of black infants]; for galactosemia, with 38 states reporting, approximately 70% of live births screened.)
    Note: As measured by the proportion of infants served by programs for sickle cell anemia and galactosemia. Screening programs should be appropriate for state demographic characteristics.
19. Achieve for all disadvantaged children and children with disabilities access to high-quality and developmentally appropriate preschool programs that help prepare children for school, thereby improving their prospects with regard to school performance, problem beaviors, and mental and physical health. (Baseline: 47% of eligible children age 4 were afforded the opportunity to enroll in Head Start in 1990.)
20. Increase to at least 30% the proportion of people age 18 and older with severe, persistent mental disorders who use community support programs. (Baseline: 15% in 1986.)
21. Increase to at least 45% the proportion of people with major depressive disorders who obtain treatment. (Baseline: 31% in 1982.)
22. Increase to at least 20% the proportion of people age 18 and older who seek help in coping with personal and emotional problems.

Special Population Target	1985 Baseline	2000 Target
People with disabilities	14.7%	30%

23. Establish and monitor in 50 states comprehensive plans to ensure access to alcohol and drug treatment programs for traditionally underserved people.
24. Reduce the incidence of secondary disabilities associated with injuries of the head and spinal cord to no more than 16 and 2.6 per 100,000 people, respectively. (Baseline: 20 per 100,000 for serious head injuries and 3.2 per 100,000 for spinal cord injuries in 1986.)
    Note: Secondary disabilities are defined as those medical conditions secondary to traumatic head or spinal cord injury that impair independent and productive lifestyles.

From the U.S. Department of Health and Human Services. (1990). *Healthy people 2000: National health promotion and disease prevention objectives. Summary report.* Washington, DC: U.S. Government Printing Office.

Note: Objectives addressing cardiac disease and cancer can be found in Chapters 16 and 17.

TABLE 25–4

Selected Chronic Conditions Causing 30% or More Limitations in Major or Outside Activity, by Percentage with Limitation, United States, 1986–88

Chronic Condition	Percentage of Persons with Limitation in Major or Outside Activity
Mental retardation	83.6
Malignant neoplasms of the lung, bronchus and other respiratory sites	75.0
Multiple sclerosis	70.2
Blindness—both eyes	61.2
Paralysis of extremities—complete or partial	57.4
Paralysis of extremities—complete	47.5
Paralysis of extremities—partial	62.8
Cerebral palsy	69.8
Other deformities or orthopedic impairments	50.0
Other selected diseases of the heart (excludes hypertension)	47.4
Emphysema	46.6
Intervertebral disk disorders	46.6
Paralysis of other sites—complete or partial	45.5
Disorders of bone or cartilage	41.1
Malignant neoplasms of stomach, intestines, colon, and rectum	39.5
Cerebrovascular disease	39.2
Malignant neoplasm of prostate	38.5
Epilepsy	35.8
Absence of lower extremities or parts of lower extremities	35.4
Orthopedic impairment of shoulder	34.7
Diabetes	33.3
Pneumoconiosis and asbestosis	32.5
Ischemic heart disease	32.2

From Collins, J. (1993). Prevalence of selected chronic conditions: United States, 1986–1988. *National Center for Health Statistics, Vital Health Statistics, 10*(182), 15.

TABLE 25–5

People with Limitations in Basic Life Activities and Those Who Get Help from Others

	Total Population (in thousands)	Percentage of Total Population Limited in Basic Life Activities	Percentage of Those With Limitations Who Get Help From Others
Total	237,890	4.0	76.7
Age			
0–17	63,900	0.3	91.3
18–44	101,609	1.5	78.5
45–54	22,427	3.8	73.1
55–64	22,046	6.0	69.9
65–74	16,886	11.8	73.4
75–84	8,750	26.5	76.8
85+	2,274	57.6	86.7

Data from LaPlante, M., & Miller, K. (1992). People with disabilities in basic life activities in the U.S. *Disability Statistics Abstract.* Washington, DC: U.S. Department of Education, National Institute on Disability and Rehabilitation Research (NIDRR); 1987 National Medical Expenditure Survey, Round 1.

TABLE 25–6

Percentage of Workers with Disability Employed Full Time

Type of Worker	1981	1986	1991
Women with a work disability	11.4	11.3	15.1
Women with no work disability	41.6	44.8	49.1
Men with a work disability	29.8	25.8	25.3
Men with no work disability	74.1	73.6	72.4

From National Center for Health Statistics. (1990). *Current estimates from the National Health Interview Survey, United States, 1990.* Hyattsville, MD: U.S. Department of Health and Human Services.

DISABILITY BY GENDER

There are gender differences related to disability and work. Among disabled adults with no work disability, almost 50% of women and 72% of men worked full time in 1991. However, only 15% of women and 25% of men with a work disability were employed full time in 1991 (Table 25–6). Although a higher percentage of disabled men work, men are more likely to be limited in the amount or kind of work they do and have a higher percentage of severe work limitations than women (LaPlante et al., 1992; National Center for Health Statistics [NCHS], 1990a).

Injury and chronic disease patterns also vary by gender. Among adolescents and young adults who sustain traumatic injuries, males are twice as likely to sustain severe injuries than their female counterparts. Such injuries most often result from vehicular accidents and assaults.

When examining the causes of disability among older adults, one must be cognizant of the fact that women continue to live longer than men. Therefore, it is no surprise that women experience more strokes than men. Men continue to have more heart attacks than women, but as more women join the work force, smoke, or encounter stresses equal to or greater than those encountered by their male counterparts, there may soon be little difference between incidence rates.

Legislation

Legislation to protect and promote the rights of individuals with disabilities is a critical component of rehabilitation. The following sections discuss major legislative initiatives that have helped to expand the employability and integration of individuals with disabilities in the community.

EMPLOYERS' LIABILITY LAWS

In 1911 the first Workmen's Compensation laws were enacted in this country to provide financial support for workers unemployed because of work-related injuries. In 1920 the first civilian rehabilitation program was established via the Smith-Fess Act (Civilian Rehabilitation Act). This program provided vocational rehabilitation services through state boards of vocational rehabilitation to people disabled in industry (Van de Bittner, 1987).

VOCATIONAL REHABILITATION ACTS

The Social Security Act of 1935 established permanent authorization for vocational rehabilitation. It also established old age insurance, aid to the blind, and services for crippled children. Amendments to the Vocational Rehabilitation Act have been enacted periodically. In 1943 the Vocational Rehabilitation Program was broadened to include emotionally disturbed and mentally retarded persons and to provide maintenance monies for living expenses and occupational tools. Training grants were authorized for the preparation of professional rehabilitation personnel in 1954. These amendments also authorized federal support for research.

During the 1960s the Council of State Governments published the Workmen's Compensation and Rehabilitation Law, which contained detailed provisions governing vocational rehabilitation services for injured employees. Other amendments passed during this decade provided federal assistance to plan, equip, and initially staff rehabilitation facilities and workshops; authorized funds to determine rehabilitation potential; and mandated follow-up services to clients and families.

In 1975 mandatory vocational rehabilitation laws began in California and followed in most states. Currently all states have Workers' Compensation laws that require employers to assume the cost of occupational disabilities without regard to any fault involved. Employers therefore are spared civil lawsuits involving negligence (Van de Bittner, 1987).

REHABILITATION ACT OF 1973

One of the most critical reforms affecting the rehabilitation movement was the Rehabilitation Act of 1973. This act required state rehabilitation agencies to develop an individualized, written care plan for each client. This plan is to be designed jointly by the rehabilitation team and the client; it states long- and short-term goals and spells out the terms under which services are offered. The Rehabilitation Service Administration was established within the U.S. Department of Health, Education, and Welfare to administer all aspects of the rehabilitation programs authorized by the act.

Section 501 required development of Affirmative Action programs for employment of disabled individuals in departments and agencies of the executive branch of the federal government. Section 502 established the Architectural and Transportation Barriers Compliance Board to develop standards for compliance with regulations to overcome architectural, transportation, and communication barriers in public facilities.

Other sections include the following key points:

- Discrimination against otherwise qualified disabled persons in any federally assisted program or activity is forbidden.
- Children with disabilities are entitled to a free, appropriate public education in the least restrictive setting.
- Qualified people with disabilities may not be denied, or discriminated against in, recruitment or admission to postsecondary educational and vocational programs.
- Employers may not refuse to hire individuals who are disabled when applying for positions if they meet the job requirements.
- Preemployment inquiries about disabilities may not be made.
- All federally assisted programs must provide facilities that are accessible and usable.
- All new facilities built with federal funds must be barrier free (Van de Bittner, 1987).

CATASTROPHIC CARE ACT

When it was enacted, the Medicare Catastrophic Coverage Act of 1988 was described as historic health care legislation that provided the largest expansions in the Medicare program since its inception in 1966. However, just 6 months later, Congress repealed the majority of the Act after senior citizens' groups waged vigorous protests against the income-based surtax imposed on middle- and upper-income retirees. In addition, the law failed to provide insurance for the cost of long-term nursing home care.

Several aspects of the Act were retained, however, including the mandate for states to expand Medicaid coverage to include not only low-income elderly, but also low-income pregnant women and children, and the requirement that states increase the amount of income and assets that may be kept by a person whose spouse's nursing home costs are being paid by Medicaid.

Some sections of the Act that were eliminated would have benefited elderly disabled individuals. Unlimited coverage of hospital and physician costs once out-of-pocket costs reached certain limits, outpatient prescription drug coverage, and extended nursing home coverage were not retained (Spears, 1990a).

The issue of catastrophic health care coverage continues to be addressed. Community health nurses are in unique positions to document the need for and to advocate for health care legislation for those with disabilities.

TECHNOLOGY-RELATED ASSISTANCE ACT

The Technology-Related Assistance for Individuals with Disabilities Act of 1988 (P.L. 100–407), known as the "Tech Act," offers grant monies to states interested in establishing programs for informing the public about the benefits of assistive technologies for individuals with disabilities. These programs are required to be statewide, and the activities initiated with the federal funding are to be eventually funded by state and local resources. The following six provisions are to be addressed in each program:

1. *Conduct a needs assessment.* Each state is required to survey the potential needs individuals with disabilities might have for assistive technologies.
2. *Identify resources.* The delivery of assistive technology services must be coordinated between public and private agencies.
3. *Provide assistive technology devices and services.* Each state must provide assistive devices and related services directly to consumers; provide funding to consumers, enabling them to purchase the product or service they desire; and establish facilities to loan equipment and/or provide funding to individuals who make assistive devices for individuals with disabilities. (Examples include wheelchairs, computers, and modified eating utensils.)
4. *Disseminate information.* Strategies are required to inform the public about the benefits and availability of assistive technologies. Computer databases and print and electronic media should be utilized.
5. *Provide training and technical assistance.* States must teach consumers and professionals how to use assistive technologies.
6. *Support public and private partnerships.* States must encourage the public and private sectors to work more closely together to meet the assistive technology needs of the community.

AMERICANS WITH DISABILITIES ACT

In 1990 the Americans with Disabilities Act (ADA) was enacted. It provides protection from discrimination to the 43 million Americans with disabilities. This Act extends the protection of civil rights to people with physical and mental handicaps and chronic illnesses (ADA Consultants, Inc., 1992; Spears, 1990b; Watson, 1990).

The Americans with Disabilities Act deals with access to employment, government services, public accommodations and transportation, and telecommunications. Five key provisions of the Americans with Disabilities Act are as follows:

1. All state and local governments and businesses open to the public must make their services available to people with disabilities unless the cost to do so is excessive. The reasonableness of the costs must be decided in each instance.
2. Interstate and commuter rail systems and local and intercity bus lines must accommodate passengers in wheelchairs.
3. All businesses with 15 employees or more are required to disregard handicaps in hiring decisions.
4. All telephone companies are required to provide special services for people with speech or hearing impairments.
5. Food industry employers can reassign workers with diseases that are transmitted through contact with food (e.g., salmonellosis).

FAMILY AND MEDICAL LEAVE ACT

The Family and Medical Leave Act of 1993 provides an employee with up to 12 weeks of unpaid leave per year to care for a newborn or recently adopted child; a foster child; or the employee's spouse, parent, or child with a serious health condition, or for the employee's own serious health condition. This law applies to all public and private employers with 50 or more employees and is enforced by the Department of Labor.

Although not everyone can afford unpaid leave, the Act allows family members to care for each other during times of serious health conditions, such as recuperation from surgery for correction of congenital defects or recovery from a spinal cord injury. Health care insurance continues during the worker's absence, and the worker is guaranteed his or her job or an equivalent job on return to work.

In summary, legislation affecting the civil rights of individuals with disabilities should be part of the knowledge base of all nurses. To truly advocate clients' rights, nurses should lobby actively for health care legislation that protects all health care consumers and advances the employability and accessibility of disabled persons in the community.

Conditions Necessitating Rehabilitation

IMPACT OF AN INCREASING LIFE SPAN

Approximately 31 million Americans, or 12.5% of the population, are 65 years of age or older (U.S. Bureau of the Census, 1992). By the year 2030, 55 million Americans, or nearly one person in five, will be over the age of 65 years. Thus, the elderly population is the fastest-growing age group in the country. It is also the age group in which chronic illness is most prevalent (Avillion and Mirgon, 1989).

Persons who are disabled as a result of a chronic illness comprise the majority of patients requiring rehabilitation services (Avillion and Mirgon, 1989). Arthritis, atherosclerosis, and osteoporosis are just a few of the conditions that influence an older person's ability to perform the activities of daily living.

The incidence of sudden, critical illnesses such as heart attacks and strokes also increases as an individual ages. In addition, the survivors of heart attacks and strokes are often left with residual effects. After a heart attack, diet and mobility may have to be altered. Fear of another heart attack may inhibit a person's ability to work, enjoy leisure activities, or have a satisfying sexual relationship. After a stroke, mobility, manipulation, speech, and elimination functions, and safety awareness may all be affected. After rehabilitation within a rehabilitation facility, additional community follow-up involving various therapies is often recommended. Home health care, clinic services or nursing homes may be needed. Respite care may be helpful for family members who are caregivers.

Both of these critical events influence nearly all aspects of clients' and their families' activities of daily living. Role changes, fear, anxiety, and the ability to provide adequate care must be assessed in the community environment. Safety issues such as the ability to summon help if left alone at home, crime prevention, and cognitive abilities (such as judging whether water is too hot in which to bathe, or remembering how to transfer from a wheelchair to a toilet without falling) are of critical importance. If there are steps in a home, is the cardiac client able to mount them without compromising respiratory status? Is there an adequate family or social support system for these clients? These questions indicate that the integration of these clients into the community environment is an ongoing process.

Following through with medical treatment regimens is of critical importance in those with chronic diseases. The community health nurse may be notified of problems only after complications develop from a chronic condition. These difficulties often result from a failure to understand the treatment regimen (e.g., medication administration or nutritional needs). Cost factors may also influence a person's ability to adhere to necessary health care practices.

Individuals who experience a sudden onset of a critical illness may have to learn a regular regimen of medications. Compliance with diets and medication schedules and the reestablishment of sexual and social relationships must be considered.

TRAUMATIC INJURIES

As a result of significant advances in health care technology and practice, more persons are surviving severe traumatic injuries. These individuals are usually young men (Avillion and Mirgon, 1989).

The residual effects of traumatic injuries often require many lifestyle adaptations. A polytrauma client—for example, one who has experienced multiple fractures, contusions, and lacerations—may have to deal with chronic pain for the rest of his or her life. Traumatic amputation, or amputation owing to an inability to maintain or restore adequate circulation, may result from these injuries. Mobility, ability to work, sexual identity, and self-concept are affected. Wound healing and the ever-present threat of infection may exist for an indefinite period of time depending on the complexity of the injuries. Financial hardship may result if the client is unable to work and/or health insurance coverage is inadequate.

According to the National Head Injury Foundation (1983), each year 50,000 people under the age of 30 years survive a head injury as a result of a motor vehicle or sports accident. The severity of the injury influences the degree of residual deficit and the person's subsequent need for medical and social support services in the community. Individuals who sustain head injuries may have permanent functional deficits in one or more of the following areas: cognition, activities of daily living, manipulation, mobility, speech, vision, and behavior.

Many areas must be assessed to facilitate community reintegration for persons who sustain catastrophic injuries. The extent of community services the individual requires must be determined. It is also important to determine the degree of supervision or care needed and who will provide the supervision. Family, friends, and paid caretakers must be considered. The rehabilitation nurse may be responsible for teaching the appropriate, safe physical care needed and referring the client for financial and other assistance.

Psychosocial issues also are critical. The client's educational and vocational interests must be explored. The individual with a head or spinal cord injury may be unable to return to a former occupation or academic course of study. Family roles may have to be altered to accommodate the person's disability. Spouses of those with spinal cord injury experience more role change than do parents of the injured; new ways to express sexuality may have to be learned (Killen, 1990). The issue of substance abuse should also be explored, as alcohol or other drug abuse is often a contributing factor in accidents resulting in traumatic injury.

Each year about 8000 persons in the United States sustain a spinal cord injury; client needs in this population are extensive and vary with the level and type of injury (i.e., complete or incomplete nerve damage). Does the client have use of his or her hands? How has fine motor control been affected? To what extent is he or she capable of performing activities of daily living, such as bathing, dressing, and toileting, and managing emergency situations?

Traumatic injuries influence all physical and psychosocial aspects of the lives of clients and their families and friends. The same may be said of persons and families affected by chronic illnesses. After returning to the community, rehabilitation clients may be in danger of being "lost" by the health care system. Follow-up health care appointments may be infrequent, and problems may develop between visits and worsen. Clients may choose not to seek or maintain health care contacts because of depression or anger, or they may fail to recognize (or refuse to acknowledge) a problem's existence. To be effective, the rehabilitation community health nurse must be available over a period of time to reassess the client's readiness to accept rehabilitative care. Instead of waiting for the client to seek care, care must be offered where the client lives, works, or plays.

Responsibilities of the Rehabilitation Nurse

The responsibilities of the community health nurse in rehabilitation are varied and challenging. As in any nursing specialty, the role of caregiver is important. However, when dealing with clients who must adapt the ways in which they carry out every aspect of their lives, the nurse must develop flexible and creative interventions and an acceptance of patients' rights to determine their care as never before.

TEAM MEMBER AND CASE MANAGER

The rehabilitation nurse is a member of a health care team of which the client is the "captain." A client may choose a treatment option of which the nurse disapproves. For instance, a client may elect to use a wheelchair for mobility rather than an artificial limb. The team must respect the client's wishes and assist him or her to an optimal state of wellness as defined by the client. The nurse must avoid imposing her or his own attitudes and cultural values on the client.

Another important aspect of this role is the ability to work collaboratively with other health care professionals. Occupational, physical, speech, and recreational therapists and vocational counselors are just a few of the specialists working to enhance the rehabilitation process. If a community health nurse is assessing a client's ability to self-administer medications in the home and notices that the client is not utilizing the dressing techniques as taught by the occupational therapist, the nurse should reinforce the proper method. The occupational therapist may have to be notified, and additional home visits may be necessary. Thus, the nurse must be aware of all treatment interventions advocated by the team and support continuity of interdisciplinary care.

It is a fairly simple matter to be a team player when problems are recognized and clients and their families have access to and make use of needed health care services. But what about the rehabilitation client who is unable or unwilling to seek health care? How does the rehabilitation nurse find those persons who are "lost" by the health care industry?

There is no easy answer to this question. Referrals by family or friends are often excellent ways for the client to enter the health care system. However, client reluctance may be a problem. A client cannot be forced to accept health care. Community health nurses must constantly be alert to information about clients who have no family or friends to serve as advocates. Perhaps the family or friends do not know how to gain entry into the health care system. There are many stumbling blocks to successful community interventions. As the number of persons who survive traumatic illnesses and injuries grows, community health practitioners will become more and more critical to successful community reintegration. The rehabilitation nurse must fulfill responsibilities other than those of caregiver and team member if rehabilitation clients are to achieve optimal wellness.

EDUCATOR AND CASE-FINDER

The rehabilitation nurse assists the client and family to learn new skills that must be used continuously in all components of daily living. Common nursing diagnoses used by rehabilitation nurses for care with individuals appear in Table 25–7. Functions such as walking or speaking may be taken for granted, but when an illness or injury forces a person to relearn these skills, the emotional stress is great. The client who has access to a rehabilitation team also has access to necessary support for community reintegration.

Rehabilitation nurses employed by insurance companies and home health care agencies use additional nursing diagnoses that focus more on issues of community reintegration (Table 25–8) (Sawin and Heard, 1992).

The role of case-finder is useful in locating clients who need help and are "outside" the health care system. Financial concerns may keep clients from receiving health care services and adhering to good health practices. The promotion of free health screening clinics is often helpful

TABLE 25–7

Frequent Nursing Diagnoses for Rehabilitation
Impaired physical mobility
Self-care deficit
Alteration in urinary elimination pattern
Impaired skin integrity
Alteration in bowel elimination pattern
Potential for physical injury
Knowledge deficit
Impaired verbal communication
Decreased activity tolerance

Adapted from Sawin, K., & Heard, L. (1992). Nursing diagnoses used most frequently in rehabilitation nursing. *Rehabilitation Nursing, 17*(5), 256–259.

TABLE 25–8

Rehabilitation Diagnoses Focusing on Community Reintegration

Ineffective individual coping
Noncompliance
Ineffective family coping
Health management deficit
Impaired thought processes

Adapted from Sawin, K., & Heard, L. (1992). Nursing diagnoses used most frequently in rehabilitation nursing. *Rehabilitation Nursing, 17*(5), 256–259.

in locating persons with disabilities who are not receiving health care services. A blood pressure screening clinic not only gives the nurse a chance to assess the actual blood pressure, but also provides opportunities for education regarding medication compliance, proper nutrition practices, and psychosocial support. Such clinics should be offered as frequently as possible and in a variety of easily accessible locations.

Screening clinics are not the only means of fulfilling the casefinding and educator roles. Senior citizens centers, parent–teacher organizations, and support groups for survivors of devastating illnesses and injuries are other places where an active community health nurse could offer to speak on health care topics such as rehabilitation and community reintegration. In this way vital information is brought to the community. By being easily accessible, the nurse may learn of persons needing help who are unable or unwilling to attend such activities. The nurse should make a point of asking those present if they know of potential clients or families who are in need of rehabilitation services. The role of educator is effective only if the information is presented to those in need.

CLIENT ADVOCATE

Many of the diagnoses used by rehabilitation nurses in individual care plans focus on the limitations and difficulties of the person with the disability. However, often his or her frustration and difficulties stem from inadequate community resources, such as financially inaccessible health care or a lack of public transportation, or from discriminatory attitudes. The nurse has an obligation to advocate for the promotion of accessible health care for all citizens.

The nurse as advocate initiates and supports community and legislative activities that promote the civil rights and community reintegration of individuals with disabilities (Hanlon and Sharkey, 1989). There are no common denominators for the disabled population as a whole. Problems range from obvious physical limitations (loss of a limb or use of a wheelchair for mobility) to no visible sign of disability (such as cognitive deficits following a head injury). The nurse as advocate must have knowledge of current laws, especially regarding financial entitlement and existing support services. She or he must also know what services are needed but unavailable. For example, a community health nurse may assist several persons with disabilities to form their own support group.

Formal mechanisms for advocacy, such as legislative lobbying and working through professional health care organizations, are excellent means of promoting the rights of individuals with disabilities. However, day-to-day experiences also have the potential to influence civil rights issues. For example, during a routine shopping trip a nurse may notice many instances of barriers to the activities of daily living.

Are there adequate parking facilities for the disabled at local shopping malls, grocery stores, churches, and schools? If so, are these parking spaces occupied by cars that do not have "handicapped" license tags? Such vehicles should be reported to the facility's management immediately. Do public buildings advertise themselves as being accessible to individuals with disabilities but have heavy doors that are difficult to open even by able-bodied persons? A wheelchair ramp to a doorway is useless if the doors cannot be opened by an individual with limited upper body strength or coordination.

As health care professionals go about their daily lives, they should review the environment for barriers to persons with disabilities. A letter to management identifying such barriers will carry more clout if it contains not only a complaint but a statement that the writer will no longer do business at the offending establishment until barriers are removed. (Of course, this may not be realistic in small communities.)

Other sources of help for advocacy activities are government, voluntary, and professional organizations such as the Association of Rehabilitation Nurses (Table 25–9). Such organizations have the potential to be sources of strength in the community.

PROFESSIONAL DEVELOPMENT

The Association of Rehabilitation Nurses (ARN) was founded in 1974 and recognized as a specialty nursing organization by the American Nurses' Association in 1976. Its major purposes include advancing the quality of rehabilitation nursing services, offering educational opportunities to promote interest and awareness in rehabilitation, and to facilitate the exchange of ideas in rehabilitation programs.

In 1975 ARN developed a journal, *Rehabilitation Nursing,* as a vehicle for sharing information and rehabilitation nursing research. The organization initiated certification for specialty practice as a means of recognizing a level of rehabilitation nursing expertise. Certified nurses use the title certified rehabilitation registered nurse (CRRN).

In 1994, there were 9000 ARN members and over 9900 certified rehabilitation registered nurses. The organization

TABLE 25–9

Resources for Rehabilitation Clients

Administration on Developmental Disabilities
U.S. Department of Health and Human Services
200 Independence Ave. SW
Washington, DC 20201–0001
(202) 245–2980

American Association of Retired Persons
601 E St. NW
Washington, DC 20049
(202) 434–2277

American Cancer Society
90 Park Ave.
New York, NY 10016
(212) 599–3600

American Civil Liberties Union
132 W. 43rd St.
New York, NY 10036–6599
(212) 944–9800

American Diabetes Association
1600 Duke St.
Alexandria, VA 22314–3447
(800) ADA–DISC
(703) 549–1500

Association of Rehabilitation Nurses
5700 Old Orchard Rd., 1st Floor
Skokie, IL 60077–1057
(708) 966–3433

Clearinghouse on Disability Information
Office of Special Education and Rehabilitation Services
Room 3132, Switzer Bldg.
330 C St. SE
Washington, DC 20202
(202) 732–1723
(800) 346–2742

Federation for Children with Special Needs
95 Berkeley St., Suite 104
Boston, MA 02116
(617) 482–2915

Information for Individuals with Disabilities
Fort Point Place
27–43 Wormwood St.
Boston, MA 02210
(617) 727–5540

Mainstream, Inc.
1030 15th St. NW, Suite 1010
Washington, DC 10005
(202) 898–1400

National Amputation Foundation
12–45 150th St.
Whitestone, NY 11357
(718) 767–0596

National Center for Youth with Disabilities
University of Minnesota
Box 721
420 Delaware St. SE
Minneapolis, MN 55455
(800) 333–6293

National Clearinghouse on Postsecondary Education for Individuals with Disabilities
HEATH Resource Center
One Dupont Circle NW
Washington, DC 20036
(800) 544–3284

National Council on Disability
800 Independence Ave. SW
Washington, DC 20591
(202) 267–3846

National Rehabilitation Information Center (NARIC)
8455 Colesville Rd., Suite 935
Silver Spring, MD 20910
(800) 34–NARIC
Publishes the *Directory of National Information Sources;* houses the organization and computer data base called ABLEDATA that provide information about commercial rehabilitation products; is a clearing-house on disability information)

Office of Vocational and Adult Education
U.S. Department of Education
Policy Analysis Staff
Room 4525, Switzer Building
330 C St. SE
Washington, DC 20202–0001
(202) 732–2251

continues to grow, facilitating educational, research, and professional advancement opportunities for rehabilitation nurses. Members are active in promoting the civil rights of individuals with disabilities and their families and in lobbying for legislation that provides an accessible environment for all its citizens (Van de Bittner, 1987).

Community Reintegration Issues

Wellness may be defined as being sound in body, mind, and spirit. It is an ongoing, dynamic process, and the ultimate responsibility for wellness rests with the client. As the rehabilitation client adapts within and modifies the environment, the nurse must be aware of factors in the community that facilitate or inhibit successful community reintegration. Table 25–10 presents a guide for assessing health problems and barriers for persons with disability in the community. Access to health care, availability of physical and interpersonal resources, safety, psychosocial concerns, and promotion of a barrier-free environment are essential for well-being.

Promotion of health among those with disabilities fosters optimal use of personal strengths and resources and prevents further disability. New or existing resources must be evaluated for availability, accessibility, and acceptability. Community health nurses in rehabilitation can propose new services and modifications to existing ones.

TABLE 25–10

Guidelines for Assessing Community Reintegration Needs of Persons with Disabilities

Access to Health Care

- Are health care facilities architecturally accessible?
- Does the client have access to either private or public transportation that may be used by a person with his or her specific disability?
- Are needed health care programs available? (Substance abuse treatment programs may not be accessible or available.)
- Are needed health care programs financially accessible?
- Are negative attitudes on the part of the client, family, or health care professionals prohibiting adequate health care? (Feelings regarding sexuality counseling or employment capability may have a major impact on community reintegration.)
- Does the client want to promote his or her own wellness?

Community Resources

- Are community resources financially, attitudinally, and architecturally accessible?
- Are the sources used credible?
- Does the client/family know how to locate resources? This may be a particular problem in a rural area where resources and transportation may be limited.
- The telephone book may be a valuable resource for locating community resources. Does the client/family have the necessary reading and verbal skills to utilize this method?
- Has the rehabilitation team investigated community resources available in the client's environment, and have they notified both the client and the resources?
- Does the health care professional make it a point to network with key community resource personnel?

Safety

- Has the home been assessed for potential safety problems?
- Does the client and family know how to assess workplaces, schools, and recreational areas for potential problems?
- Does the client have a plan in the event he or she must summon help? (For example, how will a person with a communication disorder report an emergency situation over the telephone?)
- Has crime prevention been addressed? An individual using a wheelchair may be especially vulnerable to street crime.

Psychosocial Issues

- What role changes have taken place as a result of the client's disability?
- What are the financial resources and what effects do they have on wellness?
- If the person with a disability requires assistance with activities in daily living, are other members of the family unit feeling neglected by the caregiver?
- Is the caregiver given a chance to grieve? Is he or she devoting all energy to the person with the disability and in danger of compromising his or her own wellness?
- Has the family been assessed for adequate coping skills?
- Does the client have emotional as well as physical support systems?
- Are the developmental tasks of the client and family being addressed?

Promotion of a Barrier-Free Environment

- What attitudinal barriers exist in the client's environment? Are there feelings that individuals with disabilities cannot adequately work, attend school, or enjoy leisure activities?
- How is the client's sexuality viewed by him- or herself and others?
- Does the client have a negative outlook? Does he or she avoid interpersonal relationships or refuse to maintain wellness, look for a job, attend school, or interact with the health care system?
- Is there adequate housing for individuals with disabilities?
- Is there barrier-free public and/or private transportation?
- If the client requires 24-hour caregivers, how are these persons located, evaluated, and trained?
- Is the client's place of worship, school, work setting, and shopping facilities accessible?
- What advocacy groups exist in the community? What barriers exist to these groups?
- Do health care providers have feelings that negatively influence their ability to provide adequate care for the disabled?
- Has the client/family been taught to plan ahead when going to a new setting for the first time? Are schools, restaurants, and stores assessed before attending?
- What provisions are available for travel and vacations?

Safety is a concern not only in the home, but also in the workplace, academic setting, and leisure setting. Some communities offer self-defense classes especially for those with disabilities.

The rehabilitation client has experienced loss of a variety of skills. The parents of an infant or child recently diagnosed with an impairment or disability mourn the loss of a child with full functioning. It is important that both the client and the family be given the opportunity to grieve. The nurse helps them acknowledge their losses, allows expression of grief, provides information about the disabling condition, and fosters realistic expectations and hope for the future.

Throughout this chapter barriers to the successful community reintegration of the rehabilitation client have been discussed. The community health nurse in rehabilitation, indeed the entire rehabilitation team, must accurately assess and diminish barriers to the community.

KEY IDEAS

1. Rehabilitation is a dynamic process that aids a person with disabilities to successfully achieve well-being. This process must also involve successful community integration.
2. Society in general and health care professionals in particular have a long history of treating citizens with disabilities as second-class people. A key component of any rehabilitation specialist is the belief in quality of life and the right of all persons to live satisfying, productive lives.
3. As a member of an interdisciplinary team, the rehabilitation nurse must have the ability to collaborate with a variety of health care professionals.
4. The nurse must be a client advocate, aware of legislation and community factors that affect the disabled person's ability to integrate successfully into the community.
5. Part of this advocacy role includes being able to assess barriers to wellness that affect both the client and his or her family.
6. One of the biggest barriers to successful rehabilitation is the possibility of a client getting "lost" in the health care system. The rehabilitation client must be able to access the health care system, especially after returning home from an inpatient setting. The rehabilitation community health nurse must be aware of ways to keep the door to wellness open.

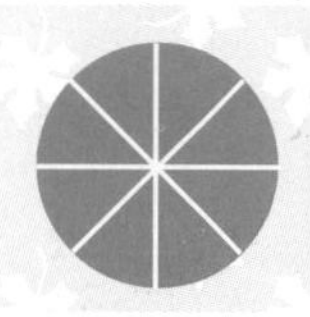

CASE STUDY: *Advocating for Rehabilitation Clients*

A community health nurse is attending a small state university part time. She is working on a master's degree and has a particular interest in individuals with disabilities. On the first evening of class she is surprised to find that the class location has been moved from one building to another. The first location was close to the parking lot, next to the library, and a popular classroom setting for students and professors. The new location is a considerable distance from the parking lot and is referred to in a negative manner by the majority of students and faculty. It is "too far from everything," parts of it are still under construction, and the heating system isn't working properly.

The nurse listens to her classmates grumble as they walk to the new building. It seems that there is a student who uses a wheelchair for mobility, and the class had to be relocated to the newer, wheelchair-accessible building. She tries to point out that communities have an obligation to provide barrier-free academic settings, but no one really wants to listen. The majority of the students in this business class are not health care professionals and are not happy about being inconvenienced. This class is an elective for the nurse, who hopes to enhance her budgetary skills. The nurse believes she will also have an opportunity to be a client advocate.

The disabled student is about one-half hour late for class. She seems nervous and uncomfortable when she arrives. The professor comments that the class has undergone considerable inconvenience on her behalf, and she should plan to arrive on time in the future. The student is a paraplegic who must do wheelchair pushups several times an hour to relieve pressure on her sacrum. This causes several giggles from watching classmates and another comment from the professor about distracting the class. At break time the disabled student's leg bag bursts, and she wheels herself from the room in tears.

The nurse attempts to follow the student but finds that there is no wheelchair-accessible bathroom on this floor. It is still being constructed. The only accessible bathroom is two floors down. The nurse finds the student, introduces herself as a nurse, and offers to assist her. She is surprised when the student angrily refuses her help with the comment, "You nurses don't understand what it's like to be this way!" The student does not return to class after break.

As a community health nurse and client advocate, what actions would be appropriate to take?

The nurse may approach the professor privately and discuss the need for successful community reintegration. She may also point out the need for the wheelchair pushups and the importance of wheelchair-accessible bathrooms. The nurse may also share this information with her classmates. She should probably examine her own feelings in this situation, as she did not intervene until after the disabled student left the class in tears. For example, the nurse may also be feeling resentful at being inconvenienced.

The nurse also could contact the campus office responsible for implementing the Americans with Disabilities Act to report her observations and make suggestions. She might also involve some of her classmates in touring the campus and classroom building to identify barriers to wheelchair mobility. It is likely that some of them will continue to hold negative attitudes, but a practice- oriented illustration of barriers may be more effective than verbal arguments. She should also find out about the existence of advocacy groups for disabled persons on campus.

Finally, the nurse may help the disabled student gain access to appropriate assistance for community reintegration. This is a particularly difficult issue. The student has already refused assistance. If she does not return to class the nurse may attempt to find her via friends or student health services. The student with the disability may benefit from help in planning her activities of daily living. She may need help in assessing new situations for potential barriers. If the student with the disability is not found or if she continues to refuse assistance, the nurse cannot ethically pursue the matter. However, she can continue to work to promote a barrier-free environment in her academic setting.

The success of the plan does not depend totally on the ability of students and professors to acknowledge the barriers present and eliminate them. Realistically, the nurse must evaluate her impact on the academic setting by both long-term and short-term changes. If, as a result of this nurse's efforts on campus, awareness of the rights of persons with disabilities has been increased and acknowledged, then the nurse has been an effective client advocate. An important factor is the realization that nursing takes place in all settings and at all times, not merely within the professional work setting.

GUIDELINES FOR LEARNING

1. As you go about your day, take time to imagine what life would be like if you used a wheelchair for mobility. Attend class, go shopping, and attend a movie, all from the viewpoint of a person with a disability. What barriers did you encounter? How would you attempt to eliminate these barriers? How do you feel about living with a disability?
2. Visit a supervised living arrangement such as senior housing or a group home. Identify the criteria for residency, the services available, and the home's ambiance. What nursing care is available and from whom?
3. Explore a supply store or catalog that sells equipment for environmental adaptation and assistive devices for the disabled. Notice what equipment and devices are available and their prices.
4. Participate with a rehabilitation nurse, physical therapist, occupational therapist, or vocational rehabilitation counselor as they make their assessment and plan care.
5. Recall a time you felt uncomfortable in the presence of someone with a disability. Role play alternative ways of relating to the person that emerge from different attitudes.

REFERENCES

ADA Consultants. (1992). *What every rehab professional in the USA should know about the ADA.* South Miami, FL: Author.

American Heart Association (1989). *Fact sheet on heart attack, stroke, and risk factors.* Dallas: Author.

American National Standards Institute. (1983). *Specifications for making buildings and facilities accessible to and usable by physically handicapped people.* New York: Author.

American Nurses' Association and Association of Rehabilitation Nurses. (1988). *Rehabilitation nursing: Scope of practice, process and outcome criteria for selected diagnoses.* Washington, DC: American Nurses' Association.

Avillion, A. E., & Mirgon, B. B. (1989). *Quality assurance in rehabilitation nursing: A practical guide.* Rockville, MD: Aspen.

Carlson, C. E. (Ed.). (1987). *Spinal cord injury: A guide to rehabilitation nursing.* Rockville, MD: Aspen.

Collins, J. (1993). Prevalence of selected chronic conditions: United States, 1986–1988. *National Center for Health Statistics, Vital and Health Statistics, 10*(182), 1–87.

Dittmar, S. (1989). Scope of rehabilitation. In S. Dittmar (Ed.), *Rehabilitation nursing process and application* (pp. 2–15). St. Louis: C.V. Mosby.

Fidler, G. S., & Fidler, J. W. (1979). Doing and becoming: Purposeful action and self-actualization. *American Journal of Occupational Therapy, 32,* 305–310.

Hanlon, D., & Sharkey, E. L. (1989). Professional practice of rehabilitation nursing. In S. Dittmar (Ed.). *Rehabilitation nursing process and application* (pp. 73–82). St. Louis: Mosby–Year Book.

Hickey, J. (1992). *The clinical practice of neurosurgical nursing.* Philadelphia: J.B. Lippincott.

Killen, J. (1990). Role stabilization in families after spinal cord injury. *Rehabilitation Nursing, 15*(1), 19–21.

LaPlante, M. (1988). *Data on disability from the National Health Interview Survey, 1983–1985.* Washington, DC: National Institute on Disability and Rehabilitation Research.

LaPlante, M. P., & Miller, K. S. (1992). People with disabilities in basic life activities in the U.S. *Disability Statistics Abstract.* Washington, DC: U.S. Department of Education, National Institute on Disability and Rehabilitation Research (NIDRR).

LaPlante, M. P., Miller, S., & Miller, K. (1992). People with work disability in the U.S. *Disability Statistics Abstract.* Washington, DC: U.S. Department of Education, National Institute on Disability and Rehabilitation Research (NIDRR).

Mumma, C. (Ed.). (1987). *Rehabilitation nursing: Concepts and practice, a core curriculum* (2nd ed). Evanston, IL: Rehabilitation Nursing Foundation.

National Center for Health Statistics (NCHS). (1990a). *Current Estimates from the National Health Interview Survey, United States, 1990.* Hyattsville, MD: U.S. Department of Health and Human Services.

NCHS. (1990b). *Health, United States, 1989 and prevention profile.* Hyattsville, MD: U.S. Department of Health and Human Services.

National Committee for Injury Prevention and Control. (1989). Injury prevention: Meeting the challenge. *American Journal of Preventive Medicine, 5*(3 suppl), 1–303.

National Head Injury Foundation (1983). *The silent epidemic.* Framingham, MA: National Head Injury Foundation.

National Institute on Disability and Rehabilitation Research. (1989). *Chart book on disability in the United States.* Washington, DC: Author.

Rice, D. P., Mackenzie, E. J., & Associates. (1989). *Cost of injury in the United States: A report to Congress.* San Francisco, CA: Institute for Health & Aging, University of California, and Injury Prevention Center, The Johns Hopkins University.

Rosen, E., & Fox, I. G. (1972). *Abnormal psychology.* Philadelphia: W.B. Saunders.

Ross, B. (1992). The impact of reimbursement issues on rehabilitation nursing practice and patient care. *Rehabilitation Nursing, 17*(5), 236–238.

Rusk, H. (1972). *A world to care for.* New York: Random House.

Russel, H. (1973). *Affirmative action for disabled people.* Washington, DC: Government Printing Office.

Sawin, K., & Heard, L. (1992). Nursing diagnosis used most frequently in rehabilitation nursing practice. *Rehabilitation Nursing, 17*(5), 256–260.

Spears, J. (1990a). Legislative department. *Rehabilitation Nursing, 15*(2), 98.

Spears, J. (1990b). Legislative department. *Rehabilitation Nursing, 15*(4), 220.

Task Force on Medical Rehabilitation Research. (1990). *Report of the Task Force on Medical Rehabilitation Research.* Bethesda, MD: National Institutes of Health.

U.S. Bureau of the Census. (1992). *Statistical abstracts of the United States.* Washington, DC: Author.

U.S. Department of Education. (1988). *Summary of existing legislation affecting persons with disabilities.* Washington, DC: Government Printing Office.

U.S. Department of Health and Human Services. (1990). *Healthy people 2000: National health promotion and disease prevention objectives. Summary report.* Washington, DC: Government Printing Office.

Van de Bittner, S. (Ed.). (1987). Reintegration of client into the community. In C. Mumma (Ed.). *Rehabilitation nursing: Concepts and practice, a core curriculum* (2nd ed.) (pp. 1–25). Evanston, IL: Rehabilitation Nursing Foundation.

Watson, P. (1990). The Americans with Disabilities Act: More rights for people with disabilities. *Rehabilitation Nursing, 15*(6), 325–328.

World Health Organization, Expert Committee on Disability Prevention and Rehabilitation. (1981). Disability prevention and rehabilitation, Technical report series 668. Geneva: World Health Organization.

SUGGESTED READINGS

Atkinson, I. (1992). Experiences of informal carers providing nursing support for disabled dependents. *Journal of Advanced Nursing, 17*(7), 835–840.

Center for Functional Assessment Research, Department of Rehabilitation Medicine. (1990). *Guide for use of the uniform data set for medical rehabilitation including the Functional Independence Measure (FIM).* Buffalo: State University of New York.

Des Rosier, M., Catanzaro, M., & Piller, J. (1992). Living with chronic illness: Social support and the well spouse perspective. *Rehabilitation Nursing, 17*(2), 87–91.

Graham, P., Weingarden, S., & Murphy, P. (1991). School reintegration: A rehabilitation goal for spinal cord injured adolescents. *Rehabilitation Nursing, 16*(3), 122–127.

Kaatz, J. (1992). Enhancing the parenting skills of developmentally disabled parents: A nursing perspective. *Journal of Community Health Nursing, 9*(4), 209–219.

Talley, B., & Coleman, M. (1992). The chronically mentally ill: Issues of individual freedom versus societal neglect. *Journal of Community Health Nursing, 9*(1), 33–41.

Watson, P. (1990). The Americans with Disabilities Act: More rights for people with disabilities. *Rehabilitation Nursing, 15*(6), 325–328.

Chapter 26

Children in the Community

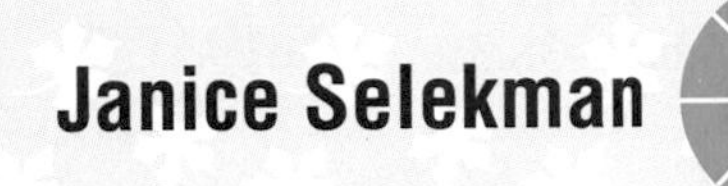

Janice Selekman

Focus Questions

What are common health care needs of children from birth through adolescence?

Who are the children "at risk" who require community health nursing interventions?

What is the impact of poverty on child health?

What is the role of the community health nurse in meeting the needs of a child with a chronic condition?

What community resources are available to promote the health of children?

How do the various health care funding programs affect the community health nurse's role with children?

Children in the United States

DEMOGRAPHICS

The population of children younger than 19 years in the United States is approximately 72 million. This constitutes 27.4% of the population in the United States (*Statistical Abstracts,* 1992). In 1990, approximately 4,179,000 children were born, which is a 4% increase from 1989 (Wegman, 1991). The percentages of children in each age group are identified in Table 26–1. Approximately 74% of American children are white; 15% are black; and 12% are Hispanic. The Hispanic population is very young—38.3% are younger than 19 years of age (*Statistical Abstracts,* 1992).

In the 1980s, the number of children living in poverty increased by 21% (National Center for Health Statistics, 1991). In 1970, 14.9% of all children lived in poverty. Currently 20% of children live in poverty, and by the year 2000, 25% of all children are expected to be poor (*Statistical Abstracts,* 1991). Minority children are at special risk. According to the Children's Defense Fund (1989), 45.8% of black children and 39.8% of Hispanic children are poor. Children living in female-headed households are especially vulnerable to poverty. In 1988, 56% of black families and 38% of white families with children younger than 18 years of age in female-headed households were classified as living below the poverty level (*Infant Mortality,* 1990).

Viewed in perspective, the Children's Defense Fund provides some startling and disturbing news about the status of children who are expected to be the first high school graduation class of the 21st century (Table 26–2). These children are currently at significant risk of poverty and related outcomes (e.g., inadequate child care and health insurance) and are at greater risk of dropping out of school and of becoming teenage parents (see Chapter 22). Community health nurses devote considerable time and energy to addressing these concerns in an effort to have an impact on the health care and health status of children.

TABLE 26–1

Percentage of the U.S. Population in 1991 for Pediatric Age Groups

Age (Years)	Percent of Total Population	Number in Thousands
< 5	7.3	19,222
5–9	6.9	18,237
10–14	6.7	17,671
15–19	6.5	17,242
Total	27.4	72,372

From: *Statistical Abstracts of the United States, 1992.* U.S. Department of Commerce, Bureau of the Census. Washington, DC: US Government Printing Office.

TABLE 26–2

Risks for Children Projected to Graduate in the Year 2000

1 in 5 is living in poverty
1 in 5 is at risk of teen parenthood
1 in 5 has no health insurance
1 in 7 risks dropping out of school
1 in 2 has working mother, but many lack affordable daycare

Data from Children's Defense Fund. (1989). *The Children's Defense Fund looks at America from a special point of view.* Washington, DC: Author.

IMPACT OF POVERTY ON CHILD HEALTH

Poverty results in decreased nutritional intake, which contributes to a variety of health problems and increased risk of infant mortality. There is an increased incidence of anemia and other nutrition-related diseases and a possible decrease in cognitive or physical growth. Poverty also results in increased delinquency and dropping out of school. A hungry person primarily focuses on basic survival needs. Infants born to teenage mothers are at greater risk of lifetime poverty than are infants whose mothers waited until they were older than 20 years of age to have children (National Center for Health Statistics, 1991).

Poor children also have less access to health care services. One in three of these children has never been to a dentist. One in five poor children does not see a physician during the year. Uninsured children have fewer child health visits and are less likely to receive immunizations than are those with health insurance (Children's Defense Fund, 1988).

The National Commission on Children (1991) recommended a universal system of health insurance coverage for pregnant women and children up to 18 years of age. The insurance coverage would include a basic level of health care services in order to improve the quality of health care available to poor children.

In poor families, the focus is on basic survival; health care is crisis-oriented rather than preventive. This is especially true when there are so many barriers to health care services. Social service agencies have lengthy eligibility processes. Once a family is eligible, it may receive services from several sources, such as Aid to Families with Dependent Children and Medicaid. Because of the involvement of multiple agencies, fragmentation of services can occur. One important responsibility for community health nurses is to ensure access to services and to coordinate services for families in need.

LEGAL PARAMETERS GUIDING THE CARE OF CHILDREN

Because children are considered to be minors, decisions regarding anything that affects their lives must be made legally by their parents or guardians. The guardian is to act as a protector of the child's best interests and should be the child's advocate. Faced with a variety of family constellations and potential health care situations, the legal system has made a number of judgments in an attempt to clarify who can make decisions for the child and when the child can be considered "mature."

American society and its various cultures have had multiple measures of what constitutes adulthood. At 13 years of age, the Jewish child has a bar or bat mitzvah to signify the beginning of adulthood; however, this role is only practiced within the religious institution. The age at which one can obtain a driver's license ranges from 15 to 18 years of age. Voting and enrollment in military service can occur at age 18 years, but alcohol consumption in many states is not allowed until the person is 21 years of age. The age at which a child can be tried in court as an adult depends on the state but ranges from 14 to 18 years of age (Committee on Child Psychiatry, 1989).

The issue of what constitutes legal age depends on state laws and is more closely related to chronological age than maturational or mental age. General policies on age are made to fit children into slots, which is especially true of the age at which children may start school. The cutoff is usually based on the *month* of the year and not necessarily on the child's readiness for school.

The largest group of "mature" children are called *emancipated minors*. "An emancipated minor is one who is legally under age but is recognized as having the legal capacity of an adult under circumstances prescribed by state law" (Whaley and Wong, 1993, p. 1103). The situations resulting in a young person becoming emancipated vary from one state to another but usually include any female who becomes pregnant and anyone experiencing high school graduation, marriage, military service, or living independently (English, 1990).

Although not emancipated, some teenagers may still consent to a variety of medical and surgical procedures without notifying their parents or guardians. The types of services vary from state to state, but frequently include treatment for sexually transmitted diseases, pregnancy, drug and alcohol problems, outpatient mental health counseling, and emergency situations as well as contraceptive counseling (English, 1990).

Children receiving care at home or in the community should be participants in the decision-making process regarding their health care from the time when they are preschoolers. Health care providers frequently make decisions for younger children. However, as appropriate to children's maturation, community health nurses should allow children the opportunity to express their opinions about a decision that affects them *before* that decision is finalized. In addition, a child whose parents refuse lifesaving measures for that child based on religious practices (e.g., blood transfusions) has the legal right to petition the court.

HISTORY OF COMMUNITY HEALTH CARE FOR CHILDREN

Since the 1880s, a major role of community health nurses has been to assist new mothers to care for their newborn children. This early role was an attempt to decrease high infant mortality rates as well as the incidence of child neglect. Initially, nurses visited mothers on the day after a child was born to teach child care measures that would foster and maintain health. Home visits included information on sanitation and nutrition (Malinowski, 1989).

In the early 1900s, infection was the primary killer of children. Sick children were cared for in the home. Community health nurses played a vital role in infection control through home visiting; they assessed families for the risk of infection, taught prevention control and care of the sick to parents and other caregivers, and monitored quarantined families until the quarantine was removed. One important point is that almost all children who would have required sophisticated medical treatment to survive died, because the technology had not yet been invented.

By the mid-1930s, the family was recognized for its important role in the growth and development of children, and the focus of community health nurses expanded. In 1932 the National Organization of Public Health Nursing identified family health as the primary focus for public health nursing practice.

Health care services as well as community support services for children with significant disabilities were usually minimal. Prior to World War II, these children were either placed in institutions or kept at home. If families chose to take care of them at home, they coped on their own.

By the late 1950s, immunization programs prevented many communicable diseases and screening programs had begun to identify students with special needs. When it was possible, these children were placed in "special education" classes in the schools in order to receive some degree of education. The entire focus of educational rights and services for children with disabilities changed dramatically with the enactment of Public Law (P.L.) 94–142 (Education for All Handicapped Children Act) in 1975. This law guarantees free and appropriate education for all children with disabilities in the least restrictive environment.

The development and implementation of high technology care in the 1970s and 1980s have resulted in an entirely new population for the community health nurse. "The number of children surviving the perinatal period with significant impairment has grown rapidly with a corresponding rise in the need for programs that can maximize human potential and minimize the economic costs associated with such disability" (Gallagher et al., 1989, p. 170). The technology-dependent or medically fragile child is now a health care challenge. Providing optimal care in the home, while promoting normal growth and development for these children in the schools and communities, introduces new problems and avenues for problem solving. For example, how is a school experience provided for ventilator-dependent children?

In general, however, the goals of community health nursing today are only slightly changed from what they were 100 years ago—health promotion, disease prevention, and risk reduction for the child, the family, and the community. The resources available are diverse and vary from one state to another. It remains the responsibility of the community health nurse to assess the child and family and to plan interventions utilizing appropriate available resources.

FINANCING HEALTH CARE FOR CHILDREN

Availability of health care is, to a great extent, related directly to funding sources. In addition, confusion arises with regard to who shall pay, what resources are available, and who has access to health insurance (see Chapter 5). It is estimated that 12 million children younger than 18 years of age have no health insurance nor government funds for health care. Another few million children are underinsured, with funds only available for major acute illnesses and trauma, not for preventive (well-child) care (*Assuring Children's Access* . . ., 1989; Oberg, 1990).

For those who cannot afford health care, the federal government has attempted to establish resources in two ways. One method "uses grants to invest in the availability of specific health care services such as maternal and child health services, immunizations, community and migrant centers, and physician services" (*Faces of the Uninsured*, 1990, p. 2). The second method is the Medicaid program (Title XIX of the Social Security Act) and is aimed at providing health care for the poor.

Medicaid is the single largest public funding program of health care for children (see Chapter 5). Enrollment in Medicaid-sponsored programs is not automatic and can be quite a lengthy and difficult process. It is usually done by personnel in the local department of social services.

The primary groups of children covered under Medicaid are those covered under Aid to Families with Dependent Children (AFDC) and those physically or mentally disabled children covered by federal Supplemental Security Income (SSI). SSI provides a monthly stipend to eligible families to defray costs related to their child's disability, such as adaptive equipment and special clothing (Nelson, 1989).

There is a discrepancy in the expenditure of Medicaid funds. More money is spent on care for the elderly than for poor children. Half of all poor children who need financial assistance for health care do not have Medicaid ("Assuring Children's Access," 1989).

A great concern exists regarding the decrease in health care insurance for teenagers. Without health insurance many pregnant teenagers are unable to have access to and use prenatal care. Fifty-nine percent of 15 to 19 year olds have no insurance for maternity care. The result is a higher rate of neonatal mortality and morbidity (Oberg, 1990). The lack of health insurance coverage prevents teenagers from having access to other medical services as well.

The Early and Periodic Screening, Diagnosis, and Treatment Program (EPSDT) is a federally mandated program enacted in 1967. Its purpose is to provide preventive screening and health services for children receiving Medicaid benefits. Some health care services included in this program are a comprehensive health assessment, including vision, dental, and hearing care; immunizations; and treatment for any conditions discovered during the assessment (Oberg, 1990). This also includes some home care services, such as outreach, transportation, private duty care, medical equipment and supplies, and therapies (McCoy and Votroubek, 1990). The EPSDT promotes the concept of preventive health care within a crisis-oriented health care system. Unfortunately, not all states include EPSDT as a resource to their constituency.

Ten percent of severely disabled children use up to 50% of all physician services provided to children. A large gap exists between the services needed and the funds available. Children with chronic conditions constitute a special group who frequently have private or Medicaid funds to pay for inpatient services but have difficulty receiving funds for home care services. A series of waivers exists in the Medicaid system to allow states to offer home- and community-based services for special groups of children. For example, Regular 2176 Waivers can pay for mentally retarded, developmentally disabled, or mentally ill children who would otherwise require inpatient treatment in a skilled care facility. Model 2176 Waivers provide these services for a limited number of disabled children who would have been eligible for Medicaid only if they received care in an institution. For community health nurses unfamiliar with the procedure, medical social workers can often be helpful in obtaining waivers.

Children with Special Health Care Needs (CSHCN), formerly called the Crippled Children's Services, provides clinic-based services for children with chronic health problems. This funding source covers a large number of children with chronic conditions from asthma and diabetes to epilepsy, attention deficit disorder, ventilator dependency, and acquired immunodeficiency syndrome (AIDS). Although the services vary among states, they also include "skilled nursing care, extended home care services, outpatient visits, medications, supplies, and equipment" (McCoy and Votroubek, 1990, p. 38).

Private health insurance as well as governmental funding agencies are more frequently oriented toward the individual and to treatment for existing conditions. They are not family oriented nor do they focus on health promotion and disease prevention (except for selected health maintenance organizations [HMOs]).

Health care reform initiatives are expected to include greater emphasis on health promotion and disease prevention. It is up to the community health nurse and the nursing profession to promote family health. One way nurses can do this is to conduct empirical research to support the cost savings evidenced by prevention measures and early interventions to decrease morbidity and mortality.

Common Health Needs of Children

HEALTH PROMOTION/DISEASE PREVENTION

One of the primary goals of community health nursing is to promote health and prevent disease. In many communities, these services are provided through the public health sector. One role of the community health nurse is to work with children in their normal state of health to maintain that health and promote wellness. This is accomplished by way of counseling, education, and anticipatory guidance.

Families with newborn infants have numerous health promotion and primary prevention needs. Well child care (e.g., bathing, feeding, holding, and diapering) as well as interpreting the communication cues of the infant are important for all new parents to know. In addition, parents are learning and adjusting to their new roles. Community health nurses usually find that parents welcome and eagerly solicit support and advice.

Parents need information on normal growth and development and how to promote physical, psychosocial, and cognitive development throughout childhood. This includes knowing what age-appropriate developmental tasks to expect, suggestions on how to implement age-appropriate stimulation (Table 26–3), and how to recognize and handle the physical health problems common to young children (Table 26–4). An explanation of the recommended immunization schedule and an understanding of the diseases that they prevent are essential for promoting health (see Chapter 19). It is important to encourage immunization of children not only to prevent disease in the child and its spread to other family members but also to protect the community.

Adjustment to the parenting role and knowledge of the needs of children are not isolated to the family with a newborn infant. It takes just as much support and information to adjust to becoming the parent of a toddler or a teenager. Parents continually need to understand the physical, psychosocial, cognitive, and nutritional needs of their children as well as how to prevent dental decay, accidents, and contagious disease (especially when they begin nursery school or day care).

Healthy young children have more episodes of illness than do healthy adults. It is normal for young children to have six to nine respiratory infections per year. This is the result of increased contact with others at risk (peers) in their environment as well as an immature immune status. Children's immune systems develop over time as they come in contact with a variety of illnesses.

TABLE 26–3

Age-Appropriate Play

Age	Play
Birth–3 mo	Rocking, singing, talking to the infant, touching
3 mo	Observes the face and the mobile; listens to musical sounds
4 mo	"Busy box" on the cribside or a "cradle gym" across the crib top to encourage reaching out
6 mo	Textured toys
	Household objects: plastic cups, pot lids, spoons, clutch ball, and squeaky toys
9 mo	Teething toys
	Likes image in mirror
	Nesting toys
	Jack-in-the-box
12 mo	Cloth books
	Motion toys
Toddler	Imitative play
	Parallel play
	Push-pull toys to master walking
Preschool	Role play
	String large beads
	Water play
	Sandbox
	Crayons/fingerpaint
	Clay
	Read stories
School age	Collections
	Games
	Group activities
	Bike
	Skates
	Sports

From Selekman, J. (1993). *Pediatric nursing*. Springhouse, PA: Springhouse.

ENVIRONMENTAL SAFETY

A priority for young children is a safe environment. Nurses who make home visits are the first line of defense in assessing the homes for safety and making prevention-focused recommendations to the family. Safety needs change as children grow and their mobility, dexterity, and curiosity mature. The nurse can assist the parents to identify and alleviate risks in the home environment and the community. A list of suggested measures for home safety is provided in Table 26–5.

Accidents are the main cause of death for children from 1 to 18 years of age, especially motor vehicle accidents (see Chapter 24). Most accidents occur in or near the home, and most can be prevented. Safety-proofing the home, as well as increasing supervision for infants, toddlers, and preschoolers, will decrease the incidence of injury. An assessment of the environment for lead-based paint on

TABLE 26–4

Common Health Problems in Young Children

Problem	Comments	Interventions
Teething	Begins around age 6 months when lower central incisors arrive Molars arrive during toddlerhood Caries develop mostly during preschool/school age	Teething biscuits Hard teething toys Acetaminophen for irritability Use fluoride until age 12 Brush teeth from age 3 Prevention: annual dental checkups from age 5 Encourage brushing after meals
Bottle mouth syndrome	Results from sleeping with juice/milk-filled bottle and having long-term contact between the nipple and the teeth	Give the bottle of water or have the child finish the bottle and take an empty or clean bottle to bed
Toddler does not begin to speak		Assess hearing Assess the amount that the child is spoken to at home
Iron deficiency anemia	Child's iron supply from birth is depleted by age 4–6 mo	1. Begin iron supplements or iron-enriched foods at 4–6 mo of age 2. Limit milk or formula intake to no more than 30 oz/day
Temper tantrums	Common and normal during toddlerhood Prevent by keeping routines simple and consistent; set reasonable limits; provide choices	1. Provide a safe environment during a tantrum 2. Help the child regain control; attempt distraction; remove the child to a neutral area until control is achieved 3. Do not reason, threaten, promise, or hit 4. Respond consistently
Streptococcal pharyngitis		Throat culture is needed to confirm Antibiotics are essential to prevent development of rheumatic fever or glomerulonephritis Treatment of a sore throat is dependent on age
Urinary tract infections	May be related to poor hygiene, fecal contamination, or sexual abuse	Assess for frequency, burning, foul-smelling urine, fever, irritability Refer for treatment with antibiotics Teach the child to wipe from front to back Avoid bubble baths Promote use of cotton underwear
Diaper rash		Change diaper frequently; clean skin with water at each changing and then dry skin well; avoid plastic coverings; use a thin layer of A&D ointment or zinc oxide; wash diapers thoroughly with mild soap and rinse well; expose diaper area to air if possible during the day
Constipation	Defined as hard consistency to the stools; not related to straining or grunting during defecation	1. Increase liquids in the diet 2. Add Karo syrup (1 tsp to 3 oz of formula or milk)
Upper respiratory infection	6–9/year is normal	Increase fluid intake; cool mist vaporizers; use a bulb syringe to remove nasal mucus; acetaminophen
Otitis media	The child may exhibit irritability, fever, and pulling on the ear lobe	Refer for treatment with antibiotics and decongestants

windows, toys, and old baby furniture; installation of gates across high-risk areas (steps); and keeping medications and toxic substances in their original containers and out of the reach of children (locked cabinets) will provide a safer environment for children. In addition, encouraging the use of child car seats and helmets when using bicycles and skateboards will decrease a significant amount of vehicular mortality and morbidity.

For older children and adolescents, accidents and injuries are frequently related to substance abuse. To be effective, school and other community nurses should plan risk-reduction interventions that are straightforward and informative, and, whenever possible, incorporate the use of peers. High school students in groups (e.g., Students Against Drunk Driving) can use peer pressure and peer education to reinforce the dangers of drinking and driving, as well as the need for seat belts.

The increase in homicides and suicides in the adolescent population is correlated with the use of alcohol and illegal drugs (Potter-Efron and Potter-Efron, 1990). Because of

TABLE 26–5

Safety Measures for Infants and Young Children

SAFETY MEASURES FOR INFANTS
Support the infant's head
Keep the crib rails up
No pillows in the crib
Never leave an infant unattended on the dressing table
Do not prop bottles
Use bumper pads in the crib
Use approved car seats
Never leave an infant unattended in the bathtub
No pins, plastic, or small objects in a child's environment
No hanging electrical cords
No bean bag toys
SAFETY MEASURES FOR TODDLERS
Safety plugs in all electrical outlets
Gates across stairways
Locked cabinets for medication and cleaning agents/poisons; keep poisons in original containers
Remove dangerous plants from the child's environment
When the child begins to climb over the crib rails, it's time for a bed
Put pot and cup handles away from the edges of the table or the stove
Keep medication in child-proof containers and out of reach
No toys with sharp edges or small parts
Reinforce that pills are not candy
No peanuts or popcorn
GENERAL ENVIRONMENTAL SAFETY
Decrease cigarette smoke in the child's environment
No lead paint on windows, toys, or furniture
Decrease use of powder or aerosols in the child's environment
Screens in the windows
Play areas should be clear of debris
Food storage is appropriate for the foodstuffs
Damp dust
Keep insect, rodent traps, and poisons out of the reach of children
Smoke detectors
Keep matches out of the reach of children
Keep guns out of the reach of children

the increased violence, teaching nonviolent conflict resolution and the association between weapons and risk of injury also become important learning needs (see Chapter 20).

PSYCHOSOCIAL WELLNESS

In addition to the physical and safety needs for children, emphasis must be placed on their emotional needs. Consistency in their care will promote the young child's development of trust and a sense of control over his or her environment. As children grow, their need to have someone to talk to and to share their feelings with increases. Parents need to be available and to keep lines of communication with their children open.

Community health nurses who teach parenting skills should emphasize the important roles that emotional support, encouragement, and listening have in child development. Parents should encourage and even initiate discussion on sensitive topics. The nurse can help parents to role play sensitive conversations, such as those regarding sex education and values clarification. Some nurses may be uncomfortable with these topics themselves and may need to practice role playing with their professional peers before attempting parental interventions.

Communication is the key to enhancing a strong family system for the family with adolescents. Promoting communication and providing information on sexuality and the risks involved, drug and alcohol use, automobile safety, as well as promoting quality mental health for teenagers are essential. Freedom within age-appropriate limits, support, and authoritative rather than punitive relationships is associated with higher self-esteem in children and adolescents.

Adolescents must know that their family is available to them in times of crisis or just to help in problem solving. Parents may benefit from suggestions as to how to help their children develop a positive self-image. Empowering parents to set limits on their children and to check to see if responsible adults are present when their children visit others is appropriate. Encouraging parents to meet and share their frustrations and concerns assists in this empowerment. With the increased number of working parents, many parents have difficulty finding extra time to discuss their child-rearing issues with others.

When working with adolescents, the nurse should plan to talk separately with the teenagers and their parents. Teenagers will frequently share information with the nurse that they do not want to share with their parents. They may seek information on where to obtain birth control counseling, where to be tested for the AIDS virus or other sexually transmitted diseases, how to obtain an abortion, or share how depressed they are. The nurse must *not* impose his or her values on the young person but can certainly teach and promote information on health and healthy behaviors. It is important to help the teenager solve problems in a way that is acceptable to his or her culture and is age-appropriate. Whenever possible, the nurse should encourage the teenager to share the situation or health concern with his or her parents. Community health nurses frequently find themselves acting as a bridge for communications between the parent and the child.

HOME HEALTH VISITING TO THE FAMILY-INFANT UNIT

Successful maternal-child home visiting programs have been aimed at health promotion and primary prevention (Chamberlin, 1989; Malinowski, 1989; Olds et al., 1986; Powell and Grantham-McGregor, 1989). Some of the specific populations served were women who were reluctant to use the traditional health care system; families who were considered high risk for developing future problems, such as pregnant teenagers and those from low-income areas; and families in which an infant had been born prematurely and was now being discharged to the home (see Chapter 22).

Chamberlin (1989) reports that positive outcomes can be identified from home visits that occur at least weekly (during the initial period of time), occur over a 1-year period, and are carried out by individuals who provide both education and support. In addition, these visits must focus on the "whole" family and incorporate the family into any plans that are developed.

Despite research that repeatedly demonstrates that early intervention measures decrease mortality and morbidity in infants, these visits are rarely reimbursable by private third-party payers. Public health clinics do operate successfully in many communities, but they require the families to come to the centers, rather than visits occurring in the families' homes.

In the mid-1980s federal amendments to Medicaid expanded services to low-income pregnant women. As a part of case-management for these women, many states now reimburse for home visits by nurses employed by local health departments or health centers (see Chapter 5).

A second aim of home health visits by community health nurses is early identification and treatment of illness and handicapping conditions. Use of skills such as developmental and family assessments can help to identify children at high risk for future problems. Some of the interventions appropriate for community health nurse home visits include teaching parents to implement measures to promote growth, development, and safety; ensuring that the child is being provided with proper nutrition; and addressing the child's and family's health care for its adequacy and accessibility.

Families and Communities with Children

CHILDREN AND THEIR FAMILY CONSTELLATIONS

Children live in almost every conceivable form of family constellation. Although many children still experience the traditional nuclear family (husband, wife, and their children, adopted or natural), many may experience an alternative family environment at some point during their childhood. As divorces and remarriages increase, the number of children in blended families with step-parents, step-siblings, and extra sets of grandparents also increases (Bradshaw, 1988).

Approximately 16.4 of every 1000 children younger than 18 years are involved in divorced family situations (*Compilations of Data . . .*, 1990). Many of these children must make an additional adjustment when one or both of their parents remarries. Blended or reconstituted families are the fastest growing family constellation.

The extended family includes the nuclear family and adds blood relatives or those related by marriage. It is not uncommon today to find children being raised by grandparents or being raised with their cousins. In such situations, this will increase or change the individuals with whom the nurse interacts regarding health education. For example, the teenage mother frequently brings her child home to be raised by the baby's grandmother, who also needs to be included in all teaching about the child's care.

TABLE 26–6

Presence of Parents in Homes with Children Younger than 18 Years Old

Race	% Living with Both parents	% Living with Only Mother	% Living with Only Father	Neither Parent	Total
All races	72	22	3	3	100
White	79	17	3	2	100
Black	36	54	4	7	100
Hispanic	66	27	3	4	100

From: *Statistical Abstracts of the United States, 1992.* U.S. Department of Commerce, Bureau of the Census. Washington, DC: US Government Printing Office.

The family constellations for all children younger than 18 years of age in 1989 demonstrated that 72% lived with both parents, 22% lived with only their mothers, and a very small percentage lived with their fathers or with neither parent ("Statistical Abstracts," 1992). There is a marked difference across racial lines, with more white children living in two-parent homes than black or Hispanic children (Table 26–6).

While these are the most common situations in which American children live, it cannot be overlooked that some children live in communal families, in which multiple "families" share common ownership of property and goods, and homosexual households, in which the child is raised by a same-sex couple.

Two other groups of children and their families who are in need of a great deal of community resources and support are those who are homeless and those children who are placed in foster care. Finding health care services for these children is a concern for the community health nurse. Questions arise regarding who is responsible for their health care. Who ensures that they receive the proper nutrition, preventive dental care, prevention against disease via immunizations, and treatment for illness? Who is responsible for their health care as well as their continuity of care? Many homeless and foster care children are eligible for Medicaid and other community services. The community health nurse should act as the child's advocate, seeking appropriate community sources and coordinating care among different agencies.

DEVELOPMENTAL TASKS OF FAMILIES

Developmental tasks have long been associated with childhood. Accomplishment of physical tasks (e.g., sitting alone and walking), cognitive tasks (e.g., learning concepts of time, numbers, and letters), and psychosocial tasks (e.g., development of trust and a sense of self) are necessary for children to progress toward maturity (Table 26–7). Using

TABLE 26–7

Developmental Tasks for Infants and Children (Includes Physical, Psychosocial, and Cognitive)

	Age	Task
Infancy	3 mo	• Decrease in primitive reflexes except protective and postural reflexes
		• Social smile (indicates development of memory traces)
	4 mo	• Laugh
	5 mo	• Birth weight doubles
		• When prone, can push up on arms
		• Rolls over
	6 mo	• Teething begins
		• Sits with support
		• Exhibits "stranger anxiety" (is wary of strangers and clings to mother)
	8 mo	• Sits alone
		• Crawls
	9 mo	• Pincer grasp
		• Holds own bottle
	10 mo	• Stands with support
	12 mo	• Birth weight triples
		• Takes first steps alone
		• Develops trust
		• Speaks 5 words
		• Claps hands; waves bye-bye
Toddlerhood	13 mo–2.5 yr	• Masters walking
		• Climbs stairs
		• Feeds self (autonomy)
		• Language (increases to 400 words and 2- to 3-word phrases)
		• Toilet training/bowel and bladder control
		• Separation anxiety (screams when the mother leaves)
Preschool	2.5–4 yr	• Increased vocabulary; uses sentences
		• Alternates feet on steps
		• Copies circles and lines
		• Builds a tower of blocks
		• Concepts of causality, time, and numbers begin
		• Body image develops
		• Role plays
		• Enculturation begins
		• Development of conscience begins
		• Fears loss of body integrity
School age	5–12 yr	• Vision matures by age 6 yr
		• First baby tooth is lost at age 6 yr; all permanent teeth except final molars are in by age 12 yr
		• Develops peer relationships
		• Enjoys activities/groups/teams
		• Morality develops
		• Cognitive development: concepts of time/space, reversibility, conservation, parts/whole
		• Can classify objects in more than one way
		• Reading/spelling and math concepts develop
		• Puberty begins: age 9 yr for girls; age 11 yr for boys
		• Sense of industry
Adolescence	13–19+ yr	• Secondary sex characteristics develop
		• Attains adult growth
		• Adjusts to body changes
		• Menses begin
		• Abstract thought develops
		• Develops an identity
		• Fantasizes role in different situations
		• Increased heterosexual interests
		• Increased peer influences

From Selekman, J. (1993). *Pediatric nursing.* Springhouse, PA: Springhouse.

this developmental approach, the family also has been assigned developmental tasks. Developmental tasks of families involve the interaction among family members toward enhancing the growth and development of all family members as well as strengthening the family unit (Bradshaw, 1988). These include aspects of physical requirements, cultural practices, and development of the family's values and aspirations.

Duvall (1977) identified eight stages for families based on the age and school placement of the oldest child. The four stages that affect the family with children younger than 18 years of age include stages II through V. These include families with infants and toddlers (II), preschoolers (III), school-age children (IV), and adolescents (V). Critics of her model note that these were developed for "two-parent families" and are neither appropriate nor accurate for other family constellations, families who have a child with a chronic condition, or for some cultural groups (see Chapter 8).

Developmental tasks for the early childbearing family (II) include the development of parenting skills and new communication patterns and the task of managing time and energy (Bomar, 1989). Parents and grandparents accommodate to their new roles, and the infant is integrated into the family unit. Throughout this process, the parents are attempting to maintain and strengthen their marital bond (Friedman, 1986; Whaley and Wong, 1993).

Families with preschoolers are often deciding whether or not to have more children and are working through this process. Three- and 4-year-old children may begin preschool, and parents and the child must learn to deal with the separation. Childhood illnesses are common, and the resultant family stress as well as alternative child care arrangements are issues that must be dealt with. Children become socialized to their home values and cultural practices while adult members of the family attempt to meet their own needs for privacy and make employment decisions (Bomar, 1989). This is the time when identification of the child with their same-sex parent occurs; therefore, the availability of an adult of the child's same sex is thought to be important.

Parents of school-age children are adjusting to the influence of a third party—the school—on their child's life and must adjust to the impact of the child's peers and teachers. The focus for the child is now on school achievement while at the same time parents are trying to develop a satisfying marital relationship. Parents of adolescents must deal with their child's increasing autonomy and independence. During this time parents begin to refocus on their own marital and career issues and their concern for the older generation (Whaley and Wong, 1993).

Because of the multiple variables that can interfere with these tasks, generalizations are hard to make. For example, a teenage mother who is living with her mother may find herself in multiple stages at the same time.

Community health nursing is family health nursing. The nurse is in an ideal position to identify the strengths of the family as well as its needs. Communication is basic to family functioning. The nurse can enhance communication skills among family members and support the concept of meeting group needs as well as individual ones. Parenting is a learned (not innate) skill. Multiple issues and problems related to parenting develop at each developmental stage and must be addressed; thus parents can grow with their children.

CULTURAL/ETHNIC INFLUENCES ON HEALTH CARE

Community health care is culturally sensitive care. Cultural sensitivity is a much greater challenge for the community health nurse because of the increasing diversity of our population and because interventions and teaching provided in the home and community must be appropriate and acceptable to that cultural group (see Ethics Box VIII).

Because individuals from specific ethnic backgrounds are likely to develop certain health problems, screening is very important. Genetic inheritance is no one's "fault" nor is it a cultural weakness; however, certain groups have a genetic predisposition to certain inherited childhood conditions. Whites are at a greater risk for inheriting cystic fibrosis; Ashkenazic Jewish families are at risk for Tay-Sachs disease; blacks are prone to sickle cell anemia, and individuals of Mediterranean descent are at risk for inheriting beta-thalassemia. Prenatal screening and early detection can either prevent the occurrence or decrease the morbidity from these conditions.

Child-rearing practices may also differ among the different groups. Asian Americans may insist on breastfeeding their children until their fifth birthday (Whaley and Wong, 1993). Cultures vary in whoever is the major decision-maker in child rearing. It is important to know the child-rearing practices and to identify the "key" decision-maker so that teaching and planning will incorporate all persons responsible for the child's care (see Chapter 6).

How children are expected to behave varies in different cultures. Questions that consider a cultural viewpoint might be, "Are children allowed to express their opinions? What are the expectations of the child at a particular age?" It is important for the community health nurse to ascertain how children are viewed in the community. The culture of childhood is also included within the concept of culture. Childhood chants and games are handed down from one generation of children to another. Jump rope, stick ball, swapping baseball cards, and tag are only some of the many components of childhood. These experiences (with some modifications) should also be provided whenever possible for children with chronic conditions.

Children at Risk

Children at risk are those with biophysical or psychological conditions or in environmental situations that place

Ethics Box VIII

Gail A. DeLuca Havens, M.S., R.N., C.N.A.

Cultural Differences

The monthly immunization clinic is always busy. Since it opened 4 months ago, the number of new enrollees at this site in the eastern part of the city has continued to rise each month. It pays to advertise, thinks Martin, a Pediatric Nurse Practitioner who practices at the Eastside Primary Care Center. No doubt providing immunizations at no cost, or for a nominal fee, is an influential factor too.

Martin enters an examination room to begin a visit with his next patients, 9-month-old twin infants and their preschool siblings, ages 3 and 4. Their mother, Mrs. Flores, converses in Spanish. Since all employees of the primary care center speak both English and Spanish, Martin is able to talk directly with Mrs. Flores. He learns that her native tongue is the language of the Ojibways, but that she has learned Spanish since her marriage.

Mrs. Flores has brought her preschoolers to the clinic to begin their routine immunizations. However, when asked about the twins, she refuses to give permission for their routine immunization series. When talking with Mrs. Flores, Martin learns that the mother's tribal beliefs include not "poisoning" babies with man-made medicines. She relates, also, that her neighbor's baby became very ill 2 months ago, after receiving his first set of routine immunizations, and that he is still "not right." Martin attempts to explain to Mrs. Flores that her twins are at greater risk without their routine immunizations. Without alarming her, he tries to impress upon Mrs. Flores that now is a particularly bad time to leave her twins unprotected, because of the increase in confirmed cases of "whooping cough" in this section of the city during the past 3 months. He explains that the disease is very contagious and severe. Martin acknowledges that there are risks with immunizations as well, but that, particularly regarding "whooping cough," the risks related to the disease far outweigh those associated with immunization (Frank et al., 1984).

Mrs. Flores disagrees that her babies are unprotected because she is breast-feeding them. She recounts the beliefs of her tribe about the physical and social misfortunes that befall members later in life who do not acknowledge, by their actions at the beginning of life, their belief in the protective power of the natural, traditional ways of nurturing the well and treating the sick. Since these actions fall to parents on behalf of their children, she is frightened for her babies' future well-being, if she allows them to be immunized with "bad medicine" before they are 2 years old. Martin acknowledges Mrs. Flores' confidence in traditional ways as being necessary and sound but tells her that her breast milk will not prevent her twins from getting "whooping cough" (Frenkel, 1990). Mrs. Flores is adamant and, after having her preschoolers immunized with the first series of vaccines, she leaves the clinic without the twins having been immunized.

What should Martin do? Should he simply document Mrs. Flores' refusal and file the twins' records, forgetting about the conversation? What, if any, obligation does Martin have to the twins? Should he continue to try to convince Mrs. Flores to have them immunized? If Martin chooses to follow up, how can he be most effective in working with Mrs. Flores to find a culturally acceptable approach to immunizing her babies?

If Martin decides not to follow-up with Mrs. Flores and her twins, he would be practicing within the parameters of his position at the primary care center. His responsibilities do not include community outreach, but the provision of primary care to those who come to the center seeking it. Attempting, although unsuccessfully, to convince Mrs. Flores to accept immunizations for her twins has fulfilled his job-related obligation. In this situation, Mrs. Flores is acting on behalf of her children, the clients, when deciding against immunizations. In fact, the Code for Nurses (American Nurses' Association, 1985) states that "clients have the moral right to determine what will be done with their own person; to be given accurate information, and all the information necessary for making informed judgments; to be assisted with weighing the benefits and burdens of options in their treatment; to accept, refuse, or terminate treatment without coercion" (p. 2).

An alternative course of action is for Martin to follow up with Mrs. Flores and her twins. Although Martin respects the autonomy of the twins as expressed by their mother, he is motivated to continue dialogue with Mrs. Flores. The Code for Nurses (American Nurses' Association, 1985) describes the

(Continued)

nurse's respect for the worth and dignity of the individual human being as extending to all those who require the services of the nurse for the promotion of health and the prevention of illness. It does not qualify the nurse's respect by indicating that it applies only when the client is in the nurse's practice setting. Perhaps the twins will not contract pertussis before it is culturally acceptable for them to be immunized; however, given the growing incidence of pertussis in this part of the city, they could contract the disease and even be left with extreme and irreversible brain damage due to the hypoxia associated with prolonged coughing spasms (Frenkel, 1990). He believes that cross-cultural differences have resulted in conflicting views about how to prevent harm to the twins.

The American Nurses' Association's Code for Nurses (1985) describes the need for health care as "transcending all national, ethnic, racial, religious, cultural, . . . differences" (p. 3), which is Martin's specific interest in this situation. Recognizing the complex factors that influence behaviors surrounding states of health and illness within cultures is fundamental to competent nursing practice (Anderson, 1990). Martin perceives it to be his personal responsibility to maintain competency in his practice. A consultation with colleagues practicing in the community ought to give Martin some insight into how best to approach Mrs. Flores. Perhaps they could identify people in the community who are culturally sensitive to Native American value systems and who might be willing to collaborate with him in approaching Mrs. Flores about the immunization of the twins or help him better understand her perspective. Enlisting the assistance of a respected member of a specific cultural community is often an effective strategy in negotiating over health beliefs with a client from that culture. In this situation, such action could be helpful to the twins, Martin, and Mrs. Flores.

References

American Nurses' Association. (1985). *Code for nurses with interpretive statements.* Kansas City, MO: Author.

Anderson, J. M. (1990). Health care across cultures. *Nursing Outlook, 38,* 136–139.

Frank, T., Parks, B., & Fischer, R. G. (1984). Pertussis immunizations? *Pediatric Nursing, 10,* 360.

Frenkel, L. D. (1990). Routine immunizations for American children in the 1990s. *Pediatric Clinics of North America, 37,* 531–548.

them at risk for alterations in physical, cognitive, or psychosocial development. For some children, it is possible that a single factor may place them at risk for future developmental problems, whereas for other children, multiple factors must be considered.

BIOPHYSICAL RISK FACTORS

Infants and Young Children

Risks resulting from biophysical situations can occur before, during, or after the birth of the infant. These risks include smoking and drug and alcohol use by the mother prior to and during the pregnancy, congenital and chromosomal anomalies, central nervous system deficits, prematurity, and serious illness during early infancy. More than 3700 infants are born annually with fetal alcohol syndrome (Garwood and Sheehan, 1989), and approximately 375,000 American infants are born annually to mothers who have used drugs (*Faces of the Uninsured,* 1990). The emphasis has been on the dramatic increase in the number of infants born to cocaine-abusing mothers.

As advances are made in medical science, children are being saved from illness and other conditions that only a few years ago would have resulted in death. However, with the increase in these life-supporting measures comes an increase in morbidity and chronic conditions. It is quite common to see premature infants develop respiratory distress syndrome. Many of these children survive and go on to develop bronchopulmonary dysplasia and dependency on oxygen or ventilators in childhood, putting them at increased risk for chronic respiratory problems for life.

The number of child survivors from neonatal drug withdrawal, serious conditions related to prematurity, chronic childhood illnesses, and brain tumors has increased. These may be some of the multiple causes in the significant increase in the number of children being diagnosed with learning disabilities and attention-deficit hyperactivity disorder (Selekman, 1991).

As the illicit drug abuse epidemic grows, more and more infants are being born to women who carry the human immunodeficiency virus (HIV) (American Hospital Association, 1991). AIDS is now the leading cause of death for children between 1 and 4 years of age. By December 1993, 5234 children younger than 13 years of age had been diagnosed with AIDS (Centers for Disease Control and Prevention [CDC], 1994). The CDC estimates that over 10,000 children are infected with HIV. By March 1992, 4406 adolescents had been diagnosed with AIDS; in later data, adolescents are included with adults, and adolescents with AIDS are not reported separately (CDC, 1992).

Community health nurses play a major role in facilitating community services to infants and children with HIV disease. They have also been instrumental in reducing community anxiety about exposure to children with HIV disease. Community health nurses provide public education forums to inform citizens about HIV and AIDS and answer questions of concern, including the risk associated with casual contact.

Infant Mortality Rate. The infant mortality rate is used as an indicator of the health status of the nation. Infant mortality is defined as death that occurs during the first year of life. While the average infant death rate is approximately 10 per thousand live births, the disparity across groups is great. For infants born to unmarried mothers, the numbers are much higher: 13.1 per thousand live births for whites and 19.6 per thousand live births for blacks (*Infant Mortality,* 1990).

Although the infant mortality rate in the United States compares poorly with other industrialized nations (see Chapter 3), the infant mortality rate in 1989 of 9.8 per thousand live births was the lowest ever recorded. In 1990, 38,100 infants died before 1 year of age (Wegman, 1991). Massachusetts had the lowest infant mortality rate (6.8 per thousand live births) and Washington, District of Columbia, the highest (23.2 per thousand live births) (*Statistical Abstracts,* 1991). The rate of infant death is much higher among infants born to black mothers than to white mothers (17.7 vs. 8.2 per thousand live births) and is higher in the southern states than in other areas of the United States (*Infant Mortality,* 1992). The year 2000 National Health Objective for infant mortality set a goal to reduce deaths to 7 per thousand live births (Table 26–8).

Low-Birth-Weight Infants. Low birth weight (LBW) is a major factor of infant mortality. "A low-birth-weight infant is almost 40 times more likely to die in the first four weeks of life than a normal-birth-weight infant, and two thirds of all deaths during the first month are attributable to low birth weight" (Oberg, 1990, p. 827).

There is an increase in the numbers of children being born who are of low birth weight. In 1985 6.8% of all infants were born weighing less than 5 lb 8 oz (2500 gm). This included 5 of every 100 white infants and 12 of every 100 black infants. With improved technology, 90% of infants born weighing between 1000 and 1500 gm survive (*Technology-Dependent Children,* 1987), resulting in a greater number of chronic sequelae. The morbidity associated with low birth weight includes mental retardation, cerebral palsy, seizure disorders, developmental delay, decreased school achievement, learning disabilities, attention-deficit hyperactivity disorder, visual and hearing deficits, and autism. It is estimated that one of three drug-exposed infants has a low birth weight. The sequelae for these children include physical and neurological damage and developmental delay (*Faces of the Uninsured,* 1990).

Early prenatal care is correlated with decreasing low-birth-weight risk for infants. Nevertheless, half of all pregnant women do not receive adequate prenatal care. According to the Children's Defense Fund, "the high proportion of women who receive either no prenatal care or none until after the sixth month of pregnancy represents one of the most serious health problems facing the nation" (*Maternal and Infant Health,* 1990, p. 14). Other factors that contribute to low birth weight include inadequate nutrition and maternal smoking during pregnancy.

Primary Causes of Infant Death. The primary causes of mortality from birth to 1 year of age are listed in Table 26–9. The community health nurse can initiate preventive measures for conditions over which there is control; for conditions for which there is no control, nurses need to understand the frequency of their occurrence and anticipate the supportive measures that the family may need.

Adolescents

Adolescents, because they are less likely to consider health risks realistically, represent a high-risk population. The three main causes of mortality among teenagers are accidents, especially motor vehicle accidents, suicide, and homicide. In addition, approximately a half million babies are born to teenagers each year (Children's Defense Fund, 1989) (see Chapter 22). The majority of these teenagers are unmarried.

ENVIRONMENTAL RISK FACTORS

Environmental risks for children include the quality of care a child receives, inappropriate amounts of physical or environmental stimulation, or an unsafe environment. Additional environmental risks include maternal deprivation; parents who are teenagers (single or divorced); inadequate nutrition; and inadequate social supports for the family.

Although morbidity is usually considered in its physical context, the emotional effects of living in poverty, with chronic illness, or in abusive homes must also be considered. Conditions such as failure to thrive are often related to poor quality of parenting. Maladaptive coping mechanisms and delinquency have become more prevalent among school-age children and adolescents. More and younger juveniles are becoming involved in violence, and more children are bringing weapons to school. Firearm injuries are the third leading cause of death among youngsters aged 10 to 19 (*Unintentional Firearm-Related Fatalities,* 1992). These problems are thought to be related to the increased availability of guns, the increasing drug problem in the United States, and, for some, having abusive parents as role models.

HEALTHY PEOPLE 2000

TABLE 26–8

Healthy People 2000 Objectives for Children

1. Reduce the infant mortality rate to no more than 7 per 1000 live births (baseline: 10.1 per 1000 live births in 1987).
2. Reduce low birth weight to no more than 5% of live births (a 28% decrease).
3. Reduce the fetal death rate (20 weeks or more of gestation) to no more than 5 per 1000 live births plus fetal deaths (baseline: 7.6 per 1000 live births plus fetal deaths in 1987).
4. Increase first trimester prenatal care to at least 90% of live births (an 18% increase).
5. Increase to at least 95% the proportion of newborns screened by state-sponsored programs for genetic disorders and other disabling conditions and to 90% the proportion of newborns who have a positive test result for disease and who receive appropriate treatment (baseline: For sickle cell anemia, with 20 states reporting, approximately 33% of live births screened [57% of black infants]; for galactosemia, with 38 states reporting, approximately 70% of live births screened).
6. Increase to at least 90% the proportion of babies aged 18 months and younger who receive recommended primary care services at the appropriate intervals.
7. Reduce growth retardation among low-income children aged 5 and younger to less than 10% (baseline: up to 16% among low-income children depending on age and race/ethnicity).
8. Reduce the prevalence of serious mental retardation in school-age children to no more than 2 per 1000 children (baseline: 2.7 per 1000 children aged 10 in 1985–1988).
9. Reduce iron deficiency to less than 3% among children aged 1 to 4 (baseline: 9% for children aged 1 to 2, 4% for children aged 3 to 4 in 1976–1980).

Special Population Targets

Iron Deficiency Prevalence	*1976–1980*	*2000 Year Target*
Low-income children aged 1–2 yr	21%	10%
Low-income children aged 3–4 yr	10%	5%

10. Reduce the prevalence of blood lead levels exceeding 15 μg/dl and 25 μg/dl among children aged 6 months to 5 years to no more than 500,000 and zero, respectively (baseline: An estimated 3 million children had levels exceeding 15 μg/dl, and 234,000 had levels exceeding 25 μg/dl, in 1984).
11. Reduce asthma morbidity, as measured by a reduction in people hospitalized due to asthma to no more than 160 per 100,000 people (baseline: 188 per 100,000 in 1987).

Special Population Targets

Asthma Hospitalizations (per 100,000)	*1987 Baseline*	*2000 Year Target*
Blacks and other nonwhites	334	265
Children aged ≤ 14 yr	284	225

12. Reduce residential fire deaths to no more than 1.2 per 100,000 people (Age-adjusted baseline: 2.1 per 100,000 in 1987).

Residential Fire Deaths (per 100,000)	*1987 Baseline*	*2000 Year Target*
Children aged ≤ 4 yr	4.4	3.3

13. Reduce nonfatal poisoning to no more than 88 emergency department treatments per 100,000 people. (Baseline: 103 per 100,000 in 1986.)

Special Population Target

Nonfatal Poisoning (per 100,000)	*1986 Baseline*	*2000 Year Target*
Among children ≤ 4 yr	650	520

14. Reduce nonfatal head injuries so that hospitalizations for this condition are no more than 106 per 100,000 people (baseline: 125 per 100,000 in 1988).
15. Enact in 50 states laws requiring that new handguns be designed to minimize the likelihood of discharge by children (baseline: 0 states in 1989).
16. Provide academic instruction on injury prevention and control, preferably as part of quality school health education, in at least 50% of public school systems (grades K to 12).
17. Increase to at least 50% the proportion of primary care providers who routinely provide age-appropriate counseling of safety precautions to prevent unintentional injury.

From USDHHS. (1990). *Healthy people 2000: National health promotion and disease prevention objectives. Summary report.* Washington, DC: US Government Printing Office.

TABLE 26–9

Causes of Infant Deaths, 1980 and 1991

Causes of Death	% of Deaths in 1980	% of Deaths in 1991
Congenital anomalies	20.3	20.9
Sudden infant death syndrome	12.1	14.5
Respiratory distress syndrome	11.0	7.0
Disorders related to short gestation and low birth weight	8.0	11.3
Newborns affected by maternal complications of pregnancy	3.5	4.2
Intrauterine hypoxia and birth asphyxia	3.5	1.6
Infections specific to prenatal period	3.3	2.4
Accidents	2.1	2.6
Newborns affected by complications of placenta, cord, and membranes	2.2	2.6
Pneumonia and influenza	2.2	1.7
All others	32.9	31.2

Data from 1980 *Statistical Abstracts of the United States, 1992.* U.S. Department of Commerce, Bureau of the Census. Washington, DC: US Government Printing Office; Infant Mortality—United States, 1991. (1993) *MMWR, 42*(48), 926–930.

Child Abuse and Neglect

One to two million child abuse and neglect cases are reported annually (see Chapter 20). Abuse or neglect may be perpetrated by anyone—a parent, a babysitter, or a teacher. Community health nurses are in a prime position to observe for abusive behavior, because they come in contact with babysitters, licensed and unlicensed daycare settings, and other child care arrangements.

Observing how a caretaker holds the children or interacts with them, assessing the children for signs of abuse or neglect, and assessing the environment for safety and hygienic conditions are often the first steps. Reporting suspected child abuse and neglect to the police or the child protective service agency is mandatory in *all* states for *all* health professionals.

Families in abusive situations need parenting role models and a support system during periods of stress. Hotline or crisis phone numbers can be one way to provide help for people in stressful situations. Some examples of these types of services are Parents Anonymous and the National Abuse Hotlines.

SUPPORT SERVICES

Resources

In many areas of the United States multiple services are available to the family at risk. Traditional health services are those that offer screening and well child care. These include public clinics and private medical practices that provide immunizations, developmental screening, and parent education (e.g., parenting skills, safety practices, and nutritional and developmental stimulation needs). Pediatric nurse practitioners are experts in providing primary care and are employed in community agencies. Community health nurses provide anticipatory education to parents and also child health screening. If a child is not completing appropriate developmental tasks, the community health nurse should assess the child, the family, and the environment. The assessment should be geared toward determining needs, initiating appropriate referrals for further diagnosis and treatment, and teaching the family members appropriate care measures.

Child Watch or Child Find programs are screening programs that occur during preschool or grade school admission. For younger children, especially those who are poor, nurses in well child clinics and on home health visits can perform screening under the services of Early Periodic Screening, Diagnosis, and Treatment. This testing includes vision and hearing screening, lead detection, developmental assessments, and routine physical examinations.

Other health promotion services include foster grandparents programs (intergenerational supports) or big brother and sister programs to provide someone who cares and who is a role model; preschool education; Special Olympics; and creative programs for adolescents. Adolescent pregnancy prevention programs have included the use of incentives to stay in school; job training programs; and access to information on sex, sexually transmitted diseases, AIDS, and birth control. A nonprofit organization of families, health professionals, and educators devoted to supporting and facilitating home care for technology-dependent children is Sick Kids (Need) Involved People, Inc (SKIP).

Promotion of nutrition for families who are poor is a challenge. Food stamps are available to all who meet the eligibility criteria, but the Women, Infants, and Children (WIC) program is specifically for pregnant women, mothers, and young children. Provision of healthy food to pregnant women increases the chance that their children will be healthy and of a normal weight. If proper nutrition is provided to young children, this will promote normal growth, both neurological and physical. WIC has proved to be effective both in financial savings of hospital care for newborns and in improving the health of high-risk infants ("Further Evidence," 1985).

One of the premier advocacy groups for children is the Children's Defense Fund. This private organization serves as an advocate for children, especially poor, minority, and handicapped children. Their goal is to "educate the nation about the needs of children and encourage preventive investment in children before they get sick, drop out of school, or get into trouble. (They) focus on programs and policies that affect large numbers of children (and) monitor the development and implementation of federal and state policies" (Children's Defense Fund, 1989).

Children with disabilities and those with chronic conditions are even more in need of support services than are other children. These special children require regular health care as well as special care during periods of exacerbation or stress. Many of the specific conditions have their own support organization that can assist parents to find information and services. Table 26–10 includes some of the numerous organizations serving children with special needs and their families.

In addition to these disease-specific services, the Indian Health Program, developmental disabilities programs, Children with Special Health Care Needs, National Easter Seal Society, March of Dimes Birth Defects Foundation, services for the blind and deaf, mental health/mental retardation services, and local departments of social services are additional resources (Gallagher et al., 1989). These agencies provide financing for health services, support services, and educational information for children and parents.

McCoy and Votroubek (1990) and Ahmann (1986) have provided more comprehensive lists as have many health departments and social service agencies. Another resource is the National Information Center for Children and Youth with Handicaps (NICHCY) (see Table 26–10).

Parents who provide continuous care for a child with special needs benefit from frequent breaks in their routines to maintain their own mental health. Respite care offers parents a break from the routine, continuous care of the child, either for a short period each day or for a more prolonged time. This care may be offered in the home or in another facility. Respite allows parents time to be together as well as allowing parents to do activities with their other children. Some health insurance plans will pay for respite care. If that is not an option, community health nurses can look for volunteers, charitable funding, or, in some circumstances, public funding for respite care.

Early Intervention for Children at Risk

In 1975, the federal government recognized that handicapped children had a constitutional right to a free public education in the least restrictive environment (P.L. 94–142, Education for All Handicapped Children Act). The least restrictive environment refers to an environment that can handle the demands of children with disabilities. Whenever possible, children are encouraged to become integrated into the normal school environment. The law mandates nondiscriminatory individualized testing, classification, and placement of the children as well as an emphasis on the participation of parents in the decision-making process.

This law includes children with physical impairments, learning disabilities, and mental and emotional disabilities. It requires schools to develop an individualized education plan (IEP) for each child that states the short- and long-term goals and describes the services that would be provided in the school. One limitation was that most children had to be of school age to obtain services.

Prior to this act, children with chronic conditions and disabilities were taught at home without peer contact, were taught in separate classrooms or schools where all special needs children were taught as a group, received an inadequate education, or received no education at all. During the 1985 to 1986 school year, special education and related services were provided to 3.7 million children and youths (Garwood and Sheehan, 1989).

Mainstreaming, or attempting to integrate children with special needs with peers of the same age in a regular classroom, is now referred to as *normalization.* Although there may still be a need for some children to have separate special education classes, this practice is not the one most desired. "A 1985 report to Congress noted that, during 1982–83, 68% of all children across the nation who were identified as disabled attended classes with their nondisabled peers for at least part of the time" (Gallagher et al., 1989, p. 34).

In addition to education, P.L. 94–142 requires schools to provide "related services" to these children at no additional expense to the parents. These services are the supports needed by the child to benefit from the educational system. Physical and occupational therapies may be needed to provide mobility and devices that allow the child to participate in classroom activities. Speech therapy or development of a method of communication is necessary in order for learning to be successful in the classroom. Special transportation arrangements are also included as well as counseling or psychiatric services.

Debate over what services are considered to be the responsibility of school districts is becoming more common in the courts. Whereas one court has ruled that a child who needs intermittent catheterization during school hours should be the responsibility of the school in order to maintain school attendance, another court has stated that "services that are medically extensive, expensive, continuous, and require the competence beyond that of a school nurse are likely to be ruled excludable" (Vitello, 1989, p. 38).

P.L. 94–142 was amended in 1986 through P.L. 99–457 and expanded coverage for high-risk children *from birth.* P.L. 99–457 (the Education for All Handicapped Children Act Amendments of 1986) authorizes a discretionary state grant program focusing on comprehensive early intervention for high-risk children from birth through school age, with the intent of providing financial incentives to states to develop and implement comprehensive, coordinated, multidisciplinary, and interagency programs. This law is among the first proactive measures adopted by Congress.

TABLE 26–10

Resources

The Alliance of Genetic Support Groups
38th and R St. N.W.
Washington, DC 20057
(202) 331–0942

American Cancer Society
90 Park Ave.
New York, NY 10016
(212) 599–3600

American Heart Association
National Center
7320 Greenville Ave.
Dallas, TX 75231–4599
(214) 373–6300

American Juvenile Arthritis Organization
1314 Spring St. N.W.
Atlanta, GA 30309
(404) 872–7100

Association for Children and Adults with
Learning Disabilities
4156 Library Rd.
Pittsburgh, PA 15234
(412) 341–1515

Association for the Care of Children's Health
7910 Woodmont Ave., Suite 300
Bethesda, MD 20814
(301) 654–6549

Association of Birth Defects in Children
Orlando Executive Park
5400 Diplomat Circle, Suite 270
Orlando, FL 32810
(407) 629–1466

Association of Retarded Citizens
500 E Border St., Suite 300 (location)
P.O. Box 1047 (mailing)
Arlington, TX 76010
(817) 261–6003

Asthma and Allergy Foundation of America
1125 15th St. N.W., Suite 502
Washington, DC 20036–2005
(202) 466–7643

Candlelighters Childhood Cancer Foundation, Inc.
7910 Woodmont Ave., Suite 460
Bethesda, MD 20814
(301) 657-8401

Children's Defense Fund
122 C St. N.W., Suite 400
Washington, DC 20015
(202) 628–8787

Children's Hospice International
901 N. Washington St., Suite 700
Alexandria, VA 22314
(703) 684–0330

Cystic Fibrosis Foundation
6931 Arlington Rd.
Bethesda, MD 20814
800-FIGHT CF
or
(301) 951–4422

Disabilities Clearinghouse
National Center for Youth with Disabilities
Box 721, 420 Delaware St. S.E.
Minneapolis, MN 55455
(800) 333–6293

Easter Seal Society for Crippled Children and Adults
70 East Lake St.
Chicago, IL 60601
(800) 221–6827
or
(312) 726–6200

Epilepsy Foundation of America
4351 Garden City Dr.
Landover, MD 20785
(800) 332-1000
or
(301) 459–3700

Juvenile Diabetes Association
432 Park Ave. S.
New York, NY 10016
(212) 889–7575

March of Dimes Birth Defects Foundation
1275 Mamaroneck Ave.
White Plains, NY 10605
(914) 428–7100

Muscular Dystrophy Association
3300 E. Sunrise
Tucson, AZ 85718
(602) 529–2000

National Association for Down Syndrome
P.O. Box 63
Oak Park, IL 60303
(708) 325–9112 (office hours 9 AM–1 PM)

National Hemophilia Foundation
110 Greene St., Suite 303
New York, NY 10012
(212) 219–8180

National Hotlines
Parents Anonymous 1–800–421–0353
National Abuse Hotline 1–800–422–4453

National Information Center for Children and Youth with Handicaps
(NICHCY)
P.O. Box 1492
Washington, DC 20013
(800) 999–5599
or
(703) 893–6061

Pediatric AIDS Foundation
2407 Wilshire Blvd.
Suite 613
Santa Monica, CA 90403
(213) 395–9051

Sick Kids Need Involved People (SKIP)
216 Newport Dr.
Severna Park, MD 21146

United Cerebral Palsy Association, Inc.
1522 K. St. N.W., Suite 1112
Washington, DC 20005
(800) USA–5UCP

It includes Title I—Program for Infants and Toddlers with Handicaps (birth up through 2 years of age), and Title II—Preschool Grants Program (ages 3 to 5 years). Title I is also referred to as Part H of the law. It focuses on enhancing development and minimizing developmental delay for handicapped infants and toddlers in order to decrease their need for special education and related services, including institutionalization, later in life. Title II is an extension of P.L. 94–142 that provides free and appropriate education to handicapped children beginning at 3 years of age.

P.L. 99–457 recognizes the unique and important role of the family in the development and implementation of a plan of care for their child. It emphasizes the importance of multiple disciplines helping families to meet the special needs of their young children with handicaps (Committee on Education and Labor, 1986). In order to provide family centered care, an important component of P.L. 99–457 requires the development of an Individualized Family Service Plan (IFSP) for each eligible child and family. This IFSP must contain a multidisciplinary assessment that includes parent participation; the *individualized* and specific early intervention plan, including the major expected outcomes; the services necessary for this child; the projected dates for treatment; and the identification of a case manager to coordinate the services. The plan must contain an assessment of the child's present level of development in the physical, cognitive, language, and psychosocial parameters.

Family involvement is required in these early intervention initiatives. Perhaps the most positive focus of the IFSP is the requirement of identification of the family's strengths in addition to their needs in order to enhance the child's development. The plan for intervention should build on these strengths. The law also mandates performance and updating evaluations once a year, with a review occurring every 6 months; Child Find activities to locate eligible children and families; and the establishment of a state Interagency Coordinating Council, appointed by the governor of that state, that would coordinate services (Smith, 1988).

It is up to each state whether it chooses to develop an early intervention program. The state can decide who the special "at risk or handicapped" population will be. Eligibility criteria and the definition of developmental delay differ from one state to another, but the law does specify services to children who are, or may be, as a result of a current condition, developmentally delayed. Prior to P.L. 99–457, schools serving disabled children older than 5 years had to report children according to predetermined categorical labels (e.g., mildly retarded, learning disabled). "P.L. 99–457 does not require states to report children ages 3–5 by disability labels, thus allowing for noncategorical approaches to child identification" (Gallagher et al., 1989, p. 103).

However, because schools now service very young children, the community health nurse is challenged to develop new tools to assist in early developmental screening of infants and young children. The goal is to identify young children at risk for language, speech, psychosocial, physical, or mental conditions that may result in developmental delay.

The federal government enacted this law but did not provide funding for its implementation. Funding these services is the responsibility of the individual states. The federal government did indicate that funds for this program may not be used for services that are already covered under other medical and social programs. Most states have begun the process of developing this early intervention system. The law does not require states to develop new services; rather it involves coordination of existing services and a plan to deliver those services to children. The law made clear that any state funds used for the treatment of any child are *not* to result in a reduction of medical or other assistance available to this child and family.

In 1991, P.L. 94–142 and P.L. 99–457 were renamed the Individuals with Disabilities Education Act (IDEA). Implementation of IDEA requires a great deal of leadership to enhance communication among service providers and organizations to prevent replication of services and yet provide comprehensive care (see Chapter 28). The community health nurse is in an ideal position to participate in this case management process, especially with Part H (programs for infants and toddlers with disabilities). Nursing has been slow to develop its role in this law (Hansen et al., 1990). If nursing does not develop and promote its strengths in this early intervention program, we will lose an opportunity to have a key role in the team effort to improve child health.

Daycare and Nursery School

"Early childhood educational programs were first established in the United States in the late 1800s" (Hanson and Lynch, 1989, p. 5). The initial intent of nursery school programs was to enhance the child's ability to learn, promote social skills, and provide "catch-up" learning time, if needed. Typically, it served children 3 and 4 years old and met from a few mornings a week to full-day, 5-day-a-week sessions.

Structured programs of early intervention services for preschool children considered high risk for future cognitive delay began in the mid-1960s with community programs such as Head Start and Follow Through. Their purpose was to help disadvantaged children be prepared for and cope with regular school programs (Hanson and Lynch, 1989). Head Start and Home Start are two programs that involve empowering parents to spend increased time with their children. Head Start involves the parent in programmed activities in a formal school program. Home Start provides parents with guidance, suggested learning activities, and positive reinforcement to encourage stimulating the child's learning in the home environment. Both programs are effective in enhancing school readiness and have been widely studied (Steinmetz, 1988).

Daycare programs developed as an alternative to home babysitting services for parents who were not in the home during the day. Their intent was not necessarily educational, but rather an alternative for child care services. The terms "nursery school," "preschool," and "daycare" have now become blurred and are frequently used synonymously. Some states even license in-home daycare.

Parents are now seeking daycare for their child as young as a few weeks of age. It is difficult in many areas of the United States to obtain quality child care in facilities that are licensed and have high standards of care and small staff:children ratios. Adequate child care is expensive and many families must make do with substandard arrangements. Child care for one child costs about half of the wages for a full-time worker making minimum wage. For that reason, many children are left unsupervised. The estimate is that approximately 2 million children are left alone while their parents work (Children's Defense Fund, 1991).

Several additional demands for specialized daycare have now emerged. A need has been identified for "sick" daycare, to which parents can bring a child who is ill, so that they (the parents) will not have to miss a day of work in order to care for the child. With an increase in the number of working parents, additional need exists for "afterschool care" or "older child daycare" for school-age children whose parents are not at home at the end of the school day. By the year 2000, 70% of all preschool children will have mothers in the labor force (Children's Defense Fund, 1989).

Community health nurses can help parents ensure that their children are placed in safe, approved child care environments. These programs promote health practices, such as handwashing before meals and after toileting, brushing teeth after meals, and proper disposal of soiled clothes and diapers; provide role models for the children; implement environmental safety measures; and enhance social interaction and language skills, especially for children from non–English-speaking homes. They should have a diversity of equipment that is cleaned daily and small groups of the same-age children. Above all, the environment should be one of love and acceptance.

Community health nurses can act as consultants and on-site care providers in daycare and preschool settings. They can teach the aforementioned content to daycare staff, facilitate parent group sessions, have sessions with the older children, and, in some areas, may have a role in daycare licensure that involves monitoring implementation of standards and regulations.

One of the prime concerns for children in daycare is the easy spread of pathogens which is, in part, due to the young age of the children and their normally high risk for developing contagious diseases, the increased amount of bodily contact among young children, and their decreased ability to control their body functions. Therefore, infection control in this environment is essential. Implementation of precautions, including the use of gloves when changing diapers, the cleansing of the changing table and toys between children, and policies regarding how and where sick children will be handled, must be implemented consistently.

Community Health Care for Children with Special Needs

Children with chronic conditions are increasingly requiring interventions by community health nurses. Newacheck (1989) estimates that 30% of all children younger than 18 years of age have some form of chronic physical or mental condition. It is estimated that 2.2% of children younger than 5 years of age (403,000) and 6.2% of children ages 5 to 17 are limited in their activity by a disability. The Disability Statistics Bulletin states that 4.4% of school-age children (5 to 17 years) attend special schools or special classes, and 0.3% of children in this age group need help with their activities of daily living (*Prevalence of Disability in Childhood,* 1988).

Children with chronic conditions are often the primary recipients of services of the community health nurse, especially children requiring technological care at home. High-technology home care is the special domain of the community health nurse. "The same medical technology responsible for saving children's lives has also made children dependent on technology for their survival" (Raulin and Shannon, 1986, p. 338). One complex condition requiring home care is the child who requires a ventilator.

Less than 10 years ago, the only place where care could be provided to a child who required life-sustaining technology was in a hospital setting, and that was often in an intensive care setting. These children would often spend years of their lives in this high-technology setting. In the early 1980s, an effort began to improve the quality of life for these children. Home routines and family interactions were considered more beneficial than the stress of the hospital setting (and for parents of visiting the hospital daily). Home care seeks to create a more normal environment for them.

The hospital setting is *not* an appropriate environment in which to raise a child. A child in a hospital has an increased risk of contracting nosocomial infections because of an increased number of invasive procedures, multiple caretakers, and increased contact with organisms from other children and staff. Altered environments due to an increased noise level, constant lighting, and large number of circulating individuals result in sensory overload, sleep deprivation, and decreased learning opportunities. This environment is not conducive to growth and development (Jackson, 1986).

Children with chronic conditions have a right to grow up in a home with a family; home care provides them with access to this right. Home care promotes the concepts of normalization and self-care. Home care for children dependent on technology begins during the inpatient stay. Ongoing involvement and teaching of parents will make the discharge process smoother. Intensive discharge planning is needed before these children can go home. Collaboration and communication between hospital nurses and home care nurses are a necessity.

In the home, the parents resume the role of the primary caretaker, a role that they may otherwise never have assumed. This requires some adjustment, because the child has been "raised" and cared for by multiple health care providers and the parents have only been "visitors." The goal for this family is to promote attachment and confidence. Parents often have feelings of anger at others for knowing their child better than they do or feelings of incompetence regarding their child's care. Community health nurses can facilitate the goal of attachment and improved parental confidence by treating the parents as equal partners in planning care and by acting as a mentor as parents gain the technical skills needed to provide care. Above all, the nurse should remind parents that the experiences of private interaction with their child will be different and special (Jackson, 1986).

While home care for some children with chronic conditions has many positive assets, several drawbacks also pertain. Often a disruption in the home environment occurs. Living space may be taken up by special equipment and sometimes requires structural adjustments to the home. The needs of siblings must be addressed because they may become an additional caretaker for their sibling or parents may not be able to take them to their activities because of the time and equipment needed by their sibling. The family may feel isolated and have difficulty finding babysitters or caregivers in order to pursue their careers.

Pediatric home care can range from one visit or intervention to a long-term team approach, but it is the family members who must control the home environment. The parents need to be empowered to be the child's advocate and participate fully in decisions regarding the child. It is *not* the intention of home care to create another hospital environment in the home.

Perhaps the greatest impediment to providing high-technology care in the home is the difficulty in obtaining funding. "The funding process involves long waiting periods, negotiations, and evidence that the discharge is well planned" (McCarthy, 1986, p. 333). While third-party payers may pay 100% for inpatient care, that is usually not the case for the same care in the home. Numerous studies have documented the fact that home care is cost effective, yet third-party payers, including governmental agencies, are slow to acknowledge these data.

As equipment manufacturers have responded to the home care needs of children, equipment has become smaller and more portable. This will continue to decrease the most negative component of home care: that of restricting the family to the confines of the home. Portable ventilators, backpacks to carry continuous infusion pumps for toddlers, and motorized wheelchairs for children have opened the community to the child and family. The cost of equipment rental or purchase; the cost of supplies, cleaning agents, and electricity; as well as vender service contracts must all be factored into the cost of home care.

The community health nurse must remember that chronically ill children and children with chronic conditions still need well-child or regular preventive care. In addition interventions and services put in place one year may be totally inappropriate the next—for example, when an infant becomes a toddler. Therefore, the care plan must be revised continually. Nurses need to assess the expectations of the parents. If they are unrealistic, clarification and perhaps more education are needed. Nurses above all must remember that their role is one of partnership with the family. The nurse is a primary resource and the coordinator of the care; the nurse is *not* the primary caregiver.

Home care for children with chronic conditions must provide flexible scheduling in order to allow children to participate in age-appropriate activities. Depending on the situation, school hours may take up half of a child's waking hours; therefore, home treatments need to be scheduled before and after school hours. Another option is to arrange treatments in the child's school environment during nonessential periods.

SPECIFIC CONDITIONS REQUIRING HOME CARE

Children who are considered technology dependent or medically fragile are a growing target population for community health nursing services. Their chronic conditions and needs are multiple and varied. The nursing literature speaks to the special needs of the following groups:

- Terminal hospice care for children with cancer, including family support before, during, and after the death.
- Infants born with spina bifida for whom no surgical correction will be performed.
- Children who are the siblings of children who died of sudden infant death syndrome and who are now on an apnea monitor.
- Children requiring peritoneal dialysis.
- Children with hemophilia receiving cryoprecipitate.
- Children requiring assistance with diabetes control, especially children older than 12 years of age who are ready to learn self-injections and self-blood glucose monitoring.
- Children requiring pain control at home, where routine pain assessments are needed.

Children receiving parenteral nutrition, nasogastric or gastrostomy feedings, or intravenous antibiotics.

THE CHILD REQUIRING USE OF A VENTILATOR

The ventilator-dependent child requires more community and home health services than does almost any other child. There are more than 3000 ventilator-supported children in the United States (Lynch, 1990). Only those who are medically stable and have a motivated family with the time and resources to meet the child's needs are appropriate candidates for care at home. Some areas of the United States do not have licensed home care agencies or qualified nursing personnel who can support ventilator care in the home.

There are benefits to home care for ventilator-dependent children. These children have fewer infections, improved nutrition, increased socialization, and improvement in their motor skills than do children cared for in institutions. However, there is always the risk of an accidental death (Schreiner et al., 1987).

The community health nurse should assist families to maintain a home-like rather than intensive care atmosphere. Keeping the environment safe, simple, and accessible will help to normalize the environment for the child. The increased amount of electrical equipment requires an adequate amount of grounded outlets. It is best that families have two ventilators in case one fails and to increase mobility of the child from one part of the house to another.

In addition to the ventilators, the family must have a suction machine and suction catheters, tracheotomy tubes, and strings as well as vent tubing. For safety, the community health nurse should ensure that the following community services have been informed of this child's status: local fire and rescue units; gas, electric, and telephone companies; the emergency room in the closest hospital; city or township services to ensure street clearing in bad weather; and, if appropriate, the child's school.

For some children dependent on technology, the cost of their home care can decrease health care costs 78 to 87% (Hazlett, 1989; Lynch, 1990). The average length of time that a child is on a ventilator is 1 year; however, many children are dependent on them for years (Schreiner et al., 1987). Costs include the equipment, supplies, oxygen, nursing care, special diets, and therapies. Many cost-related studies, however, do not address the family's out-of-pocket expenses. These expenses may include structural changes to the house to accommodate the child's needs, an intercom system, and the fact that the utility and water bills are frequently two to three times higher. After taking these secondary costs into account, there may not be a significant cost savings. However, the family is together and the child definitely benefits. The child is in a familiar environment surrounded by his family, friends, and pets and can take a greater role in participating in his or her activities of daily living.

Some problems related to home health care have been identified by parents, and these include the lack of parental support groups, the lack of privacy related to home nursing care, the restrictions placed on the parents' travel or social activities, stressful time schedules, disrupted sleeping patterns, insufficient financial assistance, physical and mental exhaustion, and the stress involved in dealing with these conditions (Hazlett, 1989). The result may be marital stress for these families.

Families want to be respected by health care providers for their ability to take care of their child. Parents who are overwhelmed by their required role and who fear being inadequate may have "parent drop-out syndrome" (Byers and Fabian, 1988). These parents may be relieved if the health care worker will "do" the care. The parents may actually become dependent on the community health nurse. This family needs a great deal of support and encouragement to assume its role in the child's care.

Community health nurses should be alert for signs of increased stress and burnout. Sometimes just the simple act of acknowledging the parents' responsibilities can re-energize caretakers. Community health nurses should be aware of any respite care service opportunities in their community and should encourage parents to take advantage of them.

Trends in Child Health Services

Economic trends will continue to have a significant impact on the availability and quality of health care provided to children. Health care services for both wellness and illness need to be available and accessible. Early screening and developmental assessments must be available to *all* children to prevent further disabilities. The provisions of P.L. 99–457 should be available in *all* states and not just those that are financially solvent. These needs are directly related to funding options. Governmental trends must focus on finding sufficient funding for federal and state programs for home care and child care.

One of the primary needs of families is the availability of quality child care resources. In 1987, 60% of women enrolled in AFDC could not take advantage of employment and training programs because of a lack of affordable child care (Frager, 1990). Long-range plans must be developed to assist those families dependent on governmental subsidies to become productive and self-sufficient. An extension of child care includes the need for developing medical daycare facilities.

Improved treatment modalities and survival rates will continue to increase the number of children requiring community home health care services. Community health care agencies must respond to this expanding population. This can be accomplished by having nursing staff who are knowledgeable in growth and development, family dynamics, and public policies affecting children as well as competent in nursing care for acute and chronic illnesses and disabling conditions.

Nursing must be involved as states continue to develop their programs related to the implementation of PL 99–457. Nursing has a long history of working with children with disabilities and children at risk. Nurses are the ideal professionals to coordinate care for these children.

Community health care services cannot just focus on the child with chronic conditions. A refocusing on provision of immunizations to all children is mandatory in light of the recent measles epidemic in the United States (*Measles,* 1990). Public health initiatives and creative community health approaches to decrease the risk factors that result in mortality and morbidity for children are needed. Various tools exist to screen infants and young children for developmental delays.

The role of parents as decision-makers in controlling the care of their children will continue to grow. Parents are recognized as part of the health care team, but many still have not fully taken advantage of their strengths.

The increased emphasis on normalization of children with chronic conditions will enhance the role of school nurses (as per P.L. 94–142). It will also promote home care services for the medically fragile or technology-dependent child (see Chapter 29). The cost effectiveness of home care must continue to be empirically supported, and then the information must be used to change public policy related to third-party funding for home care. The United States must focus on providing sufficient services for child care, home care, and health care for children and adolescents.

Finally the needs of special groups of children must be addressed. Improved quality foster care and adoptions, especially for technology-dependent children, must be developed. Affordable and available group homes and respite facilities must be available to support families to provide continuing quality care for their children as well as be able to meet their own needs. The community health nurse will need to act as a family advocate to encourage the development of an adequate support network.

Community Health Nursing Responsibilities

A primary goal of nursing is to attain, regain, or maintain health for children and their families. This involves the responsibilities of care provider, educator, coordinator, advocate, and developer of public policy.

Provision of direct care requires a knowledge base in child development, family development, and acute and chronic care needs of children. The nurse must have the ability to assess the child's growth and developmental level, identify family strengths and needs, and assess the environment. This information will assist the nurse in planning comprehensive care. Interventions include measures to promote normal growth and development; enhance the nutritional, dental, and immunological status of the child; provide a safe environment; and promote healthy family interactions. As a direct care provider, community health nurses must be able to identify and locate children and families eligible for community resources. It is a challenge for the community health nurse to reach those who are reluctant to use existing health care services.

The responsibility of nurse as educator includes not only teaching parenting skills but also educating the community and schools of their role in PL 99–457. Teaching others to adapt the environment for children with disabilities (*The More We Do Together,* 1985), providing information and resources to parents providing home care to their children, and modifying technology for the home are additional teaching activities. It is also the responsibility of the community health nurse to coordinate education at the time of hospital discharge with information regarding home care needs.

Nurses cannot promote home care without advocating for funds to make it possible. They must participate in health policy development and also identify sources to fund the programs. Community health nurses must be able to identify appropriate sources of services and to provide cost-effective health care. This advocacy role for nursing includes helping parents advocate to get services for their children, ensuring access to quality services and initiating referrals, ensuring public awareness of home management issues, and promoting accessibility of schools and playgrounds for children with disabilities.

The coordinating responsibility is more important for the community health nurse than for the nurse in an acute care setting. In the community, it is important to coordinate comprehensive services by promoting interagency communication and training. As nurses become more involved in developing their roles in P.L. 99–457, this mandated case management role will continue to expand. Because nursing recognizes the changing needs of children, community health nurses recognize the need to update the plan of care on a routine basis as the child develops and his or her chronological age changes.

Nurses cannot only deal with the physical concerns of children; they must also provide emotional support. This includes empowering caretakers, dealing with the fears and home changes affecting siblings, and informing families of available support groups. Nursing will continue to develop new and creative approaches to address the home, educational, and community needs of children.

KEY IDEAS

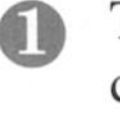
The responsibilities of community health nurses in child health include health promotion, disease prevention, risk reduction efforts, and case manage-

ment as well as home health care for the ill and disabled.

2. Community health nursing care is culturally sensitive and supports the physical, cognitive, psychosocial, and environmental needs of children and their families.

3. Children in the community have many health problems, both chronic and acute. Some of these problems include infectious diseases, chronic illness such as asthma, and environmental risks such as lead exposure and injury. Accidents are the main cause of death of children from 1 to 18 years of age.

4. Children in poverty are at greater risk of health problems (e.g., low birth weight and infant mortality), and exposure to environmental and safety hazards than are children of other income groups. They may also have less access to health care services.

5. Primary prevention and early identification and intervention services are targeted to groups of children and adolescents who are especially at risk of poorer health: children living in poverty, those with chronic illnesses and disabilities, and teenage parents.

6. Public funding for child health services is variable. Eligibility criteria are state determined; thus, children with similar needs may receive funding in one state but may not in another.

7. Children with special needs require multiple resources and services from a variety of agencies. Home care for those children is the most desirable placement. Community resources are not always available to support home care.

8. Community health nurses need to be knowledgeable about resources available within the community to support children and their parents.

9. PL 94–142 and PL 99–457 (now called IDEA) established educational and health care services rights for children with disabilities. These laws provided for public education, school support services, and early screening and interventions to reduce developmental delays and encourage the mental, physical, and emotional development of children with special needs.

10. At present, there is not enough adequate and safe daycare for children of working parents. The need is expected to continue to increase, as well as the need for afterschool care for school-age children of working parents.

11. Community health nurses involved with children's services need to advocate for improved funding, the expansion of existing services, and the creation of policies and additional support services to help families to maximize the health and well-being of their children.

12. Above all, the community health nurse must remember that regardless of age, environmental situation, or physical and mental ability, children are children first. Caregivers should take care to allow them as many of the delights of childhood as possible.

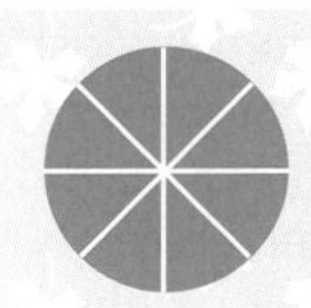

APPLYING THE NURSING PROCESS: *A Developmentally Delayed Child*

Daniel is 6 years old. He lives with his mother and two younger sisters. His parents are divorced, and his mother wants to return to her job as a waitress if she can find affordable child care. Daniel was born with a large myelomeningocele (spina bifida) that was repaired shortly after birth, leaving him paralyzed from the waist down. At 3 months of age he received a ventriculoperitoneal (VP) shunt for hydrocephalus. He has just received his first wheelchair. Home care visits are requested because he has been having frequent urinary tract infections, possibly because he is catheterized every 4 hours. His mental development is slightly delayed (mental age of 5 years), but he is continuing to progress. Daniel is about to start regular school.

Assessment

- Assess the mother's technique for catheterization as well as the technique of significant others who perform the task on Daniel.
- Assess the physical, psychological, and social needs of the child and family.
- Assess the home environment for wheelchair accessibility and safety.

- Assess the school environment for readiness to accommodate the special needs of this child.
- Explore the readiness of Daniel to learn to assist with intermittent clean catheterization.
- Assess the specific health promotion and maintenance activities of the mother and two siblings.

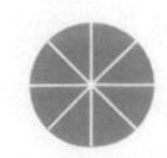

Nursing Diagnosis	Goals	Interventions
Knowledge deficit regarding catheterization by mother as evidenced by increased urinary-tract infections in Daniel.	Daniel's mother will demonstrate improved asepsis when performing a catheterization.	Demonstrate the correct technique for catheterizing a 6-year-old male.
Impaired physical mobility related to new assistive device for lower limbs.	Daniel will adapt to his wheelchair.	Provide anticipatory guidance related to the growth and development needs of the child entering school, as well as his physical, psychological, and cognitive needs. Collaborate with physical therapist.
Impaired home maintenance management related to an environment that is not wheelchair accessible.	Daniel's mother will obtain resources to make the necessary modifications in the home.	Coordinate access to community resources related to finding child care and obtaining resources for home modifications.
Altered role performance related to the inability of the mother to find adequate child care that would allow her to return to work.	Daniel's mother will identify community resources relating to child care for her two younger children.	
Knowledge deficit of school system related to its role in educating a child with a chronic condition.	The school will successfully integrate Daniel into the educational program.	Participate in the development of an individualized education plan with school personnel and the mother. Empower the mother to be her child's advocate by educating her about the rights of children with disabilities.
Possible altered health-seeking behaviors.	The mother and siblings will have current knowledge of immunizations and will have received age-appropriate screening, referral, and anticipatory health guidance.	Teach about home safety, health promotional activities, and the need for immunizations, as appropriate based on the assessment. Refer the mother and Daniel's siblings to financially accessible health care providers.

Evaluation

Effectiveness is measured by:

- The number of urinary tract infections experienced by Daniel will decrease.
- Daniel will demonstrate the ability to utilize his wheelchair.
- The home environment will be modified to be accessible to a wheelchair.
- The mother will find acceptable child care and will return to work.
- Daniel will demonstrate adjustment to the school environment.
- The home environment will be safe for preschoolers and Daniel.
- Daniel's mother and siblings will have current immunizations and will have received age-appropriate screening and referral for treatment of any abnormal findings.

GUIDELINES FOR LEARNING

1. When you were a child, whom did you know who had a chronic condition? How were their needs addressed in your school? How were their needs addressed in the community? What supports were available to their families? How did you and your peers respond to the child with a chronic condition?
2. Interact with and assess a child with a chronic condition. Does he or she appear to focus more on the illness and disability or on the common concerns of childhood?
3. How would you feel if your own child was born prematurely, developed bronchopulmonary dysplasia, and was now ready to be discharged to your home on a ventilator?
4. How would you counsel an unmarried, poor, 16-year-old female who is now pregnant with her second child and who is using cocaine? What anticipatory guidance would you provide, and what community resources would be appropriate for her use?
5. Consider how you might resolve the conflict of promoting health care and preventive measures with poor homeless families who share one room for two families and have no physical resources or utilities? Explore your community's resources. Identify any resources that might meet the needs of this family.

REFERENCES

Ahmann, E. (1986). *Home care for the high risk infant.* Rockville, MD: Aspen Publishers.

American Hospital Association, Section for Maternal and Child Health (1991). *Women, children, and AIDS.* Chicago: Author.

Assuring children's access to health care: Fixing the Medicaid safety net. (1989). Alexandria, VA: National Association of Children's Hospitals and Related Institutions.

Bomar, P. (1989). *Nurses and family health promotion.* Baltimore: Williams & Wilkins.

Bradshaw, M. (1988). *Nursing of the family in health and illness.* Norwalk, CT: Appleton & Lange.

Byers, J., & Fabian, A. (1988). The parent drop-out syndrome. *Caring,* June, 36–38.

Centers for Disease Control and Prevention. (1992). *HIV/AIDS Surveillance report,* 1–18. Atlanta: Author.

Centers for Disease Control and Prevention. (1994). *HIV/AIDS Surveillance report,* 17. Atlanta: Author.

Chamberlin, R. (1989). Home visiting: A necessary but not in itself sufficient program component for promoting the health and development of families and children. *Pediatrics, 84*(1), 178–180.

Children's Defense Fund. (1988). *Annual Report.* Washington, DC: Author.

Children's Defense Fund. (1989). *The Children's Defense Fund looks at America from a special point of view.* Washington, DC: Author.

Children's Defense Fund. (1991). *Outside the dream: Child poverty in America.* Washington, DC: Author.

Committee on Child Psychiatry. (1989). *How old is old enough? The age of rights and responsibilities: Group for the Advancement of Psychiatry, Report No. 126.* New York: Brunner/Mazel.

Committee on Education and Labor, U.S. House of Representatives. (1986). *Education of the Handicapped Act Amendments of 1986.* Report 99–860. 99th Congress, 2nd Session. Washington, DC: U.S. Government Printing Office.

Compilations of data on natality, mortality, marriage, divorce, and induced terminations of pregnancy (May, 1990). *Vital and Health Statistics,* Series 24: Number 1. Hyattsville, MD: U.S. Department of Health and Human Services.

Duvall, E. (1977). *Marriage and family relationships.* Philadelphia: J.B. Lippincott.

English, A. (1990). Treating adolescents: Legal and ethical considerations. *Medical Clinics of North America, 74*(5), 1097–1112.

Faces of the uninsured: Children as the dream deferred (March 18, 1990). Alexandria, VA: The National Association of Children's Hospitals and Related Institutions.

Frager, B. (1990). A national child care crisis: Action for the 90s. *Journal of Pediatric Nursing, 5*(3), 229–231.

Friedman, M. (1986). *Family nursing: Theory and Assessment.* Norwalk, CT: Appleton-Century-Crofts.

Further evidence on the value of the WIC program. (1985). *American Journal of Public Health, 75*(8), 828–829.

Gallagher, J., Trohanis, P., & Clifford, R. (1989). *Policy Implementation and P.L. 99-457.* Baltimore: Paul H. Brookes Publishing Co.

Garwood, S. G., & Sheehan, R. (1989). *Designing a Comprehensive Early Intervention System: The challenge of Public Law 99-457.* Austin, TX: Pro-Ed, Inc.

Hansen, S., Holaday, B., & Miles, M. (1990). The role of pediatric nurses in a federal program for infants and young children with handicaps. *Journal of Pediatric Nursing, 5*(4), 246–251.

Hanson, M., & Lynch, E. (1989). *Early intervention: Implementing child and family services for infants and toddlers who are at risk or disabled.* Austin, TX: Pro-Ed, Inc.

Hazlett, D. (1989). A study of pediatric home ventilator management: Medical, psychosocial, and financial aspects. *Journal of Pediatric Nursing, 4*(4), 284–293.

Infant mortality by marital status of mother—United States 1983 (1990). *Morbidity and Mortality Weekly Reports, 39*(30), 521–523.

Infant mortality—United States, 1989. (1992). *Morbidity and Mortality Weekly Report, 41*(5), 81–85.

Infant mortality—United States, 1991. (1993). *Morbidity and Mortality Weekly Report, 42*(48), 926–930.

Jackson, D. (1986). Nursing care plan: Home management of children with BPD. *Pediatric Nursing, 12*(5), 342–348.

Lynch, M. (1990). Home care for ventilator-dependent children. *Children's Health Care, 19*(3), 169–173.

Malinowski, A. (1989). Maternal-child preventive health home visiting. *Holistic Nursing Practice, 3*(2), 26–29.

Maternal and infant health: Key data (1990). Special Report 1. Washington, DC: Children's Defense Fund.

McCarthy, M. (1986). A home discharge program for ventilator-assisted children. *Pediatric Nursing, 12*(5), 331–335, 380.

McCoy, P., & Votroubek, W. (1990). *Pediatric Home Care.* Rockville, MD: Aspen.

Measles—US, 1989 and first 20 weeks 1990. (1990). *Mortality and Morbidity Weekly Reports, 39*(21), 353–363.

National Center for Health Statistics, 1989. (Dec. 12, 1991). *Monthly Vital Statistics Report, 40*(85).

National Commission on Children. (1991). *Beyond rhetoric: A new American agenda for children and families.* Washington, DC: U.S. Government Printing Office.

Nelson, R. (1989). Community services for children with mental retardation. *Pediatric Annals, 18*(10), 615–621.

Newacheck, P. (1989). Chronically ill children and their health care needs. *Caring,* 4–10.

Oberg, C. (1990). Medically uninsured children in the United States: A challenge to public policy. *Pediatrics, 85*(5), 824–833.

Olds, D., Henderson, C., Chamberlin, R., & Tatelbaum, R. (1986). Preventing child abuse and neglect: A randomized trial of nurse home visitation. *Pediatrics, 7*(1), 65–78.

Potter-Efron, R., & Potter-Efron, P. (1990). *Aggression, family violence, and chemical dependency.* New York: Haworth Press.

Powell, C. & Grantham-McGregor, S. (1989). Home visiting of varying frequency and child development. *Pediatrics, 84*(1), 157–164.

Prevalence of disability in childhood. (Spring, 1988). *Disability Statistics Bulletin,* Number 1. San Francisco: Institute for Health and Aging, University of California.

Raulin, A., & Shannon, K. (1986). PNPs: Case managers for technology-dependent children. *Pediatric Nursing, 12*(5), 338–340.

Schreiner, M., Donar, M., & Kettrick, R. (1987). Pediatric home mechanical ventilation. *Pediatric Clinics of North America, 34*(1), 47–60.

Selekman, J. (1991). Primary care of children with learning disabilities. In P. Jackson, & J. Vessey (Eds.). *Primary care for children with chronic conditions.* St. Louis: Mosby–Year Book.

Selekman, J. (1993). *Pediatric nursing.* Springhouse, PA: Springhouse.

Smith, B. (Ed.). (1988). *Mapping the future for children with special needs: PL-99-457.* Iowa City, Iowa: The University of Iowa.

Statistical Abstracts of the United States 1991. (1991). U.S. Department of Commerce: Bureau of the Census. Washington, DC: U.S. Government Printing Office.

Statistical Abstracts of the United States 1992. (1992). U.S. Department of Commerce, Bureau of the Census. Washington, DC: U.S. Government Printing Office.

Steinmetz, S. (1988). *Family and support systems across the life span.* New York: Plenum Press.

Technology-dependent children: Hospital and home care—a technical memorandum (1987). Washington, DC: U.S. Congress, Office of Technology Assessment, U.S. Government Printing Office.

The more we do together. (1985). New York: World Rehabilitation Fund.

Unintentional firearm-related fatalities among children and teenagers—United States 1982–1988. (1992). *Morbidity and Mortality Weekly Reports, 41*(25), 442–445.

USDHHS. (1990). *Healthy people 2000: National health promotion and disease prevention objectives. Summary report.* Washington, DC: U.S. Government Printing Office.

Vitello, S. (1989). The Detsel case: Limitation of school health services for special education students. *Journal of School Health, 59*(1), 37–38.

Wegman, M. (1991). Annual summary of vital statistics—1990. *Pediatrics, 88*(6), 1081–1092.

Whaley, L., & Wong, D. (1993). *Nursing care of infants and children.* St. Louis: Mosby–Year Book.

SUGGESTED READINGS

Chamberlin, R. (1989). Home visiting: A necessary but not in itself sufficient program component for promoting the health and development of families and children. *Pediatrics, 84*(1):178–180.

Children's Defense Fund. (1992). *The state of America's children.* Washington, DC: Author.

Frager, B. (1990). A national child care crisis: Action for the 90s. *Journal of Pediatric Nursing, 5*(3), 229–231.

Hansen, S., Holaday, B., & Miles, M. (1990). The role of pediatric nurses in a federal program for infants and young children with handicaps. *Journal of Pediatric Nursing, 5*(4), 246–251.

Johnson, C.M. (Ed.), (1991). *Child poverty in America.* Washington, DC: Children's Defense Fund.

Johnson, C.M. (Ed.). (1992). *Vanishing dreams: The economic plight of America's young families.* Washington, DC: Children's Defense Fund.

National Commission on Children. (1991). *Beyond rhetoric: A new agenda for children and families.* Washington, DC: U.S. Government Printing Office.

Robins, L., & Mills, J. (Eds.). (1993). Effects of in utero exposure to street drugs. *American Journal of Public Health,* Suppl. *83*(12), 1–32.

Chapter 27

Elderly Persons in the Community

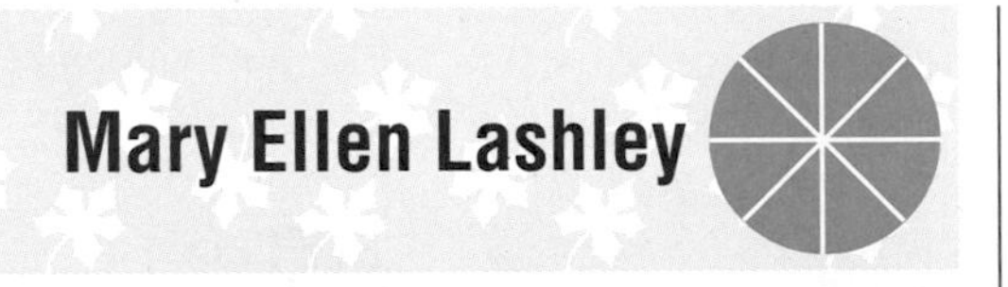

Mary Ellen Lashley

Continued

Focus Questions

What does it mean to be old?

What crises do aging families experience?

What are the common health care needs of elderly persons?

What support systems are available to meet the needs of an aging society?

How have community resources been organized and developed to promote a coordinated and comprehensive system of care for elderly persons?

What are the responsibilities of the community health nurse in meeting the needs of an aging population?

Case Management
Advocacy
Teaching and Counseling
Collaboration

With the growing population of individuals 65 years and older, complex and unique health care needs have emerged that call for knowledge and expertise in the field of gerontology. *Gerontology* has been defined as the study of aging persons and of the process of aging (Borenstein, 1983). The term gerontology is derived from the root word *gera* or *geron* meaning "great age" or "privilege of age" (Spicker et al., 1978).

In 1988 12.4% of the U.S. population was age 65 years or older. It is projected that by the year 2000 13% of the population will be 65 years or older. By the year 2030 approximately 22% of the population will be 65 years or older (U.S. Department of Health and Human Services [USDHHS], 1992). In addition persons 85 years and older are expected to increase seven times by the middle of the 21st century and are projected to be the fastest-growing segment of the U.S. population (USDHHS, 1990a; *Senior Power,* 1987).

Since the profession of nursing comprises the greatest number of health care providers to elderly persons (Ross, 1983), nurses need to be knowledgeable about the unique health care needs of an increasingly aging population. It is particularly important for community health nurses to understand the needs of elderly persons, since 75% of all persons 65 years and over remain independent in the community (Cohen, 1988).

This chapter explores the role of elderly persons in the family and community in light of developmental and sociocultural influences, unique crises experienced by aging families, and need for support systems to assist families coping with the crises of aging. Common health care needs of elderly persons in the areas of nutrition, medication, mobility, and social isolation are reviewed. The influence of poverty is examined in view of its impact on the health of older Americans and the ability of older Americans to secure needed health care services.

Recent trends in legislation for health care and social services for elderly persons that have arisen in response to the changing demography of the U.S. population are examined. These political trends greatly influence the development and organization of community resources for elderly persons. The patterns of organization, the role of the state and local governments, and the social actions taken for the welfare of elderly persons have resulted in the development and organization of nationwide services for them. Finally the responsibilities of the community health nurse as facilitator-collaborator, advocate, teacher, and case manager in working with the elderly client in the community are explored.

Aging

MEANING

What does it mean to be old in contemporary Western society? Is one "old" when he or she reaches the age of 65 years? In 1935 the age of 65 years was adopted by the federal government as the official threshold of "elderliness."

Aging has been defined as a universal human experience that defines human finitude (Lashley, 1989). Aging is a dynamic state of existence that changes with one's perspective. Meanings of old age are based on societal views of aging, cultural beliefs about the meaning of being old, and values associated with old age.

MYTHS

Common myths about elderly persons are that they are frail, senile, unhealthy, unhappy, set in their ways, irritable, lacking in interest in matters of sexuality, and ineffective and undependable as workers (Palmore, 1984). In fact 80% of older persons are healthy enough to engage in normal activities. Although reaction time slows with age, the majority of older persons are not senile and do not have serious memory deficits. Older people are not set in their ways. In fact most have had to adapt to such major life events as retirement, having children leave home, and declining health.

Studies also show that older working Americans work as effectively as their younger counterparts. They change jobs less frequently, have fewer job-related accidents, and have lower rates of absenteeism. The majority of elderly persons also report that they feel relatively satisfied most of the time. Overall elderly persons experience frequent social contacts with friends or relatives, participate in church-related activities or voluntary organizations, and continue to have interest in and a capacity for sexual relations (Palmore, 1984) (Table 27–1).

TABLE 27–1

Some Facts about the Elderly

Some Facts about the Elderly
Three of four elderly persons (75%) live independently in the community; only 5% live in nursing homes
Persons 65 years of age can expect to live for more than 16 more years
Two of three older workers retire before age 65 years
Half of elderly women are widows, many of whom live alone
Elderly persons consume 30% of all prescription medications
Approximately 40% of noninstitutionalized elderly persons have some activity limitation, most frequently related to arthritis
Informal networks of family, friends, and neighbors provide the majority of health and social services to elderly persons

CHRONOLOGY

Chronology is a poor measure of aging, as persons 65 years and over may span an age range of 40 or more years and may experience diverse and unique needs during this time. For this reason some theorists make a distinction between the *young-old* and the *old-old.* The old-old have been defined as persons 85 years and older and the young-old as persons between the ages of 65 and 74 years (*Senior Power,* 1987). Other theorists argue that aging should be defined not in terms of chronology, but in terms of biopsychosocial functioning (Ebersole and Hess, 1990). However aging is defined, a growing aging population is a demographic reality with definite health care implications. An increase in the prevalence of chronic diseases and functional impairments (i.e., the ability to perform activities of daily living) can be expected. The need for health care services for chronically ill persons will increase. An increase in chronic illness and residual disability will necessitate more long-term care. Medical care expenditures will increase in proportion to the greater number of elderly persons in need of health care services. These trends will require that health care providers have a thorough understanding of the unique health care needs of a growing aging population (Andreopoulous and Hogress, 1989).

Role of Elderly Persons in the Family and the Community

Since 1930 the life expectancy at birth has increased approximately 12 years for males and 16 years for females. Since the mid-1960s the older population has grown at a rate twice that of the general population (*Senior Power,* 1987). On the average persons 65 years and older can expect to live an additional 16.4 years. However it is estimated that only 12 of these years will be spent in a state of good health (USDHHS, 1990a).

DEVELOPMENTAL TASKS AND CRISES OF AGING FAMILIES

As persons age they face new challenges, new life experiences, and new life crises. Erikson and co-workers (1986) conceive of the primary developmental task of old age as the achievement of integrity over despair. *Integrity* refers to a sense of wholeness and meaning in one's past and present experiences. *Despair* involves a sense of dread and hopelessness and the feeling that life lacks meaning and purpose. The developmental task of old age includes the reaffirmation of meaning in life and the acceptance of the inevitability of death (Erikson et al., 1986).

Maintaining a sense of wholeness and purpose may represent a challenge in the midst of declining health and significant alterations in major life roles and relationships. Such major developmental life events as retirement, loss of significant others, and the dependency incurred by declining health produce multiple role changes and may precipitate a major life crisis (Ebersole and Hess, 1990; Palmore, 1984).

Retirement as a Developmental Task

Role changes that accompany the aging process are often abrupt and undesired (Ebersole and Hess, 1990). A person's occupation represents a significant societal role that may be interrupted by illness or retirement, both of which may be viewed as undesirable. *Retirement* is a withdrawal from a given service in society; operationally retirement is measured by counting those who are no longer employed full-time (Palmore, 1984). Approximately 26 million persons over 65 years in the United States are retired (Palmore, 1984). Approximately two thirds of older workers retire before age 65 years ("Senior Power," 1987).

Advantages of retirement include freedom from work, greater leisure time, and the eligibility to collect retirement benefits or pensions. Despite these advantages persons may feel useless, unproductive, or worthless on losing this significant role. Men, in particular, who retire unwillingly are at a significant risk for alcoholism, depression, and suicide. For this reason it is important that persons receive adequate support and counseling in preparation for retirement. The community health nurse is uniquely prepared to provide this service. The occupational health nurse can engage in pre-retirement planning with clients in the middle years, long before retirement becomes a reality.

Although federal legislation prohibits mandatory retirement based on age, most workers in private or government sectors may still be encouraged to leave work through early retirement incentive programs (American Association of Retired Persons [AARP], 1988). The community health nurse may be responsible for coordinating pre-retirement planning programs. These programs should include information on attitudes toward retirement, retirement benefits, legal aspects of retirement, the effects of retirement on family relationships, and possible uses of leisure time. AARP, a national organization devoted to the needs of older Americans, publishes a package of training materials for coordinators of pre-retirement programs.

Loss and the Elderly Population

Sixty percent of persons 65 years and older are women (U.S. Bureau of the Census, 1989). Fifty percent of elderly women are widows (AARP, 1989a; *Senior Power,* 1987). The death of a spouse or loss of another significant person through death or relocation (e.g., children leaving home) represent major life crises that require support and intervention. The loss of a loved one is an important predictor of physical and emotional decline in the elderly client. Clients who experience the loss of a spouse or significant other may grieve not only for the lost person, but also for the loss of multiple roles provided by that individual (e.g., loss of a lover, a homemaker, a comforter, a provider). Widows are less likely to remarry than widowers, since elderly women significantly outnumber elderly men. In addition the loss of a spouse may necessitate relocation, which further contributes to the sense of loss and the disruption of integrity in one's life.

As persons age they are likely to experience the death of significant others of their own age and cohort. The loss of a significant other represents the loss of a part of one's past and of life history. The experiences shared with the lost member and the ability to fondly recall memories together is partially lost when the co-creator of these memories is no longer present. Anger, guilt, loneliness, and depression are common outcomes.

The community health nurse may provide support by encouraging reminiscence (i.e., by acknowledging meaningful past experiences and times of distress and by assisting the client to identify past coping mechanisms), assessing for signs of depression and suicidal intention, and assisting clients to grieve. Clients may be referred to support groups in the community that provide an opportunity to share experiences, to draw on others for support, and to establish new relationships.

Declining Health. The multiple losses experienced with aging are represented not only through the loss of significant others but also through the experience of declining health. Although the majority of elderly persons are healthy and rate their health as excellent or good (*Vital Statistics,* 1988), the chance of experiencing a health impairment increases with age. In 1987, approximately 38% of noninstitutionalized persons 65 years and over had some activity limitation owing to chronic illness (*Vital Statistics,* 1988). Twenty-four percent were limited in major activities such as bathing and dressing (U.S. Bureau of the Census, 1989).

Dependency. The likelihood of increased disability with age also increases the likelihood of dependency on others (Weissert, 1985). This increased dependency may produce feelings of guilt, anger, frustration, and depression in clients and their families.

Research indicates that 80% to 90% of health and social services required by the elderly population are provided by informal support systems (e.g., family, friends, or neighbors) (Brody, 1986). Approximately 72% of caregivers are women family members. One third of caregivers live at or near the poverty level and rate their health as fair or poor. Two of three caregivers provide care for at least 1 year. Four of five are involved in caregiving activities 7 days a week. This intense level of caregiving often requires either significant readjustment in employment or job resignation, which may lead to financial burden and a significant alteration in family relationships (AARP, 1988). Since most caregivers are women, they often must balance multiple and competing demands in the family. This problem is compounded by the scarcity of services available to support family caregivers. Finally, the network of informal caregivers (e.g., family and friends) is likely to continue to decrease owing to societal trends such as divorce, fewer children, and geographic mobility (AARP, 1988) (see Ethics Box IX).

With the increase in life expectancy, middle-aged persons may find that four generations are ultimately dependent on them (i.e., young children, grandchildren, parents, and grandparents). In fact, with older age comes changes in family roles and relationships.

Intergenerational dependency and support of the aging family is greatly influenced by marital and health status, culture and ethnicity, and quality of family relationships. Family members need to be recognized as highly significant in promoting the health of older clients. The community health nurse should assess the family support system, anticipate future needs and crises, and help families to plan ahead for potential crises. Family members should be encouraged to discuss their concerns and their past and present coping behaviors. The dependent elderly client should be incorporated into the family's plans as much as possible. The community health nurse can also explore with the family the available resources in the community to meet client and family needs. Common problems encountered in working with an elderly dependent family member include a lack of awareness of services in the community, the need for respite care for families assuming caregiving responsibilities, and the guilt, resentment, and frustration that arise in attempting to provide care and support to the elderly client.

SUPPORT SYSTEMS FOR AGING FAMILIES IN THE COMMUNITY

Since families provide the majority of caregiving to elderly persons, programs for respite and support are needed to improve caregiver coping and to support a continued willingness to care for elderly persons (Koff, 1988). A variety of support systems are available in the community that may assist in meeting the diverse needs of dependent elderly persons and their families (Table 27–2 consists of a directory of national resources specific to the needs of the elderly population). Elderly persons who receive social support are able to function independently for much longer than those who lack these needed services.

Long-Term Care

Long-term care refers to a comprehensive range of health, personal, and social services that are coordinated and delivered over a period of time to meet the changing physical, social, and emotional needs of chronically ill and disabled persons. Long-term care may be delivered in the home, in the community, or in an institutional setting

Ethics Box IX

Gail A. DeLuca Havens, M.S., R.N., C.N.A.

When Roles Reverse: Caring for a Parent

Nancy waves to Mrs. Costello, as she does each day when she passes the older woman sitting on the porch of her daughter's home. Today, though, Mrs. Costello doesn't respond. Puzzled, Nancy finishes her walk. Nancy, a community health nurse clinical specialist and a certified gerontological nurse, practices in the state agency for the aging. Mrs. Costello is the mother of one of her best friends and long-time neighbor, Peggy. After dinner, Nancy telephones Peggy and asks if she may come visit for a few minutes. Peggy sounds welcoming, but her voice is somewhat hesitant.

Nancy is shocked to see the change in Mrs. Costello since she last saw her 2 weeks ago. She is disheveled and smells of urine. Her clothing is stained with food and she appears to have lost weight. Both of her arms are wrapped in elastic bandages and suspended in slings, which explains why she couldn't wave to Nancy this afternoon. Peggy explains that her mother fell this morning and, according to their family doctor, sprained both of her arms. Mrs. Costello looks downward, seemingly to avoid even nonverbal communication with Nancy. Nancy recalls that any unusual trace of what one might consider fear exhibited by an elder in the presumed safe atmosphere of his or her home, or in the presence of a familiar caregiver, is a cue for further assessment (Anderson and Thobaben, 1984). Peggy shows little interest in talking any longer, so Nancy leaves.

The next day Nancy keeps remembering Mrs. Costello's appearance and affect. She is unnerved as she begins to recall other instances of "accidents" that Mrs. Costello has had over the past few months. Nancy realizes that it is possible that Mrs. Costello is being abused by her family. Before Nancy starts out on her walk that evening, she calls Peggy to see whether she would like to join her. Peggy agrees.

During their walk Nancy raises the subject of Mrs. Costello's accidents. Initially Peggy denies any recollection of Mrs. Costello having multiple accidents. She is evasive and becomes somewhat hostile. Then as their walk draws to a close, Peggy begins to cry. She is overwhelmed by the multiple responsibilities in her life. Her mother is requiring increasingly more care and supervision. Peggy's husband is not as understanding of the constraints placed on their spousal relationship by Peggy's responsibility to care for her mother as he was when Mrs. Costello first moved in with them 2 years ago. Peggy tells Nancy that she has far less patience with her mother than she used to have. "It is so frustrating to have to care for a parent as if she were your child. It makes me resentful and angry. And, now that my mother's memory is really beginning to fail, I find that I have much less tolerance for her behavior than I ever did. Nancy, I realize that I am not treating my mother well. You are an expert in caring for the elderly. Would you please help me?"

"Peggy, have you been the cause of the accidents that your mother has had?"

"Yes, but I realize that I have been very wrong in treating her in the way that I have. That's behind me now. I just need help coping."

What should Nancy do?

How should Nancy respond to her friend's call for help? Should she work with Peggy and introduce her to strategies for coping with her mother, give her ongoing support and encouragement, and hope that a positive relationship will be re-established between Mrs. Costello and her family in the process? Or should Nancy talk with Mrs. Costello to determine her wishes in this matter? Should Nancy, even though the problem is unrelated to her work responsibilities, report her findings to the elder ombudsman at the Council on Aging, advocating as she would for any elderly client in the context of her work?

Since family dysfunction can occur gradually over a prolonged period of chronic stress, it is important in a situation of this nature that deliberation be thoughtful and not precipitous (Williams-Burgess and Kimball, 1992). Nancy could talk with Mrs. Costello. It is her right to choose what will happen to her (American Nurses' Association, 1985).

There would be several advantages in a decision that would include Nancy's helping her friend learn

(Continued)

how to cope with her mother. Most important, it would allow Mrs. Costello to continue to live with her family. When the suspicion of elder abuse is reported, removal of the elder to a nursing home often occurs. If Mrs. Costello agreed, having her remain at home, supported emotionally and cared for by her family, would be to her benefit (Anderson and Thobaben, 1984). Helping Peggy would develop skills Peggy needs to cope constructively with the ongoing care of an elder. This expertise would have long-term benefits for Mrs. Costello, as it would enable Peggy, her primary caregiver, to become more skilled in caring for her. This strategy would serve as well to bolster Peggy's self-confidence and belief that she can care for her mother appropriately. Finally such a decision would avoid having to expose Peggy to legal penalties resulting from reported abuse, which would help to maintain the psychological equilibrium and integrity of the family unit. A disadvantage of such a strategy would be the need for Nancy to maintain objectivity in such a situation. Is the successful separation of professional and personal roles a realistic expectation?

Mrs. Costello, however, needs an advocate. She is being physically harmed by her daughter. Given her physical appearance and her affect it is also likely that she is a victim of active neglect, that is, the intentional omission of caregiving activities (Williams-Burgess and Kimball, 1992). Nancy's reporting Mrs. Costello's situation to Adult Protective Services would trigger an investigation and eventual protection of Mrs. Costello from further physical and psychological harm. But would it be in Mrs. Costello's best interest, considering that such protection would most likely be accomplished by removing her from the family unit? Nancy recalls how delighted Mrs. Costello was 2 years ago when she moved into her daughter's home. Nancy must decide what is the greater harm. Another consideration in choosing to report the abuse is the enduring psychological trauma Mrs. Costello and Peggy will experience knowing that mother and daughter must be separated in order to avoid repeated episodes of abuse. Finally, there is the matter of Peggy confiding in Nancy and asking for her help. Is the nature of Peggy's communication with Nancy confidential? If so, given this situation, what obligation does Nancy have to maintain confidentiality?

Another alternative to be considered is respite care for Mrs. Costello combined with counseling for Peggy and/or Peggy and her husband (Patwell, 1986). This approach contains the advantages of removing Mrs. Costello, temporarily, from Peggy's home and of focusing on the family as a unit (Williams-Burgess and Kimball, 1992). Counseling with an expert, other than Nancy, who is not personally involved in the situation could then begin. Since Nancy is familiar with respite and counseling services in the area, she could make recommendations to Peggy from a professional perspective. This strategy has several advantages. It removes Mrs. Costello from harm but on a temporary basis. All things being equal this is a positive intervention, as the plan includes Mrs. Costello eventually returning to her daughter's home. It gives the family the opportunity to receive counseling without the pressure of caring for Peggy's mother. This ought to be a therapeutic arrangement as well as a constructive one, because Mrs. Costello likely will return to her family's care when they become better prepared to cope with the demands and the stress of caring for an elder. Finally such a strategy clarifies Nancy's roles in the situation and avoids the difficulties that often occur when one attempts to blend professional and personal roles. Nancy decides that if Peggy does not seek respite care and counseling, Nancy can then report the situation to Adult Protective Services.

References

American Nurses' Association. (1985). *Code for nurses with interpretive statements.* Kansas City, MO: Author.

Anderson, L., & Thobaben, M. (1984). Clients in crisis. *Journal of Gerontological Nursing, 10*(12), 6–10.

Patwell, T. C. (1986). Familial abuse of the elderly: A look at caregiver potential and prevention. *Home Healthcare Nurse, 4*(2), 10–13.

Williams-Burgess, C., & Kimball, M. J. (1992). The neglected elder: A family systems approach. *Journal of Psychosocial Nursing and Mental Health Services, 30*(10), 21–25.

(AARP, 1988). Long-term care services may be provided to clients who exhibit a degree of functional impairment that necessitates assistance with activities of daily living (e.g., bathing, dressing, toileting, eating) or instrumental activities (e.g., meal preparation, housework, shopping). Twenty-five percent of elderly persons possess at least a mild degree of functional disability or difficulty carrying out personal care and home management activities. Fifty percent of persons 85 years or older have some degree of functional disability (AARP, 1988). Long-term care services focus on assisting the client to maintain independent functioning to the fullest extent possible.

TABLE 27–2

Selected Community Resources for the Elderly

U.S. Department of Health and Human Services
Administration on Aging
330 Independence Ave. S.W.
Washington, DC 20201
(202) 619–0724

Alzheimer's Association
919 N. Michigan Ave., 10th Floor
Chicago, IL 60611
(312) 335–8700

American Association of Homes for the Aging
901 E St. N.W., Suite 500
Washington, DC 20004
(202) 783–2242

American Association of Retired Persons
601 E St. N.W.
Washington, DC 20049
(202) 434–2277

American Association for Geriatric Psychiatry
P.O. Box 376A
Greenbelt, MD 20770
(301) 220–0952

American Geriatric Society
770 Lexington Ave., Suite 300
New York, NY 10021
(212) 308–1414

American Public Health Association
(Section of Gerontological Health)
Suite 300, 1015 15th St. N.W.
Washington, DC 20005–2699
(202) 789–5600

American Society on Aging
833 Market St., Suite 512
San Francisco, CA 94103–1824
(415) 882–2910

American Speech and Hearing Association
10801 Rockville Pike
Rockville, MD 20852–3279
(301) 897–5700

Arthritis Foundation
1314 Spring St. N.W.
Atlanta, GA 30309–2898
(404) 872–7100

Gerontological Society of America
1275 K St. N.W., Suite 350
Washington, DC 20005–4006
(202) 842–1275

Gray Panthers
2225 Pennsylvania Ave. N.W., Suite 820
Washington, DC 20006
(202) 466–3132

The Institute of Retired Professionals
The New School of Social Research
66 W. 12th St., Room 502
New York, NY 10011
(212) 229–5600

National Association for Home Care
519 C St. N.E.
Washington, DC 20002
(202) 547–7424

National Caucus of the Black Aged
1424 K St. N.W., Suite 500
Washington, DC 20005–2410
(202) 637–8400

National Council of Senior Citizens
1331 F St. N.W.
Washington, DC 20004

National Citizen's Coalition for Nursing Home Reform
1224 M St. N.W., Suite 301
Washington, DC 20005
(202) 393–2018

National Institute on Aging
National Institutes of Health
9000 Rockville Pike
Bethesda, MD 20892–0001
(301) 496–4000

National Senior Citizens Law Center
1302 18th St. N.W., Suite 701
Washington, DC 20036
(202) 887–5280

and

1052 W. 6th St., Suite 700
Los Angeles, CA 90017
(213) 482–3550

Older Women's League
National Office
666 11th St. N.W., Suite 700
Washington, DC 20001
(202) 783–6686

Home Care

Because support systems in the community may be confusing, fragmented, or unknown to the family, the community health nurse needs to coordinate in-home and community services to meet family health care needs (AARP, 1988). *Home care* refers to a range of health and supportive services provided in the home to persons who need assistance in meeting health care needs. These services, provided through home health agencies, hospitals, or public health departments, include skilled nursing care, occupational therapy, physical therapy, speech therapy, personal care (e.g., bathing, dressing, toileting), assistance with meals, meal preparation, and housekeeping. The National Association for Home Care represents the facilities and organizations that provide home care services. Various types of home care services are summarized in Table 27–3. The reader is directed to Chapter 29 for an in-depth discussion of home care.

Respite Care

Respite care refers to the provision of temporary, short-term relief to family caregivers (Heckheimer, 1989; AARP, 1985). Trained personnel care for the elderly client while the caregiver is away for a period of hours, days, or even weeks. Respite care services may be sponsored by churches, synagogues, nursing homes, home health agencies, volunteer agencies, or for-profit agencies (AARP, 1985).

Adult Daycare. Adult daycare may serve as an out-of-home form of respite care for family caregivers. Adult daycare centers offer a variety of services for persons who require some assistance but not 24-hour care (AARP, 1985). The centers may provide health and physical care and recreational, legal, and financial services. Transportation is usually provided to the program. Adult daycare provides a structured program for dependent community-based elders who have difficulty performing activities of daily living or who require attention or support during work hours when significant others are not available. Adult daycare programs may provide hot meals, assistance with medications and personal care, counseling, therapy, and recreational activities. The National Institute of Adult Day Care is the national organization representing adult daycare programs. Daycare may be offered through community centers including local senior citizen centers, religious organizations, retirement homes, nursing homes, or hospitals (AARP, 1985, 1986).

TABLE 27–3

Types of In-Home Services

Home-Delivered Meals. Provides hot meals to senior citizens who are housebound or unable to cook.

Friendly Visiting Services. Provides routine home visits to elderly clients who need companionship.

Emergency Response Systems. Provides an immediate and accessible way of notifying appropriate authorities in case of medical emergency.

Telephone Reassurance Programs. A program in which volunteers make daily calls to elderly persons living alone.

Personal Care Services. Provision of household and personal care (such as homemaker and home health aide services) under the direction of a health professional.

Chore Services. Provides help in home maintenance, minor repairs, housecleaning, and yard work.

Data from American Association of Retired Persons (AARP). (1985). *The right place at the right time.* Washington, DC: Author.

Adult daycare may be classified according to its primary objective. *Medical daycare* programs are closely affiliated with hospitals or nursing homes and are aimed at providing comprehensive rehabilitation and/or support services, frequently to clients who have recently been discharged from a hospital. The objective of medical daycare is to restore or maximize physical and mental functioning to the fullest extent possible. *Social daycare* programs are designed to meet the needs of chronically disabled clients and to provide an opportunity for socialization, recreation, monitoring, and other social services. The goal of these types of programs is to maximize physical and social well-being and to prevent or delay hospitalization (Pegels, 1988).

Multipurpose senior centers are community centers that provide lunch programs, home-delivered or congregate meals, socialization, recreational activities, health counseling and screening, information and referral services, and legal and financial counseling services to elderly persons and their families (Heckheimer, 1989; AARP, 1985). Senior centers attempt to meet the needs of both well and frail elderly persons in the community. A senior center often offers adult daycare programs to frail elderly clients.

Community-Based Living Arrangements

Other forms of community-based support systems include *foster care,* in which the elderly client is cared for in a personal residence by a family licensed through a social service agency to provide meals, housekeeping, and personal care services. *Group homes* provide shared living arrangements for a group of older adults who are jointly responsible for food preparation, housekeeping, and recreation. *Congregate housing* describes a variety of group housing options for the elderly in which housing is supplemented by services such as 24-hour security, transportation, recreation, and meals (Koff, 1988). *Life care communities* are one form of congregate housing that provides comprehensive health and social services to the elderly. Residents move from one level to another within the community as their health care needs change (Heckheimer, 1989). Life care communities usually require that the client have financial assets to pay for entry into the community.

Nursing Homes

Although only 5% of the elderly population lives in nursing homes, approximately 20% to 30% of individuals will require nursing home care at some time in their lives. Nursing homes provide continuous nursing care, rehabilitation, social activities, supervision, and room and board in state licensed facilities. Considering nursing home placement is often a painful and traumatic experience for both the client and the family. Families may feel guilt and despair at being unable to maintain their elderly loved one at home. It is important that the older person be involved as much as possible in the decision-making process. The AARP publishes valuable consumer information to assist families in choosing a nursing home that will best meet their needs (AARP, 1985) (Table 27–4 presents a tool for assisting families in making decisions about nursing home placement).

SOCIOCULTURAL INFLUENCES

As a group, the elderly population represent a diversity of beliefs, values, and cultural practices. Differences in beliefs and values may be attributed to ethnic, cultural, and generational influences. Culture is a learned way of thinking and acting. The behavioral, intellectual, and emotional forms of life expression represent a cultural heritage that is passed on from generation to generation.

A *cohort* refers to a group of people who share similar characteristics. People born in the same time period (i.e., within approximately 10 years) represent an *age cohort.* Individuals growing up in different historical eras have lived through similar major life events (e.g., World War II, the Great Depression). These events, however, may affect persons differently depending on their age at the time the events were experienced. Differences in age ranges among elderly persons may span as much as 40 years, indicating that the elderly population is a heterogenous group of people who have lived through a diversity of life experiences that have helped to shape them in unique and unpredictable ways. Therefore when working with elderly clients and their families, the community health nurse should approach each person as unique.

The community health nurse can assess the influence of the client's ethnic and cultural heritage on beliefs, values, and health care practices. Specific areas affected by ethnic and cultural orientation include perception of women's roles, social responses to a growing aging population (changes in legislation, creation of federal programs, emergence of special interest groups), and changes in role performance and opportunities (Matteson and McConnell, 1988). Other significant sociocultural influences include family relationships, customs, and habits; religious practices; diet; work and leisure activities; beliefs about pain, illness, and death; forms of verbal and nonverbal expression; and the ethnic and cultural orientation of the surrounding community. Family rituals and practices that are meaningful to the client and do not pose a threat to health or safety should be respected (Ebersole and Hess, 1990).

A community with similar cultural practices, beliefs, and values tends to reinforce the client's and family's cultural heritage. Foreign-born elderly persons who recently immigrated to the United States may have difficulty communicating in English and may live in a community that is foreign to their cultural orientation. Foreign-born residents may require assistance in locating and utilizing needed community resources including a support network of persons who share in their ethnic heritage and reinforce their cultural practices. The community health nurse may also advocate for the needs of these non–English-speaking persons by increasing community awareness of the need for bilingual service providers, publications, and community announcements (Lacayo, 1984). Services most acceptable to elderly members of ethnic groups are usually those provided in their community by persons who are conversant in their native language and are sensitive to their cultural practices and beliefs (Heckheimer, 1989). (See Chapter 6 for a detailed discussion of cultural influences.)

In general, when examining social and cultural influences, the community health nurse requires knowledge of the historical and cultural traditions that have shaped and influenced the personal life experiences of elderly clients and families. These experiences will exert a significant impact on the client's physical, psychological, social, and economic well-being.

Common Health Needs of Elderly Persons

Four of five elderly persons experience at least one chronic condition, and many suffer from multiple chronic diseases. The likelihood of disability increases with age. Approximately 40% of persons 65 to 74 years and 60% of persons 85 years and older experience some activity limitations as a result of chronic illness (USDHHS, 1990b). A national health objective for the year 2000 is to reduce to no greater than 90 per 1000 population the proportion of persons 65 years and older who have difficulty performing two or more personal care activities; this is intended to preserve the independence of this group (USDHHS, 1990a).

Persons 65 years and older average 32 disability days per year compared with 13 days for persons younger than 65 years. Overall elderly persons account for 884 million days of disability a year. These figures represent days when persons have to reduce their normal activities because of illness or injury, days of confinement to bed, as well as days lost from work or school (U.S. Bureau of the Census, 1989).

The prevalence of chronic disease and disability in elderly persons produces a number of health care needs. Preventive care is also needed for elderly persons who are healthy to maintain wellness and prevent the onset of illness or disability. The community health nurse should encourage such health promotion behaviors as a balanced diet, regular exercise, stress management, routine medical and dental evaluations, monthly breast or testicular self-examination, annual mammography, and influenza (annually) and pneumonia (one time only) immunizations. The reader is directed to Chapters 16 and 17 for an in-depth discussion of health promotion and screening.

TABLE 27–4

Checklist for Selecting a Nursing Home

A: ______________________________

Name of Facility

____

Address

____

City, State, ZIP

____

Telephone Number

B: ______________________________

Name of Facility

____

Address

____

City, State, ZIP

____

Telephone Number

Nursing homes are regulated by both federal and state authorities, but their general atmosphere, policies, and programs vary. The better ones welcome visits and inspections, and the staff should be willing to answer your questions. After you have narrowed your choice to a few homes, the final decision should be based on how well the home matches your (or your relative's) health and social needs. Some of your major considerations in choosing a particular home should be:

- Your need to be close to family, friends, and doctor
- Your need for specific kinds of treatments and services
- The nursing home's accommodation to your personal habits and lifestyle
- The cost and financial situation of the nursing home

Licensing and Certification

A	B	
☐	☐	The nursing home is licensed by the state and is a member of the American Health Care Association or the American Association of Homes for the Aging.
☐	☐	The home is certified for Medicare/Medicaid reimbursement if this coverage is needed.

Services and Fees

A	B	
☐	☐	The nursing home offers the level of care, intermediate or skilled, that is needed.
☐	☐	The home provides complete information on its fees and a sample list of services offered and their costs.
☐	☐	The contract states clearly which services are provided in the basic fee and which are provided at extra cost.
☐	☐	The contract states what action the nursing home will take, if any, if your personal financial resources are depleted and you become eligible for Medicaid. The nursing home assists privately paying residents who have used up their personal resources in making application for Medicaid.

Living Environment

A	B	
☐	☐	The buildings are in good repair and the grounds are well-kept. There are places to walk and sit outside. The nursing home is pleasantly and tastefully decorated. The residents' rooms are well-lighted and comfortably furnished. There is ample drawer and closet space, and toilet and bathing facilities.
☐	☐	The kitchen is well-equipped. Menus are varied and individual food preferences are considered.
☐	☐	There is a warm atmosphere in the residents' dining room. The staff graciously assists residents who need help.
☐	☐	Nurses and attendants are highly visible and treat residents with dignity and respect. The staff is cheerful and helpful.
☐	☐	Good custodial care is provided to residents who require it.

Resident Activities

A	B	
☐	☐	There is an active social director and a varied program of recreational and social activities. Residents' birthdays and holidays are celebrated. Volunteers come to entertain, instruct, and work with residents.
☐	☐	Residents seem to be neat, comfortably dressed, and active (playing games, watching television, reading, writing, knitting, doing handicrafts, visiting each other, walking, and exercising).
☐	☐	There are planned trips to concerts and exhibits. Transportation is available for residents who want to go to religious services or out shopping.
☐	☐	There are religious services of the resident's choice and opportunity for contact with clergy.

From AARP. (1985). *The right place at the right time: A guide to long-term care choices* (pp. 46–47). Washington, DC: Author. Reprinted with permission.

TABLE 27–4

Checklist for Selecting a Nursing Home *Continued*

Emergency Care

A	B	
□	□	Nurses are on hand 24 hours a day to follow doctors' instructions and to handle emergencies.
□	□	A physician is available in an emergency.

Residents' Rights

A	B	
□	□	The "Residents' Bill of Rights" is prominently displayed.
□	□	There is an active resident council or committee to represent the interests of residents.

Staff and Training

A	B	
□	□	The nursing home has, in addition to an administrator, a director of nursing, a full-time social worker, and an activities' director.
□	□	The home requires nursing aides to be trained and provides additional training while on the job.

NUTRITIONAL NEEDS

Nutritional needs in elderly persons may be affected by normal physiological changes associated with aging and psychosocial and environmental factors that affect nutrition (Table 27–5).

Dietary planning should take into consideration cultural preferences, religious observances, behavioral patterns (e.g., timing of meals), and special dietary needs (e.g., low-fat, cholesterol, diabetic, low-salt). Eliciting a diet history may help the community health nurse to identify dietary patterns and habits. General nutrition education should stress adherence to a balanced diet; maintenance of ideal body weight; limited intake of alcohol, fats, and sugars; increased intake of dietary fiber; and avoidance of excessive salt intake (USDHHS, 1990a).

TABLE 27–5

Factors Influencing Nutrition in Elderly Persons

Physiological Factors

Decrease in digestive enzymes and in intestinal motility
Activity reduction
Dental problems (e.g., poorly fitting dentures may limit intake and predispose to nutritional deficiencies)
Sensory losses (e.g., decreased taste, vision, hearing)
Physical illness

Psychosocial Factors

Inadequate income to purchase nutritional foods
Lack of motivation to prepare balanced meals (e.g., client lives alone)
Inadequate knowledge of basic nutrition
Depression
Grief
Substance abuse

Environmental Factors

Accessibility of shopping areas
Adequacy of space and equipment to store and prepare food

Data from Morton, P. (1983). *Health assessment in nursing* (2nd ed.). Springhouse, PA: Springhouse; Heckheimer, E. (1989). *Health promotion of the elderly in the community.* Philadelphia: W.B. Saunders; and AARP. (1987b). *How does your nutrition measure up?* Washington, DC: Author.

Decreases in hearing, vision, and taste may decrease food appeal. In addition, clients may be unwilling to eat in noisy, public places. When eating out, quiet, well-lit dining areas should be sought to enhance the dining experience (Heckheimer, 1989).

Decreases in intestinal motility may predispose clients to constipation and overuse of laxatives. Fluid and fiber should be incorporated into the diet to compensate for decreases in intestinal motility. For clients who prefer not to cook for themselves or who have difficulty getting to the store, the community health nurse may wish to investigate home delivery services provided through neighborhood groceries, home-delivered meal services (e.g., Meals on Wheels), or congregate eating programs. The local senior center may provide transportation for shopping or "eating together" programs in which seniors gather for a hot meal in a group setting. Clients experiencing financial difficulties may be eligible for the federal food stamp program. Nutritional information for seniors is available through the National Institute on Aging and the AARP.

MEDICATION USE

Elderly persons consume approximately 30% of all prescription medication and pay more than $9 billion annually for prescription drugs (AARP, no year; Santo-Novak and Edwards, 1989). Older clients are at a higher risk for adverse drug reactions because of (1) normal aging changes that affect the absorption, distribution, metabolism, and excretion of drugs in the body; (2) conditions such as bed rest, dehydration, congestive heart failure, and stress that affect the body's response to drugs; and (3) the use of multiple drug regimens to treat concurrent health problems (Heckheimer, 1989; Santo-Novak and Edwards, 1989).

Elderly persons usually take drugs over long periods for chronic conditions. About 25% to 50% of elderly persons who take prescription medications are noncompliant (Jenike, 1989). The reasons for noncompliance are numerous and include the following:

- Lack of finances
- Lack of knowledge of the reason for taking medications or the nature of the illness
- Conflicts with cultural or religious beliefs
- Sense of hopelessness about getting better
- Inaccessibility of pharmacy services
- Complexity of drug regimens
- Inadequate supervision
- Inability to open drug container owing to sensory-motor impairments
- Desire to avoid unpleasant side effects
- Fear of drug dependency
- Failure to discard discontinued or outdated medications
- Pill sharing
- Failure to report self-medication with over-the-counter drugs

Among persons misusing over-the-counter drugs, laxative dependency is most common (Heckheimer, 1989; Jenike, 1989; Patsdaughter and Pesznecker, 1988).

Drug misuse may occur through errors in prescription, the use of prescription drugs without physician supervision, or physician overprescription. In addition lack of knowledge of how to take medications properly, self-medication without physician consultation, or receiving medications from multiple physicians without each provider's knowledge may contribute to drug misuse. Age- and disease-related conditions and multiple drug regimens also compound the problem and may lead to adverse drug reactions or drug overdose (Jenike, 1989; Lamy, 1986).

To improve patient compliance the community health nurse working with the elderly client should assess all prescription and over-the-counter drugs in use, including vitamin and mineral supplements, by obtaining a thorough drug history. Elderly clients should be monitored for adverse drug reactions, potential interactions between drugs, and compliance with prescribed regimens. The community health nurse should teach the client and family about the purpose, use, appropriate dosage, and side effects of all drugs. Instructions should be given verbally and in writing to facilitate retention of information. For clients with memory impairment a calendar or schedule may be developed for taking medications; times for taking medications may be associated with daily activities, such as meals or bedtime (Ebersole and Hess, 1990; Ascione and Shimp, 1988; Haynes et al., 1987).

The client may be advised to select pharmacies that are able to monitor the client's complete medication profile and alert the client and health care provider to potential adverse drug interactions. Providers are also responsible for explaining drug use and seeking validation of client understanding. Clients may request large-print medicine labels to facilitate readability and flip-off (versus child-proof) caps to allow for ease of opening. The community health nurse may also investigate pharmacies that offer discounts to senior citizens and generic drugs to decrease the cost of medications.

In addition to medication misuse owing to lack of knowledge or physical or cognitive impairment, the elderly client may abuse drugs in an attempt to cope with depression and loss. Substance abuse is difficult to identify in the elderly client, because family members may attempt to protect the client by covering up the problem. The problem may only become visible when the behavior of an individual living alone begins to draw the attention of others. For example neighbors may become concerned when basic home repairs are not made, or family members, on visiting the client, may find their loved one unkempt or poorly nourished. The community health nurse can develop outreach programs to reach older persons who are drug-dependent and to educate the public and health professionals about the unique causes and manifestations of substance misuse and abuse in the elderly population (Ascione and Shimp, 1988; Haynes et al., 1987). (See Chapter 21 for a detailed discussion of substance abuse in the community.)

MOBILITY

Each year approximately 150,000 elderly persons injure themselves in falls; 9500 die as a result. The risk of falling is increased in elderly persons owing to confusion, disturbances in gait, alterations in musculoskeletal functioning, medication side effects, unfamiliarity with new surroundings, poor eyesight, and orthostatic hypotension, which may produce dizziness and syncope (Berryman et al., 1989).

Arthritis is the leading cause of morbidity in persons 65 years and older (USDHHS, 1992). Approximately 53% of noninstitutionalized persons 65 years and older suffer from arthritis (U.S. Bureau of the Census, 1989). The loss of muscle strength, painful joints, and stiffness affect gait and limit range of motion (Morton, 1993).

Osteoporosis is a condition that is prevalent in postmenopausal women and in men older than 80 years. Estrogen deficiency accelerates the loss of bone mass associated with aging and may lead to back pain, deformity, or loss of height due to osteoporotic bone changes. Clients with osteoporosis are at a greater risk of sustaining fractures with little or no trauma.

Activity limitations imposed by chronic illness serve to further compromise mobility in the elderly client. Approximately 19% of persons 65 years and older experience gait disturbances. Ten percent have difficulty going outside. Twenty-four percent are limited in major activities such as bathing and dressing (U.S. Bureau of the Census, 1989).

The community health nurse may assist the elderly client to maintain flexibility, muscle strength, and bone mass through counseling about sound nutritional practices and urging adoption of exercise programs that strengthen muscle and improve cardiovascular functioning. Walking, calisthenics, water aerobics (calisthenic exercises performed in a swimming pool), or cycling on a stationary bicycle are examples of activities that provide an excellent form of exercise with a minimum degree of stress on joints (Graham, 1991). Active, passive, and resistive range-of-motion exercises may be employed to promote activity in clients who are bed-bound.

All five senses become less acute with age. Sensory impairment affects both perception and the ability to move around in the environment. Approximately 20% of all persons 65 years and older report visual difficulties (Heckheimer, 1989). One of every 20 Americans 85 years or older is legally blind (Salmen, 1988). The leading causes of blindness in persons 65 years and older include glaucoma (increased intraocular pressure), macular degeneration (which leads to loss of central vision), cataracts (a clouding or opacity of the lens of the eye), and diabetic retinopathy. These conditions may lead to a decrease in visual acuity, a decrease in depth perception, a decrease in peripheral vision, a decreased tolerance to glare, and a decreased ability of the lens of the eye to focus on objects. Visual and hearing impairments may mask warning signs in the environment, predisposing elderly persons to accidental injury. When caring for clients who have sensory impairments that may compromise mobility, the community health nurse needs to identify hazards in the environment, teach the client and the family about home safety, and promote an environment that encourages both independence and safety (Heckheimer, 1989).

Information about transportation services for elderly clients may be gotten by contacting the local office on aging or the local senior center. The area agency on aging may contract with a local taxi company to provide transportation to seniors at a discounted rate. In some localities mass transit buses and subways receive federal funding from the Department of Transportation and provide discounted rates for senior citizens (Heckheimer, 1989; Pegels, 1988). These discounts may be available on a 24-hour basis or restricted to non–rush-hour times. Medicare cards may enable the elderly client to ride at half fare, or reduced fare cards may be obtained from the local office on aging. The American Red Cross may provide emergency transportation when an elderly client is discharged from a hospital or emergency room (Heckheimer, 1989). Local governments or community agencies may also sponsor "senioride" programs, which provide door-to-door transportation to elderly persons at a minimal cost.

SOCIAL ISOLATION

It is estimated that 31% of persons 65 years and older live alone (AARP, 1984). The high percentage of elderly persons living alone coupled with the prevalence of sensory-perceptual and mobility impairments, cognitive impairment, and chronic illness place the elderly client at a higher risk for social isolation.

Mental Health Disorders

Social isolation may be a symptom of a mental health disorder. Depression and dementia are the two most common mental health disorders in elderly persons.

Depression. It is estimated that 10% to 65% of elderly persons may experience depression. Depression may be characterized by a persistent sad or depressed mood (i.e., at least 2 weeks), loss of pleasure in previously enjoyable activities, impaired thinking and concentration, or recurrent thoughts of death or suicide. Depressed clients may also experience insomnia or hypersomnia (increase in sleep), early morning awakening, loss of interest in activities, feelings of guilt, fatigue, loss of appetite, weight gain or loss, agitation, and feelings of helplessness or hopelessness (Blazer, 1989; Jenike, 1989).

Geriatric depression may be brought on by actual or perceived losses, environmental stresses, neurological or endocrine disorders, adverse effects of medication, or infection (Jenike, 1989). Treatment of depression in elderly persons may be delayed or never pursued, since sadness and loss are often thought to be a normal consequence of aging. Depression may also be inappropriately regarded as a normal consequence of senility. Depression may not be identified early in clients who live alone and have few social contacts. Elderly depressed clients may report anxiety, physical symptoms such as chronic pain or worries about the body, or a loss of concentration and difficulties with memory.

The elderly population accounts for 17% to 25% of suicides in the United States (Brant and Osgood, 1990). Men 65 to 74 years of age have the highest suicide rate in the United States (USDHHS, 1990a). Elderly persons who live alone, perceive themselves as friendless, have few meaningful attachments to the community, and have little social support are more vulnerable to psychiatric illness, depression, and suicide (Osgood, 1988). Warning signs of suicidal intent include verbal clues indicating a desire to commit suicide (e.g., "others would be better off without me"), behavioral clues such as getting personal affairs in order or changing one's will, and situational clues (e.g., significant loss, death of spouse, diagnosis of illness, recent undesired move, family conflict) (Osgood, 1988).

It is important for the community health nurse to monitor for signs and symptoms of depression and to refer clients to the appropriate resources for medical evaluation, counseling, and support. Clients who are struggling with feelings of worthlessness and low self-esteem may also benefit from therapeutic reminiscence. Reminiscence may be helpful in assisting persons to come to terms with previous painful life experiences (Lashley, 1993). The notion of *reminiscence* or *life review* involves a reflection on past life experiences with the goal of building self-esteem and understanding, stimulating thinking, transmitting a cultural heritage, and finding meaning, worth, and acceptance in life. Reminiscence is, in essence, the sharing of one's life story (Lashley, 1992; Nussbaum et al., 1989; Ryden, 1981).

A story recounts the joys and struggles of human experience and links the different ways in which a person comes to perceive events (Novak, 1971). Persons may be assisted in telling their stories through involvement in activities that invite storytelling (e.g., sharing memorabilia and family pictures; participating in reminiscence support groups; constructing family trees or scrapbooks; writing or audiotaping a personal autobiography; creating safe, supportive environments that permit disclosure; and demonstrating a nonjudgmental, open, accepting attitude to the client's disclosures) (Lashley, 1992; Ryden, 1981) (Fig. 27–1). The community health nurse can teach the family the value of reminiscence and techniques for facilitating reminiscence, and can thereby assist persons in finding meaning in their memories and coming to terms with unresolved life conflicts.

Dementia. Dementia is a serious cognitive impairment involving thought, memory, or personality (Jenike, 1989). Dementia is prevalent in approximately 5% to 10% of persons older than 65 years and in 20% to 40% of persons who have reached the age of 80 years (USDHHS, 1990a). Dementia may be caused by a variety of diseases (Leroux, 1986).

The term *pseudodementia* describes cognitive deficits that mimic organic mental disorders but that are reversible when the underlying condition is treated. Pseudodementia may be caused by depression, social and environmental stresses, sensory-perceptual impairment, or side effects of medications (Jenike, 1989). Often clients with depression are inappropriately diagnosed as having dementia because of the memory impairments that may accompany the depressed state.

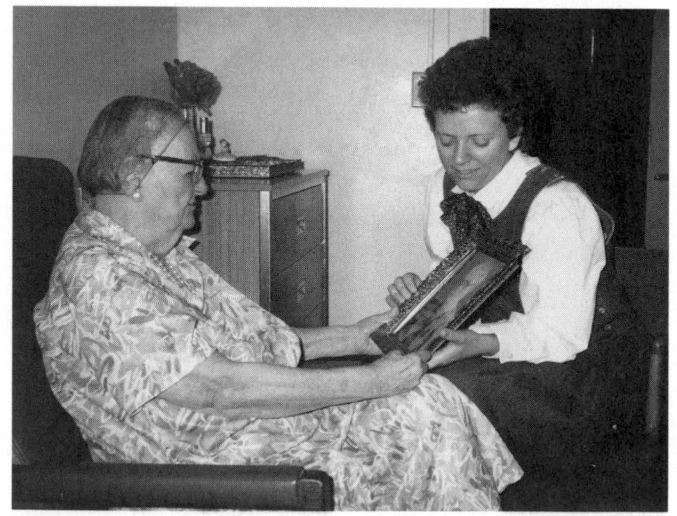

Figure 27–1 ● A community health nurse reminisces with a client. (Courtesy of Dr. Edna Fordyce, Associate Professor of Psychiatric-Mental Health Nursing, Towson State University, Towson, Md.)

More than $10 billion spent on nursing care in 1982 was spent on clients with dementing illnesses. Approximately 50% of nursing home beds are occupied by clients with dementia (Jenike, 1989). The most common form of irreversible dementia in the elderly person is senile dementia of the Alzheimer type (SDAT) or Alzheimer's disease. This disease affects approximately 5% to 7% of all persons aged 65 years and older and approximately 20% of persons aged 80 years and older (Jenike, 1989; Whitbourne, 1985). Alzheimer's disease is the leading cause of cognitive impairment in elderly persons and is the fourth leading cause of death in adults (USDHHS, 1990a; Leroux, 1986).

The exact cause of Alzheimer's disease is unknown. The diagnosis is established by ruling out all other possible causes of dementia. Ultimately the diagnosis can only be positively confirmed at autopsy, at which time distinct changes in the brain may be evident. The disease is progressive, presenting initially with subtle changes in memory and personality (e.g., decrease in attention span, forgetfulness, losing or misplacing items). The disease progresses over a period of years to complete disorientation, extreme agitation or apathy, incontinence, complete loss of self-care ability, and loss of language (Heckheimer, 1989; Jenike, 1989).

Respite care and eventual nursing home placement may need to be considered for the client with Alzheimer's disease. Unfortunately, not all nursing homes are able to accommodate clients with Alzheimer's disease. The Alzheimer's Association is a family-established, volunteer-operated, national organization that provides family support, education, advocacy, referral services, and research funding. Local chapters within the community sponsor family support groups.

Families caring for clients with Alzheimer's disease will also likely require legal and financial consultation. Legal consultation is needed to assist the family in getting the client's legal affairs in order before he or she is no longer competent to make legal decisions regarding medical care and handling of property and assets. Financial consultation is needed to assist the family in preparing for the financial burden likely to be incurred as the client's condition deteriorates and he or she requires greater assistance in meeting personal and health needs. The Alzheimer's Association may supply families with referrals for these important services. Referrals for legal services may also be obtained through the local department on aging, the local legal aid society, the local bar association, or legal clinics in law schools (Heckheimer, 1989).

Hearing Loss

Hearing loss may contribute to social isolation because of the embarrassment or frustration that sensory-impaired persons experience when they are unable to hear and respond appropriately in social settings or because of the stigma associated with hearing loss. Approximately 30% to 50% of persons 65 years and older experience hearing loss significant enough to interfere with their ability to communicate (Calvani, 1985). The community health nurse may assess for the presence of a hearing impairment and refer the client for audiological evaluation and treatment. The community health nurse provides support, counseling, and advice on locating affordable resources (e.g., funding for a hearing aid that is not covered by Medicare) and securing appropriate intervention.

Incontinence

Incontinence, or the involuntary loss of urine or stool, is a significant cause of disability and dependency in the elderly population. Fifteen percent to 30% of noninstitutionalized elderly persons experience urinary incontinence. Incontinence may contribute to social isolation through embarrassment, feelings of loss of control, low self-esteem, and infantilization ("Reaching a Consensus," 1989). The community health nurse works with the older client and family to assist them in coping with this serious problem. Interventions may include encouraging regular toileting, teaching Kegel exercises (a series of exercises that strengthen the pelvic floor), or investigating pharmacological options with the client.

Victimization

Elderly persons are vulnerable to being victimized. Because of increased dependency and the potential for chronic health impairment, elderly individuals may be placed in situations in which they are less able to advocate for their own needs. Elderly persons may be abused or neglected by caregivers or be victims of criminal practices.

Elder Abuse and Neglect. Families experiencing the stress of caring for a chronically ill member are at a high risk for elder abuse or neglect. More than 1 million elderly persons in the United States are victims of abuse. One of every 25 elders are abused in the United States each year. Elderly persons rarely report acts of abuse. This failure to report abuse or neglect may be due to physical or mental impairment; fear of injury, retaliation, or abandonment; or fear of not being believed or taken seriously (Heckheimer, 1989). (See Chapter 20 for a detailed discussion of family violence.)

Criminal Victimization. Concerns over criminal victimization may contribute to social isolation in the elderly by breeding suspicion, mistrust, and fear of leaving home. Although the incidence of crime is no higher in the elderly population than in the general population, the consequences of criminal victimization may be greater (Ebersole and Hess, 1990). For example a client who has been physically assaulted may sustain a hip fracture during a fall. Recovery may involve bed rest or other mobility limitations that may increase the client's risk of developing pneumonia.

Crime is a major concern of the elderly because of their heightened sense of vulnerability (Garcia and Luck, 1987). Elderly clients who are frail and live in inner city neighborhoods where the incidence of crime is high are often prime targets for criminal victimization, such as robbery and assault. The most frequently performed crimes against elderly persons are purse snatchings, fraud, thefts of checks from the mail, vandalism, and harassment (Heckheimer, 1989). The community health nurse works with older clients in the community to educate them about crime prevention, protection from fraud and harassment, and sources of emotional, financial, and legal assistance should they experience criminal victimization (Garcia and Luck, 1987).

Impact of Poverty on Elderly Persons

In the last decade the income status of the elderly population has improved owing to an increase in Social Security benefits (i.e., the National Retirement Income Supplement Program) and improvements in private pension plans. Even so, on retirement the elderly may experience a 40% to 60% drop in income (Streib, 1984). In the final report of the 1981 White House Conference on Aging, the federal government acknowledged the importance of older persons receiving income sufficient to maintain at least a minimum level of comfort and dignity.

Approximately 13% of elderly individuals live at or near the poverty line (Grau, 1988). Poverty levels are higher for minorities, women, and persons 85 years and older (AARP, 1984, 1988). Elderly widows are primary victims of poverty. Three of four elderly poor persons are women. Both elderly men and elderly women may have inadequate pension income due to prior limited employment opportunities, frequent job changes, or low-wage jobs with no employer-sponsored pension plans. In addition women may experience lower pension income due to interruption in work history as a result of child-rearing or cessation of pension related to death of a spouse (AARP, 1988; Streib, 1984).

Since elderly persons often have inadequate cash income available for immediate expenses they may deprive themselves of needed goods and services to avoid selling their homes (Ebersole and Hess, 1990). In addition few pensions protect against inflation, an economic reality that significantly affects income adequacy over the years (AARP, 1988). Fortunately Social Security benefits are indexed for cost of living. However benefits are reduced if the recipient earns in excess of a certain amount of money. This practice has been called into question as an unfair penalty for older workers (AARP, 1988). Finally some pension plans may place a ceiling on the maximum years of credited service (AARP, 1988).

For many elderly persons 65 years and older, Social Security payments constitute the sole source of income. The elderly population constitutes the heaviest users of health services, and health care spending in this group accounts for a third of the personal health care expenditures in the nation. Despite the benefits of Medicare, elderly persons spend approximately 15% of their income on medical care (AARP, 1988). As discussed in Chapter 5, Medicare does not cover costs and services such as deductibles, co-insurance premiums, additional charges when Medicare rates are not accepted as full payment, and charges for noncovered services such as long-term care, dental care, eyeglasses, hearing aids, and preventive care (Pegels, 1988). Often older persons must purchase additional supplemental insurance (referred to as "Medigap" policies) to cover the gaps in Medicare coverage. Consequently elderly persons who cannot afford to pay for services not covered by Medicare or for Medigap policies may be denied access to needed services. In addition many elderly poor do not qualify for Medicaid, which is the joint federal and state health care program for low-income persons, because some states set Medicaid eligibility requirements below the federal poverty line (AARP, 1988).

Although new legislation in recent years has allowed elderly persons to maintain a portion of their assets and remain eligible for Medicaid, many nursing home residents still must deplete their financial assets and become financially destitute before receiving federal aid. Costly long-term nursing home stays often leave both the client and his or her spouse impoverished (AARP, 1988). Persons at greatest risk of "spending down" their economic assets to reach Medicaid eligibility levels include those suffering from chronic debilitating illness who are of moderate income and lack informal family support to assist in their care (Grau, 1988).

Poor elderly persons may lack available, affordable health care services, the transportation needed to reach these services, or the knowledge of where to look for services. Services that are fragmented, inadequately covered, and inaccessible leave significant gaps in health care. Since elderly persons often demonstrate multiple health care needs they require a comprehensive continuum of services that are integrated and coordinated (AARP, 1988).

An encouraging trend in federal initiatives for low-income elderly individuals is legislation that went into effect on June 12, 1992. Under the Omnibus Reconciliation Act of 1990, reimbursement is provided for health promotion and screening activities for Medicare patients through federally qualified health centers (FQHC) in medically underserved, low-income areas. Preventive services amenable to reimbursement include physical examinations, immunizations, cholesterol checks, urinalyses, thyroid function tests, hearing screening, and counseling related to diet and exercise, substance abuse, and injury prevention ("Federal Register," 1992).

Development and Organization of Community Resources

Community resources have been established historically through federal, state, and local initiatives that have effected needed social action for the welfare of elderly persons. Several pieces of important legislation have been passed to assist in meeting the needs of older Americans.

SOCIAL SECURITY ACT

In 1935 the Social Security Act was passed in response to economic hardships arising from the Great Depression (White House Conference on Aging, 1981). This act provided for a national retirement income system and a system of federal grants to assist states in providing support to aged, disabled, and blind persons and to dependent children (Pegels, 1988).

In 1965 *Title 18* of the Social Security Act established Medicare, a federal program providing hospital and medical insurance to persons entitled to social security. Nearly all members of the nation's elderly population are covered by Medicare (White House Conference on Aging, 1981). *Title 19* of the Social Security Act was enacted to provide health care coverage for low-income persons. Finally, *Supplemental Security Income* is a federally funded program that ensures a minimum monthly income to aged, blind, and disabled persons who are not covered by Social Security or for whom Social Security is insufficient (White House Conference on Aging, 1981).

OLDER AMERICAN'S ACT

The Older American's Act (OAA), enacted in 1965, constituted an important piece of federal legislation in promoting the welfare of elderly persons. This legislation set forth congressional policies related to aging, defined responsibilities of state and local governments, and provided for demonstration projects, research, and training programs (Pegels, 1988). The OAA called for better coordination of resources and state assistance in developing new programs for elderly persons; it established a network of state and local *area agencies on aging* (AAAs), which are responsible for planning, coordinating, and funding local services and programs for persons 60 years and older (AARP, 1987a).

In 1981, an amendment to the OAA mandated the development of a *State Ombudsman Program* to provide liaison services between nursing home residents and their families and nursing home administration. The state-appointed ombudsman investigates problems and complaints in skilled nursing, residential care, and other health-related facilities and works with the health care administration to resolve grievances. Currently every state must have an ombudsman to investigate grievances and monitor long-term care (AARP, 1989).

Title 2 of the OAA established the *Administration on Aging* (AOA) as a division of the federal Department of Health and Human Services. The focus of the AOA is the development and coordination of federal programs for elderly persons.

Title 3 of the Older Americans Act provided for programs for elderly persons to be established at a state level. The *State Unit on Aging* (SUA), an office within each state government, was established to develop a statewide plan for providing services to elderly persons.

The OAA, then, laid the foundation for the development of a *National Network on Aging* (NNOA). The NNOA is a program for establishing and maintaining a coordinated, nationwide system of services for elderly persons. It is nationally coordinated and funded, but it is locally administered and organized (Pegels, 1988).

SPECIAL INTEREST GROUPS

In addition to federal, state, and local government initiatives, special interest groups and organizations may serve as advocates in effecting needed social action for the welfare of older Americans. The most notable group is the AARP, the nation's largest nonprofit, nonpartisan organization of individuals 50 years and older. The AARP offers a variety of membership benefits and educational and community service programs that are provided through a national network of volunteers and local chapters. In addition AARP is an effective lobbying group at both the federal and the state levels (AARP, 1987a).

Other senior advocacy and political action groups, such as the Gray Panthers, the National Council of Senior Citizens, the National Retired Teachers' Association, and the National Caucus on the Black Aged, work independently or in cooperation with other organizations to advocate for the needs of the elderly population and to promote legislation that preserves and protects the rights of older Americans. Because a higher percentage of elderly persons vote than do their younger counterparts, the elderly population is recognized as a powerful political force.

Trends in Health Care Services for Elderly Persons

America has witnessed tremendous changes in health care policies and priorities as the number of older Americans has continued to grow. Major social policy issues and concerns, centering on the aging of the "baby boom" population (i.e., those born from 1945 to 1964) and the reduced birth rate of succeeding cohorts necessitate that younger people bear a heavier burden in paying for retirement, Social Security, and health benefits for aged persons in the future. The condition of the economy is also likely to affect the ability of older Americans to care for themselves and the ability of the government to provide needed support. Finally the need for long-term care will continue to escalate as the population ages. Current problems in long-term care include fragmentation of services, high cost of services, difficulty locating and utilizing appropriate resources, limited funding for long-term care, insufficient community-based alternatives to nursing home care, and inadequate support to family and informal support networks that provide the greatest amount of long-term care to elderly persons (White House Conference on Aging, 1981).

NATIONAL CONFERENCES ON AGING

In the wake of these concerns and in response to the changing demography of the population, the White House has sponsored four National Conferences on Aging. The most recent National Conference on Aging was held in 1981. Major recommendations from this conference are summarized in Table 27–6.

TABLE 27–6

Summary of White House Conference on Aging 1981 Recommendations

1. Strengthen the Social Security system
2. Enact legislation to prohibit mandatory retirement
3. Increase the availability of home- and community-based care
4. Improve long-term care alternatives and facilitate continuity of long-term care
5. Place greater emphasis on preventive health care through programs aimed at health promotion and disease prevention. Suggested health promotion activities include:
   a. Supporting persons against social isolation and loneliness
   b. Providing appropriate recreational and social facilities
   c. Fostering knowledge of multiple medication regimens
   d. Screening for early detection and treatment of disease
   e. Supporting research on preventive approaches that ameliorate the need for long-term care

Data from White House Conference on Aging. (1981). *Final report of the 1981 White House Conference on Aging,* Vol. 1–3. Washington, DC: Author.

OMNIBUS RECONCILIATION ACT

On December 20, 1987, President Ronald Reagan signed into law the Omnibus Reconciliation Act (P.L. 100–203). This act was aimed at improving the standards of nursing home care. The act calls for expanded coverage by registered and licensed practical nurses in nursing homes and requires formal training, in-service education, and competency-based evaluation of nurses' aides working in nursing homes (Gebhart, 1988). The Omnibus Reconciliation Act produces a greater demand for nurses to be employed in skilled nursing and intermediate care facilities to improve and monitor the quality of nursing home care.

PATIENT'S SELF-DETERMINATION ACT

The Patient's Self-Determination Act is a federal law adopted under the Omnibus Reconciliation Act of 1990.

TABLE 27–7

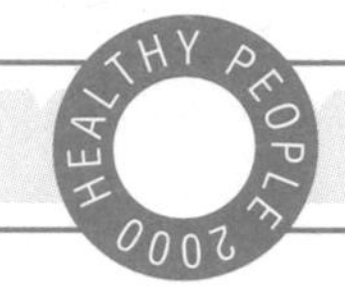

Selected Healthy People 2000 Objectives for Elderly Persons

Physical Activity

Reduce to no more than 22% the proportion of people aged 65 years and older who engage in no leisure time physical activity. (Baseline: 43% in 1985.)

Safety

1. Reduce suicides in white men aged 65 years and older to no more than 39.2 per 100,000 persons. (Baseline: 46.1 per 100,000 in 1987.)
2. Reduce deaths from falls and fall-related injuries to no more than 14.4 per 100,000 persons aged 65 to 84 years and 105 per 100,000 persons aged 85 years and older. (Baseline: 18 per 100,000 and 131.2 per 100,000, respectively, in 1987.)
3. Reduce hip fractures among persons aged 65 years and older so that hospitalizations for this condition are no more than 607 per 100,000 persons. (Baseline: 714 per 100,000 in 1988.)
4. Increase to at least 50% the proportion of primary care providers who routinely provide age-appropriate counseling on safety precautions to prevent unintentional injury.
5. Reduce residential fire deaths to no more than 3.3 per 100,000 persons aged 65 years and older. (Baseline: 4.4 per 100,000 in 1987.)

Chronic Disabling Conditions

1. Reduce to no more than 90 per 100,000 persons the proportion of all people aged 65 years and older who have difficulty in performing two or more personal care activities, thereby preserving independence. (Baseline: 111 per 100,000 in 1984–1985.)
2. Increase years of life to at least 65 years. (Baseline: An estimated 62 years in 1980.)
3. Reduce significant visual impairment to a prevalence of no more than 70 per 1000 persons aged 65 and over. (Baseline: 87.7 per 100,000 in 1986–1988.)
4. Reduce significant hearing impairment among persons aged 45 years and older to a prevalence of no more than 180 per 1000 persons. (Baseline: 202.5 per 100,000 in 1986–1988.)

Health Promotion and Screening

1. Increase to at least 40% the population of adults aged 65 years and older who have received, as a minimum within the appropriate interval, all of the screening and immunization services and at least one of the counseling services appropriate for their age and gender as recommended by the U.S. Preventive Services Task Force.
2. Increase immunization levels as follows: pneumococcal pneumonia and influenza immunization among institutionalized chronically ill or older people to at least 80%.
3. Increase to at least 80% the receipt of home food services by people aged 65 years and older who have difficulty in preparing their own meals or are otherwise in need of home-delivered meals.
4. Increase to at least 90% the proportion of people aged 65 years and older who had the opportunity to participate during the preceding year in at least one organized health promotion program through a senior center, life care facility, or other community-based setting that serves older adults.
5. Increase to at least 60% the proportion of people aged 65 years and older using the oral health care system each year. (Baseline: 42% in 1986.)
6. Increase to at least 60% the proportion of providers of primary care for older adults who routinely evaluate people aged 65 years and older for urinary incontinence and impairments of vision, hearing, cognition, and functional status.
7. Increase to at least 90% the proportion of perimenopausal women who have been counseled about the benefits and risks of estrogen replacement therapy (combined with progesterone when appropriate) for prevention of osteoporosis.

(Also see Chapters 16 and 17 for additional health promotion and screening objectives.)

From U.S. Department of Health and Human Services. (1990a). *Healthy people 2000: National health promotion and disease prevention objectives. Summary report.* Washington, DC: Government Printing Office.

This act applies to all Medicare and Medicaid provider organizations and requires that each health care facility maintain written policies and procedures for advance directives (i.e., directions given in advance to a health care provider articulating a patient's wishes regarding health care decisions). Under this law each patient has the right to make his or her own health care decisions, refuse medical treatment, and establish advance directives. Advance directives may take the form of living wills or durable powers of attorney. *Living wills* enable persons to document in advance their decisions regarding medical care should the time come when they are incapable of expressing their wishes. The living will defines under what conditions, if any, life-sustaining measures may be instituted. A *durable power of attorney* is a written document giving another adult the right to make health care decisions on one's behalf, in the case of incompetence or inability to render these decisions independently (Torchia, 1992). The Patient Self-Determination Act will have a great impact on elderly persons, who are more vulnerable to chronic and long-term illness and are more likely to have to face difficult health care decisions.

HEALTHY PEOPLE 2000

Finally, the recently published document entitled *Healthy People 2000: National Health Promotion and Disease Prevention Objectives* sets forth a national agenda for promoting and protecting the health of the American people. In this document, major health needs of the older adult are identified, and national objectives for promoting the health of the American people, including the nation's elderly population, are articulated (USDHHS, 1990a) (Table 27–7).

Responsibilities of the Nurse in Working with the Elderly Client in the Community

The community health nurse may function as a *facilitator-collaborator, advocate, teacher,* and *case manager* in assisting the elderly client and family in the community to maintain and improve health and well-being. The responsibilities of the community health nurse are carried out using the nursing process. The community health nurse assesses the client, family, and community to determine actual or potential health care needs and resources. A comprehensive assessment should include physical, psychosocial, spiritual, functional, developmental, and environmental factors (Matteson and McConnell, 1988). Data from the comprehensive assessment are used to develop nursing diagnoses that are individual-, family-, and community-focused.

CASE MANAGEMENT

Based on a comprehensive assessment of needs, the community health nurse collaborates with the client and family in jointly setting mutually acceptable goals. A nursing care plan is developed and implemented to meet family health promotion goals. In implementing the plan of care, the CHN needs to function as a *case manager,* referring the client and family to appropriate resources and monitoring and coordinating the extent and adequacy of services to meet family health care needs. (See Chapter 29 for an in-depth discussion of home health care.)

Case management is the process by which services are organized and coordinated to meet client needs. In working with frail elderly clients with multiple health problems, case management is an essential service that is frequently required over a long period of time. In addition the need for case management may increase in intensity and complexity as individual and family needs change. For example an elderly client returning home from the hospital after experiencing a stroke may require a variety of services. The community health nurse functions as a case manager by locating and coordinating resources in the community to meet client needs. Services may include in-home personal care, transportation, assistance in restructuring the home environment to facilitate mobility and wheelchair accessibility, physical therapy, or speech therapy. In this example evaluation of case management is based on the client's adjustment to the home environment once resources are in place, improved access to needed services such as physical and speech therapy, and avoidance of repeated hospitalization or the need for nursing home care.

Services should be appropriate to meet a client's changing health care needs over time. The community health nurse should work to ensure that services are not overutilized or underutilized. The nursing care plan may require modification in response to changing needs (Koff, 1988).

Case management programs for elderly persons are offered in many states through the local health department or office on aging. *Geriatric Evaluation Service* (GES) is an example of a program that provides assistance to elderly and functionally disabled adults who are at risk of institutionalization. The goal of GES is to maintain the individual in the community or in the least restrictive environment and to promote the highest possible level of independence and personal well-being. GES teams, located in local health departments, assess the health status and psychosocial needs of the individual and develop a plan of care to address these needs. The GES team is usually composed of a nurse, a social worker, and, as needed, a psychiatrist and a psychologist. Following this comprehensive assessment, case management services are provided to assist the individual in obtaining needed community resources (Maryland Department of Health and Mental Hygiene, 1991).

Under the Nursing Home Reform Act of 1987, GES personnel are also federally mandated to conduct preadmission screening and annual resident reviews of persons seeking nursing home placement or of persons currently residing in a nursing home who are suspected of having a diagnosis of mental illness or mental retardation. GES evaluates these individuals annually to determine whether nursing home placement is the most appropriate health care setting to meet the client's needs. Finally GES evaluates persons 65 years and older who are referred for admission to a state psychiatric facility to determine what is the least restrictive environment appropriate for the client (Bureau of Patient Care, 1992).

ADVOCACY

Effective case management requires a broad knowledge base of the diversity of health, social, and supportive community resources. By having a case manager, the confusion that may come from having contact with multiple persons in the health care team is eliminated (Koff, 1988). To function effectively as a case manager, the community health nurse must assume a strong *advocacy* role.

Key elements of the advocacy role include a sensitivity to the needs of the client and family, a broad knowledge base of available community resources and supports, and the ability to communicate a professional assessment of client and family needs to the appropriate service providers (Bremer, 1989). Persistence is also needed when acting on behalf of the family, since much time and patience are often required to locate and channel the client into the appropriate resource or support service. For example home care services are often fragmented and decentralized, preventing elderly persons from easily making arrangements to safely remain at home. Frail elderly clients who require multiple home care services often find coordinating needed services complex and overwhelming. Families may consider nursing home placement, simply because it is easier to arrange, than it is to unravel the complex and fragmented mix of community support services. By assisting frail elderly persons to locate and receive services that enable them to carry out activities of daily living and remain independent in the community, nursing home placement may be delayed or avoided (Grassi, 1988).

TEACHING AND COUNSELING

Teaching and counseling are also essential responsibilities of the community health nurse in working with aging families. Clients and families often require teaching related to the disease processes being experienced, management of symptoms, mobility, medications, diet, bowel and bladder function, normal health promotion activities, and recommendations for health screening. Counseling includes the provision of family and caregiver support, assistance in coping with and adjusting to the normal consequences of aging, assistance with the grieving process and coping with loss, and improvement of interpersonal communication between family members (Bremer, 1989). Clients should also be counseled on how to locate appropriate community resources and what questions to ask in investigating agencies. The AARP publishes valuable consumer information to assist clients and caregivers who are investigating community resources (AARP, 1986).

Bremer (1989), in a study of 16 elderly clients who had health or functional deficits that placed them at a high risk of institutionalization, found that 25% to 70% of all teaching and planning interventions by community health nurses and 50% of all counseling interventions were directed toward the caregiver. In addition 25% of all community health nursing interventions were directed to case management activities. Teaching and counseling to caregivers focused on acceptance of respite care and in-home services, planning and anticipating future health care needs and services, and teaching caregiving and assessment skills. The author concludes that community health nurses are uniquely qualified to conduct comprehensive assessments and to bridge the gap between social and health care needs and services in the population. In addition the community health nurse as case manager is uniquely qualified to decrease fragmentation of services and to refocus services from an acute illness model to a preventive model of care (Bremer, 1989).

COLLABORATION

Through teaching, counseling, advocacy, and case management roles, the community health nurse may collaborate with the family and other providers to facilitate improved health and well-being. Collaboration involves working together with others to meet a common goal. On a broader scale the community health nurse may collaborate with local and state governments to provide more comprehensive services for elderly persons by acting as a representative of consumer interest groups before state regulatory bodies and local health planning commissions and by lobbying for legislation that promotes expanded services for the elderly person. The community health nurse may work with a coalition of providers and citizen groups to advocate for the needs of the elderly population or may participate in AAA hearings to advocate for greater community-based long-term care services.

The community health nurse may also engage in such valuable community services as coordinating the preparation of a directory of community resources for elderly persons, developing telephone hotlines to provide information on long-term care, holding public education forums and seminars on the needs of the elderly population in the community, educating the community about long-term health care coverage, conducting surveys and publicizing price information on long-term care in the community, and meeting with corporations to explore long-term care and retirement options for employees. The community health nurse may also be responsible for organizing, coordinating, or supervising paid or volunteer programs (such as Friendly Visitors), family respite care, or self-help and support groups (AARP, 1985).

The community health nurse may also be involved in supporting federal policies that provide and finance care for elderly persons, such as legislation that provides greater financial protection against catastrophic costs not covered by Medicare. Finally, through mass screening efforts, the community health nurse can promote preventive health education, screening, and referral services to elderly persons. Through teaching, counseling, case management, advocacy, and collaboration with the client/family and other providers, the community health nurse can effect needed social change for the welfare of elderly persons.

KEY IDEAS

1. As the number of older Americans continues to grow the need for health care services for the elderly population will escalate.
2. Since the majority of elderly Americans live independently in the community, community health nurses are responsible for delivering health care services to a large segment of the elderly population.
3. As society continues to age the amount of chronic disease and functional impairments in the population will increase.
4. The community health nurse is responsible for facilitating utilization of needed resources by collaborating with service agencies; coordinating care to ensure systematic, comprehensive delivery of needed services; and advocating for the needs of older Americans. Advocacy is accomplished through community education and support of legislation that promotes a healthy, vital, and meaningful aging experience for elderly persons.
5. Through concerted efforts at the local, state, and federal levels to address the needs of older Americans, the nation's health care system may move to a more comprehensive and holistic vision for improving quality of care throughout the life span.
6. Through teaching, counseling, case management, advocacy, and collaboration with the client/family and other providers, the community health nurse can effect needed social change for the welfare of elderly persons.

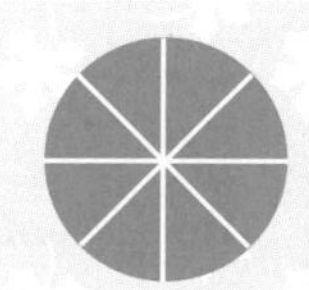

APPLYING THE NURSING PROCESS: *An Elderly Couple at Home*

Mr. W. is an 80-year-old client who lives with his 76-year-old wife. Mrs. W. has been suffering from Alzheimer's disease for 5 years. She has been experiencing progressive memory impairment, forgetfulness, and difficulty in naming objects. Recently she has begun to wander at night. Mrs. W. becomes highly anxious when she is unable to perform a task and requires a great deal of reassurance and encouragement. Mrs. W. denies awareness of a decline in cognitive functioning. She is ambulatory and can dress and feed herself with minimal assistance.

Mr. W. has become increasingly frustrated and overwhelmed with caregiving activities. Mr. W. states he does not understand what is happening to his wife and adds "You work all your life and for what? It doesn't make sense."

Mr. and Mrs. W. have two adult children and six grandchildren who live in a 5-mile radius. Regarding his family, Mr. W. notes "My children do not want to visit, because they don't want to see their mother acting that way."

On her initial home visit to this family, the community health nurse noted that both Mr. and Mrs. W. appeared disheveled and unkempt. Mr. W. complained of chronic fatigue and repeatedly made the statement "We would both be better off dead."

Assessment

Based on a thorough assessment of individual and family needs, the community health nurse developed a mutually acceptable plan of care with the family. The nursing assessment included:

- Assessing physical, psychological, social, spiritual, and environmental needs of individual/family.
- Assessing for the presence of depression, suicidal intentions, social isolation, ability to meet nutritional needs, compliance with medication, and self-care behavior.

- Assessing degree of family and social supports available to assist individual/family through crisis of coping with chronic illness (e.g., transportation, financial assistance, legal assistance, caretaking, respite care).
- Assessing for presence of abuse or neglect due to ineffective family coping (see Chapter 20).
- Assessing potential for injury as a result of Mrs. W.'s declining cognitive function and night wandering.

The community health nurse formulated *nursing diagnoses* and *goals* based on assessed needs. Nursing diagnoses and goals for this family included the following:

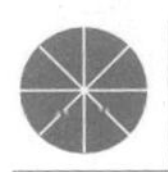

Nursing Diagnosis	Goals
Ineffective family coping related to chronic illness of family member and caregiver stress.	The individual/family will utilize respite services to attain additional caregiver support. The individual/family will communicate to the community health nurse and to each other their feelings and concerns in coping with the experience of chronic illness. The individual/family will verbalize knowledge of disease process and sources of caregiver support.
Potential for injury to wife related to her cognitive impairment.	The individual/family will identify and reduce the number of home hazards that have the potential to increase the risk of falls or accidental injury. Mrs. W. will not experience accidental injury.
Disturbance in self-concept related to chronic disease.	Mrs. W. will ventilate feelings and concerns regarding declining mental capacities.
Impaired social interaction related to chronic illness of family member.	The individual/family will experience meaningful social interaction with informal and formal support networks.
Alterations in thought processes related to progressive dementia.	Mrs. W. will be assisted by caregivers in remaining oriented to her surroundings. The individual/family will identify and demonstrate communication and environmental restructuring techniques that help to orient family member.
Potential for spiritual distress related to crisis of chronic dementing illness in family member.	The individual/family will openly express feelings of hopelessness, meaninglessness, and despair. The individual/family will experience a sense of meaning and purpose in the midst of the crisis of chronic illness.

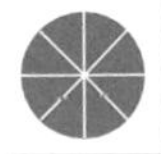

Interventions	Outcome
Assisting the individual/family in identifying and securing needed support services. Initiating appropriate referrals. Referring the individual/family for counseling and mental health evaluation to assess for depression, potential threat of self-harm, and potential for abuse or neglect.	The local office on aging was contacted for information and referral services. The department of social services offered social work consultation and family services. Even so, the husband denied the need for mental health services stating "I don't need a shrink."

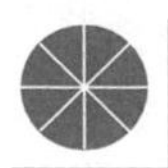

Interventions	Outcome
Referring family to local Alzheimer's Association chapter support groups for family support, respite care, and consumer information.	The husband did agree to attend a family support group two times a month. He reported, "What a relief to know I'm not alone."
Investigating homemaker and chore services for assistance in food preparation, housekeeping, laundry, and minor housing repairs. Investigating home health aide services to meet client's personal care needs, home-delivered meal programs (Meals on Wheels), Friendly Visitors, adult daycare, or live-in attendant to provided needed socialization and respite care. Investigating sources of spiritual support (church, synagogue, clergy).	Church members and pastoral care staff were mobilized and began weekly visits to offer support and counsel. Family accepted Meals on Wheels and homemaker services three times a week. Husband reported satisfaction with services and improved coping.
Encouraging complete geriatric evaluation (medical, psychological, and social testing) and mental health evaluation for client through private source of care or through local health department or department of aging.	Evaluation conducted. Diagnosis of Alzheimer's disease confirmed.
Providing anticipatory guidance to assist individual/family in identifying and planning for potential needs likely to occur in future (e.g., financial, legal). Investigating legal services to inform family of options and provide information on wills, guardianships, power of attorney.	Local Legal Aid Society assisted family in preparing and securing durable power of attorney for husband.
Assisting family to secure needed transportation services.	Senioride mobilized for medical visits. Neighbor offered to take husband to support group meeting. Clients' family agreed to offer assistance.
Teaching individual/family environmental modifications to promote safety and decrease risk of falls or accidental injury by confused family member (e.g., using night lights, removing furniture and loose rugs in path, making bathroom accessible to bedroom, developing fire escape plan, placing emergency numbers near telephone, ensuring smoke alarm is present and operable, having patient wear identification).	Modifications made. No accidents or injuries reported in 6-month period.
Teaching family and caregiver techniques of reality orientation (e.g., visible clocks, calendars, signs pointing to common objects) to assist client in remaining oriented to surrounding environment. Encouraging stability in environment. Surrounding client with familiar objects, pictures, memorabilia.	Mrs. W.'s recent memory improved slightly. Decreased agitation noted.
Supporting individual/family to share family stories. Involving Mrs. W. in activities that support reminiscence to facilitate a sense of meaning and purpose in the midst of painful life experiences.	Both husband and wife verablized satisfaction and meaningfulness. AARP volunteer provided one-on-one therapeutic reminiscence in home.

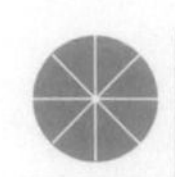

Interventions	Outcome
Supporting individual/family in maintaining self-care practices to promote health and prevent illness (e.g., routine health examinations, adequate nutrition, exercise, rest, meaningful social interactions, opportunities for personal development).	Husband still reports difficulty "getting to my doctors."
Discussing possible need for nursing home placement in future.	Husband agreed nursing home placement may be indicated in future. Began investigating options.
Supporting individual and family through grief journey and assisting family members with adjustments to role reversals due to chronic illness of family member.	Family members verbalized concerns and understanding regarding need for role reversals.
Supporting legislation and community resources that advocate for and provide needed services to elderly persons.	Family agreed to write their legislators to support expanded services for elderly in the community.

Evaluation

In general the evaluation of the effectiveness of community health nursing interventions is based on the following client outcomes:

- Reported decrease in agitated and confused behavior of client with Alzheimer's disease.
- Family reports improved communication between members. (Children resumed visits after meeting with community health nurse and learning about Alzheimer's disease.)
- Decreased feelings of frustration, hopelessness, and helplessness. No suicidal ideation.
- Satisfaction with and acceptance of available community resources for respite and support.
- Improved family participation in care of ill member. (Children became more active in visiting and assisting mother with activities of daily living and providing respite for father.)
- Absence of evidence of abuse, neglect, or accidental injury.
- Improvements in home maintenance, personal hygiene, and self-care behavior.
- Decreased episodes of night wandering.
- Satisfaction of family members with social relationships, spiritual supports, and sense of meaning and purpose in past and present life experiences.
- Expanded community resources to meet the needs of the elderly population. (Although the community health nurse did not directly witness this outcome, the family was mobilized to write to local legislators to support expanded services for the elderly in the community.)

GUIDELINES FOR LEARNING

1. Assess your home environment for the presence of safety hazards. What modifications would need to be made in your home if you suddenly needed to assume care for a frail, dependent, elderly family member?
2. Institute a dialogue with an elderly client or family member. Encourage him or her to share a part of his or her life story. Storytelling may be enhanced by sharing family pictures or memorabilia, asking open-ended questions that invite reminiscence, taking a family history, and supporting past recollections (Ryden, 1981). Empathize with and acknowledge positive and negative feelings that the person may experience as his or her life story is shared. In what way does past experience influence who the person is today (e.g., choices, beliefs, and values)?
3. Ask an elderly parent and an adult child to recall a shared past experience. Compare the perceptions between generations. In what ways are the life stories similar? In what ways are they different? What might influence the storytellers' perceptions? In

what way do you become a part of the life story by sharing in past and present experiences? How is your life story changed by being with the clients?

4. Reflect in writing on your perceptions of old age. What do you think it is like to be old? Share your reflections with an older family member or significant other.
5. Take time to review old family photographs, scrapbooks, or memorabilia. Reflect on the changes you can see in yourself over the years. What patterns do you see emerging in your past? In what ways are you the same or different? What do you think you will be like as you grow older?
6. Interview an elderly client or family member regarding the most difficult choices he or she has had to make in life. What were the conditions surrounding these choices? How was a decision made? How does the person feel about the decisions he or she made?

REFERENCES

American Association of Retired Persons (AARP). (1988). *Aging in America: Dignity or despair?* Washington, DC: Author.

AARP. (1984). *A profile of older Americans.* Washington, DC: Author.

AARP. (1987a). *Before you buy: A guide to long-term care insurance.* Washington, DC: Author.

AARP. (no year). *Getting the most for your money: A survey of local pharmacy services and drug prices.* Washington, DC: Author.

AARP. (1987b). *How does your nutrition measure up?* Washington, DC: Author.

AARP. (1989). *Making wise decisions for long term care.* Washington, DC: Author.

AARP. (1986). *Miles away and still caring: A guide for long distance caregivers.* Washington, DC: Author.

AARP. (1985). *The right place at the right time.* Washington, DC: Author.

Andreoli, K., Musser, L., & Reiser, S. (Eds.). (1986). *Health care for the elderly: Regional responses to national policy issues.* New York: The Hawarth Press.

Andreopoulos, S., & Hogress, J. (1989). *Health care for aging society.* New York: Churchill Livingstone.

Ascione, F., & Shimp, L. (1988). Helping patients to reduce medication misuse and error. *Generations, 12,* 52–55.

Berryman, E., Gaskin, D., Jones, A., Tolley, F., & Macmullen, J. (1989, July/August). Point by point: Predicting elders' falls. *Geriatric Nursing,* pp. 199–201.

Borenstein, A. (1983). *Chimes of change and hours: Views of older women in 20th century America.* Cranbury, NJ: Farleigh Dickinson University Press.

Blazer, D. (1989). Affective disorders in late life. In E. Busse & D. Blazer (Eds.). *Geriatric psychiatry* (pp. 369–402). Washington, DC: American Psychiatric Press.

Brant, B., & Osgood, N. (1990). The suicidal patient in long-term care institutions. *Journal of Gerontological Nursing, 16*(2), 15–18.

Bremer, A. (1989). A description of community health nursing practice with the community-based elderly. *Journal of Community Health Nursing, 6,* 173–184.

Brody, E. (1986). Institutional versus community health care of the elderly: The delicate balance of social policy position paper. In K. Andreoli, L. Musser, & S. Reiser (Eds.). *Health care for the elderly: Regional responses to national policy issues* (pp. 113–129). New York: The Hawarth Press.

Bureau of Patient Care. (1992). *Patient assessment and care planning division.* Baltimore: Baltimore County Health Department.

Busse, E., & Blazer, D. (Eds.). (1989). *Geriatric psychiatry.* Washington, DC: American Psychiatric Press.

Calvani, D. (1985). How well do your clients cope with hearing loss? *Journal of Gerontological Nursing, 11*(7), 16–19.

Cohen, E. (1988, Spring). The great, gray wave. *Maryland Today,* pp. 8–9.

Ebersole, P., & Hess, P. (1990). *Toward healthy aging: Human needs and nursing responses* (3rd. ed.). St Louis: Mosby–Year Book.

Erikson, E., Erikson, J., & Kivnick, H. (1986). *Vital involvement in old age.* New York: WW Norton.

Gebhart, R. (1988, March/April). Government briefs. *Nursing Homes,* pp. 9–13.

Garcia, E., & Luck, R. (1987). Crime and the older adult. *Aging Network, 3*(12), 4.

Graham, C. (1991, May). Exercise and the aging. *Diabetes Forecast,* pp. 34–37.

Grau, L. (1988). Illness-engendered poverty among the elderly. *Women and Health, 12*(3/4), 103–117.

Grassi, L. (1988, July/August). The frail elderly: The challenge to long term care management. *Nursing Homes,* pp. 11–15.

Haynes, R., Wang, E., & Gomes, M. (1987). A critical review of interventions to improve compliance with prescribed medications. *Patient Education Counsel, 10,* 155–166.

Heckheimer, E. (1989). *Health promotion of the elderly in the community.* Philadelphia: W.B. Saunders.

Jenike, M. (1989). *Geriatric psychiatry and psychopharmacology: A clinical approach.* Chicago: Year Book.

Koff, T. (1988). *New approaches to health care for an aging population.* San Francisco: Jossey-Bass.

Lacayo, C. (1984). Hispanics. In E. Palmore (Ed.). *Handbook of the aged in the United States* (pp. 253–267). Westport, CT: Greenwood Press.

Lamy, P. (1986). Drug interactions and the elderly. *Journal of Gerontological Nursing, 12*(2), 36.

Lashley, M. (1989). *Being with the elderly in community health nursing: Exploring lived experience through reflective dialogue.* Unpublished doctoral dissertation, University of Maryland, Baltimore.

Lashley, M. (1992). The painful side of reminiscence. *Geriatric Nursing, 14*(3), 138–141.

Lashley, M. (1992). Reminiscence: A biblical basis for telling our stories. *Journal of Christian Nursing, 9*(3), 4–8.

Leroux, C. (1986). Coping and caring: Living with Alzheimer's disease. Washington, DC: AARP.

Maryland Department of Health and Mental Hygiene. (1991). *Geriatric evaluation services.* Baltimore: Author.

Matteson, M., & McConnell, E. (1988). Gerontological nursing: Concepts and practice. Philadelphia: J.B. Lippincott.

McConnell, E., & Matteson, M. (1988). Psychosocial aging changes. In M. Matteson & E. McConnell (Eds.). *Gerontological nursing: Concepts and practice* (pp. 445–475). Philadelphia: J.B. Lippincott.

Morton, P. (1993). *Health assessment in nursing* (2nd ed.). Springhouse, PA: Springhouse.

Novak, M. (1971). *Ascent of the mountain: Flight of the dove.* New York: Harper & Row.

Nussbaum, J., Thompson, T., & Robinson, J. (1989). *Communication and aging.* New York: Harper & Row.

Osgood, N. (1988, April). Suicide in the elderly. *Carrier Foundation Letter,* No. 133. (Cited in Jenike, M. (1989). *Geriatric psychiatry and psychopharmacology: A clinical approach.* Chicago: Year Book.)

Palmore, E. (Ed.). (1984). *Handbook on the aged in the United States.* Westport, CT: Greenwood Press.

Patsdaughter, C., & Pesznecker, B. (1988). Medication regimens and the elderly home care client. *Journal of Gerontological Nursing, 14*(10), 30–34.

Pegels, C. (1988). *Health care and the older citizen.* Rockville: MD: Aspen Publishers.

Reaching a consensus on incontinence. (1989, March/April). *Geriatric Nursing,* pp. 78–80.

Ross, M. (1983). Learning to nurse the elderly: Outcome measures. *Journal of Advanced Nursing, 8,* 373–378.

Rules and regulations. (1992). *Federal Register, 57,* 24966–24972.

Ryden, M. (1981). Nursing interventions in support of reminiscence. *Journal of Gerontological Nursing, 7,* 461–463.

Salmen, J. (1988). *The doable, renewable home.* Washington, DC: AARP.

Santo-Novak, D., & Edwards, R. (1989, March/April). Rx: Take caution with drugs for elders. *Geriatric Nursing,* pp. 72 75.

Senior power: America's newest untapped natural resource. (1987). Towson, MD: Baltimore County Association of Senior Citizen Organizations.

Simpson, C., & Dickinson, G. (1983). Exercise. *American Journal of Nursing, 4*(1), 273–274.

Spicker, S., Woodward, K., & Tassel, P. (Eds.). (1978). *Aging and the elderly.* Atlantic Highlands, NJ: Humanities Press.

Streib, G. (1984). Socioeconomic strata. In E. Palmore (Ed.). *Handbook on the aged in the United States* (pp. 77–92). Westport, CT: Greenwood Press.

Tedrick, T. (1985). *Aging: Issues and policies for the 1980's.* New York: Praeger.

Torchia, D. (1992). Advance directives. *Physician Assistant, 16*(5), 79–87.

U.S. Bureau of the Census. (1989). *Statistical abstracts of the United States: 1989* (109th ed.). Washington, DC: Author.

U.S. Department of Health and Human Services. (1990a). *Healthy people 2000: National health promotion and disease prevention objectives. Summary report.* Washington, DC: Government Printing Office.

U.S. Department of Health and Human Services. (1990b). *Prevention 89/90: Federal programs and progress.* Washington, DC: U.S. Government Printing Office.

Vanderbilt, M. (1989, October). Nurses asked to support rural nursing bill. *The American Nurse,* p. 2.

Vital Statistics of the United States 1986. Vol II: Mortality. Part B. (1988). Hyattsville, MD: Center for Health Statistics.

Weissert, W. (1985). Long term care: Current policy and directions for the 1980's. In T. Tedrick (Ed.). *Aging: Issues and policies for the 1980's* (pp. 61–82). New York: Praeger.

Whitbourne, S. (1985). *The aging body: Physiological changes and psychosocial consequences.* New York: Springer-Verlag.

White House Conference on Aging. (1981). *Final report of the 1981 White House Conference on Aging,* vol 1–3. Washington, DC: Author.

SUGGESTED READINGS

Beadleson-Baird, M., & Lara, L. (1988). Reminiscing: Nursing actions for the acutely ill geriatric patient. *Issues in Mental Health Nursing, 9,* 83–94.

Hardy, V., & Riffle, K. (1993). Support for caregivers of dependent elderly. *Geriatric Nursing, 14*(3), 161–164.

Kligman, V., & Pepin, E. (1992). Prescribing physical activity for older persons. *Geriatrics 47*(8), 33–44.

Kurlowicz, L. (1993). Social factors and depression in late life. *Archives of Psychiatric Nursing, 7*(1), 30–36.

Pfister-Minogue, K. (1993). Enhancing patient compliance: A guide for nurses. *Geriatric Nursing, 14*(3), 124–132.

Puntil, C. (1991). Integrating three approaches to counter resistance in a noncompliant elderly client. *Journal of Psychosocial Nursing, 29*(2), 26–30.

Schiff, M. (1990, May/June). Designing environments for individuals with Alzheimer's disease: Some general principles. *The American Journal of Alzheimer's Care and Related Disorders Research,* pp. 4–8.

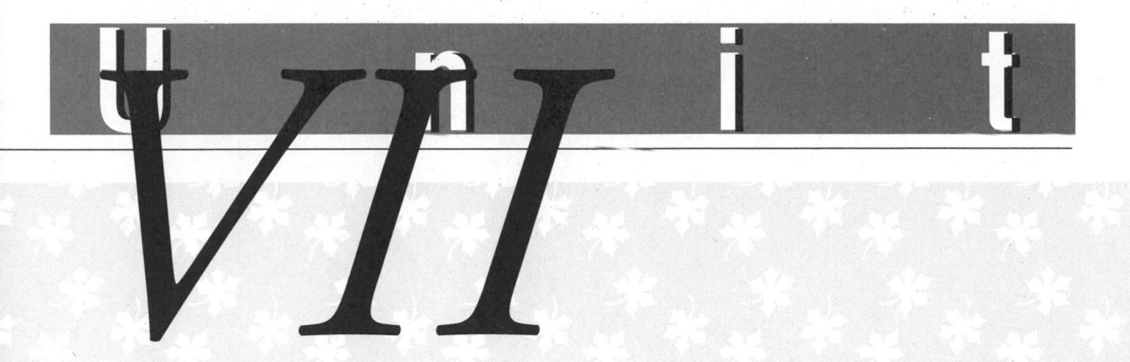

Settings for Community Health Nursing Practice

Chapter 28

School Health

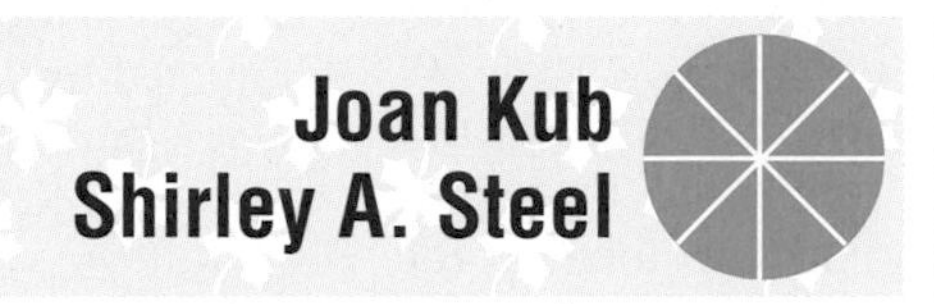

Joan Kub
Shirley A. Steel

Continued

Focus Questions

What is "comprehensive" school health for the 1990s and beyond?

What new models provide a framework for school health?

How are school health programs organized and regulated?

What are the various roles of the school nurse?

What professional standards guide the practice of school nurses?

What is the relevance of health promotion to the delivery of health services and health education and the provision for a healthy environment?

What are the common health concerns of school-age children, and what interventions are provided within school settings?

What are the future trends in school health?

How can schools contribute to the accomplishment of the objectives set forth in *Healthy People 2000?*

The health problems facing American children have changed dramatically since World War II. Instead of contagious diseases, children are currently threatened with problems that are primarily related to their own behavior. These include drinking and driving, tobacco and drug use, poor nutrition, inadequate physical activity, violence, unintended pregnancy, and sexually transmitted diseases (Cohen, 1992). In one report, *Code Blue: Uniting for Healthier Youth,* the National Commission on the Roles of the School and the Community in Improving Adolescent Health (NCRSCIAH) declared an adolescent health crisis: "For the first time in the history of this country young people are less healthy and less prepared to take their places in society than were their parents. And this is happening at a time when our society is more complex, more challenging, and more competitive than ever before" (NCRSCIAH, Executive Summary, 1990).

The important role that schools can play in the promotion of health of school-age children has been recognized since the early 1900s. In 1927 the American School Health Association was founded and has since worked to solve school health problems (Stone and Perry, 1990). The traditional school health approach has included the three broad areas of health services, health education, and the environment.

In preparation for the 21st century, an even broader, more comprehensive school program is being advocated (DeFriese et al., 1990; Kirby, 1990; Nader, 1990). This comprehensive school health program consists of a broad spectrum of school-related activities and services that will provide students and families with cognitive, affective, and skill development opportunities with respect to health (DeFriese et al., 1990). Some additional components of this comprehensive approach for the future are school and community linkages, physical instruction, and employee wellness programs (Wiley et al., 1991).

Historical Perspectives of School Nursing

To have a clear understanding of the current status of school health services, it is helpful to examine the evolution of this specialty. The beginnings of school health services can be traced back to the 19th century, when nurses provided their services in schools in Europe. The attention of these nurses was focused on both nutritional problems and improvement of sanitary conditions (Wold and Dagg, 1981).

In the United States, communicable diseases were influential in the development of school nursing. School health services were initially established in Boston schools in 1894 for the purpose of identifying and excluding students with communicable diseases (Wold and Dagg, 1981). With the evolution of a demonstration project initiated by Lillian Wald in New York City in 1902, there was a shift in the focus of school nursing. At this time there was a growing concern for the increasing numbers of school absences. When Lina Rogers Struthers, the first school nurse, was placed within a school to provide follow-up for children, school absences decreased significantly. This resulted in the placement of more school nurses in the schools of New York City and provided an example of the importance and value of health education to children and families.

During the 1920s and 1930s, the focus of school health was threefold. Initially attention was focused on medical inspections for the sole purpose of preventing the spread of contagious diseases. With time, medical examinations for all children were recognized as being important to ensure child health. The incorporation of health education into the curriculum in turn evolved into the goal of teaching students responsible health behaviors (Wold and Dagg, 1981).

During the 1940s and 1950s, school nursing became more public health oriented; approximately half of all public health nurses were employed in school health at that time (Wold and Dagg, 1981). This public health orientation resulted in a more family-centered approach to care, and the role of the nurse was one of providing health guidance and consultation with an overall emphasis on health promotion. In addition, the importance of the health team evolved during this period, supporting the importance of collaboration between nurses and teachers.

The years since 1970 have been times of innovation as well as of confusion and precariousness (Wold and Dagg, 1981). The school nurse practitioner concept was developed in Denver in 1970 and allowed for an expansion of the nurse's skills in the areas of history taking, physical appraisal, and developmental assessment (Igoe, 1975). Currently, school nurses are providing more case management services and have responded to the multiple changing health needs of children. Such innovations clearly define the role of the school nurse, but in times of budgetary cutbacks, the future continues to be somewhat precarious.

Since the early 1900s, the development of school health has been influenced by multiple external forces. These forces have included developments within public health, nursing, pediatrics, and education. Social and legislative initiatives have also shaped the development of this specialty. All of these factors are likely to continue to influence the scope of school nursing. In addition, the future of school nursing will depend on the ability of nurses to respond to the new opportunities that will undoubtedly arise.

Current Status of School Health

During the first part of the 20th century, the roles of the school nurse and the school health team evolved out of the needs of school-age children. The same principle has held for the latter half of the century. Children's needs for health services, health education, and a safe and healthy environment have guided the development of school initiatives and school health programs.

HEALTH SERVICES

Health services generally include initial health screening and referral activities, record keeping regarding compliance with state laws (e.g., immunizations) and special needs, provision for first aid, and counseling and education for individual students and teachers (Stone and Perry, 1990). School nurses typically serve as providers of health services. The recommended nurse-to-student ratio is 1:750 for healthy populations, 1:250 for children with disabilities in regular classrooms, and 1:125 in severely/profoundly disabled populations (American Nurses' Association [ANA], 1983).

Some schools have established clinics either within the schools or within close proximity. The number of schools in the United States offering comprehensive health services has grown from one in 1970 to more than 200 (Baker, 1992).

The role of the school nurse practitioner has gradually grown since the early 1980s. The first pilot program for school-based primary care with school nurse practitioners was begun in 1969. A position statement on the role of the school nurse practitioner was subsequently developed by public health, school health, and medical associations. In the 1980s the Robert Wood Johnson Foundation funded school projects that showed the effectiveness of school-based diagnosis and treatment by school nurse practitioners within schools (Igoe and Giordano, 1992).

HEALTH EDUCATION

The second component of a school health program is health education. The development of health education in schools has paralleled the changing nature of disease in children. In the earlier part of the 20th century, health programs in schools stressed hygiene, communicable disease control, and medical inspections (Smith et al., 1992). More recent instruction has focused on health promotion and the effects of individual behavior on health status.

There is an emphasis on comprehensive health education, which is a planned program of experiences for students in kindergarten through grade 12 and teaches important information, skills, and positive attitudes toward health (DeFriese et al., 1990). The curriculum should include instruction in physical, mental, social, and emotional health and should address topics such as stress, exercise, diet, alcohol and drug use/abuse, sexuality, human relationships, family health, nonviolent conflict resolution, safety, smoking, and environmental health.

ENVIRONMENTAL HEALTH

The third component of a school health program is environmental health. The school environment has both physical and psychosocial aspects. Physical concerns include sanitation, heating and lighting, and safety issues. Safety concerns are always an important issue for nurses, teachers, and administrators. The presence of asbestos or lead in the school building, for example, is of great concern to students' well-being.

Psychosocial aspects of the environment are of equal importance. These concerns might include the effects of community or school violence on the safety of the children in the schools. There may be a need for preventive educational programs regarding safety (Nader, 1990). There may be a need to improve the social environment by measuring the morale of students and teachers and evaluating attitudes regarding apathy, powerlessness, or hostility (Comer, 1988).

Other environmental concerns include the availability of special programs and attempts to modify the existing environment. The school lunch program may need modification to ensure the availability of good nutritious foods. The establishment of smoke-free schools and teacher health promotion programs are examples of other attempts to achieve healthy environments (Nader, 1990).

Conceptual Models of School Health

The traditional school health triad of service, education, and environment has guided the development of school health programs during the 20th century (Stone, 1990). Although this model remains relevant, a new definition and model are being advocated for the 1990s and the 21st century (Fig. 28–1). Nader (1990) proposed this model, which builds on previous work in the school health field. In this model a child's health status and educational achievement are placed at the apex of a triangle consisting of family, school, and community.

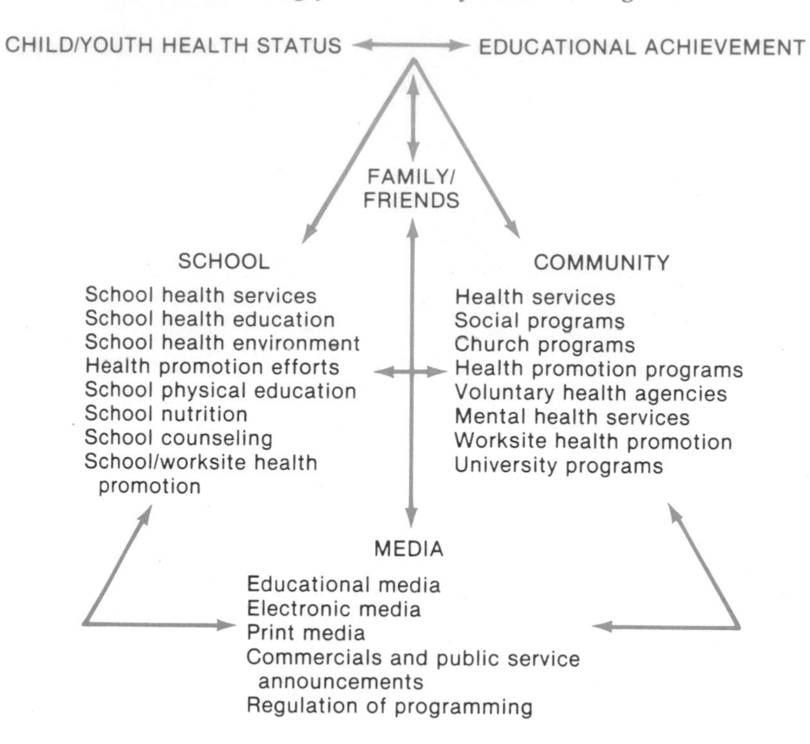

Figure 28–1 ● A school health model for the 1990s. (Adapted from Nader, P. R. (1990). The concept of "comprehensiveness" in the design and implementation of school health programs. *Journal of School Health,* 60(4), 133–138.)

A child's health status and educational achievement are interrelated. A child with a disability may need a modified learning environment; a child with a more acute illness may be absent from school and require home teaching. The reverse is also true: educational achievement affects health status. For example, adolescents who succeed in school tend to stay in school and have lower rates of pregnancy and substance abuse.

Nader's (1990) model recognizes that family and friends have the greatest influence on a student's health status and academic achievement. School-based programs, community services, and the media also play a role. The media is included because of the influence it has on health-related behavior (Flynn et al., 1992). This influence, however, flows in both directions, indicating reciprocal effects of each component on each other.

This new model suggests that numerous health and educational activities are conducted within the school by many individuals. The school health program includes health services, health education, a healthy environment, health promotion efforts, physical education, nutrition, counseling, and school/worksite health promotion.

Nader (1990) has identified five steps to implementation of this model: providing links to the community, performing needs assessments, developing or modifying school health services, developing or modifying school health education, and developing or modifying the school environment. This model describes an institution-based problem-solving model for working with school populations that is similar to the phases of the nursing process.

Organization and Administration of School Health

PATTERNS OF ORGANIZATION

An understanding of the organizational system of school health requires an initial understanding that public education is decentralized. Most nations have centralized systems in which a national ministry prescribes curriculum. In the United States, education remains the primary responsibility of local and state governments. Consequently, education is the legal responsibility of the states, which have delegated the operational responsibilities for schools to nearly 15,000 local school boards (Usdan, 1990).

Management of the School Health Program. At the local level, the school health program consists of a school health team. No single discipline can meet the needs of all children, so this team may consist of teachers, principals, consultants, homebound teachers, social workers, screening technicians, volunteers, physical therapists, speech therapists, school psychologists, and nurses. An organizational diagram of Rustia's (1982) school health program model illustrates the school health team and the targets, mission, and objectives of the program (Fig. 28–2).

To ensure that a school health program receives the support it needs, planning for school health should be a joint endeavor involving members of a school health council (Igoe and Speer, 1992). This council should be composed of teachers, school nurses, parents, students,

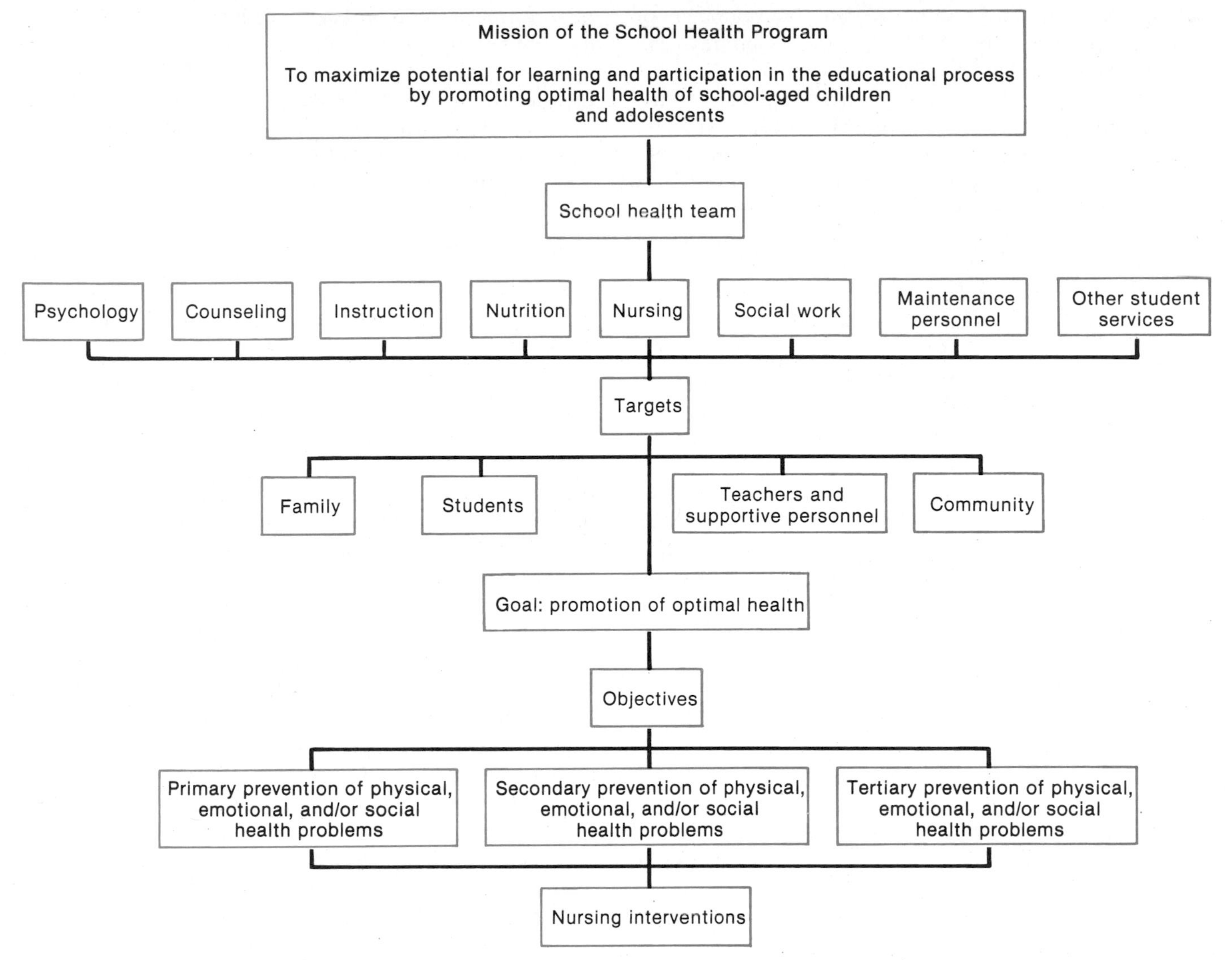

Figure 28–2 ● Rustia's school health promotion model: organization. (From Rustia, J. (1982). Rustia school health promotion model. *Journal of School Health,* 52(2), 109. Copyright 1982, American School Health Association, Kent, OH.)

administrators, and community leaders. The role of the council is to set the goals of the school health program and to check the consistency of these goals with those of the school district and the larger community.

Patterns of Nursing Services. Many administrative patterns exist for providing nursing services in schools. Community health nurses in school health are most often employed by either boards of education or boards of health. In addition, nurses hired through boards of health may be assigned to specialized services in schools or to generalized nursing services with occasional assignments in the school setting. Some innovative approaches to hiring also include the use of agency nurses to fill school nurse positions, hiring of school nurses by parent–teacher associations, and the assignment of special project nurses as a result of industry or government grants. All school nurses have some accountability to school administrations, as well as to the organization responsible for their hiring.

LEGISLATIVE AND ADMINISTRATIVE REGULATIONS

State Variation

The status of school health varies markedly across the United States. This is largely due to the fact that school health at the state level is determined by state mandates and laws.

A national survey of school health conducted in 1989 provides some documentation of the legal status of health services, health education, and a healthy environment (Stone and Perry, 1990). A legal basis for school health services exists in almost two thirds of the states. Some mandated responsibilities of health service programs include immunizations, health screenings, development of nursing care plans for children with disabilities, and provision of emergency care.

A legal basis for health education exists in more than three fourths of the states. Almost all states require certification of teachers in secondary health education, but only one state requires certification for elementary health education. Forty-four states (88%) have a state administrative office that directly supervises health education in public schools.

Almost four fifths of the states have a legal basis for a healthy school environment. The required standards most often address kitchen fires, fire safety, accessibility for disabled individuals, safety glass, vermin control, heating/cooling, and lighting.

In addition to state laws, mandates, and codes, there are also some federal laws that have an impact on school health. The National School Lunch Act of 1946, for example, resulted in the placement of food service programs in the schools. The goals of the school food service are to provide nutritionally adequate meals and health and nutrition education.

Schools are also subject to occupational and safety concerns. Federal regulations approved in 1991 are designed to protect school personnel from all occupational exposure to blood or other potentially infectious materials. Some of the requirements of this standard include (1) universal precautions and compliance to prevent contact with blood or potentially infectious materials, (2) engineering controls and work practice controls that would be used to eliminate or minimize exposure to employees at these facilities, and (3) hepatitis B vaccination for all employees who may have exposure to blood or potentially infectious materials and postexposure evaluation and follow-up.

Federal Laws for Students with Disabilities

In 1975 the Education for All Handicapped Children Act (EHA), known as Public Law (P.L.) 94–142, was enacted. This law gives all students between the ages of 6 and 18 years the right to a "free and appropriate public education" in the least restrictive environment possible regardless of physical or mental disabilities. The 1986 amendments to P.L. 99–457 expanded the eligible population to include preschool students 0 to 5 years of age. This law created two new federal programs: the Handicapped Infant and Toddler Program and the Preschool Grants Program. The Handicapped Infant and Toddler Program, for children 0 to 3 years of age, was established to reduce the potential for developmental delays, minimize institutionalization of children with disabilities, help families meet the special needs of their children, and reduce the cost to society. Incentive funding for this program is being used to plan and implement early intervention programs. Under the Preschool Grants Program, state educational agencies must provide free and appropriate education for all children with disabilities beginning at age 3.

In 1991 additional amendments to the EHA were signed into law. In the general provisions the EHA was renamed the Individuals with Disabilities Education Act (IDEA) (P.L. 101–476). The text of IDEA reflects both person-first language (infants and toddlers with disabilities) and the use of the term *disability* instead of *handicapped.*

Advances in science and technology have made it possible to provide extended life to infants who formerly would have died at birth or shortly thereafter. The higher survival rates of trauma victims have also led to increases in the number of children with long-term health care needs (U.S. Congress, Office of Technology Assessment, 1987). This phenomenon has created special challenges for school health professionals, as the numbers of these children are increasing significantly. Before the 1980s, children with special needs were cared for in hospitals or long-term care facilities. However, federal and state deinstitutionalization policies, cost considerations, and advocacy groups have placed these children back in the home and the public schools. However, who pays for the health care costs incurred during school attendance? Also there is the question of who performs these highly technical procedures, as most school systems do not have a full-time school nurse. In a national survey of state health and education agencies conducted to determine the existence of guidelines for such specialized procedures as catheterization, colostomy/ileostomy care, tube feeding, seizure management, medication administration, respiratory care, and positioning, only six states had written guidelines for all eight procedures. Twenty-six states had no guidelines or had guidelines for medication only (Wood et al., 1986).

A multidisciplinary task force consisting of representatives from both health and education was convened in 1988 by the American Federation of Teachers (AFT) to examine issues related to special health care needs in the school. As a result of the task force efforts, a document entitled *The Medically Fragile Child in the School Setting* (AFT, 1992) offered recommendations regarding role delineation for those providing special health care in the school setting. This document was published along with a survey of state nurse practice acts that described delegation and supervisory practices for nurses.

> School personnel, by and large, have no training in health related fields. Moreover, most have never anticipated ever having to perform health care procedures when they prepared to become teachers or school employees. Many have struggled with their anxieties over this additional responsibility, as they work to provide high standards of education for their students. Since school staff are with the students the majority of the day, and are the primary caretakers, it is imperative that all members of the team are trained to participate in appropriate procedures, activities, and know when to get the school nurse or secure emergency assistance (AFT, 1992, p. 8).

The school nurse helps this multidisciplinary team coordinate activities that will meet the needs of students with disabilities. To ensure that this is accomplished, the task force made the following recommendations for the medically fragile child in the school setting (AFT, 1992, p. 8):

- Develop a procedure or policy manual and update it on a regular basis.
- Establish a uniform recording system, with standardized forms, for use by all staff.
- Train staff on (appropriate) procedures and routinely assess individual's ability to perform those procedures safely.
- Keep a documented list of trained staff, when they were trained, and your assessment of their capabilities.
- Develop emergency procedures/evacuation plans and train and evaluate staff in these areas.
- Arrange for or provide inservice training on basic first aid and cardiopulmonary resuscitation training.
- Arrange for or provide inservice programs on current health issues.
- Arrange for or provide inservice programs on universal precautions and the appropriate disposal of contaminated waste.

Under IDEA (P.L. 101–476) students must be enrolled in special education to be eligible for related services. However, another federal law, Section 504 of the Rehabilitation Act of 1973 (P.L. 93–112), may broaden a student's eligibility for related services. The Office of Civil Rights is responsible for overseeing compliance with Section 504. The law ensures that federally assisted programs and activities are operated without discrimination on the basis of disabilities and that reasonable accommodations to the disability of students and employees are made. A free and appropriate education must meet the individual needs of students who qualify as handicapped and can consist of special or regular education. Section 504 defines the handicapped person in a broader context than its IDEA counterpart. All students who are handicapped under IDEA will generally be considered handicapped for the purposes of Section 504; however, not all handicapped persons under Section 504 are also handicapped for the purposes of IDEA. Some examples of conditions that meet the definition under Section 504 but not necessarily under IDEA are attention deficit/hyperactivity disorder (ADHD), acquired immunodeficiency syndrome (AIDS), pregnancy with complications, obesity, and drug addiction. The severity of a 504 handicap must result in a substantial limitation of one or more major life activities.

Many school districts face seemingly insurmountable tasks in meeting their responsibilities for providing related services to school-age children with disabilities. Districts are deterred by a lack of adequate funds and a shortage of trained personnel. Clear documentation of the specific needs of the student in the individual education plan (IEP) is imperative, and parents and schools must become partners in developing strategies for increased funding to provide services for students. Interdisciplinary and interagency collaboration must be achieved, and new, creative planning must be accomplished to utilize all school and community resources to help students with disabilities feel valued as members of the community.

Responsibilities of the School Nurse

SCOPE OF PRACTICE

The practice of school nursing has been significantly influenced by the evolution of specialty practices within the broad field of nursing. Nurses within a specialty develop a philosophy, goals, and qualification and education requirements needed by its practitioners. School health nursing makes an important contribution to the support of the educational process for children and adolescents. In one of the most cost-effective community settings for the delivery of health services to the school-age child and families, professional school nurses provide an important link between the school and the community health system.

Traditionally the school nurse has been viewed from a limited perspective as a case-finder and provider of basic health services to the student population. However, more recently a new paradigm for the school nurse, one that creates a totally new value structure of prevention and enhances the enormous diversity of the role and function of the practicing school nurse, has begun to emerge. This expanded role includes program management, interdisciplinary collaboration, health education, health counseling, school–community coordination, and research.

Economic changes, legislation, and the growing costs of health care have led a large segment of our population to begin to view the school nurse in a different light. As health care requirements increase relative to family income, the school nurse is pressed into service as the primary health care provider. Changes in public law have "mainstreamed" students with disabilities who previously would have been educated in a special environment. This array of classroom dynamics must be addressed both for the special needs student and for the school population in general.

Thus, school nurses find themselves in an expanding role to ensure optimum health awareness and wellness of the student population, the faculty, and the community. No longer can this nursing specialty operate as the singular advocate of healthy children. Collaboration and cooperation with other health specialties and with education professionals are critical to a successful school health program.

The school nurse practitioner, functioning in the school setting in collaboration with the school nurse, may manage a comprehensive school-based wellness center to provide more extensive primary care services to students who do not have access to preventive and restorative health care. Nearly 12 million American children under 18 have no health insurance coverage (American Medical Association Council on Scientific Affairs, 1990). The inclusion of children into insurance programs does not guarantee that they will receive adequate health care. Often, well child care, developmental examinations, and immunizations are not covered by private insurance (Newacheck, 1990). Therefore, the school nurse and/or the school-based wellness center can provide a model for the delivery of health services not only to the underserved population and the entire audience of children and adolescents ages 0 to 21, but also to the adult population within the school setting who provide for educational needs and support services.

In an American Nurses' Association publication, *Expanding School Health Services to Serve Children, Youth and Families* (Igoe and Giordano, 1992), the *family health center* is described as an innovative approach to community-oriented primary health care. "The fundamental principles of this proposal are the emphasis on family, the convenient delivery of primary health care, the utilization of a grass roots institution, the school, as the health care delivery site, and a proposed role shift that empowers consumers by increasing their ownership of their own health care and the exchange of information with professionals" (Igoe and Giordano, 1992 p. vii). School nurses are essential to implementing such a plan. These proposed family centers at or near schools reflect the belief that society has some responsibility for helping parents and families meet the needs of their children and elders (Igoe and Giordano, 1992). School-based family health centers will be designed to offer an extensive selection of services to meet the needs of school-age children and youths, their siblings, their parents, and other family members living within the school service areas. Collaboration and cooperation with community resources, private health care facilities, and colleges and universities will help the family health center function as a primary health care focal point for the community.

The proposed services would include diagnosing and treating common illnesses early in the course of the disease or condition, screening and referral of more complex health problems requiring more extensive diagnostic and therapeutic interventions, preparing consumers to become their own care coordinators, monitoring chronic disease, and providing individual and group health counseling about health practices and health promotion for higher level wellness (Igoe and Giordano, 1992).

EDUCATIONAL PREPARATION AND CERTIFICATION

School nurses should have academic credentials comparable to those of other faculty members in the school. *The Standards of Community Health Practice* (ANA, 1986) and the *Guidelines for a Model School Nursing Services Program* (Proctor, 1990) both cite a baccalaureate degree in nursing as the minimum educational background for the practitioner whose functions relate to school health nursing. Nurses also should meet the certification requirements in their individual state (Wold and Dagg, 1981). These teaching requirements vary from state to state and are administered by the state department of education. There are two national certification examinations for school nurses that validate a body of knowledge and practice within the field of school nursing. These are offered by the National Association of School Nurses (NASN) and the ANA.

Because school nursing is a subspecialty, the baccalaureate program in nursing does not totally prepare individuals for a career in this field. Therefore, it is imperative that the school nurse's background include courses in community health, public health, school law, educational theories and methods, school health administration and management, health assessment, growth and development, communication skills, advanced first aid, psychology, and sociology. Some of these courses must be obtained at the graduate level.

STANDARDS OF PRACTICE

School nurses function according to a set of standards. The purpose of the standards of school nursing practice is to fulfill the profession's obligation to provide a means of improving the quality of care. Generic nursing standards developed by the ANA "are authoritative statements by which the nursing profession describes the responsibilities for which its practitioners are accountable. Consequently, standards reflect the values and priorities of the profession. Standards provide direction for professional nursing practice and a framework for the evolution of practice" (ANA, 1991, p. 1).

Current school nursing standards (Proctor et al., 1993) have been published by the NASN. These standards evolved over a 20-year period from numerous documents published by the ANA, the NASN, and the Western Interstate Commission on Higher Education (Fig. 28–3). Proctor and colleagues (1993) identify specialty standards of practice for the school nurse under the auspices of generic standards of clinical practice that relate to all nurses, concentrating on role synthesis and role actualization (Table 28–1).

LEGAL ISSUES

Delegation of tasks and maintenance of appropriate medical records are legal issues for school nurses. Each school nurse functions under a nurse practice act in the particular state in which she or he is employed. These acts, which govern the scope of practice, vary from state to state. In some school districts, school nurses have responsibilities

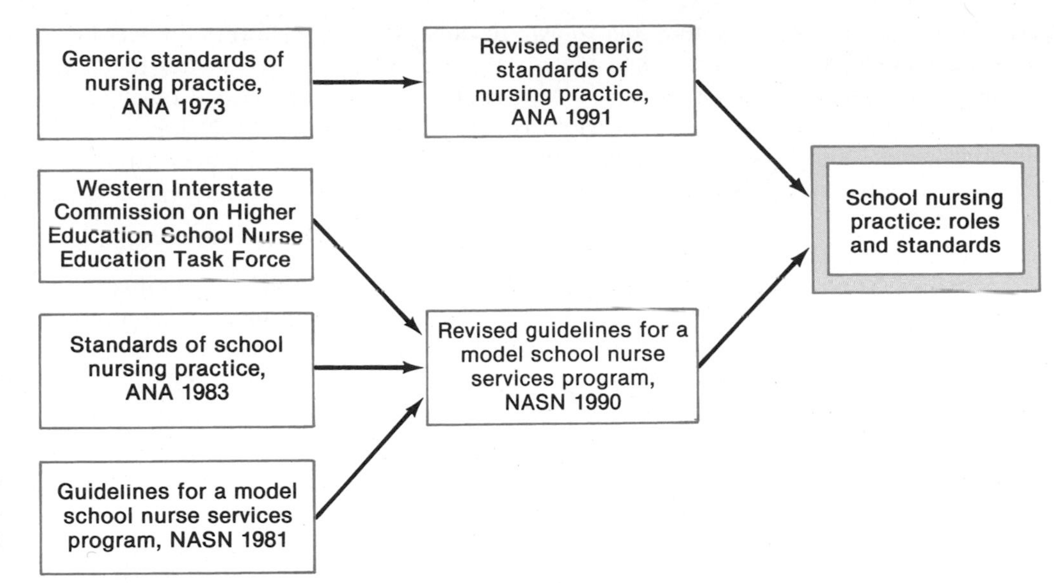

Figure 28–3 ● Evolution of the standards of school nursing practice. (Adapted from Proctor, S., Lordi, S., and Zaiger, D. (1993). *School nursing practice: Roles and standards.* Scarborough, ME: National Association of School Nurses.)

for many different schools and so must delegate tasks. It is critical that the delegation of care to an unlicensed person is appropriate within the requirements of both the nurse practice act and the administrative policy of the district (AFT, 1992). The following four points can serve as guidelines in helping the nurse determine appropriate delegation (Neumann, 1989):

1. *Safety:* Student safety must be paramount. If the health-related task is too complex for the skill level of the caregiver, it should not be delegated.
2. *Staffing:* The skill levels and capabilities of all team members should be known and tasks assigned appropriately.
3. *Schooling:* All educational components in the caregivers' background should be considered. Proper instruction and observation, once the task is assigned, are critical.
4. *Supervision:* The caregiver must be adequately supervised periodically, and documentation of the observation must be recorded.

Confidentiality is an important issue in school health that often results in ethical and legal concerns. The issues are complex because health records are considered part of the education record and fall under the Federal Educational Rights and Privacy Act (FERPA). Under FERPA, a parent or guardian of a student under the age of 18 years has the right to inspect and review the education records of the student. Consequently, school nurses must be aware of the laws and use judgment in recording information obtained from the student. It should be noted that school-based health clinic records, records connected with treatment of a student in a federally assisted program for drug or alcohol abuse, and records connected with child abuse or neglect

TABLE 28–1

School Nursing Practice: Roles and Standards

- *Role Concept 1: Clinical knowledge:* The school nurse utilizes a distinct clinical knowledge base for decision making in nursing practice.
- *Role Concept 2: Nursing process:* The school nurse uses a systematic approach to problem solving in nursing practice.
- *Role Concept 3: Clients with special needs:* The school nurse contributes to the education of the client with special health needs by assessing such clients, planning and providing appropriate nursing care, and evaluating the identified outcomes of care.
- *Role Concept 4: Communication:* The school nurse uses effective written, verbal, and nonverbal communication skills.
- *Role Concept 5: Program management:* The school nurse establishes and maintains a comprehensive school health program and contributes to the formulation of school health policy.
- *Role Concept 6: Collaboration within the school system:* The school nurse collaborates with other school professionals, parents, and caregivers to meet the health, developmental, and educational needs of clients.
- *Role Concept 7: Collaboration with community health system:* The school nurse collaborates with members of the community in the delivery of health care and utilizes knowledge of community health systems and resources to function as a school–community liaison.
- *Role Concept 8: Health education:* The school nurse assists students, families, and the school community to achieve optimal levels of wellness through appropriately designed and delivered health education.
- *Role Concept 9: Research:* The school nurse contributes to nursing and school health through innovations in practice and participation in research or research-related activities.
- *Role Concept 10: Professional development:* The school nurse identifies, delineates, and clarifies the nursing role; promotes quality of care; pursues continued professional development; and demonstrates professional conduct.

From Proctor, S., Lordi, S., & Zaiger, D. (1993). *School nursing practice: Roles and standards.* Scarborough, ME: National Association of School Nurses.

are not considered part of the educational records. In addition, ethical issues also arise when adolescents share or confide certain problems that include contemplation of suicide, statements about harming another person, or thinking about running away. These will most likely require notification of parents, thus resulting in a breech of student confidentiality.

ROLES OF THE SCHOOL NURSE

The roles of school health nurses are numerous and include educator, consultant/researcher, liaison, advocate, case manager, health screener, provider of nursing procedures (e.g., medication administration), provider of emergency care, and manager. School nurses provide interventions directed toward all levels of prevention (Fig. 28–4). Positive health outcomes are expected among students, teachers and other school personnel, and families of the students. Nursing interventions can also strengthen the larger community health system.

The School Nurse as Educator

The school nurse has a unique opportunity within the educational setting to facilitate maintenance or change in health attitudes, values, beliefs, and behavior in a captive audience. Health education may occur in a formal setting as in a classroom, or an informal setting on a one-to-one basis, as during a health suite visit by a student. Each interaction the school nurse has with students or staff

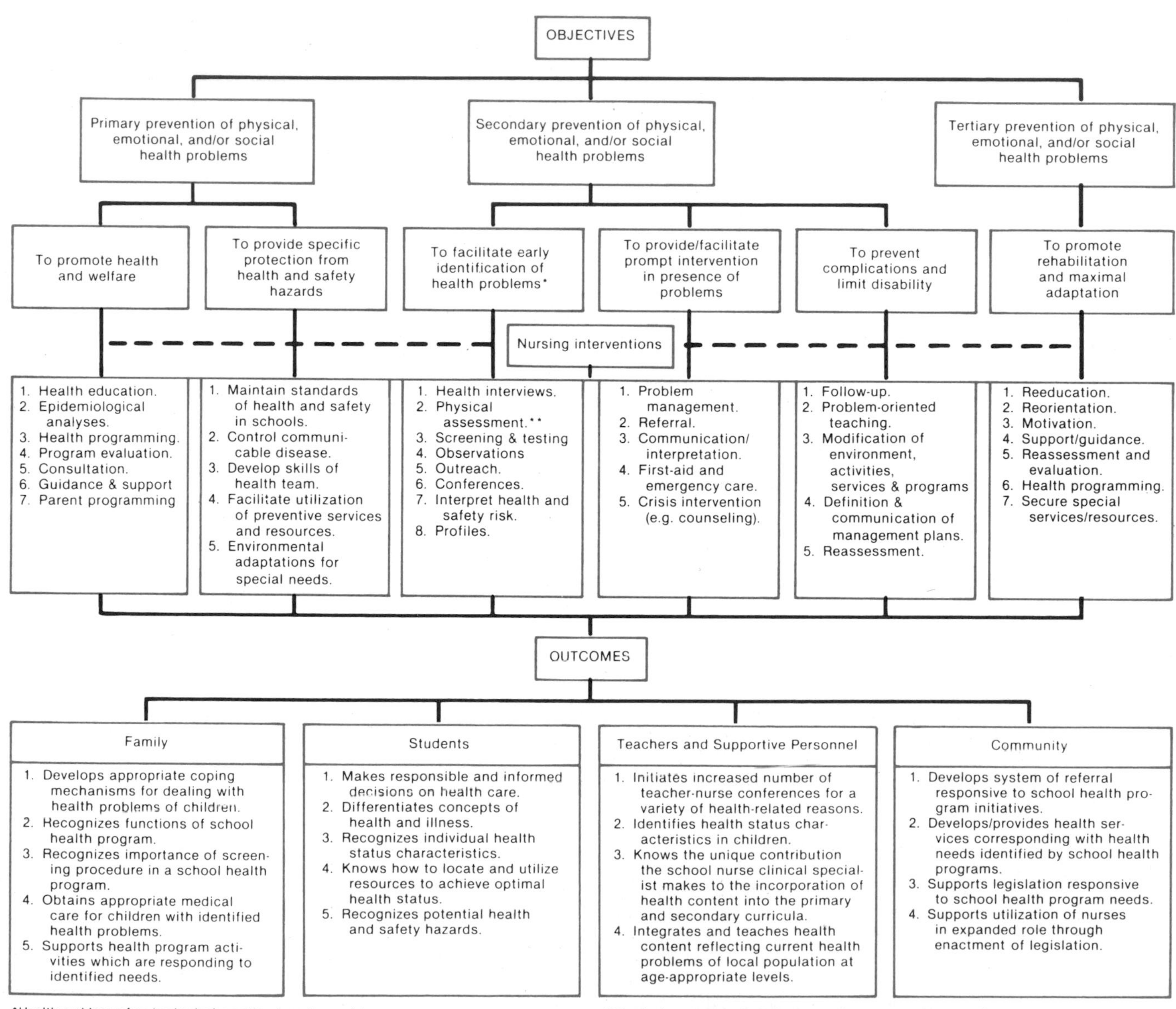

Figure 28–4 ● Rustia's school health promotion model: interventions and outcomes. (From Rustia, J. (1982). Rustia school health promotion model. *Journal of School Health,* 52(2), 110. Copyright 1982, American School Health Association, Kent, OH.)

members has the potential for health teaching that can maintain health, prevent disability, and promote a higher level of wellness.

The school nurse identifies student and staff requirements for health education by conducting a needs assessment, observing health practices, and gathering and assessing statistical data on health room visits (see Unit III). Using all of the information collected, the school nurse employs learning principles and appropriate teaching methods to link health information with positive, healthy behavior changes. School nurses also serve as a professional resource to the staff by implementing health education curricula.

The following examples describe the school nurse's participation both formally and informally in relation to the delivery of health education to students and staff:

- *Informal health teaching with students, staff, and parents.* A student is identified with pediculosis (head lice). The school nurse advises the student that sharing combs and caps is a prime method for spreading the infestation. The parent is called, and instructions are given concerning the application of a pediculocidal shampoo and the removal of nits. School staff can be taught to screen for pediculosis and to observe students who scratch their heads more than usual. All persons involved should be informed that lice infestation is not a major health threat but a nuisance condition that often creates embarassment and panic within the community.
- *Formal health teaching.* Pregnant adolescents are taught the normal physiology of pregnancy, including prenatal care, expectations of labor and delivery, and child care in a class on education for responsible parenthood. The class is team taught with the home economics instructor.
- *Health teaching as a support to the classroom teacher.* Materials and resources are provided to the classroom teacher to enhance a particular subject or learning unit. A nurse who has special expertise in growth and development helps the biology teacher prepare for a class presentation by providing posters featuring the growth and development of a fetus.
- *Formal in-service health education.* The 1991 federal standard from the Department of Labor, Occupational Health and Safety Administration (OSHA) mandates that all staff members who may be at risk for occupational exposure to bloodborne pathogens be instructed annually on universal precautions. An in-service program can be planned and implemented by the school nurse, with demonstrations, handouts, and a film on universal precautions in the school setting. The delivery of this formal health education material will help allay concerns and fears about dealing with body fluid spills.
- *Curriculum planning and development.* Health education can be addressed by integrating it throughout the curriculum (kindergarten through grade 12) or by developing specific courses. A combination of the two is probably the most effective method. In developing a high school health course, the nurse is a valuable resource in helping to apply the health belief model (Rosenstock, 1974) to at-risk behavior such as smoking, drug and alcohol abuse, and obesity.

School nurses engage in health education on many levels. Informal activities capitalize on the *teachable moment* when a student expresses a desire or need to learn about wellness, whereas the formal approach to health education is a systematic process of assessment of learner needs, exploration of learner readiness, development of planned outcomes, development and implementation of a teaching plan, and evaluation of learner outcomes and teacher effectiveness (see Chapter 18).

The School Nurse as Consultant/ Researcher

As managers of the school health program, school nurses have specific knowledge and expertise to share with the school community. In assisting with the planning, implementing, and evaluating of a school health program, the nurse uses and applies knowledge of nursing, health, and education as related to the delivery of health care and prevention strategies to students and staff. School nurses collect information and data germane to the type of services needed and wanted within the school community. They are uniquely able to identify the resources and appropriate budgetary shifts necessary to deliver an effective program while maintaining good patterns of communication as they interact with parents, students, school staff, and community agencies. The ability to gain cooperation, trust, and acceptance is dependent on this approach (Wold and Dagg, 1981).

For students with special needs, the school nurse is knowledgeable and conversant concerning the federal laws that afford these students a free and appropriate education in the least restrictive environment. They function as advocates for students and families while facilitating normalization of the student's educational experience. School nurses also know about the health needs of children with specific illnesses and disabilities.

School nurses develop and implement policies and procedures concerning the health of students and staff. It is school nurses who interact with a variety of agencies regarding public school policy, legislation, and funding (Proctor et al., 1993). This political role is necessary to ensure collaboration among all elements of the school health model.

Working within the school system itself requires a knowledge of the goals, philosophy, and mission statement of the educational system. Health objectives must dovetail with educational goals. A good working knowledge of the role and function of each player (professional as well as ancillary) within the health team is imperative for the school nurse to appropriately focus consultative efforts.

In the collaboration with community agencies, the school nurse can enhance communication between the health care provider and the family in terms of health progress; compliance with, barriers to, and effectiveness of treatment; and gaps in resources. "The most effective school nurses see themselves as community health professionals. It is nursing without walls" (Proctor et al., 1993). They represent the conduit between the school, the family, and the community resources.

As consultants to classroom teachers in the area of health promotion, school nurses participate in assessment, implementation, and evaluation of the health education curriculum. They also have an active role in the selection of materials for classroom instruction, counseling activities, and health suite displays. The school staff and parents may benefit considerably from health promotion through workshops and inservice activities initiated and/or conducted by the school nurse.

In research activities, "school nurses are the most advantaged of all nurses because their work is a natural place in which to study health problems, measure the effectiveness of programs and to contribute to a growing body of knowledge about nursing" (Proctor et al., 1993). School nursing research is necessary to justify its practices and develop new knowledge. If school nurses use their unique skills and expertise to initiate research studies and to test new approaches and concepts, they will clarify and strengthen their contributions in the area of school health.

The School Nurse as Liaison

The school nurse has the opportunity to engage in community liaison activities that enhance the delivery of health services to students. Of primary concern to the school nurse working with students and families are the mores, belief systems, values, and resources of the community in which these students and families live. The health status of children is affected by disease, injury, behavior, and social and educational problems, sometimes referred to as the "new morbidities" and outlined in Table 28–2 (Igoe and Giordano, 1992). School nurses must form partnerships with parents, health care and social services agencies, religious institutions, law enforcement and judicial systems, civic organizations, business and industry, and the media to provide a framework within which these devastating statistics can be reversed (National School Boards Association, 1991–1992).

A successful school nurse seeks community input at each level of health services program planning. Community groups are more interested in supporting initiatives if they have participated in the planning of the program. Conversely, the school nurse can gain a greater appreciation of community problems and different viewpoints if community input is sought. However, an overriding challenge for the school nurse as a community liaison may be to "convince a critical mass of citizens and leaders that the child poverty, drug abuse, violence, and family neighborhood disintegration pose as much of a threat to American prosperity, security, competitiveness, and moral leadership in the new decade as any other enemy outside or inside our borders; . . . [and to] push Americans in all walks of life to

TABLE 28–2
The New Morbidities

- In 1989, almost 20% of the nation's children lived in a family with an income below the poverty level. This 20% represents 12.6 million children, an increase of 2.5 million over the previous decade.
- In 1989, 52% of all poor families were headed by single women. More than half of all children currently will spend some time growing up in a single-parent home.
- In 1988, 7% of all births were of an infant weighing 5.5 lb or less; these low-birth-weight infants are at greater risk for long-term developmental problems than infants weighing more at birth. Early and adequate prenatal care could diminish the problem of low birth weight and associated learning difficulties, but only 76% of women received such care in 1988.
- In 1989, 2.2 million children were reported abused or neglected, a 147% increase over the figures for 1979.
- More than half of all adolescents between the ages of 15 and 19 are sexually active.
- In 1988, 34.7% of youth indicated having five or more drinks in the previous 2 weeks.
- Between 7 and 10 million children and teenagers have emotional problems, but only 20% of them are getting any help.
- In 1988, 15% of children and youths under the age of 21 had no health insurance coverage.
- In 1990, there were more than 30,000 cases of measles, mumps, and whooping cough—all of them preventable by adequate immunization. Only half of all American children are fully immunized before age 2.
- Poor children are twice as likely as more affluent children to have health or mental health problems that impair their daily functioning. These are the students who often are at highest risk for absenteeism and academic failure.
- Poor children are four times as likely as more affluent children to miss school because of their ailments; upper respiratory infections, dental decay, allergies, injuries, and skin disorders are frequent ailments of poor children.

From Igoe, J., & Giordano, B. (1992). *Expanding school health services to serve families in the 21st century.* Washington, DC: American Nurses' Association.

TABLE 28–3

Case Management Role Functions

- Coordinating care and services, including coordination of care and service providers responsible for furnishing services needed by a given client and, in many models, of all payment sources that reimburse providers for those services.
- Case-finding and screening to identify appropriate clients for case management.
- Comprehensively assessing the client's goals, as well as his or her physical, functional, psychological, social, environmental, and financial status.
- Assessing the client's informal and formal support systems.
- Analyzing and synthesizing all data for formulating appropriate nursing diagnostic and/or interdisciplinary problem statements.
- Developing, implementing, monitoring, and modifying a plan of care through an interdisciplinary and collaborative team process in conjunction with the client and his or her caregiver.
- Linking the client with the most appropriate institutional or community resource, advocating on behalf of the client for scarce resources, and developing new resources if gaps exist in the service continuum.
- Procuring services, including eligibility decisions and authorizing hospitalization and home care (essential in some programs).
- Problem solving.
- Facilitating access.
- Providing direct patient care in some programs.
- Providing liaison service.
- Educating client, family, and community support services; facilitating the goal of self-care by the client and his or her family.
- Facilitating communication.
- Documenting.
- Monitoring the client's progress toward goal achievement and periodically reassessing changes in health status.
- Monitoring the plan to ensure the quality, quantity, timeliness and effectiveness of services; providing periodic reassessment to assure that services are appropriate and cost effective and do not increase the client's dependence.
- Monitoring activities to ensure that services are actually being delivered and meet the needs of the client.
- Evaluating client and program outcomes to determine whether the client should be discharged or assigned inactive service.

From Bower, K. (1992). *Case management by nurses* (p. 222). Washington, DC: American Nurses Publishing.

confront and clarify their values and commitment to working together, rather than just talking about protecting and nurturing children" (Children's Defense Fund, 1991, pp. 7–9).

The School Nurse as Student, Family, and Staff Advocate

It is fitting for the school nurse to advocate for the health rights of students, families, and school staff. The nurse functions as a facilitator who is able to see the health care needs of these clients and provide support and resources as the clients themselves make the actual arrangements for the particular service needed. The role of the school nurse is to help these clients develop the necessary skills to become self-confident and self-reliant in arranging their own health care (Wold and Dagg, 1981). The school nurse then becomes a change agent for participatory decision making to increase the client's level of wellness. School nurses must recognize that education and health are inextricably intertwined, and achieving the mission of education—helping each student to become a productive member of society—will require advocacy for the health needs of the school-age population (NCRSCIAH, 1990).

It should be noted that the role of the school nurse as an advocate for students and families does not stop at the local school level but continues at the state and federal levels to lobby for legislation that may have an impact on school health services, school health education, and a healthy environment for American children.

The School Nurse as Case Manager

The case management concept provides an excellent opportunity for school nurses to act as advocates for their clients. Case management in nursing originated with service coordination in public health nursing during the turn of the 20th century. The primary functions of case management, as noted in Table 28–3, are performed by school nurses. One function, procuring services, including eligibility decisions and authorizing hospitalization and home care (Bower, 1992), is not appropriate for the school nurse. The function of case management confirms the need for the minimum preparation provided by a baccalaureate degree in nursing for the school nurse. School nursing currently has an identifiable population for case management owing to the "mainstreaming" of students who are developmentally disabled into the regular classroom setting. Other students who benefit from case management include those with the human immunodeficiency virus or AIDS, previous closed head injuries, or transplants; students who are technologically dependent; and students who are severely compromised by an acute illness or an acute exacerbation of a chronic illness. High-risk infants 0 to 3 years of age are currently being served by schools under P.L. 99–457 through the Handicapped Infant and

Toddler Program (Education of the Handicapped Amendments, 1986). Although these students are considered a priority group for case management, at one time or another, groups within the generally well population of the school may require this model. Examples of these students include obese children and pregnant adolescents.

The School Nurse as Health Screener

There are two conditions under which health screenings occur in the school setting. First, there are vision, hearing and scoliosis screenings, which are mandated by most states to detect disease conditions. Second, screenings for blood pressure, cholesterol, dental disease, lead absorption, and tuberculosis are often initiated to identify chronic or infectious diseases in the school community. They are performed to identify asymptomatic individuals who may unknowingly have a problem, and should not be substituted for medical examinations. Screenings are presumptive and require a follow-up to confirm diagnosis. Many times children who are at risk are omitted because of absence from school or refusal by parents to allow screening. Screening programs for preschool children such as Early and Periodic Screening, Diagnosis, and Treatment (EPSDT); Head Start; and Child Find are related to public laws. In planning a state-mandated program, the school nurse should be familiar with the laws governing the screenings, with the disease conditions themselves, and with the goals and benefits of the screening program. Schools are ideal places to conduct health screenings because of the "captive audience" available and the opportunity for easy detection, diagnosis, and treatment of the identified health conditions (see Chapter 17).

"School Health Programs have relied on economical mass screening to detect common health problems between periodic physical examinations or in place of periodic physical exams" (Kornguth, 1991, p. 272). However, data from the National School Health Services Program funded by the Robert Wood Johnson Foundation Program suggests that school health programs should include both mass screening programs and regular physical examinations because the two methods do not overlap. The number of problems diagnosed by physical examination has been shown to predict a child's absenteeism from school; having two or more diagnosed problems was found to be associated with an absentee rate of 24% (Kornguth, 1991). Children whose mothers had a less than complete high school education, who came from low-income families, who had minority status or government insurance versus private insurance were more likely to be absent as a result of illness (Kornguth, 1991). Absenteeism is a critical issue for school nurses, as it is related to various risk behaviors and a low level of wellness in students. Absenteeism is also an important issue for educators, as it creates disruption in the classroom and reduces teacher efficiency, thus impeding the learning process for all students.

The School Nurse as Provider of Emergency Care

It is appropriate that the school nurse take the lead in the management of medical emergencies that occur in the school setting. Many school systems hire nurses primarily to care for the ill or injured student or faculty member. However, it should be remembered that in the school setting, students and staff are considered basically a well population and the emphasis of the school nurse should not be on emergencies, but rather on prevention of illness and injury.

Many emergencies occur in the school, and the school nurse must be knowledgeable about first aid, management of emergencies, community resources, and referral and follow-up procedures. In many school sites, the school nurse may not be available when an emergency arises. Therefore, teachers or other appropriate school personnel should be trained in first aid and cardiopulmonary resusitation and should know how to activate the emergency medical system in their community. School staff should also be trained in universal precautions. Protective equipment such as latex gloves, goggles, and sharps containers must also be provided.

The School Nurse as Manager of Programs for Aggregates in the School Setting

A school community is made up of various groups within its population. These groups may be identified as "at risk" for potentially contracting illness or injury because of certain activities in which they engage. The population groups are aggregates of persons who have one or more shared personal or environmental characteristics.

In the school community the school nurse, using biostatistical data to determine the extent and distribution of specific health problems, can set priorities for program planning. "Health promotion strategies are those related to individual lifestyles—personal choices made in a social context—that can have a powerful influence over one's health prospects. These priorities include physical activity and fitness, nutrition, tobacco, alcohol and other drugs, family planning, mental health and violent and abusive behavior" (U.S. Department of Health and Human Services [USDHHS], 1990, p. 6). "Health protection strategies are those related to environmental or regulatory measures that confer protection on large population groups. These strategies address issues such as unintentional injuries, occupational safety and health, environmental health, food and drug safety, and oral health" (USDHHS, 1990, p. 6). All of these strategies require assessment of the needs and problems of aggregates and the planning of a school-wide intervention program for aggregates.

Health Curricula

The purpose of a comprehensive school health education curriculum is to provide students with planned, systematic, and ongoing learning opportunities designed to help them make personal health decisions that will promote growth and health in their lives (Seffrin, 1990). This mission of a comprehensive school health curriculum is critical to school-age children and to our nation, as our most serious health problems relate to personal decision making and lifestyle. In addition, many of these lifestyle factors and individual behaviors are developed in the school years (Seffrin, 1990).

We are currently experiencing a time of reform or "restructuring" in the educational arena. These changes have implications for both health educators and health education curricula. Restructured schools, for example, are focused on outcome-based education. In considering outcomes, health educators might suggest that students become involved in peer education, local environmental campaigns, or school-wide health fairs as part of the curriculum (Cleary, 1991).

Integration of curricula is another trend that will have implications for health education. Time allocation and available resources are important considerations in planning health content.

There are several national initiatives to promote school health education. The NCRSCIAH has been established (DeFriese et al., 1990) by the National State Boards of Education and the American Medical Association for the purposes of examining the potential of school and community partnerships. At the federal government level, partnerships have developed among the Office of Disease Prevention and Health Promotion, the Centers for Disease Control and Prevention, the U.S. Department of Education, the American School Health Association, and other organizations focused on school health (McGinnis and DeGraw, 1991).

Schools represent a key to attaining the *Healthy People 2000* objectives. More than one third of the 300 objectives for the year 2000 can either be directly attained by schools or advanced by the schools (McGinnis and DeGraw, 1991). The key objectives that relate to school health education are listed in Table 28–4.

CRITERIA AND CONTENT

National organizations have established criteria that can be used in assessing the comprehensiveness of the health curriculum within a school (Seffrin, 1990). Some specifically selected criteria are as follows:

- Instruction should be intended to motivate health maintenance and promote wellness, not merely to prevent disease.
- Activities should be designed to develop decision-making competencies.
- Curriculum should be planned and sequential from pre-kindergarten through grade 12.
- Opportunities should be present for all students to develop knowledge, attitudes, and practices.
- There should be an integration of the physical, mental, emotional, and social dimensions of health in the curriculum.
- Specific goals and objectives and a means of evaluation should be present.

In general there is a core body of knowledge that is recommended for comprehensive health education (Seffrin, 1990). This core consists of community health, consumer health, environmental health, family life, growth and development, nutritional health, personal health, prevention and control of diseases and disorders, safety and accident prevention, and substance use and abuse. The specific nature of the curriculum should accommodate the unique local needs and preferences of each community (e.g., the inclusion of nonviolent conflict resolution).

TEACHING METHODS

In designing a curriculum for health education, critical thought must be given to which teaching strategies will be effective in increasing knowledge, changing attitudes, and influencing health-related behavior. Some characteristics of more effective techniques include (1) the use of discovery approaches, with opportunity for "hands on" experiences; (2) the use of student learning stations, small work groups, and cooperative learning techniques (Nastasi and Clements, 1991); (3) cross-age and peer teaching, especially regarding drug use; (4) positive approaches that emphasize the value of good health and normal growth and development; and (5) emphasis on the affective domain (e.g., self-esteem and self-efficacy) (Seffrin, 1990).

MATERIALS

Selection of materials for curricula should be based on a broad framework. In 1984, the National Professional School Health Organizations asserted that, "comprehensive school health instruction provides the cognitive information, behavioral skills, and affective experiences necessary for students to more effectively decide which behaviors they will choose. The focus is on the processes the student encounters or participates in as well as the final behavioral outcomes" (Elias, 1990, p. 157).

The selection of curriculum material should reflect the link of affect, cognition, and social relationships to health

TABLE 28–4

Healthy People 2000 Objectives Related to School Health Education

1. Increase to at least 75% the proportion of elementary and secondary schools that provide planned and sequential quality school health education from kindergarten through 12th grade.
2. Increase to at least 75% the proportion of schools that provide nutrition education from preschool through 12th grade, preferably as part of quality school health education.
3. Establish tobacco-free environments and include tobacco use prevention in the curricula of all elementary, middle, and secondary schools, preferably as part of quality school health education. (Baseline: 17% of school districts banned smoking in 1988; antismoking education existed in 75% of elementary schools, 81% of middle schools, and 78% of secondary schools.)
4. Increase the proportion of high school seniors who perceive social disapproval associated with the heavy use of alcohol, occasional use of marijuana, and experimentation with cocaine.

Behavior	1989 Baseline	2000 Target
Heavy use of alcohol	56.4%	70%
Occasional use of marijuana	71.1%	85%
Trying cocaine once or twice	88.9%	95%

Note: Heavy drinking is defined as having five or more drinks once or twice each weekend.

5. Increase the proportion of high school seniors who associate risk of physical or psychological harm with the heavy use of alcohol, regular use of marijuana, and experimentation with cocaine.

Behavior	1989 Baseline	2000 Target
Heavy use of alcohol	44%	70%
Regular use of marijuana	77.5%	90%
Trying cocaine once or twice	54.9%	80%

Note: Heavy drinking is defined as having five or more drinks once or twice each weekend.

6. Provide to children in all school districts and private schools primary and secondary school educational programs on alcohol and other drugs, preferably as part of quality school health education. (Baseline: 63% provided instruction, 39% provided counseling, and 23% referred students for clinical assessments in 1987.)
7. Increase to at least 85% the proportion of people ages 10 through 18 who have discussed human sexuality, including values surrounding sexuality, with their parents or have received information through another parentally endorsed source, such as youth, school, or religious programs (baseline: 66% of people 13 through 18 had discussed sexuality with their parents in 1986).
8. Increase to at least 50% the proportion of elementary and secondary schools that teach nonviolent conflict resolution skills, preferably as a part of quality school health education.
9. Provide academic instruction on injury prevention and control, preferably as part of quality school health education, in at least 50% of public school systems.
10. Increase to at least 95% the proportion of schools that have age-appropriate HIV education curricula for students in 4th through 12th grade, preferably as part of quality school health education (baseline: 66% of school districts required HIV education in 1989).
11. Include instruction in sexually transmitted disease prevention in the curricula of all middle and secondary schools, preferably as part of quality school health education (baseline: 95% of schools reported offering at least one class on sexually transmitted diseases in 1988).
12. Increase to at least 50% the proportion of school physical education class time that students spend being physically active, preferably engaged in lifetime physical activities (baseline: 27% of class time in 1984).

From U.S. Department of Health and Human Services. (1990). *Healthy people 2000: National health promotion and disease prevention objectives. Summary report.* Washington, DC: U.S. Government Printing Office.

knowledge and behavior. Critical issues in curriculum selection have been outlined by Elias (1990) and include the following:

- The materials should convey wellness as a priority and value.
- The curriculum should prepare students to access school health services as well as other health services.
- The materials should emphasize health promotion.
- The curriculum should specify ongoing roles for parents, including parent education and involvement.
- The curriculum should link to age levels and be built on multiyear sequencing. The first year in the sequence would focus on knowledge and attitudes, whereas subsequent sequences would focus on application.

Curricular focusing is one approach to organizing and selecting materials. Curricular "hubs" can be established and might include areas such as self-care, relationship with parents and siblings, communication, nutrition, heart health, drug use, or sexuality (Elias, 1990). These hubs can then be based on well-developed curriculum materials which might include Growing Healthy (Smith et al., 1992), Life Skills Training (Botvin, 1985), or Project Star (Pentz et al., 1986), to name a few.

HealthPACT is an example of curriculum materials designed specifically for health instruction (Igoe, 1991). This curriculum is designed to prepare children to communicate effectively with health professionals. It teaches them to talk with the health provider; listen and learn; ask questions; decide what to do, with help from the provider; and follow through. These materials emphasize the important role of the consumer as a partner in health care. One of the roles of the school nurse is to help students develop their own skills in coordinating their own health care needs.

Health Promotion

"Although one can trace the idea of health promotion back to ancient times, the term itself has become prominent only in recent years. Current thinking on health promotion stems mainly from two roots: (1) the remarkable improvements in health during the 20th century and the ensuing opportunity to focus on health in a positive as well as negative (disease control) sense, and (2) increasing recognition that medicine constitutes only one factor in the advance of health that a complete strategy for health must embrace" (Breslow, 1990, p. 6). Health promotion currently is being used in reference to a wide range of activities undertaken by government, industry, private practitioners, health institutions, and schools to maintain or improve the level of wellness of individuals (see Chapter 16). It is the science and art of helping people change their lifestyle to move toward a state of optimal health (O'Donnell, 1986). In *Healthy People 2000,* educational and community-based programs are challenged to address lifestyles and personal health practices as well as to improve the health aspects of the physical and social environment (USDHHS, 1990).

There is a growing consensus that health promotion and education efforts should be centered in and around schools. The schools are the "workplace" for nearly one fifth of the U.S. population of children and adults. It is clear that the school environment affects the lives of students' families as well as the entire community. Therefore, it is imperative that a school health program provide health promotion activities to address health and social problems that adversely affect learning and productivity (Lavin et al., 1992a,b).

Successful school health programs can be the key to providing health promotion programs for the school-age child that will significantly affect wellness behaviors. Society clearly benefits from having healthier people. A healthy work population produces more, needs fewer benefits, and is generally more satisfied on the job. It is to society's advantage to promote wellness in homes, schools and the workplace.

Common Health Concerns of School-age Children

School nurses are in a unique position to help children achieve and maintain a high level of wellness. Injury-related deaths are the predominant cause of mortality in school-age children, whereas violent deaths and accidents account for the majority of deaths in adolescents. Common causes of morbidity in school-age children include asthma and school adjustment disorders, including phobia and learning difficulties. For adolescents, substance abuse, sexually transmitted diseases, and pregnancy are common problems.

DRUG AND ALCOHOL USE

Illegal use of drugs continues to be a problem in school-age children. The prevalence of this problem has been documented since 1975 by yearly surveys conducted by the University of Michigan Institute in the Monitoring the Future Project. The 1990 survey found the following percentages of students who had used each drug at least once during the previous month: alcohol, 57%; cigarettes, 29%; marijuana, 14%; and cocaine, 2% (McGovern and DuPont, 1991) (see Chapter 21).

School nurses can be instrumental in implementing comprehensive programs to address these problems. One role is that of case-finder. It is important to survey the extent of the problem within the school and community, to identify those children at risk, and to appropriately intervene. Within the school setting, some common childhood risk factors for adolescent drug use include academic failure, a low degree of commitment to education, and low level of attachment to teachers and schools.

One mechanism for early identification, intervention, referral, and follow-up of at-risk students is the Student Assistance Program (SAP) (McGovern and DuPont, 1991). SAPs have existed since 1978 and were derived and adapted from Employee Assistance Programs. One way to implement an SAP is to have a single coordinator who is responsible for counseling, assessment, and interventions within the school. The other approach is to train a team of school personnel (nurses, counselors, teachers) who collaborate and may work with community experts in providing services to the students. Implementation of the program consists of identification, data collection, intervention, referral, and follow-up.

Drug abuse prevention programs are also common in schools (Table 28–5), but the effectiveness of these programs must be consistently evaluated. Early approaches of providing only knowledge have given way to programs that address psychosocial and life skills (Synovitz, 1992). There is a need to continue to evaluate the appropriateness of interventions and to possibly design interventions that

TABLE 28–5

Examples of School-Based Alcohol and Drug Prevention Curricula

Curriculum	Description
Here's Looking at You 2000 (Ogden & Germinario, 1988).	A curriculum that teaches refusal, assertiveness, problem-solving, risk assessment, and self-control skills. A cognitive/affective component assists students in identifying personal and others' strengths.
Here's Looking at You—Two (Tricker & Davis, 1988)	A curriculum that includes participatory activities designed to enhance self-esteem and improve decision-making and coping skills.
Project STAR (Students Taught Awareness and Resistance) (Pentz et al., 1986)	Teaches resistance, social, and communication skills.
From Peer Pressure to Peer Support	An alcohol and drug use prevention curriculum for grades 7–12 that emphasizes working in groups to develop life skills.
Facts, Feelings, Family, Friends Series	A K–12 alcohol and drug use prevention curriculum that emphasizes learning about emotions, building friendships, and improving decision making.
Project Direction	A peer-led initiative that teaches refusal, coping, and decision-making skills as well as cognitive strategies.

From Synovitz, L. (1992). Alcohol education through schools: A psychosocial perspective. *Journal of School Health, 62*(2), 69.

are gender specific and address unique psychosocial predictors (Clayton, 1991). There is also a need to begin preventive interventions early, even as early as in the preschool years (Hahn and Papazian, 1987).

The use of legal substances is also an important concern of the health team. Preventing tobacco use should be a focus of all school health programs. Although smoking and snuff use have declined among youths, the smoking prevalence rate has remained at about 20% (Glynn, 1989). However, between 1990 and 1992, the proportion of adolescent girls aged 12 to 17 years who reported smoking within the past month rose slightly (Ernster, 1993).

An advisory panel of the National Cancer Institute has identified the following essential elements of school-based smoking prevention programs (Glynn, 1989):

- *Program focus:* The program may have a smoking-only or a multicomponent health focus.
- *Program content:* Minimum components should include information about social consequences and short-term physiological effects of tobacco, information about social influences on tobacco use, and training in refusal skills.
- *Program length:* Minimum length should be two blocks of five sessions delivered in separate school years between sixth and ninth grade.
- *Age at intervention:* Ideally, the program should be in all grades. If not, then it should focus on students in grades 6 through 9.
- *Peer involvement:* This can enhance program efficacy. The most effective involvement has consisted of a peer leader who assists a trained teacher in specific portions of the program.
- *Parent involvement:* This is important to the effectiveness of the program.
- *Implementation:* Community norms and needs, the interest of the educational community, smoking policies, costs, needs of the curriculum, and ease of implementation all must be considered.

SEXUALLY TRANSMITTED DISEASES

Several population-based surveys have documented the extent of sexual behavior among adolescents. The national school-based Youth Risk Behavior Survey in 1990 revealed that in a representative sample of 11,631 students in grades 9 through 12, 54% reported having had sexual intercourse and 39% had had intercourse in the 3 months preceding the survey (Centers for Disease Control and Prevention [CDC], 1990).

This behavior places adolescents at risk for unwanted pregnancies and sexually transmitted diseases (STDs). Of the STDs, human papillomavirus (HPV) is the most common in sexually active adolescent girls (Coupey and Klerman, 1992). STDs in females can result in pelvic inflammatory disease that can lead to infertility and sterility; *Chlamydia trachomatis* is the most common organism found in association with pelvic inflammatory disease. The prevalence of HIV infection is also rising in teenagers (Coupey and Klerman, 1992) (see Chapter 19).

Prevention efforts and health education regarding STDs are important activities in working with school-age children. AIDS/HIV education is particularly important. Guidelines for effective HIV education have been written by the CDC (1988). There has also been an emphasis on the need to use a developmentally based education approach (Walsh and Bibace, 1990). The focus of AIDS/HIV education, for example, can move from alleviating fear in younger age groups, to identifying and differentiating causes and myths about transmission of HIV in the intermediate age groups, to articulating strategies for AIDS prevention in older age groups.

School nurses can play a key role in meeting the challenges of the AIDS epidemic. To do so, the nurse must be prepared to provide leadership in planning the care of students or staff with HIV, manage the school attendance of HIV-infected students or staff, and act as a change agent in dealing with the epidemic (Brainerd, 1989). In particular, the nurse must use knowledge about HIV disease to teach, counsel, and refer students and staff and to change risky behaviors.

TEENAGE PREGNANCY

Childbearing during adolescence is another potential consequence of high-risk sexual behavior (see Chapter 22). One theoretical approach to pregnancy prevention is based on the development of self-confidence and life skills necessary to obtain an education and enter the labor force as an alternative to parenthood. Effective strategies for pregnancy prevention are abstinence and contraceptive use. Examples of some school-based interventions are listed in Table 28–6.

In addition to school-based interventions, there have been joint efforts between school and community-planned programs. For example, in South Carolina, a School/Community Sexual Risk Reduction Program for Teens was begun (Vincent, 1990). In addition to an emphasis on school education, considerable educational interventions are conducted for clergy, parents, and youths in the community.

School-based clinics are another approach for working with school-age children in middle and high schools. However, school-based clinics have not yet proved to be effective in pregnancy prevention (Dryfoos, 1992). Only 10% to 20% of the students report using clinics for family planning services. Community health nurses and nurse practitioners are continuing to evaluate health outcomes of those who attend such clinics.

Although many interventions are focused on primary prevention, they are not limited to this. If a pregnancy has occurred, the role of the nurse is one of assisting the student to define the most appropriate way of handling the pregnancy. Prenatal counseling by the school nurse has been shown to be effective for health outcomes (Chen et al., 1991).

VIOLENCE AND ACCIDENTS

Between 1933 and 1985, death rates from natural causes for Americans age 10 through 19 decreased significantly, but death rates from violence and injury increased over this same time period (Gans, Blyth, and Elster, 1990). Homicides in 15- to 19-year-olds increased by 74% from 1985 to 1990 (Jenkins and Bell, 1992). Homicide is the leading cause of death in black males age 15 to 19. Suicide is the third leading cause of death among those age 15 to 24 years (Tishler, 1992). Abuse and neglect of teenagers have increased 74% since 1980 (Gans et al., 1990) (see Chapter 20).

Violence prevention programs have been established in some schools and neighborhoods (Jenkins and Bell, 1992). One example is a Boston-based project in which the curriculum addresses three broad issues: the role of anger in violence and ways of addressing the anger without violence, risk factors associated with youth homicide, and nonviolent conflict resolution techniques.

Children and adolescents at risk for interpersonal violence can be identified by the health team. Living in dysfunctional and abusive families is a risk factor, and violence prevention should be stressed with these students.

Child maltreatment is another form of violence that has also reached epidemic proportions. Such maltreatment can consist of physical and/or psychological abuse and neglect and/or sexual abuse. The school nurse is key in the early identification of abuse, reporting of actual or suspected cases, and early intervention.

MENTAL HEALTH

Mental health programs within a school can include a range of programs focused on adolescent development, self-esteem, depression, suicide, and coping. With the multiple pressures and stresses affecting children, many potential needs can be identified within the school setting. Teachers may observe for decreased attendance and performance or attitude problems. Teenagers may display behavior problems, withdrawal, or somatic complaints (Puskar et al., 1990).

An important area for primary prevention is suicide, a leading cause of death among adolescents. There were 237 deaths by suicide among 10- to 14-year-olds in 1988

TABLE 28–6

Examples of School-Based Pregnancy Prevention Curricula

- *Postponing sexual involvement:* Helps young people to identify and develop skills to resist peer pressure to become sexually active.
- *Life skills counseling:* A social skills program designed to teach problem-solving and assertiveness skills related to sexual behavior.
- *Life planning curricula:* Combines materials on vocational guidance with exercises to decrease risk taking.
- *Teen outreach program:* Group life planning class and counseling sessions and weekly volunteer community service assignments.

Data from Dryfoos, J. (1992). School- and community-based pregnancy prevention programs. *Adolescent Medicine, 3*(2), 241–255.

(USDHHS, 1990). Suicide prevention programs are often established to (1) increase awareness in the school/community of the incidence of teenage suicide, (2) train school personnel in strategies for teenage suicide awareness/prevention, (3) develop and implement school-based preventive programs, and (4) utilize community resources in the implementation of teenage suicide prevention programs (Maryland Department of Education, 1989).

The three components of one suicide prevention program in Maryland consist of prevention, intervention, and postvention. Prevention is focused on services and activities that help students, school families, and communities to develop an awareness of the problem and identify students at risk. This phase consists of suicide awareness education training for youths, local school personnel, parents, and the community. Intervention consists of services and activities that are appropriate for students at risk. These services include the provision of crisis intervention by school counselors. Postvention services and activities help students, school staff, families, and the community to cope with the aftermath of a student's attempted or completed suicide (Maryland Department of Education, 1989).

DERMATOLOGICAL DISORDERS

Skin conditions remain a significant part of school nursing practice. It is important that school nurses maintain current information on skin conditions and be knowledgeable in nursing assessment and management of the school-age child who presents with such conditions. Nurses must allay fears among school personnel, students, and parents concerning the communicability and transmission of these conditions while providing emotional support. Assisting the student and the family to comply with medical treatment may reduce the severity of the condition. It is important for school nurses as well as other staff members to recognize the sensitivity students have concerning any skin disorder that may affect their physical appearance or their exclusion from school.

Public health laws in most states require exclusion of students who may have conditions or symptoms that are suspected as being communicable. However, school health professionals recognize that there are degrees of contagiousness, and discretion is used in complying with these laws or regulations. In conditions such as the common cold, sore throats, tinea capitis, impetigo, and herpes virus types 1 and 2, it is not usually necessary to immediately exclude the student from school. The school nurse should communicate with parents through notes or telephone calls at the end of the school day, requesting that the student be seen by his or her usual source of medical care before returning to school (Newton, 1989). Scabies and pediculosis present no emergency to the child or the school population. However, because of the emotional reactions associated with these nuisance conditions, it may be prudent to exclude the child immediately until treatment is completed. No other contagious conditions seem to incite as much fear, anger, and shame in parents and teachers than scabies and head lice.

If examined closely, no two skin disorders look exactly alike. Most of them have some characteristic primary lesions, which are the presentation at the onset of the skin disorder. Secondary lesions appear as a result of excessive scratching, infection, or excessive treatment. Frequently both primary and secondary lesions occur (Sauer, 1985).

Fungal Infections

"Fungi are known to be present as a part of the asymptomatic normal flora of the skin or as abnormal inhabitants" (Sauer, 1985, p. 91). The abnormal or pathogenic inhabitants can invade the skin superficially or deeply. Superficial skin invasions are most commonly seen in the school-age child and may be due to the more common sharing of objects such as caps, combs, socks, and shoes. Superficial fungal infections affect various sites of the body and require individualized therapy. The fungal condition tinea in the school-age child is most often seen in the scalp (tinea capitis) or the feet (tinea pedis).

Tinea pedis ("athlete's foot") is characterized by blisters, maceration, and fissures. It presents as a chronic scaly type of infection that itches and burns. Males are more susceptible than females. Tinea capitis (ringworm of the scalp) is primarily a disease of prepubertal children (ages 2 through 10) rather than adults. The lesions are characterized by the presence of broken-off hairs; inflamed, circumscribed, pustular or scaly dry patches; and possibly even bald areas. Multiple patches are common. The epidemiology of tinea capitis has changed. In the past, most cases were caused by microsporum organisms, but currently *Trichophyton tonsurans* is the major etiological agent. The Woods lamp is no longer effective for screening, as *T. tonsurans* organisms do not fluoresce (Shapiro, 1990). Treatment consists of selenium sulfide shampoos for tinea capitis. Treatment for tinea pedis includes systemic and topical antifungal agents (griseofulvin, tolnaftate) as well as aluminum acetate or acetic acid soaks followed by application of glucocorticoid cream (Whaley and Wong, 1987).

Bacterial Infections

The skin normally harbors a variety of bacteria. The degree of their pathogenicity depends on variables such as the integrity of the skin, the immune and cellular defenses of the host, and the toxigenicity and invasiveness of the organism. Impetigo is an example of a bacterial infection caused by *Staphylococcus aureus* or group A beta-hemolytic streptococci, which can appear after minor trauma or another skin lesion. The resulting infection is characterized by pruritus with crusted lesions. The lesions tend to spread peripherally (Chauvin, 1989). Treatment includes careful removal of the crusts with soap and water and topical application of a bacterial ointment. Systemic administration of antibiotics may be used in extensive lesions.

Viral Infections

Some viral infections common to the school-age child include verruca (warts), herpes simplex virus types 1 (cold sore) and 2 (sexually transmitted lesion), herpes zoster (shingles), rubeola (10-day measles), rubella (3-day measles), and varicella zoster (chickenpox). Most of the communicable diseases of childhood and adolescence are associated with rashes, and each rash is characteristic. Treatment is usually symptomatic for pain and discomfort. The goal of therapy in viral illnesses is to prevent secondary infection. Various topical applications are used as palliative therapy. Steroid ointments should not be used, but antibiotic ointment may be used if secondary infection occurs. The antiviral drug acyclovir (Zovirax) has been used in the treatment of herpes simplex types 1 and 2. Aspirin should not be given for viral infections because of the potential for the development of Reye's syndrome. Verruca may be surgically removed or treated with caustic solutions. They sometimes disappear spontaneously.

Allergic Conditions

Atropic dermatitis (eczema) is an inflammatory skin response to internal or external factors that occurs in acute forms. The primary symptoms are pruritus and acute epidermal/dermal edema, with vesicles on the face, scalp, trunk, and limbs. Chronic changes of dry, flaky skin, secondary fissures, or lichenification are found (Chauvin, 1989). Contact dermatitis is an inflammatory reaction of the skin to direct contact with a chemical substance that evokes an allergic hypersensitivity. In both types of dermatitis the causative agent should be eliminated if possible, or the student may need medical desensitization therapy. Treatment of the lesions consists of topical corticosteroid gel for prevention or relief of inflammation. Oral corticosteroids may be needed for extensive reactions (Whaley and Wong, 1987).

RESPIRATORY CONDITIONS

Acute conditions of the respiratory tract are a common cause of illness in the school-age child. The lower respiratory tract consists of the structures contained in the chest related to the flow of air to and from the lungs (e.g., the trachea, bronchi, and bronchioles). The upper respiratory tract consists primarily of the nose and the pharynx and can be subjected to a variety of infective organisms. The type of illness and the physical response are related to factors such as the type of infectious organism, the age of the child, and the integrity of the child's defense mechanisms.

Most upper respiratory infections are caused by viruses and may be self-limiting. However, secondary infections such as otitis media, acute bronchitis, influenza, and pneumonia can cause serious complications. Asthma causes more absences from school, more hospital admissions, and more emergency department visits than any other chronic childhood illness. It occurs in approximately 7.5% of all children in the United States and is most common in black, inner city children. Allergies, viral infections, cigarette smoke, exercise, and changes in weather can trigger asthma (Evans, 1991). During the 1980s the prevalence rate of asthma increased by 29%, and the death rate for asthma as the first listed diagnosis increased 31% (National Institutes of Health, 1991). The reasons for these alarming increases are unclear, but increased exposure to environmental irritants and pollutants may be the major culprits. Environmental factors that frequently trigger asthmatic episodes can be addressed in the home, but addressing such factors in the school setting may present difficulty, as air temperature, humidity, and odors from hair sprays, perfumes, and chemicals are not as easily controlled. Guidelines for air flow and maintenance of heating and air conditioning units are available to help prevent and resolve indoor air quality problems (U.S. Environmental Protection Agency, 1991).

Asthma is characterized by obstruction of the airways or the bronchioles in the lungs, persistent airway inflammation, and airway hyperresponsiveness to various stimuli. The obstruction of the airway is responsible for the clinical manifestations (e.g., wheezing, dyspnea, and cough). These symptoms can occur insidiously or can develop abruptly.

An asthma attack is an episode or flare-up of symptoms that interrupts normal activities. It can also be embarrassing to the child and affect the child's self-esteem. Because asthma can be unpredictable, parents are often concerned about the health of their child. If asthma is not well controlled, it can cause disruptions to school and home life. Sports and social activities may also be interrupted by sudden attacks.

The foremost goal in the management of asthma is to keep the child free of symptoms and maintain participation in activities of life. This may require reducing or avoiding exposure to allergic and irritant triggers, such as pollens from ragweed, grasses, and trees and dust. Chemical irritants such as perfume, tobacco smoke, air pollution, insecticides, paints, varnishes, and cleaners can also trigger an asthma attack and should be avoided. Keeping in good physical health enables the body to resist viral infections such as the common cold or upper respiratory bacterial infections that may precipitate the asthma response. However, exercise may reduce the humidity of inhaled cool air, thus triggering bronchospasms (Mendoza et al., 1989).

To aid in the management of asthma, peak flow monitoring of air expelled from the lungs can predict when an asthma episode is likely to occur. This can be accomplished by using an inexpensive, hand-held device that indicates the asthma status of a person. The peak flow meter is an invaluable tool in the school setting. It provides information to the school nurse and the student concerning the patency of the larger airways. It also gives an objective assessment of whether the asthma is under control, whether medication is needed to prevent an "attack," or whether the medication is effective. Peak flow monitoring allows the student to alter exercise levels in physical education classes to prevent attacks. Periodic monitoring of the peak flow helps also to assess trends in the school-age child and to reassure parents when risk of an asthma attack is present.

The technique of peak flow monitoring is easy to learn. The meters and disposable mouthpieces are inexpensive and offer a cost-effective means of preventing absenteeism and maintaining the student's health while he or she is attending class (Mendoza et al., 1989). Ideally, each child should have his or her own peak flow meter. However, one meter may be sufficient for all students as long as individual disposable mouthpieces are used. The instrument and mouthpieces should be washed and air dried between uses.

The school nurse should become involved in the management of asthma in the school-age child. He or she can promote a close, cooperative relationship with the student, the family, and the usual source of medical care, which will enhance the student's ability to benefit from his or her educational experience.

The following four care principles in a self-management program (Whaley and Wong, 1987) are effective when the child and parent are active participants:

1. Asthma is a common, annoying disease in which psychological aspects are a response rather than a cause.
2. Persons with asthma can live an active and full life.
3. Compliance with therapy is important, because asthma is much easier to prevent than treat.
4. The emphasis is on managing the condition rather than curing it.

These principles are also relevant to other chronic diseases such as diabetes mellitus and epilepsy.

NUTRITIONAL CONSIDERATIONS

"Dietary factors are associated with 5 of the 10 leading causes of death: coronary heart disease, some types of cancer, stroke, non-insulin dependent diabetes mellitus, and atherosclerosis" (USDHHS, 1990, p. 114). Therefore, there is great interest in changing behavior to protect school-age children from future illnesses. Children who learn good nutrition practices at an early age will be able to take an active part and be responsible in developing a healthy body. Proper nutrition also plays an important role in the mental development of individuals.

Children are receiving mixed messages concerning diet and nutrition. Families and some school systems encourage children to "stay healthy and eat right" but provide meals that are high in fat and cholesterol and low in needed complex carbohydrates and dietary fiber. Vending machines in schools often provide limited nutritional choices. Television networks advertise foods that contain empty calories during programming for children. With little or no parental supervision, children fill up on "junk food." Because children usually develop the eating habits of their families, the quality of their diet relates directly to their family's pattern of eating. In many families, both parents work, and the number of one-parent families has increased. Some children find themselves responsible for preparing their own meals. Developmentally, both physically and socially, children may not be ready to make proper decisions about food choices. They will tend to satisfy their hunger with foods that are convenient. Therefore, "the once-prevalent nutrient deficiencies have been replaced by excesses and imbalance of some food components in the diet" (USDHHS, 1990, p. 114).

The federal government, in response to nutrition problems, established the National School Lunch Program and the School Breakfast Program in many areas. The meals are free or at a reduced price and are planned to meet specific nutritional requirements and provide at least one third of the recommended daily allowance for children in the United States. Low family income is necessary for eligibility (U.S. Congress, OTA, 1991b).

In *Healthy People 2000,* dietary practices to minimize the risk of chronic diseases and premature death are recommended. These recommendations include maintaining desirable weight; increasing intake of complex carbohydrates and fiber-containing foods; reducing sugar intake, total fat and cholesterol, total saturated fat, and sodium intake; and increasing calcium intake (USDHHS, 1990). Diet and physical activity started at an early age must be emphasized. This belief must be nurtured in the home and reinforced in the school setting. Schools can provide healthful foods in the school breakfast and lunch programs; physical education can teach fitness activities that can be maintained for life; and classroom instruction can address knowledge, attitudes, and beliefs (Kolbe, 1982). However, parents appear to have the greatest influence in changing poor eating behaviors, as they have control over food purchasing, food preparation, peer support among family members, and modeling positive eating behaviors. "Parental knowledge is important in a behavior change model, because accurate knowledge about food consumption and health consequences of certain eating patterns is needed before parents can teach and model positive behaviors" (Crockett et al., 1988, p. 56). School nurses can teach parents about healthy nutrition.

Obesity in the school-age child is one of the most prevalent health problems. Obesity in childhood or adolescence, coupled with a sedentary lifestyle, may persist into adulthood and increase the risk for chronic physical and psychological conditions (USDHHS, 1990). In a survey concerning childhood obesity, school nurses reported that poor eating habits and excessive caloric intake, coupled with a lack of nutritional knowledge, were major factors in the development of childhood obesity (Price et al., 1987). Schools are in a position to assist in the prevention of childhood obesity. Nutrition information should be integrated into the curriculum for kindergarten through grade 12, and school nurses must take a leadership role in assisting the classroom teacher to deliver the appropriate message to both parents and children.

Eating disorders in adolescents primarily include anorexia nervosa and bulimia. These conditions are psychological problems with severe physical results. These individuals must have psychotherapy as well as medical help, and proper nutrition is a prime concern.

Anorexia nervosa is characterized by an intense fear of becoming obese and a refusal to eat, which leads to a significant weight loss (U.S. Congress of the United States, OTA, 1991b). In the school setting, the anorectic student may be identified as one with a marked disturbance in body image but who regards this appearance as normal. These students attempt to hide their appearance by wearing clothing that is bulky. However, they may be preoccupied with food (e.g., hoarding snacks, preparing food for others, and obsessively conversing about food). They tend to increase their physical activity, and females may have primary or secondary amenorrhea.

The incidence of anorexia has doubled in the United States since the mid-1970s. It is more often seen in white females from middle or upper class families and usually occurs between the ages of 12 and 14 or 17 and 18 years (Herzog and Copeland, 1985). These young people tend to isolate themselves and withdraw from peer relationships. They continually strive for perfection and are overachievers.

This condition is one of the most difficult of all adolescent disorders to treat. The approach must be multidisciplinary, with input from the primary physician, psychiatrist, school nurse, nutritionist, family members, and peers. The focus must include reinstitution of normal nutrition, resolution of the disturbed patterns of family interactions, and individual psychotherapy to correct deficits and distortions in psychological functions.

Bulimia is characterized by binging and purging the body by self-induced vomiting or the use of laxatives and is seen more frequently in older female adolescents and young adults (U.S. Congress of the United States, OTA, 1991b). This disorder is characterized by binging on large amounts of high-calorie foods in a brief period of time. There are repeated attempts to lose weight by self-induced vomiting or the use of laxatives. There may be wide fluctuations in weight accompanied by depression and overconcern about body weight and shape (Whaley and Wong, 1987). Bulimic females may have a history of childhood maladjustment and family psychiatric disorders; often there is history of rejection and blame (Humphrey, 1988). Bulimia appears to be a disorder of regulating affect and impulse control (Yates, 1989).

In the school setting the adolecent may present with symptoms related to gastrointestinal problems (e.g., pain, bloating, reflux, sore throat, and difficulty swallowing). Tooth enamel may be eroded from repeated vomiting of stomach acid (Whaley and Wong, 1987).

Therapies similar to those discussed in the treatment of anorexia may be initiated. A team approach to address the nutritional as well as the psychological aspects of the disorder must be considered. School health personnel must be patient and understanding and provide opportunities for acceptance and the development of a positive self-image. Physical manifestations should be monitored in bulimic students, as serious illness or death can occur. School nurses are a link joining the student, parent, treatment team, and teachers.

DENTAL HEALTH

The incidence of dental caries has declined steadily since the 1940s, leaving only one half of school-age children with some decay in their permanent teeth (USDHHS, 1990). Fluoridation of the water supplies, initiated in 1945 in the United States, is probably responsible for this decline among children and adolescents (U.S. Congress of the United States, OTA, 1991a). However, there are more than 100 million people in the United States, a large percentage of whom are school-age children, who do not have fluoridated water available. For this segment of the population, dental sealants and topical fluoride treatments have been promising in the attempt to reduce dental caries (USDHHS, 1990). Dental caries may also be caused by eating foods high in sugars, omiting brushing and flossing, eating foods that adhere to the teeth between meals, and the use of some liquid medications.

There is a great need for dental health education. Parents are still considered the main support for children's wellness behavior and ability to make appropriate decisions about behavior change. Role modeling by parents concerning good oral health practices also greatly influences these decisions. Many physicians do not conduct basic examinations of the mouths of children or provide parents with counseling and referral to a dentist for care. For these reasons, it has been suggested that by the year 2000, 90% of all children entering school programs for the first time should undergo oral health screening, referral, and follow-up for the necessary diagnostic, preventive, and treatment services (USDHHS, 1990). Because this goal is largely dependent on the family commitment to the prevention of dental disorders, school health personnel must address and improve dental health education and services in the schools. The school nurse who is educated in health, child development, and interdisciplinary collaboration will be able to strengthen positive parental influence on children's dental health behavior through the dissemination of information to parents at workshops or in a one-to-one parent conference (Scanlan, 1991).

The school nurse can also assist in the promotion of dental health by encouraging regular dental checkups; by providing instruction on good oral hygiene, including proper brushing and the use of dental floss; by encouraging sound nutrition practices, including restricting cariogenic foods; and by preparing children for dental services in a way that will provide a positive experience. Dental health behaviors (e.g., keeping dental appointments and following through on recommended treatments and practices) should be developed and perpetuated into adulthood.

Another dental health problem facing school health personnel is tooth trauma, which constitutes a large percentage of all injuries in schools. It has been estimated that 1 in 200 school-age children will experience tooth trauma that involves avulsion. Almost any avulsed tooth can be replanted and retained, with a 90% success rate. However, avulsion causes pain, embarrassment, expense, and loss of time from school or sports activities. In addition, it presents a scenario for possible legal suits related to injury (Krasner, 1992).

The avulsed tooth should be replanted and stabilized as soon as possible, preferably within 30 minutes and by a dentist. However, the tooth may also be stored and transported to a dentist, who will then replant and splint the tooth. The tooth should be washed with clear running water only, carefully holding it by the crown. It may then be placed either in the mouth of the child, under the tongue, or in cold milk. The best storage medium is a cell culture preserving fluid that can keep the cells viable for up to 96 hours (Krasner, 1992).

In remote areas or when a dentist is not available, the student or the school nurse may replant the tooth. School nurses may not alway be available when trauma or tooth avulsion occurs. Therefore, it is important for other school staff to be trained in emergency procedures related to the implantation of an avulsed tooth and the proper method of storing the tooth until the child sees a dentist. The procedure used for implantation and storage of the tooth between the time of accident and proper care determines the ultimate prognosis (Krasner, 1992). Consideration must also be given to the emotional trauma as well as the physical trauma experienced by the child.

Future Trends and Issues in School Health Programs

Increasing optimism has developed about the role of schools in promoting the health of children, with emphasis on creating comprehensive school health programs. The role of the federal government in promoting health in the schools appears to be expanding. What can be expected for the future? First, we can expect an increase in school-linked services that integrate education, health, and social services for children. "In a school-linked approach to services for children, (a) services are provided to children and their families through a collaboration among schools, health providers, and social service agencies; (b) the schools are among the central participants in planning and governing the collaborative effort; and (c) the services are provided at, or are coordinated by personnel located at the school or a site near the school" (Center for the Future of Children, 1992, p. 7).

We can also expect increased collaboration with many components of the community and an increased interest in policy (Usdan, 1990). At the federal level, legislation and funding for schools are being linked with issues such as AIDS, drugs, child care, and youth training. The *Healthy People 2000* objectives are providing guidance to schools on how to ensure healthy students in the future. There will be an increased emphasis on building coalitions with businesses and churches for addressing the health needs of students.

The following questions outlined by Kirby (1990) will most likely have to be addressed:

- What are the most effective strategies for educating the community about the health needs of the community's youth and motivating it to take a leadership role?
- How can school and community programs, especially school and public health programs, become more integrated and reinforcing?
- What are the effective methods of involving parents, employers, youth-serving agencies, and churches?

In general, there seems to be a call for a broad perspective on school health. One approach is an expansion of the concept of school health from an approach consisting of school health services, health education, and health improvements in the environment, to a more comprehensive approach that includes nutrition, physical education, guidance, and health promotion for students and faculty. Some authors are calling for the development of family health centers (Igoe and Giordano, 1992).

It is an exciting time of change. The curricula, goals, and structure of the public education system are in flux. There is a need for change in addressing the educational, psychosocial, and health needs of students in this time of "new morbidities." It is both a necessity and an opportunity for nurses to participate in redesigning the school health programs for the future (Baker, 1992).

In this period of optimism and time of change, however, there is also a need to address the reality of budgetary cuts. Since the 1970's school nurses have been faced with budgetary cuts that have resulted in a loss of job security (Wold and Dagg, 1981). This trend became especially prevalent in the early 1990s with budgetary deficits at all levels of the government and in the private sector. Efforts are being made to reduce the increasing costs of health care. In a cost containment environment, school nurses are not exempt from further cutbacks.

If school nursing is to survive and continue to grow, efforts must be made to secure funding and to justify the existence of school health programs. Funding will have to be sought in the public sector through lobbying efforts at the federal, state, and local levels. In the public and private sectors, efforts must also be made to creatively seek funding to address the special needs of children.

Innovative programs and responses to opportunities can help not only to secure funds, but also to provide the means to evaluate creative approaches to meeting the needs of children. Research is essential to the survival of school nursing. Answers will be needed to the following questions:

- Is nursing care making a difference?
- How are the children and adolescents most in need being served?
- What are the goals of the health program?
- How can school nurses most effectively address the "new morbidities"?

The future of school nurses will depend on innovativeness, research, and the ability of school nurses to convince communities of the value of their interventions to children and adolescents, who are often forgotten and underserved.

KEY IDEAS

1. Comprehensive school health programs must play an important role in the health promotion of children and adolescents. This comprehensive approach will have to include factual knowledge, attitudes, and skill development with respect to health. Additional components of a comprehensive approach for the 21st century will include school and community linkages and employee wellness programs.
2. Three key components of a school health program continue to be health services, health education, and provision of a safe and healthy environment.
3. School health is largely under the jurisdiction of state mandates and laws, which results in variation among school health programs across the United States.
4. The responsibilities of the school nurse have evolved from a limited perspective to expanding roles that include school nurse practitioners, managers of school-based clinics, providers of comprehensive wellness centers, and providers of extensive case management.
5. School nurses function according to standards that can be found in *School Nursing Practice: Roles and Standards* (Proctor et al., 1993). These standards provide direction and a framework for professional school nursing practice.
6. Common roles of the school nurse include educator, consultant/researcher, liaison, advocate, case manager, provider of screening and emergency services, and manager of health programs.
7. It is imperative that school health programs provide health promotion activities to children and families. More than one third of the 300 objectives from *Healthy People 2000: National Health Promotion and Disease Prevention Objectives* (USDHHS, 1990) can be directly attained or advanced by schools.
8. School nurses influence mortality and morbidity of children. Problems that must be effectively addressed by school nurses include violence, mental health, substance abuse, accidents, sexually transmitted diseases, pregnancy prevention, and physical and chronic health problems. Interventions must focus on reduction of high-risk behavior and promotion of healthy lifestyles.
9. There is increasing optimism about the role of schools in promoting the health of children. As we approach the 21st century, there is an opportunity for change and innovation in establishing partnerships among schools, families, and communities. This will result in an increased emphasis on policy planning and the need to creatively approach financing for school health programs.

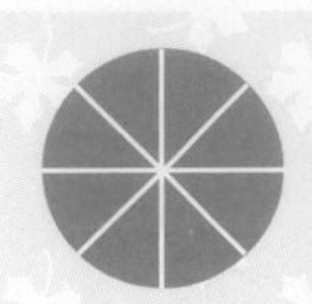

CASE STUDY

*Experiences as a School Nurse**

Mr. W., a social studies teacher, has just finished going over a classroom drill when he notices Susan is not looking well. As he moves toward her desk she begins to jerk her arms and legs. He quickens his pace to keep her from falling out of her chair. As he reaches her desk and provides support, he calls to John to press the intercom button at the front of the room. The office asks what is wrong; Mr. W. states that the school nurse is needed immediately. In a calm voice he reassures the class that Susan will be fine.

In the back of his mind he is thinking how fortunate he is to have received a lecture at the faculty meeting 3 months earlier. "Don't try to stop the movements; protect the student from injury; remain calm," he recalls the school nurse saying. The policy on Care of a Student Having a Seizure was just redistributed at midyear. He remembers thinking that he would never use it but is glad he read it.

The school nurse arrives at the classroom door, assesses the situation, and instructs Mr. W. to help place Susan on her side on the floor. Mr. W. then instructs the class to move to an adjacent vacant classroom. Susan's color is poor, but her respirations are within the normal rate. Fortunately, the last student leaves the room before Susan loses bladder control. After 2 minutes, Susan's seizure stops, and she is moved to the health suite. Although the nurse is aware of Susan's diagnosis of epilepsy, this is her first seizure during school.

Susan is assessed at regular intervals during her recovery period. Susan's mother is notified and assured that her daughter is in no danger. Arrangements are made for a change of clothing to be brought to the school. After about an hour Susan is alert; her main concern is what her classmates are going to think about her. Arrangements are made to provide information about epilepsy to her classmates during the next period, and the school nurse and Susan will allow her classmates an opportunity to talk. Susan is glad that her classmates did not witness her loss of bladder control and asks how Mr. W. knows so much about epilepsy. The school nurse uses material designed by the Epilepsy Foundation to educate Susan's peers. About a week later the school nurse sees Susan in the lunchroom, and with a subtle wave, Susan indicates she is doing well.

Mrs. H., an English teacher, is waiting to have her blood pressure checked. During the faculty wellness blood pressure screening program, Mrs. H. was referred to her physician. Since that time, she has been placed on antihypertension medication. Routine blood pressure checks by the school nurse assist Mrs. H. in maintaining her level of wellness. The faculty wellness program is a natural adjunct to the health services program, as a healthy faculty provides students with a better educational program.

As the nurse finishes recording Mrs. H.'s blood pressure, in walks Thomas, a student with asthma. Thomas is acutely short of breath, diaphoretic, pale, and anxious. The school nurse takes a reading with the peak flow meter and administers the prescribed medication by inhaler. As for all children with a chronic health condition, the nurse, in collaboration with the primary health care provider and the parents, has developed a plan of care. After the medication begins to take effect, an additional peak flow reading is obtained. Thomas's condition improves, he becomes less anxious, and within 30 minutes returns to class.

The preceding examples illustrate the role of the school nurse in meeting the health needs of a varied school population. It is important to visualize the school nurse in the roles of caregiver, health counselor, advocate, consultant, collaborator, educator, and researcher to realize her or his value to the school community. Because new models for school health are evolving, school nurses must document and promote their services to students, parents, school staff members, and local and state legislators who may control funding sources. The school nurse remains the most cost-effective community resource for maintaining a high level of wellness in school-age children.

* By Robert Mehl, B.S.N., R.N., School Nurse, Baltimore County Public Schools, Baltimore, MD.

GUIDELINES FOR LEARNING

1. Spend a day with a school nurse or school nurse practitioner. Observe the nurse interacting with children of various ages. Note the health problems of the students identified by the nurse. What interventions did the nurse provide?
2. Interview a school nurse regarding her or his perception of the role of the nurse in the school. What frustrations and rewards does the nurse experience?
3. Interview school-age children to determine their perception of health/wellness and their perception of health promotion within their school. What services are provided? How satisfied are these children with their school health program? How do their perceptions of health/wellness vary with age?

4. Write an essay on your perception of the concept of "comprehensive school health." What do you think the components of a comprehensive school health program should include? Share your reflection with a school health team member to compare your ideas with an existing program.
5. Interview a school nurse to discuss ethical problems that arise within the school setting. How are ethical issues resolved?
6. Interview a school nurse regarding care of high-risk children within the school setting (e.g., children with AIDS or disabilities). What barriers exist in caring for these children? How is the nurse involved in educating the school/community regarding the needs of these children?
7. Review the health curriculum for a local school system. How does the curriculum address the new morbidities and the *Healthy People 2000* objectives?
8. Review current federal, state, or local legislation related to school health services, education, or environment.

REFERENCES

American Federation of Teachers. (1992). *The medically fragile child in the school setting.* Washington, DC: Author.

American Medical Association, Council on Scientific Affairs. (1990). Providing medical services through school-based health programs. *Journal of School Health, 60*(3), 87–91.

American Nurses' Association (ANA). (1983). *Standards of school nursing practice.* Kansas City, MO: Author.

ANA. (1986). *Standards of community health practice.* Kansas City, MO: Author.

ANA. (1991). *Standards of clinical practice.* Kansas City, MO: Author.

American School Health Association. (1983). *Standards of school nursing practice.* Kent, OH: Author.

Baker, C. (1992). Every child in America needs a professional school nurse. *Reflections, 18*(2), 23.

Botvin, G. J. (1985). The life skills training program as a health promotion strategy: Theoretical issues and empirical findings. In J. Zins, D. Wagner, & C. Maher (Eds.), *Health promotion in the schools* (pp. 9–23). New York: Haworth. pp. 9–23.

Bower, K. (1992). *Case management by nurses.* Washington, DC: American Nurses Publishing.

Brainerd, E. (1989). HIV in the school setting: The school nurses's role. *Journal of School Health, 59*(7), 316–317.

Breslow, L. (1990). A health promotion primer for the 1990's. *Health Affairs, 9*(2), 6.

Centers for Disease Control (CDC). (1988). Guidelines for effective school health education to prevent the spread of AIDS. *Journal of School Health, 58*(4), 142–148.

CDC. (1990). Sexual behavior among high school students. *Morbidity and Mortality Weekly Report, 40,* 885–888.

Center for the Future of Children. (1992). *The future of children.* Los Altos, CA: The David and Lucille Packard Foundation.

Chauvin, V. (1989). Common skin rashes in children and adolescents. *School Nurse, 5*(1), 23–38.

Chen, S.-P., Fitzgerald, M., DeStefano, L., & Chen, E. (1991). Effects of a school nurse prenatal counseling program. *Public Health Nursing, 8*(4), 212–218.

Children's Defense Fund. (1991). *The state of America's children 1991.* Washington, DC: Author.

Clayton, S. (1991). Gender differences on psychosocial determinants of adolescent smoking. *Journal of School Health, 61*(3), 115–120.

Cleary, M. (1991). Restructured schools: Challenges and opportunities for school health education. *Journal of School Health, 61*(4), 172–175.

Cohen, W. (1992). The role of the federal government in promoting health through the schools: An opening statement. *Journal of School Health, 62*(4), 126–127.

Comer, J. (1988). Educating poor minority children. *Scientific American, 259,* 42–48.

Coupey, S., & Klerman, L. (1992). Preface to adolescent sexuality: Preventing unhealthy consequences. *Adolescent Medicine, 3*(2), ix–xii.

Crockett, S., Mullis, R., & Perry C. (1988). Parent nutrition education: A conceptual model. *Journal of School Health, 58*(4), 53–57.

Crossland, C., MacPhail-Wilcox, B., & Sowers, J. (1990). Implementing comprehensive school health programs: Prospects for change in American schools. *Journal of School Health, 60*(4), 182–187.

DeFriese, G., Crossland, C., Pearson, C., & Sullivan, C. (1990). Comprehensive school health programs: Their current status and future prospects. *Journal of School Health, 60*(4), 127–128.

Department of Labor, Occupational Safety and Health Administration. *Occupational exposure to bloodborne pathogens; Final rule.* 29 CFR 1910.1030. December 6, 1991.

Dryfoos, J. (1992). School- and community-based pregnancy prevention programs. *Adolescent Medicine, 3*(2), 241–255.

Elias, M. (1990). The role of affect and social relationships in health behavior and school health curriculum and instruction. *Journal of School Health, 60*(4), 157–162.

Ernster, V. (1993). Women and smoking. *American Journal of Public Health, 83*(9), 1202–1204.

Evans, R. (1991). What you should know about asthma. *Advance,* Washington, DC: Asthma and Allergy Foundation of America.

Flynn, B. S., Worden, J. K., Secker-Walker, R. H., Badger, G. J., Geller, B. M., & Costanza, M. C. (1992). Prevention of cigarette smoking through mass media intervention and school programs. *American Journal of Public Health, 82*(6), 827–834.

Gans, J., Blyth, D., & Elster, A. (1990). *America's adolescents: How healthy are they?* Vol. 1. Chicago: American Medical Association.

Glynn, T. (1989). Essential elements of school-based smoking prevention programs. *Journal of School Health, 59*(5), 181–187.

Hahn, E. & Papazian, K. (1987). Substance abuse prevention with preschool children. *Journal of Community Health Nursing, 4*(3), 165–170.

Herzog, D. B., & Copeland, P. M. (1985). Eating disorders. *New England Journal of Medicine, 313,* 295.

Humphrey, L. L. (1988). Relationships within subtypes of anorexics, bulimics, and normal families. *Journal of American Academy of Child and Adolescent Psychiatry, 27,* 544.

Igoe, J. (1991). Empowerment of children and youth for consumer self-care. *American Journal of Health Promotion, 6*(1), 55–64.

Igoe, J. B. (1975) The school nurse practitioner. *Nursing Outlook, 23,* 381.

Igoe, J., & Giordano, B. (1992). *Expanding school health services to services to serve families in the 21st century.* Washington, DC: American Nurses' Association.

Igoe, J., & Speer, S. (1992) The community health nurse in schools. In M. Stanhope & J. Lancaster (Eds.), *Community health nursing.* St. Louis: Mosby–Year Book.

Jenkins, E., & Bell, C. (1992). Adolescent violence: Can it be curbed? *Adolescent Medicine: Psychosocial Issues in Adolescents, 3*(1), 71–86.

Kirby, D. (1990). Comprehensive school health and the larger community: Issues and a possible scenario. *Journal of School Health, 60*(4), 170–177.

Kolbe, L. (1982). What can we expect from school health education? *Journal of School Health, 52*(3), 145–150.

Kornguth, M. (1991). Preventing school absences due to illness. *Journal of School Health, 61*(6), 272–274.

Krasner, P. (1992). Management of tooth avulsion in the school setting. *The Journal of School Nursing, 8*(1), 20.

Lavin, A., Shapiro, G., & Weill, K. (1992a). *Creating an agenda for school-based health promotion: A review of selected reports.* Harvard School Health Project, Department of Health and Social Behavior. Boston: Harvard School of Public Health.

Lavin, A., Shapiro, G., & Weill, K. (1992b). Creating an agenda for school-based health promotion: A review of 25 selected reports. *Journal of School Health, 62*(6), 212–228.

Maryland Department of Education. (1989). *Youth suicide prevention school program.* Baltimore: Author.

McGinnis, J. M., & DeGraw, C. (1991). Healthy schools 2000: Creating partnerships for the decade. *Journal of School Health, 61*(7), 292–297.

McGovern, J., & DuPont, R. (1991). Student assistance programs: An important approach to drug abuse prevention. *Journal of School Health, 61*(6), 260–264.

Mendoza, G., Garcia, M. K., & Collins, M. (1989). *Asthma in the school: Improving control with peak flow monitoring.* Cedar Grove, NJ: Health Scan, Inc.

Nader, P. R. (1990). The concept of "comprehensiveness" in the design and implementation of school health programs. *Journal of School Health, 60*(4), 133–138.

Nastasi, B., & Clements, D. (1991). Research on cooperative learning: Implications for practice. *School Psychology Review, 20*(1), 110–131.

National Commission on the Roles of the School and the Community in Improving Adolescent Health. (1990). *Code blue.* Alexandria, VA: National Association of State Boards of Education.

National Institutes of Health (1991). *Executive summary: Guidelines for the diagnosis and management of asthma* (NIH Publication No. 91-3042A). Bethesda, MD: Author.

National Professional School Health Organizations. (1984). Comprehensive school health education. *Journal of School Health, 54*(8), 312–315.

National School Boards Association. (1991–1992). *School health: Helping children learn.* Vol. 1 and 2. Alexandria, VA: Author.

Neumann, T. (1989). A nurse's guide to fail-safety delegating. *Nursing '89, 19*(9), 63–64.

Newacheck, P. W. (1990) Improving access to health care for children and youth and pregnant women. *Pediatrics, 86*(4), 626–635.

Newton, J. (1989). *The new school health handbook.* Englewood Cliffs, NJ: Prentice-Hall.

O'Donnell, M. (1986). Definition of health promotion. *American Journal of Health Promotion, 1*(1), 4.

Ogden, E., & Germinario, V. (1988). *The at-risk student.* Lancaster, PA: Technomic Publishing Co.

Pentz, M., Cormack, C., Flay, B., Hansen, W., & Johnson, C. (1986). Balancing program and research integrity in community drug abuse prevention: Project Star approach. *Journal of School Health, 56*(9), 389–393.

Price, J. H., Desmond, S. M., Ruppert, E. S., & Stelzer, C. M. (1987). School nurses' perceptions of childhood obesity. *Journal of School Health, 57*(8), 332–336.

Proctor, S. (1990). *Guidelines for a model school nursing services program.* Scarborough, ME: National Association of School Nurses.

Proctor, S., Lordi, S., & Zaiger, D. (1993). *School nursing practice: Roles and standards,* Scarbaurough, Maine: National Association of School Nurses.

Puskar, K., Lamb, J., & Norton, M. (1990). Adolescent mental health: Collaboration among psychiatric mental health nurses and school nurses. *Journal of School Health, 60*(2), 69–71.

Rosenstock, I. M. (1974). Historical origins of the health belief model. *Health Education Monographs, 2,* 325–328.

Rustia, J. (1982). Rustia school health promotion model. *Journal of School Health, 52*(2), 109.

Sauer, G. (1985). *Manual of skin diseases.* Philadelphia: J.B. Lippincott.

Scanlan, B. (1991). An holistic approach to school dental health. *The Journal of School Nursing, 7*(4), 12–15.

Seffrin, J. (1990). The comprehensive school health curriculum: Closing the gap between state-of-the-art and state-of-the-practice. *Journal of School Health, 60*(4), 151–156.

Shapiro, S. (1990). *Adolescent medicine.* Philadelphia: Hanley and Belfus.

Smith, D., Redican, K., & Olsen, L. (1992). The longevity of Growing Healthy: An analysis of the eight original sites implementing the school health curriculum project. *Journal of School Health, 62*(3), 83–87.

Stone, E. (1990). ACCESS: Keystones for school health promotion. *Journal of School Health, 60*(7), 298–300.

Stone, E., & Perry, C. (1990). United States perspectives in school health. *Journal of School Health, 60*(7), 363–369.

Synovitz, L. (1992). Alcohol education through schools: A psychosocial perspective. *Journal of School Health, 62*(2), 67–69.

Tishler, C. (1992). Adolescent suicide: Assessment of risk, prevention, and treatment. *Adolescent Medicine Psychosocial Issues in Adolescents, 3*(1), 51–60.

Torre, C. (1981). Nutritional needs of adolescents. In S. Wold (Ed.). *School nursing: A framework for practice.* North Branch, MN: Sunrise River Press.

Tricker, R., & Davis, L. (1988). Implementing drug education in schools: An analysis of the costs and teacher perceptions. *Journal of School Health, 58*(5), 181–185.

U.S. Congress, Office of Technology Assessment. (1987). *Technology dependent children: Hospital vs home care—a technical memorandum.* OTA -TM-H 38. Washington, DC: U.S. Government Printing Office.

U.S. Congress, Office of Technology Assessment. (1991a). *Adolescent health: Volume I: Summary and policy options.* OTA-H-468. Washington, DC: U.S. Government Printing Office.

U.S. Congress, Office of Technology Assessment. (1991b). *Adolescent health: Volume II: Background and the effectiveness of selected prevention and treatment services.* OTA-H-466. Washington, DC: U.S. Government Printing Office.

U.S. Congress, Office of Technology Assessment. (1991c). *Adolescent health: Volume III: Cross-cutting issues in the delivery of health and related services.* OTA-H-467. Washington, DC: U.S. Government Printing Office.

U.S. Department of Health and Human Services. (1990). *Healthy people 2000. Summary report.* Washington, DC: Public Health Service.

U.S. Environmental Protection Agency. (1991). *Building air quality: A guide for building owners and facility managers.* Washington, DC: U.S. Government Printing Office.

Usdan, M. (1990). Restructuring American educational systems and programs to accomodate a new health agenda for youth. *Journal of School Health, 60*(4), 139–141.

Vincent, M. (1990). Additional considerations in the development of comprehensive school health programs: A commentary. *Journal of School Health, 60*(4), 149–150.

Walsh, M., & Bibace, R. (1990). Developmentally-based AIDS/HIV education. *Journal of School Health, 60*(6), 256–261.

Wiley, D., James, G., Jonas, J., & Crosman, E. (1991). Comprehensive school health programs in Texas public schools. *Journal of School Health, 61*(10), 421–425.

Whaley, L., & Wong, D. (1987). *Nursing care of infants and children.* St. Louis: Mosby–Year Book.

Wold, S., & Dagg, N. (1981). School nursing: A passing experiment? In S. Wold (Ed.), *School nursing.* North Branch, MN: Sunrise River Press.

Wood, S., Walker, D., & Gardner, J. (1986). School health practices for children with complex medical needs. *Journal of School Health, 56*(6), 215–217.

Yates, A. (1989). Current perspectives on the eating disorders: I. History, psychological, and biological aspects. *Journal of the American Academy of Child and Adolescent Psychology, 28,* 813.

SUGGESTED READINGS

Dougherty, D., Eden, J., Kemp, K., Metcalf, K., Rowe, K., Ruby, G., Strobel, P., & Solarz, A. (1992). Adolescent health: A report to the U.S. Congress. *Journal of School Health, 62*(5), 167–174.

Igoe, J., & Campos, E. (1991). Report of a national survey of school nurse supervisors. *School Nurse, 7*(2), 8–20.

Jones, M. E., & Clark, D. (1993). What school nurses really do: A study of school nurse utilization. *Journal of School Nursing, 9*(2), 10–17.

Kosarchyn, C. (1993). School nurses' perceptions of the health needs of Hispanic elementary school children. *Journal of School Nursing, 9*(1), 37–42.

McGovern, J., & Dupont, R. (1991) Student assistance programs: An important approach to drug abuse prevention. *Journal of School Health, 61*(6), 260–264.

Pacheco, M., Powell, W., Cole, C., Kalishman, N., Benon, R., & Kaufman, A. (1991) School based clinics: The politics of change. *Journal of School Health, 61*(2), 92–94.

Richardson, N., & Zrebiec, D. (1990). A student run health fair. *School Nurse, 6*(4), 11–13.

Chapter 29

Home Health Care

Paula Milone-Nuzzo

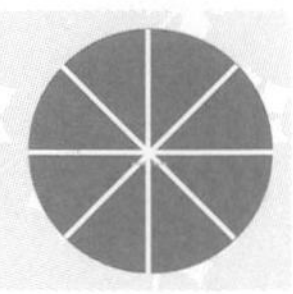

Focus Questions

What is the relationship between public health nursing, community health nursing, and home care nursing?

What are the responsibilities of the home care nurse relative to other members of the home care team?

What are the major sources of reimbursement for home health care?

In what ways do third-party payers influence care that is provided in the home?

How does the application of universal precautions in the home differ from such application in the hospital?

What are rights of individuals and their families who receive home health care?

Home care is the fastest growing aspect of community health nursing and, in fact, of all nursing. Between 1988 and 1992, the number of nurses working in home care increased by 50%. However, home care is not a new concept to the health care system. Community health nursing began with services offered to sick poor persons in their homes. As early as 1859 William Rathbone of Liverpool, England, set up a system of visiting nurses after a nurse cared for his wife at home before her death. With the help of Florence Nightingale, Rathbone started a school to train visiting nurses at the Liverpool Infirmary; the graduates prepared to help the sick poor in their homes.

In the late 1800s the United States experienced rapid urban growth fueled by large waves of immigration to America. Poor living and working conditions gave rise to problems of hygiene and communicable diseases. Visiting nurse associations (VNAs) were developed in the United States by philanthropists, usually wealthy women who wanted to assist the poor to improve their health. Like their counterparts in England, VNAs focused their services almost exclusively on ill individuals who were poor.

The first VNA in the United States was established in 1885 in Buffalo, New York, followed closely by VNAs in Boston and Philadelphia. At this time, agencies operated on private contributions. By the early 1900s care of the ill and the disabled in their home was the traditional form of health care for most people (Spiegel, 1987).

In the 1940s hospitals began taking a more serious interest in home health care because of the increased number of chronically ill individuals. In New York the Montefiore Hospital Home Care Program, which began in 1947, was a comprehensive home care program that focused on posthospital acute care (Mundinger, 1983).

From the late 1800s to the mid-1960s, VNAs were established across the country in major cities and small towns alike (see Chapter 2). In 1965 the face of home health care changed dramatically with the passage of Medicare legislation through the Social Security Act. VNAs that had previously served the health needs of the poor were used more frequently, as home health care was a benefit provided to all elderly patients who participated in Medicare. The passage of the Medicare legislation thus forced home health care to change from a "mom-and-pop" industry to a business. No longer did agencies rely on the charitable giving of wealthy businessmen and women for the money needed to provide care. Also, care was no longer provided primarily to the sick poor. Medicare legislation changed the populations who received home health care as well as the system of paying for that care.

In 1967 there were about 1750 Medicare-participating home health care agencies in the United States; the majority of these were VNAs and public agencies. In 1992 there were more than 6100 Medicare-certified home health care agencies, and the largest percentage of these were proprietary agencies (free-standing, for-profit home health care agencies). Currently only 10% of all home health care agencies in the United States are VNAs (Table 29–1).

Although the growth of the home health care system was initiated by the passage of Medicare legislation, it has since been fueled by economic, technological, and societal factors. In the early 1980s, in an attempt to curb the increasing cost of hospitalization, the nationwide system of diagnostic-related groups (DRGs) was phased into hospitals over a 4-year period. A significant result of the DRG system was a decrease in the client's length of hospital stay and an increased demand for home health care to provide care to clients while they were still recovering from surgery or illness.

Home health care continues to be viewed as not only the most preferred way to provide care to clients, but also the most cost effective. The Nursing Home Without Walls (NHWW) program in New York state was designed to provide home health care services to eligible clients to prevent institutionalization in nursing homes. The costs of services for clients in the NHWW has consistently been half of the cost of corresponding institutional care (National Association for Home Care [NAHC], 1992a).

Medical technology has been developed so that clients can receive more complex, high-technology care at home. Bulky equipment that was difficult and impractical for use

TABLE 29–1

Number of Medicare-Certified Home Health Agencies by Sponsor, 1967, 1987, and 1992

Sponsor	1967		1987		1992	
	No.	*%*	*No.*	*%*	*No.*	*%*
VNA	642	36.6	551	9.5	604	9.9
Public	939	53.6	1073	18.5	1149	18.7
Proprietary	0	0.0	1846	31.9	1953	31.9
Private, not-for-profit	0	0.0	766	13.2	594	9.7
Hospital-based	133	7.6	1439	24.9	1688	27.5
Other	39	2.2	110	1.9	141	2.3
Total	1753	100.0	5785	100.0	6129	100.0

From NAHC. (1992). *Basic statistics about home care.* Washington, DC: Author.

in the home has been modified so that it is smaller, portable, and user friendly (Humphrey and Milone-Nuzzo, 1991). For example, clients can receive continuous parenteral nutrition using a feeding system that is stored in a pouch resembling a backpack. Patient-controlled analgesia pumps that resemble a beeper can be worn by clients on their belt straps. For some clients, this new technology has resulted in being able to maintain daily activities, including work and school.

Finally, clients and caregivers have recognized the positive therapeutic effect that home care can have on the client. No matter how receptive hospital staff try to be, the environment is foreign and antiseptic. Adults who are ill may be comforted by the familiarity of their home and the control over their environment. For children, the ability to remain an integral part of the family in the presence of severe illness is critical to their development.

By the year 2030, one of five Americans will be older than 65 years. Chronic illnesses are common in the elderly and the need for long-term care, including home health care, will grow as this segment of the population increases (U.S. Department of Health and Human Services [USDHHS], 1991). To address the increasing needs of all populations, home health care must continue to grow and diversify to meet the changing needs for services.

For some clients, home care prevents admission to a hospital or nursing home. Other clients enter an inpatient setting from their home and return to their home to receive home care after hospitalization. An understanding of the home health care system is essential to effectively assist clients through the continuum of care from home to hospital and back to home again.

Definitions

The term *home health care* conjures up a variety of images. Many professional organizations involved in home health care, such as the NAHC, have developed their own definition of home health care. Traditionally, home health care includes an arrangement of services provided to people in their place of residence. The following comprehensive definition has been offered by Warhola (1980).

> Home health care is that component of a continuum of comprehensive health care whereby health services are provided to individuals and families in their places of residence for the purpose of promoting, maintaining, or restoring health, or of maximizing the level of independence, while minimizing illness. Services appropriate to the needs of the individual patient and family are planned, coordinated and made available by providers organized for the delivery of home care through the use of employed staff, contractual arrangements, or a combination of the two patterns.

Home health care services can be classified into two broad categories: professional and technical. *Professional home health care* is practice driven—that is, the boundaries of practice are determined by legal and professional standards with a basis in scientific theory and research. This type of home care is provided by professionals with licenses, certifications, or special qualifications (Humphrey, 1988). Home health care nursing is an example of professional home health care.

Technical home health care is product driven, sometimes with a zeal for bottom-line profits. These providers do not always have standards or regulations that guide their practice. Instead, they follow reimbursement guidelines outlining their payments (Humphrey, 1988). Technical home health care providers include durable medical equipment suppliers.

Both types of home health care providers are necessary to ensure comprehensive care to clients. If a client needs oxygen therapy in the home, a supplier is needed to provide equipment such as the oxygen tank and nasal cannula and to service the equipment on a regular basis. The home health care nurse makes home visits to assess the client's respiratory status and observe for any side effects of the therapy. The home health care nurse is also involved in instructing the client and family about the special precautions that must be taken when a client is on oxygen in the home. Either provider alone could not meet the client's total health care needs. Through collaboration, however, the client can be maintained safely and effectively in his or her own home.

The root of home health care nursing can be found in the proud heritage of public health nursing. The initial focus of the American public health nurse was on caring for the sick in the home and preventing disease. An emphasis on health promotion and disease prevention with groups rather than individuals began to emerge in the 1930s. Grounded in the concepts and theory of public health, a specialty called *community health nursing* developed. The American Nurses' Association has defined community health nursing as more than generic nursing carried out in a nonhospital setting. It is a "synthesis of nursing practice and public health practice applied to promoting and preserving the health of the population" (American Nurses' Association [ANA], 1974). Inherent in the practice of community health nursing is health promotion and disease prevention to population groups, with a family-centered focus. Consideration is given to the environmental, social, and personal factors that affect the client's health.

The theory and principles that form the foundation for the practice of community health nursing also are foundational to home care nursing. The family, which can be defined as any significant other, is an integral part of home health care. Family-centered care is critical as the home care provider shifts the responsibility for care from the professional to the patient or the significant other. The individual client as a part of the family is influenced by the activities of the family. In addition, the client's illness in some way affects all other members of the family. *Home care nursing,* as a subspecialty of community health nursing, is defined as the provision of nursing care to acute and chronically ill clients of all ages in their homes while integrating community health nursing principles that focus on the environmental, economic, cultural and personal health factors affecting an individual's and family's health status (Humphrey and Milone-Nuzzo, 1991).

Standards and Credentialing

The ANA (1986) has developed standards of practice for home health care to fulfill the profession's obligation to provide a means for assessing quality of care and to develop measures for improvement of care. Standards reflect the current state of knowledge in the field and are the basis for characterizing, measuring and providing guidance in achieving quality care. The home health care standards are grounded in the nursing process and are based on the ANA standards of community health nursing. The standards, without their interpretive statements, can be found in Table 29–2.

The standards reflect two levels of practice: the generalist prepared at the baccalaureate level and the specialist prepared at the master's level. The role of the generalist includes teaching, providing direct care to clients, managing resources needed to provide care, collaborating with other disciplines in the provision of that care, and supervising ancillary personnel. The role of the specialist in home care includes such activities as direct care, consultation with other providers, development and evaluation of agency policy, and staff development. The specialist role focuses on supporting and developing the system in which home care services are delivered (ANA, 1986).

Certification is a means to provide recognition to professional nurses' accomplishments in well-defined clinical or functional areas of nursing. The ANA offers certification in four areas: generalist, nurse practitioner, clinical specialist, and nursing administration. Each one of these areas has a specific focus, and the examinations are based on content from that area of specialization.

In 1992 the American Nurses Credentialing Center approved a new certification in home health care at the generalist level of practice (Morgan, 1991; Cary and Galten, 1992). Currently this is the only area of home health care practice in which a certification examination is available. This certification is based on the scope of practice established in 1991 by the Congress on Nursing Practice in *A Statement on the Scope of Home Health Nursing Practice* (ANA, 1992). The first certification examination was offered in 1993.

TABLE 29–2

The American Nurses' Association Home Care Nursing Standards

Standard I: Organization of Home Health Services

All home health services are planned, organized, and directed by a master's-prepared professional nurse with experience in community health and administration.

Standard II: Theory

The nurse applies theoretical concepts as a basis for decision in practice.

Standard III: Data Collection

The nurse continuously collects and records data that are comprehensive, accurate, and systematic.

Standard IV: Diagnosis

The nurse uses health assessment data to determine nursing diagnosis.

Standard V: Planning

The nurse develops care plans that establish goals. The care plan is based on nursing diagnoses and incorporates therapeutic, preventive, and rehabilitative nursing actions.

Standard VI: Intervention

The nurse, guided by the care plan, intervenes to provide comfort; to restore, improve, and promote health; to prevent complications and sequelae of illness; and to effect rehabilitation.

Standard VII: Evaluation

The nurse continually evaluates the client's and family's responses to interventions to determine progress toward goal attainment and to review the data base, nursing diagnosis, and plan of care.

Standard VIII: Continuity of Care

The nurse is responsible for the client's appropriate and uninterrupted care along the health care continuum and therefore uses discharge planning, case management, and coordination of community resources.

Standard IX: Interdisciplinary Collaboration

The nurse initiates and maintains a liaison relationship with appropriate health care providers to assure that all efforts effectively complement one another.

Standard X: Professional Development

The nurse assumes responsibility for professional development and contributes to the professional growth of others.

Standard XI: Research

The nurse participates in research activities that contribute to the profession's continuing development of knowledge of home health care.

Standard XII: Ethics

The nurse uses the code for nurses established by the American Nurses' Association as a guide for ethical decision making in practice.

From American Nurses' Association. (1986). *Standards of home care nursing practice.* Washington, DC: Author. Reprinted with permission.

Current Status of Home Health Care

Although home health care providers have been providing high-quality health care to clients in their homes since the late 1800s, most growth in home health care nursing has taken place since 1970. As described earlier, this growth has been due in part to the enactment of Medicare legislation in 1965. There are many different types of home care agencies that provide various services to clients in their homes. The regulations for operation of such an agency differ from state to state and are dependent on the type of services provided by the agency. Of the 50 states, Puerto Rico, and the District of Columbia, only 39 states require licensure for home care agencies (NAHC, 1992a). Through licensure law, these states set specific rules and requirements for staffing, policies, and practices and set minimal operating standards for various programs and services. If the home health agency meets the legal conditions set out in the licensure law, it is granted a license; if not, it cannot operate in that state.

In some states only those agencies that provide professional services are required to have a license. For example, agencies that provide skilled nursing or physical therapy services would need a license, while those agencies that provide unskilled nursing service or custodial care (e.g., companion services) would not need a license for operation.

For an agency to be reimbursed by Medicare for services provided to clients, it must be Medicare certified. *Medicare certification* means that an agency meets the *conditions of participation,* which include rules, standards, and criteria established by the federal government. These regulations dictate such things as type and number of personnel, agency structure, and billing methods. For example, the administrator of a home health agency must be a licensed physician or a registered nurse with at least 1 year of supervisory experience in a home health agency. Because it is a federal program, the requirements for Medicare certification remain constant across the country. Medicare certification is required even in those states that require licensure for home care agencies. To maintain Medicare certification, an agency is periodically subjected to an unannounced site visit by an external evaluator who reviews the agency's records and makes home visits to determine that the conditions of participation are being maintained.

State licensure laws are usually written to identify the minimum standard for patient safety and quality of care that an agency must achieve. Medicare certification standards are slightly more rigorous than licensure standards and regulations. Agencies that want to further define the quality of their services to their clients and the community may also seek voluntary *accreditation,* which is a rigorous process in which an agency seeks to be evaluated on the basis of comprehensive criteria that influence the quality of care. The cost of this process is assumed by the home health care agency. An agency that is accredited seeks to demonstrate to consumers that it far exceeds the minimum standards for operation and has achieved a standard of excellence that is superior to that of its nonaccredited competitors.

There are two accreditation programs for home health care agencies throughout the country: the Community Health Accreditation Program (CHAP), administered through the National League for Nursing (NLN) (Mitchell, 1992), and the Home Care Accreditation Program of the Joint Commission on Accreditation of Healthcare Organizations (JCAHO) (Rooney and Biere, 1992). Both programs require the agency to conduct a thorough self-evaluation based on identified objectives and to compile a self-evaluation report that is reviewed by a group of professionals. An unannounced, on-site survey is also conducted by peer reviewers as part of the review process. Based on review of the self-evaluation report and the site visit, which includes home visits to clients, the accrediting agency (either CHAP or JCAHO) makes a determination as to whether the agency will be accredited.

A home health care agency accredited by CHAP or JCAHO is considered to have *deemed status,* which refers to the Medicare conditions of participation. Because accreditation standards are more rigorous than the Medicare conditions of participation, an accredited agency is deemed to have met the Medicare standard as well. Therefore, an accredited agency would have to undergo only the accreditation site visit and not the Medicare site visit.

TYPES OF AGENCIES

Currently there are many different types of home health care agencies. In the early days of home health care, services were likely to be delivered by a nurse from a VNA. In some parts of the country this continues to be true. In most of the country, the mix of home care agencies more commonly includes other types of agencies such as official, proprietary, and hospital-based agencies.

Official Agencies. Official or public agencies are supported by tax dollars and are given power through statutes enacted by legislation. An example of an official agency involved in home health care would be a state or local health department with a nursing division. Home health care services (care of the sick) and traditional public health nursing services (preventive care) may be combined in the same nursing division of the health department.

There has been a gradual decline in the number of local health departments with certified home health care agencies. Increased competition from other agencies left health departments with the task of caring only for those people unable to pay for services. More importantly, the growth of public health problems such as the acquired immunodeficiency syndrome (AIDS) and high-risk mother–child health have necessitated that official agencies focus their energy and resources on the public health needs of the community.

Voluntary Agencies. Voluntary home health care agencies are governed by a volunteer board of directors and are supported primarily with nontax funds such as donations, endowments, United Way contributions, and reimbursements from third-party payers (e.g., Medicare, Medicaid, and private insurance). They are considered to be community based because they provide services within a well-defined community or geographic location.

Voluntary agencies are nonprofit and therefore are tax exempt. Nonprofit status is not exactly what the name implies. An agency that is nonprofit must operate in a fiscally responsible manner designed to either break even or end the year with a surplus. Nonprofit status means that the accrued profit goes back into the functioning of the agency in the form of free client care, staff development, or capital expenditures. A nonprofit agency that continually runs a fiscal deficit will soon be out of business. An example of a voluntary agency is a VNA.

Private Agencies. Private home health care agencies can be either for-profit or not-for-profit. Private, not-for-profit home health care agencies are governed either by a board of directors or by the agency's owner.

The majority of private agencies are proprietary in nature, which means they plan to make a profit on the home care they provide. Proprietary agencies make up the largest percentage of home health care agencies in the country. These agencies can be locally owned or part of a national or international chain. Unlike voluntary agencies, the profit made on the home care goes either to the stockholders of the corporation or the owners of the company and therefore is not tax exempt. There is no requirement that the profits be returned to the agency. The stockholders or the owner determine how these profits will be allocated.

Hospital-based Agencies. Hospitals began entering the home health care industry in large numbers in the 1980s to maintain clients within their health care system, provide a more comprehensive program of health services, and increase revenue. The hospital-based home health care agency is governed by the sponsoring hospital's board of directors and receives the majority of its referrals from the sponsoring hospital.

Home Care Aide Agencies. A home care aide agency provides paraprofessional services such as homemaking, companionship, or custodial care to clients. These agencies are usually privately owned and receive direct payment from a client or a private insurance company.

Certified Hospice Agencies. Many communities have home health care agencies that provide hospice care to the terminally ill in the community. These agencies have received certification from the federal government as a Medicare hospice provider. Hospice home care has grown as a result of a trend toward providing terminal care in the home. Some hospice agencies are free standing and serve only hospice clients, whereas others are part of a larger organization such as a VNA. Reimbursement for hospice care is provided by Medicare and private insurance companies.

TYPES OF SERVICES

Home care services are traditionally divided into three categories of service: care of the ill, public health (also known as preventive care), and specialized home care services (e.g., high-technology care). Although each category is unique, the categories are not mutually exclusive either in theory or in practice. In theory they are not mutually exclusive because high-technology care such as for a ventilator-dependent client may be also part of the program for care of the ill. In practice, when a home care nurse visits a 50-year-old women who needs wound care, the nurse will provide instruction about the need for routine preventive health care measures (e.g., mammograms and Pap smears) in addition to performing the wound care.

Care of Ill Persons. The care of the ill program is the largest program in home health care. As the term implies, these individuals are ill and require services to improve their health outcome or prevent hospitalization. Most of this care for qualified clients is covered by a third-party payer such as Medicare, Medicaid, or a private insurance company.

Public Health Services. Public health services focus on the promotion of health and the prevention of disease. They include such services as teaching a new mother to care for an infant, physical examinations for children, and diet teaching for the elderly. Although VNAs were founded on the principles of public health services, most home health care agencies do not provide public health services. Third-party payers do not reimburse home health care agencies for care that is exclusively preventive in nature. The home care agencies that do provide public health services usually fund these programs through monies donated to them from the jurisdiction in which the services are provided or through private donations or grants.

Specialized Home Care Services. Specialized home care practice includes such programs as high-technology home care, pediatric care, psychiatric mental health care, and hospice care. High-technology home care has grown in direct response to shortened hospital stays of clients and the need to reduce health care costs related to treatment in the hospital. Technology that was previously available only in the hospital has been adapted for use in the home. For example, clients who would previously have had to remain hospitalized to receive long-term antibiotic therapy currently can receive it in the home as a result of changes in infusion technology.

However, not all clients or situations are suited for high-technology home care. Discharging a high-technology client to the home requires thorough assessment of the client, the caregiver, and the home environment. This can be accomplished through the collaborative efforts of the discharge planner in the hospital and the home care nurse who will be involved after discharge. Before the client is discharged, decisions must be made and plans developed. To evaluate the client's suitability for discharge home, the following questions should be discussed by the home health care nurse and the discharge planner in the hospital before the client is discharged (Humphrey and Milone-Nuzzo, 1991):

1. What is the client's and caregiver's understanding of the specified therapy, and what are their roles in performing the therapy?
2. Is the therapy safe to be performed in the home, and does the client have the means to perform the therapy safely?
3. Are the client and family willing and committed to become involved in the client's therapy?
4. What is the availability of equipment, supplies, and expertise?
5. What is the availability of financial resources to pay for the proposed services?

Pediatric programs can focus on providing short-term care to the acutely ill child (e.g., total parenteral nutrition for a child after bowel surgery) or providing long-term care to the chronically ill child (e.g., home ventilator care for a child with a respiratory condition). Whatever the need, there is significant benefit to providing care to children in the home rather than in an institution. Unlike in the hospital setting, a child's development at home tends to advance, even in the presence of a debilitating or chronic illness (Humphrey and Milone-Nuzzo, 1991). In addition, children at home have fewer infections and socialization occurs more rapidly (Donar, 1988; Handy, 1989). The appearance of normalcy has a positive impact on the ill child as well as on other family members. Funds for pediatric home care come from Medicaid, private insurance carriers, local community organizations, and private foundations or state entitlement programs. (See Chapter 26.)

Some home health care agencies deliver psychiatric/mental health services to clients in their homes. Because Medicare guidelines for the reimbursement of care for psychiatric clients are extremely rigid, many home health care agencies have developed alternative care programs. These programs are usually funded through a private foundation or grant and are likely to be limited in scope according to client diagnosis, age, or previous medical history. For example, a home health care agency received a grant from the Connecticut Department of Mental Health to provide psychiatric home care to clients over 65 years of age with dementia. The objective of this program was to prevent institutionalization in this population. Because this program was funded by a grant, it was not constrained by the regulations set forth by Medicare for psychiatric care in the home.

Hospice is a philosophy of care rather than a place of care. Thus, hospice programs are designed to provide palliative care to the terminally ill in both the home and inpatient institutions. In 1983, legislation resulted in the development of a Medicare Hospice Benefit for the terminally ill. Clients who meet specific admission criteria are allowed to waive their traditional Medicare benefit and receive the Hospice Medicare Benefit, which provides funding for services that more closely meet the needs of the terminally ill.

In addition to teaching caregivers about physical care and providing such care, hospice nurses focus on psychological, social, and spiritual needs of the terminally ill. Hospice services assist terminally ill persons, their caregivers, other family members, and friends to "accept the diagnosis, adjust to life with illness, and prepare for approaching death" (Callahan and Kelley, 1993, p. 40).

REIMBURSEMENT MECHANISMS

Home health services are reimbursed by both commercial and government third-party payers as well as by private individuals. Government third-party payers include Medicare, Medicaid, the Civilian Health and Medical Program of the Uniformed Services, and the Veterans Administration system. These government programs have specific conditions for the coverage of services. Commercial third-party payers include insurance companies, health maintenance organizations (HMOs), preferred provider organizations (PPOs), and case management programs. Commercial insurers often allow for more flexibility in their requirements than does Medicare. For example, the home care nurse may negotiate with an insurance company to obtain needed services for the client in the home based on the cost-effectiveness of the home care plan.

Regardless of the third-party payer, home care is reimbursed after the services are provided (i.e., retrospective reimbursement). That is, an agency makes a determination about the client's care needs, provides the needed care within the agency's interpretation of the guidelines of the third-party payer, and then bills the payer for the services provided. At times third-party payers will question or deny payment for the care provided. If it is determined that the provided care is not reimbursable, the agency must assume financial responsibility for that care.

Medicare. Medicare is a federal insurance program for elderly (over 65 years old) and disabled persons in the United States. Because it is a federal program, procedures and qualifying criteria should not vary significantly from state to state. To be eligible for this program, an individual must be over 65 years of age or have received Social Security disability payments for more than 24 months. Ninety-three percent of elderly persons in the United States are covered by Medicare (Commerce Clearing House [CCH], 1991). The Health Care Financing Administration (HCFA), a department of the federal government, regulates payments for services under Medicare (HCFA, 1989). The rules developed by HCFA that guide the Medicare program are detailed in the *Health Insurance Manual-11* (HIM-11). The HCFA contracts with insurance companies to process the Medicare claims submitted by home care agencies; these insurance companies are called *fiscal intermediaries*

(FIs). The United States is broken into 10 geographic regions, each with its own FI.

The home care agency sends the FI a bill each month, accompanied by specific clinical information for the services provided the previous month. Professionals at the FI review the information to determine whether the client and the home health care service meet the coverage criteria for home care. If the information clearly meets the specified criteria, the bill is paid. If there is any question regarding the need for the services provided or the client's eligibility, the FI will request more information. Decisions regarding reimbursement are based on the additional information provided. If the FI denies payment for the services, an appeal can be initiated by the home care agency.

Criteria for Reimbursement under Medicare. There are five criteria a client must meet to be eligible for Medicare home care services:

1. *Reasonable and necessary.* Under Medicare, services provided to a client must be considered "reasonable and necessary." This term refers both to the nursing care clients receive to effect a positive health outcome and the frequency with which that care is provided. Medicare does not give a clear definition of the term; the decision as to whether this criterion is met is based on the client's health status and medical needs as reflected in the plan of care and the medical record. For example, daily visits may not be deemed reasonable for a client who requires twice-weekly blood glucose level determinations. Similarly, if a care plan has been ineffective over a long period of time, continuation of that care plan would not be considered reasonable. Therefore, comprehensive documentation by the home care nurse is essential to validate that the care provided was both reasonable and necessary.
2. *Homebound.* A client must be considered essentially homebound to be eligible for home care benefits under Medicare. This means that the client has difficulty in mobility and leaves the home only for medical appointments. The client is considered homebound if home absences are rare and of short duration or attributable to the need to receive medical treatment (HCFA, 1989). Homebound criteria may also be considered met if the client attends adult daycare, if the purpose is related to the client receiving medical care.
3. *Completed Plan of Care.* The plan of care for Medicare clients must be completed on HCFA forms 485, 486, and 487. These forms, provided by the federal government, require very specific information regarding the client's diagnosis, prognosis, functional limitations, medications, and types of services needed. The home health care nurse often has the primary responsibility for ensuring that these forms are completed appropriately.
4. *Skilled service.* To qualify for home care services under Medicare, the client must be in need of a skilled service. In the home, skilled services are provided by a nurse, a physical therapist, or a speech therapist. Medical social work and home care aide services are considered to be dependent services and therefore will be reimbursed under Medicare only if they are combined with one of the skilled services. Occupational therapy is not considered a skilled service for initiating care. However, after the skilled service has discharged the client, occupational therapy can serve as the qualifying service for other dependent services in the home. Reimbursement for occupational therapy in the home is dependent on the inherent complexity of the service and the condition of the client.

   Skilled nursing service encompasses three major areas: skilled observation and assessment, teaching, and skilled procedures. Skilled observation and assessment may include assessment of a congestive heart failure patient for the early signs of pulmonary edema. Teaching, one of the most common interventions performed by the home care nurse, may include instructing a new diabetic patient about his or her diet. The teaching plan must include new information, not just a reinforcement of material on which the client has been instructed. Skilled procedures include such interventions as wound care or dressing changes.
5. *Intermittent/part-time service.* Medicare specifies that home care services be provided on an intermittent basis, usually a few hours per day for several days per week for a specified length of time. It is anticipated that clients requiring more than intermittent/part-time care could be cared for more cost effectively in a setting other than the home (e.g., a nursing home).

Medicaid. Medicaid is an assistance program for poor individuals and some disabled persons and children. Unlike Medicare, Medicaid is jointly sponsored by the federal government and the individual states; therefore, Medicaid coverage differs from state to state. These differences can often be dramatic and in some cases are dependent on the state's financial health. Eligibility for Medicaid is based on income and assets and is not contingent on any previous payments to the federal or state government.

Unlike Medicare, Medicaid covers both skilled and unskilled care in the home and does not require that the client be homebound. To qualify for home care benefits under Medicaid, clients must meet income eligibility requirements and have a plan of care signed by a physician, and the plan of care must be reviewed by a physician every 60 days.

Commercial Private Payers. Many commercial insurance companies are involved in health insurance for individuals or groups. These local or national companies often write policies that include a home care benefit. Commercial insurers often cover the same services covered by Medicare in addition to covering preventive, private duty, and supportive services such as a home health aide or homemaker (discussed later).

Commercial insurance often has a maximum lifetime benefit as part of the policy. The high cost of high-technology care forces more patients to reach this maximum and face the loss of coverage. This has resulted in the development of case management programs administered by insurance companies. The case manager projects the long-term needs and costs to care for the client and develops a plan with the client to meet those needs in a cost-efficient manner. Consideration is given to the life expectancy of the client in relationship to the maximum lifetime benefit.

TYPES OF HOME CARE PROVIDERS

Interdisciplinary collaboration is a hallmark of home health care practice. The home health care team is made up of several, if not all, of these home health care providers. The client's needs mandate the home care providers that will be part of the home health care team. The standards of home health nursing practice indicate that the home care nurse is responsible for initiating collaboration with other providers (ANA, 1986). In addition, collaboration is mandated in the conditions of participation for those agencies that are Medicare certified ("Medicare Conditions of Participation," 1989).

The role of the professional in home health care involves both the provision of direct care to clients and consultation with other professionals and paraprofessionals involved in care. For example, a client needing skilled nursing service for a dressing change and assessment of a leg wound may also need some range-of-motion exercises for the affected extremity. If this is an uncomplicated clinical situation, the home care nurse may ask the physical therapist to suggest some exercises that can be done by the client instead of having the physical therapist make a home visit.

Home Care Nurse. Nursing services are the most frequently provided skilled service in the home. Nursing care in the home is provided by a registered nurse or a licensed practical nurse, is authorized by a physician, and is based on the client's needs. A nurse may make an initial visit to a client to obtain an assessment without a physician order but must receive physician approval and direction for follow-up care to be delivered.

Primary Physician. Clients in the home must be under the current care of a physician or an osteopath. Although home visits were once a widespread practice, currently physicians rarely make them. The current role of the physician in home care is to provide information to the home care provider regarding the medical condition of the client, to serve as a resource to other home care providers, and to certify a plan of treatment. A plan of treatment must be reviewed by the physician at least every 60 days, with more frequent review if a change in the client's situation warrants it.

Physical Therapist. The focus of physical therapists in the home is on improving the client's ability to use his or her large muscle groups. Physical therapists provide maintenance, preventive, and restorative treatment in the home for clients of all ages with varying diagnoses. The body systems most associated with the need for home physical therapy are the musculoskeletal, neurological, and cardiopulmonary systems. Physical therapists focus on gross motor skills, the lower extremities, and the respiratory system. For example, a client with chronic obstructive pulmonary disease may have home visits by the physical therapist for postural drainage.

Occupational Therapist. The occupational therapist helps the client acquire the skills necessary to perform activities of daily living. Occupational therapists focus most of their interventions on the client's upper extremities and on the fine muscle skills needed to perform functional activities such as eating and dressing. In addition to teaching self-care activities, the occupational therapist is involved in assessing the home for safety and suggesting modifications for improving the client's ability to function independently. These modifications may include installation of adaptive equipment, such as a grab bar in the bath tub, or modification of existing structures in the home to make self-care possible. For example, the occupational therapist may suggest modifications to a kitchen to allow the client to prepare his or her own meals; these might include installation of a sink that allows a wheelchair to fit under it or cabinets that have easily accessed pulls.

Speech Therapist. Speech therapists work with clients who have difficulty with communication, both expressive and receptive. The speech therapist's goal is to assist the client's development of optimal communication skills. Speech therapists may also be involved with clients who are experiencing difficulty in swallowing.

Medical Social Worker. The medical social worker helps clients and families deal with the social and emotional issues associated with illness and long-term care. Often families are unprepared for the adjustments required to care for an ill member. The social worker can be helpful in easing this transition to the caregiver role. Traditionally, social workers have helped clients identify health and social service needs and have made referrals to community agencies that address those needs. In home care, the social worker also assists with applications for services and provides financial assistance information.

Home Care Aide. The home care aide is a paraprofessional involved in services ranging from basic housekeeping to complex personal care. Services performed by the home care aide typically include ensuring a clean, healthy home environment; shopping and preparing meals; and grooming, bathing, and other personal care services. To facilitate long-term care planning, three levels of home care aide have been identified, each with its own focus:

- *Home care aide I:* The home care aide I assists with environmental services such as housekeeping and home-making to preserve a safe, sanitary, healthy home; he or she is not involved in providing any personal care to clients (NAHC, 1992b).
- *Home care aide II:* The home care aide II can perform nonmedically directed personal care in addition to all the duties of the home care aide I. The home care aide II is not to be assigned duties related to medication administration and wound care (NAHC, 1992b).
- *Home care aide III:* The home care aide III can perform all the duties performed by home care aides I and II. In addition, the home care aide III works under a medically supervised plan of care to assist the individual/family with household management and personal care. Activities that may be part of the medically supervised plan of care include nonsterile wound care, assistance with self-administered medications, and assistance with prescribed exercises and rehabilitation activities (NAHC, 1992b). The home care aide III may be certified or uncertified. To be certified, a home care aide must complete a course of study that includes instruction on the personal care of clients and household management skills. Medicare will reimburse the home health care agency only for care provided by a certified home care aide.

Supervision of paraprofessionals such as home care aides is the responsibility of the home care nurse. If the home care nurse is not directly involved in the client's care, he or she can delegate the responsibility to professionals such as the physical therapist or speech therapist. Medicare mandates that the home care aide III be supervised every 2 weeks, which means that the home care nurse makes a visit to the client's home either when the home care aide is present to observe the aide providing care, or when the aide is absent to assess the relationship between the aide and the client ("Medicare Conditions of Participation," 1989). Licensure requirements vary from state to state regarding frequency of supervision for those clients not under Medicare.

Business Office Staff. Business office staff include the bookkeepers, clerks, and computer operators who prepare bills, track reimbursements, and maintain the agency's data base. The business office is integral to an agency's ability to deliver home care services to clients. A home health agency cannot function without an efficient business office staff that works effectively with the clinical staff. The relationship between the business office staff and the clinical staff is unique in home care. Professional staff must have an understanding of the financial aspects of the client's care and provide information to the business staff so that reimbursement can be obtained for the services provided.

Responsibilities of the Home Care Nurse

Although there is a great deal of similarity between the roles and functions of inpatient care nurses and those of home care nurses, there are some unique aspects of practice in the home. This section will focus on the differences in nursing practice between home care and inpatient care.

DIRECT CARE

Direct care is defined as the actual nursing care that is provided to clients in their homes (Humphrey and Milone-Nuzzo, 1991). Nursing care may involve assessment of physical or psychosocial status, performance of a skilled intervention, and teaching. In performing assessments and skilled interventions, the home care nurse must give consideration to the 24-hour needs of clients. Integration of the individual client, family, and caregiver into the care plan is essential to ensure continuity of care during the time the nurse is not in the home. Home care nurses provide care on a short-term, intermittent basis. Most care provided in the home is the responsibility of someone other than the nurse. Thus, teaching becomes the most common intervention performed by home care nurses. Nurses are responsible for providing the client and family with the necessary knowledge and skills to provide safe care between home visits by nurses and after discharge from the home care agency.

The home care nurse is not routinely involved in the client's personal care (e.g., bathing, hair washing, or changing linen). Although these activities are considered essential to the client's recovery, the responsibility for performing these tasks on a routine basis is assigned to the home care aide or the client's family member. However, this does not mean that the home care nurse never provides personal care to the client. For example, there will be times when the home care nurse will make a home visit to a client who is in need of help with his or her personal hygiene. The nurse performs these tasks in addition to performing the skilled care that was the visit's purpose. The home care nurse, together with the client, then makes a determination as to whether continued personal care assistance is needed. If so, the nurse would make arrangements for those needs to be met.

DOCUMENTATION

Documentation of care is just as important as the direct service role of the home care nurse. The time and effort a home care nurse must spend on documentation to meet reimbursement and regulatory requirements are difficult to comprehend. In addition to addressing the regulatory and reimbursement requirements, the purpose of documentation is to convey the clinical course of care for the client. As an indication of the magnitude of the problem, the NAHC has developed a task force of administrative and clinical experts to examine methods of reducing the documentation burden for home care providers. Many agencies already have developed strategies to reduce the amount of time a home care provider must spend on documentation. These include the use of dictaphones for charting home visits, computerized care plans, and the use of flow sheets or standardized care plans.

Documentation in home health care serves several purposes. As in the inpatient setting, the documentation in the record is a written account of the client's history, status, and progress. The written record is the basis for planning individualized care and serves to communicate information to all health professionals involved in the client's care. Specifically in home care, third-party payers use the client record as a tool to justify payments. The payer not only will inspect the record for the number of home visits made, but also may examine the services provided to determine whether they were appropriate to meet the determined goal. Also, the home care record is one of the many documents examined in the total quality improvement program of an agency. Record reviews are an important tool for assessing the quality of care provided by the home health care team. Finally, accurate documentation is the key to the nurse's and agency's protection from liability. If there is a question about the type, amount, or quality of care a client received, the written record is viewed as the best indicator of what occurred, as it was written at the time care was given.

COORDINATION OF SERVICES AND CASE MANAGEMENT

The home care nurse is responsible for coordination of the other professionals and paraprofessionals involved in the client's care. Central to the role of case manager is the ability to assess the client's needs, determine priority of needs, identify how those needs can be met, and implement a plan for meeting the identified needs. In addition, the home care nurse is the primary contact with the client's physician, reporting changes in the client's condition and securing changes in the plan of care ("Home Care Nursing Services," 1988).

As the care coordinator, the home care nurse must have current information regarding the services provided by all caregivers in the home and the response to those services. Case conferences are conducted regularly among professionals and paraprofessionals to share information, discuss problems, and plan a course of action to effect the best possible outcome for the client. Medicare mandates that case conferences occur every 60 days when more than one discipline is involved in the client's care. A written summary of each client's case conference must be sent to the primary physician for review. At times the client or caregivers are included in the case conference. Case conferences can occur over the telephone with professional caregivers who are not affiliated with the home care agency from which the client is receiving most of his or her care (known as the primary home care agency).

Many times clients will need services not provided by the primary home care agency. As coordinator of care, the home care nurse must be knowledgeable about the many community resources existing to meet the needs of clients in their homes. A *community resource* is any agency, organization, program, or individual that delivers a service to residents in the community. To keep a record of the many resources there are in a community, a home care nurse may begin a community resource file. This file consists of a small box in which the home care nurse will collect information about community resources on 3 × 5 index cards. When a resource is identified, the home care nurse records information about the name of the agency, contact person, hours of operation, telephone number, eligibility requirements, and cost of services. These cards can be filed in the box according to the service provided for future reference with clients. Sources of information about community resources can be found in the Yellow Pages of the local telephone directory or the directory of organizations and services for the community. National resources also provide useful information regarding home health nursing practice and client care (Table 29–3).

DETERMINATION OF FINANCIAL COVERAGE

A unique aspect of the role of the home care nurse is involvement in the financial aspects of delivering care to the client. The home care nurse must know who is going to pay for services from the first visit to the time of discharge. At the time of admission, the home care nurse determines the type of services needed based on the assessment and the physician's orders. The home care nurse must also determine the payment source (Medicare, Medicaid, private insurance, or client) for the necessary care. If the client does not have a fee source for the care needed, it becomes the responsibility of the agency to determine whether the client will receive the care free of charge or at a reduced cost. Many agencies have a sliding fee scale, which means that the charge for the services is based on the client's ability to pay. Determining the ability to pay includes a review of the client's income and assets.

DETERMINATION OF FREQUENCY AND DURATION OF CARE

The home care nurse is responsible for determining both the frequency and the duration of client care. *Frequency of*

TABLE 29–3

National Home Care Resources

National Association for Home Care
519 C St. N.E.
Washington, DC 20002
(202) 547–7424

Visiting Nurse Association of America
3801 E. Florida Ave.
Suite 900
Denver, CO 80210
(303) 629–8622

National League for Nursing
Community Health Accreditation Program
350 Hudson St.
New York, NY 10014
(800) 669–1657

Joint Commission on the Accreditation of Healthcare Organizations
1 Renaissance Blvd.
Oakbrook Terrace, IL 60181
(708) 916–5600

Public Health Service AIDS Information Hotline
(800) 342–AIDS
(202) 245–6867 in AK, HI only (call collect)

Occupational Safety and Health Administration
Office of Public and Consumer Affairs
U.S. Department of Labor
Room N3637
200 Constitution Ave. N.W.
Washington, DC 20210
(202) 523–8148

National Clearinghouse for Drug Abuse Information
P.O. Box 416
Kensington, MD 20795
(301) 443–6500

Alzheimer's Disease and Related Disorders Association, Inc.
700 E. Lake St.
Chicago, IL 60601
(312) 853–3060
(800) 621–0379
(800) 572–6037 in IL only

American Foundation for the Blind, Inc.
15 W. 16th St.
New York, NY 10011
(212) 620–2000

American Cancer Society
90 Park Ave.
New York, NY 10016
(212) 599–3600

Clearinghouse on Child Abuse and Neglect Information
P.O. Box 1182
Washington, DC 20013
(301) 251–5157

National Hospice Organization
301 Maple Ave. W.
Suite 506
Vienna, VA 22180
(703) 938–4449

National Institute on Adult Day Care
National Council on the Aging
600 Maryland Ave. S.W.
Washington, DC 20024
(202) 479–1200

American Association of Retired Persons
1909 K St. N.W.
Washington, DC 20049
(202) 872–4700

National Gerontological Nursing Association
1818 Newton St. N.W.
Washington, DC 20010

National Clearinghouse for Family Planning Information
P.O. Box 2225
Rockville, MD 20852
(301) 251–5153

National Rehabilitation Information Center (NARIC)
8455 Colesville Rd.
Suite 935
Silver Spring, MD 20910
(800) 34–NARIC

Independent Living for the Handicapped
Department of Housing and Urban Development
HUD Building
Washington, DC 20410
(202) 755–5720

Clearinghouse on Health Indexes
National Center for Health Statistics
Division of Epidemiology and Health Promotion
3700 East-West Highway
Room 2-27
Hyattsville, MD 20782
(301) 436–7035

American Public Health Association
1015 15th St. N.W.
Washington, DC 20005
(202) 789–5600

National Clearinghouse for Mental Health Information
National Institute of Mental Health
5600 Fishers Ln.
Room 11A33
Rockville, MD 20857
(301) 443–4517

American Heart Association
7320 Greenville Ave.
Dallas, TX 75231
(214) 373–6300

National Hearing Aid Helpline
(800) 521–5247
(313) 478–2610 in MI only

High Blood Pressure Information Center
National Institutes of Health
Bethesda, MD 20205
(301) 496–1809

American Diabetic Association
Journal of the American Dietetic Association
430 N. Michigan Ave.
Chicago, IL 60611
(312) 899–0046

National Multiple Sclerosis Society
205 E. 42nd St.
New York, NY 10017
(212) 986–3240

TABLE 29–3

National Home Care Resources *Continued*

Poison Control Branch Food and Drug Administration Parklawn Building Room 15B-23 5600 Fishers Ln. Rockville, MD 20857 (301) 443–6260	Rehabilitation Services Administration Office of Special Education and Rehabilitative Services Department of Education 330 C St. S.W. Room 3431 Washington, DC 20202 (202) 723–1282
National Center for the Prevention and Control of Rape Parklawn Building Room 6C-12 5600 Fishers Ln. Rockville, MD 20857 (301) 443–1910	Sex Information and Education Council of the United States 32 Washington Pl. New York, NY 10003 (212) 673–3850
	National Injury Information Clearinghouse 5401 Westbard Ave. Room 625 Washington, DC 20207 (301) 492–6424

care is defined as how often home visits are made to the client in a specified period of time; *duration of care* is defined as the length of time the client receives home care services. In collaboration with the physician, the home care nurse must determine whether the client needs daily, biweekly, weekly, or monthly home visits. As the care is provided and the client's clinical status improves, the home care nurse, in collaboration with the physician, must determine whether the frequency of visits should be reduced and when to discharge the client from the agency. The condition of the individual client, the needs of the client and the family, and any reimbursement regulations are significant variables in determining frequency and duration of care.

CLIENT ADVOCACY

Although the role of advocate is not unique to home care nursing, the context in which the home care nurse does this requires additional knowledge about health care finance. Many client advocacy responsibilities center around assisting clients to negotiate the complex medical care system. This may involve assisting clients in interpreting their hospital bill or organizing their receipts for submission to their insurance company. Although this may not seem significant, the stress caused by these financial matters may prohibit the client from learning the information necessary for successful recovery from his or her illness.

Issues in Home Care

INFECTION CONTROL

Universal precautions are as important in the provision of care to clients in the home as they are in the intensive care unit of the hospital. As a result of shortened hospital stays, many clients with communicable diseases and multiple invasive devices currently are being cared for in the home by home care nurses. Two major concerns for the home care nurse in caring for any client in the home are as follows:

1. How can infection be prevented in clients who are debilitated and may be immunocompromised?
2. How can the nurse, family, and community be protected from a client who has a communicable disease?

The home setting provides some unique challenges for the control of communicable disease and the prevention of infection. In some cases the home may lack the facilities to implement optimal infection control measures; for example, a client with hepatitis A may live in a rooming house with shared bathroom facilities. In other cases family members may be unwilling or unable to implement the necessary precautions to protect themselves from a communicable disease. The unique nature of the home as the setting of care necessitates the development of unique solutions to the problems faced by the home care nurse.

Universal Precautions. The Centers for Disease Control and Prevention (CDC) (1989) recommends the use of universal precautions by all health professionals to prevent transmission of the human immunodeficiency virus (HIV) and the hepatitis B virus (Table 29–4). Because the medical history or physical examination is unreliable in identifying those clients with a bloodborne pathogen, universal precautions should be used consistently with all clients, regardless of diagnosis. Universal precautions apply to blood, other specified body fluids, and any body fluids containing visible blood (Table 29–5).

Measures to Control the Spread of Communicable Disease. The presence of a family member with a communicable

TABLE 29–4

Principles of Universal Precautions to Prevent Transmission of HIV and Hepatitis B Virus

1. Assume that all patients are infectious for HIV and other blood-borne pathogens.
2. Be immunized for hepatitis B virus.
3. Wash hands frequently.
4. Use protective barriers to prevent percutaneous exposure to blood and other potentially hazardous body fluids.
5. Properly disinfect work areas, equipment, and clothing.
6. Properly dispose of contaminated waste.
7. Document exposure and report to employer, who is required to report occupational injuries to the Federal government.

Data from Centers for Disease Control. (1989). Guidelines for prevention of transmission of human immunodeficiency virus and hepatitis B virus to health-care and public-safety workers. *Morbidity and Mortality Weekly Report, 38*(S-6), 1–37.

disease need not be a hazard for the other members of the household or the community. The role of the home care nurse is to instruct the client and family regarding measures to control the spread of the communicable disease and to provide information to allay the fears of the family in the caregiving process. Isolation precautions in the home should be based on common sense and an understanding of the method of transmission of the communicable disease. The guidelines in Table 29–6 can be used in the home to control the spread of communicable disease.

Measures for the Immunocompromised. In an effort to reduce the possibility of a nosocomial infection, the immunocompromised client is often cared for in the home setting. The inability of the client to fight off infection may be caused by many conditions, including AIDS, chemotherapy, or genetic absence of an antibody. The following special precautions can be taken in the home to prevent the development of infectious diseases:

1. Avoid contact with family members or visitors who have a contagious disease (Berg, 1988).
2. Avoid raw foods (e.g., salads and fruit), raw eggs (as in eggnog), and unpasteurized milk (Berg, 1988).
3. Use precautions when caring for pets (e.g., do not allow the patient to empty litter boxes or clean bird cages and aquariums) (Berg, 1988).
4. Use small containers for the storage of food and make only enough for one serving to prevent leftovers (Humphrey, 1986).
5. Provide clients with their own eating utensils, dishes, and glasses (Humphrey, 1986). A dishwasher is the ideal method for cleaning dishes. If a dishwasher is unavailable, soap and hot water rinsing of the client's eating utensils will suffice.
6. Avoid cut flowers and house plants. Water standing for long periods of time can be a medium for the growth of bacteria (Humphrey, 1986). If cut flowers are in the home, changing the water and cleaning the vase frequently will reduce the chance of infection.

TABLE 29–5

Body Fluids That Do and Do Not Require Universal Precautions to Prevent Transmission of HIV and Hepatitis B Virus

FLUIDS THAT REQUIRE PRECAUTIONS
Blood
Semen
Vaginal secretions
Amniotic fluid
Pericardial fluid
Peritoneal fluid
Pleural fluid
Synovial fluid
Cerebrospinal fluid
Any body fluid visibly contaminated with blood
FLUIDS THAT DO NOT REQUIRE PRECAUTIONS
Feces
Nasal secretions
Sputum
Sweat
Tears
Urine
Vomitus

Data from Centers for Disease Control. (1989). Guidelines for prevention of transmission of human immunodeficiency virus and hepatitis B virus to health-care and public-safety workers. *Morbidity and Mortality Weekly Report, 38*(S-6), 1–37.

QUALITY OF CARE

While the home care industry has become more business-like, creating new financial arrangements that maximize income-generating potential, interest in the quality of care has remained paramount. As the number of home care agencies has increased, competition has become intense, particularly in urban areas. Home care agencies are seeking to excel in this competitive market through accreditation or other visible means of ensuring excellence in the care they provide. This competitive climate has had a direct impact on the examination of quality care in the home care arena.

In the assessment of the quality of care, home care agencies must first identify who is the customer and who is the consumer of care. In home care these are often different individuals. The *customer* is the person who refers the client to the home care agency. This may be the client's physician, the family of the client, or the discharge planner in the hospital that discharged the client. In some cases the customer may be the individual client. The *consumer* is the recipient of the home care. This is the individual client, family, or significant other who receives the care provided by the home care agency (Peters, 1992). Recognizing that the consumer and the customer are often different, the home care agency must demonstrate quality care to both.

TABLE 29–6

Measures to Control the Spread of Communicable Disease in Homes

1. The most appropriate and effective method of disease prevention is hand washing.
2. Excessive isolation practices in the home, in addition to being impractical and inappropriate, may compromise the quality of patient care in the home and socially isolate the client.
3. Client wastes (feces, urine, blood, contents of suction canisters, etc.) can be flushed safely down the toilet. Waste matter of clients with AIDS can be disposed of in the same manner and does not need special treatment.
4. Disposable dishes are not indicated for home care clients with infectious diseases. The client's dishes and eating utensils can be washed, along with the family dishes, in hot, soapy water or in the family dishwater on the hot cycle.
5. Sharing personal articles (e.g., combs, razors, towels, toothbrushes) among client and family members should be avoided.
6. Clients and caregivers should be educated to use clean gloves when changing the dressings of infected or draining wounds. The importance of hand washing, even though gloves are worn, must be emphasized.
7. Soiled dressings, used gloves, disposable equipment, and so forth should be saturated with bleach, placed in plastic bags, tied, and discarded in the trash can. This method is also appropriate for discarding patient care items used for AIDS clients.
8. Soiled linens and clothing (including those used by AIDS clients) can be laundered in the family washer using the hot cycle, detergent, and one cup of bleach and then dried in the family dryer on the hot cycle.
9. Blood spills and other body secretion spills should be cleaned with a good household disinfectant (e.g., alcohol, peroxide, bleach, or Lysol, diluted as directed). Gloves should be worn to protect skin from disinfectant and body fluids.
10. Home clients with enteric disease should not be allowed to assist in food preparation until symptoms resolve or until results from two consecutive cultures taken at least 24 hours apart are negative. The client should practice scrupulous hand washing at all times. If it is not possible to exclude the client from food preparation, the client must be educated to practice strict hand washing and hygiene during food preparation.
11. Clients with enteric infections do not require a private bathroom if they practice good hygiene. If the client is unable to practice good hygiene, a private bathroom should be considered. (*Note:* In homes with one or no bathroom, the best approach is to clean fecal contamination immediately with a household disinfectant.) If the client uses a commode, the wastes can be flushed safely down the toilet and the commode cleaned with a household disinfectant.
12. Clients with respiratory infections should be instructed to cover all coughs and sneezes with a tissue and discard the tissue in a designated receptacle. Clients should also wash their hands after coughing and sneezing.

From Humphrey, C., & Milone-Nuzzo, P. (1991). *Home care nursing: An orientation to practice* (pp. 27–28). East Norwalk, CT: Appleton & Lange.

Perceptions of quality of care may differ between the consumer and the customer. For example, the physician (customer) may be mainly interested in avoiding rehospitalization or infection, while the client (consumer) may define quality in terms of the promptness of the home care aide for the scheduled visit. Customer and consumer satisfaction is essential to a home care agency's survival. Quality care means meeting or exceeding customers' and consumers' expectations in every encounter (Shamansky, 1991).

Development of the mechanisms to assess quality of care in the home care setting has been slow compared with such development in the institutional setting. The following issues affect the ability to assess home care quality:

1. Home care providers are limited in their ability to influence the patient care environment.
2. Home care patients typically receive other types of care in the community in addition to formal home health care.
3. Clients goals vary considerably among clients, even among those with like conditions or illnesses.
4. Data for quality measurement in home care are difficult to acquire, as large-scale studies are impractical to do in the home (Shaughnessy, Bauman, and Kramer, 1990).

Despite these obstacles, the need to quantify the quality of care has resulted in the development of patient classification systems (Daubert, 1979; Martin and Scheet, 1992), outcome scales (LaLonde, 1988), and taxonomies that categorize home care patients (Shaughnessy et al., 1990). The new focus on quality represents a shift in focus from assessment and monitoring to customer and consumer satisfaction and outcomes of care.

Total Quality Improvement

Total quality improvement (TQI) is a system in which all aspects of the organization are examined for the purpose of improvement of the organization and of the quality of care provided. The focus of TQI is on identification of strengths and weaknesses in the system for the purpose of improving patient care (Sherman, 1991). Three aspects of an agency are examined in the TQI system: structure, process, and outcome.

Structure. Structure is the setting or framework under which the nurse–client relationship exists. It is the employing agency, not the home in which the actual nurse–client interaction takes place. Assessment of structure includes an examination of the mission and philosophy of an agency, its objectives, organizational structure, staffing patterns, employment criteria, available resources, and communication patterns.

Process. The process aspect of TQI focuses exclusively on the activities of the care provider (e.g., the home care nurse, physical therapist, or home care aide). It involves an assessment of the clinical performance of the care provider, including the degree of skill, the interactions between the client and the care provider, and the degree of involvement of the client in the care provided. There are many ways in which information about the activities of the care provider can be measured. The most common type of process evaluation is the record audit, which is a method of appraisal of the care given as reflected in the client care record. Other types of process evaluation include supervisory evaluation of staff performance through joint home visits and client questionnaires.

Outcome. The third and most significant phase of the TQI process centers on the assessment of outcomes. Outcome measures examine the end result of care and determine behavioral changes in the client. These measures of outcome are based on specified preestablished criteria, such as standards of care or client goals. A second aspect of outcome measures relates to the assessment of client satisfaction with care. Client satisfaction with care can be determined through interviews and surveys.

The interrelationship of these three dimensions is critical to the assessment of quality of care. Examination of the care provided is of little value if the client made no real progress toward his or her goal. Similarly, exclusive examination of the outcome of care gives little information about the impact the care provider has had on the achievement of that outcome. Perhaps improvement in the client's condition had little to do with the care given.

The collection of data is merely the beginning of the TQI process. The benefits of TQI are seen in the use of such data to improve the system for the provision of care. As information is collected about difficulties in the agency and client problems, modifications are made in the system to improve the care provided. As strengths in the system are identified, those strengths are nurtured and improved on to enhance quality. The circular nature of data collection and system change is the foundation of the TQI process.

For example, an outcome audit for a home care agency revealed that there was very little change in clients' ability to cope with their illness as a result of the nursing care provided. After reviewing patient care records, it was determined that the nursing staff spent little time in assisting their clients in the psychosocial adaptation to their disease. Consultation with the nursing staff revealed that the nurses did not feel comfortable with that aspect of providing care to clients. Based on all these data, the agency implemented a series of in-service programs for the home care nurses on providing psychosocial care to clients. Reassessment of this outcome measure was conducted to determine whether the in-service programs resulted in a change in the nurses' ability to provide psychosocial care to clients and in the clients' response to that care.

HOME HEALTH CARE AND *HEALTHY COMMUNITIES 2000*

Home health care is traditionally thought of as illness care in the home. Although the majority of care provided to clients is precipitated by an acute illness, treatment of the presenting problem is only part of the responsibilities if the home care nurse. Although home care is provided primarily for care of the ill, health promotion, disease prevention, and early diagnosis should be a part of each contact with an individual client or family.

In the early 1990s the United States Department of Health and Human Services developed *Healthy People 2000,* a statement of the nation's health objectives for the year 2000. Accompanying that document was *Healthy Communities 2000,* which provides comprehensive goals and objectives to encourage community leaders to work together to improve the health, environment, and quality of life in communities (American Public Health Association [APHA], 1991).

Objective 21 of *Healthy Communities 2000* relates to clinical preventive services in the community. The model goal for this objective states:

> The community will promote, achieve, and maintain optimum health for all residents through the provision of primary health care services, including clinical preventive primary health care services and home health care (APHA, 1991).

This objective deals specifically with many aspects of home health care, including the availability and accessibility of all types of high-quality home care services for all members of the community. Community awareness of the multidisciplinary home health care services that are available is also included in this objective. The importance of providing home care that is responsive to the many different populations in the community (e.g., hospice clients, chronically ill persons, and elderly individuals) is defined by this objective.

Home care nurses are in the position of operationalizing this objective and the *Healthy People 2000* objectives in their clinical practice with individual clients and families in the community (Table 29–7). Based on the developmental needs or situational issues the individual client is confronting, the home care nurse can include relevant health promotion teaching or guidance in the care plan (Knollmueller, 1993).

Even though patients receiving home care are required to have a medical provider, not all physicians routinely assess for risky health behaviors and provide appropriate counseling and referral (USDHHS, 1990). Professional home health nurses can routinely include these assessments in the patient histories taken on admission to home health

TABLE 29–7

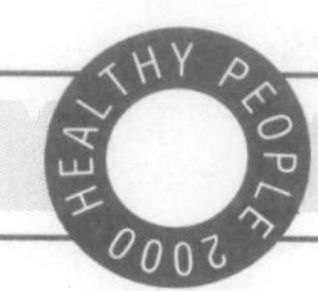

*Healthy People 2000: Selected Objectives for Assessment, Counseling, and Referrals by Home Care Nurses**

1. Increase to at least 75% the proportion of primary care providers who:
   a. Provide nutrition assessment and counseling and/or referral to qualified nutritionists or dietitians (baseline: 40% to 50% of physicians in 1988).
   b. Routinely advise cessation and provide assistance and follow up for all their tobacco-using patients (baseline: 52% of internists reported counseling more than 75% of their patients in 1986).
   c. Screen for alcohol and other drug use problems and provide counseling and referral as needed.
   d. Elicit occupational health exposures as a part of patient history and provide relevant counseling.
   e. Routinely review with their patients age 65 years and older all prescribed and over-the-counter medicines taken by their patients each time a new medication is prescribed.
2. Increase to at least 60% the proportion of primary care providers who routinely evaluate people age 65 and older for urinary incontinence and impairments of vision, hearing, cognition, and functional status.
3. Increase to at least 50% the proportion of primary care providers who:
   a. Routinely review their patients' cognitive, emotional, and behavioral functioning and the resources available to deal with any problems that are identified.
   b. Provide age-appropriate counseling on safety precautions to prevent unintentional injury.
4. Increase to at least 60% the proportion of people age 65 and older using the oral health care system during each year (baseline: 42% in 1986).
5. Increase to at least 40% the proportion of people with chronic and disabling conditions who receive formal patient education, including information about community and self-help resources.

Adapted from U.S. Department of Health and Human Services. (1990). *Healthy people 2000: National health promotion and disease prevention objectives. Summary report.* Washington, DC: U.S. Government Printing Office.

*See Chapter 17 for additional screening objectives.

services. For example, the home care nurse may include teaching about the need for mammography for all female clients and their female caregivers over the age of 35. The nurse may include in the teaching a brochure listing all the community agencies that provide this service and the related cost. Another example of health promotion would be to include diet teaching regarding fat reduction for all clients and their caregivers.

The concept of family-focused care goes beyond integrating the family into the established care plan of the individual client. To integrate the *Healthy People 2000* objectives into the community, the home care nurse may identify specific needs of family members and address those needs during a home visit to the identified patient. For example, while making home visits to a woman for wound care, the home care nurse may observe that the spouse is a heavy smoker. Discussion of smoking cessation may reveal that the spouse desires to stop but feels he needs assistance. The home care nurse may provide the necessary information and external motivation for seeking help with smoking cessation.

The use of the *Healthy People 2000* objectives is consistent with professional home care. Ethically, there may be a conflict between the professional care needed by the client and the efficient, reimbursable care demanded by the home care agency. The professional nurse can use the standards of home care practice (ANA, 1986) as a guide for assessing the types of interventions that are appropriate in the home care setting. Nurses must remain committed to prevention as an integral part of their nursing care of the ill at home (Knollmueller, 1993).

ADVANCE MEDICAL DIRECTIVES

There is growing evidence that clients should have a voice in decision making regarding treatment options and the refusal of medical care (Annas and Glantz, 1986; ANA, 1986). This is uncomplicated when people are alert and can make their wishes known to their primary care provider. In January 1993, the advance medical directive was initiated to clearly identify a course of medical action in a situation in which the client is unable to make decisions and communicate those decisions to the primary care provider.

The *advance medical directive* is a document that indicates the wishes of the client regarding various types of medical treatment in representative situations (Emanuel and Emanuel, 1989). There are two types of advance medical directives: living wills and health care proxies, also called durable power of attorney for health care. Either type of directive would come into effect only if the client became incapacitated and unable to make decisions; both are subject to change at any time.

Living wills are usually used by people to record their decision to decline life-prolonging treatment if they become hopelessly ill. The living will indicates the circumstances for its implementation and the care that should be provided if these circumstances arise. A *health care proxy* (*durable power of attorney*), on the other hand, focuses on naming someone who will make health care decisions if the client becomes unable to make them. The proxy also incorporates knowledge of the client's wishes regarding care.

Each state has its own laws governing the circumstances, content, and procedures for completing advance directives. Tables 29–8 and 29–9 are examples of forms that are legal in Maryland and may be completed without an attorney, if desired. Home care nurses should become aware of the law governing advance directives in the specific state in which they practice.

In 1990 the federal government passed the Patient Self-Determination Act (U.S. Code, 1990). This act, which was part of the Omnibus Reconciliation Act of 1990, required that hospitals, skilled nursing facilities, home health agencies, health maintenance organizations, and hospices provide written information to patients about their option to accept or refuse medical or surgical treatment and to formulate advance directives in compliance with state law. This act also mandates that the health care provider document in the medical record whether clients have executed advance directives. A copy

TABLE 29–8

State of Maryland Living Will

On this _______day of _______________________(month, year),

I, ____being of sound mind, willfully and voluntarily direct that my dying shall not be artificially prolonged under the circumstances set forth in this declaration:

If at any time I should have an incurable injury, disease, or illness certified to be a terminal condition by two (2) physicians who have personally examined me, one (1) of whom shall be my attending physician, and the physicians have determined that my death is imminent and will occur whether or not life-sustaining procedures are utilized and where the application of such procedures would serve only to artificially prolong the dying process, I direct that such procedures be withheld or withdrawn, and that I be permitted to die naturally with only the administration of medication, the administration of food and water, and the performance of any medical procedure that is necessary to provide comfort care or alleviate pain. In the absence of my ability to give directions regarding the use of such life-sustaining procedures, it is my intention that this declaration shall be honored by my family and physician(s) as the final expression of my right to control my medical care and treatment.

I am legally competent to make this declaration, and I understand its full import.

SIGNED ____

ADDRESS ____

Under penalty of perjury, we state that this declaration was signed by

____in the presence of the undersigned who, at

___________request, in ___________presence, and in the presence of each other, have hereunto signed our name as witnesses this

___________day of _______________________19____. Further each of us, individually, states that: The declarant is known to me, and I believe the declarant to be of sound mind. I did not sign the declarant's signature to this declaration. Based upon information and belief, I am not related to the declarant by blood or marriage, a creditor of the declarant, entitled to any portion of the estate of the declarant under any existing testamentary instrument of the declarant, entitled to any financial benefit by reason of the death of the declarant, financially or otherwise responsible for the declarant's medical care, nor an employee of any such person or institution.

________________________________ ________________________________

ADDRESS

____

________________________________ ________________________________

ADDRESS

____

From Department of Legislative Reference, General Assembly of Maryland. (1993). *State of Maryland—The living will and the durable power of attorney for health care: A guide to Maryland law on advance medical directives.* (Forms are included.) Annapolis, MD: General Assembly of Maryland.

TABLE 29–9

State of Maryland Durable Power of Attorney for Health Care

1. Designation of Health Care Agent

I, ____ hereby appoint

____________________ NAME | ____________________ HOME ADDRESS

____________________ HOME TELEPHONE NUMBER | ____________________

____________________ WORK TELEPHONE NUMBER | ____________________

as my agent to make health care decisions for me as authorized in this document.

If the person named as my agent is not reasonably available or is unable to act as my agent, then I appoint the following person to serve in that capacity:

____________________ NAME | ____________________ HOME ADDRESS

____________________ HOME TELEPHONE NUMBER | ____________________

____________________ WORK TELEPHONE NUMBER | ____________________

2. Creation and Effectiveness of Durable Power of Attorney for Health Care

With this document I intend to create a durable power of attorney for health care, which shall take effect when and if two physicians, one of whom is my attending physician, certify that I am disabled because I lack sufficient understanding or capacity to make or communicate decisions with respect to my own health care. The power shall continue in effect during my disability.

3. General Statement of Authority Granted

Except as indicated in Section 4, below, I hereby grant to my agent named above full power and authority to make health care decisions on my behalf, including the following:

(1) To request, review, and receive any information, verbal or written, regarding my physical or mental health, including, but not limited to, medical and hospital records, and to consent to the disclosure of this information;
(2) To employ and/or discharge my health care providers;
(3) To consent to and authorize my admission to and discharge from a hospital or related institution;
(4) To give consent for, or to withhold consent for, x-ray, anesthesia, medication, surgery and all other diagnostic and treatment procedures prescribed (ordered) by or under the direction of a licensed physician, dentist or podiatrist. This authorization specifically includes the power to consent to measures for relief of pain.
(5) To direct the withholding or withdrawal of life-sustaining procedures or measures when and if I am terminally ill or permanently unconscious. Life-sustaining procedures or measures are those forms of medical care which only serve to artificially prolong the dying process, and may include mechanical ventilation, dialysis, antibiotics, artificial nutrition and hydration, and other forms of medical treatment which stimulate or maintain vital bodily functions. Life-sustaining procedures do not include care necessary to provide comfort or alleviate pain.
(6) To take any lawful actions that may be necessary to carry out these decisions, including the granting of releases of liability to medical providers.

of the advance medical directive must be maintained in the client record.

In response to this legislation, home care agencies have provided education regarding advance directives to their direct care staff. As part of the admission process to a home care agency, the home care nurse must discuss advance directives with the client, their meaning, and their use. During this discussion the nurse must be careful not to influence the client in any way with regard to his or her choices and decisions. Each time a client enters a health

TABLE 29–9

State of Maryland Durable Power of Attorney for Health Care *Continued*

4. Special Provision and Limitations

In exercising the authority under this durable power of attorney for health care, the authority of my agent is subject to the following special provisions and limitations:

____

____

____

____

5. Guardianship Provision

If it becomes necessary for a court to appoint a guardian of my person, I nominate my agent or successor agent named above to be the guardian of my person.

6. Signature of Principal

By signing here I indicate that I understand the purpose and effect of this document.

SIGNATURE ______________________ DATE ____________

7. Signature of Witnesses

I declare that the person whose signature appears on this document signed or acknowledged the document in my presence and that I am not the person appointed as agent by this document.

FIRST WITNESS

Signature: ______________________

Home Address: ______________________

Print Name: ______________________

Date: ______________________

SECOND WITNESS

Signature: ______________________

Home Address: ______________________

Print Name: ______________________

Date: ______________________

From Department of Legislative Reference, General Assembly of Maryland. (1993). *State of Maryland—The living will and the durable power of attorney for health care: A guide to Maryland law on advance medical directives.* (Forms are included.) Annapolis, MD: General Assembly of Maryland.

care organization (hospital, nursing home, home care agency), he or she is asked whether advance medical directives exist. Collaboration between providers will reduce the frequency with which a client will have to communicate his or her wishes about care.

PATIENT RIGHTS AND RESPONSIBILITIES

The Medicare conditions of participation require that the home health agency provide the client with written

TABLE 29–10

Home Care Bill of Rights*

Home care clients have a right to be notified in writing of their rights and obligations before treatment begins. The client's family or guardian may exercise the client's rights when the client has been judged incompetent. Home care providers have an obligation to protect and promote the rights of their clients, including the following rights.

Clients and Providers Have a Right to Dignity and Respect

Home care clients and their formal caregivers have a right to not be discriminated against based on race, color, religion, national origin, age, sex, or handicap. Furthermore, clients and caregivers have a right to mutual respect and dignity, including respect for property. Caregivers are prohibited from accepting personal gifts and borrowing from clients.

Clients Have the Right:

- to have relationships with home care providers that are based on honesty and ethical standards of conduct;
- to be informed of the procedure they can follow to lodge complaints with the home care provider about the care that is, or fails to be, furnished, and regarding a lack of respect for property. (To lodge complaints with us call ______________________________);
- to know about the disposition of such complaints;
- to voice their grievances without fear of discrimination of reprisal for having done so; and
- to be advised of the telephone number and hours of operation of the state's home health "hot line," which receives complaints or questions about local home care agencies. The hours are ______________________________ and the number is ____________.

Decision Making

Clients Have the Right:

- to be notified about the care that is to be furnished, the types (disciplines) of the caregivers who will furnish the care, and the frequency of the visits that are proposed to be furnished;
- to be advised of any change in the plan of care before the change is made;
- to participate in the planning of the care and in planning changes in the care, and to be advised that they have the right to do so;
- to be informed in writing of rights under state law to make decisions concerning medical care, including the right to accept or refuse treatment and the right to formulate advance directives;
- to be informed in writing of policies and procedures for implementing advance directives, including any limitations if the provider cannot implement an advance directive on the basis of conscience;
- to have health care providers comply with advance directives in accordance with state law requirements;
- to receive care without condition on, or discrimination based on, the execution of advance directives; and
- to refuse services without fear of reprisal or discrimination.

The home care provider or the client's physician may be forced to refer the client to another source of care if the client's refusal to comply with the plan of care threatens to compromise the provider's commitment to quality care.

Privacy

Clients Have the Right:

- to confidentiality of information about their health, social, and financial circumstances and about what takes place in the home; and
- to expect the home care provider to release information only as required by law or authorized by the client.

Financial Information

Clients Have the Right:

- to be informed of the extent to which payment may be expected from Medicare, Medicaid, or any other payer known to the home care provider;
- to be informed of the charges that will not be covered by Medicare;
- to be informed of the charges for which the client may be liable;
- to receive this information, orally and in writing, before care is initiated and within 30 working days of the date the home care provider becomes aware of any changes in charges; and
- to have access, upon request, to all bills for service the client has received regardless of whether the bills are paid out-of-pocket or by another party.

notification of his or her rights either before furnishing care to the client or during the initial evaluation visit. In addition, the home health agency must keep written documentation showing that the agency has complied with this requirement ("Medicare Conditions of Participation," 1989). The National Association for Home Care has established a Bill of Rights for clients and families to inform them of the ethical conduct they can expect from home care agencies. This document is widely used by such agencies (Table 29–10).

TABLE 29–10

Home Care Bill of Rights* *Continued*

Quality of Care

Clients Have the Right:

- to receive care of the highest quality;
- in general, to be admitted by a home care provider only if it has the resources needed to provide the care safely and at the required level of intensity, as determined by a professional assessment; a provider with less than optimal resources may nevertheless admit the client if a more appropriate provider is not available, but only after fully informing the client of the provider's limitations and the lack of suitable alternative arrangements; and
- to be told what to do in the case of an emergency.

The Home Care Provider Shall Assure That:

- all medically related home care is provided in accordance with physicians' orders and that a plan of care specifies the services and their frequency and duration; and
- all medically related personal care is provided by an appropriately trained home care aide who is supervised by a nurse or other qualified home care professional.

Client Responsibility

Clients Have the Responsibility:

- to notify the provider of changes in the condition (e.g., hospitalization, changes in the plan of care, symptoms to be reported);
- to follow the plan of care;
- to notify the provider if the visit schedule needs to be changed;
- to inform providers of the existence of, and any changes made to, advance directives;
- to advise the provider of any problems or dissatisfaction with the services provided;
- to provide a safe environment for care to be provided; and
- to carry out mutually agreed responsibilities.

*To satisfy the Medicare certification requirements, the Health Care Financing Administration requires that agencies:

1. Give a copy of the Bill of Rights to each patient in the course of the admission process.
2. Explain the Bill of Rights to the patient and document that this has been done.

To minimize confusion, the National Association for Home Care recommends that agencies have clients sign *one form* that shows that the client acknowledges all of the agency's policies and procedures (e.g., release of medical information, billing procedures).

Some home care agencies have adapted this Bill of Rights to include other rights specifically applicable to their clients. Others have added a list of responsibilities the patient and family must assume to receive home care, such as notifying agency personnel of changes in health status or providing care in the absence of the home care nurse.

Home health care agencies and home care nurses often face difficult ethical dilemmas about the delivery of care to clients. At times a client will require or desire more care than Medicare or private insurance will pay for. The home care agency has to decide whether it will provide care to the client even if there is no reimbursement. Home care agencies have written policies to guide the decision-making process. It may be the responsibility of the home care nurse to find another community agency that can meet the client's needs at a cost the client can afford. Home care agencies are prohibited from discharging clients from care because they are unable to pay for the service they need. If the client needs service for which he or she is unable to pay and there is no other agency willing to provide that care, the agency must continue to provide care until the client no longer needs care or referral can be made to another agency.

Summary

Home health care, as part of the health care system, has grown significantly. It is anticipated that this growth will continue in response to current health care reform initiatives. Home care nursing as a specialty area of practice has also grown in response to the changes in the health care system and the increasing desire by clients to be cared for in their homes. Home care nurses provide restorative and maintenance care to clients and families to promote independence and improve the quality of life of clients in the community. In addition to providing illness care to clients, professional home care nurses include health promotion and disease prevention education in their care plans for all clients.

KEY IDEAS

1. Home care nursing practice has its foundation in the theory and concepts that guide community health nursing. Home care nurses provide family-

focused care to acutely and chronically ill clients of all age groups.

2. Many types of agencies can provide home care services to clients in the community. Some home care agencies provide both professional and paraprofessional services, while others provide exclusively paraprofessional services.
3. Home care services can include care of the ill client in the home, health promotion or disease prevention, or specialized home care services such as high-technology care, pediatric care, or hospice care.
4. Several factors must be considered in making the decision to discharge a technology-dependent client from the hospital to home care.
5. Home care agencies are reimbursed for the services they provide by Medicare, Medicaid, private insurance companies, client self-payment, other public funds, and private donations. For a home care agency to receive reimbursement from Medicare, the client receiving care must meet certain eligibility requirements.
6. Although many professionals and paraprofessionals are members of the home care team, the home care nurse is responsible for case management and coordination. That is, the home care nurse is responsible for the coordination of the other professionals and paraprofessionals in the home to ensure that the client's health care needs are being met.
7. The ANA has developed standards of home care practice that are designed to guide the delivery of home care nursing service at both the generalist and specialist levels.
8. Infection control in home care involves two major concepts. Home care providers must protect themselves from communicable diseases of clients and protect the individual/family/community from the spread of communicable disease.
9. Total quality improvement involves the customers and consumers of home care services and the outcomes of care provided in the home.
10. Home care nurses can operationalize the *Healthy People 2000* objectives in their clinical practice through the inclusion of health promotion and disease prevention interventions in all care plans for acutely and chronically ill clients and their families.

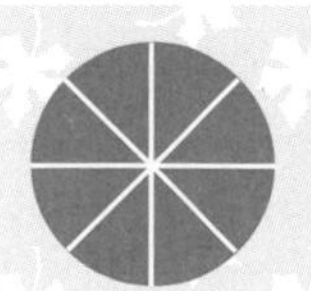

CASE STUDY
A Day in the Life of a Home Care Nurse

Jane Jones is a home care nurse at the Hill Valley VNA, a nonprofit home health care agency serving a suburban population. She has worked in home care for 4 years. Before that she was assistant head nurse on a cardiothoracic floor in the local community hospital. She left the hospital because she felt unable to practice nursing the way she believed it should be practiced. She found home care to be an exciting alternative to the hectic pace of the acute care institution.

Jane arrives at the home care agency at 8:00 A.M. and reviews the cases she has scheduled. Her caseload for today includes five visits: two visits to perform daily dressing changes, one visit to perform a cardiac assessment for a client who is seen weekly, one visit to supervise a home care aide, and an admission visit to a client who is newly diagnosed with diabetes. Given that she has to do a new admission with all the accompanying paperwork, she considers five visits as her maximum for today. On days when she does not have a new admission or her scheduled visits are short, she will often make a sixth home visit, as the agency expects the nurses to make an average of 5.5 visits per day.

To plan her day, the first piece of information Jane needs is the time the home care aide will be in the home. Her other visits must be scheduled around this time, as Jane must supervise the home care aide at the client's home. Jane calls the home care aide supervisor and finds out that the aide is assigned to the client from 11 A.M. to 1 P.M. Jane believes that she can make the two home visits to do the dressing changes and then be at the client's home to supervise the home care aide by 11:30 A.M. Thus the admission visit to the newly diagnosed diabetic and the home visit to the client in need of a cardiac assessment are scheduled for the afternoon. If all goes as planned, Jane believes that she will be back in the office at 3 P.M. to do her paperwork and make the necessary telephone calls.

Before she leaves, she calls all her clients and tells them the approximate time she will arrive at their homes. She also asks them if there have been any changes since her last home visit. This helps her to determine whether she needs to plan anything different for today's home visit. She assembles all the equipment she will need, as she will not return to the agency until the end of the day. Today she will need the agency's glucometer for the new diabetic and the scale for the cardiac client. She stocks her bag with extra gloves, paper towels, and aprons. On the way out the door of the agency, she leaves the receptionist with the list of clients she will be seeing today, the approximate time of the home visit, and the client's telephone number, so that anyone who needs to contact her can call her at the client's home at which she is scheduled. At the home care agency, she removes a pen and some change from her purse and locks it in the trunk, as she does not take her purse into the client's home or leave it visible in her car.

Her first two home visits are relatively uneventful and are conducted as planned; the home care aide supervision is scheduled for the third visit. However, when the home care aide reached the client's home, the client was having difficulty breathing. The aide helped the client to a sitting position, which helped slightly. Jane arrives shortly after the home care aide. Assessment of the client reveals severe dyspnea, elevated pulse, widening pulse pressure, and cyanosis around the mouth and in the nailbeds. On auscultation, crackles are heard in all lung fields, and the client expectorates frothy sputum. The client has a history of congestive heart failure. After reassuring the client and making her as comfortable as possible, Jane calls the primary physician. Jane relays the physical symptoms to the physician and asks if the client should be sent to the emergency department or the physician's office. Given the client's condition, the physician states that the emergency department is more appropriate. Because the client has no one to transport her, an ambulance is called. While waiting for the ambulance, Jane asks the home care aide to collect some of the client's personal belongings that she will need if hospitalized and pack them in an overnight bag. The home care aide also makes sure the client has her Medicare card and the card from her supplemental insurance policy. Jane remains with the client, monitoring her physical status. The house is prepared for the client's absence by making sure all appliances are turned off and turning on some lights. Jane and the home care aide stay with the client until the ambulance arrives. After the client leaves in the ambulance, Jane provides support to the home care aide for her activities with this client.

After her lunch break, Jane proceeds with the two home visits scheduled for the afternoon. Both visits occur as planned, and Jane is ready to return to the home care agency by 3:00 that afternoon. After her return to the agency, the major tasks of completing the paperwork and case coordination begin. Her first task is to call the primary physician for the client she admitted to the home health care agency today. The client had been discharged from the hospital with orders for skilled care to teach him about his diabetic diet. During her visit with the client, Jane noted that he needs assistance with his personal care because of his weakness and instability. The physician is notified of this problem, and a home care aide is requested for 2 hours per day, twice a week. Jane also needs to call the state subsidized pharmacy program on behalf of her cardiac client. During her home visit today, the client informed Jane that she received a letter stating that she would no longer be eligible for her medication subsidy. Without the subsidy, the client will be unable to afford the expensive cardiac medications she is taking. The client tried several times to find out why her subsidy was discontinued but did not understand the reason for this change. Jane said she would try to find out why the client's subsidy was changed. Jane also calls the hospital emergency department to see if her client was admitted to the inpatient facility.

Jane tries to reach the physical therapist involved with one of her clients. Jane changes the dressing to the large burn on the leg, and the therapist provides gait training and range of motion to the affected extremity. During her home visit today, Jane noted that the client was not using his crutches correctly. Because the therapist is at the agency, she and Jane have a case conference regarding this and determine that the therapist will instruct the client again on the proper use of crutches.

After making her telephone calls and having a case conference with the physical therapist, Jane completes the paperwork that is a large part of her job. An admission visit requires completion of HCFA forms 485 and 486, the social and physical data base, and many other forms that provide data for subsequent visits. She also must document the home visits, the telephone calls made, and the case conference in her clients' service records. Finally, she completes her time sheet for the day and is ready to leave the office. Before she leaves, Jane looks at her calendar for tomorrow; seven visits are scheduled. It looks like she will need some help tomorrow, so she informs her supervisor of this before she leaves.

GUIDELINES FOR LEARNING

1. Arrange to spend a day with a home care nurse. Notice the types of clients for whom care is provided, the family-centered approach to care, and the interventions used by the nurse. Identify the unique aspects of providing care to clients in their homes.
2. Interview an elderly client who has recently received home care to assess his or her perceptions of the experience. Try to determine what services were needed that were not covered by Medicare. Also assess the client's perceptions of the benefits of home care.
3. Review the health care records used in a home health agency. Specifically identify the standard Medicare HCFA forms 485, 486, and 487. Identify ways nurses in that agency have increased the efficiency of their recording.
4. Interview a legislator from your state who is interested in health care reform. Discuss the future role of home care in the proposals for reforming the

American health care system. Discuss how these changes will affect the delivery of health care in general and home health care specifically.

5. Ask a home care nurse to discuss a clinical situation in which she or he had to make a difficult ethical decision. This may include a decision to discharge a client who is unsafe in the home, to discharge a Medicare client who continues to need nursing care but is no longer homebound, or to terminate services because of inability to pay. Discuss the process the nurse went through to make the decision and its impact on her or his professional development.
6. Explore your state's laws governing advance directives. Obtain or develop forms for a living will and a durable power of attorney for health care that are consistent with state law. Consider whether you desire to complete such forms for yourself. Do you need any additional information before completing them? If so, from whom?

REFERENCES

American Nurses' Association (ANA). (1974). *Standards of community health nursing practice.* Washington, DC: Author.

ANA. (1986). *Standards of home care nursing practice.* Washington, DC: Author.

ANA. (1992). *A statement on the scope of home health nursing practice.* Washington, DC: Author.

American Public Health Association. (1991). *Healthy communities 2000: Model standards* (3rd ed.). Washington, DC: Author.

Annas, G. J., & Glantz, L. H. (1986). The right of elderly patients to refuse life-sustaining medical treatment. *Milbank Quarterly, 64* (suppl 2), 95–162.

Barkauskas, V. H. (1990). Home health care. *Annual Review of Nursing Research, 8,* 103–132.

Berg, R. (1988). *The APIC curriculum for infection control practice.* Iowa: Kendall Hunt.

Callahan, M., & Kelley, P. (1993). *Final gifts: Understanding the special awareness, needs, and communications of the dying.* New York: Bantam Books.

Cary, A. H., & Galten, R. E. (1992). *Nurses of distinction: The debut of home health nurses' specialty practice. Presented at the National Association for Home Care Annual Meeting,* New Orleans, October 1, 1992.

Centers for Disease Control and Prevention. (1989). Guidelines for prevention of transmission of human immunodeficiency virus and hepatitis B virus to health-care and public-safety workers. *Morbidity and Mortality Weekly Report, 38*(S-6), 1–37.

Commerce Clearing House. (1991). *Medicare and the American health care system.* No. 658, Part II, June 24, 1991.

Daubert, E. (1979). Patient classification system and outcome criteria. *Nursing Outlook, 27*(7), 450–454.

Donar, M. (1988). Community care: Pediatric home care. *Holistic Nursing Practice, 2*(2), 68–80.

Emanuel, L. L., & Emanuel, E. J. (1989). The medical directive: A new comprehensive advance care document. *Journal of the American Medical Association, 261*(22), 3288–3293.

Handy, C. (1989). Patient-centered high technology home care. *Holistic Nursing Practice, 3*(2), 46–53.

Health Care Financing Administration. (April, 1989). *Medicare home health agency manual Pub II.* Washington, DC: Author.

Home Care Nursing Services. (1988) *Caring, 7*(12), 8–9.

Humphrey, C. J. (1986). *Home care nursing handbook.* Norwalk, CT: Appleton-Century-Crofts.

Humphrey, C. J. (1988). The home as a setting for care. *Nursing Clinics of North America, 23*(2), 305–314.

Humphrey, C. J., & Milone-Nuzzo, P. (1991). *Home care nursing: An orientation to practice.* East Norwalk, CT: Appleton & Lange.

Knollmueller, R. (1993). The role of prevention in home healthcare nursing practice. *Home Health Care Nurse, 11*(1), 21–23.

LaLonde, B. (1988). Assuring the quality of home care via the assessment of client outcomes. *Caring, 7*(11), 20–24.

Martin, K., & Scheet, N. (1992). *The Omaha system.* Philadelphia: W.B. Saunders.

Medicare conditions of participation: Home health agencies. (1989). *Federal Register, 54*(155).

Mitchell, M. K. (1992). Nursing's legacy of leadership. *Nursing and Health Care, 13*(6), 297–295.

Morgan, K. J. (1991). National certification for home care RNs. *Nursing Management, 22*(9), 63–64.

Mundinger, M. (1983). *Home care controversy: Too little, too late, too costly.* Rockville, MD: Aspen.

National Association for Home Care (NAHC). (1992a). *Basic statistics about home care.* Washington, DC: Author.

NAHC. (1992b). *National uniformity for paraprofessional title, Qualifications and supervision.* Position paper. Washington, DC: Author.

Peters, D. (1992). Consumer oriented quality assurance in home care. *Pride Institute Journal of Long Term Home Care, 10*(2), 8–13.

Rooney, A. L., & Biere, D. M. (1992). Demonstrating excellence in home care through joint commission accreditation. *Journal of Nursing Administration, 22*(9), 31–36.

Shamansky, S. L. (1991). QI, CQI, QM, TQM, TQI, AYE, AYE, AYE. *Public Health Nursing, 8*(3), 145–146.

Shaughnessy, P., Bauman, M., & Kramer, A. (1990). Measuring the quality in home health care. *Caring, 9*(2), 36–39.

Sherman, C. V. (1991). Total management, not total quality management. *Journal of Quality Assurance, 27*(1), 26–31.

Spiegel, A. (1987). *Home health care,* Owings Mills, MD: National Health Publishing.

U.S. Code, Title 42, Section 1396a(w), Public Law 101-508, Section 4751. (1990). Patient self-determination act.

U.S. Department of Health and Human Services (USDHHS). (1990). *Healthy people 2000: National health promotion and disease prevention objectives.* Washington, DC: U.S. Government Printing Office.

USDHHS. (1991). *Aging in America: Trends and projections.* Publication No. 7C OA-28001. Washington, DC: U.S. Government Printing Office.

Warhola, C. (1980). *Planning for home health services: A resource handbook.* Washington, DC: U.S. Department of Health and Human Services.

SUGGESTED READINGS

Albrecht, M. (1992). Research priorities for home health nursing. *Nursing and Health Care, 13*(10), 538–541.

Arblaster, G., Brooks, D., Hudson, R., & Petty, M. (1990). Terminally ill patients' expectations of nurses. *Australian Journal of Advanced Nursing, 7*(3), 34–43.

Burke, S. M. (1990). Home health challenges: Paperwork vs. peoplework. *Nursing Management, 21*(11), 64.

Carr, P. (1990). Visit notes. *Home Healthcare Nurse, 8*(3), 47–48.

Cloonan, P. A., & Shuster, G. F. (1990). Care coordination: A resource intensive component of home health nursing practice. *Public Health Nursing, 7*(4), 204–208.

Collopy, B., Dubler, N., & Zuckerman, C. (1990). The ethics of home care: Autonomy and accommodation. *Hastings Center Report, 20*(2), 1–16.

Dellasega, C. (1991). Caregiving stress among community caregivers for the elderly: Does institutionalization make a difference? *Journal of Community Health Nursing, 8*(4), 197–205.

Hanley, R. J., Wiener, J. M., & Harris, K. M. (1991). Will paid home care erode informal support? *Journal of Health Politics, Policy and Law, 16*(3), 507–521.

Hekelman, F. P., Stricklin, M. L., Brown, K., & Alemagno, S. (1992). Clinical research in home care. *Journal of Nursing Administration, 22*(1), 29–32.

Jaffe, K. B. (1989). Home health care and rehabilitation nursing. *Nursing Clinics of North America, 24*(1), 171–178.

Myers, M. B. (1988). Home care nursing: A view from the field. *Public Health Nursing, 5*(2), 65–67.

Nadwairski, J. A. (1992). Inner-city safety for home care providers. *Journal of Nursing Administration, 22*(9), 42–47.

Ralph, I. (1993). Infectious medical waste management: A home care responsibility. *Home Healthcare Nurse, 11*(3), 25–33.

Simmons, M. D., Trusler, M., Roccaforte, J., Smith, P., & Scott, R. (1990). Infection control for home health. *Infection Control Hospital Epidemiology, 11*(7), 362–370.

Stern, T. E. (1991). An early discharge program: An entrepreneurial nursing practice becomes a hospital-affiliated agency. *Journal of Perinatal and Neonatal Nursing, 5*(1), 1–8.

Stulginsky, M. (1993). Nurses' home health experience: Part I. The practice setting. *Nursing and Health Care, 14*(8), 402–407.

Stulginsky, M. (1993). Nurses' home health experience: Part II. The unique demands of home visits. *Nursing and Health Care, 14*(9), 476–485.

Zelewsky, M. G., & Deitrick, E. P. (1987). Rx for caregivers: Respite care. *Journal of Community Health Nursing, 4*(2), 77–84.

Chapter 30

Local Health Departments

Lucile H. Maher

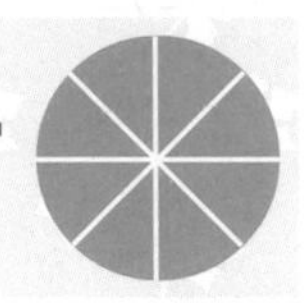

Focus Questions

What health services and populations have traditionally been a focus of public health nursing?

What funding sources does public health nursing use to support client services?

How is nursing in local health departments organized?

What are the various responsibilities of the public health nurse in the local health department?

How can the Assessment Protocol for Excellence in Public Health (APEX-PH) and the *Healthy People 2000* objectives be used to plan nursing services for populations?

What are future trends for nursing in local health departments?

The previous chapters have dealt with the definition and scope of community health nursing and its many facets for nursing practice. Community health nurses make up the largest percentage of health care workers in more than 2200 local health departments (National Association of County Health Officials [NACHO], 1990; Zerwekh, 1993). This has been true since the 1920s, when many local governments (counties, cities, or multicounty regions) developed health departments to promote the health of the people residing in their jurisdictions. Although the terms *community health nurse* and *public health nurse* are used interchangeably, nurses working for government-sponsored (public) entities often prefer the original name *public health nurse* (see Chapter 2).

Evolution of Public Health Nursing in Official Agencies

Public health nursing preceded the widespread development of local health departments. In the late 1800s Lillian Wald coined the term public health nurse. This term was appropriate not only because the nurse worked on behalf of the public, but also because "she was to create a public sphere that drew upon the diversity of cultural beliefs and societal demands of the populace" (Reverby, 1993, p. 1662). Local health departments expanded in part because of the successes of both public health nurses working in voluntary agencies and sanitary reformers. Local governments desired to provide such services for their residents and to protect the health of the public.

Public health nurses were and are professionals who attempt to develop healthful communities. These community health nurses employed by local health departments continue to use population-based planning to determine priorities for nursing programs. Their specific functions are determined by the societal demands of the time (Salmon, 1993).

Early public health work focused on environmental and sanitation problems to control the spread of communicable diseases. Local health departments with full-time employees to address these issues were established in Baltimore in 1793. Other cities, notably Philadelphia, New York, and Indianapolis, formed health departments during the 1800s (Pickett and Hanlon, 1990).

Public health nursing, at its inception, focused on the sick and those living in poverty and on indigent pregnant and postpartum women and their newborns. These nurses worked primarily in visiting nurse associations and were not affiliated with those first health departments.

Los Angeles (in 1898) and New York City (in 1908) began to employ nurses who would formally carry out public health nursing responsibilities (Pickett and Hanlon, 1990). This work continued to center on the poor and on control of communicable diseases, such as tuberculosis. Public health nurses performed nursing assessments, health and social histories, and health and risk reduction education and provided home health care.

With the passage of the Shepard-Towner Act in 1921 providing for complete birth registration (Last and Wallace, 1992), maternal and child health services became a mainstay of public health nursing in state and local health departments. In the intervening years, numerous programs and services have been added.

Structure and Responsibilities of Local Health Departments

A local health department has been defined by the NACHO (1990) as "an administrative or service unit of local or state government concerned with health and carrying some responsibility for the health of a jurisdiction smaller than the state."

Statistics from a 1990 survey done by NACHO indicate the following:

1. There are 2932 local health departments in 46 states.
2. Two thirds of the local health departments serve jurisdictions of less than 50,000 people, and 4% serve populations of 500,000 or more (Fig. 30–1).
3. Forty-six percent of the respondents have fewer than 10 full-time employees, while 10% have 100 or more.
4. Ninety percent report employing full- or part-time registered nurses either directly or through contracted services.

Under the U.S. Constitution, states retain the power to protect the health and welfare of their residents. Local health departments obtain their authority through state law and additional local ordinances.

Each state has a designated public health agency, but the structures of these agencies vary dramatically (Institute of

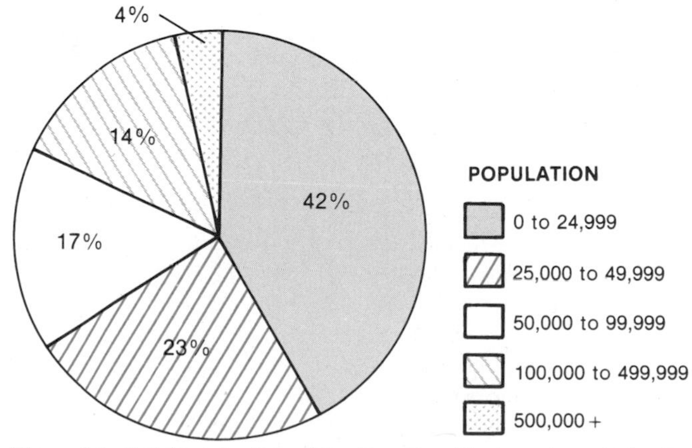

Figure 30–1 ● Distribution of the local health departments by the reported population of their jurisdiction (N = 2263). (Redrawn from National Association of County Health Officials. (1990, July). *National Profile of Local Health Departments.* Washington, DC: Author.)

Medicine [IOM], 1988). Some states have health agencies that include environmental and mental health; other states have separate agencies for each. Each state specifies its relationship with local health departments, with some states being more centralized than others. Whatever the organizational structure, it is local health departments that directly provide public health services to the residents.

Each local health department carries out three core functions: assessment and surveillance of the health status of its residents as well as of existing health resources; policy development and leadership to provide equitable distribution of health resources and to complement health activities in the private sector; and assurance that personal health care services and public health protection are available to all (IOM, 1988). The *Healthy People 2000* objectives acknowledge these core functions for local health departments (Table 30–1).

The local health department may have as few staff as one public health nurse, one environmentalist (sanitarian), and a part-time health director, or it may employ hundreds of employees to meet major city/jurisdiction health and environmental needs. The staff may be comprised of public health nurses, nurses in expanded roles (e.g., nurse practitioners), nutritionists, environmentalists, health educators, a biostatistician, clerical and laboratory staff, nursing or home health aides, counselors for alcohol and substance abuse, the health director, physicians, and various administrative staff. States also vary regarding whether or not the chief administrative officer is required to be a physician.

Environmental sanitarians are concerned with safe air, water, food, and housing (Miller, 1992). They conduct routine sampling of air and private water sources and inspect restaurants, dairies, and food processing sites. Sanitarians provide environmental education, enforce environmental laws, and respond to complaints. They may collect residential paint samples for lead analysis and address noise, unsafe dwellings, rodent control, and hazardous wastes.

Biostatisticians and *epidemiologists* apply their knowledge of statistics and the natural history of diseases to describe the health of communities, explore the causes of specific disease outbreaks, predict health hazards, and evaluate interventions. These health specialists are employed primarily at the state level or by larger local health departments.

Environmental issues and communicable disease control remain local health department mandates and priorities. Food and water sanitation and vector control exist alongside such modern concerns as hazardous waste management and swimming pool inspections. When a food- or water-borne disease is reported, the public health nurse and environmentalist work together to discover the source, follow-up with people reporting illness or symptoms, refer them for medical treatment, and bring the problem under control.

Public health nurses continue to address communicable disease control, including multidrug-resistant tuberculosis, the human immunodeficiency virus (HIV), and diseases of childhood such as polio, diphtheria, and measles (see Chapter 19). New vaccines for *hepatitis B* and *Haemophilus influenzae type B* offer protection for the future. However, each generation must be educated to maintain appropriate levels of immunity in susceptible populations. Detection, risk factor education (including HIV education and testing), treatment, and contact follow-up for sexually transmitted diseases are equally important.

Providing public information and education are critical aspects of public health nursing. Education about risk factors motivates individuals and groups to modify health-related behaviors (U.S. Department of Health and Human Services [USDHHS], 1990). Health education is expanding to include issues such as violence prevention.

A health department may be a *combined agency,* having both wellness services and home health services for the ill and disabled. Combined agencies may employ or contract for physiotherapists, home care aides or nursing assistants, nutritionists, social workers, speech or occupational therapists, and others.

In addition to control of communicable diseases and injuries, promotion of wellness and reduction of risks to health, and provision of home health care, community data may also dictate the need for primary care. *Primary care* is the provision of personal health services to individuals and family members, including screening and referral, health maintenance, long-term management of chronic disease, and care for acute illnesses. Primary care services imply a point of first contact with the health care system, as well as the source of continuing care.

Assuring the provision of basic health services is a part of public health. In response to the economic hardships of

TABLE 30–1 HEALTHY PEOPLE 2000

Healthy People 2000 Objectives for Local Health Departments

Increase to at least 90% the proportion of people who are served by a local health department that is effectively carrying out the core functions of public health. Core functions include the following:

1. Assessment of the population
2. Policy development
3. Assurance (including assuring access to essential clinical preventive services)

Adapted from U.S. Department of Health and Human Services. (1990). *Healthy people 2000: National health promotion and disease prevention objectives. Summary report.* Washington, DC: Government Printing Office.

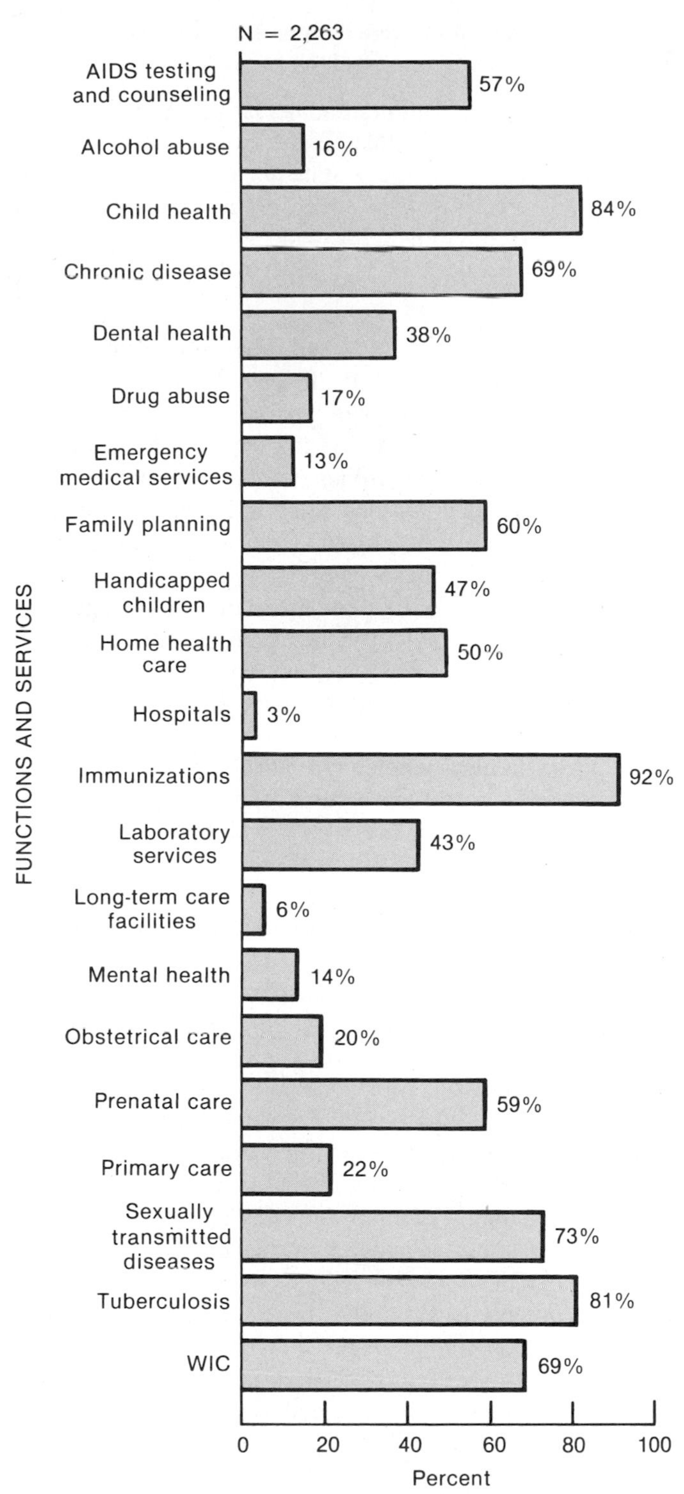

Figure 30–2 ● Percentage of local health departments that reported being active in personal health assurance functions and services (N = 2263). (Redrawn from National Association of County Health Officials. (1990, July). *National Profile of Local Health Departments.* Washington, DC: Author.)

the early 1980s and the increases in the number of medically uninsured and underinsured people, more health departments became directly involved in providing primary care services. This generated financial reimbursement for health department services but also diverted emphasis away from health promotion efforts (Felton and Parker, 1990; Zerwekh, 1993). Home visitation to vulnerable families was reduced as nurses worked more in primary care clinics (Anderson, O'Grady, and Anderson, 1985).

Public health nurses provide a broad array of services that vary with the specific health needs of the public. Most local health departments have immunization, communicable disease, child health, chronic disease, family planning, prenatal, and home health programs (Fig. 30–2). However, the specific services vary with each health department.

External Influences on Public Health Nursing

Public health nursing services have expanded and become more comprehensive as population needs have changed and as nursing's knowledge and skills base have broadened. Other influences are financial, political, legislative, and geographic.

Public health nursing services are financed through a variety of sources: local taxes; state and federal appropriations, grants, and contracts; fees and reimbursements for services; and private grants and donations. In one proposal for health care reform, federal public health allocations to states would be based on size of populations served, poverty rate, and rate of premature death (i.e., years of productive life lost) (White House Domestic Policy Council [WHDPC], 1993). States would continue to distribute these monies to local health departments to use for state programs. Additional federal funds would continue to be designated to specific health programs.

FUNDING SOURCES

Local Funds

Most local health departments have several funding sources, with the majority of revenue coming from local taxes or a levy (IOM, 1988). A *levy* is a mechanism for raising money through the ballot box. It is similar to a bond issue in that it is a determined percentage of the local property tax or a local income tax approved by voters.

Public health professionals desire to acquire adequate revenues to achieve public health goals. Because general tax monies fluctuate with the strength of business and industry in the community, a levy must be placed on the ballot periodically for voter approval. As the renewal time nears, the staff of the levy-supported health departments provide extensive community education about their services, the numbers of people served, and the successful outcomes for individuals and the community because of these services. Influential citizens are frequently asked to assist with community education; this may increase voter support for the levy.

Many states have a legislatively allocated local health department subsidy of a few cents to a few dollars per capita. This subsidy is derived from a states's general fund, which comprises taxes, fees collected, and grant monies that do not have a specified expenditure. This is not sufficient to support local health department programs but is important in the total financial scheme.

Although 75% of local health departments collect fees, these fees account for a small portion of the total budget (IOM, 1988; NACHO, 1990). The larger the local health department, the more likely it is to collect fees for services (Fig. 30–3).

Fees are collected for most health, environmental, counseling, and birth and death registration services. Many nursing services also have a service fee. *A sliding fee scale* is used to determine what percentage of the fee the client will pay based on the client's financial assets. Generally service fees are not sufficient to fully cover the cost, but if a client cannot pay, service is not denied. If a client has a third-party payer (e.g., Medicaid or private health insurance), some departments will bill that source or provide the client with a receipt to file for reimbursement. Fees may be used within the department to partially support health and environmental services. Such monies may also become part of the jurisdiction's general funds.

Federal and State Funds

State and federal monies account for almost 50% of local health department funds (IOM, 1988). The most common federal funding programs will be discussed here, but it must be remembered that types of appropriation and funds change over time. Federal and state governments may appropriate monies differently during each legislative session. As health care reform evolves, some or all of the following funds will change by title, how appropriated, and how incorporated into new plans.

Department of Agriculture Monies for the Women, Infant, and Children (WIC) Supplemental Food Program. These monies are funneled through state departments of health to local health departments or other community agencies that administer the program and provide the services. The WIC program has resulted in healthier mothers, infants, and children.

Centers for Disease Control and Prevention (CDC) Funds. Federal and state funds are allocated for biologicals for childhood immunization programs and for influenza vaccines for elderly persons. Health departments may pay a nominal cost for the influenza vaccine; immunization is generally limited to medically indigent elderly individuals and those with chronic lung and heart diseases. In 1993, Medicare began payment for influenza vaccine for all individuals with Medicare part B coverage. Arrangements were made for health departments to bill Medicare for immunizations provided. The state usually does not charge for biologicals used to immunize children.

Acquired immunodeficiency syndrome (AIDS) and HIV education and screening programs receive funding through state or federal competitive grants or direct appropriation. Interested community groups or agencies are encouraged to form cooperative agreements or consortia to avoid duplication of services (Table 30–2). Much of these monies fund HIV laboratory costs and the test materials necessary to obtain blood specimens and transport them to the laboratory. The monies also support AIDS/HIV counselors who assist HIV-positive clients with support and access to additional evaluation.

In some states and health departments, CDC monies fund disease investigation staff who track contacts of persons infected with specific sexually transmitted diseases (STDs), including syphilis, gonorrhea, and HIV. Contact follow-up is important epidemiologically for STD treatment, but reductions in federal and state funds and investigator staff have altered this component. State laws and health department regulations may also preclude investigations. Treatment medications for gonorrhea or other STDs may also be provided.

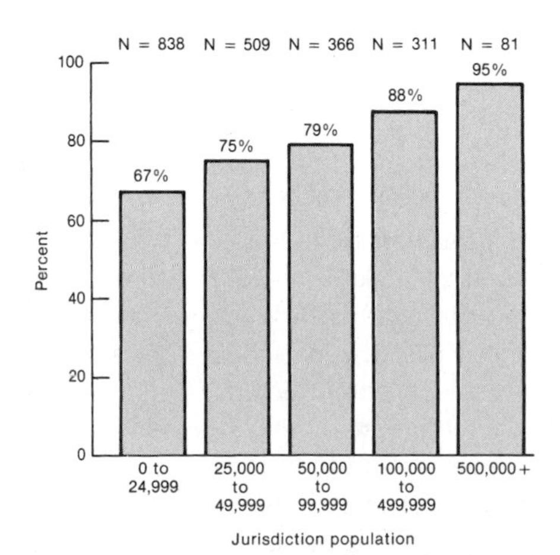

Figure 30–3 ● Percentage of local health departments that charge for personal health services by jurisdiction population. Overall, 75% reported charging for services (N = 2105). (Redrawn from National Association of County Health Officials. (1990, July). *National Profile of Local Health Departments.* Washington, DC: Author.)

TABLE 30–2

Types of Partnerships

Consortia: Two or more agencies, groups, or communities that work together toward a goal and share the costs and/or funds that support the pursuit of the goal.

Cooperatives: Two or more agencies, groups, or communities that work together to support and achieve a common goal, but without sharing the costs. Each agency supports its own staff and whatever activities and meetings are necessary to achieve the goal.

Tuberculosis monies have been increased since the 1980s as the incidence and prevalence of this disease have increased. The most affected populations have been clients with AIDS or HIV disease, homeless persons, and refugees who did not have access to prophylactic or treatment medications or did not complete the regimen. Tuberculosis is still a controllable disease, but extensive efforts to reach at-risk populations for diagnosis and appropriate treatment cost more than the $20.6 million appropriated in 1992. Accordingly, Congress is being asked by the CDC and interested health groups to increase funding to 14 times that amount.

Health and Human Services Funds. Health promotion/risk reduction monies have generally been competitive funds used for high blood pressure screening, referral, and follow-up; smoking cessation; and other risk assessment activities. These monies are targeted for health education initiatives and frequently are used to provide financial support to targeted community groups for professional counseling services.

Federal substance/alcohol abuse program funds have been available for some years and are generally augmented by state monies. The funds may come through the state health department or the state department of mental health. Some states have combined alcohol and substance abuse programs into a separate department of alcohol/mental health. Certainly both mental and physical factors influence how well an individual and the family succeed in efforts to end substance abuse. Extensive community education is an important component of these programs, both to prevent the development of abusive behaviors and to assist the client, family, and community in dealing with substance abuse. Public health nurses, psychologists, counselors, and health educators form the nucleus for intervention (see Chapter 21).

Maternal/Child Health (MCH) Block Grant. Federal Child and Family Health Services monies are funneled through state health departments and may be augmented by state MCH funds. The goal is to support comprehensive health assessment services, appropriate education and counseling, referrals, and follow-up for pregnant women and their infants and children. The monies may go to the health department, to other agencies, or to consortia/cooperatives formed between local agencies and the health department. Monies are limited; the greater the number of agencies involved, the more limited the support is for any one component or agency. Comprehensive services are defined by the grantor and vary from state to state. Grants must be renewed annually, and the grant award usually does not keep pace with inflation.

Health care reform discussions allude to changes for maternal and child funds. In 1994, federal monies were added for childhood immunizations. Medicaid waiver plans in some states may be a forerunner of managed care.

Special initiative MCH funds also require competitive grant proposals, which allow any interested state, local health department, or appropriate agency to apply for these monies. Each year a focus is selected, such as adolescent pregnancy or early childhood intervention. The emphasis of the intervention is based on community and/or agency perceptions of local health problems and innovative ideas to address them. The federal or state agency administering the monies reviews the submitted proposals and selects those to be funded. These are time- and amount-limited monies. They are not intended to subsidize established services but may be used to add a new service to a population presently being served or to begin a completely new program targeted to a special population.

Crippled/Handicapped Children's program monies became available in the mid-1930s to support detection, medical treatment, and ongoing follow-up of a broad range of physically and medically handicapping conditions in newborns and children up to 21 years of age. Orthopedic appliances, orthodontic devices (after cleft palate repair), hearing aids, and any therapist consultations necessary for appropriate treatment are some of the services available with this program. The program has been renamed Services for Children with Special Health Care Needs. There are financial and other eligibility criteria, which are generally determined by the state health department. Public health nurses often provide case management for these children and their families. Some states have expanded funding to pay for all services public health nurses provide to eligible families. Public health nursing visits to homes, schools, or other places are currently being reimbursed at rates commensurate with the degree of comprehensiveness, assistance, and advocacy necessary for the family and/or child with a disability.

Lead Poisoning Program funds come from the federal government through the state for education (of family, community, and local health department personnel), detection, and limited emergency housing abatement for childhood lead poisoning. Many child health programs include blood lead screening for children, ages 9 months to 6 years, and parent education. Some local health departments are designated teaching centers. A public health nurse and an environmentalist work with local health department personnel in designated counties to help establish blood lead screening and education programs.

Other Funds. There have been federal and state monies for other health department programs, such as air quality control and care at corrections facilities. Public health nursing may be involved, depending on the services to be provided. Medicaid and Medicare reimburse for specific services to individuals. Federal programs, including Medicaid, the Civilian Health and Medical Program of the Uniformed Services (CHAMPUS), and Medicare Part B, reimburse for nursing services provided by nurse practitioners and certified nurse midwives, especially in rural areas.

Medicaid. Title XIX monies consist of both federal and state funds on which the majority of health departments rely for service reimbursement (Fig. 30–4). The client must meet financial and other eligibility criteria. Medicaid reimbursement to service providers for medical or wellness-centered care may vary by state. The priority populations are pregnant women, infants, and children (2 through 18 years old), and some older adults who need chronic disease treatment or nursing home care. These priority populations were selected because they are unable to afford health care and are vulnerable to conditions that are expensive to treat if not prevented. For example, provision of prenatal care and nutrition increases the likelihood of a healthy infant and reduces the need for expensive neonatal intensive care services. Medicaid funds are frequently administered through state departments of human services with health maintenance services monitored by state health departments. Plans for managed care as proposed with health care reform, or proposed by states seeking Medicaid waivers, may change, incorporate, or eliminate Medicaid as it exists in 1994.

The Early Periodic Screening, Diagnosis, and Treatment (EPSDT) program is an example of Medicaid-funded health promotion services for children. Infants and children are entitled to physical examinations, immunizations, screening tests, health histories, nutrition assessment (referral to WIC and/or interim WIC visits as appropriate), and anticipatory guidance at specified age levels from birth to 18 years.

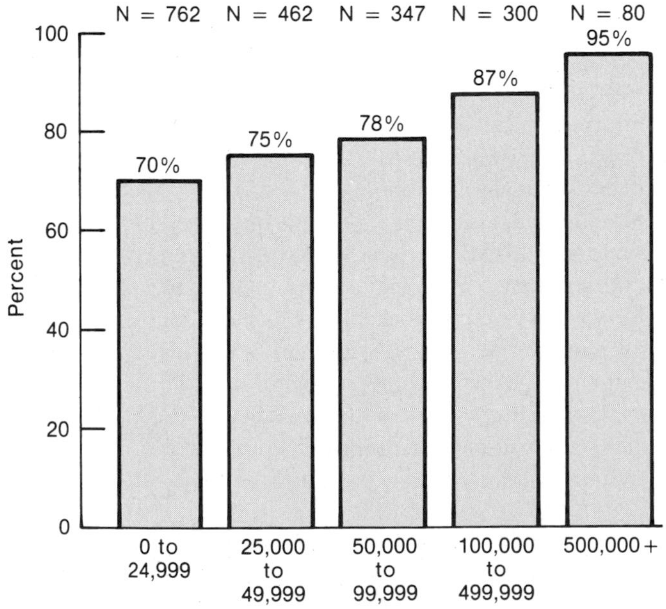

Figure 30–4 ● Percentage of local health departments that accept Medicaid reimbursement by jurisdiction population. Overall, 76% reported accepting Medicaid reimbursement (N = 1951). (Redrawn from National Association of County Health Officials. (1990, July). *National Profile of Local Health Departments.* Washington, DC: Author.)

CHAMPUS. The CHAMPUS program is the health insurance program for military personnel and their families. It mirrors EPSDT in its services but not in the age limits for those serviced.

Medicare. Medicare monies are a reimbursement source for combined agencies providing home health care. Physician-ordered services provided by public health nurses; physical, occupational, and speech therapy; and home health aide services are reimbursable for specified time periods at specified payment levels.

Medicare funds reimburse physician-provided primary care, specified diagnostic tests, and hospitalization for elderly persons. In 1992 Congress broadened Medicare coverage to pay for mammograms at specified intervals for women age 65 years and over.

Foundations. Foundations are philanthropic groups (formed by businesses, individuals, or industries) that support research and service proposals reflecting the emphases of the foundation. They may be national in focus, such as the Kellogg and Robert Woods Johnson trusts, or local. Foundations encourage competitive proposals that must meet certain guidelines. They can be excellent sources of funds for research or small local efforts.

IMPACT OF FUNDING VARIATION

Most local health departments rely on several funding sources; some may use all the types of funding previously listed. The cost to the department of the restrictions and accountability imposed by the grantor may exceed the benefits obtained with the money. Staff hired with grant monies are technically to work only on that program, or the work time of the numbers of people providing part-time services must equal the full-time equivalent. When monies are no longer available or are cut, jobs paid by those funds may be lost. Some funds cannot be used for rental space, building, or equipment purchases. If equipment can be purchased, those items may be claimed by the funding sources when monies end. Reports and data for federal or state monies, which must be collected and reported in a set format, frequently duplicate data collected at the local level—all in a different format. This leads to more pressure as a result of nursing time spent in paperwork rather than attention to a client.

Local health department costs—salaries, supplies, equipment, and benefits—increase annually. However, the amount of appropriations often remains the same over time or is reduced. Thus the degree to which these monies actually support local services decreases. In the difficult economy of the 1990s, the demand for public health nursing services is increasing. Local health departments are continually challenged to be innovative, creative, flexible, and available.

At one time nursing tried to avoid having staff on time-limited, or "soft," monies, but currently staff may be paid by two or three funding sources. This is where the full-time-equivalent factor enters the equation. Community health nursing administrators address difficult questions as they modify budgets. What components of a perinatal or child health program can be financed by other monies when a funding source ends or decreases? When child health funds do not keep pace with costs, how can sufficient child health services be incorporated into the WIC program? Similar questions arise for all public health nursing services. With flexible hours and flexible staffing, two part-time employees can fill a full-time position. If possible, other types of employees, such as nursing assistants, may be hired to perform nonnursing tasks and allow more efficient use of nursing time.

LEGISLATION

The funding sources discussed previously are considered legislative, except for foundations. State and federal agencies and programs have evolved through legislation. The appropriations are made or withheld based on state and federal budget emphases, the interests and power of legislators, and the demands of lobbying groups and constituents.

Both congressional and state legislatures are skilled in passing health-related bills without appropriate funds to implement the program. One example involves a Federal Medicare influenza study conducted from 1989 to April 1992 (Fedson, 1990). The U.S. Public Health Service determined to increase the influenza immunization level for elderly and high-risk individuals from 32% to at least 60% in 1990 and 1991. Eleven states across the country participated and increased influenza immunization levels by offering free vaccine to all Medicare Part B recipients. Vaccine purchased with federal monies was widely distributed in these states, not only health departments, but also to physicians, first-response and emergency care centers, and any other care source for elderly persons. Special clinics were also held. The percentage of susceptible people immunized improved greatly, meeting the 60% projection and more. At the end of the study period, no plan was made for free vaccine for the 1992–93 influenza season. Discussions and efforts from April to August 1992 produced promises of limited vaccine to meet some of the immunization demand. In 1993, Medicare began reimbursement for influenza vaccine.

Public health employees have become effective working with legislators. Public health nurses, environmentalists, administrators, and other staff working with programs such as substance/alcohol abuse, HIV testing, and AIDS case coordination organize networks to initiate, support, or oppose legislation that will adversely affect local health departments and communities. For example, in a number of states, public health professionals have been highly effective in guiding and supporting specific HIV testing and AIDS legislation. The bills afford protection for health care workers by the availability of HIV tests and employment security if that test is positive. Public health advocates have been equally effective in opposing broad AIDS legislation that would compromise an individual's privacy, employment, and/or health insurance coverage.

GEOGRAPHIC VARIATIONS

As noted earlier, the majority of local public health programs serve populations of 50,000 or less. All the factors noted within this chapter heavily influence the needs of and services for rural areas and small towns in the United States.

Medical personnel and health services are often concentrated in urban areas. Last and Wallace (1992) have discussed the growth of group medical practices in the United States. Group practices afford individuals access to the care they may need, be it family medicine, internal medicine, or other specialty represented in a group practice. This sounds beneficial to the client. However, the geographic maldistribution of physicians leads to inner-city and rural areas being medically underserved. These areas may attract only the single-specialty physician, who may practice alone in communities with great needs. Some communities with populations of 15,000 to 30,000 have only one physician. Even the state health department may not have clinics in inner-city areas or some rural communities. Transportation problems and appointment times that conflict with employment can be added barriers (see Chapter 31).

Public health nurses in rural communities and city health departments provide wide-ranging wellness care and health screening to detect potential problems. Education regarding health promotion and lifestyle adaptions that reduce risks to good health is an important component. Nurse practitioners monitor and/or treat illnesses and chronic diseases depending on the support of the department's medical director and on community needs.

Many public health nurses are long-term residents of their community. They know their community, and they are often available for consultation any hour of the day or night. These nurses may not have at hand all the social, medical, and other consultative sources available in cities. They are skilled in their assessment and teaching abilities and can guide clients to appropriate resources as needed.

Some state health departments, through maternal and child health programs, may provide itinerant multidisciplinary teams of specialists for diagnosis and treatment of infants and children with disabilities. The local public health nursing staff provide follow-up, case management, and continuing family/client support and guidance.

Public Health Nursing Practice

Public health nurses have demonstrated professional competencies that continue to be relevant (Table 30–3). Public health nurses have experience in seeking out those who have health needs but are not actively involved with the health care system. Because of their knowledge of family and community theory and their firsthand experiences with both, public health nurses are leaders in addressing contemporary public health problems.

EDUCATIONAL PREPARATION

The theory and practicum of public/community health courses in baccalaureate nursing programs begin the foundation for public health nursing practice. A baccalaureate degree in nursing is preferred by most local health departments. However, the diploma or associate degree remains the nursing education base for the majority of practicing public health nurses.

Other qualifications may include some knowledge of the practices and objectives of public health and of social and economic forces within communities and families. The nurse should be able to work effectively with colleagues and the public and to show initiative, enthusiasm, and the ability to work independently.

Baccalaureate and higher nursing education remains economically and geographically inaccessible for many nursing candidates, but opportunities for such education are growing for diploma or associate degree nurses who desire baccalaureate or master's level education. Equally important have been continuing education opportunities that include subjects pertinent to community health, such as environmental assessments, community assessment, health education strategies, and case management. These programs may be sponsored by collegiate nursing continuing education departments. Community health nursing faculty and local health department staff are often the speakers or leaders for these programs that address public health nursing issues.

Management and supervision in public health nursing usually require master's preparation; this preparation can be in nursing or public health, either alone or in combination with management or business courses. Again, geographic availability, local health agency funding, governmental personnel policies, and politics all can impede hiring people with these degrees. The national nursing organizations (National League for Nursing [NLN] and American Nurses' Association [ANA]) encourage advanced practice and advanced degrees. Both staff public health nurses and management must advocate more fully and appropriately for qualified public health nurses.

TABLE 30–3

Public Health Nurses' Strengths

1. Public health nurses have a special role in policy making because they can "translate" among scientists, the public, and other policy makers (Salmon, 1993).
2. Public health nurses have always been flexible, creatively adjusting to meet the changing needs of clients (Salmon, 1993).
3. Public health nurses have a long history of successful outreach to find people within communities who are in need of all levels of preventive health care (Salmon, 1993; Zerwekh, 1992, 1993).
4. Public health nurses have experience with culturally appropriate preventive care (Reverby, 1993).
5. Public health nursing care to vulnerable populations, especially with elderly persons at home, pregnant women, and young children, has been demonstrated to be cost effective (Reverby, 1993).
6. Public health nurses are health professionals who have much experience with human responses to everyday situations. For this reason, public health nurses can lead a return to neighborhood-centered practice (Schorr, 1989; Zerwekh, 1993).

STANDARDS OF PRACTICE

Public health nurses function within the ANA standards for community health nursing discussed in Chapter 1. In selected states general public health standards have been developed. These may or may not have a legislative mandate or a funding incentive. How well standards are met depends on local health department capability and willingness to participate in the standards implementation and review process and whether there are incentives for maintenance of standards.

POPULATION-BASED PLANNING

Healthy People 2000 Objectives. With the advent of the *Healthy People 2000* objectives (USDHHS, 1990), national objectives covering all areas of health and the environment challenge public health personnel to involve their state and local communities in exploring what good health and wellness mean. The objectives cover traditional facets of public health, as well as the concerns of AIDS and HIV infection, violence in the community, and dental care.

There are more than 300 objectives. Certainly no one health department can address all of them, and for some objectives there is no mechanism for collecting data that would demonstrate accomplishment. Small local health departments, in conjunction with state health departments, and larger local health departments are to assess the health status of their residents and the existing resources. Each community can compare its status relative to the targets within *Healthy Communities 2000* (APHA, 1991).

State and local health departments are to choose objectives pertinent to their communities and develop action plans and methods to accomplish the objectives. These plans contribute to development and maintenance by communities, families, and individuals of behaviors and lifestyles to achieve and maintain healthy lives.

TABLE 30–4

Management By Objectives: A Nursing Plan to Detect and Control Hypertension

OBJECTIVE:

To provide high blood pressure detection, evaluation, education, referral, and/or treatment services for 5000 clients during 1992 at a cost not to exceed $101,900.

METHODS:

1. Develop a uniform plan by June 1992 to educate all new clients enrolled in the high blood pressure program regarding risk behaviors.
2. Blood pressure screening and related services will be available to Adult Health Clinic clients, and no less than 55% of all clinic clients will be screened.
   Percentage screened: ______________________.
3. Clinic clients will complete a hypertension screening form at the time of clinic registration.
4. Accept referrals of clients needing blood pressure re-screening or other clinic services.
   Number of clients referred from community programs:______________________.
5. Promote heart health services to medically under- or noninsured clients who require assistance to restore or maintain normal blood pressure status.
   Number of clients who receive regular monitoring of blood pressure status in the clinic while receiving primary care from a private medical source:______________________.
   Number of clients with blood pressure under control:______________________.
   Number of clients receiving assistance with obtaining medication at the Akron Health Department (AHD) Clinic while receiving primary care from a private medical source:______________________.
   Number of clients with blood pressure under control:______________________.
   Number of clients receiving all primary medical care for hypertension at AHD Clinic:______________________.
   Number of clients with blood pressure under control:______________________.

From Division of Public Health Nursing. (1992). *Management by objectives.* Akron, OH: Akron Health Department.

Management by Objectives. Management by objectives and results is one mechanism by which many health departments take components of the *Healthy People 2000* objectives and translate them into manageable action plans for their own locale (Table 30–4).

Example. Heart disease and cerebral vascular accidents were the leading causes of adult deaths in Akron, Ohio. As good public health practice, nurses performed blood pressure checks for most adult clients along with the services requested by the clients. Over the years, the health department has also made blood pressure screening available at the Bureau for Employment Services, the county department of human services, barber shops in African-American neighborhoods, health fairs, and other sites where high-risk populations can be screened. Those with elevated blood pressure are referred to the health department for additional blood pressure monitoring and referral, diagnostic workup, treatment, and follow-up as appropriate. The objectives and methods for this hypertension program have developed as the program evolved over 7 to 8 years. The program is ongoing. Objectives and methods are reviewed quarterly and revised annually by the nursing management staff and the director of health.

Assessment Protocol for Excellence in Public Health (APEX–PH). Another tool for community and organizational assessment that may allow better definition of local needs and development of more practical objectives is APEX-PH (NACHO, 1991). APEX-PH has two components: internal assessment of the agency and community assessment of health needs.

Internally, the APEX-PH process helps a local health agency look at its organizational structure and its relationship within the community as viewed by the staff. Examples of the organizational structure of a local health department and a flow chart for assessing organizational capacity are shown in Figures 30–5 and 30–6. The APEX-PH process is voluntary, and all staff have the opportunity to be involved. APEX-PH can lead to an ongoing evaluation process with practical plans and actions to respond to identified internal concerns. It can also lead to better understanding of the agency's mission, the populations being served, the support systems in the agency and community, and the mechanisms for agency/program accountability.

A second part of APEX-PH is a community assessment of health needs (Fig. 30–7). In this part of the program, community leaders and consumers must be involved in priority setting, policy development, and assurance that identified needs are met. The assessment considers the health department's relationships with social, health, and related community agencies, both local and state. This affords the health department greater visibility and a cooperative role with the community in the work of the department, which is the health of its people. In these times of "doing more with less," APEX-PH is an opportunity for nurses to recognize their public health successes and join with the community to meet daily new challenges.

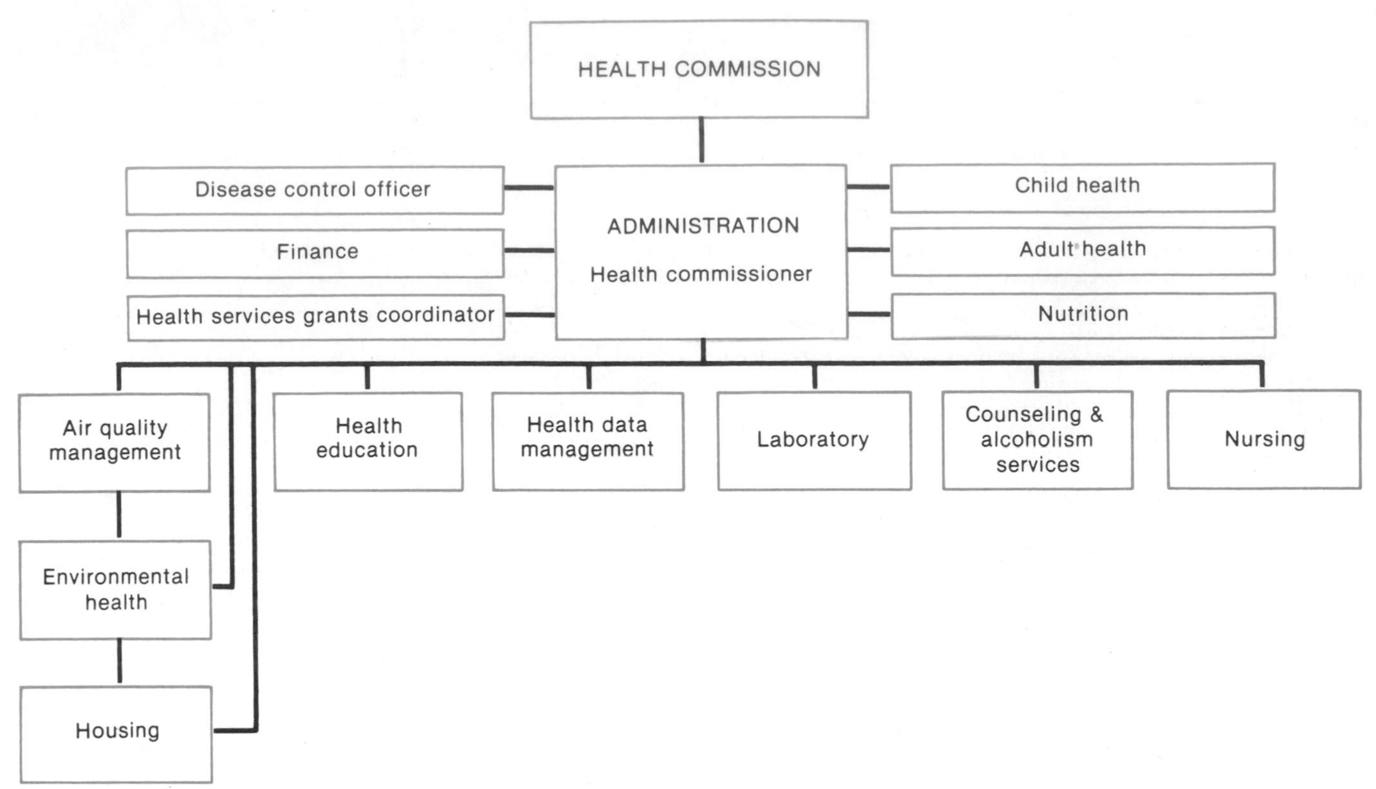

Figure 30–5 ● Organizational chart: local health department. (Redrawn from Akron Health Department. (1992). *Akron Health Department organizational chart.* Akron, OH: Author.)

ORGANIZATION OF SERVICES AND STAFF

Figure 30–5 depicts a health department organization chart showing public health nursing in the scheme of the department as a whole. Depending on agency staffing size, there may or may not be formal organizational charts for the health department or for nursing. An example of a formal public health nursing chart is provided in Figure 30–8.

Nursing assignments in local health departments are determined by the agency and community needs, complexity of services, numbers of nursing programs, the number of staff, and availability of grant funds. Public health nurses may be assigned as generalists across several health department programs or as specialists in one specific program, such as child health or adult health.

Generalized Practice. Traditionally, nurses in local health have been generalists. All nurses were oriented in and responsible for all services. This remains fairly true in small departments with limited staffs. Public health nurses provide the clinic, home visit, community education, school, and civic activities within their jurisdiction. They participate in community needs assessments and in quality assurance activities, and serve as case managers with families and the varied resources involved in client care. Assignments may be geographically determined according to the available public health nurses among the population served. Each public health nurse has greater expertise and interest in some programs than in others; colleagues collaborate with each other for consultation and assistance.

Program-Specific Practice. As public health nursing practice becomes more comprehensive and specialized, generalization in work assignments is less feasible. Nurses may elect assignments or be assigned by specific population group; by geographic area; by programs such as adult, maternal, or child health services or home health care; or by combinations of these. Expanded practice nurses in pediatrics, geriatrics, and family health have also found a niche in many public health agencies, particularly large ones. The variety of public health nursing activities and settings are discussed later.

The wisdom of using nurses' special interests and skills has led some agencies to pay part or all of the costs of nurse practitioner education or to develop job classifications for the expanded role nurse. This contributes to the enrichment of that nurse's skills and work, thereby enhancing the services and care for the client.

ACTIVITIES AND RESPONSIBILITIES

Public health nurses in local health departments are responsible for working with other professionals and community residents to assess the health needs of the

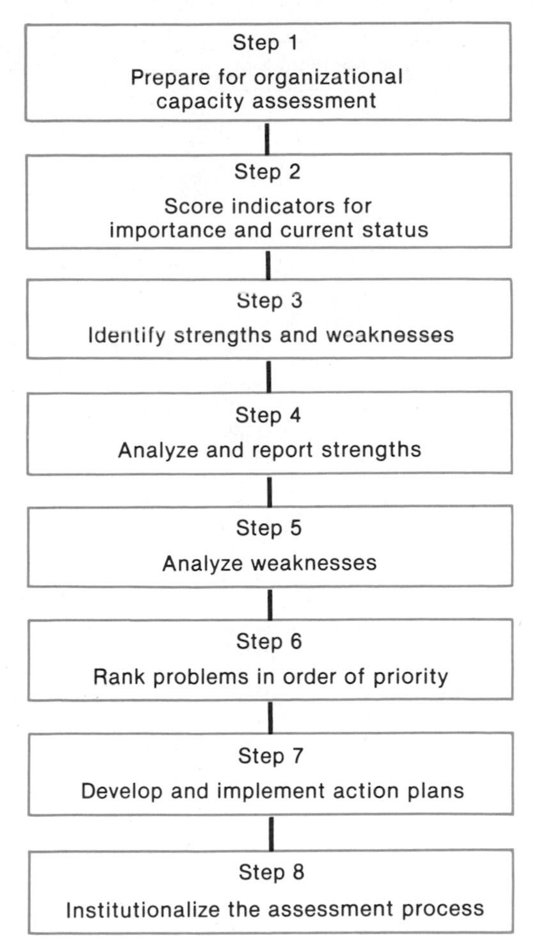

Figure 30–6 ● Flow chart of steps in assessing organizational capacity. (Redrawn from National Association of County Health Officials. (1991). *Assessment Protocol for Excellence in Public Health (APEX-PH).* Washington, DC: Author.)

population within their jurisdiction. They describe the population's health status and identify the degree to which there are resources available to address the health problems and issues. Public health nurses are experts in identifying health needs that can be addressed through nursing care. They develop, implement, and evaluate nursing services for primary, secondary, and tertiary levels of prevention (Table 30–5).

All of the responsibilities discussed in Chapter 1 are carried out in some measure by public health nurses. Education, screening and case-finding, advocacy, and the development of new services all occur in partnership with the community.

Nurses in local health departments have traditionally focused on health promotion; health protection; lifestyle adaptation to maintain health; and detection, referral, and treatment for health problems. Specific interventions may be focused on an individual, on the community as a whole, or on vulnerable populations, such as elderly persons, pregnant adolescents, or males susceptible to hypertension. In larger health departments, education efforts are frequently multidisciplinary, with staff from nursing, health education, and nutrition and/or other health department staff providing expertise.

SETTINGS AND POPULATIONS

Public health nurses have always worked in homes, occupational settings, schools, and clinics. Currently public health nurses continue to work in these sites, as well as recreation centers, prisons, medical daycare centers, and wellness centers. Public health nursing services also are provided in group or transitional housing for people with physical disabilities or developmental delays or those returning to the community after hospitalization for mental illness, imprisonment, or other social and health problems.

Clinics. Traditionally, public health nurses have targeted populations who are underserved or who have higher than average morbidity and mortality. Health department clinics usually target specific populations such as women of childbearing years (maternity and family planning clinics), children and adolescents (well-child clinics and clinics for children with disabilities), and adults (primary care and wellness centers). Such clinics may complement private

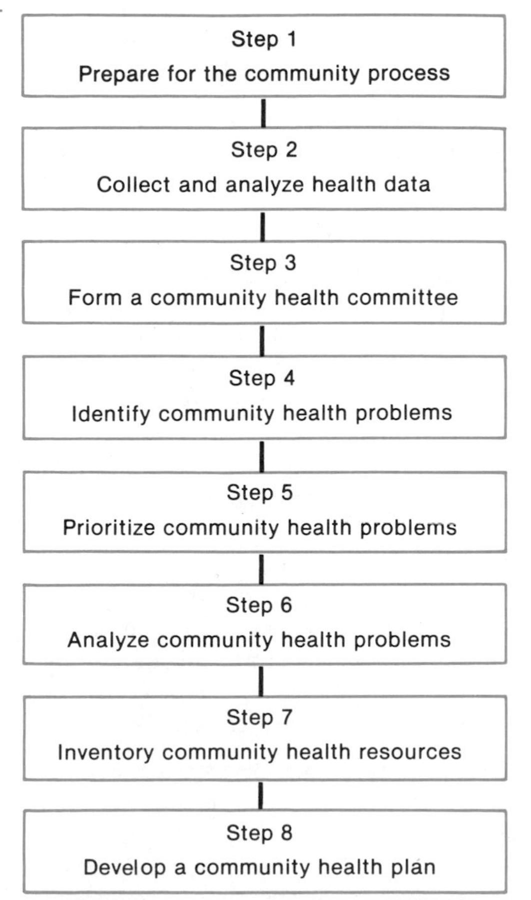

Figure 30–7 ● Flow chart of steps in the APEX-PH community process. (Redrawn from National Association of County Health Officials. (1991). *Assessment Protocol for Excellence in Public Health (APEX-PH).* Washington, DC: Author.)

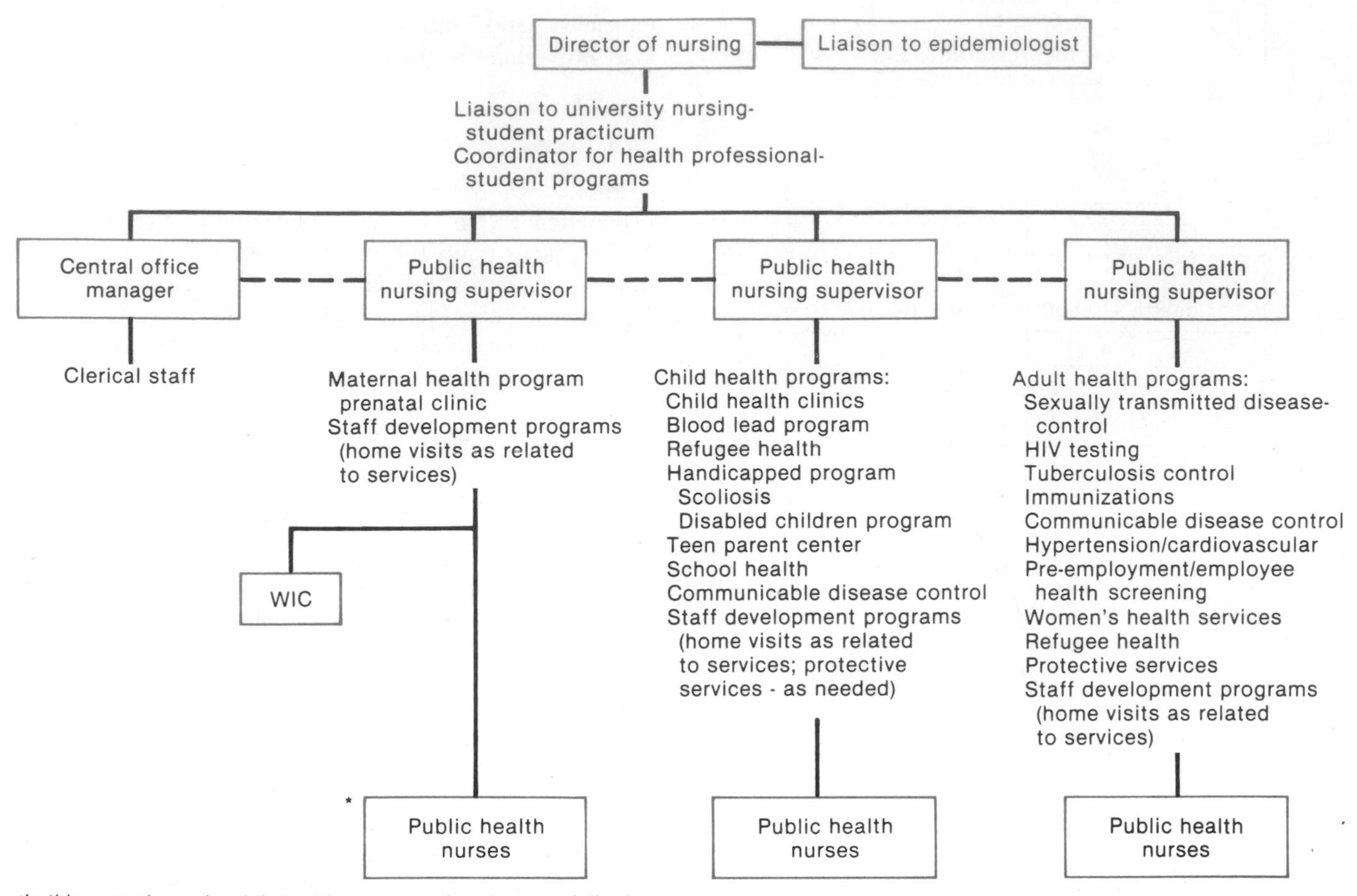

Figure 30–8 ● Organizational chart: local health department, division of public health nursing. (Adapted from Akron Health Department. (1992). *Organizational chart.* Akron, OH: Author.)

sector personal health services or be the only health services in medically underserved communities.

Public health nurses often manage these clinics as well as provide direct client services. They also organize and evaluate nursing services, supervise nursing assistants and volunteers, document patient records and collect information about the numbers of persons served at the site, and collaborate with other professional personnel. Table 30–6 lists some direct care activities performed by public health nurses in primary care clinics.

Nurses consider the whole person and, where appropriate, how that person fits within a family and the community. They look at how that person's health affects others. Public health nurses observe, listen, interact, and record how clients respond to questions, teaching, and counseling.

Prison Facilities. Health services for prisoners may be provided by the health department. Services may be provided at the prison facility as part of broad community services or through a contract for public health nursing, physician, or other practitioner time. Nursing and physician services include a physical assessment or full examination on incarceration; a health history, including any history of specific chronic diseases, alcohol or substance abuse, or risk factors for HIV and other communicable diseases. The nurse performs appropriate screening tests, which may include a tuberculin test; obtains blood and other body fluid specimens for tests and cultures; and checks vision and hearing. Immunizations, minor illness treatment, and medications for control of health problems (hypertension, epilepsy) are provided as ordered by the physician or nurse practitioner.

The environmental staff provide food service inspections. A health department nutritionist may work with food preparation staff on menus that provide appropriate calories and nutrition within the food budget. The nutritionist may also provide menus for medically ordered diets.

Work Sites. Some local health agencies are involved with industries and businesses (see Chapter 24). Nursing and health education staff provide education, risk assessment, and screening programs to promote healthier employee lifestyles and reduce employees' health risks. Employees benefit personally and sometimes by a reduction in their copayment for health insurance. Employers benefit through better health insurance coverage, perhaps at a reduced cost, and less employee time away from work owing to illness or injury. The types of service provided

TABLE 30–5

Public Health Nursing Services by Levels of Prevention

PRIMARY PREVENTION

Prenatal care clinics
Family planning clinics
Health education for health promotion and risk-reduction
Identification of those at risk for communicable diseases
Identification of those at risk for alcohol and drug abuse and other mental health problems
Immunizations (education campaigns and clinics)
Anticipatory guidance for parents regarding child care and parenting
Safety and environmental education
Home visits for health promotion for pregnant women, new parents, and frail, elderly individuals
School health promotion, especially regarding substance abuse, pregnancy, and violence prevention
Worker health promotion programs
Inspection and licensing (nursing homes and daycare centers)

SECONDARY PREVENTION

Health screening, case-finding, and referral (i.e., hypertension and communicable diseases)
Health screening, case-finding, and referral for alcohol and drug abuse and other mental health problems
Health screening, case-finding, and referral for children with developmental delays and disabilities
Outreach during home visits and at work sites and schools to identify targeted populations, such as pregnant women, adolescents, and chronically ill and disabled persons
Contact investigation for communicable diseases
Clinics for sexually transmitted diseases
Clinics for tuberculosis
Treatment for specific illnesses (i.e., medication for sexually transmitted diseases based on medical orders and treatment protocols)
Primary care clinics
Clinics for the homeless
Environmental surveillance

TERTIARY PREVENTION

Case management for disabled children
Case management for disabled adults
Case management for frail, elderly individuals
Home health care
Geriatric evaluations prior to institutional placement
Adult medical daycare

Compiled by Smith, C. M. University of Maryland.

depend on employer–employee decisions and the content of the contract or letter of agreement with the local health department.

Other Service Sites. Shelters for the homeless, nutrition sites for elderly persons, and daycare or Head Start centers are also places where public health nursing may take place. This may involve obtaining health and risk assessment histories or providing group teaching or one-on-one counseling. Specific screening and immunization services may be provided, such as tuberculin tests and blood pressure screening for staff and clients in a homeless shelter or blood pressure screening at a senior citizen meal center. Immunizations may include hepatitis B, influenza, pneumococcal or tetanus–diphtheria vaccines. With expanded role nursing, primary care in shelters, apartments for elderly persons, or group homes for developmentally delayed clients has become possible through agency contracts or volunteer programs.

One area not often a part of general public health nursing involves mental health counseling and care. Nurses recognize persons with mental disorders and use the resources of their community for education, referral, and/or networking (see Chapters 21 and 23). If the health department has an alcohol and/or substance abuse program, one or some of the counselors may be licensed psychologists, psychiatric social workers, or psychiatric mental health nurse specialists. Public health nurses find these colleagues to be good consultants for assistance in developing alternatives for and with their clients. With the number of people needing mental health services steadily growing and local agencies stretched to their maximum, alternative service avenues must be explored. Additional preventive mental health programs are needed to address public health concerns such as substance abuse, teenage pregnancy, violence, mental illness, and the stresses of homelessness.

TABLE 30–6

Public Health Nursing in a Primary Care Clinic

- Interview to learn the reason for the visit and determine the severity of the problem.
- Obtain a health history, including sexual activity and birth history as appropriate.
- Review affected body systems.
- Obtain appropriate blood and body fluid specimens for laboratory analysis.
- Conduct a risk assessment (see Chapter 17).
- Discuss screening tests that are relevant based on risk assessment and standard recommendations, such as:
  - Pelvic examination and Pap smear for women who have not had these done in a year or more.
  - Breast examination and breast self-examination teaching as necessary with mammogram education and/or referral.
  - Testicular examination education.
  - Discussion of HIV/AIDS risks and anonymous or confidential blood test.
  - Tuberculin skin testing as appropriate.
  - Blood pressure screening and history of hypertension, medication, and/or care source.
- Administer medication or other treatments as medically ordered.
- Discuss contraindications, possible reactions, and any accompanying food or lifestyle adaptations while on medications or participating in other treatment.
- Obtain feedback from the client to determine what he or she has understood about the diagnosis, treatment, education, and planned follow-up.
- If this is a clinic visit for a communicable disease, especially a sexually transmitted disease, provide a time for a test of cure and the clinic telephone number so the client may call and, with a coded request, receive culture test results. For specific illnesses, home visits may be conducted to trace contacts.

The clinical psychiatric/mental health nurse specialist is an asset to community public and mental health agencies, as he or she can guide the nurses or other staff in ways to detect, approach, and assist those with mental illnesses to seek and use counseling and treatment programs. The nurse specialist has skills for individual and group counseling and for working with the staff of group homes or homeless shelters in concert with other professionals. Programs focus on ways to help individual clients achieve socially appropriate behavior, a feeling of self-worth, and greater independence.

Future Trends and Issues in Local Health Department Nursing

Predicting the role of local health departments and public health nursing in 5, 10, 20, or more years currently is as difficult as it has ever been. The changing program emphases and efforts to make services more comprehensive with more services available at any one visit have already been noted. The Institute of Medicine (1988) has provided a picture of the political, financial, and leadership problems that affect public health nationwide.

Fishman (1992, p. 16) has discussed the plight of the state of Connecticut and the dearth of public health services in the richest state (based on per-capita income) in this country. She asks the question, "Should not any national health program include access to primary prevention services, if it is to be national HEALTH rather than a national medical care program?" She calls on public health nurses to become more proactive in developing appropriate services, particularly the basic ones. She also challenges the government to rethink its expenditure priorities.

Public health nursing is, and will continue to be, instrumental in the continuation, development, and enhancement of client and community-centered services. The public health nurse collects community needs information determined by tools such as APEX-PH (1990) and the *Healthy People 2000* objectives (USDHHS, 1990) and develops strategies, along with professional colleagues and the community, to empower the community and individual clients in resolving those needs. National government agencies and professional organizations are resources (Table 30–7). Local public health nurses will become more visible community change agents, facilitators, case-finders, and case managers, as well as service providers.

Medically underserved areas will see better and more utilization of clinical nurse specialists for primary care in local health departments. These may be employees of the health department providing perinatal care, pediatric specialists in child health–sick child care, or specialists in gerontology to work with the growing aged population. Their goal is to help people maintain good health and delay the onset of illness or chronic diseases, problems that compromise the productive lives of a community's population.

TABLE 30–7

Resources
American Nurses' Association 600 Maryland Ave. S.W. Washington, DC 20024 (202) 554–4444
American Public Health Association 1015 15th St. N.W. Washington, DC 20005 (202) 789–5600
Centers for Disease Control and Prevention Atlanta, GA 30333 (404) 329–3311
National Association of County Health Officials 440 First St. N.W. Washington, DC 20001 (202) 783–5550
National League for Nursing 350 Hudson St. New York, NY 10014 (212) 989–9393

In areas with access to basic personal health services, the focus of public health nurses will return to "assessment, surveillance, policy, health promotion and disease and injury prevention activities" (Salmon, 1993, p. 1647). Even after health care reform and universal access to comprehensive personal health care become realities, there will still be a mission for the public health sector. Public health funds can be shifted from direct primary care and treatment to development of services systems and focusing on population-based services (Table 30–8).

As noted earlier, nursing will be involved in more multidisciplinary or multiagency cooperatives or partnerships. These cooperatives will seek funds, develop programs, and focus on defined community needs, such as assistance for elderly or mentally ill individuals; hepatitis B, HIV, AIDS, and tuberculosis education, intervention, and control; community education for violence/accident/injury control; and intervention to break the cycle of substance abuse in communities.

Because many current public health problems are linked with social behaviors, public health nurses will return to family-focused care within communities. Vulnerable groups can be empowered within these communities (Zerwekh, 1993). Integrated services to strengthen families and community support networks have the potential to decrease such problems as teenage pregnancy, substance abuse, and violence (Schorr, 1989).

Nurses and others in public health can enable the community as a whole, as well as individual neighborhoods, to accept responsibility for ensuring its residents a reasonable standard of living, which includes health and access to health services.

TABLE 30–8

Examples of Future Public Health Nursing Functions

- Special focus on women, adolescents, and children for HIV/AIDS prevention.
- Targeted education and directly observed medication therapy to control tuberculosis.
- Collaboration with law enforcement, education, and recreation personnel to reduce alcohol misuse, injuries, and violence.
- Comprehensive school health, including mental health.
- Outreach to prevent infant mortality and morbidity, including "targeted public education, programs of home visiting, case management for children with special needs, and child and spouse abuse services" (White House Domestic Policy Council, 1993, p. 167).
- Target nursing outreach to the following populations that previously have been underserved and have not used preventive services:
  - Those with low income and low education levels
  - Those who speak languages other than English
  - Residents of medically underserved urban and rural areas
  - Homeless individuals
  - Migrants
  - Adolescents
  - Those with severe disabilities or illnesses such as chronic mental illness, substance abuse, and HIV/AIDS.

Data from White House Domestic Policy Council. (1993). *The president's health security plan.* New York: Time Books.

Zerwekh (1993), a leader in revealing the underlying themes of current public health nursing practice, challenges public health nurses to "imagine the neighborhood nurse as a health care generalist responsible for a neighborhood or region" (p. 1667).

KEY IDEAS

1. Public health nursing is multifaceted, providing assessments, service, advocacy, counseling, and caring for individuals, families, and the community.
2. The emphases for nurses in a local health department vary according to community needs; what is already available for specific populations; federal, state, and local mandates; and funds for service provision.
3. Funds for local health department programs predominantly consist of local tax monies, but varied federal, state, and private funds may also be used. These change with new federal, state, and local administrations; politics; general economic conditions; and the desires of the people.
4. Laws play a major role in health department planning, be they financial appropriations, mandates for service, or laws that influence the community or individuals who seek health department services.
5. Nursing competence in history taking, assessment, observation, counseling, teaching, caring, and advocacy are imperative to public health nursing. Public health nurses participate in community assessments and planning to develop population-focused interventions to meet specific health objectives.
6. The ability to be flexible, independent, and a thoughtful decision maker are also imperative.
7. Communicable disease control was a major emphasis in the formative days of public health nursing. Some diseases are no longer a threat, while others remain so. New diseases, such as HIV, have evolved. Control, education, investigation, and prevention will remain key emphases.
8. Because of experience provided in family- and community-focused care, the baccalaureate nursing degree will be essential for public health nursing in the future. With the growing trend for primary care in local health, the clinical nurse specialists will also play a major role.
9. The standards of public health nursing and the components/concepts of this nursing specialty will continue to be reviewed and updated to make them relevant to the changing responsibilities of the public health nurse.
10. Public health nursing is becoming more comprehensive and the sites for services more varied than the traditional homes, schools, and clinics of the past.

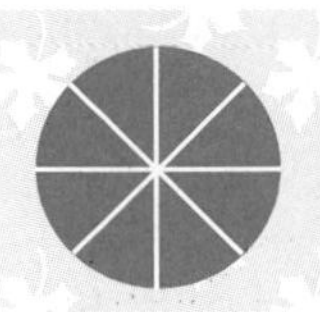

CASE STUDY
A Week in the Life of a Public Health Nurse

One way to envision the activities and varied settings of public health nursing is to consider a typical week's schedule. The following schedule occurs in an agency that provides generalized public health services but not home health care.

Monday. Check in at office for mail or messages, pick up biologicals and client records for clinic, or go directly to child health clinic for a half or full day, with 15 to 40 clients, depending on services, staffing, and clinic location. Clients are generally 3 weeks to 6 years old, although children of all ages are eligible for services. The nurse may provide the following as appropriate for each child: measurements; screening tests (vision, hearing); developmental screening; nutrition history and WIC referral; immunizations and education; blood lead and hematocrit screening; and anticipatory guidance for health, safety, development, and/or parental concerns. If clinic is a half day, the nurse may make home visits after clinic or spend time in the office evaluating the child health records for completeness, preparing for home visits, or making client contacts for advocacy and client follow-up.

Tuesday. Prenatal clinic from 8:00 A.M. to 12:30 P.M. Jane S. is a new client for whom the nurse provides nursing assessment; health and previous pregnancy history; blood and urine specimen collection for initial baseline data; one-on-one or group education appropriate to history and assessment findings; information about handling emergencies and telephone contact for questions; referrals to WIC (if not part of the clinic) or social services; and date for next appointment. If these are follow-up visits the program may combine public health or expanded role nursing visits with those of the physician so that the physician sees the clients with problems, while nurses see other clients at intervals during the pregnancy. At these interval visits the public health nurse conducts an interim history and all other components of the complete prenatal or postpartum visit.

The afternoon may consist of record keeping or home visits (known clients), determining priorities among new neonate referrals, and receiving a referral from Meals on Wheels for assessment of an elderly client with apparent health needs and no known care.

Wednesday. The morning includes an in-service education program developed and given by the nursing staff for themselves or as an informational program for all agency staff. The supervisors provide updates on agency programs or policies and discuss matters brought up by the nurses.

In the afternoon an immunization clinic is specifically planned to meet school entry requests from parents whose children do not need full child health services. The clinic lasts until 7:00 P.M. to provide accessibility for people whose work hours mirror those of the health department.

Thursday. Record keeping, telephone calls, informal supervisor conferences, and networking with other staff may fill the morning. Brainstorming ideas for revision of forms, planning an upcoming continuing education program, or an APEX-PH planning meeting may also be part of the morning.

Several school activities are planned for the afternoon. Scoliosis screening may be conducted for sixth graders. There may be a health education session planned jointly with a class teacher. An education session with pregnant teenagers about the emotional and physiological changes that occur during pregnancy may be combined with time for individual conferences with some of those teenagers. This conference may include a discussion of health history, pregnancy progress, care source, and pattern of attendance at appointments; referrals for social service needs and Lamaze or infant care classes; and plans for home visits as needed.

Friday. Adult health programs may encompass clinic clients needing screening for or treatment of sexually transmitted disease, teachers or health care employees needing tuberculin skin tests for work, some new or continuing hypertension clients, pre- or posttest HIV counseling, adult travel immunizations, and/or some communicable disease investigations conducted by telephone or home visit.

Individuals targeted for adult health services are those without a regular source of health promotion or monitoring, those who may have contracted a reportable communicable disease, and any adult member of the community who seeks assistance.

The nurses provide the same types of service as provided in maternal and child health programs (e.g., health histories, assessment of the presenting problem or request, extensive health teaching about risks pertinent to the client's concern, and education regarding lifestyle adaptations for risk reduction). Appropriate blood or other specimens are collected; screening tests are completed, and treatment is provided.

GUIDELINES FOR LEARNING

1. Contact your local health department and ask what programs exist, what services are offered, how the department reaches out to the community, how its work is funded, and what fees are charged for services.
2. Talk with your legislators and determine what they know about pending health legislation and about state and local health department mandates, funding, and personal health services. Become a resource for the legislators.
3. Select an objective from *Healthy People 2000* (USDHHS, 1990) and develop an intervention plan.
4. Obtain an entry level public health nurse job description from a local health department. Consider what the qualifications are; if you have questions about them, ask for clarification.
5. Explore your own prior feelings and knowledge about local health departments. Did you know there was a health department? Did you know the populations it serves? What can be done to increase the visibility of public health nurses to the public?

REFERENCES

American Public Health Association. (1991). *Healthy communities 2000: Model standards.* Washington, DC: Author.

Anderson, M., O'Grady, R., & Anderson, I. (1985). Public health nursing in primary care: Impact on home visits. *Public Health Nursing, 2* (3), 145–152.

Fedson, D. S. (1990). The Influenza Vaccination Demonstration Project: An expanded policy goal. *Infection Control and Hospital Epidemiology, 11*(7), 357–361.

Felton, B., & Parker, S. (1990). The resource dependence of a county nursing department: Efforts to thrive in the 1980s. *Public Health Nursing, 7*(1), 45–51.

Fishman, R. U. (1992). What is APHA's future in public health? *Journal of Public Health Policy, 13*(1), 14–17.

Institute of Medicine, Committee for the Study of the Future of Public Health. (1988). *The future of public health.* Washington, DC: National Academy Press.

Last, J.M., & Wallace, R.B. (1992). *Public health and preventive medicine* (13th ed.). Norwalk, CT: Appleton & Lange.

Miller, D. (1992). *Dimensions of community health.* Dubuque, IA: William C. Brown.

National Association of County Health Officials (NACHO). (1990). *National profile of local health departments.* Washington, DC: Author.

(NACHO). (1991). *Assessment protocol for excellence in public health (APEX-PH).* Washington, DC: Author.

Pickett, G., & Hanlon, J. (1990). *Public health administration and practice* (9th ed.). St. Louis: Times-Mirror/Mosby College Publishing.

Reverby, S. (1993). From Lillian Wald to Hillary Rodham Clinton: What will happen to public health nursing? *American Journal of Public Health, 83*(12), 1662–1663.

Salmon, M. (1993). Editorial: Public health nursing—The opportunity of a century. *American Journal of Public Health, 83*(12), 1674–1675.

Schorr, L. (1989). *Within our reach: Breaking the cycle of disadvantage.* New York: Anchor Books.

U.S. Department of Health and Human Services. (1990). *Promoting health preventing disease: Year 2000 objectives for the nation. Summary report.* Washington, DC: Government Printing Office.

White House Domestic Policy Council. (1993). *The president's health security plan.* New York: Time Books.

Zerwekh, J. (1992). Laying the groundwork for family self-help: Locating families, building trust, and building strength. *Public Health Nursing, 9,* 15–21.

Zerwekh, J. (1993). Commentary: Going to the people—public health nursing today and tommorrow. *American Journal of Public Health, 83*(12), 1676–1678.

BIBLIOGRAPHY

Freeman, R. (1957). *History of public health nursing.* Philadelphia: W. B. Saunders.

Gardner, M. S. (1936). *Public health nursing* (3rd ed.). New York: Macmillan.

Green, L., & Anderson, C. L. (1986). *Community health* (5th ed.). St. Louis: Times-Mirror/Mosby College Publishing.

Kristjanson, L., & Chalmers, K. (1990). Nurse-client interactions in community based practice: Creating common ground. *Public Health Nursing, 7*(4), 209–214.

Riordan, J. (1991). Prestige: Key to job satisfaction for community health nurses. *Public Health Nursing, 8*(1), 59–64.

Sovie, M. (1990). Redesigning our future: Whose responsibility is it? *Nursing Economics, 8*(1), 21–26.

Tappen, R. M., Sanchez-Murrell, M., Hopkins, S., Donovan, G., Dolan, J., & Moore, N. (1990). Challenges for continuing education for public health nurses in Florida. *Public Health Nursing, 7*(4), 236–242.

SUGGESTED READINGS

Aiken, L. & Fagin, C. (1992). *Charting nursing's future: Agenda for the 1990's* (pp. 255–269). Philadelphia: J.B. Lippincott.

American Nurses' Association. (1986). *Standards of community health nursing practice.* Washington, DC: Author.

Focus on children's health. (1991). *American Journal of Public Health, 81*(8), entire issue.

Masson, V. (1992). Progress notes: Mindset. *American Journal of Nursing, 92*(8), 10.

Chapter 31

Rural Health

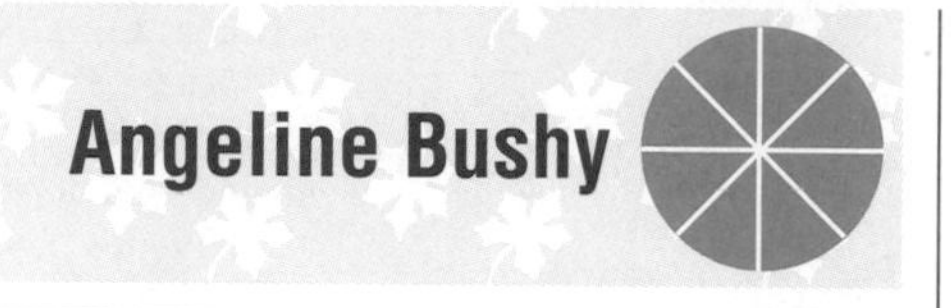

Angeline Bushy

Focus Questions

What do the terms *urban, rural, frontier, metropolitan, nonmetropolitan,* and *Health Professional Shortage Area* mean?

What at-risk populations live in rural areas? What are some of their special nursing care needs?

What factors affect accessibility, availability, and acceptability of health care services for rural residents?

What significant economic, social, and cultural factors affect rural community nursing?

How does rural community nursing differ from practice in more populated settings?

How does a community health nurse build a partnership with residents of a rural community?

According to the United States Bureau of Census (1992) approximately one fourth of all Americans live in rural communities. The United States General Accounting Office (USGAO, 1989) reports that 31 states have designated more than 60% of their counties as rural (Fig. 31–1). Concerns about rural health care services, especially in regions with insufficient numbers of all types of health care providers (designated as Health Professional Shortage Areas [HPSAs]), are becoming a national priority. Those concerned with rural health delivery issues are aware of the problems in recruiting and retaining qualified health professionals, but relatively little research on rural practice has been published. Only relatively recently has information become available on the special challenges, problems, and opportunities of community health nursing in geographically large, sparsely populated areas (Bushy, 1991a; Case, 1991; Davis, 1991; DeLao, 1992; Davis and Droes, 1993).

Definitions

The term *rural* is not easy to define, as it means different things to different people (Lee, 1991). This diversity is a concern among policy makers and health care providers, because it hampers a coordinated approach to understanding the demographics, epidemiology, and health problems of rural communities. The U.S. Office of Rural Health Policy currently is working to develop a definition of *rural* that will be useful to researchers to enable a more coordinated approach for describing clinical problems and addressing health care delivery issues (Hewit, 1989; USGAO, 1989). As evidenced in this chapter, most individuals include geographic and population factors as well as subjective perceptions in their notion of *rural* versus *urban*.

GEOGRAPHIC REMOTENESS AND SPARSE POPULATION

Several commonly used definitions for *rural* refer to the geographic size of an area in relation to its population density or the number of people per square mile (Table 31–1). To establish some consensus of viewpoints, one pair of descriptors used by policy makers and program developers is *metropolitan* and *nonmetropolitan.* A *metropolitan area* is defined as a city or adjacent area having a total of 50,000 or more residents. Using this criterion, 79.4% of the U.S. population lives in a metropolitan area (U.S. Bureau of Census, 1992).

Another set of definitions distinguishes among urban, suburban, rural, farm, and nonfarm residency. In these, *rural* refers to a community having fewer than 20,000 residents, and any community having a greater population is considered *urban.* Of the total U.S. population, approximately 25% live in rural areas, but only 5% live in towns of 2500 residents. Less than 2% of the total U.S. population live on a farm (Fig. 31–2).

Yet another set of definitions considers urban, rural, and frontier regions. In some ways these terms better illustrate the problems that are encountered by people living in a large geographical region.

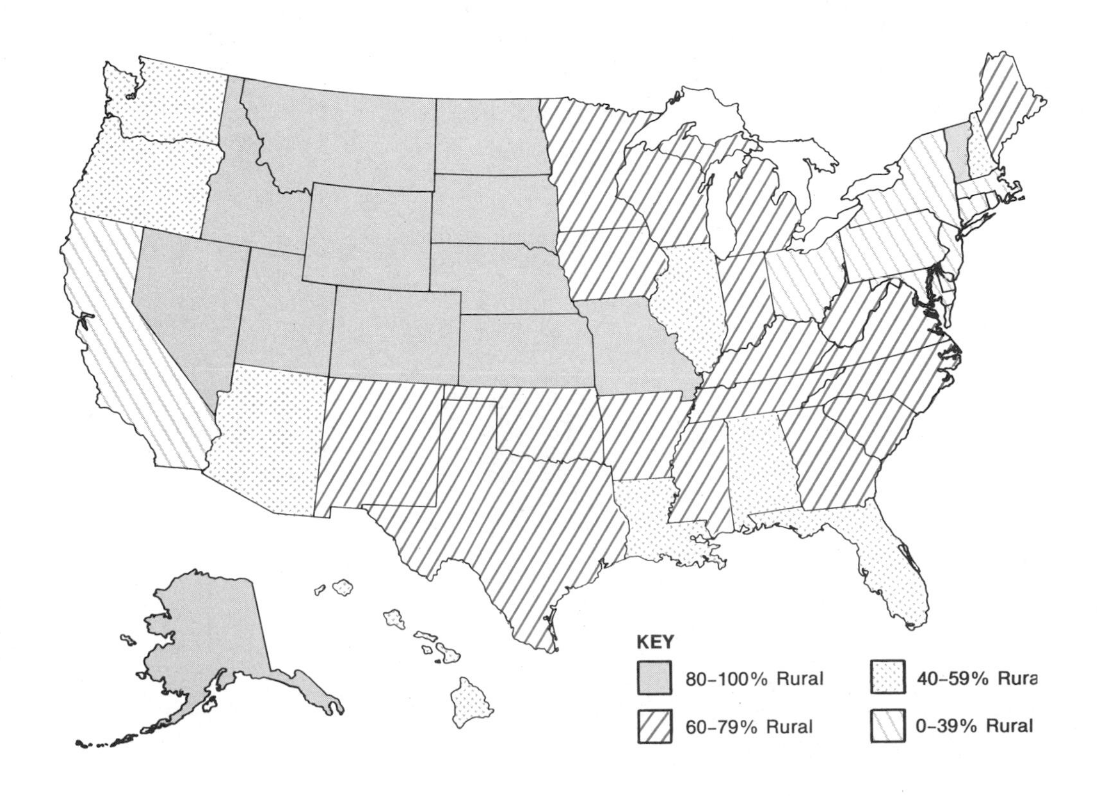

Figure 31–1 ● Percentage of rural counties by state. If 80% or more of a state's counties are rural (per our definition), that state falls into the first category—80% to 100% rural. The other categories are similarly defined. Of the 50 states, 13 are in the 80% to 100% category, 18 are in the 60% to 79% category, 9 are in the 40% to 59% category, and 10 are in the 0% to 39% category. (From U.S. General Accounting Office. (1989). *Rural development: Federal programs that focus on rural America and its economic development* (Publication No. GAO–RCED–89–56BR). Washington, DC: Author.)

TABLE 31–1

Summary of Terms and Definitions

Metropolitan: An area having 50,000 or more residents.
Nonmetropolitan: An area having fewer than 50,000 residents.
Urban: An area having more than 99 persons per square mile.
Rural: An area having less than 99 but more than 6 persons per square mile.
Frontier: An area having fewer than 6 persons per square mile.
Farm residence: A rural residence outside city limits involved in an agriculturally related occupation.
Nonfarm residence: A rural residence inside city limits.
Suburban residence: A residence near an area designated as a metropolis.

A more specific definition accounts for the distance and/or time to commute to an urban area to access health care services (e.g., greater than 30 minutes or more than 20 miles). However, the time factor to determine access to services also may be applicable to residents who live in inner city or suburban areas (Elsion, 1986; Williams, 1983; U.S. Senate, 1990).

SUBJECTIVE PERCEPTIONS OF "RURAL"

Some Americans perceive rural areas as not having access to cable television, while others think that any town having a major discount store is an urban center. However, some rather grim rural scenes are often hidden from view. On Indian reservations impoverishment is comparable to that of third world countries. In migrant labor camps, one-room shanties shelter two or more Mexican-American families, toilet facilities are lacking, and workers suffer intense exposure to highly carcinogenic herbicides and pesticides. "Boom towns" that spring up overnight in energy-rich (i.e., coal, oil, or precious metals) regions of the United States are not prepared to handle the social problems stemming from the massive influx of outsiders into long-established agricultural communities.

The "typical rural town" is hard to describe because of wide population and geographic diversity. A rural town in North Dakota is quite different from one in Oregon or Tennessee. Likewise, there can be many differences among towns in the same state. Legislators' understanding of a rural area is usually based on the district they represent.

Another classification of rural areas created by the federal government provides greater specificity concerning a rural area's economic climate based on the principal industries in that area (Rogers and Burdge, 1986; Lee, 1991). The seven classes of nonmetropolitan counties, based on economic dependencies, are farming-dependent, manufacturing-dependent, mining-dependent, specialized government, persistent poverty, federal lands, and retirement. For example, manufacturing-dependent counties are characterized by a larger and more dense population, a higher proportion of households with a female head, and a greater proportion of black residents. In contrast, farming-dependent counties are characterized by a smaller population, fewer persons per square mile, fewer households with female heads, and a higher proportion of elderly persons. This set of terms based on demographic characteristics may also indicate a community's health problems (e.g., elderly individuals with chronic illness, lower average population age with higher fertility rates, and specific types of occupational hazards and environmental risks such as farming and ranching with an increase in skin cancer). This

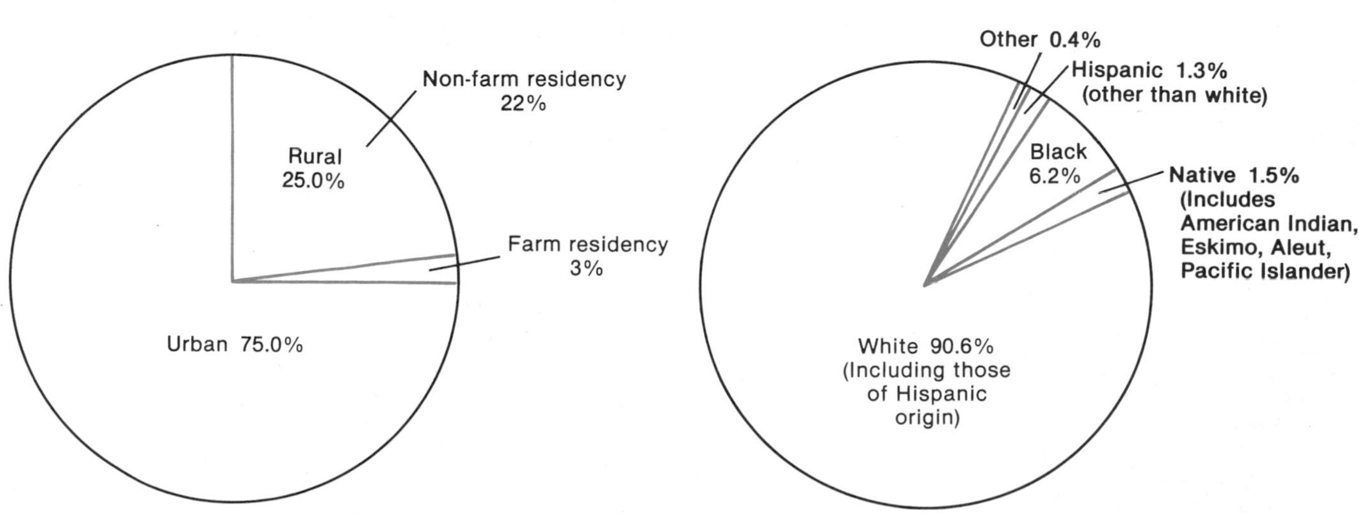

Figure 31–2 ● Summary of U.S. rural population. *A*, Percentage of population by place of residence. *B*, Profile by race of rural residents living in towns having a population of 2500 or less. (Data from U.S. Bureau of the Census. (1992). *Statistical Abstracts of the United States: 1990 National general population characteristics.* Hyattsville, MD: Author.)

kind of classification, however, can falsely lead to a perceived homogeneity of the community because little consideration is given to subpopulations (underrepresented groups) who live there as well.

Little is known about rural residents in general, and even less is known about subgroups within the major culture in either rural or urban areas. Most health information about rural populations focuses on maternal, infant, and elderly populations; such information is easier to assess and monitor because of existing public services. The various terms used to understand rural residency are relative in nature. For instance, "small" communities with more than 25,000 population have some features that one expects to find in a large city, and residents in a community of less than 2000 perceive a town with 10,000 people as a city. Residents in geographically remote areas may not feel isolated, because they perceive having urban services within easy reach either through telecommunication or dependable transportation.

RURAL DEMOGRAPHICS

In general, rural areas can be described as "bipolar"—that is, most residents are either under age 17 or over 65 years. The economic recession of the early 1990s, however, has resulted in major demographic shifts in many small towns. For instance, there has been an "in-migration" of urban residents to rural areas experiencing an economic boom, while in economically depressed communities, there has been an "out-migration" of families to seek employment elsewhere. Both phenomena produce problems that, in many instances, a small town cannot solve because of the lack of resources. Population shifts disrupt long-established informal "helping networks," creating a need for unusual kinds of human services for localities, such as support services for abused women, parenting classes, and crises intervention teams. Despite these needs, however, public health programs, community nursing, and mental health services are not available, accessible, or acceptable to target groups in rural areas.

Status of Health in Rural Populations

RURAL INITIATIVES: *HEALTHY PEOPLE 2000*

The *Healthy People 2000* initiatives (U.S. Department of Health and Human Services [USDHHS] 1990) have important implications for rural areas. A significant number of at-risk populations mentioned in this document reside in rural settings. For this reason, a number of states are developing a plan that mirrors the national Healthy People initiatives. Each state considers its own demographic patterns and the health status and pertinent health risks of its vulnerable populations. Compared with urban Americans, rural people have:

- Higher infant and maternal and morbidity rates
- Higher rates of chronic illnesses, such as hypertension and cardiovascular disease
- Problems unique to rural occupations, such as machinery accidents, skin cancer from sun exposure, and breathing problems from exposure to chemicals and pesticides
- High rates of mental illness and stress-related diseases (in the rural poor)

In addition, American Indians, Native Alaskans, Native Hawaiians, migrant workers, southern blacks, and rural homeless persons have their own set of health problems. For instance, rural homeless persons often are families from the community who had their farm foreclosed. Sometimes they are able to continue living in their house, according to the law, but they no longer have a means of livelihood and thus are without any income to purchase food or services. Other rural homeless persons are seasonal workers who travel from work site to work site to seek a job, living and sleeping in their automobiles.

Poverty is on the rise in the United States, and racial and ethnic minorities have a higher incidence of poverty and lower health status than whites. Economically depressed areas definitely affect the health status of communities. For instance, unemployment and underemployment have left millions of Americans unable to afford medical insurance, perpetuating the incidence of uninsured and underinsured families. More than 50% of the medically underinsured live in nonurban areas. Forty percent of all rural families live below the poverty level. Thus, even though minority children represent only 20% of the rural population, they experience poverty to a greater degree than do their urban counterparts. These children experience substandard housing, poor sanitation, inadequate nutrition, contaminated water, and lack of public health services, particularly prenatal care, immunizations, health screening, and health education (Children's Defense Fund, 1991; Monheit and Cunningham, 1992; Perloff, 1992; USDHHS, 1990, 1991).

Overall, rural adults are less likely than urban adults to engage in preventive behaviors such as regular blood pressure checks, Pap smears, or breast examinations. Also, higher percentages of rural adults engage in risk behaviors such as smoking and not wearing seat belts, which have implications for their overall health status (Fig. 31–3) (Frame, 1992; U.S. Office of Technology Assessment [USOTA], 1990; Wagenfeld and Wagenfeld, 1990; Wakefield, 1990).

FAMILY SERVICES

Family planning and maternal, perinatal, and infant/child health care services are lacking in rural areas. Like the larger health system, maternal and infant health services in

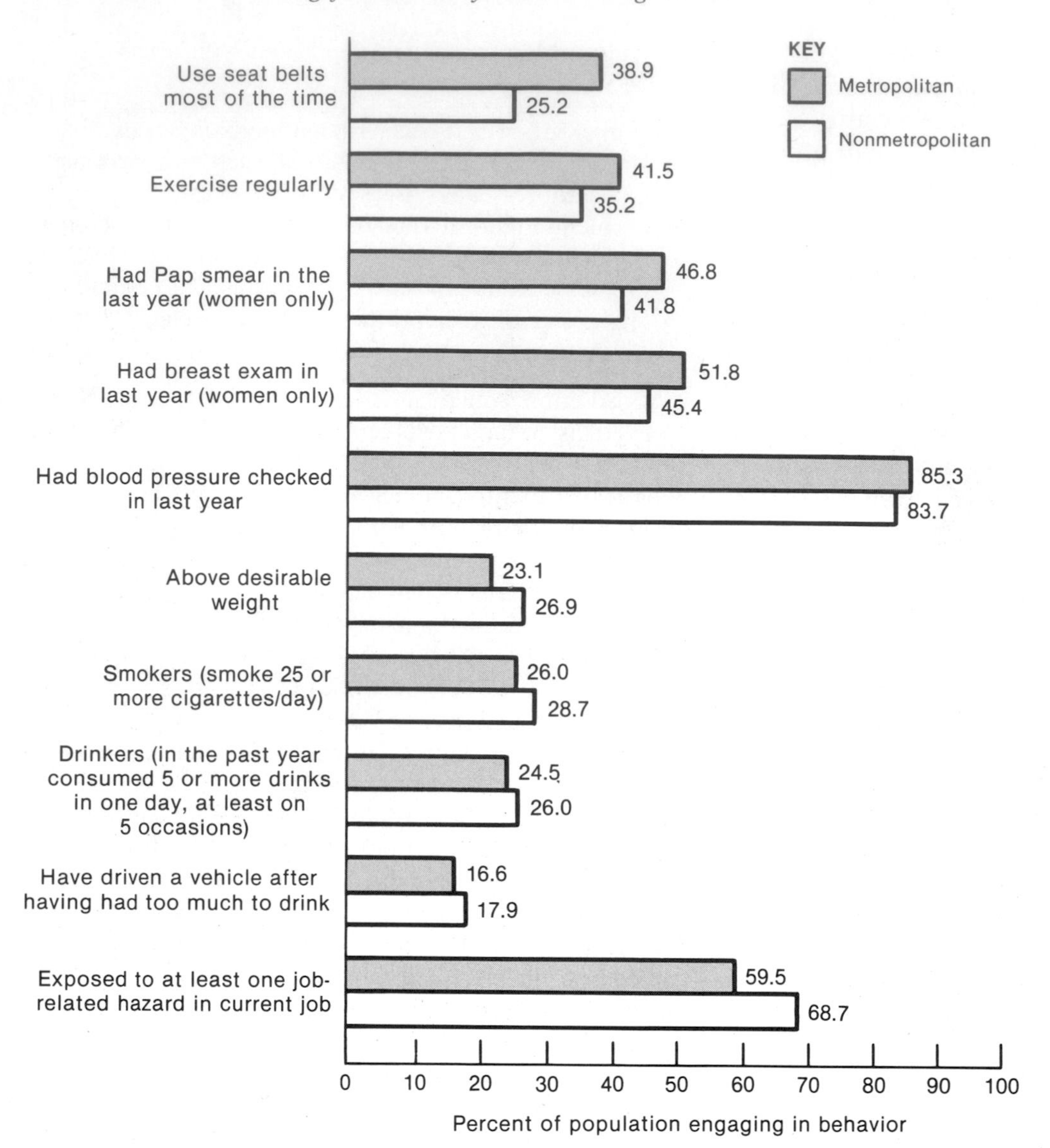

Figure 31–3 ● Comparison of metropolitan and nonmetropolitan residents on selected preventive behaviors and risk exposures. (Data from U.S. Office of Technology Assessment. (1990). *Health care in rural America* (Publication No. 052–003–01205–7). Washington, DC: U.S. Government Printing Office.)

the United States are an ironic mixture of superb medical care for some segments and inadequate care for many minorities and economically deprived individuals. Like their metropolitan counterparts, poor rural families face significant barriers to adequate maternal and infant health care. However, rural families face additional problems, including greater travel distances and difficulty in maintaining comprehensive health services, especially for pregnant women, infants, and children (Ahern, 1980; American Academy of Pediatrics, 1986).

Although many regional differences exist, generally there are higher rates of maternal and infant mortality and morbidity in rural areas than in urban areas; this is a reflection of many social, genetic, economic, and environmental factors. For instance, social factors include a group's religious belief system regarding the appropriate time for a pregnant woman to seek professional prenatal services. A genetic factor is exemplified by the predisposition of blacks to sickle cell anemia. Environmental factors include contaminated water or air pollution to which a pregnant woman may inadvertently be exposed. Some of the poor pregnancy outcomes, however, can be attributed to impaired access and availability of obstetrical and pediatric providers and services.

Since the early 1980s there has been a marked reduction in the number of family planning, abortion, and maternal child care providers and services in nonmetropolitan areas (Hughes and Rossenbaum, 1989; USGAO, 1990a). Despite an overall increase in the number of obstetricians, pediatricians, and family/general practitioners in the United States, many children and pregnant women experience a shortage of providers and services. This can be attributed partly to the high cost of malpractice insurance and partly to the fact that health care providers are not equitably distributed in rural geographical areas. This leaves some areas of the United States without any, or with an insufficient number of, health professionals (American Medical Association [AMA] 1987; Nasbitt et al., 1990;

U.S. Bureau of Health Professions [USBHP] 1990; USOTA, 1990). In eastern Montana, for example, some pregnant women must travel more than 150 miles one way to obtain care from an obstetrician (Bushy, 1991a). Traveling long distances also may be required for children with disabilities who live in rural environments, as specialists usually practice in urban areas. Consequently, pregnant women living in rural areas are less likely to initiate care during the first trimester, and their children with special needs are less likely to have rehabilitative and restorative care (Henshaw and VanVort, 1991; McManus and Newacheck, 1989; McManus, Newacheck, and Greany, 1990; Monheit and Cunningham, 1992: Perloff, 1992).

The closure of rural hospitals and their obstetrical units also has had an adverse effect, not only on access to services, but also on pregnancy outcomes. (Closures are attributed to depressed rural economies and inequitable prospective reimbursement policies associated with diagnostic-related groups [DRGs].) Consequently, women who live in communities with relatively few obstetrical providers are less likely to deliver in their local community hospital than those who live in communities with a higher ratio of providers. Moreover, women who must leave their "high-outflow" communities to deliver have been found to have a higher rate of complicated and premature births. Often this is attributed to delays in seeking prenatal care early in their pregnancy and because they have not had adequate health education.

Mothers and infants living in professionally underserved areas remain in the hospital longer after delivery than do those who have better access to obstetricians and pediatricians. Because of the distance involved and the potential need for emergency services, these patients are not discharged as quickly as those who live closer. For example, a new mother who lives more than 100 miles from the hospital and must contend with ice and snow on the highway to reach her home likely will not be discharged with her new infant after 24 hours, as will a patient who lives in the same town in which the hospital is located (Bronstein and Morrisey, 1991; Hoffmaster, 1986).

However, these higher rates of maternal and perinatal mortality and morbidity among rural individuals cannot be attributed entirely to geographical distances and delays in securing health care. As mentioned earlier, rural areas suffer from higher rates of poverty and lower percentages of families with health insurance. Rural states often have more restrictive qualification criteria for Aid to Families with Dependent Children (AFDC) programs and are less likely to adopt eligibility and service options not required by the federal government for needy families (Children's Defense Fund, 1991). For instance, in some states, a family cannot qualify for public assistance when there is a male present in the home, even if he is the head of the household and unemployed. These factors also contribute to the overall health status of rural women and their children (USDHHS, 1992).

MAJOR HEALTH PROBLEMS

There are regional differences in the predominant health problems in a rural community; these problems depend on environmental, genetic, industrial, and socioeconomic factors. However, when compared with urban areas, there are wider variations in rural rates of accidents, trauma, chronic illness, suicides, homicides, and the use of alcohol and drugs.

Accidents and Trauma

Trauma and violence pose serious threats for death and long-term disability in Americans, especially adolescent and young adult males. The leading cause of adolescent death is automobile accidents (25,000 per year). Annually, thousands of others are severely injured because of alcohol-related accidents. In the United States there are more than 125,000 trauma-induced paraplegics, a significant number of whom are between the ages of 15 and 24. Rural populations suffer more injuries from lightning, farm machinery, firearms, drowning, and accidents involving vehicles such as boats, snowmobiles, motorcycles, and all-terrain vehicles, although separate rural morbidity and mortality data are often unavailable for such accidents (Baker et al., 1987; Stern, 1980).

In the 1990s, the Surgeon General has focused attention on agricultural health and safety (National Safety Council, 1990–1993). Of the three most dangerous industries (agriculture, mining, and construction), agriculture has had the greatest proportional increase in occupation-related death rates, although the number of persons actively engaged in farming has decreased. Not only is agricultural work inherently dangerous, but it must also be performed under adverse conditions such as snow, mud, and extreme heat or cold, and workers must endure long hours. The agricultural labor force is extremely diverse with respect to age and work experience. Because most farm enterprises are categorized as family farms, spouses, children, and other relatives often help with the work without much regard to competency, training, or safety. Similarly, migrant workers often consist of women and children of various ages who spend long hours working in fields. For these reasons agriculture has by far the highest number of injuries and deaths in children compared to any other industry (Field and Tormoehlen, 1982; Geller, Ludtke, and Stratton, 1990; Greydanus, 1992; Purschwitz and Field, 1987).

The number of agricultural accidents among women and children and the impact on the family when the male head of household is involved in a serious injury or death are unknown. Because family businesses are small, they do not have workers' compensation insurance. Because health professionals are scarce, education regarding safety and injury prevention becomes an important responsibility of community health nurses who practice in rural communities.

Chronic Illness

Rural residents in general are characterized by a relatively low mortality rate but a high rate of chronic illness. This increase in long-term health problems can be attributed to the greater percentage of poor elderly and other at-risk populations, poorer pregnancy outcomes, and the long-term consequences of nonfatal accidents. The most critically needed services in rural areas include preventive services such as health screening clinics, nutrition counseling, and wellness education to reduce the incidence of chronic health problems. To provide care to those who have chronic health problems, there is an ever-increasing need for adult daycare, hospice and respite care, homemaker services, and meal deliveries to help chronically ill individuals who remain at home in geographically isolated areas. Community health nurses in rural areas can be instrumental in advocating such services (Weinert and Long, 1993; USOTA, 1990).

There are special challenges in providing acute care services for the chronically impaired. More than 200 rural hospitals closed between 1980 and 1988, a higher rate of closures than among nonrural hospitals. Of the remaining 2700 rural hospitals, 600 have reported financial problems that could lead to closure. Furthermore, the transfer of even one care provider, most often a physician or nurse, can mean that a small hospital must close its doors because of insufficient staff. The limited supply and increasing demand for health professionals in general, particularly nurses, will continue for some time. This shortage has a detrimental impact on providing a continuum of care to the chronically impaired who live in rural and underserved areas and creates an even greater demand for community health nurses (Nadel, 1991; Nasbitt et al., 1990).

Providing care to the chronically ill requires a move away from specialized acute curative medicine to a continuum of health care services. In rural areas, because of the current shortage of health care services, more facilities and personnel are needed to achieve an adequate level of service. Existing programs in urban as well as rural areas must become more effective by decentralizing services, providing more home services, and using mobile units. Nurses can have an important role in helping to address these concerns by providing available, accessible, and acceptable services. However, legislated provisions must be made for direct third-party reimbursement for care provided by nurses prepared at the advanced level (Luloff and Swanson, 1990; Schwab and Pierce, 1986).

Suicide and Homicide

Nationwide, among those 15 to 19 years of age, homicide and suicide are the two leading causes of death in males and the third and fourth leading causes of death in females. Each year between 3000 and 5000 youths are murdered, and nearly an equal number commit suicide. Homicide is more likely to take place in the inner city, while suicide is more prevalent in suburban and rural settings. Often, however, it cannot be determined whether a vehicular or occupational accident was truly unintentional. Even so, since the mid-1980s a sharp upsurge has occurred in the rural suicide rate, especially among male adolescents and young men.

Because of the cluster or "copycat" phenomenon related to self-inflicted death, in several towns the suicide rate has reached epidemic proportions, with three or more suicide incidents occurring in a very short time (after one suicide there is an increased incidence of additional suicides in a community). In small towns or rural areas, where most people are fairly well acquainted, a sudden death can be devastating to students and to the community as a whole. Many reasons are cited for the rise in rural suicides, including the increasing economic hardships, changing community social structures, higher drug and alcohol use, and lack of counseling and other social services (Bergland, 1988; Copan and Racusin, 1983; Wagenfeld and Wagenfeld, 1990). Community health nurses have an important role in educating the community to recognize self-destructive and risk-taking behaviors and advocating crisis interventions to prevent those activities.

Alcohol and Drug Use

The National Clearinghouse for Alcohol and Drug Information (NCADI) has provided rather unsettling information about alcohol use by Americans from 1984 to 1988. Of particular interest are the following rural trends (NCADI, 1991; USGAO, 1990b):

- Arrests for drug abuse violations increased 54%.
- Arrests for use of cocaine and heroin increased 20%.
- The majority of prison inmates in rural states abused alcohol, other drugs, or both.
- Children as young as 11 and 12 are drinking as many as 14 to 18 beers on Friday and Saturday nights.

Even so, compared with more populated areas, there are fewer health providers and services available per capita in rural areas to address chemical substance abuse (Murray and Keller, 1991). Consequently, community health nurses in rural settings should assume a proactive role with the community in planning, implementing, and evaluating primary prevention and follow-up intervention programs to educate the public about responsible alcohol consumption behaviors.

Factors Influencing Rural Health

RURAL HEALTH CARE DELIVERY ISSUES

Currently discussion is under way by policy makers on ways to equitably allocate acute and primary preventive services among all Americans, especially those living in

HPSAs, the majority of which are in either rural counties or the inner city. Community health nurses who practice in rural areas, as well as those who provide outreach services to rural communities, should be aware of the concerns surrounding the availability, accessibility, and acceptability of services (Case, 1991; Hamel-Bisel, 1992). These interrelated delivery issues have serious implications for planning, implementing, managing, and evaluating community nursing services that target rural clients.

Availability of Services

Availability refers to the existence of services and sufficient personnel to provide those services. In rural areas, there are fewer physicians and nurses in general, as well as fewer family practice physicians, nurse practitioners, and specialists, especially obstetricians, pediatricians, psychiatrists, and social service professionals. Economically speaking, a sparse population limits the number and array of services in a given region. The per-capita cost of providing special services to a few people often becomes prohibitive (Human and Wasem, 1991; National Association of Community Health Centers [NACHC], 1992; USOTA, 1990).

Accessibility of Services

Accessibility refers to whether a person has the means to obtain and afford needed services. Accessibility to health care by rural families may be impaired by the following:

- Long travel distances
- Lack of public transportation
- Lack of telephone services
- A shortage of health care providers
- Inequitable reimbursement policies (e.g., Medicare, DRGs)
- Unpredictable weather conditions
- Inability to obtain entitlements

Consider the case of a male rancher with a high income who lives in a medically underserved area and has a sudden heart attack. He may not have access to the most basic emergency care, even though he has comprehensive medical insurance.

Access to funding sources to implement public health programs also can be hampered by the lack of grantsmanship skills on the part of those seeking aid. Successful grant writing requires practice and collaborative efforts between agencies to produce a fundable project. Political forces in small towns often oppose outside help because a grant writer is unable to quantify the immediate benefits to the local community from a proposed public health program for which funds are being sought. Resistance, for example, may be evidenced by the community's explicit preference for local government interventions as opposed to the perceived meddling of federal or state bureaucracies (Human and Wasem, 1991). As another example, a grant proposal to implement an innovative program to address the community health care needs of local subpopulations may not be supported by formal and informal community leaders. Rural power structures, for instance, often are vested in an elite segment of the community. These individuals often remain unaware of the needs of the underprivileged. Sometimes an affluent minority has more power than numerically greater ethnic groups in the community. Insensitivity to others' needs on the part of leading community members can reinforce the stigma of seeking public assistance. Consequently, an individual who needs public services may avoid using them, even if they are available and accessible, out of concern that someone will tell others that he or she needs help. Community health nurses must recognize the stigma attached to using certain services such as human immunodeficiency virus (HIV) testing, family planning, and chemical dependency services.

Acceptability of Services

Acceptability refers to whether a particular service is offered in a manner congruent with the values of a target population. Considering the wide diversity among rural families, acceptability of available community nursing services can be hampered by any of the following:

- Traditions of handling personal problems (e.g., self-care practices such as using over-the-counter medications, exercising, ingestion of alcohol, resting, prayer).
- Beliefs about the cause of a disorder and the appropriate healer for it (e.g., medicine man, medicine woman, curandero, shaman).
- Lack of knowledge about a physical or emotional disorder and the value of formal services for prevention and treatment of the condition (e.g., being stoic and suffering in silence rather than seeking supportive care; only seeking care for emergencies rather than for health promotion or primary prevention).
- Difficulty in maintaining confidentiality and anonymity in a setting where most residents are acquainted.
- The urban orientation of most health professionals.

Many health professionals, including community health nurses, are educated in urban settings and have most, if not all, of their clinical experiences there. Thus, they are not exposed to rural clients. When coupled with the stress experienced by many clients when seeking publicly funded care, cultural insensitivity can exacerbate a rural individual's mistrust of health professionals. Ultimately, a nurse's attitude affects the long-term health status of a client who may be embarrassed about his or her health problems. Embarrassment often is evidenced by a client minimizing symptoms of illness and not seeking care when needed (i.e., health care is primarily sought for acute illness or in an emergency). Therefore, it is prudent for schools of nursing to expose students to the rural environment and the people who live there. Rural clinical experiences will do much to create a climate of mutual sensitivity and trust between community health nurses and rural clients.

LEGISLATION AFFECTING RURAL HEALTH CARE DELIVERY SYSTEMS

Table 31–2 highlights some of the major legislation that has affected rural health care delivery. In rural communities, the issues of accessibility, availability, and acceptability of services and providers must always be considered when legislation is implemented. A program that is highly effective in a more populated area rarely can be "lifted" and transplanted to a rural environment. In some cases, legislated programs have resulted in highly innovative approaches that serve the population well. In other cases, mandated programs simply create other barriers that deter rural populations from using a much needed service.

A successful program that serves as a good model is an immunization clinic held in conjunction with the county fair in an Appalachian community. This annual event is scheduled the week before school starts and attracts most county residents. Children's immunizations can be updated while adults undergo glaucoma and cholesterol tests. The program is promoted through word-of-mouth announcements to homemaker's clubs, in church bulletins, and in public service announcements in the local media. Since the late 1980s the community has come to expect and accept the services that are offered at that particular time, as evidenced by the increasing numbers who seek care during the county event (National Rural Health Association [NRHA], 1994).

Conversely, a poorly received program involved working with Native American children who are discharged from hospitals on apnea monitors (Bushy and Rohr, 1990). Using established protocols that were highly successful in the white community, health care providers made a dedicated effort to have young Native American mothers comply by placing their child on a monitor while sleeping. Follow-up questioning indicated that the mothers adhered to all aspects of the program as instructed. However, after completing home visits, home health aides reported that the mothers were not following instructions. The program developers speculated that the mothers' verbal reports were motivated by fear of being reprimanded by caregivers or fear that their actions would be reported to Indian Health Service (IHS) officials located on the reservation.

Unfortunately, the program planners did not consider Native American beliefs related to the interference of biotechnology with a person's spirituality, nor did they consider the inherent role of extended family in caring for a child. In this particular tribe, grandmothers and aunts often provide the primary care to children in the extended family, but they were not included in the discharge planning. Other overlooked environmental considerations include the fact that it is not unusual for homes on the reservation to be without electricity or plumbing, and many

TABLE 31–2

Legislation Affecting Rural Health Care

1954 Transfer Act: Provided that all functions, responsibilities, authorities, and duties related to the maintenance and operation of hospitals and health facilities and the conservation of Indian health were to be administered by the Surgeon General of the U.S. Public Health Service.

1957 Indian Health Assistance Act: Provided for construction of health facilities for Native Americans.

1958 Hill-Burton Act: Provided for construction of health care facilities where these were lacking. Many rural communities built hospitals with these funds. A number of these hospitals currently are experiencing economic problems and are on the verge of closing.

1962 Migrant Health Act: Authorized federal aid for clinics serving migratory agricultural workers and families.

1964 Economic Opportunity Act: Provided a legal framework for the antipoverty program.

1968 Neighborhood Health Centers: Extended grant to migrant health services.

1970 Health Training Improvement Act: Provided expanded aid to allied health professionals.

1971 Comprehensive Health Manpower Training Act: Increased federal programs for development of health manpower.

1972 Act to Establish the Health Service Corps: To encourage health professionals to practice in areas designated Health Professional Shortage Areas.

1973 Health Maintenance Organization and National Health Planning and Resource Development Act: Increased health insurance coverage for the rural population.

1975 Indian Self-Determination Act: Gave tribes the option of staffing and managing Indian Health Service programs in their communities and provided for funding for improvement for tribal capability to contract for health care services.

1976 National Consumer Health Information Act: Provided medical services in areas with an insufficient number of physicians.

1976 Indian Health Care Improvement Act: Intended to elevate the health status of Native Americans and Alaska Natives to a level equal to that of the general population by authorizing a higher budget for the Indian Health Service.

1977 Rural Health Clinics Service Act: Provided medical services in areas with an insufficient number of physicians.

1981 Planned Approach to Community Health (PATCH): Provided funding to states for delivery of preventive and health promotion to rural communities.

1981 Omnibus Budget Reconciliation Act: Consolidated various sets of categorical grant programs into block grants that served to increase state discretionary use of federal monies (block grants for maternal and child health, services for disabled and other children with special health care needs, Supplemental Security Income services for disabled children, hemophilia treatment centers, and other programs aimed at specific groups or health problems).

1986 to Present: Amendments added existing health care legislation to revise policies.

Native American families do not own a car. If the family does have access to a car, it may break down before they arrive at the hospital, or they may not be able to afford the gas. Program planners should have worked more closely with the community health nurses on the reservation to arrange transportation for families, or specialists might have taken their services to the IHS clinic on the reservation to make it easier for the women to get to the service. In brief, socioeconomic and cultural factors should always be considered when adapting a successful program to fit the needs and beliefs of a special population.

Over the years a number of approaches have been legislated by the government to create innovative programs that are available, accessible, and acceptable to vulnerable rural populations (Tables 31–2 and 31–3). Of particular interest are rural health clinics, community health centers, migrant health centers, and the Indian Health Service, because community health nurses play an active role in all these programs (Fenton, 1988; Fenton et al., 1991).

Rural Health Clinics

Rural health clinics (RHCs) (Public Law 95-210) provide comprehensive primary care to populations living in regions that are designated as medically underserved or as HPSAs through the use of midlevel providers (midwives, nurse practitioners [NPs] and physician's assistants [PAs]). An RHC may be based in the outpatient department of a hospital; it may also be a freestanding clinic or located in a physician's office. To become certified as an RHC under Medicare and Medicaid, an agency/clinic must meet the following criteria, but the law allows the services to be tailored to meet the needs of the community in which it is located (Martin and Martin, 1991; NACHC, 1992; USOTA, 1990):

- Be located in a rural setting that is federally designated as an HPSA.
- Be engaged primarily in the provision of outpatient primary medical care.
- Employ at least one physician or nurse practitioner;
- Meet applicable federal, state, and local requirements for Medicare and Medicaid health and safety requirements.
- Be under the direction of a physician, who must be on site at least once every 2 weeks.
- Have a midlevel practitioner (NP, PA, midwife) available to provide patient care services in the clinic at least 50% of the time when the clinic is open.
- Provide routine diagnostic services, including clinical laboratory services.
- Maintain health records on all patients.
- Have written policies governing the services that the clinic provides.
- Have available drugs, blood products, and other necessary supplies to treat medical emergencies.
- Have arrangements with other providers and suppliers to ensure that clinic patients have access to inpatient hospital care and to other physician and laboratory services not provided in the clinic.

Community Health Centers

The Community Health Center (CHC) Program is authorized in section 330 of the Public Health Act. To receive funding as a CHC, an agency must meet the following criteria while providing basic primary care services, with optional services that can be tailored to meet the needs of the local community (NACHC, 1992):

- Be located in a rural setting that is federally designated as an HPSA.
- Provide physician services and, where feasible, the services of PAs and NPs.
- Provide diagnostic laboratory and radiology services.
- Provide preventive health services, including family planning and prenatal and well-child care.
- Provide emergency medical services.
- Provide transportation services as needed.
- Provide preventive dental care.

In addition, CHCs may, where appropriate, provide the following supplemental health services:

- Pharmaceutical services.
- Hospital services.
- Home health services.
- Long-term services.
- Rehabilitative services.
- Mental health services.
- Therapeutic radiology services.
- Vision services.
- Public health services, including counseling, referral, and follow-up for social and nonmedical needs that affect health status.
- Ambulatory surgical services.
- Health education services.
- Other services, such as interpreters who promote the CHC's services to a large, non–English-speaking population.

Migrant Health Centers

The Migrant Health Centers (MHC) Program closely resembles the CHC Program, but the population is limited to migratory and seasonal agricultural workers and their families. Services in an MHC generally are on a fee-for-service basis. A sliding fee schedule is applied to those without insurance or who cannot pay the full charge for the services they receive. An MHC must accept patients covered by Medicare and Medicaid (Cole and Crawford, 1991; NRHA, 1986, 1994; Smith, 1986). In addition to those services provided by CHCs, and, depending on the

TABLE 31–3

Rural Health Resources

National Resources

Agriculture Health and Safety Center
University of California-Davis
Davis, CA 95616–8757
916–752–4050

American Family Farm Foundation
National Rural Crisis Response Center
Box 65
Washington, DC 20002
202–547–6767

American Farm Bureau Federation
225 Touhy Ave.
Park Ridge, IL 60068
312–399–5764

Appalachian Regional Commission
1666 Connecticut Ave. N.W.
Washington, DC 20235
202–673–7893

Center for Rural Elderly
5245 Rockhill Rd.
Kansas City, MO 64110
816–276–2181

Department of Agriculture
Office of Small Community and Rural Development
Rural Development Administration
14th Street and Independence Avenue
Washington, DC 20250
202–690–2394

Department of Health and Human Services
Office of Rural Health Policy
5600 Fishers Lane
Rockville, MD 20857
301–443–0835

Department of Veteran Affairs
Office of the Chief Medical Director
810 Vermont Ave. N.W.
Washington, DC 20420
202–233–2596
(For concerns of rural veterans)

East Coast Migrant Health Project
1234 Massachusetts Ave. N.W.
Suite 623
Washington, DC 2005
202–347–7377

Farm Safety Just for Kids
716 Main St.
P.O. Box 458
Earlham, IA 50072
703–371–5615

Indian Health Services
Park Lawn Building
5600 Fishers Lane
Rockville, MD 20857
301–443–1180

National Association for County Health Officials
440 First St. N.W.
Washington, DC 20001
202–783–5550

National Association for Rural Mental Health
c/o National Rural Health Association
301 E. Armour Blvd.
Suite 420
Kansas City, MO 64111
816–756–3140

National Center on Rural Aging
409 3rd St. S.W.
2nd floor
Washington, DC 20024
202–479–6683

National Congress on American Indians
900 Pennsylvania Ave. S.E.
Washington, DC 20023
202–546–9406

National Farmers Union
600 Maryland Ave. S.W.
Suite 202
Washington, DC 20024
202–554–1600

National Farm Medicine Center
c/o Marshfield Medical Research Foundation
1000 North Oak
Marshfield, WI 54449–5790
715–387–9298

National Migrant Resources Program
2512 South I.H. 35, Suite 220
Austin, TX 78704
512–447–0770

National Rural Electric Cooperative
1800 Massachusetts Ave. N.W.
Washington, DC 20036
202–857–9500

National Rural Health Association
301 E. Armour Blvd.
Suite 420
Kansas City, MO 64111
816–756–3140

National Rural Institute on Alcohol and Drug Abuse
Arts and Science Outreach
University of Wisconsin-Eau Claire
Eau Claire, WI 54702–4004
715–836–2031

National Rural and Small School Consortium
Western Washington University
Miller Hall
Bellingham, WA 98225
206–676–3576

National Safety Council
444 N. Michigan Ave.
Chicago, IL 60611–3991
312–527–4800

Rural Family Issues Coalition
Department of Public Institutions
P.O. Box 94728
Lincoln, NE 68509
402–872–1445

TABLE 31–3

Rural Health Resources *Continued*

UCD Agricultural Pesticide
Farm Safety Center
University of California-Davis
Occupational and Environmental Health
Davis, CA 95616
916–752–5676

Rural Information Center Health Services (RICHS)
National Agricultural Library
10301 Baltimore Boulevard, Room 304
Beltsville, MD 20705–2351
1-800–633–7701

State Resources

Senate Rural Health Caucus—established to increase the level of awareness in Congress of rural health concerns and to provide a united voice on rural health care issues before Congress. Most states have one of their elected officials (senator and/or representative) on this committee. Contact elected officials for specific information for your state.

Several states have the following organizations that also can provide information to community health nurses having an interest in rural health care issues in their particular state or region. For more information, contact your state department of health regarding these resources:

Area Health Education Centers (AHECs)
Cooperative Agreement Agencies
Nurses' Association
Office of Rural Health
Rural Health Association
Rural Health Research Center

Publications

Rural Health Resources Directory (1991)
Published by the Office of Rural Health Policy
Health Resources and Services Administration
Public Health Service
U.S. Department of Health and Human Services
Park Lawn Building, Room 14-22
5600 Fishers Lane
Rockville, MD 20857

Journal of Rural Health
c/o National Rural Health Association
301 E. Armour Blvd.
Suite 420
Kansas City, MO 64111
816–756–3140

Rural Community Health Newsletter
National Association for Rural Mental Health
c/o National Rural Health Association
301 E. Armour Blvd.
Suite 420
Kansas City, MO 64111
816–756–3140

Rural Sociology
Rural Sociological Society
Department of Rural Sociology
Texas A&M University
College Station, TX 77843

health care needs of the community, an MHC may also offer the following:

- Environmental health services (e.g., rodent control, field sanitation, sewage treatment).
- Infectious and parasitic disease screening and control.
- Accident prevention programs (including prevention of excessive pesticide exposure).

Indian Health Service

The Department of Health and Human Services, primarily through the Indian Health Service (IHS) branch of the Public Health Service, is responsible for providing federal health services to American Indians and Alaska Natives. The IHS became a primary responsibility of the Public Health Service under Public Law 83-568. The goal of the IHS is to ensure equity, availability, and accessibility of a comprehensive high-quality health care delivery system providing maximum involvement of American Indians and Alaska Natives in defining their health needs, setting health priorities for their local areas, and managing and controlling their health program. The IHS acts as the principal health advocate for Native Americans by ensuring that they have knowledge of and access to all federal, state, and local health programs to which they are entitled (USDHHS, 1991). The IHS developed and operates a health services delivery system designed to provide a broad range of preventive, curative, rehabilitative, and environmental services. The system integrates health services delivered directly through IHS facilities and staff with those purchased by IHS through contractual agreements (Fig. 31–4). The degree of involvement by individual tribes and the success of the IHS in providing comprehensive health care to Native Americans and Alaska Natives varies from one setting to another.

Overall, IHS facilities have been found to be limited in scope and underfinanced and serve less than half of the total American Indian population (USDHHS, 1990). Although IHS recruitment advertisements state that practice in their service offers a diversity of health problems and transcultural enrichment, it has been difficult to recruit and retain qualified health providers who have the potential to deliver culturally consistent health care services.

Health care providers who are culturally connected with a minority group are best equipped to provide meaningful care to them. This has not been possible, for the most part, with IHS. There is a critical shortage of Native American nurses and physicians who are adequately prepared and available to work with the Native American population in

BEMIDJI
55,742
BILLINGS
49,368
PORTLAND
109,969
ABERDEEN
84,280
PHOENIX
99,569
NAVAJO
190,946
CALIFORNIA
86,699
NASHVILLE
43,545
OKLAHOMA
CITY
218,262
TUCSON
20,702
ALASKA
85,737
ALBUQUERQUE
60,667
Note:
Texas is administered by
Nashville, Oklahoma City,
and Albuquerque.
● Area Office

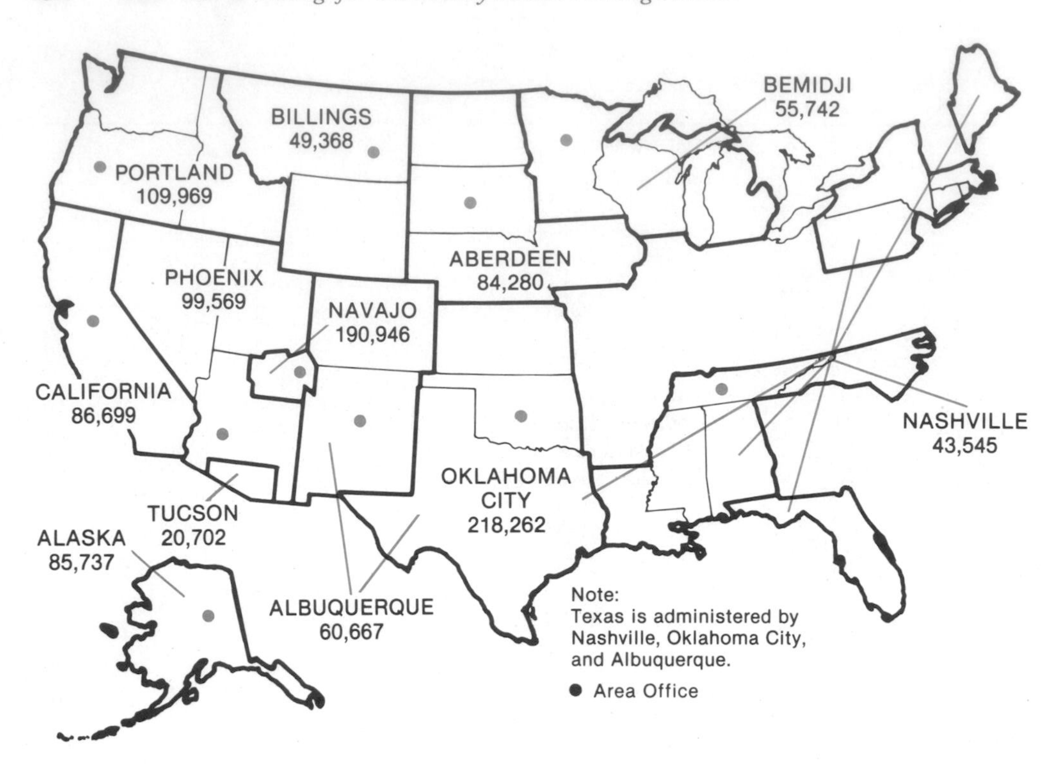

Figure 31–4 ● Indian Health Service—service population by area during fiscal year 1990 (total service population = 1,105, 486). The largest percentage of the service population, 19.7%, is located in the Oklahoma City area followed by the Navajo area, with 17.3%. The Tucson area program has the smallest percentage: 1.9%. (From U.S. Department of Health and Human Services. (1989). *Trends in Indian Health.* Washington, DC: Indian Health Service.)

general, and with the various tribes in particular. Recruited professionals usually are of non-Indian origin, which has been a source of contention (NRHA, 1994). On the one hand, IHS providers complain of treatment noncompliance, tardiness in seeking care, and broken clinic appointments on the part of Native Americans. On the other hand, Native Americans describe provider indifference and cultural intolerance toward them (e.g, verbal reprimands, impatience, inflexibility, and attitudes of superiority).

The problems become even more complex because nursing and medical personnel (who are usually white) tend to remain within the IHS only long enough to pay back National Service Corps education loans. Once these loans are paid, these individuals usually leave the IHS for more financially rewarding practice locations. Despite the legislated intent of IHS, Indian reservations are some of the least healthy areas in the United States, with a multitude of social and health-related problems, including high rates of unemployment, alcoholism, high school dropouts, poor perinatal outcomes, suicide, and homicide.

Federal Efforts to Augment Rural Health Resources

Legislation has been drafted to augment existing health resources such as RHCs, CHCs, MHCs, and the IHS, and there is a trend in state and federal funding to make the needs of rural and frontier communities, particularly HPSAs, a priority. However, the actual dollars allocated for public health programs in rural areas have decreased in many cases. Currently, the focus is on accountability and innovation of programs and is enforced through allocation of federal and state funds.

One recent trend is the linking of federal training dollars to program outcomes. For example, when tax dollars are allocated to support an educational program, certain results should be expected relative to rural health care. Questions that are being asked include: Are benefits of the program distributed to all of the state's residents, rural as well as urban? Do educational programs expose students to rural community practice? Are graduates remaining in state? How many continue to practice in areas of need? Schools preparing health professionals in general, and nurses in particular, are mandated to assume greater accountability for outcomes of funded programs. Likewise, schools applying for grants currently are required to provide student clinical rotations in underserved areas. The goal is not to simply educate professionals, but to prepare providers who are capable and willing to increase access to care for underserved and minority populations (Wasem, 1993). Community health nurses, because of their high visibility and leadership role in rural communities, must be aware of these trends, as they often are consulted regarding development and support of public health programs.

Another trend in America's agenda for health care reform is an emphasis on the use of midlevel primary care providers (NPs, PAs, midwives) in rural systems. The National Health Service Corps supports this effort through its ongoing scholarship and loan repayment program for midlevel providers. The greatest challenge will be to develop and maintain education programs in a time of federal and fiscal constraints. To effectively use declining resources, practicing health professionals and educational programs of health professionals will have to forge partnerships with rural communities to plan, implement, and evaluate programs that are available, accessible, and acceptable to populations who live there (Wasem, 1993).

Program innovation in underserved areas is another trend, and this is essential for both providers and accrediting bodies. In essence, a program must mesh with local lifestyles, values, and economic structures. Program evaluations, on the other hand, must reflect outcomes appropriate to a particular community or population. The Kellogg Foundation and the Robert Wood Johnson Foundation, for example, have led the movement by providing grants to universities to develop and take interdisciplinary education models into rural communities. Federal programs such as the Rural Interdisciplinary Health Profession Training Program have fostered similar activities to expose students and professionals to the rural environment. These models have led to exciting new interactive telecommunication technologies that enable educational institutions to deliver classes directly to students living and working in even the most geographically remote settings. Telecommunications and computers hold great promise for linking rural professionals with their urban colleagues for the purpose of seeking consultation with health care specialists.

Congress and policy developers are looking at nurses to provide vital services to rural populations. For nursing to effectively respond to this opportunity, creativity is needed to ensure delivery of services to underserved regions of the United States. Nurses, however, must be sensitive to the health beliefs of clients and then plan and provide nursing care that fits with a rural person's value systems. For instance, how is health defined by a rural group? For a group of retired coal miners with black lung disease, it may mean being able to walk about in their home with a portable oxygen tank. To an elderly woman with cancer in its late stages, it may mean being able to spend her last days in the local hospital to be near her family, rather than having chemotherapy at the medical center located in a city some distance from home.

To address the challenge most effectively, information is needed about clients' (patients') perspective. Although this may seem obvious to a community health nurse, most of the data that have been collected on rural populations are for reimbursement and policy-making purposes. We know very little about family systems of subcultures living in rural areas in terms of their health beliefs, values, and perceptions of health (Dickey and Kamerow, 1992; Hibbard et al., 1991; Long and Weinert, 1989). Pertinent information is needed on rural subpopulations to provide acceptable and meaningful community nursing programs and services to those groups.

Rural Lifestyle and Belief Systems

RURAL LIFESTYLE

What is it like to live in a small, rural town? What do nurses know about rural populations and their nursing needs? Even though each community is unique, the experience of living in a small town is similar in all 50 states (Rogers and Burdge, 1986; Stein, 1989; Williams, 1983). The "typical" rural lifestyle is characterized by the following:

- Greater spatial distances between people and services.
- An economic orientation related to the land and nature (agriculture, mining, lumbering, and/or fishing, all of which are classified as high-risk occupations).
- Work and recreational activities that are cyclic and seasonal in nature.
- Social interactions that facilitate informal, face-to-face negotiations, as most, if not all, residents are either related or acquainted.

In brief, for rural residents, a small town is the center of trade for a region, and its churches and schools usually are the centers for socialization. This has implications for planning and implementing public health and community nursing programs for rural clients (Bushy, 1991b; Davis, 1991; Davis and Droes, 1993; Long and Weinert, 1989; Scharff, 1987). In the following discussion, common themes and belief systems of rural groups will be elaborated on, particularly self-reliance and self-care practices, a work ethic that is reinforced by rural economic structures, and utilization patterns of social support services. These factors can either motivate or deter rural persons to seek care.

RURAL BELIEF SYSTEMS

Belief systems of rural people are complex and multifaceted, but common themes relate to their fatalism and subjugation to nature (e.g., rain and frost effects on crop outcome; a hard winter's effect on livestock) and an orientation to concrete places and things. Rural families tend to be more conservative politically, with a strong religious preference ("church going"), and this, too, affects their health beliefs (Bergland, 1988; Hamel-Bissel, 1992; Hardgrove and Howe, 1981).

In day-to-day activities, rural persons prefer to deal with someone they know, rather than with a stranger. The preference for extended family ("kith and kin") can be advantageous as a support network (e.g., providing child care to a family during an illness). Familiarity, however, can also create some unusual problems. For instance, because most people in a rural area are acquainted, leaks in confidentiality can have serious consequences for someone who is seeking health care or social services.

Informal community dynamics pose an even greater concern with regard to confidentiality. It is not unusual to have rural people report that even though they are well acquainted with most residents in the community, they feel there is no one they can trust and with whom they can discuss personal problems. This attitude stems from residents in small towns having a genuine interest in and questioning others about the well-being of neighbors and relatives. Public knowledge about personal problems can be devastating for all involved. In brief, social and economic structures can impose restrictions for those who desire to seek professional help for concerns having moral overtones, such as drug and alcohol dependency, an unplanned pregnancy, sexuality issues, conflicts in personal relationships, or behaviors associated with mental illness (Human and Wasem, 1991; Murray and Keller, 1991).

Self-Reliance and Self-Care Practices

Self-reliance, which includes self-care practices, is a characteristic attributed to rural residents. Historically, self-care helped people to survive in austere, isolated, and rugged environments. Self-reliance is reflected in the statement, "We take care of our own," implying a preference for receiving care from familiar people. "Neighborliness" and family support can be beneficial in promoting healthy behaviors, and a close-knit family can be highly supportive to a member who has a medical problem (e.g., chronic obstructive pulmonary disease or a pregnancy with complications). However, such support can be detrimental. For example, a member with a drinking problem may be deterred from acknowledging the problem or seeking appropriate help because of family members' enabling behaviors (Long and Weinert, 1989; National Institute of Mental Health [NIMH], 1986). Or, emotional problems may be viewed by a family as a character flaw. Secrecy is reinforced by the rule of silence: that is, what happens in the family stays in the family. To save the family integrity within the community, it becomes important not to let anyone in town know about the problem (e.g., substance abuse; domestic violence; incest; rape; emotional disorders; having a condition that may be associated with a stigma, including certain types of cancer and a positive HIV blood test; and deciding whether to terminate a pregnancy). Likewise, attempting to adhere to established family and community standards can be a source of tremendous stress for individuals who are struggling to develop their own sense of identity, especially adolescents and others with low self-esteem.

Work Ethic Reinforced by Economic Structures

Economic structures can also affect a person's health status and his or her health care–seeking behaviors. For example, family enterprises are characteristic of rural environments. Small businesses such as farms, ranches, or family-owned grocery stores and service stations generally do not provide employee benefits such as health insurance. Concomitantly, some rural people define health as "the ability to work; to do what needs to be done." This comment reinforces a work ethic and could be interpreted to mean that "illness is not being able to do one's usual work." Therefore, these people do not seek health care until they are too ill to work.

Economic structures and work ethic ultimately influence a family's choice of leisure activities, how they view mental health, and their choice of health-promoting activities as well as primary prevention behaviors. For example, children may be taken to the physician for an illness at a time that coincides with the need to purchase repair parts for a piece of machinery in town; similarly, the services provided by the parish nurse may be welcomed at church, but the services of an outreach worker at the county mental health clinic may not be welcomed.

Utilization Patterns of Social Support Services

Before implementing any kind of health care service, program planners must be sensitive to a target group's preferences regarding social support. Specifically, three levels of social support have been identified in the literature (Rogers and Burdge, 1986; Stein, 1989). The first level includes services volunteered by family and friends. Although generally this help is not paid for, there is an expectation of reciprocity. The second level includes services that are provided by a group (e.g., civic organization, homemakers club, church circle, fraternity, Chamber of Commerce, 4-H Club, or sports team). Members of the group may provide assistance to needy individuals and families in the community (e.g., volunteering time, providing food, and making financial contributions). Both of these social support systems offer a mutually understood "insurance policy" should a catastrophic event occur for others in the network. The third level of support includes formal government services, public health agencies, visiting or community nursing services, mental health centers, and school counseling services. Generally remuneration by clients is expected for those services, albeit on a sliding scale.

Comparing the utilization patterns of the three levels of social support, urban residents tend to prefer the third level, as they often do not have access to the informal systems that are more common in a small town. Historically, rural persons have learned to rely on the first two levels of social support as a way to cope with the hardships associated with geographical isolation. This pattern of help-seeking behavior has reinforced their notion of self-reliance. Demographic changes have disrupted informal support networks and forced many rural residents to rely more on public support. However, reluctance persists because outreach services to a rural community are provided by professionals who often are strangers to the people who live there (Wakefield, 1990; Turner, 1991).

Rural Community Health Nursing Practice

There is ongoing debate as to whether there is anything unique about rural nursing practice, as nursing care is similar regardless of the setting (Bigbee and Crowder,

1985). There is little information in periodicals or nursing texts on what makes community health nursing in rural settings different. Since 1990, however, most community nursing texts have included a chapter on rural nursing practice. This debate stems partly from some people interpreting "rural" as a geographic practice setting. Proponents of this view believe that nursing care is probably no different for rural clients than for other individuals, and health problems and patient care needs are similar regardless of the setting. Other nurses believe that rural practice should be designated as a specialty, or at least a subspecialty, area because of factors such as isolation, scarce resources, and the need for a wide range of practice skills that must be adapted to social and economic structures. The actual degree of uniqueness of rural nursing probably lies somewhere between these two extremes (Case, 1991; Davis, 1991; Davis and Droes, 1993; Scharff, 1987; Washington State Nursing Network, 1992). Often one or a few community health nurses provide a broad span of diverse services in rural communities (Table 31–4).

Considering the wide variations of people and geographic settings in rural communities, how can nurses best be prepared to practice in health care settings in these environments? What entices nurses to elect to practice in these settings? Nurses being prepared for rural practice must be able to assess the community health needs in a region, including the particular causes of morbidity and mortality (Aaronson, 1982; Henry and Moody, 1988; Ingram, 1985; Jamie, 1992; Lassiter and Goeppinger, 1986; Moser, 1992; Moulton, 1992). In light of current health care delivery issues, five factors emerge as salient themes for rural community health: confidentiality, traditionally defined gender role behaviors, geographic and professional isolation, scarcity of resources, and legal considerations with regard to community health nurses' scope of practice.

CONFIDENTIALITY

Confidentiality may be a concern for anyone who lives in a rural community, even those who say they enjoy being personally acquainted with others in the community. A nurse will probably know most clients as a neighbor, friend, or friend of a friend or relative. As with all facets of professional life, familiarity has advantages and disadvantages. One nurse describes the experience in these terms:

> Personally knowing a client and his or her family's lifestyle helps me to provide total care. After I provide care, I'm also able to keep track of the person's progress from direct reports by the person when I meet him or her in the store or on the street. Or, if the client is home bound, I get word-of-mouth reports from his or her family, friends, neighbors or other members of his or her church (D.R.B., personal communication, 1992).

Nurses, like physicians, usually are viewed with high esteem by the rural community, but this can make it difficult to have a life outside work, as another nurse describes:

> In an urban setting, when you leave work and drive your car out of the parking lot, you are just one more person in a city of a million people. In a rural area when you move your car out of the parking lot . . . you are the same person as when you were in the parking lot. Everywhere you go you are seen as [a nurse]. . . . This affects how you conduct yourself when you are downtown, too (Davis and Droes, 1993, p. 167).

Personally knowing a patient creates some concerns and frustrations, as illustrated by this community health nurse's remark:

> Sometimes knowing your patients well allows you to make assumptions without a really valid evaluation. . . . You can miss something that should actually have been caught. . . . I just think other emotions can get in the way when you know someone well (Davis and Droes, 1993, p. 166).

Maintaining confidentiality is often difficult, particularly when the clinic or agency is located in a public facility such as the county courthouse. Often the waiting room may be in a common hallway or area where clients are likely to be recognized. Moreover, announcements of "specialty services" such as sexually transmitted disease (STD) clinics, family planning clinics, HIV testing, the Women, Infants and Children (WIC) program, and immunization clinics are published in the local newspaper and church bulletins, announced over the local radio station, and posted in public places such as grocery stores, service stations, and grain elevators (Case, 1991; Davis and Droes, 1993). Because most people in a small town are recognized by the car that they drive, even parking lots can jeopardize confidentiality. Scheduling a clinic at a certain time also can impose problems. If an STD clinic is held on Friday mornings, for example, assumptions may be made about anyone seen in the building, even if it is not to attend the clinic. Leaks in confidentiality result from such chance encounters, which can lead to one becoming stigmatized as the information quickly becomes public knowledge through the local rumor mill (Bushy, 1991a; Davis and Droes, 1993).

Maintaining confidentiality has implications for planning, providing, and evaluating community health services such as determining an appropriate building and coordinating times to offer services. For example, prenatal or family planning clinics could be scheduled to coincide with an immunization clinic, and STD clinics and HIV testing could be offered on a walk-in basis. These suggestions may be difficult to implement, especially if there only is one nurse who is responsible for a large health district and visits the various communities in the area on a rotating schedule. Innovative approaches are required on the part of community health nurses in rural practice to address the community's concerns surrounding anonymity and confidentiality (Dickey and Kamerow, 1992).

TRADITIONALLY DEFINED GENDER ROLE BEHAVIORS

Persons in rural communities are more likely to adhere to traditional values, which often includes complying with

TABLE 31–4

A Week in the Life of a Community Health Nurse in Rural Practice

SETTING

The ______________________ District Health Unit is situated in the county seat of a county having nine small towns in a rural midwestern state. The county's population is approximately 10,000; the largest town has fewer than 1200 persons; there are seven schools in the county and a 15-bed hospital that provides obstetrical, emergency, surgical, and medical-surgical services for patients of all ages. The community health nursing office is located in the medical clinic, which is adjacent to the hospital. The office hours are 8:00 A.M. to 5:00 P.M. When there is no particular service scheduled, the community health nursing office is open to clients on a walk-in basis for services. Clinics are published in the county newspaper and announced on a radio station located in a nearby county.

STAFF

RN (Administrator): ½ time (0.5 full-time equivalent [FTE]).
Job shared with
RN (community health nurse): ½ time (0.5 FTE).
RN (community health nurse): as needed. Responsible for monthly foot clinics; occasionally assists with in-town clinics.
RN (community health nurse): as needed. Teaches prenatal classes four times each year.
Secretarial/reception services: shared with physician in the building.

COMMUNITY HEALTH NURSING SERVICES PROVIDED

- Office visits—by appointment only
- Maternal health—prenatal classes, in-hospital postpartum education classes, and follow-up home visits to new mothers and at-risk infants
- Healthy baby clinics
- Health promotion and education—by request and scheduled once each month (e.g., farm safety programs, babysitting classes, community health luncheons)
- Child/parent health nursing conferences
- Immunizations clinics
- Women's health clinics
- Senior health maintenance clinics
- Home visits—rural and city (health counseling and teaching; bedside and skilled nursing care; homemaker–home health aide referrals, maintenance nursing care)
- Screening for sexually transmitted diseases

WEEK'S SCHEDULE

Monday

8:00	Home visits
9:00	Administrative office work: • Plan community-wide senior wellness adventure scheduled in 8 weeks • Order hepatitis vaccine for social services personnel who provide homemaker services • Prepare presentation for county school administrators meeting (next week) • Plan and arrange for preschool screenings to be offered in all the schools
10:00	Immunization clinic
12:00	Lunch
1:30	Child protection team meeting
3:15	Women's health clinic

expected gender role behaviors (Long and Weinert, 1989; Scharff, 1987). In other words, there are defined ideas as to what constitutes "men's work" vs. "women's work." With regard to women's work, these activities, consistent with traditional values, are assumed to be "less important," as women generally are not monetarily compensated for their work. Activities such as managing a household and caring for and nurturing a spouse and children are defined as women's work—that is to say, it should be volunteered to maintain the family's well-being. A man, on the other hand, is expected to work for a salary and adequately support his family without any public assistance.

Nursing, too, because it is a predominantly female profession, tends to be viewed as women's work. In other words, nurses who live in a rural community may be expected to provide professional consultation at no cost to local people who drop by their homes, or respond to local traffic accidents. In one case where there was no home health agency in the county, a physician referred patients on discharge from the county hospital (located in another town) to an unemployed nurse in the patient's home community. Instead of having a salaried position, this nurse was involved in the family business. The nurse received no compensation for her professional services.

In very small communities the identity of a woman is often based on her relationship to someone else—that is, a woman is considered the wife, sister, daughter, or mother of someone else. This also holds true for nurses, who generally are women. Consequently, a new graduate who wants to work in a small town would have no identity of her own, even as a nurse. Directly and indirectly, assigned gender roles can contribute to the problems of retaining

TABLE 31–4

A Week in the Life of a Community Health Nurse in Rural Practice *Continued*

Tuesday	
8:00	Prepare puberty talks for students in schools
9:00	Present puberty talk to fifth graders in a school 15 miles from the community health nursing office
1:00	Immunization clinic
2:30	Home visits
4:15	Infant hearing and ear clinic
Wednesday	
8:00	Home visits
1:00	Preschool screening clinic for 4- to 5-year-olds (assisted by the part-time community health nurse and special education teacher)
1:30	Child parenting-nurturing meeting (in town)
2:00	School administrator's meeting (in town)
4:00	Home visit
7:30 p.m.	Presentation on sexuality to Methodist church youth group (in town)
Thursday	
8:00	Home visits
10:00	Healthy baby clinic
11:00	Women's health clinic
12:00	Give talk on farm safety at Farm Bureau luncheon meeting
1:00	Administrative office work • Prepare maternal child health (MCH) grant • Work on county health needs assessment • Call Dr. ________ for standing orders
3:00	Immunization and hearing clinic
4:00	Blood pressure clinic
7:30 p.m.	Give report at County Commissioner's Meeting
Friday	
8:00	Write article on farm safety for county newspaper
9:00	Home visits
11:00	Check ________ family for head lice
1:00	Be at senior citizens center (18 miles from community health nursing office) for monthly health maintenance clinic for 35 clients
3:00	Immunization clinic (out of town)
4:30	Get organized for next week

community health nurses in rural practice settings (Long and Weinert, 1989; Scharff, 1987).

ISOLATION

Isolation, both geographic and professional, is another salient characteristic of rural community health nursing (Carlson, 1984; Davis and Droes, 1993). Geographic isolation poses challenges to rural community health nurses, because clients probably do not live nearby, as described in the following:

> We had a situation in ______ County where we had a man coming home from the hospital after having a stroke. He was completely paralyzed on his left side. He came home one evening, and a nurse went out to the ranch the next morning to start services. We thought physical therapy and nursing and some aide services would be appropriate.
>
> When she got there about 10 o'clock in the morning and was taking the history and assessment she found out that the man had driven into [the nearest] town that afternoon before. She asked him how he had driven with his left side completely paralyzed. He said when he got home, he realized that unless they drove that pickup, they were stranded. There wasn't anybody around for miles and miles.
>
> So he thought it over, and he got a couple of his leather belts and put them together, climbed into his [stick-shift] pickup, which was a feat in itself, and got it into first gear, got out on the road, slipped the belt around his left foot and when he was ready to change gears he just reached over with his right hand, pulled his [left] foot up with the belt, dropped it [the left foot] on the clutch, put it in second [gear] and went down the road.
>
> Right away that precludes him from meeting the homebound criteria for Medicare. All those services were not available to him. We provided services some other ways, but we were not able to get any Medicare benefits for him (Davis and Droes, 1993, p. 163).

Although the nurse's account does not reveal the reason why the patient went into town, the account does suggest a degree of self-sufficiency and autonomy as a way of coping with the isolation. This phenomenon is not always understood by those who are responsible for policy making or discharge planning of rural patients from urban-based hospitals.

Professional isolation is closely related to geographic

isolation and can be perceived as positive, negative, or a combination of both. Many rural nurses enjoy the professional independence and creativity not usually found in a larger practice setting. Others find that the responsibilities in a rural community health agency can be overwhelming. Often there is no immediately accessible professional network that can provide support and consultation on a particular matter of concern. Likewise, the lack of immediately available opportunities for establishing relationships with other professionals, or not having the "central office" nearby, can reinforce feelings of isolation.

For community health nurses, professional isolation requires an outstanding ability to evaluate and prioritize needs and the types of services that can be provided to the local population. The lack of physical access to other providers, education, and technology can potentially cause considerable role strain. Individuals who are uncomfortable when working alone or lack the confidence to make independent nursing decisions probably would not fare well in a remote rural area. These individuals would likely be more comfortable in a less isolated setting (Dunbar, 1992).

Telecommunications and electronic media are used to form networks that can provide support and consultation to professionals who are practicing in remote rural areas. Rapidly evolving technology has done much to reduce professional isolation among health care providers who practice in geographically isolated areas with a scarcity of resources. For instance, a cellular telephone or computer modem can be used to consult with a tertiary medical center, satellite or interactive telecommunications provide education to stay abreast of recent developments, and lifeline telemetry helps monitor patients as a way to recognize problems before an emergency occurs.

SCARCITY OF RESOURCES

Associated with the problems of geographic and professional isolation is the ever-present scarcity of human and financial resources in rural environments. This, too, has implications for community health nursing budgeted positions, salaries, support personnel, and services offered within an agency. Often community nursing positions are part time, because in sparsely populated counties, there is little funding that can be allocated for the salary and benefits to hire a county nurse. Some involved in budget planning may rationalize that there are not enough people in the community to warrant a full-time equivalent nursing position. In some ways this view is congruent with the national trend of hiring "temporaries," but in rural areas there may be no part time nurses available for hire.

One reason for not having more community nurses in rural agencies is that qualified personnel often are unavailable to fill vacant positions. Although salaries tend to be lower, the cost of living also may be less in a rural area. To address these problems, two or more counties sometimes organize a partnership, often referred to as a *health district*. With this arrangement one community health nurse provides services to both counties. This may be an ideal arrangement when distances between communities are not great. Problems can arise when a health district spans great distances coupled with natural barriers such as mountains; forests; or a lack of roads or telephone, plumbing, or electrical services (Christensen, 1987).

LEGAL CONSIDERATIONS FOR COMMUNITY HEALTH NURSES' SCOPE OF PRACTICE

The expanded scope of practice has legal implications that a community health nurse considering rural practice must explore. Consideration and attention must be given to the state's requirements for advanced nursing practice and prescriptive privileges; the organizational relationship of the local health department to the state department of health; and specific mandates for specialty programs or services that are offered within the local health department, such as RHCs, CHCs, MHCs, or contract services with the IHS.

The best way to approach the scope of nursing practice in a geographically and professionally isolated setting with the associated scarce resources is to carefully review that state's nurse practice acts. This will provide a guide as to the activities a nurse can legally engage in. Likewise, all public agencies should have a health officer. This individual can provide additional guidelines for program goals as well as develop standing orders and protocols within an agency. In addition, it is prudent for community health nurses to establish a working rapport with other health care providers in the community. In professionally and geographically isolated communities, interdiscipline rapport can provide a backup system and a referral network should unanticipated or emergency situations occur in the community nurse's practice.

Nurses in rural practice must be aware of local resources that can be used should an emergency arise. For instance, some nurses own a citizens band radio or cellular telephone to contact a physician, hospital emergency department, or county sheriff if necessary. Others work closely with a religious congregation to organize home care for a client between nursing visits. Still other nurses encourage residents who live great distances from a health care facility to take an emergency medical training course. Finally, some rural community health nurses have assumed an active role in presenting community health needs to county commissioners or the district administrative board of a local or district health department. A number of these approaches have brought about significant improvement in the overall health status of communities (American Nurses' Association [ANA], 1991).

As for community standards of practice, these are consistent with those established by the nursing profession. Providing safe quality care is mandated in all client–nurse relationships. In rural areas, however, achieving this outcome may require an innovative approach stemming from a lack of resources or great distances. For instance, informal support services may have to be coordinated by the nurse within a community to provide continuity of care for an individual who needs skilled home care and lives a great distance from the community nursing clinic. Community volunteers, however, must be knowledgeable about how to reach emergency services should these be needed. In brief, an effective community health nurse in a rural setting enhances residents' self-reliance by anticipating the types of services they might need and then teaching them how to access those services, which may be located great distances from their home. The key to success in this endeavor is effective communication among nurses, clients, the community, and local health care providers (Andrews and Engelke, 1985).

A number of strategies have been used by community health nurses in rural settings to increase a population's self-reliance and self-care skills. Because schools and churches are viewed as a socialization center by rural residents, these facilities are an ideal setting in which to provide health promotion and health education programs. For example, programs on occupational safety, cardiopulmonary resuscitation (CPR), immunizations, and nutrition education are welcomed by most administrators and educators in local schools and church leaders. Women's clubs also provide an opportunity to present health-related education such as first aid interventions for emergencies, prenatal care, or breast and testicular self-examinations.

Men tend not to be overtly receptive to health promotion education, because women in rural environments usually make the final decision regarding their family's health. Most women are eager for information that will help them in maintaining their family's health. However, some health-related topics are readily accepted by men attending service and civic club meetings. Interests vary depending on the predominant recreational and economic focus of the community (e.g., lumbering, mining, fishing, ranching, or farming). Generally, most men are interested in education related to recreational safety (snowmobiles, firearms, boating, fishing, motorcycles), vehicle safety (trucks, automobiles, all-terrain vehicles), and prevention and treatment of occupational injuries (e.g., exposure to toxic products and first aid treatment of sports-related injuries, including CPR and immediate care of trauma victims). They also may express an interest in mental health topics, especially depression and substance abuse.

Other approaches have been used to meet the health care needs of rural residents who live in HPSAs. For instance, screening clinics and specialized services such as immunizations and mammography can be brought to a community by van. This approach usually incorporates a team of specialists who can provide comprehensive diagnosis and care to residents in remote geographical areas. To be most effective, the visit by a mobile clinic should coincide with a community event such as church bazaar, county fair, athletic tournament, or rodeo (Stranger, 1987). To initiate such an endeavor requires active professional–community partnerships to effectively plan, implement, and evaluate services and programs based on the community's needs (DeLao, 1992; Fuszard et al., 1991; Ingram, 1992; Jamie, 1992).

Building Professional–Community Partnerships

CONNECTING WITH THE COMMUNITY

There is increasing evidence that community members who are informed and active in planning their health care are more likely to use and support that system. The community decision-making model offers tools to develop partnership arrangements and a consensus as to the most appropriate solution for a local problem. It is important to stress that a partnership decision-making model in a rural area probably will be somewhat different from one in a larger community. In part this relates to the dilemma associated with most residents being personally acquainted while at the same time desiring to keep their health status confidential. The problem is even more complex because of their preference for informal (rather than formal) support services (Aitken et al., 1990; Balacki, 1988; Goeppinger, 1993; Taylor, 1982). In any setting, skills that encourage community health nurses to connect with a population will empower the community to do the following:

- Establish a community health care priority list.
- Involve large numbers of community members in considering and selecting their health care options.
- Conduct health care needs assessments.
- Incorporate business principles in social marketing.
- Measure the health system's (particularly nursing care's) local economic impact.
- Negotiate and evaluate ownership/sponsorship issues by getting local people involved in the planning.

In many cases, long-standing problems can be resolved by the combined efforts of several organizations in a small community. Community health nurses would do well to establish partnerships to plan, implement, and evaluate a program or services. Partnership models take into account a population's lifestyle, health status, belief systems, and overriding health care delivery issues. Nurses must bear in mind that rural residents are known for their resourcefulness. Despite the lack of resources, historically, most have fared rather well with self-care, neighborliness, and community support. Hence, partnership arrangements are not a new concept to rural communities.

Three terms are used to describe these collaborative models: cooperative networks, coalitions, and alliances. The models have minor structural variations but a similar overall goal: to improve the overall effectiveness of a plan of action to solve a problem through collaboration (Rubin and Rubin, 1986; NIMH, 1986). A partnership in a medically underserved community wishing to provide preventive care to adolescents can be more effective by:

- Combining resources and working together to recruit health professionals.
- Hiring and sharing the expertise of a school nurse or school counselor.
- Conducting a multicounty adolescent health needs assessment to determine the area's predominant health concerns.
- Planning among local agencies to avoid duplicating services, to augment existing services, and to reduce "professional turf" issues.

Cooperative Networks

Cooperative networks are informal partnerships formed when a group of persons becomes aware of another organization that is interested in the same concern. Often these arrangements are initiated through informal discussions among interested community members, which lead to a formal meeting between the interested groups, or individuals may simply express willingness to work together on some aspect of an activity. Cooperatives, albeit informal in nature, can implement a program more effectively than if several individuals work independently on that project. However, none of the participants in the cooperative need to compromise their autonomy, although some communication and consultation are necessary for a cooperative to effectively use available resources and reduce duplication of services.

Coalitions

Coalitions are loosely organized structures in which several groups agree to address a particular problem. For instance, a county-wide coalition focusing on primary prevention care for youths in a health district could include representatives from social service agencies, schools, mental health clinics, school athletic clubs, 4-H clubs, and church and civic groups. Members of the coalition are in a position to provide leadership in assessing the community's predominant health concerns, prioritizing the identified needs, developing a strategic plan of action, and implementing the plan for an integrated program to improve the health status of a targeted group.

Alliances

Alliances are long-term partnerships having a formal administrative structure and requiring membership dues. Consider the previous example of the multicounty commitment to improve the health care of adolescents. In this case an alliance would be composed of a number of public and private institutions as well as civic and service groups that are willing and able to pay a membership fee and to undertake more complex and costly projects. Presumably, each participating group also will have representation on the board of directors and voting power. Activities that this alliance might foster include the following:

- Implementing a primary prevention program in mental health for adolescents in the area.
- Providing community education programs for youth group leaders, teachers, and parents on child developmental theory.
- Arranging a workshop for teachers, religious leaders, athletic coaches, and leaders of youth groups on effective communication techniques and crises intervention. This information should enable them to intervene more effectively when encountering an adolescent with a problem.
- Implementing a multicounty-wide drug and alcohol awareness program.
- Initiating a local crisis intervention team to provide consultation and support to faculty, parents, students, and others in the community after any serious accident, suicide, or homicide involving a local youth.
- Developing a community-wide protocol to address issues of confidentiality associated with HIV testing.

BUILDING PROFESSIONAL–COMMUNITY PARTNERSHIPS

Because of the leadership roles community health nurses are expected to assume in rural communities, they must be familiar with the process of forming professional–community partnerships. This generally is a new experience for community health nurses and consumers alike. Where do we start, and how do we proceed? Table 31–5 highlights the goals of a professional–community partnership, and Table 31–6 summarizes the process for building such partnerships (see also Unit III). The remaining paragraphs examine the process as it applies to rural community nursing practice.

Step 1: Identify the Problem Area

After a community problem is identified, the community health nurse can recruit a team of two to five individuals

TABLE 31–5

Goals of Professional–Community Partnerships

- Educate residents regarding the important role the local health care system plays in the economic infrastructure of the community and the consequences of a system failure.
- Involve as many people as possible in the decision-making process using proven strategies for citizen participation.
- Expand awareness of the local health system's need for survival in a changing rural environment.
- Develop new local leadership and support for the community health system through training and experience in decision making.
- Support the development of a community-wide plan for the local health care system.
- Establish and foster the ongoing process to plan, implement, and evaluate pertinent health care programs and services.

Adapted from National Institute of Mental Health. (1986). *Mental health research and practice in minority communities: Development of culturally sensitive training programs.* DHHS Publ. no. ADM-86-1466. Washington, DC: U.S. Government Printing Office.

TABLE 31–6

Building Professional–Community Partnerships*

Step 1: Identify the problem area
Step 2: Assess the community's perspective
Step 3: Analyze the data
Step 4: Develop a long-range plan
Step 5: Take action
Step 6: Evaluate program

**Note:* Community involvement is critical in all steps of the above process. The community health nurse in a facilitator role must gain both active and passive support from the community by involving interested community groups and individuals to participate in an organization that represents the community at large. Enlist this representative group to accept the responsibility for identifying, developing, and evaluating solutions to the community's health care problems.

who share a common interest in addressing that concern. The issue of concern determines who will be involved in the preliminary discussions (Cook et al., 1986; Kirby, 1990). For instance, because of the central importance of churches and schools in a rural community, leaders from those two institutions often can be counted on as key figures in organizing professional–community partnerships to address problems encountered by families with youths. Likewise, leaders in various civic and service clubs can be considered a community resource to help identify potential contact persons to begin discussions. Through dialogue, the informal group often becomes aware of others in the community who have similar interests, hopefully leading to a more formal collaborative partnership (e.g., cooperative network, coalition, or alliance).

Step 2: Assess the Community's Perspective

Before developing a plan of action for a particular problem, it is wise for the group, with the guidance of the community health nurse, to undertake a community assessment pertaining to the problem. These data are useful to:

- gain the local perspective,
- assess the degree of public awareness and support for the cause,
- identify special-interest groups,
- identify existing services to avoid duplication of programs, and
- list potential barriers and resources in the community.

Data can be obtained by written or telephone surveys, personal interviews, the media, and national and state public health reports. Include the views of formal and informal community leaders, representatives from local organizations, and ordinary citizens. Their ideas are critical elements in planning an effective and acceptable course of action for the problem of interest. These preliminary contacts also are an effective strategy to create community awareness of the problem, gain community support, and "test the water" as to possible approaches to resolve the problem from the public's perspective. Essentially, seeking public input allows the community to have ownership in the project, as opposed to viewing the situation as an "outsider bringing another bureaucratic program into town."

Step 3: Analyze the Data

Once the assessment is completed, the data must be analyzed, which includes identifying and prioritizing the issues of concern. The community health nurse in a facilitator role should make a dedicated effort to involve members from the community in this activity. When planning for an acceptable and effective public health program or community nursing service, compare and contrast the listed concerns with available providers and existing community resources. Consider all the information and suggestions provided by informants. Remember that local residents probably are more in tune with the needs and resources of their community than the nurse or other professional. Solutions that may seem farfetched to the nurse often are highly appropriate for the local population. In essence, creativity is required on the part of a community health nurse to implement a model program that meshes with local preferences.

Step 4: Develop a Long-Range Plan

After completing the data analysis, the professional and community partners can begin long-range planning. For a program to be effective and accepted by the target group, the community health nurse should involve as many organizations and individuals as feasible or interested (Hardgrove and Howe, 1981). For instance, a multicounty partnership focusing on a program for the prevention and treatment of hypertension might include the following activities:

- Preparing a list of possible target groups or clients.
- Generating a list of potential community volunteers and professionals who can assist with the project.
- Purchasing necessary materials to implement the program.
- Creating an awareness of the program among target groups (e.g., individuals; families; senior centers; church and recreation groups; health care professionals; law enforcement personnel; and other religious, service, and civic clubs).
- Identifying potential funding sources to implement the program.

Step 5: Take Action

Once there is group consensus and a course of action is developed, implement the plan. Be willing to delegate responsibilities to interested community representatives. It is not unusual to find eager and willing volunteers among retired nurses, educators, social service personnel, and auxiliary members of local organizations. Remember that the best plans can go awry, especially when working with several individuals and groups. When planning and implementing a program, flexibility is critical to make changes in the process as the situation requires. This strategy will go a long way toward providing community nursing services that are accessible, available, and acceptable by the target group.

Step 6: Evaluate the Program

As the program is developed and during its implementation, plan for ongoing (formative) evaluation of the process as well as a final (summative) evaluation. Together, the two evaluation approaches are useful to measure the short- and long-term outcomes of the program and determine whether the problem has been adequately addressed. Partnership arrangements facilitate obtaining reliable and valid data, from the community's perspective, regarding the outcomes of the project.

For instance, with a community nursing service, the short-term outcome might be a certain per-capita utilization of services within a specified time frame. Long-term outcomes, however, may not be obvious for several years or more, as in the case of sex education provided to junior high students as an intervention to reduce the incidence of teenage pregnancies, a nutrition education program to prevent cardiovascular disease, and an integrated preconception program to improve pregnancy outcomes in the region. Community input is critical to assess both the short- and long-term outcomes of a project.

Trends and Issues

There are many opportunities and challenges for community health nurses and other health care providers who choose to work in rural settings and for urban providers who provide care in their agency or offer outreach services to rural populations in their catchment area. A few of the more critical issues that must be addressed by policy makers and health care providers alike include the following:

1. Develop a consistent definition for *rural. Rural* has been defined as nonmetropolitan, nonurban, frontier, and farming areas. Different definitions lead to divergent approaches in program planning. Increased consistency in the definition of *rural* could lead to decreased fragmentation of services and increased sharing of ideas and resources.
2. Complete secondary compilation and analyses of existing databases into small regional units and according to subpopulations. For example, when examining rates of chronic obstructive pulmonary disease in a state, include a more detailed analysis that considers counties, towns, and ethnic subgroups as well. More comprehensive use of existing data will lead to a deeper understanding of the particular health concerns of diverse populations living in varied rural settings. This will do much to avoid duplication of assessment activities and will facilitate program planning and evaluation that is population oriented.
3. Resolve problems related to recruitment, retention, and training of health professionals for rural communities. Of particular concern are the inadequate numbers of primary health care providers and community health nurses who deliver basic preventive health care services to vulnerable rural populations, as specified by *Healthy People 2000.*
4. Eliminate the problematic professional liability crisis in rural America. More specifically, lack of obstetrical care in rural communities as a result of malpractice costs has almost eliminated even the most basic prenatal care in some areas of the country.
5. Identify mechanisms to accurately assess the quality of health care services and programs in rural America from the perspective of the people who use those services. Typically, existing programs for quality assurance, continuous quality improvement, and program evaluation incorporate complex technological measures that are associated with large tertiary institutions. The comparatively low volume of clients who use services in a rural agency, combined with rural residents' beliefs and lifestyles, may render techniques used to measure program outcomes in larger agencies invalid and unreliable in rural settings.
6. Consider ethical issues that influence nursing care in rural communities. Potential issues center on poverty and the

subsequent inability to pay for health care, inadequate access to services, and the lack of necessary and prepared health care providers and programs to meet even the most basic primary prevention needs in rural communities.

7. Disseminate pertinent information on rural nursing practice in general and community health nursing in particular. To date, most of the information that is available focuses on populations living in rural communities in the Appalachian mountains, the Midwest, and intermountain regions. Information is critically needed about ethnic and racial minorities as well as other populations who live in other regions of the United States, especially groups living in the southeastern, northeastern, south central, and southwestern United States; Alaska; and Hawaii.

All of these issues and concerns have an impact on providing available, accessible, and acceptable community health nursing services to rural populations.

In conclusion, to resolve the overriding health care delivery issues, health care providers in general and community health nurses in particular should form partnerships with rural communities. Health care professionals must talk with rural Americans to learn about what they believe to be their most pressing health care needs. Together, as partners, effective solutions can be developed to meet rural America's public health and community nursing needs and achieve the goals specified in *Healthy People 2000.*

KEY IDEAS

1. Twenty-five percent of Americans live in rural communities that have fewer than 20,000 residents. Access to health care is a problem for many of them.
2. Compared with the total U.S. population, rural Americans tend to have higher rates of infant and maternal mortality, chronic disease, and occupational illnesses and injuries associated with agriculture, mining, and construction. Alcohol-related vehicle accidents are also a problem.
3. Many rural areas are designated as health professional shortage areas (HPSAs) because of inadequate numbers of health care providers and services.
4. Rural community health nurses are instrumental in providing a wide range of services to all age groups and addressing all levels of prevention. However, there are still insufficient numbers of community health nurses in rural communities.
5. A higher percentage of persons are medically underinsured in rural than in nonrural areas; 40% of rural families live below the poverty level.
6. Rural health clinics, community health centers, migrant health centers, and the Indian Health Service are federal initiatives to increase health care to vulnerable rural populations.
7. Community health nurses need to study the health beliefs and values of rural subpopulations to provide more meaningful nursing care.
8. Community health nurses provide culturally relevant care by honoring the values of rural residents, who tend to prefer informal support, are self-reliant, and often define health as the ability to work. It is a challenge to maintain confidentiality in areas where all residents know each other.
9. Successful rural community health nurses are those who enjoy professional independence and creativity and can manage with scarce resources.
10. Partnerships between community health nurses and community members are essential to develop accessible, acceptable health care in rural areas.

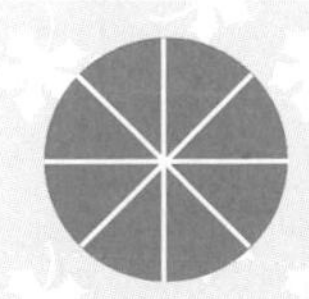

CASE STUDY
*Building a Professional–Community Partnership**

Johnson County, Tennessee, is located in the Appalachian mountains in the northeasternmost corner of the state, with borders on North Carolina and Virginia. Two-lane, winding, twisting roads offer the only vehicular access to the county. Air travel is limited by foggy weather conditions common to this eastern mountain chain. Like many rural areas, Johnson County suffered in the rural recession during the 1980s. By 1988 unemployment in the county, influenced by the closing of several small industries, had reached 35%. The farm crisis affected the agricultural base of small crop, tobacco, and

*Adapted from Edwards, J., Lenz, C., & East, J. (1993). Nurse-managed primary care: Serving a rural Appalachian population. *Family and Community Health, 16*(2), 52–57.

tree farming. Health care, once strong in the county, significantly diminished when the 60-bed Hill-Burton hospital facility in Mountain City, the county seat, closed. Only three physicians remained in the county by the end of 1988, down from a previous total of 12. The closest evening or emergency services were located at community hospitals in neighboring towns 36 miles away over dangerous mountain roads.

Step 1: Identify the Problem Area

Concerned with deteriorating economic, health, and social conditions in the county, a group of private citizens purchased at auction the equipment and supplies remaining in the defunct Johnson County Hospital and then donated the items back to the county. The group, along with the Johnson County Commission, identified accessible health care as a vital component of protecting the county population and attracting new industry and residents to the area.

Step 2: Assess the Community's Perspective

A community assessment undertaken by an outside consultant firm identified the population's health care needs and available resources. The final report noted that the rates of preventable illnesses and conditions such as diabetes, cardiovascular and cerebrovascular problems, infant mortality, cancer, suicides, and accidents were 150% to 400% higher than national and state rates. The median per-capita income in the county was $8882, compared with $17,592 nationally and $14,736 state-wide. Thirty-six percent of Johnson County high school students dropped out before graduation, further limiting economic potential in the community.

The following natural allies were identified from input to the consultants by a private–public community action group:

- The Health Science Division of East Tennessee State University, consisting of the School of Nursing, The School of Public and Allied Health, and The College of Medicine.
- The Tennessee Department of Health through the First Tennessee Community Health Agency.

Both of these agencies are headquartered in Johnson City, Tennessee, 47 miles and 1½ hours travel time away from Johnson County.

Step 3: Analyze the Data

Analysis of formal and informal community assessment data was completed by an interdisciplinary team from the Health Science Division of East Tennessee State University. Their findings strengthened the decision by community leaders to invite the participation of nursing, medicine, and public health in meeting the intense health care needs of the population. A partnership between the educational entities and the community held the potential for mutual benefit and the opening of new avenues of health care delivery appropriate to community needs. The East Tennessee State University School of Nursing, working through its Department of Family/Community Nursing, answered the expressed need of the community for primary health care during nontraditional hours.

Step 4: Develop a Long-Range Plan

The short- and long-range goals were identified and then formalized through a partnership relationship among the Johnson County Commission and the university's Health Science Division and School of Nursing. The long-term goals were to preserve the capability of the hospital to reopen and to attack the problems of joblessness and the lack of health care services.

Step 5: Take Action

With the support of key state and local leaders, the School of Nursing opened the Mountain City Extended Hours Health Center with the assistance of $176,500 in grant money from the First Tennessee Community Health Agency to help establish the community nursing practice and to offset the cost of indigent care provided by the center on a sliding scale. The Johnson County Hospital Board provided space in the vacant hospital that included two examination rooms, a waiting room, two offices, and bathroom facilities. Utilities, security, and some equipment were provided by the Johnson County Commission through the hospital board.

Site preparation for implementation of the clinic began in the summer. Trustees from the nearby Carter County Correctional Center worked with the School of Nursing project directors and the center's coordinator to prepare the long-unused site by moving equipment and furniture, cleaning, and painting. Many hours of intensive labor were required to empty, prepare, and refurbish the site.

During the preparatory months, protocols, policies, and procedures for the full range of functioning of a primary care clinic were developed. Services provided in the clinic included standard primary care options such as physical examinations, health counseling, and teaching; diagnosis and treatment of common recurring, acute, and chronic illnesses; and referral to more specialized health care providers when needed.

Application was made to and approved by the Tennessee Primary Care Board for site approval for nurse practitioner prescriptive privileges. Application was made for status as a rural community health clinic, which allows nurse practitioner care to be reimbursed on a cost-for-service basis by Medicare and Medicaid.

Step 6: Evaluate the Program

The clinic opened as scheduled, and the number of clients who seek services has increased each month. A site visit after the clinic opened confirmed that the Mountain City Extended Hours Health Center met strict federal standards and qualified for certification as a rural community health clinic. The Office of Equal Opportunity ensured that the center was in compliance with civil rights regulations. Contracts with local industry to provide employee physical examinations, employee education, and drug screening have added to the center's revenue base. Major insurance carriers also provide reimbursement of some services. Community involvement in festivals and fairs, schools, and civic groups has led to a rapidly expanding client base. Newspaper articles and radio programs have increased the center's visibility and credibility. Faculty report that their nurse-managed clinic also has provided rich clinical experiences for students enrolled in the nursing program, as well as for students in other health care disciplines. Health status outcomes are being monitored.

GUIDELINES FOR LEARNING

1. From the discussion of the first two steps of partnership building, identify Johnson County's major public health concerns (see Case Study).
2. Describe economic, cultural, and demographic factors that can influence the health status of Johnson County residents.
3. How do the goals of *Healthy People 2000* apply to the approach used to address the problem in the above case?
4. What roles and responsibilities would a community health nurse in Johnson County have in building a professional–community partnership?
5. What specific concerns are related to impaired availability, accessibility, and acceptability of health care services and providers to residents of Johnson County?
6. What approaches or measures could be used to evaluate the short- and long-term outcomes of the Mountain City Extended Hours Health Center and the effectiveness of these outcomes.
7. What strategies could a community health nurse use to address concerns related to maintaining confidentiality in this small community?
8. How is "rural" defined/perceived in your community and practice setting?
9. How do the proposed concepts of rural nursing fit rural populations in your geographic region? (If possible, cite examples.)
10. Identify challenges, opportunities, and benefits of living and practicing as a community health nurse in a small and rural community.
11. Describe potential ethical concerns in community health nursing that might emerge from rural social and economic structures. Suggest some approaches that might be used to address those concerns.
12. Identify some of the health care problems of rural residents in your state.

REFERENCES

Aaronson, L. (1982). Using health beliefs in a nursing assessment tool. In K. Babich (Ed.). *Mental health issues in rural nursing.* Boulder, CO: Western Interstate Commission for Higher Education.

Ahern, M. (1980). Health care needed for rural children. *Rural Development Perspective, 3,* 26–31.

Aitken, T., VanArsdale, S., & Barry, L. (1990). Strategies for practice as a clinical nurse specialist in a small setting. *Clinical Nurse Specialist, 4*(1), 28–32.

American Academy of Pediatrics, Committee on Community Health Services. (1986). *Rural health notebook.* Elk Grove Village, IL: Author.

American Medical Association. (1987). *The future of pediatrics.* Chicago: Author.

American Nurses Association, Council of Community Health Nurses. (1991). *Community-based nursing services: Innovative models.* Washington, DC: Author.

Andrews, A., & Engelke, M. (1985). Rural home environment assessment. Implications for community health nurses. *Home Healthcare Nurse, 3*(5), 39–44.

Baker, S., Whitfield, R., & O'Neill, B. (1987). Graphic variations in mortality from motor vehicle crashes. *New England Journal of Medicine, 316*(22), 276–279.

Balacki, M. (1988). Assessing mental health needs in the rural community. A critique of assessment approaches. *Issues in Mental Health Nursing, 9*(3), 299–315.

Bergland, R. (1988). Rural mental health: Report of the National Action Commission on the mental health of rural Americans. *Journal of Rural Community Psychology, 9*(2), 29–40.

Bigbee, J., & Crowder, E. (1985). The Red Cross Rural Nursing Service: An innovation of public health nursing delivery. *Public Health Nursing, 2*(2), 109–121.

Bronstein, J., & Morrisey, M. (1991). Bypassing rural hospitals for obstetrics service care. *Journal of Health Politics, Policy and Law, 16,* 87–118.

Bushy, A. (1991a). Rural determinants that impact family health: Considerations for community health. *Family and Community Health, 12*(4), 29–38.

Bushy, A. (Ed.). (1991b). *Rural nursing.* Vols. I & II. Newbury Park, CA: Sage Publications.

Bushy, A., & Rohr, K. (1990). The Plains Indians: Cultural considerations in the use of fetal monitors. *Neonatal Network, 8*(4), 1–6.

Carlson, L. (1984). No peers in my sphere . . . nurses working in rural community mental health centers. *Kansas Nurse, 59*(12), 10–11.

Case, T. (1991). Work stresses of community health nurses in Oklahoma. In A. Bushy (Ed.), *Rural nursing.* Vol. II. Newbury Park, CA: Sage Publications.

Children's Defense Fund. (1991). *Falling by the wayside: Children in rural America.* Washington, DC: Author.

Christensen, B. (1987). On call . . . community health nurse. *RNABC News, 19*(5), 18–20.

Cole, A., & Crawford, L. (1991). Implementation and evaluation of the health resource program for migrant women in Americus Georgia Area. In A. Bushy (Ed.), *Rural nursing.* Vol. I. Newbury Park, CA: Sage Publications.

Cook, B., Krischer, J., & Kraft, R. (1986). Health care provider and family acceptance of a rural community-based nursing service for chronically ill children. *Journal of Community Health, 11*(2), 98–110.

Copan, S., & Racusin, R. (1983). Rural child psychiatry. *Journal American Academy of Child Psychiatry, 22,* 184–190.

Davis, D. (1991). A study of rural nursing: Domains of practice—a characteristic of excellence. Unpublished thesis, Reno, NV: University of Nevada.

Davis, D., & Droes, N. (1993). Community health nursing in rural and frontier counties. *Nursing Clinics of North America, 28*(1), 159–169.

DeLao, R. (1992). A day in the life of a rural community health nurse. Tales from the trenches. *Caring, 11*(2), 10–12.

Dickey, L., & Kamerow, D. (1992, May). How to put "prevention" into practice. Paper presented at the 1992 National Rural Health Conference, Washington, DC.

Dunbar, E. (1992). Rural mental health administration. In M. Austin & W. Hersey (Eds.). *Handbook of mental health administration: The middle management perspective.* San Francisco: Jossey-Bass.

Edwards, J., Lenz, C., & East, J. (1993). Nurse-managed primary care: Serving a rural Appalachian population. *Family and Community Health, 16*(2), 52–57.

Elsion, G. (1986), Frontier areas: Problems for delivering healthcare services. *Rural Health Care, 8*(1), 3.

Fenton, M. (1988) The nursing center in a rural community: The promotion of family and community health. *Family and Community Health, 11*(2), 14–24.

Fenton, M., Rounds, L., & Anderson, E. (1991). Combining the role of the nurse practitioner and the community health nurse. An educational model for implementing community-based primary care. *Journal of the American Academy of Nurse Practitioners, 3*(3), 99–105.

Field, W., & Tormoehlen, L. (1982). *Analysis of fatal and nonfatal farm accidents involving children.* ASAE paper no. 82-5501. Chicago: American Society of Agricultural Engineers.

Frame, P. (1992). Health maintenance in clinical practice: Strategies and barriers. *American Family Physician, 43*(3), 1192–1200.

Fuszard, B., Sowell, R., Hoff, P., & Waters, M. (1991). Rural nurses join forces for AIDS care. *Nursing Connections, 4*(3), 51–61.

Geller, J., Ludtke, R., & Stratton, T. (1990). Nonfatal farm injuries in North Dakota: A sociological analysis. *Journal of Rural Health, 6*(2), 185–195.

Goeppinger, J. (1993). Health promotion for rural populations: Partnership interventions. *Family and Community Health, 16*(1), 1–9.

Greydanus, D. (1992, May). Adolescent care: Common problems and concerns. Paper presented at the National Rural Health Association 15th Annual Conference on Rural Health, Washington, DC.

Hamel-Bissel, B. (1992). On fear and courage: A first encounter with AIDs in rural Vermont. In P. Winsted-Fry (Ed.). *Rural health nursing: Stories of creativity, commitment and connectedness.* NLN Publication #21-2408. New York: National League of Nursing.

Hardgrove, D., & Howe, H. (1981). Training in rural mental health delivery. A response to prioritized needs. *Professional Psychology, 12*(6), 722–731.

Henry, B., & Moody, L. (1988). Nursing administration in small rural hospitals. *Journal of Nursing Administration, 16*(7), 37–44.

Henshaw, S., & VanVort, J. (1991). The accessibility of abortion services in the United States. *Family Planning Perspectives, 23*(6), 246–252, 263.

Hewit, M. (1989). *Defining "rural" areas: Impact on healthcare policy and research.* Washington, DC: U.S. Government Printing Office.

Hibbard, H., Netting, P., & Grady, M. (1991). *Conference proceedings—Primary care research: Theory and methods* (Publication no. 91-0011). Rockville, MD: Public Health Service—Agency of Health Care Policy and Research.

Hoffmaster, J. (1986). Rural maternity services: Community health nurse providers. *Journal of Community Health Nursing, 3*(1), 25–33.

Hughes, D., & Rossenbaum, S. (1989). An overview of maternal and infant health services in rural America. *Journal of Rural Health, 5,* 299–319.

Human, J., & Wasem, K. (1991). Rural mental health in America. *American Psychologist, 46*(3), 232–239.

Ingram, M. (1985). Some skills I thought I'd never need: When you leave a large hospital for practice in a rural community health service. *RN 1985, 48*(8), 26–27.

Jamie, D. (1992). Managing at-risk situations: Tales from the trenches. *Caring, 11*(2), 14–15.

Kirby, D. (1990). School and community relationships. *Journal of School Health, 60*(4), 170–178.

Lassiter, P., & Goeppinger, J. (1986). Education for rural community health practice. *Family and Community Health, 9*(1), 56–67.

Lee, H. (1991). Definitions of rural: A review of the literature. In A. Bushy (Ed.). *Rural nursing.* Vol. I. Newbury Park, CA: Sage Publications.

Long, K., & Weinert, C. (1989). Rural nursing: Developing a theory base. *Scholarly Inquiry for Nursing Practice, 3,* 113–127.

Luloff, A., & Swanson, L. (1990). *America's rural communities.* Boulder, CO: Westview Press.

Martin, S., & Martin, D. (1991). Nurses as primary care providers in rural America. In A. Bushy (Ed.). *Rural nursing.* Vol. II. Newbury Park, CA: Sage Publications.

McManus, M., & Newacheck, P. (1989). Rural maternal child and adolescent health. *Health Services Research, 23,* 807–818.

McManus, M., Newacheck, P., & Greany, A. (1990). Young adults with special health care needs: Prevalence, severity and access to health services. *Pediatrics, 86,* 674–682.

Monheit, A., & Cunningham, P. (1992). Children without insurance. *The Future of Children, 2*(2), 154–183.

Moser, E. (1992). The special needs of rural clients: Tales from the trenches. *Caring, 11*(2), 18–20.

Moulton, K. (1992). The frontier home care nurse: Tales from the trenches. *Caring, 11*(2), 16–17.

Murray, J., & Keller, P. (1991). Psychology in rural America: Current status and future directions. *American Psychologist, 46*(3), 220–231.

Nadel, M. (1991). *Rural hospitals: Closures and issues of access.* Testimony of U.S. General Accounting Office before U.S. House of Representatives Task Force on Rural Elderly, Select Committee on Aging, September 4, 1991.

National Association of Community Health Centers. (1992). *National health reform and access to health care.* Washington, DC: National Association of Community Health Centers.

National Clearing House for Alcohol and Drug Information. (1991). *The rural communities prevention resource guide.* Rockville, MD: Author.

National Institute of Mental Health. (1986). *Mental health research and practice in minority communities: Development of culturally sensitive training programs* (DHHS Publ. no. ADM-86-1466). Washington, DC: U.S. Government Printing Office.

National Rural Healthcare Association. (NRHA) (1986). *The occupational health of migrant and seasonal farmworkers in the United States.* Kansas City, MO: Author.

NRHA. (1994). *A shared vision: Building bridges for rural health access.* Conference proceedings on minority rural health issues. Kansas City, MO: Author.

National Safety Council. (1990–1993). *Accident facts.* (Yearly editions.) Chicago: Author.

Nasbitt, T., Connell, F., Hart, T., & Rosenblatt, R. (1990). Access to obstetrical care in rural areas. Effect on birth outcomes. *American Journal of Public Health, 80,* 814–818.

Perloff, J. (1992). Health care resources for children and pregnant women. *The Future of Children, 2*(2), 78–93.

Purschwitz, M., & Field, W. (1987). *Scope and magnitude of injuries in the agricultural workplace.* Publication no. 87-5514. Chicago, IL: American Society of Agricultural Engineers.

Rogers, E., & Burdge, R. (1986). *Social changes in rural societies.* Englewood Cliffs, NJ: Prentice-Hall.

Rubin, H., & Rubin, I. (1986). *Community organizing and development.* Columbus, Ohio: C. E. Merrill.

Scharff, J. (1987). *The nature and scope of rural nursing: Distinctive characteristics.* Unpublished thesis, Bozeman, MT, Montana State University.

Schwab, S., & Pierce, P. (1986). Assessment of clinical nursing practice in a rural decentralized case-management system . . . chronically ill children. *Public Health Nursing, 3*(2), 111–119.

Smith, K. (1986). The hazards of migrant farm work: An overview for rural public health nurses. *Public Health Nursing, 3*(1), 48–56.

Stein, H. (1989). The annual cycle and the cultural nexus of health care behavior among Oklahoma wheat farming families. *Culture, Medicine and Psychology, 6,* 81–89.

Stern, M. (1980). Adolescent medicine in rural America. *Pediatric Clinics of North America, 27*(1), 189–191.

Stranger, L. (1987). "Immunization mobile" brings protection to children in southeastern Idaho. *Public Health Reports, 102*(5), 543–545.

Taylor, J. (1982). Viewing health and health needs through many eyes. The ethnographic approach. In K. Babich (Ed.). *Mental health issues in rural nursing.* Boulder, CO: Western Interstate Commission for Higher Education.

Turner, T. (1991). Health promotion for rural black elderly: Community-based program development. In A. Bushy (Ed.). *Rural nursing.* Vol. I. Newbury Park, CA: Sage Publications.

U.S. Bureau of the Census. (1992). *Statistical abstract of the United States: 1990 National general population characteristics.* Hyattsville, MD: Author.

U.S. Bureau of Health Professions. (1990). *Seventh report to the president and congress on the status of health personnel in the U.S.* DHHS publ. no. #HRS-OD-90-3. Washington, DC: Author.

U.S. Department of Health and Human Services (USDHHS). (1986, September). *Factors influencing the geographic distribution of mental health care professionals.* Paper presented to the Health Resources and Services Administration Board, Bureau of Health Professionals, Washington, DC.

USDHHS. (1990). *Healthy people 2000: National health promotion and disease prevention objectives. Summary report.* DHHS publication no. (PHS) 91-50212. Washington, DC: U.S. Government Printing Office.

USDHHS. (1991). *Indian health services: Trends in Indian health.* Washington DC: Indian Health Service.

USDHHS. (1992). *Fifth annual report on rural health: Recommendations to the Secretary of Health and Human Services by the national advisory committee on rural health. Executive summary.* Washington, DC: Author.

U.S. General Accounting Office (USGAO). (1989). *Rural development: Federal programs that focus on rural America and its economic development* (Gao-RCED-89-56BR). Washington, DC: Author.

USGAO. (1990a). *Physician supply from the National Health Service,* (GAO/HRD 90-128). Washington, DC: Author.

USGAO. (1990b). Report to Congressional Requesters. *Rural drug abuse: Prevalence, relation to crime and programs* (GAO/PEMD-90-24, B-240854). Washington, DC.

U.S. Office of Technology Assessment. (OTA) (1990). *Health care in rural America* (OTA-H-434). Washington, DC: U.S. Government Printing Office.

U.S. Senate. (1990). Report to congressional requesters. *In Special Report by Committee on Aging.* Washington, DC: U.S. Government Printing Office.

Wagenfeld, M., & Wagenfeld, J. (1990). Mental health and rural America: A decade review. *Journal of Rural Health, 7*(6), 707–722.

Wakefield, M. (1990). Health care in rural America: A view from the nation's capitol. *Nursing Economics, 8*(2), 83–89.

Wasem, K. (1993). Interview. *Family and Community Health, 16*(10), 73–76.

Washington State Nursing Network, Celebration of Public Health Nurse Committee. (1992). *Opening doors: Stories of public health nursing.* Olympia, WA: Washington State Department of Health.

Weinert, C., & Long, K. (1993). Support systems for the spouses of chronically ill persons in rural areas. *Journal of Family and Community Health, 16*(1), 46–54.

Williams, L. (1983). How many miles to the doctor? *New Jersey Medicine, 309,* 958–963.

SUGGESTED READINGS

Bushy, A. (1991a). Rural determinants that impact family health: Considerations for community health. *Family and Community Health, 12*(4), 29–38.

Case, T. (1991). Work stresses of community health nurses in Oklahoma. In A. Bushy (Ed.). *Rural nursing.* Vol. II. Newbury Park, CA: Sage Publications.

Davis, D., & Droes, N. (1993). Community health nursing in rural and frontier counties. *Nursing Clinics of North America, 28*(1), 159–169.

Edwards, J., Lenz, C., & East, J. (1993). Nurse-managed primary care: Serving a rural Appalachian population. *Family and Community Health, 16*(2), 52–57.

Fuszard, B., Sowell, R., Hoff, P., & Waters, M. (1991). Rural nurses join forces for AIDS care. *Nursing Connections, 4*(3), 51–61.

Goeppinger, J. (1993). Health promotion for rural populations: Partnership interventions. *Family and Community Health, 16*(1), 1–9.

Lee, H. (1991). Definitions of rural: A review of the literature. In A. Bushy (Ed.). *Rural nursing.* Vol. I. Newbury Park, CA: Sage Publications.

Long, K., & Weinert, C. (1989). Rural nursing: Developing a theory base. *Scholarly Inquiry for Nursing Practice, 3,* 113–127.

Smith, K. (1986). The hazards of migrant farm work: An overview for rural public health nurses. *Public Health Nursing, 3*(1), 48–56.

Wakefield, M. (1990). Health care in rural America: A view from the nation's capitol. *Nursing Economics, 8*(2), 83–89.

Winsted-Fry, P. (Ed.). (1992). *Rural health nursing: Stories of creativity, commitment and connectedness.* New York: NLN publication no. 21-2408.

Index

Note: Page numbers in *italics* indicate illustrations; those followed by t refer to tables.

B

E

F

G

H

I

J

K

L

M

O

P

Q

R

S

T

U

V